The Veterinary Formulary

The Veterinary Formulary

Fifth edition

Edited by

Yolande Bishop

Published in association with
the British Veterinary Association

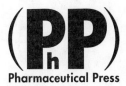

Pharmaceutical Press

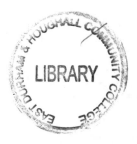

Published by the Pharmaceutical Press
1 Lambeth High Street, London SE1 7JN, UK

First edition 1991
Second edition 1994
Third edition 1996
Fourth edition 1998
Fifth edition 2001

© 2001 Pharmaceutical Press

Printed in Great Britain at The University Press, Cambridge

ISBN 0 85369 451 6

A catalogue record of this book is available from the British Library

THE VETERINARY FORMULARY
Fifth Edition

Advisory Committee

Chairman
R M Stevenson, BVMS, CertPM, MRCVS

Committee Members

A E Durham, BVSc, BSc, CertEP, MRCVS
R J Evans, MA, PhD, Vet MB, MRCVS
L A Johnson, BVMS, MRCVS, DipMan
J Marsden, BPharm, MRPharmS

Professor A M Nolan, MVB, PhD, DVA, MRCVS
H W Tasker, MRPharmS
W T Turner, BVetMed, FRSH, MRCVS
R E Vernon, BVSc, CertCHP, MRCVS

Contributors

A H Andrews BVetMed, PhD, MRCVS
M Bennett, BVSc, PhD, MRCVS
R W Blowey, BVSc, BSc, FRCVS
J C Brearley, MA, VetMB, PhD, DVA, DipECVA, MRCVS
S J Browne BVSc, MRCVS
R F Byrne BVetMed, MRCVS
S M E Cockbill LLM, BPharm, MPharm, DAgVetPharm, MCPP, MIPharmM, FRPharmS, PhD
B H Coles, BVSc, DipECAMS, RCVS Specialist in Zoo and Wildlife Medicine (Avian), FRCVS
R G Cooke, BSc, PhD
S W Cooke BVSc, MRCVS
B M Corcoran, MVB, DipPharm, PhD, MRCVS
P G G Darke, BVSc, PhD, DVR, DVC, DipECVIM, MRCVS
C Davis BVM&S, MRCVS
C E I Day, MA, VetMB, MRCVS
S J Divers, BSc (Hons), BVetMed, CertZooMed, CIBiol, MIBiol, MRCVS
J M Dobson, MA, BVetMed, DVetMed, DipECVIM, MRCVS
P W Edmondson, MVB, CertCHP, FRCVS
J Elliott MA, VetMB, PhD, CertSAC, DipECVPT, MRCVS
R J Evans, MA, PhD, VetMB, MRCVS
P A Flecknell, MA, VetMB, PhD, DLAS, DipECVA, MRCVS
T J Fletcher, BVMS, PhD, MRCVS
D H Grove-White, BVSc, DBR, FRCVS
P A Harris, MA, VetMB, PhD, MRCVS
S E Heath, BVSc, MRCVS
F M D Henson MA, VetMB, PhD, CertES(Orth), MRCVS
M E Herrtage, BVSc, MA, DVR, DVD, DSAM, DipECVIM, DipECVDI, MRCVS
Professor D E Jacobs, BVMS, PhD, FRCVS, FRCPath
L Jepson, MA, VetMB, CBiol, MIBiol, MRCVS
C B Johnson, BVSc, PhD, DVA, DipECVA, MRCVS

Professor R S Jones, OBE, MVSc, DrMedVet, DVSc, DVA, MRCA, DipECVA, FIBiol, FRCVS
J K Kirkwood, BVSc, PhD, CBiol, FIBiol, MRCVS
M Lafortune DMV
B D X Lascelles BVSc, BSc, PhD, CertVA, DSAS (ST), DipECVS, MRCVS
S A Lister, BSc, BVetMed, CertPMP, MRCVS
C A Madeiros, BVetMed, MRCVS
T S Mair, BVSc, PhD, DEIM, MRCVS
I S Mason, BVetMed, PhD, CertSAD, DECVD, MRCVS
Professor A S Nash, BVMS, PhD, CBiol, FIBiol, DipECVIM, MRCVS
Professor D E Noakes, BVetMed, PhD, DVRep, FRCVS
P-J M Noble BVM&S, BSc, MRCVS
D A L Poulter BVetMed, MRCVS
Professor D M Pugh, BVSc, MA, MSc, DrMedVet, MRCVS
G F Rendall, BVSc, MRCVS
P R Scott, DVM&S, CertCHP, DSHP, FRCVS
G C Skerritt, BVSc, DipECVN, CBiol, MIBiol, FRCVS
G G A Smith BVSc, BSc, MRCVS
L M Sommerville BVMS, MRCVS
D J Taylor MA, VetMB, PhD, MRCVS
Professor M A Taylor, BVMS, PhD, CBiol, MIBiol, MRCVS
A F Trawford, BVSc, MSc, CVMA, MRCVS
S Turner, MA, VetMB, DVOphthal, MRCVS
W T Turner BVetMed, FRSH, MRCVS
A E Wall, BVM&S, MSc, CertVOphthal, MRCVS
J P Walmsley, MA, VetMB, CertEO, DipECVS, MRCVS
W H Wildgoose, BVMS, CertFHP, MRCVS
D L Williams, MA, VetMB, PhD, CertVOphthal, MRCVS
R B Williams, BVSc, MPhil, MRCVS

Contents

GUIDANCE ON PRESCRIBING

CLASSIFIED NOTES ON DRUGS AND PREPARATIONS

APPENDICES

INDEX OF MANUFACTURERS AND ORGANISATIONS   645

British Veterinary Association

The British Veterinary Association (BVA) is pleased to continue its association with the Pharmaceutical Press, in order to support the publication of *The Veterinary Formulary*.

The BVA is the national representative body for the veterinary profession in the UK. We promote good practice by veterinarians for the maintenance of high standards of animal health, animal welfare and public health. Veterinarians require a safe and effective range of medicines to treat a wide range of animals. However, this must be balanced against the controls necessary to protect public health from any residues that might occur in those destined for the food chain. The BVA provides policy and guidance, medicines codes and pharmacy courses, and *The Veterinary Formulary* is another outlet for its wide-ranging support of best practice in all aspects of veterinary medicines.

Preface

The Royal Pharmaceutical Society has a long history of publishing veterinary medicine texts with the assistance of the veterinary profession. The first edition of *The Veterinary Formulary* was published 1991 and the second edition in 1994. The third and fourth editions, and this fifth edition are published in association with the British Veterinary Association, the national organisation representing practising veterinarians in all branches of the profession in the UK.

The British Veterinary Association is committed to making essential prescribing information available to its members. BVA Guidelines on Prudent Use of Antimicrobials and a revised BVA Code of Practice on Medicines are included in the fifth edition of *The Veterinary Formulary*. These documents are also available separately from the British Veterinary Association. The Code provides practical guidance on all aspects of prescribing and dispensing medicines and the Guidelines provide general and species-specific advice on use of antimicrobials. Discussion and debate continues over the use of medicines in animals in relation to human safety and prescribing by veterinarians, making these documents essential reading for all practitioners.

International Non-proprietary Names are used for drug names in *The Veterinary Formulary* with British Approved Names and United States Approved Names given as synonyms and indexed. A list of drug names is given on page xvi. The fifth edition includes some 60 new drug monographs and many new sections and these are listed on pages xi and xii. All the text, monographs, dosages, and drug preparations have been completely revised by some 57 Contributors who are world-recognised experts in their fields and subsequently peer reviewed by the Advisory Committee made up of veterinarians, veterinary pharmacologists, and pharmacists.

The fifth edition continues to include information on UK preparations available from veterinarians, pharmacists, agricultural merchants, and pet shops. Unlike other texts on veterinary therapeutics, in *The Veterinary Formulary*, drugs are listed under their pharmacological group rather than alphabetically. In this fifth edition, monographs and full product details are also provided in chapters 1 to 10 for preparations available in Australia, Eire, New Zealand, and the USA. Thus faciliating provision of drug information for veterinarians and pharmacists in these countries. The fifth edition contains increased text on treatment of specific conditions seen in the UK and diseases less frequently encountered but perhaps becoming more prevalent.

There continues to be a requirement for more veterinary medicines that are authorised for conditions in the target species. Until a wider range of veterinary authorised medicines are available, veterinarians will need to continue to prescribe authorised human medicines and commonly used human medicines are listed in *The Veterinary Formulary* and denoted by the symbol Ⓗ. In addition, it may be necessary to use veterinary medicines outwith the data sheet and unauthorised conditions or dosages are shown by the symbol ♦ in the text. Although recent European legislation has addressed this issue to some extent, it is important that research is undertaken and welfare issues are considered before decisions on the availability of veterinary medicines are made.

The Veterinary Formulary does not aim to contain all information necessary for prescribing. Readers should also consult specialised publications and manufacturers' current data sheets. While every effort has been made to ensure the accuracy of the contents of the book, correct prescribing, dispensing, and administration is ultimately the responsibility of the prescriber. Readers are reminded that information on medicines is constantly changing and previous editions of *The Veterinary Formulary* should be considered outdated for the purposes of prescribing in the UK.

Many individuals and organisations have assisted in the production of this fifth edition. Thanks are extended to the members of the Advisory Committee and Contributors listed on page v. The assistance of manufacturers in providing details of their products and other information is gratefully appreciated as is help given by the Veterinary Medicines Directorate and the National Office of Animal Health. Thanks are given to colleagues in the Publications Department and also the Law Department of the Royal Pharmaceutical Society. Millie Davis and Susan Shankie assisted with the publication and their help is acknowledged with thanks.

The Veterinary Formulary is intended as rapid reference text primarily for veterinarians and veterinary students but will also be valuable for pharmacists and others involved with animal health care. Comments from readers are welcome and should be sent to the Editor, The Veterinary Formulary, RPSGB, 1 Lambeth High Street, London, SE1 7JN.

Yolande Bishop
September, 2000

Tables

GUIDANCE ON PRESCRIBING

CLASSIFIED NOTES ON DRUGS AND PREPARATIONS

Additions to fifth edition

All sections have been completely revised. The following are the main changes to the fifth edition. Constant changes are made to information on medicines for animals and previous editions of *The Veterinary Formulary* should be considered outdated for the purposes of prescribing in the UK.

New monographs

Allopurinol (section 1.4.7)
Amantadine hydrochloride (section 1.3)
Ambroxol (section 5.4.1)
Amlodipine besilate (section 4.4.1.4)
Bendiocarb (section 2.2.1.3)
Beta-aminopropionitrile fumarate (section 10.2)
Bupavaquone (section 1.4.8)
Calcitonin (salmon) (section 7.7.1)
Carmustine (section 13.1.1)
Ciclosporin (section 13.2)
Cisatracurium (section 6.7.1)
Clarithromycin (section 1.1.4)
Colestyramine (section 3.10)
Desferrioxamine (Treatment of poisoning)
Desoxycortone pivalate (section 7.2.2)
Dicyclanil (section 2.2.2.3)
Diflubenzuron (section 2.2.2.1)
Dimevamide (section 3.7)
Disodium etidonate (section 7.7.2)
Docusate (section 3.2)

Docusate sodium (section 3.6.4)
Emamectin (Prescribing for fish)
Ethion (section 2.2.1.5)
Fentanyl, azaperone, and xylazine (section 6.4)
Florfenicol (Prescribing for fish)
Fluazon (section 2.2.2.1)
Fomepizole (Treatment of poisoning)
Furaltadone (section 1.1.7)
Furazolidone (section 1.1.7)
Hexastarch (section 16.2)
Indomethacin (section 10.1)
Isoniazid (section 1.1.11)
Ketorolac trometamol (section 12.3.2)
Latanoprost (section 12.5.4)
Lomustine (section 13.1.1)
Malathion (section 2.2.1.5)
Meglumine antiomonate (section 1.4.7)
Methoprene (section 2.2.2.2)
Methylcellulose (section 3.6.2
Metoprolol tartrate (section 4.4.1.2)
Methionine (section 9.2.1)
Mivacurium (section 6.71.)

Naltrexone (section 6.5)
Nizatidine (section 3.8.2)
Norethandrolone (section 7.3)
Pentamine isetionate (section 1.4.7)
Pimobendan (section 4.3.2)
Psyllium (section 3.6.2)
Pyriproxyfen (section 2.2.2.2)
Ramipril (section 4.3.1)
Rocuronium bromide (section 6.7.1)
Selamectin (sections 2.1.1.1 and 2.2.1.2)
Sodium citrate (section 9.2.2)
Sodium iodide (section 1.2)
Sodium stibogluconate (section 1.4.7)
Sotalol hydrochloride (section 4.4.1.3)
Temefos (section 2.2.1.5)
Thymol (Prescribing for invertebrates)
Tolazoline (section 6.2.1)
Tranexamic acid (section 4.7)
Triflumuron (section 2.2.2.1)
Valnemulin hydrochloride (section 1.1.10)
Vegetable/Light paraffin oils (Prescribing for invertebrates
Zafirlukast (section 5.3.3)

New sections and changes

BVA Guidelines on Prudent Use of Antimicrobials
Prescribing for equines, ruminants, and pigs divided into separate sections
Prescribing for dogs and cats divided into separate sections
Prescribing for ferrets
Table 23 Husbandry requirements for amphibians
Prescribing for geriatric animals
Table 1.1 and Table 1.2
1.1.10 Pleuromutilins
1.4.7 Dugs for leishmaniosis
1.4.8 Drugs for theileriosis
1.4.9 Drugs for trypanosomosis
2.2 Ectoparasiticides re-arranged 2.2.1 Ectoparasiticides, 2.2.2 Insect growth regulators, 2.2.3 Comound preparations for ectoparasites, 2.2.4 Sheep dips, 2.2.5 Fly repellents, 2.2.6 Environmental control of ectoparasites
2.2.1.4 Nitroguanidines
2.2.1.6 Phenylpyrazoles
4.3.1 ACE inhibitors

4.3.2 Inodilators
5.1 Treatment of respiratory infections
5.3.3 Leukotrienne receptor antagonists
6.3 Analgesics subdivided into 6.3.1 Opioid analgesics, 6.3.2 Non-opioid analgesics, 6.3.3 Compound analgesics
6.14 Artificial 'pheromones'
Prolactin antagonists listed under section 8.6
10.7 Treatment of navicular disease
12.5.4 Prostaglandin analogues
Table 13.3
14.7 Wound management
14.7.2 Preparations for wound management including 14.7.2.1 Vapour permeable adhesive films, 14.7.2.2 Foam dressings, 14.7.2.3 Hydrogel dressings, 14.7.2.4 Xerogel dressings, 14.7.2.5 Hydrocolloid dressings
17.3 Enzymes
18.2.2.4 Pasteurellosis
18.2.5.3 Samonella infection
18.2.11 Mastitis
18.3.8.4 PRRS
Appendix 5: Dosage estimation from body-weight

Arrangement of information

Guidance on prescribing

In this section, different aspects of prescribing in veterinary practice are discussed. The BVA Code of practice on medicines provides guidance on the safe use of medicines and legislation affecting the use of authorised veterinary and authorised human medicines for animals by veterinarians. Other areas included are prescription writing for medicines and medicated feedstuffs, labelling and storage requirements, and consent forms. The BVA Guidelines on prudent use of antimicrobials provides general and species-specific recommendations.

Prescribing for animals used in competitions is considered with reference to the sporting authorities, and their rules and regulations.

There are notes on prescribing for the domestic species including specific sections on prescribing for geriatrics, neonates, pregnant animals, hepatic impairment, renal impairment, and lactating animals.

There is a section providing specific information on invertebrates. The sections on exotic species such as amphibians, reptiles, and exotic birds or less frequently encountered companion animals such as fish, ferrets, rabbits, and rodents include common clinical conditions, methods of drug administration, and extensive tabular data on drug dosage including antimicrobial drugs, parasiticides, anaesthetics, and other drugs.

Information on the management of poisoning in animals, symptomatic therapy, and specific antidotes for more frequently encountered poisons are discussed in the section Treatment of poisoning.

Classified notes on drugs and preparations

The main text consists of 19 chapters each covering a particular body system, condition, or drug category. The information provided in the chapters concerns the use and administration of medicines and drugs to the domestic species including horses, cattle, sheep, goats, pigs, dogs, cats, and poultry. Each chapter is divided into numbered sections such that similar drugs are grouped together. Text on the use of these drugs in veterinary practice, mechanism of action, and adverse effects is given, and is followed by drug monographs and relevant medicines, whether generic or proprietary.

Drug monographs are listed alphabetically under each section. The **drug titles** used in *The Veterinary*

Formulary are International Nonproprietary Names (INN) wherever possible. British Approved Names (BAN) and United States Adopted Names (USAN) are given as synomyns and indexed where necessary.

The authorised **indications** for use of the drug are given. In addition, indications that are not included in the data sheet are listed and denoted by the symbol ♦. The indications under a drug monograph title may not apply to all preparations of that substance.

The **contra-indications** of the drug such as administration in certain species, specific age of animal, pregnant animals, or conditions for example renal impairment.

The **side-effects** of the drug are given. Any **warnings** associated with use of the drug in animals and cautions for humans administering the drug are listed.

The **dose** of the drug is given for domestic species. For the purposes of *The Veterinary Formulary* 'small animals' are considered to be dogs and cats; 'large animals' to be horses, cattle, sheep, and pigs. The dose is expressed in terms of the drug substance indicated by the monograph title unless otherwise specified. The doses stated in *The Veterinary Formulary* are intended for general guidance only and represent, unless otherwise stated, the usual range of doses that are generally regarded as suitable for the species indicated.

Doses are given in amounts per kilogram body-weight wherever possible. Doses of drugs to be administered in the drinking water are usually expressed as amount per 100 litres for domestic species or per litre for exotic birds. Dosages for farmed fish may be given as parts per million (ppm); see Appendix 3 for Conversions and units. Doses of drugs to be administered in the feed are usually expressed as amount per tonne of feed. It is important that drug dosage calculations are carefully checked for treatment administered via the drinking water or feed. It is advisable to establish if other drugs are included in the diet before medicating the drinking water or feed to avoid the possibility of adverse drug interactions.

The route of administration of the dose is indicated and frequency of administration.

Readers should be aware that dosages suggested for drugs that have no veterinary authorised products or for veterinary authorised products used outwith their data sheet (indicated by the symbol ♦) are commonly used doses. Such doses may not have been derived from research in the particular species being treated;

they are to be used when no suitable veterinary product is available and in accordance with the *Medicines (Restrictions on the Administration of Veterinary Medicinal Products) Regulations 1994,* as amended; the responsibility for their use lies with the veterinary surgeon.

Preparations that are authorised in the UK for use in animals are listed. In addition veterinary preparations avialble in Australia, Eire, New Zealand, and the USA are given in chapters 1 to 10, bees, and fish. Where authorised veterinary preparations are unavailable, products that are authorised for use in humans in the UK and that are commonly used in veterinary medicine are included. The latter may be easily recognised by the symbol Ⓗ and occur predominantly in the chapters and sections dealing with the Gastro-intestinal system, Cardiovascular system, Drugs used for behaviour modification, Endocrine system, and Malignant disease and immunosuppressants.

The following information is provided for preparations:

LEGAL CATEGORY **Brand Name** (Manufacturer)

Dose form, ingredients and concentration of each/unit measure (mL, g, kg, unit dose, division, etc), for *species for which the product is authorised*

Withdrawal Periods. *Species*: slaughter withdrawal period in days, milk or egg withdrawal period in days

Appendices and indexes

The appendices include Drug Interactions and Drug Compatibilities and Incompatibilities. Information is arranged under drug name, drug group name, or therapeutic category and listed alphabetically. Appendix 3 provides useful conversions of mass, volume, and temperature from Imperial to metric units, and an explanation of terms such as tonicity. Tables of conversion of body-weight to surface area for dogs and cats are also included. Appendix 4 gives a list of body-weight ranges for domestic species, exotic birds, rabbits, and rodents. Appendix 5 provides guidance on estimation of drug dosage in species for limited information is available.

The Index of Manufacturers and Organisations lists addresses, telephone numbers, facsimile numbers, and e-mail addresses of UK and overseas manufacturers whose preparations appear in *The Veterinary Formulary*. Organisations associated with veterinary practice are also included.

The general Index should be used to locate information on drugs, medicines, preparations and diseases. Brand names are listed in italics for easy recognition and the drug monograph is listed on the page number identified in bold type.

Symbols used in The Veterinary Formulary

Internationally recognised units and symbols are used in *The Veterinary Formulary* wherever possible.

(H) – authorised human preparation
°C – degrees Celsius (centigrade)
♦ – veterinary preparation or veterinary drug used for an indication that is unauthorised in the UK
> – less than
< – more than

Abbreviations used in The Veterinary Formulary

For abbreviations of names of manufacturers and organisations associated with veterinary practice see also Index of Manufacturers and Organisations on pages 645–656.

ATC – animal test certificate
Austral. – Australia
3-AV – avermectins/milbemycins
BEVA – British Equine Veterinary Association
BP – British Pharmacopoeia 1993
BP(Vet) – British Pharmacopoeia (Veterinary) 1993
Bq – becquerel
BSAVA – British Small Animal Veterinary Association
BVA – British Veterinary Association
BVetC – British Veterinary Codex and Supplement 1970
1-BZ – benzimidazoles/probenzimidazoles
CD – controlled drug
cm – centimetre(s)
CNS – central nervous system
CVL – Central Veterinary Laboratory
DANI – Department of Agriculture, Northern Ireland
DNA – deoxyribonucleic acid
DVO – District Veterinary Officer
e/c – enteric coated
EC – European Community
ECF – extracellular fluid
ECG – electrocardiogram
EFAs – essential fatty acids
EU – European Union
f/c – film coated
Fr. – France
g – gram(s)
Ger. – Germany
GSL – general sale list
HSE – Health and Safety Executive
i.co – intracoelomic
i.m. – intramuscular
i.o. – intraosseous
Ital. – Italy
i.v. – intravenous
kg – kilogram(s)
L – litre(s)
2-LM – imidazothiazoles/ tetrahydropyrimidines
M – molar
m^2 – square metres

MA – marketing authorisation
MAFF – Ministry of Agriculture, Fisheries and Food
MFS – medicated feedingstuff prescription
mg – milligram(s)
MIC – minimum inhibitory concentration
mL – millilitre(s)
mmHg – millimetre(s) of mercury
m/r – modified release
Neth. – The Netherlands
Norw. – Norway
NSAID – non-steroidal anti-inflammatory drug
NZ – New Zealand
P– pharmacy-only medicine,
pg – picogram(s)
pH – the negative logarithm of the hydrogen ion concentration
PhEur– European Pharmacopoeia
PL – product licence
PML– pharmacy merchants list
p.o. – by mouth
POM – prescription-only medicine
ppb – parts per billion
ppm – parts per million
RCVS – Royal College of Veterinary Surgeons
RPSGB – Royal Pharmaceutical Society of Great Britain
RSPCA – Royal Society for the Prevention of Cruelty to Animals
S.Afr. – South Africa
s.c. – subcutaneous
s/c – sugar coated
s/r – sustained release
soln. – solution
Swed. – Sweden
UK – United Kingdom
units – standard international units, unless otherwise stated in the text. See also Appendix 3, page 475
USA – United States of America
VMD – Veterinary Medicines Directorate

Drug names

International Non-proprietary Names (INN) are used in *The Veterinary Formulary* wherever possible with British Approved Names (BAN) and United States Approved Names (USAN) given as synonyms. The following name are used in the fifth edition.

UK name	rINN	UK name	rINN
adrenaline	epinephrine	hydroxyprogesterone hexanoate	hydroxyprogesterone caproate
alphadolone	alfadolone	hydroxyurea	hydroxycarbamide
alphaxalone	alfaxalone	indomethacin	indometacin
amethocaine	tetracaine	lignocaine	lidocaine
aminacrine hydrochloride	aminoacridine hydrochloride	methimazole	thiamazole
amoxycillin	amoxicillin	methohexitone	methohexital
amphetamine	amfetamine	methotrimeprazine	levomepromazine
amphotericin	amphotericin B	methylene blue	methylthioninium chloride
atracurium besylate	atracurium besilate	methylphenobarbitone	methylphenobarbital
beclomethasone	beclometasone	metriphonate	metrifonate
bendrofluazide	bendroflumethiazide	mitozantrone	mitoxantrone
benzhexol	trihexyphenidyl	naphthalophos	naftalofos
bretylium tosylate	bretylium tosilate	neostigmine methylsulphate	neostigmine metisulfate
busulphan	busulfan	nitroxynil	nitroxinil
butobarbitone	butobarbital	noradrenaline	norepinephrine
carbaryl	carbaril	oestradiol	estradiol
chlorfenvinphos	chlorfenvinfos	pentobarbitone	pentobarbital
chlorpheniramine	chlorphenamine	phenobarbitone	phenobarbital
cephalexin	cefalexin	phthalylsulphathiazole	phthalylsulfathiazole
cephalonium	cefalonium	polyhexanide	polihexanide
cephazolin	cefazolin	potassium clorazepate	dipotassium clorazepate
cephradine	cefradine	pralidoxime mesylate	pralidoxime mesilate
chlorbutol	chlorobutanol	procaine penicillin	procaine benzylpenicillin
chlormethiazole	clomethiazole	quinalbarbitone	secobarbital
cholecalciferol	colecalciferol	riboflavine	riboflavin
cholestyramine	colestyramine	sodium calciumedetate	sodium calcium edetate
corticotrophin	corticotropin	sodium cromoglycate	sodium cromoglicate
coumaphos	coumafos	sodium ironedetate	sodium feredetate
crotethamide	crotetamide	stilboestrol	diethylstilbestrol
danthron	dantron	sulphacetamide	sulfacetamide
dexamphetamine	dexamfetamine	sulphadiazine	sulfadiazine
diazinon	dimpylate	sulphadimidine	sulfadimidine
dichlorphenamide	diclofenamide	sulphaguanidine	sulfaguanidine
dimethicone	dimeticone	sulphamethoxazole	sulfamethoxazole
dimethyl sulphoxide	dimethyl sulfoxide	sulphasalazine	sulfasalazine
dipyrone	metamizole sodium	sulphathiazole	sulfathiazole
etamiphylline camsylate	etamiphylline camsilate	trimeprazine	alimemazine
ethinyloestradiol	ethinylestradiol	tetracosactrin	tetracosactide
ethyloestrenol	ethylestrenol	thiabendazole	tiabendazole
flumethasone	flumetasone	thioguanine	tioguanine
frusemide	furosemide	thiopentone	thiopental
glutaraldehyde	glutaral	thyroxine sodium	levothyroxine sodium
guaiphenesin	guaifenesin	tricaine mesylate	tricaine mesilate
hexamine hippurate	methenamine hippurate		

British Veterinary Association

Code of Practice on Medicines

Edited by:
Y Bishop BSc, BVMS, LLB(Hons), MRCVS

Classification of medicines
Prescribing of medicines
Dispensed medicines
Record keeping
Suspected adverse reactions
Drug residues
Disposal of medicines
Consent forms
Further information

The protection of the health and welfare of the many species under the veterinarian's care depends on the availability of sufficient veterinary medicines, which are of proven safety, quality, and efficacy for the target species. The selection of the best therapeutic is paramount. However, the rational use of medicines in veterinary practice also depends on correct handling and use by both the veterinarian and the animal owner. The professional advice the veterinarian gives in prescribing the correct medicine in a given set of circumstances is of equal importance.

The impact of European legislation and increased public concern about the use of medicines, particularly in food-producing animals, means that the veterinarian must be able to justify decisions taken in the selection and application of medical treatment. The privilege to dispense veterinary medicines rests not only on the responsible use of medicines but also on the demonstration of best accepted practice.

The aims of this Code are to provide guidance on the prescribing and dispensing of medicinal products by veterinarians in consideration of legislation and best practice. It includes information on use of medicines such as storage, labelling, sale and supply, record keeping, disposal, and suspected adverse reactions. This guidance complements that provided by British Veterinary Association (BVA) Veterinary Pharmacy courses.

Various changes have been made to the legislation and recommended best practice for prescribing and dispensing of medicines for animals since the last edition of this Code in 1998. Many individuals and BVA divisions have commented on this revised Code and their valuable contribution is acknowledged with thanks.

Classification of medicines

A 'veterinary medicinal product' means any medicinal product intended for animals and applies to veterinary medicinal products offered for sale *inter alia* in the form of proprietary medicinal products and ready-made veterinary medicinal products.

In the UK, veterinary medicines are legally classified into general sales list medicines, pharmacy medicines, pharmacy and merchants list medicines, prescription-only medicines, and controlled drugs. Other preparations, such as nutritional supplements, which are not supplied for a medicinal purpose, are classified as non-medicinal.

General sales list medicines (GSL)

All GSL medicines are listed in the *Medicines (Veterinary Drugs) (General Sales List) Order*. They may be sold without any restriction. A veterinarian can sell these to anyone, whether a client or not. However when selling the products as a retailer, the veterinarian must ensure that it is clear to the purchaser that the animal for which the medicine is sold is not under the veterinarin's care. In all other circumstances, the veterinarian may supply GSL products for animals under his/her care.

Pharmacy only medicines (P)

This is the usual category for medicines unless the licensing authority has taken statutory measures to put them into the POM, PML or GSL categories. Very few veterinary medicines fall into the P category. These medicines may be supplied by a veterinarian for administration to animals under the veterinarian's care or over the counter by a pharmacist.

Pharmacy and merchants list medicines (PML)

All PML medicines are included in the list of veterinary drugs kept by the VMD for the purposes of Article 3 of the *Medicines (Exemptions for Merchants in Veterinary Drugs) Order 1998*.

They can be supplied by a veterinarian for administration to animals under the veterinarian's care. PML medicines may also be sold in pharmacies with each sale by, or under the supervision of a pharmacist. They may also be supplied by an agricultural merchant who is registered with the Royal Pharmaceutical Society of Great Britain (RPSGB) or Department of Agriculture for Northern Ireland (DANI) and who has undertaken to observe a code of practice. A registered agricultural merchant may authorise sale of PML medicines only to persons who keep or maintain animals for the purpose of carrying on a business.

Registered agricultural merchants and saddlers may sell a small range of PML anthelmintics to horse, dog, or cat owners for animals in their care. A code of practice has to be observed.

If a veterinarian wishes to supply PML products for animals **not** under his/her care, he must register with the RPSGB as an agricultural merchant. The veterinarian may supply only to commercial keepers of animals.

Some veterinarians have taken out wholesale dealers' licences. The *Medicines (Sale or Supply) (Miscellaneous Provisions) Regulations 1980* (Schedule I) impose strict limits as to whom may be supplied in the course of wholesale dealing. A veterinarian's clients are **not** included.

Prescription only medicines (POM)

These are described in the *Medicines (Prescription Only) Order*. They may be supplied by a veterinarian for administration to animals under the veterinarian's care or supplied by a pharmacist on a veterinarian's prescription. A veterinarian is **not** normally entitled to supply POM products against a prescription issued by another veterinarian who is not in the same practice. The exception is for small quantities only of specially prepared medicines.

The veterinary prescription

A prescription is not required for the sale or supply of GSL, P, or PML veterinary medicines. A veterinarian may give a verbal or written instruction to a pharmacist for supply of GSL or P authorised human medicines.

There are legal requirements for veterinary prescriptions, which prescribe POM products and CD preparations. A veterinary prescription is used for medicines and a medicated feedingstuffs (MFS) prescription is used for POM products incorporated into feed (see below).

To avoid ambiguity it is good practice to write all prescriptions legibly in a standard manner. The following recommendations are given:

- quantities of 1 gram or more should be written as 1 g, etc.
- quantities of less than 1 gram should be written in milligrams, for example 500 mg, not 0.5 g
- quantities of less than 1 milligram should be written in micrograms, for example 100 micrograms, not 0.1 mg
- when decimals are unavoidable a zero should be written in front of the decimal point where there is no other figure, for example 0.5 ml, not .5 ml
- the terms 'micrograms', 'nanograms', or 'units' should **not** be abbreviated
- 'millilitre' (mL or ml) is used in veterinary medicine and pharmacy in preference to cubic centimetre, c.c., or cm^3.
- Names of drugs and preparations should be written clearly and **not** abbreviated. Only approved titles should be used and International Nonproprietary Names (INN) used in preference to British Approved Names (BAN).
- Directions should preferably be in **English without abbreviation**. It is recognised that some Latin abbreviations, as follows, are used when prescribing. It should be noted that the English version is not always an exact translation.
  b.d. bis die (twice daily)
  b.i.d. bis in die (twice daily)
  o.d. omni die (once daily)
  q.i.d. quater in die (four times daily)
  s.i.d. semel in die (once daily)
  t.i.d. ter in die (three times daily)

There are specific legal requirements for prescriptions for prescription-only medicines. They must be written legibly in ink or be otherwise indelible. The prescription should include:

- the name and address of the prescriber, which may be printed on practice forms.

- the name and address of the client. It is good practice to indicate the species or animal name/number and to add the words 'for animal treatment only'
- the date of prescription issue
- the name(s) and strength(s) of drug(s) to be dispensed. Usually this will be a pre-prepared formulation. Medicines may be prescribed using the generic name or specifying a proprietary preparation. In the former case only, the pharmacist may dispense any suitable product. The formulation of any preparation that needs to be extemporaneously prepared should be included. Although it is not a legal requirement to include the total amount of medicine to be supplied and the dose of the medicine, it is good prescribing practice to include this information on prescriptions
- the directions that the prescriber wishes to appear on the labelled product
- the prescriber's usual signature, in ink, and professional qualifications
- a declaration that 'This prescription is issued in respect of an animal or herd (group) under my care' or words to that effect
- any instructions for repeating the prescription.

Veterinary prescription

```
Name and address of veterinarian
Date

Name of animal
Name of client
Address of client


Name, strength, and formulation of the drug

Amount to be supplied

Dosage (amount and frequency of administration)



Instructions to appear on the label


                    For animal treatment only
                 This animal is under my care



                    Signature and qualifications
                       of veterinarian


Repeat instructions
```

A POM prescription must not be dispensed later than 6 months from the date issued and will not be repeated unless it contains a specific direction for further dispensing. If a prescription contains a direction that it is to be repeated without specifying the number of times, it will be dispensed twice only. When a prescription is to be dispensed in instalments, the number of instalments and intervals to be observed when dispensing must be specified along with the amount of drug in the instalment, and the total amount of drug to be dispensed. Exact information on the permission to issue and provisions of repeat prescriptions for a particular animal should be included in the patient's record by the veterinarian who has the animal under his/her care. This is to allow a veterinary colleague in the same practice to provide a repeat prescription if necessary. The period of time that the veterinarian may allow repeat prescriptions without re-examining the patient will be variable and dependent on the patient, the condition, the client, the medicine prescribed and the necessity to monitor clinical signs and side-effects by e.g. monitoring blood parameters or hepatic function. For guidance, the Veterinary Defence Society (VDS) suggests a time interval of 3 to 6 months (shorter for e.g. cytotoxic drugs and perhaps longer for e.g. mild cardiac disease therapy) between re-examinations. Each practice should decide general protocols for each drug; these may need to be varied in individual cases.

Controlled drugs (CD)

These are drugs that are capable of being abused. In addition to there being strict controls on use of these drugs in animals, veterinarians may themselves be vulnerable to self-use of addictive drugs. The veterinary profession operates confidential helplines, the Vet Helpline (Telephone 0941 170000), and the Veterinary Surgeons Health Support Programme (VSHSP) (Telephone 01926 315119). The Vet Helpline provides information and advice to veterinarians that contact the group on where to seek appropriate help on any problems of emotional or depressive nature, alcohol or drug abuse, and concerns over personal finance. The VSHSP helps veterinarians suffering problems of alcohol or drug abuse who contact the group or are referred to them to combat their addiction by assisting in seeking treatment and supporting them through the recovery process.

Under the *Misuse of Drugs Regulations 1985*, controlled drugs are divided into 5 schedules, in decreasing order of stringency of control.

Schedule 1 includes cannabis and hallucinogenic drugs such as LSD, which are not commonly used therapeutically. Veterinarians have no general authority to possess or prescribe them.

Schedule 2 includes some drugs that may be used in veterinary practice such as etorphine, fentanyl, morphine, pethidine, methadone, the amphetamines, and quinalbarbital (quinalbarbitone). These drugs are subject to particular requirements for prescriptions, requisition, record keeping, safe custody except quinalbarbitone (quinalbarbital), and disposal of unwanted medicines.

Prescriptions for Schedule 2 and 3 controlled drugs must be indelible and conform to particular requirements *in addition* to those for prescription-only medicines. To minimise the possibility of forgery, the prescription must be in the *veterinarian's own handwriting*, except for phenobarbital (phenobarbitone) and phenobarbital sodium (phenobarbitone sodium). Prescriptions for Schedule 2 and 3 controlled drugs must include the form and strength of drug(s) to be dispensed e.g. Pethidine Tablets, 50 mg. In addition, the total quantity, in both words and figures, to be dispensed e.g. Pethidine Tablets, 50 mg. Send 10 (ten) must be included. A pharmacist must not dispense a prescription for a Schedule 2 or Schedule 3 CD unless it complies with the above requirements and the prescriber's address is in the UK. The prescription must not be dispensed later than 13 weeks from the date of issue and repeat prescriptions for controlled drugs are not permitted. The pharmacist should be satisfied that the prescription is genuine.

A **requisition** in writing must be obtained by a supplier before delivery of a Schedule 2 drug. The requisition must be signed by the veterinarian, state the veterinarian's name, address, and professional qualifications, and specify the total quantity of the drug and the purpose for which it is required. The supplier must be reasonably satisfied that the signature is that of the person purporting to sign the requisition and the person is engaged in the occupation stated.

The **record keeping** requirements for Schedule 2 drugs indicate that they must be entered in the Register when purchased and also each time they are used. Veterinarians must make such records in the Register within 24 hours. The Register must take the form of a bound book (not a loose-leaf book) and a separate Register must be kept for each premises where controlled drugs are used. A separate part of the Register must be used for each class of drug, which must be specified at the head of each page of the Register. A class is any drug specified in Schedule 2 together with its salts, stereoisomers, and any preparation in which it is contained; e.g. a separate part of the Register must be kept for each of pethidine, morphine, and etorphine.

The layout of Registers is stipulated in the legislation :

Part 1

Entries to be made in case of obtaining a supply

FENTANYL

Date on which sup-ply received	Name address of person or firm from whom obtained	Amount obtained	Form in which obtained
(Date)	Drug Company Ltd, Market Street, Town	1 x 10 mL	Hypnorm injection

Part 2

Entries to be made in case of supply

PETHIDINE

Date on which the transaction was effected	Name address of person or firm supplied	Particulars as to licence or authority of person or firm supplied to be in possession	Amount supplied	Form in which supplied
(Date)	S Smith's dog (name), 8 Long Lane, Coxton, Surrey	Direct administration	50 mg (1 mL)	Pethidine injection

Entries must be indelible and made in chronological order. Entries must not be amended; if corrections are necessary they must be made by means of a marginal note or footnote and specify the date the correction was made. The Register must be kept for two years from the date of the last entry.

Schedule 2 controlled drugs, except quinalbarbital (quinalbarbitone), must be kept in a locked receptacle which can be opened only by a veterinarian or a person authorised by a veterinarian to do so. Schedule 2 controlled drugs may not be destroyed except in the presence of a person authorised by the Secretary of State (see Disposal of medicines).

Schedule 3 includes buprenorphine, butobarbital (butobarbitone), pentazocine, pentobarbital (pentobarbitone), phenobarbital phenobarbitone), and some minor stimulant drugs. These drugs are subject to prescription (see Schedule 2 above) and requisition requirements, but transactions do not have to be recorded in a controlled drugs Register. Phenobarbitone (phenobarbital) prescriptions are exempt from the requirement to be written by hand by the veterinarian but must comply in every other respect with prescription writing requirements. A requisition in writing must be obtained by a supplier before delivery of a Schedule 3 drug. The requisition must be signed by the veterinarian, state the veterinarian's name, address, and professional qualifications, and specify the total quantity of the drug and the purpose for which it is required. The supplier must be reasonably satisfied that the signature is that of the person purporting to sign the requisition and the person is engaged in the occupation stated.

Temazepam, diethylpropion, or buprenorphine must be kept in a locked receptacle, which can be opened only by a veterinarian or a person authorised by a veterinarian to do so; this does not apply to other Schedule 3 drugs.

Schedule 4 includes anabolic substances and the benzodiazepines. When used in normal veterinary practice they are exempt from most restrictions as controlled drugs.

Schedule 5 includes certain preparations of cocaine, codeine, and morphine that contain less than a specified amount of the drug. They are exempt from all CD requirements pertaining to veterinary practice other than the need to keep relevant invoices for two years.

A veterinarian acting in a professional capacity has authority to supply Schedule 2, 3, 4, and 5 controlled drugs. The veterinarian may administer the drug or direct any other persons to administer such drugs to patients under the veterinarian's care.

There is increased concern that some drugs that are not controlled under the *Misuse of Drugs Act 1971*, as amended, such as ketamine, may be used as drugs of abuse. The RCVS recommends that these drugs are stored in secure containers.

Medicated feedingstuffs prescription (MFS).

An MFS prescription, prescribed on the advice of a veterinarian, authorises the incorporation of a veterinary medicinal product in the form of a premix as described under the *Medicated Feedingstuffs Regulations 1998*. POM products for incorporation into feedingstuffs must be prescribed under a MFS. Anthelmintics incorporated into feed are exempt from the requirement for an MFS prescription and are classified as MFSX.

The Regulations apply to anyone who incorporates a POM in an animal feedingstuff 'in the course of business carried on by him'. Therefore, home-mixers such as farmers and keepers (of e.g. zoo animals, dogs for business purposes (packs of hounds), and farmed rabbits) are affected as well as commercial feed compounders. However, the legislation does not affect a companion animal owner administering a medicine mixed in the feed because no business is involved. The Regulations do not apply to a farmer 'top dressing' feed or medicating via the drinking water.

All feed compounders, that is commercial and home-mixers, who add medicines to feeds and all distributors of medicated feeds are required to apply to the Royal Pharmaceutical Society of Great Britain (RPSGB) or the Department of Agriculture for Northern Ireland (DANI) for approval of their premises. The RPSGB and DANI enforce the legislation and associated Codes of Practice.

Under the *Feedingstuffs (Establishments and Intermediaries) Regulations 1999* manufacturers and distributors of feedingstuffs containing vitamins, amino acids, enzymes and probiotics must be registered.

An appropriately registered person only may incorporate a POM medicine in an animal feedingstuff if the product has a relevant marketing authorisation or an Animal Test Certificate (ATC) providing specifications for incorporation. Medicines to be included in feed *must*, by law, be authorised for in-feed use, although the veterinarian may authorise use for species or conditions other than those specified in the marketing authorisation for POM products but not products under an ATC.

POM products for administration in feed will either be dispensed by the veterinarian having the animals under his/her care or dispensed under the authority of a prescription.

It is important to know of any additives that are already incorporated into the feed. The legal requirement is that it is necessary to indicate POM products on the MFS prescription but it is recommended that other feed additives already contained in the feedingstuff should also be listed. This is to impress upon the signatory veterinarian the need to ensure that no known adverse reaction between any active ingredients is likely. A veterinarian may, at his discretion and on his own responsibility, authorise combinations of medicinal feed additives unless they are specifically prohibited in the data sheet of one of the combinants.

All MFS prescriptions should follow the specified format and should include:

- the name and address of the prescribing veterinarian
- the name and address of the supplier, who should be a person registered with the RPSGB or DANI
- details of the recipient of the medicated feed
- the number and species to which the medicated feed is to be administered
- the disease to be treated (which may be written on the veterinarian's copy only)
- the amount of product to be incorporated in the feed, and how it should be used
- the withdrawal period. If a POM feed additive is to be incorporated in accordance with a product authorisation

or animal test certificate, the withdrawal period shown must be that on the data sheet of the product. When prescribing a POM outwith the recommendations specified on the current data sheet or whose data sheet does not specify a withdrawal period, the standard minimum withdrawal periods must be applied (see Drug residues). Where use involves a species indicated in the marketing authorisation, but for a different condition, the meat withdrawal period indicated on the data sheet is acceptable providing that the dosage is as given on the data sheet. Where use is for a species **not** given in the marketing authorisation, then the withdrawal period should be at least as long as the standard minimum withdrawal period

- any special precautions. It is important for the prescribing veterinarian to know of other ingredients e.g. zootechnical feed additives that may be in the feedstuff and to indicate any potential incompatibilities between these and the POM.

The MFS prescription should be personally signed and dated by the veterinarian, in respect of animals under his/her care. The MFS prescription allows a one-month supply of medicated feed and is *valid for a period of 3 months* from the date of the veterinarian's signature.

Three copies of a MFS *prescription are required*: one each for the compounder, farmer, and veterinarian.

It is essential to complete these forms accurately and legibly; otherwise the feed may be unusable. Pads of self copying MFS prescriptions are available from the Masbrooks, T G Scott (6 Bourne Enterprise Centre, Wrotham Road, Nr Sevenoaks, Kent TN15 8DG. Telephone 01732 884023. Facsimile 01732 884034. E-mail cairns@tgscott.co.uk).

Compounders and on-farm mixers who supply feedingstuffs without a MFS prescription where one is required by law, or on the basis of an invalid MFS prescription, commit an offence and become liable to prosecution and, or removal, from the register of the RPSGB or DANI.

Zootechnical Feed Additives

Previously PML feed additives, e.g. production enhancers or coccidiostats, were authorised as veterinary medicines under the *Medicines Act*. Under *The Feedingstuffs (Zootechnical Products) Regulations 1999* these preparations are no longer considered as medicines. Their use is controlled and authorised under EC legislation. Zootechnical feed additives may be incorporated in the feed at specified concentrations for particular species as indicated in the relevant Annex entry of Directive 70/524/EEC; there is no provision for incorporation in any way not in accordance with the Annex entry, for example at higher concentrations or for different species.

Homœopathic products

A homœopathic medicinal product means any veterinary medicinal product prepared from products, substances, or compositions called homœopathic stocks in accordance with homœopathic manufacturing procedure described by the *European Pharmacopoeia*, or in the absence thereof, by the pharmacopoeias currently used officially in the Member States. Products fulfilling the relevant criteria may be authorised under *The Registration of Homœopathic Veterinary Medicinal Products Regulations 1997*

Probiotics and Enzymes

Probiotics contain micro-organisms in a vegetative or arrested state, which have an effect on the environment of the gut. Enzymes enhance the digestibility of certain feed ingredients. Probiotics and enzymes are controlled under EC legislation.

Traditional remedies and chemicals

Traditional remedies and chemicals such as Epsom salts, liquid paraffin, and Stockholm tar are freely available and would not normally be considered as veterinary medicines. However, once a veterinarian supplies them for a medicinal purpose, they become medicines. They may be prescribed under *The Medicines (Restrictions on the Administration of Veterinary Medicinal Products) Regulations 1994*, as amended, as extemporaneously prepared products and as such the standard minimum withdrawal periods are applicable.

Under the *Animals and Animal Products (Examination for Residues and Maximum Residue Limits) Regulations 1997*, bees are classified as food-producing animals. The Veterinary Medicines Directorate (VMD) has advised that substances may be administered to bees if the agent is not likely to be harmful to human health if transmitted to the honey. Such products are called non-medicinal curative substances and include formic acid (60 percent and 85 percent), lactic acid, oxalic acid, thymol and other essential oils, industrial talc, and liquid paraffin, which may be administered to bees. The safety of 'frow mixture' (containing nitrobenzene, petrol, ligroin, methyl salicylate, and safrol) has not been assessed and should not be used for bees.

Prescribing of medicines

Legal requirements and provisions determine which medicines may be administered to animals or incorporated in the feedingstuffs of food-producing animals. These restrictions are of fundamental importance to veterinarians as they decide which medicines should be administered to an animal and they authorise that administration.

'Prescribing' is often taken to cover supply or dispensing. It is therefore important to remember the restrictions on supply when dispensing medicines for administration to the animal to be treated.

The *Medicines Act 1968* provides that the normal channel of retail supply of medicines should be through a retail pharmacy. There is an exception for GSL products, which may be sold freely. There is a further exception for a veterinarian, who is allowed to supply POM, PML and P products but only to be administered to animals under his/her care. The phrase 'animals under his/her care' places a restriction on the veterinarian's ability to supply POM, PML and P medicines and an understanding of this important term is given below.

Under *The Medicines (Restrictions on the Administration of Veterinary Medicinal Products) Regulations 1994* as amended, no person is allowed to administer any veterinary medicine to an animal unless the product has been granted a marketing authorisation (product licence) for treatment of the particular condition in the species being treated. *The Regulations apply to both food-producing and non-food producing animals*. There are important specific exceptions to this rule outlined in the 'cascade' method of prescribing (below). Veterinarians are reminded that if they feel that circumstances compel them to use a medicine not covered by the available legislation, they should contact the VMD.

Under the Regulations, where no authorised veterinary medicine exists for a condition in a particular species, a veterinarian, or a person acting under the veterinarian's direction, may administer to a particular animal under his /her or a small number of such animals kept on the same premises

(1) a veterinary medicine authorised for use in another animal species or for another condition in the same species ('off-label use'); or

(2) if no product as described in (1) exists, an authorised human medicine; or

(3) if no product as described in (2) exists, a product prepared extemporaneously by an authorised person in accordance with a veterinary prescription.

'Special-order' products are extemporaneously prepared products that are not commercially available such as preparations containing an usual formulation or drug concentration, or are preservative or additive free. They may be obtained from certain manufacturers or hospital manufacturing units. Where a product is authorised, the authorised preparation should be used unless a specific formulation is required.

A veterinarian should advise the owner that he or she intends to administer to the animal an authorised human preparation or an authorised veterinary preparation outwith its data sheet recommendations, and ideally obtain the client's written consent (see Consent forms). The veterinarian should prescribe from knowledge based on best current practice. Advice should be sought from pharmaceutical companies and/or consultants and such information recorded and retained.

There has been much debate over the introduction of these Regulations and the VMD have produced guidance notes for veterinarians on interpretation of the legislation (*The Medicines (Restrictions on the administration of veterinary medicinal products) Regulations 1994 (SI 1994/2987): Guidance to the veterinary profession*. AMELIA 8, March 1995). The aims of the legislation are to ensure that medicinal treatment of animals is safe and effective both for the animal, and in the case of food-producing animals safe for the consumer. The VMD advise that 'It is likely that the Regulations will be interpreted in the light of how a competent and professional veterinary surgeon would reasonably act in pursuance of these aims in a particular set of circum-

stances.' (AMELIA 8). In addition, particular issues are discussed below.

A condition in a particular species

In some instances, a product may be authorised for a condition in a particular species but be deemed to be not the product of first choice or even ineffective for the animal(s) presented. Such instances may arise due to bacterial resistance to antimicrobials and chronic infections, if the recommended dosage would be inadequate, the age and known sensitivities of the individual animal, complex conditions requiring concurrent drug treatment, unavailability of a product within a reasonable time, or owner compliance considerations provide that a formulation of an authorised product would be inappropriate. In such circumstances, the VMD indicate that 'where a veterinarian exercising his or her professional expertise and judgement in the interests of the animals under his or her care may consider that no licensed treatment exists for the condition or species to be treated ... a veterinary surgeon may prescribe another product in accordance with the cascade' AMELIA 8.

Animal under his/her care

There is no definition in the legislation of the term 'animal or herd which is under his care' - the phrase which is usually condensed to 'animals under his/her care'. The Royal College of Veterinary Surgeons (RCVS) has interpreted the meaning of the term in the *Guide to professional conduct*:

'(1) the veterinarian must have been given responsibility for the health of the animal or herd by the owner or the owner's agent

(2) that responsibility must be real and not merely nominal

(3) that the animal or herd must have been seen immediately before prescription and supply or

(4) recently enough or often enough for the veterinary surgeon to have personal knowledge of the condition of the animal or current health status of the herd or flock to make a diagnosis and prescribe

(5) the veterinary surgeon must maintain clinical records of that herd/flock/individual.

What amounts to "recent enough" must be a matter for the professional judgement of the veterinary surgeon in the individual case.'

The RCVS advice is offered for professional and ethical purposes. In a number of cases, the courts have also followed this guidance. If a veterinarian retails (or supplies under conditions corresponding to retail sale), POM, P, or PML products which are administered to animals which a court does not find to be under his/her care, the veterinarian can be convicted of an offence under the *Medicines Act 1968*.

In an emergency situation, a veterinarian may prescribe medicines, which are part of an animal's routine medicinal therapy although the animal is not usually under the care of the veterinarian (e.g. owners on holiday with their animals). The veterinarian should examine the animal and make every attempt to contact the animal's usual veterinarian to obtain the relevant case history. Only sufficient quantity of drug for the animal's immediate use should be prescribed.

Written records should be kept.

Where a client is served by more than one veterinarian or two or more veterinarians are each concerned with the same group of animals, each may properly prescribe and supply medicines to be administered to animals as part of the services provided. In order to avoid adverse reactions arising from unsuitable combinations of products, each veterinarian must keep the other(s) informed about the products he or she prescribes.

Small number of animals

The Regulations indicate that this term does not apply to non-food producing animals of minor or exotic species. 'The Directive is worded in a way which makes it clear that some companion animals are not minor or exotic species, but does not define which they are. We suggest that, as a working rule, minor and exotic species be taken to cover all companion, laboratory and zoo animals (other than any whose produce might enter the food chain) other than cats and dogs. This approach should not preclude veterinarians from concluding that in certain circumstances, certain especially sensitive breeds of cat and dog could be considered as exotic if that were to be considered necessary to treat them safely and effectively' AMELIA 8.

When treating food-producing animals the VMD consider that the 'small number' limitation would 'need to be decided on a case by case basis taking account, for example, of the method of administration, the degree of contact between the animals concerned and the condition being treated. As a general example, however, we consider that if a veterinarian wishes to sedate a deer, the deer will be treated as an individual, so in those circumstances a 'small number' would mean not more than the individual. Where, however, a veterinarian is required to treat an infectious disease in, say, farmed fish, he or she may need to proceed on the assumption that all individuals in one cage in contact with one another are all equally and identically at risk, and the interpretation of 'small number' may reflect this. What will remain unacceptable would be the indiscriminate prescription of unlicensed medicines [i.e. medicines used outwith the marketing authorisation] for use in animals and fish whose need for and propensity to benefit from treatment has not been assessed' AMELIA 8.

Food-producing animals

A food-producing animal is an animal whose flesh or products are intended for human consumption.

Veterinarians should keep adequate case records, including details of medicines used for the treatment of animals and the circumstances of their use. Records must be kept when prescribing, administering, and supplying medicines for food-producing animals under the 'cascade' (see Record keeping). Unless the product is a homœopathic medicinal product in which the level of active principles is equal to or less than one part per million, the veterinarian must specify an appropriate withdrawal period (see Drug Residues).

In addition to the above legislation, if the animal is a food-producing animal, the veterinarian or person acting under his direction may only administer a product that contains substances found in a product authorised in the UK for use in food-producing animals. This applies whichever tier of the cascade is used i.e. veterinary, human, or specially prepared medicines. Pharmacologically active substances which are not contained in products currently authorised for food-producing species, including those in products that have been withdrawn, or the active ingredient has been entered into Annex IV or for which there is no Annex entry under Regulation 2377/90/EEC, must not be administered to food-producing animals under the cascade.

This restriction may create problems for ensuring correct treatment of food-producing animals because some important therapeutic products are not authorised in these species. In particular, the VMD have issued guidance on use of anaesthetics in these species: 'at present cannot envisage the Ministry would wish to take action against veterinary surgeons prescribing and using anaesthetics and analgesics which are necessary for the health and welfare of animals in circumstances where no suitable authorised product exists and where the imposition of the withdrawal period set down in the Regulations would protect consumers' AMELIA 8.

Under EC legislation the horse is regarded as a food-producing animal. However, under recent EC legislation Equidae registered with breed societies must be accompanied with an identification document (passport) and Equidae that are intended for breeding and production also require a passport. The passport will include declarations concerning whether the animal is or is not intended for slaughter for human consumption. The purpose of these changes is to provide a means by which Equidae may be identified as to whether or not the animal may enter the food chain; consideration is currently being given to the precise way in which they will be implemented in the UK. This legislation allows continued use of medicines authorised for the treatment of Equidae that do not have Maximum Residue Limits (MRL) or withdrawal periods specified for Equidae e.g. phenylbutazone. However these products will maintain a contra-indication stating that they are *not* for use in horses intended for human consumption. The passport will include a new Annex ('Medicinal Treatment') in which to record veterinary medicines administered to the horse. Owners of Equidae not intended for human consumption will be required to sign the declaration at Part II of the new Annex and details of products that have been administered must be recorded in Part IIIB.

For Equidae that *are* intended for slaughter for human consumption, authorised medicines with equine withdrawal periods must be used. The proposed EC legislation appears to recognise that the status or purpose of Equidae may change because the authorised medicines for animals intended for human consumption includes products listed in Annex I, II, and III of 2377/90/EEC and also 'other substances'. This wording permits phenylbutazone to be used in a horses not originally intended for human consumption. Where e.g. phenylbutazone is administered to an Equidae that at a later time its status changes to that of intended for human consumption, it would appear that a minimum withdrawal period of 6 months would be required. The requirement to record all medicinal treatments in Part IIIB of the passport is therefore very important. Equidae treated with substances in Annex IV of 2377/90/EEC must *never* be slaughtered for human consumption.

Special Treatment Authorisation

Where there is no suitable authorised product animal available in the UK to treat a particular condition in a specific animal and the use of a human or extemporaneously prepared medicine is inappropriate, a veterinarian may import and supply (or use) a medicine which is authorised in another country, e.g. mitotane for the treatment of Cushing's syndrome in dogs.

The veterinarian should apply for a Special Treatment Authorisation (STA) from the VMD. This allows supply of a medicine on a named-patient basis under certain conditions. Guidelines provided by the VMD state that an STA may be issued 'to allow the treatment of individual animals suffering from conditions which cannot be treated using medicines available to the UK veterinary surgeon by normal means. They will not be issued if a suitable product is authorised and marketed in the UK for either animal or human use. Before an STA is issued, the VMD must be satisfied that the benefits of using the product will outweigh any risks and will not pose a threat to human or animal health or the environment. For these reasons, STAs may not be a suitable way of obtaining products to treat food producing animals .... [and] STAs will be issued for the importation of vaccines only in exceptional circumstances.' (VMD *Special Treatment Authorisations* AMELIA 10, November 1995).

Applications for STAs should be sent to: Information Management Section, (Special Treatment Authorisations), Veterinary Medicines Directorate, New Haw, Addlestone, Surrey KT15 3NB.

Prescribing by veterinarians established in EEA states other than the UK

The Medicines (Veterinary Medicinal Products) (Veterinary Surgeons from Other EEA States) Regulations 1994 apply to veterinarians established in EEA states other than the UK but whose practices extend into the UK. They permit such veterinarians to carry with them and use medicines (other than immunologicals) not authorised in the UK provided such medicines are authorised in the Member State in which the veterinarian is established. The Regulations specify further provisions which must be complied with and restrict the range and quantity of such medicines to those required for the daily needs of good veterinary practice.

Personal importation of veterinary medicines

The *Medicines (Restrictions on the Administration of Veterinary Medicinal Products) Regulations 1994*, as amended apply to products administered to animals whether or not they are placed on the market in the UK. They require that any product administered to animals or imported for the purposes of administration must be authorised in the UK. The VMD takes the view that a product, which is authorised in the UK, is one which is labelled for the UK market, and which bears the UK authorisation number. This would include products, which may additionally be labelled for another country's market. It must be borne in mind that a product imported into the UK is subject to the UK conditions of use, such as withdrawal period and distribution category.

There may be incidences where a product is imported for administration but which is not labelled as above. For example, a holidaymaker returning to the UK from the continent with their pet with treatment that has been prescribed by a European veterinarian. The VMD state they 'will primarily have regard to the likelihood of risks to human or animal safety. Factors which might be considered are whether the product is in fact the same as a UK authorised product, or whether there are minor differences having no effect on safety, whether the product is for food-producing or pet animals, the adequacy of the label, and its consistency with the equivalent UK label'. (VMD *Note on imports of veterinary medicinal products for administration to animals* October 1998).

Prescribing medicines for use in dart guns

The possession of weapons and ammunition designed for tranquillising and treating animals and kept for that purpose is governed by the *Firearms (Amendment) Act 1997*. This legislation will affect veterinarians who possess tranquillising dart guns in order to treat animals, and who prescribe medicines for use in dart guns or blow pipes. Drugs such as etorphine and ketamine are not authorised for food-producing animals and treated animals cannot be used human consumption.

The veterinarian or applicant must have a firearms certificate that states the purpose for which the item will be used, e.g. treating animals. (Until 1997 Secretary of State authorisation was also required.) RCVS guidance indicates that the veterinarian should ensure that the animals are 'under his/ her care'. In addition, there should be sufficient supervision considering that the medicines used are POM. The veterinarian should supply the POM only in sufficient quantity for immediate use and must instruct the user (no matter how expert the latter may be) in the use of the gun and tranquilliser. They must also direct the user as to what to do in an emergency, e.g. a person being struck by a dart. The veterinarian need not be present when the dart gun is used. It is recommended to keep this method of medication under joint review so that any additional necessary advice can be given.

The Veterinary Defence Society has produced a *Guideline for veterinary surgeons using darting procedures* and an Outline Agreement regarding the use of etorphine hydrochloride based substances by non-veterinarians, copies of which are available from the VDS (The Veterinary Defence Society Ltd, 4 Haig Court, Parkgate Estate, Knutsford, Cheshire WA16 8XZ. Telephone 01565 652737. Facsimile 01565 751079).

Dispensing medicines

Advertising and display

There are serious concerns regarding advertising of POM preparations such as antimicrobials to the general public and the possibility of the general public obtaining such products from inappropriate sources and using them without proper controls. However it may be valuable to advise clients of other products that are POM such as flea treatments because restriction on advertising could limit education, provision of information to clients, and preventative health care. For guidance POM products should not be advertised to the general public but may be advertised to clients e.g. posters in the waiting room and vaccination and flea treatment reminder cards. P, PML and GSL preparations may be displayed to the public but dummy packets for P and PML products must be used unless display cabinets are secure. The RCVS advises in the *Guide to professional conduct* that 'Medicines may be advertised to clients or to prospective clients only at their request and may not be advertised generally'.

Premises

Premises in which medicines are stored should be a building, or part of a building, of a permanent nature. Areas used for sale, supply or storage of medicines should not be any residential part of a dwellinghouse. Premises should be kept clean and vermin proof. Premises should be divided into areas to which the public have access (waiting room, surgeries, etc.) and 'staff only' areas where public access is not allowed or is controlled.

Premises in which medicines are stored and dispensed should be capable of being secured so as to exclude the public and deter unlawful entry. Insurers may require that the premises are fitted with a security alarm. Storage within the premises must also be secure and, ideally, no other activity should be allowed in storage areas. Refrigerated space must be provided for products with specific temperature requirements.

Controlled drugs and injection equipment present an attractive target not only to addicts but also to professional criminals aware of large profits to be made from illicit drug sales. The Advisory Committee on the Misuse of Drugs reviewed the security of controlled drugs in 1983. Advice should be obtained from the local crime prevention officer on the suitability of premises, receptacles, etc. for controlled drugs.

Medicines kept in consulting rooms to which the public has access should be kept to a minimum, should not be drugs of abuse, and should be kept in cupboards and drawers not readily accessible to clients. Only the minimum necessary quantities of medicines should be carried by car.

A list of key telephone numbers (doctor, hospital, fire service, poisons centre, etc.) should be prominently displayed. Appropriate safety equipment must be available. The *Control of Substances Hazardous to Health Regulations 1999* (COSHH) must be observed (contact BVA, 7 Mansfield Street, London W1M 0AT. Telephone 020 76366541. Facsimile 020 7436 2970 for further information).

There must be no smoking, eating, or storage of food for human consumption in areas where medicines are stored or dispensed. There should be notices in place to inform staff and clients accordingly.

Personnel

In all practices there must be a named person (preferably a veterinarian), who is responsible for seeing that the requirements of this code of practice are observed. It would be convenient for the same person to also be responsible for complying with COSHH requirements and waste disposal regulations. A Practice Manual should be prepared which provides staff with detailed specific instructions on practice policy including dispensing of medicines.

Anyone involved in dispensing activity (unless handling GSL products) must be suitably trained. This is particularly important for POM products. The veterinarian can supply POM products (to clients whose animals are 'under his/her care'). The qualified veterinary nurse or trained and authorised person can supply POM products provided he or she does so under the authority of the prescribing veterinarian.

All persons engaged in dispensing should observe high standards of personal cleanliness. Protective clothing should be disposable or regularly and frequently cleaned.

No person with open lesions or skin infections should be engaged in dispensing processes. Staff must report infections and skin lesions. All persons should keep any cut or abrasion on any exposed part of their person covered with a suitable waterproof dressing.

Direct contact between the operator's hands and the dispensed products should be avoided, for example by wearing gloves or by using a tablet counting device.

The dispensary

Great care should be taken to ensure safe storage of all medicines. Medicines should be stored in accordance with manufacturers' instructions. They should be protected from the adverse effects of extremes of environmental conditions, such as light, temperature, and humidity in the dispensary. Blinds, as necessary, should cover windows. Light-sensitive products should be protected from light. Sterilisers should not be sited in the dispensary because they may affect the humidity of the room. Ventilation must be adequate.

In order to avoid contamination, stocks of medicines to be supplied to clients must not be stored in toilets, laboratories, or places where animals are kept such as kennels.

Particular attention should be taken to ensure that products are stored at the correct temperature. Refrigerated space must be provided for products such as vaccines, anti-sera, and some reconstituted antibiotic solutions with specific low temperature storage requirements. Vaccines, etc. should be refrigerated as soon as received. Biological samples, food, bacteriological media, etc. should be stored in designated refrigerators. Particular care should be taken to avoid freezing or prolonged exposure to high temperatures. Refrigerators must be maintained at 2° C to 8° C and should be fitted with a means of regular daily monitoring and recording of temperatures such as a minimum/maximum thermometer and dedicated log book. An electronic device can be used to monitor temperature or manual temperature monitoring is adequate provided an accurate temperature recording is obtained and the bulb of the thermometer is placed in glycerol to reduce temperature fluctuations. A named person should check and record the temperature of each refrigerator. In-car refrigeration units are now available. Regular servicing, cleaning, and stock control should be maintained for refrigerators as for other storage areas.

Flammable products must be stored in appropriate cabinets specifically designed for the purpose.

Well-designed shelving and fittings should be installed to reduce the possibility of breakage, spillage, and stock misplacement. A named person should be responsible for stock control.

It is good practice to affix a practice label to each item before it is placed in stock. The date of first usage on multi-dose vials and date at which the vial should be discarded should be indicated. Multi-dose vials with an in-use shelf life now have a suitably labelled space for the user to insert the date for discarding the opened container. In general, medicines should be stored in the original container until required.

Dates of deliveries from manufacturers or wholesalers should be recorded, unless this information is on an invoice from the manufacturer or wholesaler, which is retained. Batches of the same product should be kept separate and older stock should be issued before new, i.e. careful stock rotation should be maintained.

Packs with defaced or damaged labels, damaged packs, or those that are date expired should be removed. Such items should not be sold.

Once stock has been dispensed, it should not be accepted back into the dispensary. No returned goods should be offered for resale because there may have been problems with storage conditions beyond the veterinarian's control. Although stock that has to be returned to a manufacturer or wholesaler should be returned without delay, there are strict regulations relating to returned stock accepted by wholesalers.

Only medicines used frequently should be carried routinely in vehicles. It is good practice to store a minimum amount of preparations in a car because the temperature within the car may fluctuate greatly and the efficacy of the products may be affected. An insulated container will provide short-term storage for some temperature sensitive items. Precautions against theft from vehicles must be taken.

Veterinarians should attempt to ensure that farmers store medicines properly and that preparations are not used beyond their expiry date or broached vial usage period (see Working with clients).

Very strict requirements operate for the storage of controlled drugs. Security is essential. Only the minimum quantity of controlled drugs should be stored consistent with routine needs and emergencies of the practice Schedule 2 and some Schedule 3 controlled drugs must be kept in a suitable locked receptacle which can only be opened by the veterinarian or by a person authorised by veterinarian to do so.

This is best implemented by having no more than one key to the receptacle per veterinarian. The keys should be kept on the person. A locked car is **not** considered to be such a receptacle within the meaning of the *Misuse of Drugs (Safe Custody) Regulations 1973* and veterinarians are advised to provide additional locked units within any vehicles used for the transport of such medicines.

Supply of human medicines for animals

A veterinarian or a person under his direction may supply an authorised human medicine for use in a particular animal (see Prescribing of medicines). A veterinarian should advise the owner that he or she intends to administer an authorised human preparation to the animal and ideally obtain the client's written consent (see Consent forms).

Some manufacturers may be reluctant to supply veterinarians directly with authorised human preparations. In such instances, veterinarians may write a prescription for supply from a pharmacist.

Guidance on the supply of an authorised human medicine for animal use by a pharmacist is given by the RPSGB. Supply may be given only with prior direction from a veterinarian. This instruction may be given verbally for GSL or P products but must be written for POM products. It is good practice for the pharmacist to record when a verbal instruction has been given by a veterinarian or for the written instruction in the form of a prescription to be entered into the prescription book in the pharmacy. The pharmacist has to be satisfied that a veterinarian has given an instruction before a supply was made. If a pharmacist is asked for an authorised human product by an animal owner for use in/on the animal, the pharmacist should refer to a veterinarian for either a recommendation or a prescription.

Containers

The RPSGB recommends that when medicines are repacked from bulk or prepared extemporaneously they must be packed in containers that are appropriate for the product dispensed and the user. All containers intended for medicinal products must be protected and free from contamination.

In general, all solid dose and all oral and external preparations should be dispensed in a reclosable child resistant container. However there are exemptions to this requirement. If the medicine is in the manufacturer's original pack such as blister-packed medicines, it may be inadvisable to change the container. Sachets and manufacturers' strip or blister-packed medicines should be dispensed in paper board cartons or wallets, or paper envelopes.

Discretion may be exercised in the use of child-proof containers. There are occasions when they are clearly inappropriate (aged and infirm clients, large animal formulations, no suitable child resistant container exists for a particular liquid preparation, etc.). A notice should be displayed in the waiting room indicating that tablets and capsules will normally be dispensed in child-proof containers but that plain containers can be supplied on request. Advice must be given to keep all medicines out of reach of children.

Tablets, capsules, and powders are often adversely affected by moisture and should be stored in the original container until required in order to protect the medicine against breakage, crushing, moisture ingress, contamination, and deterioration with the lid being properly replaced after use. In addition, adequate labelling and stock rotation should be taken into account when repackaging tablets ready for dispensing.

Paper envelopes and plastic bags are unacceptable as the *sole* container of veterinary medicines.

Under the *Medicines (Fluted Bottles) Regulations 1978* certain liquid medicinal products for external use should be dispensed in fluted bottles so that they are recognisable by touch. This requirement does not apply to containers of a capacity greater than 1.14 litres or to eye or ear drops supplied in plastic containers. However, fluted bottles may be difficult to obtain. Therefore it is recommended that preparations be dispensed as proprietary products in containers supplied by the manufacturer wherever possible.

Creams, dusting powders, granules, ointments, pessaries, powders, suppositories, semi-solids, etc. should be dispensed in wide-mouthed jars made of glass or plastic.

Medicines sensitive to light should be dispensed in an opaque or appropriately coloured container.

It is good practice to supply e.g. injectable antibacterials for administration by farmers, in 20 ml or 40 ml vials available from manufacturers (rather than in syringes).

The dispenser has a duty to ensure that the owner understands any instructions on the label (see below) and knows how to use the product safely. The owner or keeper of the animal or herd must be warned to keep all medicines out of reach of children.

Labelling of dispensed medicines

All medicines sold or supplied by a veterinarian or pharmacist in accordance with a prescription given by a veterinarian, are by definition 'dispensed medicines' and as such must be labelled correctly as given in *The Medicines (Labelling) Regulations 1976* as amended. Dispensing veterinarians should ensure that **the label uses mechanically printed lettering** (i.e. computer generated) or labels must be indelibly and legibly printed or written in accordance with statutory requirements. Biro, ballpoint or felt tip pens are acceptable for labelling; ink and pencil are not. The label must include:

- the name of the owner or keeper or the person who has control of the animal or herd (or group)
- the address of the premises where the animal or herd is kept or the address of one of such premises
- the name and address of the veterinarian
- the date of dispensing
- the words 'for animal treatment only', unless the container or package is too small for it to be practicable to do so
- the words 'keep out of the reach of children' or words having a similar meaning
- the words 'for external use only' or 'not to be taken internally' for medicines that are only for topical use

(e.g. embrocations, liniments, ear or eye formulations, lotions, liquid antiseptics or other liquid preparation or gel)

- the relevant withdrawal period should always be stated on medicines for food-producing animals. The withdrawal period, even if it is nil, should be indicated
- when writing a prescription the veterinarian may request that it be labelled with any of the following particulars (which the veterinarian would use if he or she were dispensing directly to a client): (a) the drug name, concentration and amount dispensed; (b) directions for use; (c) where appropriate, precautions relating to the use of the product to ensure operator safety. It is good practice to supply the operator with e.g. disposable gloves when dispensing griseofulvin-containing powder or granules; (d) name or description of animal(s) to be treated.

Ideally, the label should not obscure the expiry date of the preparation or important printed information on the manufacturer's label or pack. For preparations such as tubes of eye ointment, the product may be dispensed in an appropriately labelled envelope.

Specimen labels

Example 1 Dispensing 20 x 10 mg acepromazine tablets for a dog

```
Name of animal
Name and address of client
Date

      20 x 10 mg acepromazine tablets
   2 tablets by mouth, before travelling

              For Animal Treatment Only
   ─────────────────────────────────────────
        Keep all medicines out of reach of children
                  J G Bloggs MRCVS
              2 High Street, Coxton, Surrey
```

Example 2 Dispensing 50 ml x 15% framycetin injection for a cow

```
Identification number of animal
Name and address of client
Date

   50 ml x Framycetin Injection 150 mg/ml
   15 ml by intramuscular injection daily
       Withholding times:Meat 49 days
                        Milk 56 hours

              For Animal Treatment Only
   ─────────────────────────────────────────
        Keep all medicines out of reach of children
                  J G Bloggs MRCVS
              2 High Street, Coxton, Surrey
```

Apart from complying with the legislation, instructions on labels should be aimed at creating a greater awareness on the part of the end user as to the manner in which animal medicines should be stored, handled, and administered. The dispenser should bring the owner's attention to the instructions and to provide clarification or answer any questions.

Product information leaflets are often supplied by the manufacturer to supplement the information on the container and package. This additional information may prove useful to the end user and product information sheets, package inserts, or leaflets should be dispensed with the product.

Sending medicines by post

Pharmaceutical companies occasionally send medicines directly to a veterinary practice by post and wholesalers frequently use this means to forward medicines to remote practices when small items are required urgently. Veterinarians may send medicines by post to clients whose animals are under the veterinarian's care provided the medicines are not hazardous to the public, are in child resistant or manufacturer's original containers, and have been safely packed. Safe packaging is especially important for liquid medicines and the veterinarian must ensure that there should be no leakage outside the packaging if the inner container breaks; the inner container must be covered in polythene, absorbent material, etc. For the purposes of transporting CD medicines, the Home Office classifies these products as low, medium, and high risk depending on the drug and amount dispatched. In general, the usual amount of CD medicines sent by the veterinarian to a client would be classified as low risk and may be sent by post. The Home Office advises that postal services used should provide transit security or an audit trail capable of identifying where any loss has occured.

Working with clients

Under *COSHH Regulations* the veterinarian has a duty of care to ensure that an owner knows how to use a product safely and that this information is made known to the person actually using the product. The veterinarian may assist farmers with their COSHH assessment.

The veterinarian should ensure that only sufficient quantities of medicines are prescribed or supplied to the owner for the individual or group of animals being treated. In particular cases, it will be reasonable to allow selected clients to hold a small reserve of some preparations provided the veterinarian recognises a recurring need for the use and is satisfied that the client has demonstrated his reliability in all aspects of using medicines.

Clients should be advised that instructions provided should be read carefully before administering any medicine. Clients should be advised to check any warning statement and guidance given about how a medicine should **not** be used, in particular whether it can be used concurrently with any other medicines given to the animal.

Clear and concise advice should be given to clients on the safe storage and use of medicines supplied or prescribed. Clients should be advised to store medicines correctly and

in accordance with the instructions on the label. Medicines should be stored securely and should be kept out of reach of children or animals.

Part-used packs of injectable preparations should be discarded safely at the end of each daily operation or use and not re-used on subsequent days unless the data sheet specifies such a usage of opened packs. The date of first usage on multi-dose vials and date at which the vial should be discarded should be indicated. Multi-dose vials with an in-use shelf life now have a suitably labelled space for the user to insert the date for discarding the opened container. The expiry date on the label should be checked and the medicines should not be used past that date.

Clients should be reminded to use medicines only on animals recommended on the label or leaflet, unless the veterinarian has otherwise directed. The result of giving a medicine to an animal for which it is not recommended is unpredictable and may endanger the animal.

The BVA recommends that **Written Standard Operating Procedures** (SOPs) should be designed by the veterinarian attending food-producing animals to cover medicines that are used regularly on a farm. The SOPs should be under the direct supervision of the veterinarian and confidentially maintained. The reason for the use of the medicine, the dosage regimen, instructions on correct administration, storage requirements, and identification of withdrawal periods should be specified. The veterinarian should provide additional information on exactly how the withdrawal period must be followed.

During farm visits a detailed appraisal of medicinal usage on the farm should be undertaken. Discussion should take place with the stockpersons who carry out the routine day-to-tasks to ensure that the correct procedures are in use. In addition, line management on the enterprise should be observed with the owner or manager kept fully informed.

The livestock farmer has a statutory obligation to keep records (see Record keeping). A veterinarian has an ethical obligation to help the client keep such records.

Client education plays a vital role in ensuring that medicines are used correctly. The VMD publishes a *Code of Practice on the Responsible Use of Animal Medicines on the Farm*. In addition, there is a *Code of Practice for the Safe Use of Medicines on Farms* agreed by a number of organisations and a copy of this Code is included in the NOAH Animal Medicines Record Book. Regular newsletters or presentations giving clients information on issues, such as legislation affecting the manner in which veterinarians prescribe and dispense medicines, will help clients to understand any restrictions placed upon them. Open days also allow clients to observe working practices.

Supply of prostaglandins for use on the farm

Prostaglandins are very potent compounds with a wide range of physiological effects. Accidental self-injection or inadvertent inhalation of spray due to poor injection technique may cause severe reactions in humans.

Prostaglandins are used in cattle for treating unobserved oestrus, controlled breeding programmes, treatment of pyo-

Specimen form for Safe Use of Prostaglandin Products in Sows

[Practice Stamp]

SAFE USE OF PROSTAGLANDIN PRODUCTS IN SOWS

(1) I [name] understand and will carry out the following procedures for the safe use and administration of Prostaglandin [proprietary name].

(2) I have read and I understand the packaging leaflet/data sheet/my veterinarian has explained the data sheet.

(3) The handling of this product is restricted to myself and   [name] who is also bound by these rules.

(4) At ALL times the product will be stored in a nominated locked place.

(5) No other person will have access to the product or handle it.

(6) It will be administered only to sows that are my property and on my farm/farms for the induction of farrowing or other indication as directed.

(7) I will record the date of administration of each dose with the records of the sow and dose volume given together with identification of the sow in accordance with legislation.

(8) Supplies of the product will be obtained by me personally from the qualified veterinarian who has the sows under his/her care. I will sign for each consignment.

(9) Empty containers of the product will be disposed of in accordance with the agreed farm policy for disposal of pharmaceutical waste.

(10) I agree to receiving instructions as to the handling, storage, administration, and recording of the use of this product and will abide by them.

 (11) A new sterile syringe and needle will be used for each dose of the product administered. After the injection has been given the syringe and needle will be either returned to the practice or safely destroyed on the farm as agreed.

(12) Waterproof gloves will be worn by the operator handling the product; accidental spillage will be washed off the skin immediately and in the event of accidental injection, medical advice will be sought urgently.

(13) I understand that contact with prostaglandin products by women of child-bearing age or by asthmatics constitutes a particular potential hazard and is to be avoided.

(14) These rules will be displayed where the product is to be stored.

(15) I understand that failure to comply with these instructions at any time would result in no further issue of product.

Signature and date

Name and address

Telephone

Site of storage of prostaglandins if different to above

Counter signature of veterinarian   Date metra/chronic endometritis, induction of calving, hastening placental expulsion, treatment of cystic ovarian disease, and misalliance. All these indications demand accurate identification of the animals and proper veterinary examination and diagnosis.

In pig practice, prostaglandins are mainly used for the induction of farrowing. It is accepted that for logistical reasons it would not be possible to insist on veterinary administration for this purpose. If the veterinarian decides it is necessary to supply or prescribe prostaglandins for, e.g. farrowing purposes, he should ensure that the products are issued to one named person only. The guidelines given below should be followed.

Prostaglandins are POM and should be issued by a veterinarian only to a farmer who is a bona fide client, for use on his own sows, on his own farm or farms and issued on the basis that the named person/persons is individually responsible for the product storage, handling, administration and accountability, and also signs a receipt for each consignment of the product.

Records of supply and administration in accordance with legislation must be kept by the veterinarian and the farmer (see Record keeping). The veterinarian should advise the farmer that at all times the product **must** be kept in a secure locked place except as/when required for administration to sows. The on-farm storage conditions should be inspected and approved by the veterinarian.

The veterinarian should issue only sufficient product for the immediate use on the farm. Periodically the veterinarian should check the amount issued against the number of animals treated. The veterinarian should issue new stocks against the return of used or date expired packs or in accordance with amounts used as indicated by the farmer's records. The farmer should be supplied with a container in which to store sharps and syringes and needles issued with the product which should either be returned to the veterinary practice for disposal, or safely destroyed.

The client should be instructed on the safe handling of the product, the filling of syringes, the method and site of injection and warned of the risk of product exposure to women of child-bearing age and asthmatics. The packaging leaflet, copy of data sheet or copy of technical brochure should be issued to the farmer. Waterproof gloves should be worn when handling the product and any spillage should be washed off the skin immediately. In the event of accidental administration to a person, medical advice should be sought promptly.

Prostaglandins should be issued only for induction of farrowing in sows if farm records are adequate to indicate the average gestation length taking the first day of service as Day 0. The product should not be administered earlier than three days before the expected date of farrowing and it is recommended that induced farrowings be supervised.

No treated animals may be slaughtered until the appropriate withdrawal period has expired.

The BVA has compiled a form **Safe Use of Prostaglandin Products in Sows** (see above). The veterinarian is advised to request that the farmer signs the form in which he undertakes to follow a code of practice. Failure of a farmer to comply with the code of practice should result in the veterinarian withholding supply of further quantities of the product under the terms of item (15) of the undertaking (see Specimen form).

The procedure for issue of prostaglandins to a farmer client should be reviewed at regular intervals to take account of the changes in management, sow numbers, or other practical conditions on the farm.

Record keeping

It is imperative that veterinarians and all personnel involved in administration and dispensing of medicines keep permanent records. In addition to specific legal requirements for record keeping, it may be necessary to record reasons for prescribing. Under legislation, the record keeping requirements apply to administration and sale and supply for food-producing animals. However veterinarians are encouraged to maintain records of administration and sales of veterinary medicines for pets or other companion animals voluntarily especially to assist product traceability and recall should the need arise.

All necessary records should be kept in a readily retrievable manner (e.g. a handbook, files, or on a computerised data base). Where a computer is used there must be adequate precautions against inadvertent loss of data. Any discrepancies must be entered into the records.

Prescribing cards are a useful aid to record keeping and control of supply. Most small animal practices would keep this information as part of the normal case records except that the name and address of the recipient would be in the patient's record and not kept separately. There is no necessity to transfer such information to the dispensary records. For each animal or group of animals a detailed record should be kept showing what medicines are authorised to be supplied, in what quantities on each occasion, and what actual supply has occurred. A limit on the total supply should be set and no further supply can be made without the authority of a veterinarian in the practice. The cards must be checked periodically.

Records should be kept for three years to comply with the *Medicines Act 1968*. However, they should be retained for at least six years in case a civil action for damages ensues.

Administration by the veterinarian

Under the *Medicines (Restrictions on the Administration of Veterinary Medicinal Products) Regulations 1994*, as amended, a veterinarian must keep permanent records after administration of medicines to food-producing species under the 'cascade' .The following records must be kept by the veterinarian:

* date of examination of animals
* name and address of the owner
* number of animals treated
* diagnosis

- product prescribed
- dosage to be administered
- duration of treatment
- withdrawal period recommended.

The records must be kept and be available for inspection for not less than three years.

Administration by the farmer

Under the *Animals and Animal Products (Examination for Residues and Maximum Residues Limits) Regulations 1997*, a person engaged by way of business in the rearing, production or treatment of animals intended for human consumption, must keep a record of particulars relating to the administration of any veterinary medicinal product to such animals or group of animals. The record must be made as soon as practicable after administration and must include the following information:

- date of purchase
- date of administration
- identity and quantity of the veterinary medicinal product
- name and address of the supplier of the veterinary medicinal product
- identification of the animal or group of animals to which the veterinary medicinal product was administered
- the number of animals treated.
- It may also be in the farmer's interest to record
- the dates on which any withdrawal period for meat, milk, or any other animal product ended
- the date on which the treatment finished
- the name of the person who administered the medicine
- the batch numbers and expiry dates of any products used.

Records must be kept for at least 3 years.

The veterinarian has an obligation to assist clients to keep good records by e.g. supplying a medicines record book. The National Office of Animal Health (NOAH) in conjunction with the Animal Health Distributors Association (AHDA) produce an Animal Medicine Record Book, which is available from NOAH (3 Crossfield Chambers, Gladbeck Way, Enfield, Middlesex EN2 7HF. Telephone 020 83673131. Facsimile 020 8363 1155. E-mail noah@noah.co.uk) or AHDA (Gable Court, 8 Parsons Hill, Hollesley, Woodbridge, Suffolk IP12 3RB. Telephone 01394 410444. Facsimile 01394 410455. E-mail info@ahda.org.uk). The Pig Veterinary Society also produces a Veterinary Medicines Record of Administration Book (available from The Pig Journal, Southview, East Tytherton, Chippenham, Wiltshire SN15 4LX. Telephone 01249 740380. Facsimile 01249 740380. E-mail pig_journal@talk21.com). The NTF Medication Book is available from the National Trainers Federation (NTF) to assist trainers in recording the medical treatment of horses in training. Details from NTF (9 High Street, Lambourn, Hungerford, Berkshire RG17 8XN. Telephone 01488 71719. Facsimile 01488 73005. E-mail ntf@martex.co.uk).

The veterinarian should regularly examine the medicines record book to provide confirmation of the diseases and conditions requiring medication on the farm, whether the dose and regimen is as recommended, and the latest withdrawal periods.

Supply or sale of dispensed medicines by the veterinarian

Under *The Retailers' Records for Veterinary Medicinal Products Regulations 2000*, veterinarians must keep records for each incoming transaction concerning products received from wholesalers, manufacturers, etc. along with each outgoing transactions involving the sale of products to clients. In practice, the legislation applies to all PML, P, or POM products for food-producing animals; GSL medicines are not affected. Records should be made within 48 hours of the transaction, kept for a period of at least three years, and be available for inspection. Information retained must include:

- the date of the transaction
- the identity of the product
- the manufacturer's batch number
- the quantity received or supplied
- the name and address of supplier or recipient.

These Regulations also apply to pharmacists. Pharmacists supplying POM products will also have to record the name and address of the prescribing veterinarian and keep a copy of the prescription. Under the *Medicines (Exemptions for Merchants in Veterinary Drugs) Order 1998* the same record keeping requirements apply to registered agricultural merchants and saddlers.

There has been debate about the practical application of the legislation in particular recording of batch numbers. It is not possible to provide detailed guidance on the practical application of the legislation. Each practice needs to carefully consider their own situation and decide how to practically and realistically comply with the recording requirements for all medicines including those used in the day to day running of the clinic and from car boot stock. System Operating Procedures should be devised.

In addition, at least once a year a detailed audit of all transactions must be carried out. Incoming and outgoing products should be reconciled with those held in stock and any discrepancies recorded. Although small animal transactions are excluded from the Regulations, in order to perform a detailed medicines audit there is a need to account for the items used for companion animals in a mixed (large and small animal) practice, and also to account for breakages, items used in the operating theatre, and out-of-date stock.

Under the *Misuse of Drugs Regulations 1985*, veterinarians must record the purchase and administration or supply of all Schedule 2 controlled drugs in a Register within 24 hours (see Classification of medicines). Although records may be kept by electronic means for POM, P, PML, and GSL medicines, the legislation for CD specifies the method of recording and manual recording in a controlled drugs Register is required for Schedule 2 controlled drugs.

Suspected adverse reaction surveillance scheme

The Suspected Adverse Reaction Surveillance Scheme (SARSS) is a voluntary scheme mainly concerned with the collection of information on the safety of veterinary medicines in all species. The scheme also records suspected antibiotic residues in milk.

A suspected adverse reaction is a harmful and unintended reaction to a veterinary medicine when administered to an animal at its normal dosage. Any veterinary medicine, whether a drug, feed additive, or vaccine, may be associated with an adverse reaction in animals. Suspected adverse reactions in human operators are also seen. All veterinarians should accept as a serious ethical obligation the reporting of suspected adverse reactions to authorised veterinary medicines in animals or humans. Adverse reactions resulting from the use of authorised human medicines under the 'cascade' should also be reported. Any observation which might lead to suspicion of an adverse reaction should be treated with careful professional judgement.

The following categories of suspected adverse reactions are important to detect and record for all species:

- unexpected suspected adverse reaction associated with the use of an authorised product
- expected suspected adverse reaction mentioned in the data sheet but occurring more frequently than expected
- any suspected adverse reaction to a new product within the first year of marketing
- any suspected adverse reaction to an authorised veterinary medicine used outwith the data sheet ('off-label')
- lack of efficacy problems such as antimicrobial or antiparasiticidal resistance
- all suspected adverse reactions in humans possibly associated with the use of a veterinary medicine in an animal
- effects of use of authorised human medicines in animals
- effects of veterinary medicines on the environment
- suspected meat and milk drug residue problems.

A veterinarian may prescribe use of an authorised product outwith the data sheet when he or she concludes that an authorised product does not exist in a particular case because there is a likelihood of a lack of efficacy is suspected or unacceptable side-effects on the part of the authorised product. Such suspicions should be reported to the VMD where they will be recorded and monitored by the Suspected Adverse Reaction Scheme. The VMD will then assess the incidence and severity of side-effects, and the efficacy of the products and act as necessary to amend product literature.

Under the Suspected Antibiotic Residue in Milk Scheme information is collected on incidents involving provisional detection of antibiotic residues in milk of dairy cows, which have been treated with lactating or dry cow therapy to treat or prevent mastitis. Problems in individual dairy cows or bulk tank supplies may be reported. The individual animal should be identified and treatment regimens noted. In addition, information on the milking regime used on the farm such as type and servicing of the milking machine, teat-dipping protocols, the frequency of milking, and herd lactation yield should be given.

Suspected adverse reactions in animals or humans should be reported on Form MLA 252A (Rev.1/99) and suspected antibiotic residues in milk reported on Form MLA 2 (2/00) to:

> Veterinary Medicines Directorate
> FREEPOST KT 4503
> Woodham Lane, New Haw
> Addlestone, Surrey KT15 3NB

Copies of these forms are available on request from the VMD (Telephone 01932 338427. Facsimile 01932 336618), the VMD website (http://www.open.gov.uk/vmd/vmd-home.htm), and tear-out copies are included in the NOAH *Compendium of Data Sheets for Veterinary Products* and *The Veterinary Formulary*.

Identification of the product number is a vital part of the validation of a suspected adverse reaction or suspected antibiotic residues in milk report; the product number should be preceded by the PL, MA, or VM prefix. Suspected adverse reactions involving use of Animal Test Certificates or ATXs should be recorded and reported in the same way as for authorised products. Where a serious reaction occurs (especially death), the report should be sent to the VMD within 15 days of occurence.

It is also important to report a suspected adverse reaction or suspected antibiotic residues in milk to the market authorisation holder so the requisite steps can be taken where appropriate to investigate the alleged problem.

Drug residues

When treating food-producing animals, veterinarians may use only medicines whose ingredients are contained in a product authorised for use in the UK in food-producing animals. This is to ensure that residue implications have been properly and fully evaluated.

Residues of veterinary medicines are defined as pharmacologically active substances (whether active principles, excipients or degradation products) and their metabolites, which remain in foodstuffs obtained from animals that have been administered the veterinary medicine in question.

The Regulation 2377/90/EEC establishes Maximum Residue Limits (MRLs) for pharmacologically active substances used in food-producing animals. The MRL is defined as the maximum concentration of residue resulting from administration of a veterinary medicine which is legally permitted in the Community or recognised as acceptable in or on a food. Substance may be listed in one of the four Annexes to the Regulation as indicated below:

> Annex I - substances for which a full MRL has been fixed
> Annex II - substances for which an MRL is not required
> Annex III - substances for which a provisional MRL has been fixed
> Annex IV - substances for which no MRL can be fixed.

The substances listed in Annex IV are *Aristolchia* spp. and preparations thereof, chloramphenicol, chloroform, chlorpromazine, colchicine, dapsone, dimetridazole, metronidazole, nitrofurans (including furazolidone), and ronidazole. These substances are effectively banned from use in food-producing animals. In addition, substances that do not have an Annex entry (I, II, III) may not be used in food-producing animals e.g. phenylbutazone. Further information on MRLs may be found on the European Medicines Evaluation Agency (EMEA) website (http://www.eudra.org).

MRLs established under these procedures are adopted in Great Britain for surveillance and enforcement purposes under the *Animals and Animal Products (Examination for Residues and Maximum Residues Limits) Regulations 1997*. Under these Regulations a person may not sell or supply for slaughter any animal for human consumption if the withdrawal period of any authorised veterinary product, which has been administered to the animal, has not expired.

The withdrawal period is the time interval after cessation of treatment and before the animal or any of its products can be used as human food (level of residues in the tissues such as muscle, liver, kidney, skin, and fat or products such as milk, eggs, honey is lower than or equal to the MRL).

If no withdrawal period for the species concerned is indicated on the product, the veterinarian must specify a standard minimum withdrawal period of not less than the following:

7 days for eggs

7 days for milk

28 days for meat from poultry and mammals including fat and offal

$500°$ days for meat from fish (where degree days is the cumulative sum of mean daily water temperatures in degrees Celsius following the last treatment).

Whenever medicines are sold, supplied, or used for treating food-producing animals an assessment should first be made to ensure that the appropriate withdrawal period can be observed on the farm. The importance of observing a withdrawal period and its duration for the product used should be fully and clearly explained to the farmer/owner.

The UK has in place a rigorous system of statutory and non-statutory surveillance for veterinary residues in animal products at slaughterhouses and on farm. Both these programmes play a central role in ensuring that the consumer is protected against harmful residues of veterinary medicines.

The National Surveillance Scheme for residues in meat is a statutory programme designed to monitor whether residues of veterinary medicines are passing into meat for human consumption in unacceptable concentrations and fulfils the UK's obligations under Directives 96/22/EEC and 96/23/EEC. The non-statutory programme supplements the statutory programme and extends to analyte/matrix combinations not covered by it. Each year the State Veterinary Service and Meat Hygiene Service collect samples and the Veterinary Laboratories Agency on behalf of the VMD carries out analysis.

Whenever excess levels of active ingredients of authorised medicines are found, the State Veterinary Service undertakes a thorough on-farm investigation. The farmer will be advised on how to ensure that residues do not enter the food chain. Prosecution will be considered if serious shortcomings or deliberate misuse are found.

Farmer education plays a vital role in a successful residue prevention programme. The programme should not only involve the owner and his management, but also his staff and particularly the stockpersons. This can be achieved by regular farm visits, newsletters, and discussion groups.

Product withdrawal periods are subject to change. Information such as the current NOAH booklet on *Withdrawal Periods for Veterinary Products* can be available to the farmer. However some of the information may be outdated and it is important to check the current product data sheet for the appropriate withdrawal periods and ensure that the farmer is advised. Product leaflets should be left with the farmer.

Disposal of medicines

Disposal of veterinary medicines is regulated under many Acts and Regulations. Waste from medicines may be classified as clinical waste or pharmaceutical waste.

Clinical waste is defined as 'any waste which consists wholly or partly of animal tissue, blood or other body fluids, excretions, drugs, pharmaceutical products, swabs or dressings, syringes, needles or other sharp instruments, or any other waste arising from veterinary practice, investigation, treatment, care, teaching, or research'.

Drugs or pharmaceutical products such as tablets, capsules, creams, ointments, ampoules, and syringes and vials, including those containing a small amount of medicinal residue are classified as Group D clinical waste. Some clinical waste is also classified as 'special waste' and subject to controls that are over and above other waste management controls. Waste containing or consisting of POMs is classified as 'special waste'. Pharmaceutical product waste should not be included with clinical waste for disposal. Normal methods of flushing, incinerating, and local refuse collection are not appropriate. The forms required for disposal of 'special waste' are complex.

It is suggested that companies that provide a complete storage and disposal service, including sharps containers and dump-bins, should be employed to ensure safe and effective disposal of medicines; local authorities can provide information on specialist disposal service operators. In some instances, the product data sheet may indicate that the veterinarian should dispose of waste following treatment, e.g. 'Chronogest' (Intervet) or 'Veramix' (Pharmacia & Upjohn).

No person required to keep a register of transactions for controlled drugs may destroy a Schedule 2 controlled drug except in the presence of a person authorised by the Secretary of State such as police officers or Inspectors of the Home Office Drug Office. A record must be made of the date of destruction and the quantity destroyed which the authorised person must sign. Home Office legal advice indicates that destruction is taken to mean 'denatured or made not readily recoverable'. Schedule 2 controlled drugs returned by the client can be destroyed without formality and their destruction need not be entered in the controlled drugs Register. The RPSGB recommends that such destruction is documented and witnessed by a member of staff. In order to ensure that controlled drugs are denatured the RPSGB provides the following guidance. Liquid dose formulations should be added to, and absorbed by, an appropriate amount of cat litter, or similar product. Solid dose forms should be crushed and placed in bleach to which a small amount of hot water is added. The mixture should be stirred to ensure that the drug has been dissolved or dispersed. Ampoules containing parenteral formulations should be crushed with a pestle inside a plastic container. After ensuring that all ampoules are broken, a small amount of bleach or cat litter should be added. Once the controlled drug has been denatured, the resultant mixture should be added to the general pharmaceutical waste in a dump-bin.

The destruction of Schedule 3, 4, and 5 controlled drugs does not require to be witnessed by an authorised person.

In some instances, such as when an animal dies or results of diagnostic tests lead to a change in treatment, medicines may be returned. Medicines returned to the surgery should not be re-used because the condition under which the medicines have been stored will be unknown.

Once a product has reached the final user, the legislation affecting disposal no longer applies. However, a professional responsibility still exists when advising clients as to the proper disposal of dispensed medicines.

Farmers are also subject to the Regulations for the disposal of both pharmaceutical and clinical waste. Veterinarians are exempt from the need to register as carriers, provided they are carrying waste produced in the course of their business. They should consider providing a removal and disposal service for farmers for example by regularly supplying and removing a container for sharps.

Veterinarians should be aware that solutions such as spent sheep dips or pesticides should not be disposed of so as to contaminate water, including ponds, ditches, ground and surface water, public sewers or drains. The disposal of dips must be in accordance with an authorisation granted under *The Groundwater Regulations 1998*. Spent dip should be disposed of by a reputable waste disposal contractor or applied to a suitable area of land. The Environment Agency or the Scottish Environment Protection Agency should be contacted for advice. Dip concentrate should not be disposed of on the farm but should be disposed of by a reputable specialist waste disposal contractor. Farmers can contact the Environmental Services Association (154 Buckingham Palace Road, London, SW1W 9TR. Telephone 020 7824 8882. Facsimile 020 7824 8753. E-mail info@esauk.demon.co.uk) for advice on reputable waste disposal contractors.

Empty dip containers should be made safe so as to be unable to be re-used. They may be rinsed and then either buried or disposed of at licensed disposal sites depending on the original contents of the container. Rinsings should be handled as for spent sheep dips.

Consent forms

Guidance on consent forms is given by the British Veterinary Association in consultation with the Veterinary Defence Society; further information may be obtained from the VDS (The Veterinary Defence Society Ltd, 4 Haig Court, Parkgate Estate, Knutsford, Cheshire WA16 8XZ. Telephone 01565 652737. Facsimile 01565 751079). The RCVS has produced specimen consent forms in the *Guide to professional conduct* giving a suggested lay-out and allowing veterinarians to construct consent forms suitable for their own purposes bearing in mind the content of the RCVS forms.

Consent forms should be completed for all patients prescribed veterinary medicines outwith the data sheet, or prescribed authorised human medicines, or patients undergoing euthanasia, or for patients likely to require an anaesthetic (local or general) or surgery (minor or major).

It is essential that owners be advised about the risks involved with a treatment before being asked to sign a consent form. Common risks and adverse effects should be discussed appropriate for the patient's health and circumstances, and the client and then written confirmation of the client's informed consent should be sought. The owner or authorised agent of the animal should be over 18 years of age. Signed consent forms should be retained for at least two years.

Consent for medical treatment

Under *The Medicines (Restrictions on the administration of veterinary medicinal products) Regulations 1994*, as amended, a veterinarian may administer a veterinary medicine outwith the data sheet recommendations ('off-label'), an authorised human medicine, a specially prepared unauthorised medicine ('special-order product') or a medicine imported from another country under a STA under certain circumstances. A veterinarian should explain to the owner that he or she intends to administer such a preparation to the animal and ideally obtain the client's written consent.

When treating animals such as rabbits and rodents, reptiles, and exotic birds, for which there are few or no authorised products, it will be usually be necessary to use authorised human or veterinary products outwith the data sheet recommendations or specially prepared unauthorised medicines or medicines imported from another country under a STA. In order to avoid the owners having to complete a consent form for each procedure or therapeutic course, the VDS have produced a form to ensure consent of the owner for such treatment while the animal is under the care of the veterinary practice.

Consent for anaesthesia and surgery

Veterinarians may find it prudent to present a written fee estimate at the same time as obtaining written consent particularly for anaesthesia and surgical procedures. The consent form and written estimate may be included in the same document but it is advisable to obtain separate signatures for each section. When deciding on the wording, lay-out and degree to which a particular fee estimate should be itemised, the veterinarian will need to take into account the following: the animal's welfare and the need to attend promptly to an emergency; the time available for discussion with the client; the type of case e.g. acute or chronic, elective surgery, routine treatment, complex investigation followed by extensive surgery, treatment, or both; the changing profile of many disease processes; the possibility that complications may arise; the likelihood that owners will not understand the difference between an estimate and a quotation; and the need to inform owners that where cases are likely to be protracted regular updates of the fee estimate may be necessary.

The importance of maintaining good communications with clients throughout the management of a case cannot be over-emphasied.

In order to avoid unnecessarily long forms, clients may be made aware of various protocols in other ways such as practice brochures or notices in the waiting room. Such information could include the standard of supervision for in-patients, the level of care given, and practice policy on performance of procedures by a veterinary student, a listed nurse or other support staff.

Consent for medical treatment

CONSENT FORM

For the use of an authorised veterinary or human medicine outwith the data sheet recommendations (i.e. 'off label') or a specially prepared unauthorised medicine ('special-order product') or a medicine imported from another country under a Special Treatment Authorisation

[Practice Stamp]

Details of owner
Name..
Address...
Telephone Home..................Work/Mobile..........................

Description of Patient
Name ....
Species/Breed..
Colour......................... Age.................. Sex. M/F/NM/NF
Other identification (Microchip/Tattoo/Brand/Ring/etc.)............

Any relevant clinical history/special precautions.......................
....

I understand that .... is a product which is not authorised/licensed for use in .... but is acknowledged as a product useful in the treatment of ....
I have also been made aware of the possibility of side-effects and of the precautions related to its administration. In accepting its use for .... I accept any attendant risks. I am over 18 years of age.

Signature of Owner/Agent...
Name... Date..............................

If agent:
Name..
Address...
Relationship to owner..

Consent for medical treatment (life-long care)

CONSENT FORM

For the use of an authorised veterinary or human medicine outwith the data sheet recommendations (i.e. 'off label') or a specially prepared unauthorised medicine ('special-order product') or a medicine imported from another country under a Special Treatment Authorisation

[Practice Stamp]

Under UK legislation where there are no suitable drugs specifically authorised for the treatment of a particular species (the majority of small mammals, birds, reptiles, amphibia, fish and invertebrates) or a particular medical condition in that species, a medicinal product authorised for a different medical condition, or for use in another species or humans, or under certain circmstances a specially prepared unauthorised product, or a medicine imported from another country under a Special Treatment Authorisation may be used for the treatment of your animal **with your consent.** These procedures will only be used when we consider them to be the most appropriate treatment.

Details of owner
Name..
Address...
Telephone Home..................Work/Mobile..........................

Description of Patient
Name ....
Species/Breed..
Colour......................... Age.................. Sex. M/F/NM/NF
Other identification (Microchip/Tattoo/Brand/Ring/etc.)............

Any relevant clinical history/special precautions.......................
....

I understand that while the animal described above is under the care of this veterinary practice there may be occasions when it will be necessary to use authorised human or veterinary medicines (or specially prepared unauthorised medicines ot medicines imported from another country under a Special Treatment Authorisation) not authorised for use in ....(species) or which are authorised for use in this species but not for the particular condition for which the treatment will be given. I have been made aware that there may be known or unknown side-effects associated with the use of these drugs and in giving permission for their use accept any attendant risks. I am over 18 years of age.

Signature of Owner/Agent...
Name... Date..............................

If agent:
Name..
Address...
Relationship to owner..

Consent for euthanasia

It is recommended that separate consent forms for euthanasia are available. It is important that the client understands the term 'euthanasia' and that there is no misunderstanding. In the case of euthanasia of an injured horse at a sporting event, the opinion of a veterinary colleague should be sought if available.

Consent for anaesthesia

> **CONSENT FORM**
> **ANAESTHESIA AND SURGICAL PROCEDURES**
>
> [Practice Stamp]
>
> **Details of owner**
> Name..
> Address..
> Telephone Home..................Work/Mobile.........................
>
> **Description of Patient**
> Name ....
> Species/Breed...
> Colour......................... Age.................. Sex. M/F/NM/NF
> Other identification (Microchip/Tattoo/Brand/Ring/etc.)............
>
> Operation/Procedure
> ....
> The nature of these procedures have been explained to me.
>
> Any relevant clinical history/special precautions.....................
> ....
>
> I hereby give permission for the administration of an anaes-
> thetic to the above animal and to the operation/procedure
> detailed on this form, together with any other procedures which
> may prove necessary.
> I understand that all anaesthetic techniques and surgical proce-
> dures involve some risk to the animal. I am over 18 years of
> age.
> I have notified/will notify immediately the insurers concerning
> the procedures planned for this animal.
>
> Signature of Owner/Agent...
> Name.......................... Date.............................
>
> If agent:
> Name..
> Address...
> Relationship to owner...

Consent for euthanasia

> **CONSENT FORM**
> **EUTHANASIA**
>
> [Practice Stamp]
>
> **Details of owner**
> Name..
> Address..
> Telephone Home..................Work/Mobile.........................
>
> **Description of Patient**
> Name ....
> Species/Breed...
> Colour......................... Age.................. Sex. M/F/NM/NF
> Other identification (Microchip/Tattoo/Brand/Ring/etc.)............
>
> I hereby consent to the euthanasia of the animal described above.
> I am over 18 years of age.
>
> Signature of Owner/Agent...
> Name.......................... Date.............................
> If agent:
> Name..
> Address...
> Relationship to owner...

Under The *Protection of Animals Act 1911, The Protection of Animals (Scotland) Act 1912*, and the *Welfare of Animals (Northern Ireland) Act 1972* failure to destroy an animal to prevent further suffering may amount to cruelty. The veterinarian should make full records of all the circumstances supporting a decision to euthanase without the owner's consent in case of subsequent challenge. A police officer may order the humane destruction of an animal (horse, mule, ass, bull, sheep, goat, or pig) to terminate unreasonable suffering. The veterinarian should obtain a written and signed instruction to destroy from the officer in charge, including the name and identification number and the police station log number of the incident. The RCVS has provided guidance on the action to be taken for other species such as dogs and cats. If the veterinarian believes that 'immediate destruction is necessary to prevent further suffering, [he] may and should destroy the animal, even if the owner is absent or being present refuses to consent' (*Legislation affecting the veterinary profession in the United Kingdom*). In other instances, all reasonable steps should be taken to find the owner. Under the *Dangerous Dogs Act 1991*, as amended, and the *Dangerous Dogs (Northern Ireland) Order 1991*, the Court, a Justice of the Peace, or the police may order the destruction of a dog. The veterinarian should request a written and signed destruction order form from the appropriate written authorities.

Further information

Recommendations for prescribing, dispensing, and safe use of medicinal products for animals may be found in the following sources.

- BVA. *Veterinary Pharmacy Course.* For full details and a registration form contact BVA, 7 Mansfield Street, London, W1M 0AT Telephone 020 7636 6541 Facsimile 020 7436 2970 E-mail bvahq@bva.org.uk
- BVA. *Guidelines on the Prudent Use of Antimicrobials.* BVA Publications, 2000
- Bishop Y. *The Veterinary Formulary.* 5th ed. British Veterinary Assocation and The Pharmaceutical Press, 2000
- NOAH. *Animal Medicines: A user's guide.* NOAH, 1995
- National Office of Animal Health. *Compendium of Data Sheets for Veterinary Products*
- RCVS. *Guide to professional conduct.* RCVS, 2000
- RCVS. *Legislation affecting the veterinary profession in the United Kingdom*
- RPSGB. *Medicines, ethics, and practice: a guide for pharmacists*
- Tennant B. *BSAVA Small Animal Formulary.* 3rd ed. BSAVA, 1999
- VMD. *The Medicines (Restrictions on the Administration of Veterinary Medicinal Products) Regulations 1994 (SI 1994/2987): Guidance to the veterinary profession.* AMELIA 8, March 1995.
- VMD. *Special Treatment Authorisations.* AMELIA 10, November 1995
- VMD. Question and Answer Brief on Zootechnical Additives and Medicated Feedingstuffs, June 1998.

British Veterinary Association

Guidelines on the Prudent Use of Antimicrobials

Edited by:
Y Bishop BSc, BVMS, LLB(Hons), MRCVS

General guidelines
Poultry
Equidae
Pigs
Sheep
Companion animals
Cattle
Fish
Further information

The following guidelines have been produced as part of the BVA's ongoing strategy to promote the responsible use of veterinary medicines for which the Association was commended by the ACMSF (Advisory Committee on the Microbiological Safety of Food) in its recent report on Microbial Antibiotic Resistance in Relation to Food Safety: 'We particularly welcome the British Veterinary Association's expression of its willingness to adopt a leading role in informing and guiding the profession in relation to responsible veterinary prescribing through the promotion of policy, pharmacy courses, the dissemination of information, guidance on the selection and administration of antibiotics and on approaches to the treatment of individual species, and through the publication and promotion of its Code of Practice on Medicines. In view of the fact that veterinarians are a very important vehicle for the supply and administration of veterinary medicinal products, we would welcome their developing a system of self-audit of veterinary practice, with special emphasis on the use of antibiotic substances. We see this as an area where the BVA and other professional representative bodies could take a helpful lead.' (Chapter 8 'The use of antibiotics in farm animals'; paragraph 108.)

This document is set out in two sections, beginning with general guidelines on the prudent use of antimicrobials, adapted from those produced by the BVA Antimicrobials Working Party (September 1998). In addition, a series of species-specific guidelines for poultry, horses, pigs, sheep, dogs and cats, cattle and fish, have been produced in conjunction with the relevant BVA affiliated groups.

Many Association members have commented on the Guidelines and the assistance of the British Cattle Veterinary Association, British Equine Veterinary Association, British Small Animal Veterinary Association, British Veterinary Poultry Association, Fish Veterinary Society, Pig Veterinary Society and Sheep Veterinary Society is acknowledged with thanks. Contact details for those organisations that produce their own guidance and offer specialist advice on the subject of veterinary antimicrobials can be found in the further information section of this document.

GENERAL GUIDELINES

The use of antimicrobial agents provides an effective method for the control and treatment of infectious or contagious diseases caused by bacteria and certain other microorganisms. Their application in veterinary practice since the 1950s has assisted in ensuring the health of livestock and companion animals. Antimicrobial use has also contributed to improved food safety standards, by reducing the likelihood of meat, egg and milk products presenting disease problems for the consumer or those concerned with their production. In addition, freedom for animals to receive treatment for disease is incorporated in the Welfare Codes and therefore antimicrobial use is justifiable on welfare grounds.

The immediate responsibility of the prescribing veterinarian is to safeguard the health and welfare of animals under his care by controlling disease in groups and individual animals. Veterinarians must also be aware of the potential risks that this presents and show a continuous responsibility to both the animal handler, and human consumer in the case of food-producing animals.

It must be remembered at all times that the use of antimicrobials is not a substitute for efficient management, or good husbandry and that an holistic approach to disease control is preferable.

Veterinarians should be aware that these Guidelines are intended to act as an adjunct to clinical judgement. It may not be possible for every consideration to be observed in every case, but they should always form part of an automatic checklist when deciding an antimicrobial use regimen.

These Guidelines are concerned with the use of antimicrobials authorised as medicines.

Different disease conditions and management systems may affect each species. Therefore species- specific guidelines have been produced to highlight the diverse issues the veterinarian must consider when using antimicrobials in different species. The species-specific guidelines should be read in conjunction with the General Guidelines.

Principles of antimicrobial use

The appropriate use of antimicrobials in practice is a critical decision, which should ideally be based on:
- accurate diagnosis based on adequate diagnostic procedures;
- known or predictable sensitivities (antimicrobial sensitivity testing);
- known pharmacokinetics/tissue distribution to ensure the selected therapeutic reaches the site of infection;
- known status of immunocompetence;
- prognosis.

In order to minimise the likelihood of broad antimicrobial resistance developing, it is recommended that where an appropriate narrow spectrum agent is available, it should be selected in preference to a broad spectrum agent.

Routine considerations

Antimicrobial agents should only be used when it is known or suspected that an infectious agent is present which will be susceptible to such therapy.

When antimicrobial agents are used, every effort should be made to determine the origin of the problem and to ascertain the most effective treatment.

Ideally, the choice of antimicrobial for the treatment of infectious disease should be based on antimicrobial sensitivity tests wherever possible, and also on the previous history of effective antimicrobial use on the premises. Testing is particularly appropriate in relatively intensive situations where disease spread is likely and in animals where treatment failure has occurred. The decision to perform antimicrobial sensitivity testing is at the discretion of the veterinarian, based on the circumstances of the presenting case.

While therapy may need to be initiated before results of diagnostic or antimicrobial sensitivity tests are known, it will need to be reassessed as test results become available. In such circumstances, before results are known, decisions as to the choice of antimicrobial will need to be made in the light of what has previously been effective in similar types of problems, and on any knowledge of previous antimicrobial efficacy on the premises.

The efficacy of all disease treatments should be monitored and, if the livestock or pet owner is to undertake part of the treatment regimen, a check should be made to ensure that they have understood fully the instructions on dosage and duration of antimicrobial use. Quantities of antimicrobials left with the animal owner should correctly reflect the need to avoid oversupply.

Should there be recurrence of disease following successful treatment or control of an outbreak, it may need to be investigated more thoroughly depending on the situation, to ascertain the reason for recurrence and the most suitable therapy to be used.

Antimicrobials need to be used with care to maintain their efficacy. If possible, alternative methods of disease control to reduce antimicrobial use, such as vaccination, should be considered.

Antimicrobial usage should always be part of, and not a replacement for, an integrated disease control programme. Such a programme is likely to involve hygiene and disinfection procedures, biosecurity measures, management alterations, changes in stocking rates, vaccination, etc.

Continued antimicrobial use in control programmes should be regularly assessed as to effectiveness and whether use can be reduced or stopped.

Prudent use of antimicrobials is a partnership between the veterinarian and client and must involve agreement on treatment policy and veterinary involvement in ongoing disease conditions; written protocols or policies may be used. These protocols should be regularly and frequently reviewed and updated.

Written protocols or policies should be agreed and documented for treatment of all endemic conditions on the farm or other livestock rearing or production premises. These protocols should be regularly reviewed and updated.

Use of antimicrobials for the prevention of disease can only be justified where it can be shown that a particular disease is present on the premises or is likely to become so, or where other disease or treatment modalities may result in immunocompetence. In such circumstances, it should be shown that strategic use of antimicrobials would prevent clinical outbreaks of that disease. The prophylactic use of antimicrobials is never a substitute for good management.

Dosage strategy recommendations

Careful calculation of dose is always important, but in particular if an extra-label use of a product is being considered. In such cases, caution needs to be exercised regarding meat, milk, and egg withholding periods.

It is recommended that optimal therapeutic dosage strategies be used and that all efforts be made to avoid administration of sub-therapeutic dosages, which can lead to a lack of efficacy or lack of response. In general, dosage recommendations as laid down in the relevant product data sheet should be followed.

Fluoroquinolones should only be used therapeutically and not for routine prophylaxis. They should be used where clinical experience or antimicrobial sensitivity testing indicates suitability. Ideally, antimicrobial sensitivity testing should take place before or in parallel with use.

Regulatory concerns

The British Veterinary Association has produced a *Code of Practice on Medicines*, which provides guidance on the prescribing, supply, and disposal of medicines for animals. The Code gives information on medicines including prescribing under the 'cascade'; suspected adverse reaction reporting; storage, record keeping, and labelling of medicines; and administration of medicines by the animal owner or keeper. Veterinarians must comply with a range of legislative requirements when administering medicines to animals under their care and these are also addressed in the Code. The Code should be followed when using antimicrobials.

There is strict legislation in place concerning prescribing of medicines in food-producing species. Under European law, food-producing animals include horses, cattle, sheep, pigs, poultry, and fish. Veterinarians must record all medicines administered to food-producing animals. In addition, when prescribing under the 'cascade' for food-producing animals, veterinarians must use agents that are contained in medicines authorised in the UK for use in food-producing species.

It is acceptable and desirable for Quality Assurance schemes to monitor antimicrobial usage, medication documentation, and withholding period compliance. However, such schemes should not hinder the attending veterinarian from preventing suffering in the animals under his care.

There must be a commitment to Continuous Professional Development to ensure the maintenance of the depth of knowledge of all therapeutic agents and the causative microorganisms involved in disease.

A code of practice on medicines has been produced for farmers by the VMD 'Code of Practice on the Responsible Use of Animal Medicines on the Farm' and a series of guidance documents for farms, on the use of antimicrobials in major food-producing species, has been produced by the RUMA Alliance (publication to be completed in 2000). Veterinarians should be aware of these. (See Further information section for details of where to obtain copies).

GUIDELINES ON THE PRUDENT USE OF ANTIMICROBIALS IN POULTRY

Introduction

All poultry are reared, managed, and medicated as groups or flocks. In poultry production, both infected and healthy animals may need to be treated with therapeutic levels of an antimicrobial product for the recommended period. This is intended to cure the clinically affected animals, reduce the spread of disease, and prevent clinical signs appearing in the remainder.

The following guidelines are intended to be an adjunct to clinical judgement when using antimicrobial agents in poultry and are to be used by practising veterinarians as a checklist when deciding on a treatment regimen. It is not the role of these guidelines to advise the veterinarian on which antimicrobials to prescribe. The use of antimicrobials in poultry is ultimately the responsibility of the veterinarian who has the animal(s) under his care.

These guidelines should be read in conjunction with the BVA General Guidelines on the Prudent Use of Antimicrobials. Published information should also be consulted for the selection of appropriate antimicrobials for particular conditions.

Principles of antimicrobial use
Initial considerations

The selection of antimicrobials for use in poultry must be based on the General Guidelines. In addition, knowledge of specific poultry medicine, bacteriology, and antimicrobial pharmacokinetics is important.

Communication with clients

Detailed preventive medicine programmes should be documented for all companies and/or farms. These should include all routine medications such as anticoccidials, digestive enhancers, anthelmintics, competitive exclusion and probiotic treatments, and vaccines, some of which are non-prescription medicines.

Antimicrobial use

There is a legal requirement for veterinarians to record all medicines administered to food-producing animals. All medicines supplied to the farm must be recorded.

All prescribing of antimicrobials for poultry should be for animals under the care of the prescribing veterinarian and a copy of the prescription should be retained by the veterinarian for at least three years.

In an outbreak of animal disease, ideally the results of anti-microbial sensitivity testing should be ascertained before therapy is started. In disease outbreaks involving high mortality or where there are signs of rapid spread of disease among contact animals, treatment may be started on the basis of clinical diagnosis. Nevertheless, the antimicrobial sensitivity of the suspected causal microorganism should, where possible, be determined so that if treatment fails it can be changed in the light of the results of antimicrobial sensitivity testing. Antimicrobial sensitivity trends should be monitored over time and such monitoring may be used to guide clinical judgement on antimicrobial usage.

It is recognised that prophylactic medication may be appropriate in certain precisely defined circumstances in poultry production.

Each practice should develop a written policy or protocol covering the circumstances in which this is considered appropriate. The possible effects of antimicrobials on other aspects of preventive programmes should be considered.

Use of fluoroquinolones in commercial poultry outwith the data sheet recommendations is to be strongly discouraged; for example, use of these products for dipping of eggs intended for hatching chicks or poults intended for human consumption should be avoided.

GUIDELINES ON THE PRUDENT USE OF ANTIMICROBIALS IN EQUIDAE

Introduction

Equidae may be closely managed or free-grazing. The use of the animal, and husbandry systems are factors to be taken into consideration when prescribing antimicrobials in these species.

The following guidelines are intended to be an adjunct to clinical judgement when using antimicrobial agents in Equidae and are to be used by practising veterinarians as a checklist when deciding on a treatment regimen. It is not the role of these guidelines to advise the veterinarian of which antimicrobials to prescribe. The use of antimicrobials in Equidae is ultimately the responsibility of the veterinarian who has the animal(s) under his care.

These guidelines should be read in conjunction with the BVA General Guidelines on the Prudent Use of Antimicrobials. Published information should also be consulted for the selection of appropriate antimicrobials for particular conditions.

Principles of antimicrobial use

Initial considerations
The use of the horse should be considered. For horses used in competitions, some individuals become lethargic and inappetent during systemic antimicrobial treatment and this can affect training schedules. Veterinarians must also be aware of competition authority rules for administration of veterinary medicinal products and withholding times for competitions.

Current EU legislation considers the horse to be a food-producing animal and therefore the categorisation of the individual should be addressed, and antimicrobial use should take into account record keeping and withholding period requirements where this is relevant.

The selection of antimicrobials for use in horses must be based on the General Guidelines. In addition, special considerations affecting selection include the horse's size, temperament, value, competition rules, individual hypersensitivities and potential problems with adverse local or systemic reactions and side-effects. Knowledge of specific equine medicine, bacteriology, and antimicrobial pharmacokinetics is important.

The large variation in bodyweight in Equidae makes dosage estimation difficult, and may lead to problems with local adverse reactions from large volume doses. Idiosyncratic pharmacokinetics in Equidae must also be considered (for example, oral medication is often preferable to parenteral routes of administration), as should altered drug metabolism in foals.

When prescribing for animals in isolated locations where frequent administration may be impossible, preparations should be selected that have dose formulations which permit delivery of the appropriate treatment.

Communication with clients

Introduction to and communication with clients and grooms is important in order that advice aimed at addressing predisposing conditions is clearly defined.

Administration of drugs by the animal owner or keeper should be closely monitored. It should be considered unwise to dispense antimicrobials for Equidae for intravenous administration by the animal owner or keeper. Antimicrobials may be dispensed to owners for use in animals under the care of the veterinarian to be given intramuscularly, orally, or topically as appropriate. Adequate advice must be given to the owner concerning the administration and potential risks of antimicrobials.

Antimicrobial use

Where there are predisposing factors leading to the development of infectious disease, for example, damaged molar teeth with maxillary sinusitis, pneumovagina with endometritis, or a foreign body in a wound, the appropriate surgical or medical treatment should be used at the onset of antimicrobial treatment.

Antimicrobial usage should always be part of, and not a replacement for, an integrated disease control programme. Where appropriate vaccines are available, or where management strategies such as improved hygiene or quality of colostral transfer can be employed, they should be implemented in order to reduce the injudicious use of antimicrobials.

While therapy may need to be initiated before results of diagnostic or antimicrobial sensitivity tests are known, it may need to be reassessed as test results become available. Specific sampling techniques should be used, but preparations selected should not disturb the normal local microflora. Prolonged local antimicrobial treatment is to be avoided at any site unless necessary.

It should be remembered that in certain clinical situations the use of antimicrobials should be avoided because treatment may be ineffective or may lead to the development of latent carriers. For example, bacteria are seldom implicated in adult equine diarrhoea, and in cases where Salmonella infection is suspected antimicrobials can result in a carrier state and should therefore be avoided.

GUIDELINES FOR THE PRUDENT USE OF ANTIMICROBIALS IN PIGS

Introduction

Growing and finishing pigs are usually reared, managed, and medicated as a group and within each group the animals are usually of the same age, similar immune status, and have the same husbandry requirements. Both infected and healthy pigs may be present within such a group and may therefore need to be treated together. This is intended to cure the clinically affected animals, reduce the spread of disease by limiting the carriage of infection by clinically healthy animals, and prevent infection of other pigs in the group. Breeding sows and boars are normally kept in groups, and although the veterinarian may recommend herd treatment occasionally, individual treatment is more usual for these animals.

The following guidelines are intended to be an adjunct to clinical judgement when using antimicrobial agents in pigs and are to be used by practising veterinarians as a checklist when deciding on a treatment regimen. It is not the role of these guidelines to advise the veterinarian of which antimicrobials to prescribe. The use of antimicrobials in pigs is ultimately the responsibility of the veterinarian who has the animal(s) under his care.

These guidelines should be read in conjunction with the BVA General Guidelines on the Prudent Use of Antimicrobials. Published information should also be consulted for the selection of appropriate antimicrobials for particular conditions.

Principles of antimicrobial use
Initial considerations

Pigs are usually medicated on a group basis and the dose given in feed or water should be carefully calculated based on recommended doses expressed in mg/kg bodyweight. Consideration should be given to ensuring all animals in the group receive an adequate dose.

The selection of antimicrobials for use in pigs must be based on the General Guidelines. In addition, knowledge of specific porcine medicine, bacteriology, and antimicrobial pharmacokinetics is important.

Communication with clients

There should be written instructions on each farm outlining the farmer's obligations concerning his use of medications including antimicrobials. These should cover information on storage of medicines, administration techniques, record keeping, and withholding periods. Withholding periods should always be clearly conveyed to the farmer. Furthermore, for withholding periods to be correctly observed, animals must be properly identified.

Written instructions should also be specific to the farm including the correct dosage and duration of medication, the correct circumstances of use, and the correct procedures for observing withholding periods.

These written instructions should be in conjunction and coordination with a written Preventive Medicine Programme tailored to meet the needs of the pig farm and emphasising those areas of management that are likely to reduce the requirement for medication.

There should be a written procedure for a regular review of the medication prescribed to provide the opportunity to reassess the efficacy of the treatment including the medication and management. After this review and where appropriate, the medication should either be stopped or reduced in duration.

Antimicrobial use

There is a legal requirement for veterinarians to record all medicines administered to food-producing animals. All medicines supplied to the farm must be recorded.

All available practice information should be consolidated into one farm file or database, such that this centralised information should:

- allow monitoring of the level of medication used;
- contain a list of those medicines permitted for use on each farm;
- contain a list of medicine withholding periods and a system for allowing information to be updated;
- provide a record of antibacterial sensitivities, where appropriate;
- provide any comments concerning the response to medication under these circumstances.

Where the health and welfare of animals is being safeguarded by the medication of a population, the aim should be that it is used strategically, encompasses the smallest population possible, and it is used for the shortest effective duration.

Where this population includes animals not clinically affected, that is subclinical or healthy individuals, medication must be justifiable either on the grounds of the protection of the susceptible or by the reduction in the excretion of pathogens capable of producing or perpetuating clinical disease. Where such diseases are endemic, all aspects of treatment should undergo a regular routine reassessment.

GUIDELINES FOR THE PRUDENT USE OF ANTIMICROBIALS IN SHEEP

Introduction

Sheep are the category of livestock most often reared in extremely extensive conditions. However, sheep production may also comprise intensive stocking units with many animals in a single air space where spread of disease can be rapid.

The following guidelines are intended to be an adjunct to clinical judgement when using antimicrobial agents in sheep and are to be used by practising veterinarians as a checklist when deciding on a treatment regimen. It is not the role of these guidelines to advise the veterinarian of which antimicrobials to prescribe. The use of antimicrobials

in sheep is ultimately the responsibility of the veterinarian who has the animal(s) under his care.

These guidelines should be read in conjunction with the BVA General Guidelines on the Prudent Use of Antimicrobials. Published information should also be consulted for the selection of appropriate anti-microbials for particular conditions.

Principles of antimicrobial use
Initial considerations

Intensive sheep production systems encounter the same problems for mass medication as do intensive husbandry units for other production species. However, the mixed beneficial protozoal and bacterial population of the forestomach of the sheep makes oral antimicrobial therapy largely unsuitable except for the administration of some anticoccidials.

The extensive husbandry conditions of hill sheep farms present their own problems for antimicrobial therapy. It is practically impossible and economically unjustifiable for a veterinarian to be available to treat individual sheep in an extensive flock and appropriate means of justifying the allocation of stock to the veterinarian's 'real care' must be established. The veterinarian must have a real and current knowledge of the husbandry and potential bacterial infections anticipated within the flock and must have provided appropriate advice and education to shepherds to ensure that standard operating procedures for the use of prescription-only drugs are in place.

Sheep husbandry and farming is of a seasonal nature so that veterinary attention is also seasonal. Despite this, consideration should be given to ensuring that the current disease status of a flock is fully appreciated so that correct medication and advice is provided.

The selection of antimicrobials for use in sheep must be based on the General Guidelines. In addition, knowledge of specific ovine medicine, bacteriology, and antimicrobial pharmacokinetics is important.

Communication with clients

Flock Health Schemes may be adopted by sheep farmers and provide an excellent way in which advisers, veterinarians, and shepherds can interact to the benefit of the health and welfare of animals under their care.

The farmer should hold only limited stocks of medicines appropriate for the season for the treatment of his sheep. The seasonal nature of sheep farming might lead to medicines being held from one lambing season to the next and thus being used beyond the date of expiry, and/or being held in poor storage facilities. Consequently, veterinarians should decide both the type and quantity of suitable medicines that can be held by each sheep farmer. Advice on correct storage should always be given.

Where antimicrobials are to be used by a shepherd on animals under the veterinarian's care, he must have been advised on storage, handling and, in particular, aspects of antimicrobial pharmacology which could result in allergy or irritation to the person delivering the drug. Advice on the administration of the product, correct disposal, and record keeping should be given. The details on the label of medications left with the shepherd must be indelible even in farm-yard conditions. Withholding periods should always be clearly conveyed to the farmer. Furthermore, for withholding periods to be correctly observed, the animals must be properly identified.

Antimicrobial use

There is a legal requirement for veterinarians to record all medicines administered to food-producing animals. All medicines supplied to the farm must be recorded.

It is important, where possible, to establish a diagnosis before starting treatment of any description and especially so in situations that could demand extensive use of antimicrobials. For example, coccidiosis in lambs can require large scale medication with sulphonamides and diagnosis should be confirmed before commencement of treatment to avoid inadvertent over-use of these antimicrobials.

Antimicrobials are not a substitute for good management and husbandry, or for preventive medicine such as vaccination and biosecurity. For example, the repeated routine use of antimicrobials as a means of controlling certain types of ovine abortion is to be discouraged when effective vaccines are available. Similarly, the large-scale use of antimicrobials to prevent 'watery mouth' should only be employed when alternative methods are failing to prevent cases from occurring. Antimicrobial treatments should only be used when other preventive measures have failed and have been thoroughly investigated.

Where appropriate vaccines are available, or where other strategies such as improved hygiene may reduce the requirement for antimicrobial therapy, these strategies should be used. In the sheep industry, vaccines for clostridial disease, pasteurellosis, and abortion have been used very effectively and have undoubtedly reduced antimicrobial use in this animal species.

GUIDELINES FOR THE PRUDENT USE OF ANTIMICROBIALS IN COMPANION ANIMALS

Introduction

Under this section antimicrobial use in dogs and cats is considered. These species are usually kept as pets in a domestic situation but may also be kept in groups, for example, hounds used for hunting.

The following guidelines are intended to be an adjunct to clinical judgement when using antimicrobial agents in dogs and cats and are to be used by practising veterinarians as a checklist when deciding on a treatment regimen. It is not the role of these guidelines to advise the veterinarian of which antimicrobials to prescribe. The use of antimicrobials in dogs and cats is ultimately the responsibility of the veterinarian who has the animal(s) under his care.

These guidelines should be read in conjunction with the BVA General Guidelines on the Prudent Use of Antimicrobials. Published information should also be consulted for the selection of appropriate anti-microbials for particular conditions.

Principles of antimicrobial use
Initial considerations

Unlike the other domestic species, dogs and cats are not considered as food-producing animals and do not pose a potential risk for human consumption. However, potential risk to humans during handling of antimicrobials should be considered and good hygiene practices observed. The judicious use of antimicrobials is advised, in particular, over prescribing is to be avoided since cats and dogs (or their faeces) could become a source of resistant zoonotic organisms.

There is wide variation in body-weight in dog and cat breeds and ideally all animals should be weighed before treatment. Calculation of dose must be made carefully, in particular if an extra-label use of a product is made.

The selection of antimicrobials for use in dogs and cats must be based on the General Guidelines. In addition, knowledge of specific canine and feline medicine, bacteriology, and antimicrobial pharmacokinetics is important.

Communication with clients

A major consideration in the therapy of dogs and cats is owner compliance with treatment protocols. It should be emphasised to the owner/keeper that the correct dose should be given for the specified period. Veterinarians should ensure that the owner is able to administer the treatment. An alternative drug formulation should be utilised if owners are unable, for example, to give tablets to their cat.

Antimicrobial use

The efficacy of all disease treatment should be monitored and if part of the treatment regimen was undertaken by the owner, a check should be made to ensure that they have complied with the instructions on dosage and duration of antimicrobial use.

Any use of antimicrobials outside recommendations in the product data sheet or other published works (in accordance with the 'cascade') should be carefully justified, preferably as part of a written prescription. It is recommended that owners are advised of the extra-label use of a product or use of authorised human medicines and the owners' written consent is obtained.

It should be remembered that antimicrobial drug metabolism and excretion may differ in dogs and cats. In addition, certain antimicrobials may cause side-effects in dogs and cats and published information should be consulted before treatment.

GUIDELINES FOR THE PRUDENT USE OF ANTIMICROBIALS IN CATTLE

Introduction

Cattle are medicated on an individual animal basis on dairy and beef farms. Occasionally it may be necessary to medicate in-contact animals where the spread of disease may be rapid. The current legal requirements for ear tagging in cattle aid accurate animal identification and ensure appropriate withholding times are undertaken when good recording systems are in practice.

The following guidelines are intended to be an adjunct to

clinical judgement when using antimicrobial agents in cattle and are to be used by practising veterinarians as a checklist when deciding on a treatment regimen. It is not the role of these guidelines to advise the veterinarian of which antimicrobials to prescribe. The use of antimicrobials in cattle is ultimately the responsibility of the veterinarian who has the animal(s) under his care.

These guidelines should be read in conjunction with the BVA General Guidelines on the Prudent Use of Antimicrobials. Published information should also be consulted for the selection of appropriate antimicrobials for particular conditions.

Principles of antimicrobial use
Initial considerations

The selection of antimicrobials for use in cattle must be based on the General Guidelines. In addition, knowledge of specific bovine medicine, bacteriology, and antimicrobial pharmacokinetics is important.

Communication with clients

The veterinarian should communicate with the stockman or farmer to ensure that medicines are stored and disposed of correctly as given in the *BVA Code of Practice on Medicines*. A proper stock control policy, with a named person responsible, is essential to avoid situations such as old part-used bottles of medicines accumulating in cupboards. The policy may simply be a list of permitted drugs and maximum stock levels allowed, as specified by the veterinarian, along with a routine for the regular disposal of surplus or unused medicines. The details on the label of dispensed medicines must be indelible, even in farmyard conditions. BCVA has produced its *Guidelines to Good Pharmacy Practice*, which are helpful for veterinarians in this field.

It is a legal requirement for the owner or keeper of the animals to record all veterinary medicines administered to their animals. The farmer must keep records for all medicines purchased and include the identity of the animal for which they were used and the dates of use. There is no specified method of record keeping, but the NOAH *Animal Medicines Record Book* contains all the necessary details to comply with the requirements, and also includes columns for detailing meat and milk withholding periods for each individual. The veterinarian should assist the farmer to keep good records.

It is essential that the correct withholding periods, as specified on the product label, are observed. Accurate identification of the animal under treatment is essential to withhold meat and milk from treated animals and to prevent residues. There should be a farm procedure to identify and mark treated animals based on local work routines and written protocols.

All personnel involved with the medication of animals must be informed of the withholding periods and the methods of identification. Withholding periods vary according to dosage and method of administration and so there should be no assumption that familiarity with the product is adequate. Utmost care must be taken when products are used extra-label to ensure that the withholding period is adequate. The veterinarian should clearly convey to all concerned what the withholding periods are for any particular product and method of administration.

Medicinal treatments should be under the control of the attending veterinarian and, although they may be administered by farm staff, their use should be under written direction for animals under the veterinarian's care. All persons with access to the medicines should be aware of treatment and usage instructions, therefore, it is advisable to have written protocols available.

Antimicrobial use

There is a legal requirement for veterinarians to record all medicines administered to food-producing animals. All medicines supplied to a farm must be recorded.

The BCVA has consulted with some of the first purchasers of milk and dairy products to create a protocol for the investigation of antimicrobial failures in milk. Any failure should be regarded as serious and should be investigated thoroughly. A written report should be prepared. An investigation protocol is available from the BCVA office.

As a general principle, alternative methods of disease control such as attention to good husbandry practices, hygiene maintenance, good stock management, vaccination policies, and biosecurity measures should be considered before antimicrobial therapy. Treatments should only be used when these approaches fail.

Antimicrobial treatment for conditions such as mastitis should be specified by the veterinarian and be based on good clinical judgement. This may be based on bacteriological isolates, antimicrobial sensitivity testing, and previous clinical experience of the farm situation. Antimicrobial selection should be frequently reviewed and modified as appropriate.

Use of antimicrobials for enteric conditions should be based on specific diagnoses and only when clinically necessary. In addition, hygiene, management, and vaccination policies, and oral and parenteral rehydration should be considered.

Many respiratory conditions require antimicrobial therapy and should be based on good clinical practice and targeted at those conditions and animals where it would be beneficial. Management considerations should also be addressed.

Many other clinical conditions require antimicrobials and treatment should be selected on good clinical practice and used responsibly and effectively.

GUIDELINES FOR THE PRUDENT USE OF ANTIMICROBIALS IN FISH

Introduction

Farmed fish may be raised in a wide range of fresh water or salt water facilities including small indoor hatchery tanks, very large sea pens, relatively extensive earth pond systems, and highly sophisticated pumped and recirculation complexes. A variety of fish species are farmed, from 'traditional' trout and salmon production to the more recent development of halibut and cod farming. The type of facility and the species farmed will have an impact on the nature of bacterial disease seen and the course of action to be taken when using antimicrobials.

The following guidelines are intended to be an adjunct to clinical judgement when using antimicrobial agents in fish and are to be used by practising veterinarians as a checklist when deciding on a treatment regimen. It is not the role of these guidelines to advise the veterinarian of which antimicrobials to prescribe. The use of antimicrobials in fish is ultimately the responsibility of the veterinarian who has the animal(s) under his care.

These guidelines should be read in conjunction with the BVA General Guidelines on the Prudent Use of Antimicrobials. Published information should also be consulted for the selection of appropriate antimicrobials for particular conditions.

Principles of antimicrobial use
Initial considerations

The type of fish holding facility must be taken into account when treating an outbreak of disease, for example, whether the disease can be isolated to the affected population or whether there is a significant risk of spread to an associated group. The use of antimicrobials in recirculation facilities and effect on filtration systems must be taken into consideration.

To ensure correct dosage it is necessary to estimate biomass as accurately as possible using sample bodyweights, computer models, and scanning technology. It is also necessary to estimate feeding rate as accurately as possible to ensure appropriate incorporation of the antimicrobial in the feed, so that an adequate daily dose is consumed. The feeding rate estimation can be reduced slightly to ensure that all medicated feed is consumed, but not to an extent where some fish may not receive a sufficient drug dose due to feeding competition.

A Discharge Consent for the use of the antimicrobial, from the appropriate environmental protection agency, must be in place before initiation of the treatment.

The selection of antimicrobials for use in fish must be based on the General Guidelines. In addition, knowledge of specific fish medicine, bacteriology, and antimicrobial pharmacokinetics is important.

Communication with clients

Fish Quality Assurance schemes have guidelines for the use of approved antimicrobials to which reference must be made if the farm is a scheme member. It may be necessary to carry out residue analysis under the schemes if antimicrobials are used under the 'cascade'.

A written direction from the prescribing veterinarian should accompany all antimicrobial treatments; this direction should include instructions on dosage, duration of treatment, and the appropriate withholding period.

Accurate on-farm records of all veterinary medicines administered to the animals must be maintained. The farmer must keep records of all medicines purchased and used and include as a minimum the identification of the fish treated, the water temperature, and the with-holding period in degree Celsius days.

Any antimicrobials supplied to the farm must be stored under appropriate conditions and accurately labelled. An up-to-date medicinal stock record should be maintained with reference made to data sheet information for handling and safety instructions.

Antimicrobial use

There is a legal requirement for veterinarians to record all medicines administered to food-producing animals. All medicines supplied to the farm must be recorded.

Accurate diagnosis and antimicrobial sensitivity testing should be carried out in the event of an outbreak of bacterial disease. It may be necessary to initiate treatment prior to the results of sensitivity testing to prevent further development of disease and to pre-empt the inappetence which is a feature of disease in fish. The choice of antimicrobial must then be based on the previous history of bacterial disease, the monitoring of sensitivity patterns, and the effectiveness of treatment at the site. Choice of treatment should be reassessed following the results of the sensitivity testing.

Due to the limited availability of antimicrobials authorised for the treatment of fish, the prescribing 'cascade' may need to be used. Many of the authorised antimicrobials for fish are for use in Atlantic salmon and therefore the requirements of the 'cascade' must be applied if these compounds are used to treat other fish species. A minimum withholding period of 500°C days applies for any compound used under the 'cascade'. Idiosyncratic pharmacokinetics in some fish species must be considered.

Antimicrobials are not a substitute for good husbandry and their use should be minimised by the establishment of effective preventive measures such as vaccination, disinfection regimens, use of appropriate stocking densities, minimal stress and adequate fallow.

FURTHER INFORMATION

Further information and guidance on the prudent use of antimicrobials may be found in the following sources.

- **British Cattle Veterinary Association**
BCVA Office, The Green, Frampton-on-Severn, Gloucester GL2 7EP
Tel (0)1452 740816
Fax (0)1452 741117
E-mail: office@cattlevet.co.uk

- **British Equine Veterinary Association**
5 Finlay Street, London, SW6 6HE
Tel (0)20 76106080
Fax (0)20 76106823
E-mail: bevauk@msn.com

- **British Small Animal Veterinary Association**
Woodrow House, 1 Telford Way, Waterwells Business Park, Quedgeley, Gloucester GL2 4AB
Tel (0)1452 726700
Fax (0)1452 726701
E-mail: adminoff@bsava.com
Tennant B. Small Animal Formulary. 3rd ed. BSAVA, 1999

- **British Veterinary Association**

7 Mansfield Street, London, W1M 0AT

Tel (0)20 7636 6541

Fax (0)20 7436 2970

E-mail: bvahq@bva.co.uk

Bishop Y. (2000) BVA Code of Practice on Medicines
BVA Veterinary Pharmacy Course. For full details and registration form, please contact the BVA

- **British Veterinary Poultry Association**

Hon Sec Peter Cargill, BVetMed, MRCVS, c/o Merial Animal Health, Spire Green Centre, Pinnacles West, Harlow, Essex CM19 5TS

Tel (0)1432 362361

Full text of the BVPA antimicrobials guidelines may be found on the internet:
www.bvpa.org.uk/medicine/amicguid.htm

- **Federation of Veterinarians of Europe (FVE)**

Rue Defacqz, 1, B-1000, Brussels, Belgium

Tel +32 (0)2 5382963

Fax +32 (0)2 5372828

E-mail: info@fve.org

FVE (1999) Antibiotic resistance and Prudent Use of Antibiotics in Veterinary Medicine

- **Fish Veterinary Society**

c/o Dr Martin McLoughlin, 35 Cherryvalley Park, Belfast BT5 6PN

Tel/Fax (0)28 90793566

E-mail: mfmcloughlin@compuserve.com

- **National Office of Animal Health (NOAH) Ltd**

3 Crossfield Chambers, Gladbeck Way, Enfield, Middlesex EN2 7HF

Tel (0)20 83673131

Fax (0)20 83631155

E-mail: noah@noah.co.uk

- **The Pharmaceutical Press**

PO Box 151, Wallingford, Oxfordshire OX10 8QU

Tel (0)1491 824486

Fax (0)1491 826090

E-mail: pharmpress@rpsgb.org.uk

Bishop Y (2000) The Veterinary Formulary, 5th edn. Wallingford, British Veterinary Association and The Pharmaceutical Press

- **Pig Veterinary Society**

Hon Sec Nick Giles, BVSc, MRCVS, c/oVLA Winchester, Itchen Abbas, Winchester, Hampshire SO21 1BX

Tel (0)1962 779966

Fax (0)1962 842492

- **Responsible Use of Medicines in Agriculture (RUMA) Alliance**

PO Box 29066, London, WC2H 8QR

RUMA (1999) Responsible use of antimicrobials in poultry production

RUMA (1999) Responsible use of antimicrobials in pig production

RUMA (2000) Responsible use of antimicrobials in cattle production

RUMA (2000) Responsible use of antimicrobials in sheep production

- **Royal College of Veterinary Surgeons (RCVS)**

Belgravia House, 62-64 Horseferry Road, London, SW1P 2AF

Tel (0)20 72222001

Fax (0)20 72222004.

E-mail: admin@rcvs.org.uk

RCVS (2000) Guide to professional conduct

- **Royal Pharmaceutical Society of Great Britain**

1 Lambeth High Street, London SE1 7JN

Tel (0)20 77359141

E-mail: rpsgb@cabi.org

- **Sheep Veterinary Society**

SVS Secretariat, Moredun Research Institute, IRC, Pentland Science Park, Bush Loan, Penicuik, Midlothian EH26 0PZ

Tel (0)131 4455111

Fax (0)131 4456111

E-mail: svs@mri.sari.ac.uk

- **Veterinary Deer Society**

c/o British Deer Farmers' Association, Old Stoddah, Penruddoch, Penrith, Cumbria CA11 0RY

Alexander T L & Buxton D (1994) 2nd edn. Management and Disease of Deer - A Handbook for the Veterinary Surgeon

- **Veterinary Medicines Directorate**

Woodham Lane, New Haw, Weybridge, Surrey KT15 3NB

Tel (0)1932 336911

Fax (0)1932 336618

VMD (1995). The Medicines (Restrictions on the Administration of Veterinary Medicinal Products) Regulations 1994 (SI 1994/2987): Guidance to the veterinary profession. AMELIA 8

VMD (1995) Special Treatment Authorisations. AMELIA 10

VMD (1999) Code of Practice on the Responsible Use of Animal Medicines on the Farm

- **World Veterinary Association (WVA)**

Rosenlunds Alle 8, DK-2720, Vanlose, Denmark

Tel +45 38710156

Fax +45 38710322

E-mail: wva@ddd.dk

WVA Policy on Prudent Use of Antibiotics published in WVA Bulletin, vol 16, number 1, January 1999.

Prescribing for animals used in competitions

Contributors:
P A Flecknell MA, VetMB, PhD, DLAS, DipECVA, MRCVS
S A Lister BVetMed, BSc, CertPMP, MRCVS
D A L Poulter BVetMed, MRCVS
G G A Smith BVSc, BSc, MRCVS
W T Turner BVetMed, FRSH, MRCVS
R B Williams BVSc, MPhil, MRCVS

Many animals are used in competitive events. For example Greyhounds or pigeons are raced; dogs, cats, poultry, or rabbits are shown; and horses compete in racing, showing, jumping, and eventing. Drugs, including legitimate medication, can affect their performance in these competitive events. Therefore when prescribing for these species, it is important to ensure that the rules of the controlling body of the sport are not contravened.

It is the purpose of such rules to encourage fair competition with animals being judged on their inherent merits, unaided by drugs. This can present a dilemma, for there is a fine distinction between legitimate therapy and unacceptable drug administration, particularly in competitions with more than one stage taking place over time, such as Three-Day Eventing, heats and finals in the major Greyhound and Whippet racing competitions, and the various coursing events; all of which have their own rules.

Some controlling bodies allow the use of particular medications or designate threshold levels for concentrations of certain substances in body fluids, or specify appropriate vaccination programmes.

It is essential to be aware that rules need not be permanent. Legislators are conscious that approaches to therapy can change and that rules may be modified in the light of new developments and scientific discovery. Rules are available for those persons authorised under those Rules who therefore have agreed to abide by them.

Information on prescribing for animals used in competitions is included in the following sources, many of which are periodically updated.

- The Royal College of Veterinary Surgeons (RCVS). *Guide to professional conduct*
- The Jockey Club. *Rules of racing and instructions*
- Fédération Equestre Internationale (FEI). *Veterinary regulations*
- Dyke, TM. Pharmacokinetics of therapeutic substances in racehorses. *Australian Equine Veterinarian* 1989; **7** (suppl 1)
- European Horseracing Scientific Liaison Committee. *Information for veterinary surgeons on detection periods of named drugs* (available to veterinarians from the Chief Veterinary Advisor, The Jockey Club)
- Agriculture Canada Race Track Division. *Schedule of drugs*
- Australian Equine Veterinary Association. *Detection of therapeutic substances in racing horses*
- The British Horseracing Board. *Orders and instructions*
- The British Horse Society. *Endurance riding group rules and omnibus schedule*
- National Greyhound Racing Club Limited (NGRC). *Rules of racing*
- National Coursing Club. *Rules*
- The Kennel Club. *Rules and regulations*
- Governing Council of the Cat Fancy. *Rules*
- Fédération Cynologique Internationale. *Regulations*
- Royal Pigeon Racing Association. *Rules*
- Irish Homing Union. *Rules*
- North of England Homing Union. *Rules*
- North West Homing Union. *Rules*
- Scottish Homing Union. *Rules*
- Welsh Homing Union. *Rules*.

Considerations of drug administration

Ingredients. The contents of any proprietary mixture should be disclosed and the actions known. An apparently harmless tonic may contain a prohibited substance such as caffeine. Traces of caffeine metabolites have been detected in the urine for up to 10 days after administration, and it is advisable to discontinue treatment with caffeine-containing mixtures at least 14 days before competition. Proprietary injectable preparations sometimes contain unexpected substances, for example vitamin B_{12} preparations may contain a local anaesthetic. If the contents or action of any mixture or tonic are uncertain, caution should be excercised.

Ephedrine and its isomers have been detected in the urine of horses which have been treated with herbal remedies, and veterinarians must be satisfied that companies producing such remedies are exercising adequate quality control measures. Quinine and quinidine have been similarly reported to be detected after the administration of so-called 'homoeopathic' treatments. If administering oral therapy to racehorses, care should be taken when dispensing medication into feed. Hands, buckets, and utensils can be inadvertent agents of contamination, therefore medicated feedstuffs should be prepared well away from feed for other horses. Isoxsuprine has been shown to be particularly adhesive resulting in the detection of isoxsuprine in urine samples for appreciably longer than the 8-day withdrawal period generally recommended by the RCVS.

Carnivores such as Greyhounds can absorb drugs by consuming meat from animals previously treated with medication and feeding of, for example knacker meat, 24 hours before competition is prohibited. Warnings are also given regarding consumption of bread because of potential problems due to poppy seeds.

Formulation. Some drugs are specifically formulated to prolong their action. Particular care needs to be taken with hormonal implants and long-acting corticosteroid and anabolic steroid preparations. Although specific information is not available for horses or dogs, it is likely that absorption of drug from slow-release implants will be essentially complete in 6 months. However, except for certain fertility problems, the veterinarian's right to prescribe anabolic steroids for large animals (including horses) and poultry is limited by legislation in the UK under *The Animals and Animal Products (Examination for Residues and Maximum Residue Limits) Regulations 1997* (SI 1997/1729).

Despite recommendations to the veterinary profession that it is inadvisable to administer procaine benzylpenicillin to horses in training, there continue to be positive findings for procaine in post-competition samples. The drug combination is valuable for prolonging the duration of antibacterial activity, but since procaine is a basic drug its urinary concentration is governed by the pH of the urine. It may be detected in racehorse urine for several days after topical administration (even from topically applied cerate esters contained in intramammary preparations) and sporadically for over a month after injection. A course of the soluble sodium salt of benzylpenicillin should be used if treatment against penicillin-sensitive bacteria is required.

Pharmacokinetics. Delayed absorption and excretion may occur following intramuscular injection or oral administration. Since absorption is related to vascularity and lipid solubility, inadvertent injection into fatty tissue or between fascial planes may lead to prolonged excretion. In horses, acepromazine metabolites have been detected in urine many weeks after the last reported intramuscular injection and this circumstantial evidence raises the possibility that acepromazine may be sequestered and released sporadically.

Lipid-soluble substances such as corticosteroids and local anaesthetics are well absorbed following intra-articular injection and may be detected in the urine.

Absorption of drugs across mucous membranes can be rapid. Camphor and other ingredients of many traditional inhalants may be detectable in urine. Nebulisation can produce high plasma-drug concentrations due to absorption through the alveolar surface.

Consideration should be given to the content and timing of application of shampoos and other substances for skin. Caution should be exercised when applying topical NSAIDs because these substances can be absorbed through the skin of the horse or dog and consequently detected in the urine. If the epidermis is damaged, the permeable underlying dermis allows the passage of lipid-soluble and water-soluble molecules. Care must be taken with topical applications such as oil of wintergreen, which contains methyl salicylate, especially when abrasions are present.

Dimethyl sulfoxide (dimethyl sulphoxide, DMSO) possesses pharmacological properties of its own, but can also act as a vehicle for other drugs whose transcutaneous absorption may be enhanced. This is particularly applicable to substances with a molecular weight of less than 3000.

In general, the RCVS recommends the discontinuance of drugs for racehorses and Greyhounds not less than 8 days before racing, even though such a period is longer than is necessary in many instances (*Guide to professional con-*

duct. RCVS). The RCVS make it clear in issuing their advice, that they cannot accept responsibility for the possibility that an atypical horse or dog may take longer than normal to excrete a drug, even if the drug is not formulated for modified release.

In many cases, the elimination time of all components of a compound preparation may be unknown or uncertain. If such a preparation is to be administered to an animal without the certain knowledge that all residues will have been excreted before the competition or show the RCVS recommend that the owner should be advised *in writing* that the animal should not be raced or shown on the occasion in question.

Drug detection times. Member countries of the European Horseracing Scientific Liaison Committee (EHSLC) are undertaking a programme to provide detection times for drugs which are authorised for use in horses. This information is intended to assist veterinarians to give advice as to when racehorses may be raced after treatment for clinical problems.

In this programme, authorised veterinary drugs are administered to Thoroughbred horses and samples collected and analysed until the drug (or metabolites or isomers) are undetectable. The published detection times represent the longest times recorded by any of the participating European drug testing laboratories using the current methods for confirmatory analysis.

This initiative for providing drug detection information to veterinarians is complemented by an EHSLC Elective Testing programme, whereby an analytical service is offered to racehorse trainers who wish to establish before a race that drugs given in essential veterinary treatment will not give rise to positive post-race analyses.

Desensitised and hypersensitised limbs. The Fédération Equestre Internationale (FEI) states that no horse shall be allowed to compete following neurectomy on a limb nor when any limb has been temporarily or permanently desensitised by any means. Similarly under the Jockey Club rules a horse is not qualified to start a race if the animal has been the subject of a neurectomy operation.

Examination of skin for increased sensitivity may involve a clinical evaluation in addition to swabbing the limb to collect samples or the collection of bandages or other material to be analysed for prohibited substances.

Oxygen and intravenous fluid therapy. At FEI events, injections of normal nutrients such as saline fluids, electrolyte solutions, and glucose may be administered with the written approval of the Veterinary Commission or Delegate. Administration of oxygen must be made by the use of an intubation tube only, inserted into a single nostril. The use of any form of mask is forbidden. Any horse which has had oxygen or normal nutrients administered at the conclusion of Phase D at Three-day Events or after the Marathon at Driving Events must be clinically examined by the Veterinary Commission or Delegate before the next stages at these events.

Testing of animals

Forensic analysis of urine or blood samples from competing animals is undertaken at designated laboratories. Any other body fluid or biological material, such as vomit from Greyhounds, may also be examined if necessary. For samples taken from racehorses, the procedures involved in the analysis and counter-analysis (confirmatory analysis undertaken by a different approved laboratory) are subjected to scrutiny by independent review bodies before a sample can finally be declared positive.

Typically, samples are collected after performance but rules do not preclude examination at any stage of competition and animals may be tested more than once during multi-stage competitions under FEI regulations. Under NRGC rules, Greyhounds are randomly chosen by a steward of the NRGC at a race or trial meeting and subjected to sampling. A pre-race positive result may lead to the animal being withdrawn.

Generally, the amount of a substance found in a sample taken from a competing animal is irrelevant in determining whether or not there has been a breach of the rules, except for those substances with threshold concentrations specified in the Jockey Club, FEI, and Hurlingham Polo Association rules (see below). FEI regulations state that if a prohibited substance is detected on analysis, its presence is assumed to be the result of a deliberate attempt, on the part of the person responsible, to affect the performance of the horse. NGRC Rules put the onus of responsibility on the trainer in charge of the Greyhound.

Horses

Medication in equine competitions

Several autonomous bodies produce their own rules on medication control based on a list of prohibited substances. In essence these can be regarded as variations on the rules of the Jockey Club (*Rules of racing and instructions*) or of the Fédération Equestre Internationale (FEI) (*Veterinary regulations*). An exception to this is the Hurlingham Polo Association Directive *The welfare of ponies and the misuse of drugs*, which includes a list of permitted substances (see below).

The Jockey Club and FEI describe a prohibited substance as a substance originating externally whether or not it is endogenous to the horse and which is contained in the list of Prohibited Substances. 'Substance' includes the metabolites of the substance and the isomers or biological indicators (including their metabolites) of such substance.

Maximum permitted concentrations have been established for certain substances that are commonly detected in equine urine samples. Such substances may occur in ordinary diets, or may be endogenous to the horse, or may arise as a result of contamination.

Salicylic acid can be derived directly from ingested plant materials. Lucerne, in particular, is rich in salicylic acid and this feedstuff has also been incriminated in the findings of significant quantities of **dimethyl sulfoxide** in forensic samples from racehorses.

Theobromine and **arsenic** can arise as a result of feed contamination. Theobromine from cocoa products is often introduced into compound feeds during manufacture.

The adrenal cortex secretes **hydrocortisone** (cortisol) in physiologically significant amounts, and a threshold in urine for this substance has been set. Urinary levels of this substance can be affected by the administration either of corticosteroids or of specific releasing hormones.

The estranediol:estrenediol ratio in urine is used to distinguish between endogenous **nandrolone** (detectable in normal stallion urine) and administered nandrolone. If a sample exceeds the threshold set for **testosterone** or other endogenous substance, the horse may be submitted for further examination to establish whether the amount of the substance could be produced naturally by the animal.

In a departure from the normal procedure of establishing thresholds in post-race blood or urine samples, the quantitation of **available carbon dioxide** can be undertaken using pre-race samples.

Occasionally a prohibited substance has been found in the urine of a horse and the source of the substance has not been established. Therefore the Jockey Club recommends that trainers retain samples of feedstuffs used for the particular horse and any coding details that appear on the feed packaging. This advice is particularly important because maximum permitted concentrations have not yet been established for all prohibited substances that can arise from dietary sources, for example, the sympathomimetic **hordenine** derived from some barley products, the opioid **morphine** from poppies, and the alkaloid **hyoscine** and its isomers from soya bean meal.

Jockey Club list of maximum permissible concentrations of prohibited substances

Drug	Maximum permissible concentration
Total arsenic	0.3 micrograms/mL in urine
Dimethyl sulfoxide	15 micrograms/mL in urine *or* 1 microgram/mL in plasma
Hydrocortisone	1 microgram/mL in urine
Nandrolone (free and conjugated)	5α-estrane-3ß, 17α- diol to 5(10)-estrene-3ß, 17α-diol in urine at a ratio of 1
Salicylic acid	750 micrograms/mL in urine *or* 6.5 micrograms/mL in plasma
Theobromine	2 micrograms/mL in urine
Available carbon dioxide	37 millimoles/L in plasma
Testosterone (free and conjugated)	0.02 micrograms/mL in urine from geldings free and congugated testosterone to epitestosterone in urine from fillies and mares at a ratio of 12

Jockey Club list of prohibited substances

Substances acting on the nervous system
Substances acting on the cardiovascular system
Substances acting on the respiratory system
Substances acting on the digestive system
Substances acting on the urinary system
Substances acting on the reproductive system
Substances acting on the musculoskeletal system
Substances acting on the blood system
Substances acting on the immune system other than those in licensed vaccines
Substances acting on the endocrine system; endocrine secretions and their synthetic counterparts
For the purposes of clarity these include:
Antipyretics, analgesics and anti-inflammatory substances
Cytotoxic substances
Antihistamines
Diuretics
Local anaesthetics
Muscle relaxants
Respiratory stimulants
Sex hormones, anabolic agents and corticosteroids
Substances affecting blood coagulation

FEI list of maximum permissible concentrations of prohibited substances

Drug	Maximum permissible concentration
Total arsenic	0.3 micrograms/mL in urine
Salicylic acid	750 micrograms/mL in urine *or* 6.5 micrograms/mL in plasma
Theobromine	2 micrograms/mL in urine
Nandrolone (free and conjugated)	5α-estrane-3ß, 17α- diol to 5(10)-estrene-3ß, 17α-diol in urine at a ratio not exceeding 1
Dimethyl sulfoxide	15 micrograms/mL in urine *or* 1 microgram/mL in plasma
Hydrocortisone	1 microgram/mL in urine
Available carbon dioxide	37 millimoles/L in plasma
Testosterone (geldings)	0.02 micrograms free and unconjugated testosterone/mL in urine
Testosterone (fillies and mares)	free and congugated testosterone to epitestosterone 12:1 in urine

FEI list of prohibited substances

Substances acting on the nervous system
Substances acting on the cardiovascular system
Substances acting on the respiratory system
Substances acting on the digestive system
Substances acting on the urinary system
Substances acting on the reproductive system
Substances acting on the musculoskeletal system
Substances acting on the skin (eg hypersensitising agents)
Substances acting on the blood system
Substances acting on the immune system other than those in licensed vaccines
Substances acting on the endocrine system, endocrine secretions and their synthetic counterparts
Anti-infectious substances other than exclusively anti-parasitic substances
Antipyretics, analgesics and anti-inflammatory substances
Cytotoxic substances

The Hurlingham Polo Association list of permitted substances

Antibiotics except procaine penicillin
Flunixin
Isoxsuprine
Phenylbutazone
Regumate [altrenogest]
Sputolosin [dembrexine hydrochloride]
Ventipulmin [clenbuterol hydrochloride]
Vi-Sorbin [iron and vitamin B substances]
The following drugs are only permitted if prior declaration of their administration has been made:
Diuretics
Local anaesthetics

The Hurlingham Polo Association list of maximum permissible concentrations

Drug	Maximum permissible concentration
Phenylbutazone with oxy-phenbutazone	10 micrograms/mL in plasma
Flunixin	10 micrograms/mL in plasma

Note. If phenylbutazone and flunixin are used together the concentration of either must be less than 5 micrograms/mL

Vaccination of horses

All competing horses should be protected against tetanus, although this is not a mandatory requirement under any rules. However, the Jockey Club and the FEI insist that horses or ponies that compete under their regulations are vaccinated against equine influenza.

Many showgrounds require entrants to be adequately vaccinated against influenza, whether or not such a requirement is incorporated into the rules of the organising authority. This also applies to any horse or pony entering property owned, used or controlled by the horseracing authorities, unless the property is common ground. Foals less than 4 months old are exempt, providing the dam is fully vaccinated before foaling.

There must be irrefutable evidence that the vaccination record applies to the animal presented and all entries must be signed and stamped by a veterinarian. For racehorses, the Jockey Club require entries to be endorsed in the horse's passport, and does not accept entries which have been altered in any way. An incorrect endorsement must be completely deleted and a new endorsement of the whole entry made.

FEI and Jockey Club rules differ, but any vaccination programme which follows the vaccine manufacturer's recommendations will satisfy both sets of rules.

Jockey Club rules. Two injections for primary vaccination must be given not less than 21 days and no more than 92 days apart. Horses should have received a booster between 150 and 215 days after the second injection of the vaccine. Following the initial course (primary vaccination and first booster), a booster injection must be given each year.

FEI rules. Two injections for primary vaccination must be given no less than 21 days and no more than 92 days apart. A booster injection must be given each succeeding 12 months, subsequent to the second injection of the primary course.

Under both sets of rules, vaccinations given by a veterinarian, who is the owner of the horse at the time of vaccination, are not accepted. The Jockey Club extend this to exclude vaccinations given by a veterinarian who is the trainer or who is named on the Register of Stable Employees as being employed by the trainer of the horse.

No horse may compete or enter competition premises until 7 days after vaccination. When calculating this interval, the day of vaccination should not be included. Horses need only have completed a primary vaccination course before competition. It is not necessary to wait until after the first booster. Annual boosters may be given on the same day in consecutive years.

The above are minimum requirements. Both the primary vaccination course and first and subsequent booster vaccinations should be given according to the manufacturer's recommendations, which will fall within the above ruling. In some cases, it is advisable to give booster vaccinations at intervals of less than 12 months.

Greyhounds and coursing hounds

Medication in canine competitions

Drug use in racing Greyhounds is controlled by the National Greyhound Racing Club (NGRC). The NGRC *Rules of racing* do not specifically prohibit particular substances, however, their rules prohibit the administration to a Greyhound, for any improper use, any quantity of any substance which by its nature could affect the performance or prejudice the well-being of the Greyhound, the origin of which cannot be traced to normal and ordinary feeding or care. The Rules also state that it is an offence to have in one's charge a Greyhound which showed the presence of any such substance. Some Greyhounds may show positive to traces of anti-inflammatory agents, barbiturates, and antibacterials that have come from consumption of knacker meat. It is generally accepted practice to feed such meat to Greyhounds (but not less than 24 hours before a competition) and it is hoped that the NGRC will issue a list of permissible drug concentrations.

Professional and owner trainers must maintain their Trainer's Treatment Book, in which any tonic, medicament, or other substance administered or applied to a Greyhound must be recorded.

Except for preparations that are specifically authorised for the suppression/postponement of oestrus and are used under the authority of a veterinarian, no substance should be used for at least 7 days before an official trial or race. This rule is an attempt to avoid the possibility of the constituents of tonics or other medicaments being excreted in the urine, and interfering with the interpretation of any tests. With regard to oestrus control, it is important to note that only products that are specifically authorised may be used. Products authorised in the UK include Androject (Intervet), Delvosteron (Intervet), Durateston (Intervet), Orandrone (Intervet). Anabolic steroids, that have been used for oestrus control, are not included.

Medication control in coursing hounds is based on prohibited substances.

National Coursing Club list of prohibited substances

Substances acting on the central nervous system
Substances acting on the autonomic nervous system
Substances acting on the cardiovascular system
Substances affecting the gastro-intestinal function
Substances affecting the immune system and its response
Antibiotics, synthetic and anti-viral substances
Antihistamines
Anti-malarials
Antipyretics, analgesics and anti-inflammatory substances
Diuretics
Local anaesthetics
Muscle relaxants
Respiratory stimulants
Sex hormones, anabolic agents and corticosteroids
Endocrine secretions and their synthetic counterparts
Substances affecting blood coagulation
Cytotoxic substances.

Vaccination of Greyhounds

The NGRC requires that all Greyhounds in authorised kennels are fully vaccinated against distemper, viral hepatitis, *Leptospira canicola*, *Leptospira icterohaemorrhagiae*, parvovirus, and any other required vaccination as may be notified from time to time. Vaccines authorised in the UK must be used. Documentary evidence of the vaccinations must be provided for subsequent entry in the identity book. Booster vaccinations are required at 12-monthly intervals from the date of the initial puppy inoculations.

Pigeons

Racing pigeons that are kept for racing and showing are subject to *The Diseases of Poultry Order 1994*, as amended, and to the rules of the six controlling organisations: the Royal Pigeon Racing Association, Irish Homing Union, North of England Homing Union, North West Homing Union, Scottish Homing Union, and Welsh Homing Union.

There are no requirements or restrictions on the medication and vaccination of other flying breeds of pigeons, birds kept for display flying and showing, or for pigeons kept solely for showing.

Vaccination of racing pigeons

Under *The Diseases of Poultry Order 1994*, as amended, an organiser of a show or race which takes place wholly or partly in Great Britain must ensure that all racing pigeons entered for the show or race have been vaccinated against paramyxovirus 1 and a record is kept. A record must be made by the person who owns or keeps racing pigeons of every race or show for which a bird is entered. The rules for the Royal Pigeon Racing Association and the five Homing Unions all contain a strict code of practice for paramyxovirus vaccination.

Medication of racing pigeons

The Royal Pigeon Racing Association rules prohibit the use of 'anabolic steroids, corticosteroids, and beta-agonists' in birds used for racing. The five Homing Unions have no written rules regarding medication of racing pigeons but they would take appropriate action, including testing of birds, where the use of these substances for racing are suspected.

Show animals

Medication and vaccination for show animals

The Kennel Club consider that nothing may be done which is calculated to deceive. No substance which alters the natural colour, texture, or body of the coat may be used in preparing a dog for exhibition. Dogs are judged against a 'Breed Standard' and action may be taken should a dog act in a way markedly different from that described as its normal temperament. Although no specific vaccination programmes are cited, dogs should not have had a communicable disease in the previous 6 weeks.

Similarly, the Governing Council of the Cat Fancy prohibits any artificial preparation of any exhibit which is likely to change the animal's appearance relative to the 'Standard of Points'. Any treatment, including sedation, causing temporary or permanent change in the normal appearance or physical reaction of the exhibit is prohibited. All cats must have a certificate of current vaccination against cat flu and feline enteritis issued by a recognised veterinary practice.

At major livestock shows, similar rules apply and action will be taken against any exhibitor who is found to have administered, or permitted the administration of, any tranquilliser or other drugs, which may in any way affect the performance of the animal, or have the effect of making it behave in the show in a manner which is not natural.

Prescribing for equines

Contributors:
A F Trawford BVSc, MSc, CVMA, MRCVS
F M D Henson MA, VetMB, PhD, CertES(Orth), MRCVS

Horses, ponies, and donkeys are the most common species from the genus *Equus* that are kept in a domestic situation. This section provides general and specific advice on prescribing for these species; lack of reference to a particular drug does not necessarily imply safety and efficacy because species, breed, and individual variation should be considered. The conditions affecting these species and their requirements will differ according to the area, housing environment, and management system used.

In the EU, horses constitute food-producing animals providing meat for human consumption. Withdrawal periods for meat stated by the manufacturer should be adhered to. If no withdrawal periods are given, standard withdrawal periods should be applied. Under *The Medicines (Restrictions on the Administration of Veterinary Medicinal Products) Regulations 1994* (SI 1994/2987), as amended, if the animal is a food-producing animal, the veterinarian or person acting under his direction may *only* administer a product that contains substances found in a product authorised for use in food-producing animals.

In some countries, such as the UK and Ireland, horses are bred for performance and leisure activities and are not usually intended for human consumption. Under recent EC legislation, registered horses and those intended for breeding and production must be accompanied by a passport, which includes declarations whether the animal is or is not intended for human consumption and a section in which to record medicines administered to the animal. This legislation provides a means of use of medicines that do not have a MRL in Equidae. See *British Veterinary Association Code of practice on medicines* for further information.

Drug administration. In horses, ponies, and donkeys drugs are usually prescribed for individual animal treatment and can be administered via a number of routes.

For parenteral administration, injections may be given subcutaneously, intramuscularly, intravenously, or intra-articularly. Particular care should be taken when injecting drugs intra-articularly because the consequences of intra-articular sepsis are particularly severe in equines; an aseptic technique should always be used. When injecting intramuscularly, the hindquarter musculature (gluteals, semimembranous, or semitendinous), pectoral musculature, or cervical musculature may be used. Not more than 30 mL volume should be administered at any one site if given by intramuscular injection.

Horses are particularly sensitive to components of parenteral preparations and oil-based formulations or unbuffered solutions or suspensions may cause irritation and tissue damage at the site of injection. Donkeys are less sensitive than horses in this respect.

A limited number of drugs are available for oral medication including anthelmintics, some antibacterials, and some NSAIDs. These can either be administered in the feed or as an oral paste.

Drugs can also be administered by nebulisation and by topical application in equines.

Drug absorption and metabolism. In horses, an orally administered drug such as phenylbutazone may be partly absorbed from the small intestine with further absorption occurring 8 to 12 hours later from the large intestine. Absorption of some drugs administered in the feed or after feeding can be delayed and shows a biphasic pattern because unabsorbed drug may be conveyed to the large intestine where further absorption takes place.

Variation in distribution, clearance, or half-life between horses and donkeys has been shown for all drugs which have been investigated. These pharmacokinetic differences are of clinical significance for drugs that are eliminated mainly by the liver or that undergo enterohepatic circulation, such as oxytetracycline. Phenylbutazone, flunixin, and ketamine in particular have increased volume of distribution and more rapid clearance times in donkeys than in horses; phenylbutazone clearance is approximately 10 times higher than in horses.

Antimicrobial therapy can cause severe disturbances of bacterial fermentation in the colon and caecum of adult equines. Whenever such a reaction occurs, it is recommended that the antimicrobial be withdrawn. If severe colitis ensues, aggressive medical and fluid therapy may be required. Any antimicrobial can potentially cause such a disturbance, however, oral oxytetracycline or erythromycin should be avoided in adult horses. Colitis has also been recognised associated with the peri-operative use of ceftiofur particularly in stressed animals.

The use of lincosamide and macrolide antibacterials should be avoided in horses, with the exception of oral administration of erythromycin estolate in conjunction with rifampicin for the treatment of *Rhodococcus equi* infection in foals. Fluoroquinolones should not be administered to skeletally immature horses because these drugs may damage growth cartilage. Aminoglycosides, particularly gentamicin, are routinely used for treatment in horses. Gentamicin is potentially nephrotoxic and should be used with care in horses with impaired renal function. Ingestion of feed containing tylosin, tiamulin, or monensin may be fatal to horses and other equidae.

NSAIDs are used extensively to treat pain, oedema, and tissue destruction in inflammatory conditions in horses. Phenylbutazone is widely used in horses but has a narrow margin of safety and only recommended dosages should be given. Some authorities consider carprofen to be less ulcerogenic and is therefore the NSAID of choice for foals. Corticosteroids are occasionally used in equines for conditions such as allergic respiratory disease; they are reported to induce laminitis in susceptible animals.

The majority of sedatives and analgesics have wide safety margins however all sedatives can cause marked cardiovascular alterations. The alpha$_2$-adrenoceptor agonists (xylazine, romifidine, and detomidine) are useful sedatives and analgesics with xylazine having the shortest duration of action. Atipamezole has been used successfully in horses ◆ to reverse excessive sedation and ataxia resulting from inadvertent overdosage. Phenothiazines such as acepromazine should be used with caution in male horses and should not be used in breeding stallions because these drugs may cause paralysis of the retractor penis muscle. The opioid analgesic butorphanol is frequently used in combination with alpha$_2$-adrenoceptor agonists for sedation. It is recognised that butorphanol administration can very occasionally cause extreme excitation.

There are limited drugs authorised for use in donkeys. The table provides dosages for commonly used medicines.

Table 1 Doses of drugs for donkeys[1]

Drug	Dose	Condition
Acepromazine	2.5 mg/50 kg body-weight i.v. followed by 25 mg/50 mg p.o. twice daily	laminitis
Acepromazine + Detomidine + Ketamine	1.5 mg/50 kg + (after 30 minutes) 1.5 mg/50 kg + (after 5 minutes) 110 mg/50 kg i.v.	field anaesthesia
Clenbuterol	160 micrograms/kg p.o. twice daily (maximum dose) 320 micrograms/kg i.v	respiratory disease
Griseofulvin[1]	10 mg/kg p.o. daily	ringworm
Ivermectin[1]	200 micrograms/kg p.o.	roundworms, in particular *Dictycaulus arnfieldi*
Mebendazole[1]	5–10 mg/kg p.o.	roundworms
	15–20 mg/kg p.o. daily for 5 days.	*Dictycaulus arnfieldi*
Permethrin[1]	0.1 mL/kg by 'pour-on' application	*Culicoides*, lice
Phenylbutazone	500 mg p.o. twice daily 500 mg i.v. daily	laminitis
Triclabendazole	12 mg/kg p.o.	flukes

[1] drug doses for preparations that have a marketing authorisation for use in this species in the UK. Therefore, unless marked [1], the drug or doses stated are not authorised for this species

Prescribing for ruminants

Contributors:
A H Andrews BVetMed, PhD, MRCVS
T J Fletcher BVMS, PhD, MRCVS

Ruminant species that are farmed include cattle, sheep, goats, and deer.

This section provides general and specific advice on prescribing for these species; lack of reference to a particular drug does not necessarily imply safety and efficacy because species, breed, and individual variation should be considered. The conditions affecting these species and their requirements will differ according to the area, housing environment, and management system used. Limited preparations are authorised for deer in the UK. Drug dosages for deer are given in Table 2. Other drugs are authorised for deer in other counties; information is given in chapters 1 to 10.

Different species and breeds are used for different purposes: sheep and goats may be kept for fibre production; cattle, sheep, goats, and deer constitute food-producing animals providing meat, milk, or both for human consumption. Withdrawal periods for milk and meat stated by the manufacturer should be adhered to. These are specific for the stated dose and duration of therapy given in the manufacturer's data sheet. Usage outwith this treatment regimen will necessitate application of standard withdrawal periods. If no withdrawal periods are given, standard withdrawal periods should be applied. Wild and park deer may be culled and enter the human food chain with relatively few controls and consideration should be given to this when administering drugs to deer, for example care should be taken when deer that have been captured with a tranquilliser are released into the wild.

Under *The Medicines (Restrictions on the Administration of Veterinary Medicinal Products) Regulations 1994* (SI 1994/2987), as amended, if the animal is a food-producing animal, the veterinarian or person acting under his direction may *only* administer a product that contains substances found in a product authorised for use in food-producing animals (but see also prescribing for food-producing animals). This can create problems for animal welfare, for example general anaesthetics. In addition, the use of drugs and medicines in these species may be restricted or prohibited. For example, use of chloramphenicol in food-producing species is not possible because potential residues in human food may lead to bacterial resistance and aplastic anaemia in humans. The administration of stilbenes is confined to companion and laboratory animals, and farm animals kept for research purposes because of possible carcinogenicity in humans.

Drug administration. Drugs may be prescribed as group medication for administration in the feed or drinking water or for individual animal treatment. For parenteral administration in these species, injections may be given subcutaneously, intramuscularly, or intravenously. Not more than 20 mL should be administered at any one site if given by intramuscular injection in adult cattle and proportionally smaller volumes should be given at one site for other ages and species.

The rate of drug absorption can vary with the location of the intramuscular injection site. Wherever there is a choice of injection site, then the area used should be one which is not, or little used, for human consumption. When administering drugs by dart to deer especially during late summer, operators should be aware that there may be several centimetres of subcutaneous fat especially over the gluteal mass.

Ruminal boluses that provide continuous or pulsatile release of a drug over a prolonged period have been developed for use in cattle and sheep for the delivery of anthelmintics, trace elements, and magnesium; they are also used in deer♦. Ruminal boluses should not be given to cattle weighing less than 100 kg body-weight, that do not have a functional rumen, or are less than 3 months of age. Operators should be trained in the correct method of administration of boluses and suitable restraint.

'Pour-on' formulations are available for use on cattle, sheep, pigs, and are also used on deer♦.

Drug absorption and metabolism. There is wide variation in drug absorption and metabolism among these species. Absorption from the gastro-intestinal tract in ruminant species is influenced by the volume and pH of the ruminal contents and whether the drug is subject to metabolism by ruminal micro-organisms. Deer have greater gastric and intestinal motility than cattle and sheep and there is some evidence that orally administered drugs should be given at a higher dose to deer.

Drugs that are extensively metabolised by hepatic microsomal oxidative reactions are, in general, metabolised more rapidly in ruminant animals and horses than in pigs. Phenylbutazone is a notable exception in that the half-life of this drug in cattle♦ is many times longer than in horses. The dose of xylazine administered to cattle is one-tenth of that used in horses and in other ruminants the dose per kg body-weight is less.

The half-life of some drugs that are eliminated mainly by hepatic metabolism is, in goats, about half that for sheep. Therefore, in general, a dose 1.5 to 2.0 times the ovine anthelmintic dose is recommended for goats. However idiosyncratic reactions to levamisole have been noted in individual fibre-producing goats. Pygmy goats metabolise sulphonamides, chloramphenicol, and probably other drugs that are metabolised by hepatic microsomal enzymes more rapidly than other breeds. Some intramammary preparations for milking cows have a longer duration of activity within the udder of goats.

Deer may metabolise some anthelmintics more rapidly than other ruminants and the recommendation has been made that anthelmintics should be given at 2 times the dose for cattle and sheep regardless of the route of administration. No adverse effects have been reported using this regimen. 'Pour-on' preparations are prefered for use in deer. It has been shown that diethylcarbamazine and levamisole are much less effective in controlling lungworms in red deer than they are in cattle.

Whenever practicable the oral administration of antimicrobials to ruminants should be discouraged. Orally administered penicillins or broad-spectrum antimicrobials may disturb bacterial fermentation in the rumen in animals with a functional rumen resulting in severe digestive disturbances. Following oral antibacterial administration in ruminants, the ruminal microflora should be re-established by cud transfer or administration of a proprietary preparation. Probiotics may be helpful. An alternative is to ensure that drugs are delivered directly into the abomasum via the reticular groove mechanism. This can be achieved by adding the medicant to the milk of pre-weaned ruminants. In adult sheep, prior administration of copper sulphate produces groove closure. In cattle, oral administration of 60 mL of sodium bicarbonate 10% is effective in achieving groove closure. Reticular groove closure may however be counterproductive. Spontaneous closure in some individuals given oral benzimidazoles can result in a proportion of the drug being transferred into the abomasum, thus reducing the efficacy of the drug.

Tetracyclines are the drug of choice for treating deer with *Yersinia pseudotuberculosis* and in order to minimise stress in newly weaned calves, the drug is often incorporated into the ration. In cattle, rapid intravenous injection of tetracyclines may cause cardiovascular collapse due to chelation of calcium in heart muscle, with consequent vasodilation and myocardial depression.

Response to tranquillisers by darting, often used to capture deer, varies greatly between the different species, for example there is evidence that isolated populations of red deer differ in their responsiveness to xylazine.

For some species now used for production of meat, milk, or fibre there is only limited information available on the breed differences in reactions to certain drugs. **It is important that any adverse drug reactions are reported**.

Table 2 Doses of drugs for deer[1]

Drug	Dose
Antibacterial drugs	
Oxytetracycline[1]	red deer, 20 mg/kg i.m., repeat after 2–4 days
Other antibacterial drugs	in general, use at same dosage as for cattle
Parasiticides	
Endectocides	use at about 2 times dosage for cattle
Tranquillisers	
Acepromazine + Etorphine[1] (Large Animal Immobilon)	tame deer, 0.5 mL/50 kg i.m. (reduce dose by 30% in pregnant hinds) rutting or wild deer, up to 1 mL/50 kg i.m. *Reversal* Diprenorphine[1,] volume equal to total volume of Immobilon previously administered, i.m ♦, i.v.
Detomidine + Ketamine	capture of reindeer, fallow deer by dart, 60–90 micrograms/kg + 1–2 mg/kg *Reversal* Atipamezole, volume 3–7 times volume of detomidine previously administered
Ketamine + Xylazine[2]	fallow deer, 2–3 mL/50 kg
Xylazine 20 mg/mL	for sedation of red deer in yards or pens, 0.5–1.5 mg/kg, i.m. (should not be used as sole agent for capture of free ranging deer by dart) *Reversal* Yohimbine, 250 micrograms/kg i.v.
Minerals	
Copper supplements	female adult red deer, 1 Copacaps Cattle
Vaccines	
Polyvalent Clostridial vaccines	hinds, 2 times dosage for sheep

[1] drug doses for preparations that have a marketing authorisation for use in this species in the UK. Therefore, unless marked [1], the drug or doses stated are not authorised for this species
[2] dose is in mL/kg of a mixture ('Hellabrun mixture') made up of 4 mL ketamine 100 mg/mL added to xylazine 500 mg powder for reconstitution

Prescribing for pigs

Contributor:
D J Taylor MA, VetMB, PhD, MRCVS

This section provides general and specific advice on prescribing for pigs. Lack of reference to a particular drug does not necessarily imply safety and efficacy because species, breed, and individual variation should be considered. The conditions affecting this species and their requirements will differ according to the area, housing environment, and management system used. For example, a wallow should be provided for pigs kept outdoors in order to give protection against sunburn. In the UK, the Farm Animal Welfare Council publishes information and reports on aspects of animal welfare.

Pigs constitute food-producing animals providing meat for human consumption. Withdrawal periods for meat stated by the manufacturer should be adhered to. If no withdrawal periods are given, standard withdrawal periods should be applied. Under *The Medicines (Restrictions on the Administration of Veterinary Medicinal Products) Regulations 1994* (SI 1994/2987), as amended, if the animal is a food-producing animal, the veterinarian or person acting under his direction may *only* administer a product that contains substances found in a product authorised for use in food-producing animals (but see also Prescribing for food-producing animals).

There is a growing trend to keep miniature pig breeds, for example the Vietnamese pot-bellied pig, as companion animals. Veterinarians are reminded that movement of these pigs (for example from the owner's home to hospital premises) requires a licence from the DVM and treatment records should be retained for the requisite period (see Record keeping). Behavioural problems such as aggression may arise when pigs are kept as pets and owners should be warned of potential hazards.

Drug administration. Drugs may be prescribed as group medication for administration in the feed or drinking water or for individual animal treatment. For parenteral administration in these species, injections may be given subcutaneously, intramuscularly, or intravenously, or by intraperitoneal injection in piglets.

Drug absorption and metabolism. Pigs are omnivorous monogastric animals and drug absorption takes place mainly from the small intestine.

Drugs that are extensively metabolised by hepatic microsomal oxidative reactions are, in general, metabolised more rapidly in ruminant animals and horses than in pigs. In pigs, the defect in sulphate conjugation is compensated for by alternative metabolic pathways such as glucuronide synthesis.

Procaine benzylpenicillin may cause shivering in pigs. Pot-bellied pigs may be prone to hypothermia following anaesthesia.

There is limited information on breed differences in reactions to particular drugs in pigs. **It is important that adverse drug reactions are reported under the Suspected Adverse Reaction Surveillance Scheme (SARSS) at the VMD**.

Prescribing for dogs

Contributor:
W T Turner BVetMed, FRSH, MRCVS

This section provides general and specific advice on prescribing for dogs; lack of reference to a particular drug does not necessarily imply safety and efficacy because breed and individual variation should be considered.

Dogs and cats are considered as companion animals. In the UK, prescribing of medicines for these species is under *The Medicines (Restrictions on the Administration of Veterinary Medicinal Products) Regulations 1994* (SI 1994/2987), as amended. The VMD have indicated that for the purposes of interpretation of the Regulations 'in certain circumstances, certain especially sensitive breeds of cat and dog should be considered as exotic' *Medicines (Restrictions on the administration of veterinary medicinal products) Regulations 1994: Guidance notes for the veterinary profession.* AMELIA 8 published by the VMD.

Dogs should always be weighed before being medicated and especially with the larger breeds calculation of the total dose should be based at the lower end of the recommended range.

Drug administration. Drugs may be administered by mouth, via the food, by injection, or in certain circumstances by absorption through intact skin or mucous membranes. Owner compliance should be considered when prescribing medicines for dogs.

Drug absorption and metabolism. Dogs are monogastric and drug absorption takes place mainly in the small intestine. In dogs, the acetylation process for aromatic amines such as sulphonamides is absent. This does not decrease the overall rate of sulphonamide elimination because alternative metabolic pathways compensate; acidic urine favours sulphonamide reabsorption and increases half-life.

Sulphonamides, sulphasalazine, mesalazine, and olsalazine, administered systemically, may cause keratoconjunctivitis sicca. Potentiated sulphonamides may cause an immune-mediated polyarthritis particularly in larger breeds such as Dobermanns. Tetracycline antibacterials may cause permanent staining of the dental enamel if given to puppies before eruption of the permanent dentition or to the dam during pregnancy.

NSAIDs may cause gastric ulceration, particularly at high doses or if given in combination with corticosteroids. These are potent drugs and patients may show individual susceptibilities to toxic effects. Dose-dependent liver failure is encountered in dogs given excessive doses of paracetamol.

Phenothiazines such as acepromazine should be used with caution in Greyhounds and other coursing hounds and in brachycephalic breeds. In the Boxer in particular fainting may be precipitated. Phenothiazines may cause paradoxical excitement in some dogs. Xylazine may initially cause emesis in dogs. Some breeds including Basset Hounds, Great Danes, and Irish Setters, appear susceptible to bloat after xylazine administration. Thiobarbiturates such as thiopental may have prolonged action in coursing hounds due to limited redistribution of the drug into fatty tissue or decreased plasma-protein binding. Greyhounds appear particularly sensitive in this respect and some authorities suggest that use of thiopental in this breed is contra-indicated.

The unusual sensitivity of some breeds to ivermectin may be due to genetic differences in permeability of the blood-brain barrier, the release of gamma-aminobutyric acid in the CNS, or both. In dogs, severe adverse reactions to ivermectin (including fatalities) may occur. In the UK, injectable praziquantel (Droncit) is not recommended for use in hounds.

Pharmaceutical adjuvants may also induce adverse reactions in some species. Polyoxyl 35 castor oil, the solubilising constituent of Saffan (alfaxalone and alfadolone acetate), causes the release of histamine and histamine-like substances in dogs and therefore the preparation should not be used in this species.

For both dogs and cats limited information is available on breed differences in reactions to particular drugs. **It is important that adverse drug reactions are reported under the Suspected Adverse Reaction Surveillance Scheme (SARSS) at the VMD.**

Prescribing for cats

Contributor:
W T Turner BVetMed, FRSH, MRCVS

This section provides general and specific advice on prescribing for cats; lack of reference to a particular drug does not necessarily imply safety and efficacy because breed and individual variation should be considered. Cats should be weighed before being medicated.

Dogs and cats are considered as companion animals. In the UK, prescribing of medicines for these species is under *The Medicines (Restrictions on the Administration of Veterinary Medicinal Products) Regulations 1994* (SI 1994/2987), as amended. The VMD have indicated that for the purposes of interpretation of the Regulations 'in certain circumstances, certain especially sensitive breeds of cat and dog should be considered as exotic' *Medicines (Restrictions on the administration of veterinary medicinal products) Regulations 1994: Guidance notes for the veterinary profession.* AMELIA 8 published by the VMD.

Drug administration. Drugs may be administered by mouth, via the food, by injection, or in certain circumstances through absorption through intact skin or mucous membranes. Owner compliance should be considered when prescribing medicines for cats.

Drug absorption and metabolism. Cats are monogastric and drug absorption takes place mainly in the small intestine.

The cat has a relative deficiency in hepatic microsomal glucuronyl transferase activity and therefore drugs that are metabolised by this pathway will usually be eliminated at a slower rate. Organophosphorus compounds, aspirin, chloramphenicol, phenytoin, and griseofulvin may be toxic unless the appropriate dosage regimen is carefully applied. Such drugs should be used with caution.

Paracetamol should not be administered to cats because they are particularly susceptible to intoxication. Paracetamol may cause death in cats as a result of profound anaemia with methaemoglobinaemia due to the accumulation of toxic metabolites.

Antiseptic and disinfectant agents such as iodine and its derivatives, benzyl benzoate, phenols and cresol are particularly toxic to cats. This results from a combination of drug ingestion due to the animal's grooming habits together with slow drug metabolism.

Overdosage of opioid analgesics including morphine, butorphanol, etorphine, pethidine, and pethidine derivatives such as diphenoxylate hydrochloride (an ingredient of Lomotil) may cause violent excitatory activity in cats. Phenothiazines such as acepromazine may cause paradoxical excitement in some cats. Xylazine causes emesis in cats.

Cats are particularly susceptible to ototoxicity caused by aminoglycoside antibacterials such as gentamicin, streptomycin, and neomycin. Tetracycline antibacterials may cause permanent staining of the dental enamel if given to kittens before eruption of the permanent dentition or to the queen during pregnancy.

Phosphate-containing rectal enemas cause severe hyperphosphataemia in cats and their use is contra-indicated in this species.

For both dogs and cats limited information is available on breed differences in reactions to particular drugs. **It is important that adverse drug reactions are reported are reported under the Suspected Adverse Reaction Surveillance Scheme (SARSS) at the VMD.**

Prescribing for birds

Contributors:
R F Byrne BVetMed, MRCVS
C Davis BVM&S, MRCVS
S A Lister BVetMed, BSc, CertPMP, MRCVS
C A Madeiros BVetMed, MRCVS
G G A Smith BVSc, BSc, MRCVS

This section deals with prescribing for poultry, game birds, pigeons, and ostriches. Although similar diseases and conditions may affect these species, methods of housing and rearing and whether the birds are farmed for production of meat, eggs, leather, or feathers, or kept for exhibition or racing, lead to varying treatment regimens. Withdrawal periods for meat and eggs stated by the manufacturer should be adhered to. Otherwise standard withdrawal periods should be applied.

Information on other birds such as psittacines and raptors is provided in the section entitled Prescribing for exotic birds.

Poultry

Poultry are farmed domestic birds, which include chickens, ducks, geese, and turkeys. Preparations that are authorised for poultry are not necessarily safe or suitable for use in all species, for example salinomycin is toxic in turkeys.

When investigating a disease problem, management procedures should be examined before medicating the flock. An undesirable environment can nullify the benefits of medication, may be the cause of illness, and should be corrected at the same time as instigating any medication. In some circumstances it may be more economical to slaughter the flock earlier than planned because the cost of treatment would be excessive or the welfare of the birds may be compromised.

The management system can have a significant effect on the pattern of infection. Viral diseases spread via the respiratory route or in the faeces can be especially important where large numbers of birds are kept together. On multi-age sites, younger birds may be exposed to infections which are endemic in older birds on site. In cage systems, birds are removed from contact with their own faeces and the lack of interaction between birds may result in slow dissemination of certain infections within a house. This may lead to a more protracted disease as the infection spreads across the house and may make therapy more problematic.

In birds kept on litter, strategic anticoccidial regimens are required to prevent clinical coccidiosis due to the birds' exposure to the parasite on the litter. Coccidiostats are zootechnical feed additives and must be used in accordance with the relevant Annex entry of Directive 70/524/EEC (*The Feedingstuffs (Zootechnical Products) Regulations*

1999); there is no provision for the veterinarian to alter prescribing from that given in the manufacturer's data sheet. Treatment programmes are often designed to allow birds to build up natural resistance to such parasites and therefore early withdrawal of medication. This is especially significant for birds destined for litter or free range conditions as adult laying birds. Such birds should not be cage reared. Natural immunity is taken a stage further with birds kept in free range conditions where there is access to land which may be contaminated by the birds themselves, wild birds, or vermin. Control of coccidia and nematodes depends on strategic therapy and paddock rotation if the land is to be prevented from becoming 'fowl sick'.

Drug administration. Drugs may be given in the drinking water, feed, or by injection. Administration via the drinking water is usually preferable because domestic poultry will drink when they will not eat. However, fluid intake by the birds may vary due to the weather, to the ease of access or hygiene of drinking water dispensers ('drinkers'), or to the unpalatability of the medicated water. Care must be taken that the medication does not block the water system. Conversely, care should be taken to ensure that drinkers do not overflow because surrounding damp bedding could potentially encourage coccidial oocyst sporulation. Water contamination and hygiene problems may arise as a result of poor mixing and preparation, or from fungal proliferation in certain dextrose carriers present in the formulation. Drinker lines should be sanitised before drug incorporation and especially after drugs in a sucrose or similar basis have been used. They should be cleaned regularly as part of the routine terminal house disinfection.

Alternatively, the feed may be medicated. This is convenient for the farmer but it may take time getting feed mixed at the mill and mills may find making special mixes uneconomical. Absorption of the drug may be unpredictable because of binding to feed ingredients. Some birds may have a reduced feed intake and may require adjustment of the drug concentration in their feed.

Treatment by injection is the most predictable method of drug administration but is only practicable where there are sufficient staff available and the birds are of high monetary value such as turkeys and breeding stock. Intramuscular injection is usually given into the thigh or breast muscle in adult birds. In day-old chicks intramuscular vaccinations are given into the thigh or neck muscle. Aseptic procedures must be strictly observed.

The most accurate method of dosing is in direct relation to body-weight. Most preparations can be administered as mg of drug per kg body-weight. The calculated mg/kg dose can then be given as a daily loading pulsed dose or as divided amounts throughout the day.

Antimicrobial therapy. A number of antibacterials are authorised for use in poultry for the treatment of enteric and respiratory disease or systemic bacterial infection. Specific therapy must be related to accurate diagnosis of the primary cause and any secondary (usually bacterial) sequelae. The choice of medication is dependent on a number of variables including knowledge of the site of action, spectrum of activity, and distribution of the drug in tissues. If possible, the first stage in the decision process is antimicrobial sensitivity tests. In cases of high mortality, it may be necessary to medicate using the drug most likely to be effective, while awaiting laboratory results. Further medication can then be adjusted in the light of these results. In addition, other factors such as ease of use of the product may be of significance, especially in relation to the management system in operation. For example, for birds on a nipple line water system it is essential that a highly soluble product is used to prevent blockage of the water system.

Certain drugs appear especially effective against specific conditions. For example, amoxicillin is well absorbed from the gastro-intestinal tract and is effective against acute septicaemic conditions and also arthritis and tenosynovitis associated with staphylococcal infection. Amoxicillin is also active against Gram-positive micro-organisms and is the drug of choice in clostridial enterotoxaemia of broilers and turkeys. Drugs such as neomycin are not absorbed from the gastro-intestinal tract. Tylosin attains high bone levels and is reported to be effective in cases of osteomyelitis associated with femoral head necrosis. Sulfaquinoxaline and enrofloxacin appear especially effective against *Pasteurella* infections. Tylosin and enrofloxacin have specific activity against mycoplasma. Information on dosage and preparations available for poultry is found in section 1.1.1.

Coccidiosis, mainly caused by *Eimeria* spp., is a common infection in poultry flocks and medication is usually administered prophylactically to control the disease (see section 1.4.1). Anticoccidials such as monensin, narasin, or salinomycin should not be administered concurrently with tiamulin as toxic effects are often fatal. Erythromycin and sulphonamides have also been reported to cause toxic effects when administered with monensin. Anticoccidials should not be used in laying hens because of possible drug residues in eggs intended for human consumption. Chickens may be vaccinated against coccidiosis (see section 18.6.1), which avoids problems of drug resistance and continuous medication.

The British Veterinary Poultry Association has published guidelines on the use of antimicrobials in poultry.

Parasiticidal therapy. Infection with the gapeworm, *Syngamus trachea*, and intestinal nematodes such as *Capillaria*, *Heterakis*, and *Ascaridia* may be treated with authorised preparations including flubendazole. Lice, mites, and fleas may affect poultry and preparations authorised for treatment include cypermethrin (see section 2.2). Poultry houses should also be treated to ensure insect eradication (see section 2.2.2.7).

Other drugs. Some antibiotics may be used as production enhancers (see section 17.1).

Vaccines. Many vaccines are available to provide protection against poultry viruses, bacteria such as *Erysipelothrix* and *Pasteurella*, and also coccidiosis; these are described under section 18.6.

Game birds

Game birds include grouse, guinea fowl, quail, partridges, and pheasants. Many of the comments in the above section on poultry also relate to game birds. Grouse management is largely left to nature. However, *Trichostrongylus tenuis* and louping ill may cause serious losses and veterinarians may be consulted for advice on worm and tick control and vaccination programmes. The breeding, rearing, and management of pheasants and partridges is now highly specialised and intensive. Although the diseases of game birds are not unique, management practices do have an influence on the occurrence and type of diseases observed in these species. In general, parasitic diseases are common as a result of comparatively large numbers of birds being reared and released on small areas of land over a period of years.

Few medications are authorised for use in game birds, which are classified as food-producing species. Many diseases in these species present with similar clinical signs and full laboratory back up is commonly required in order to diagnose individual conditions. The correct use of medication in game birds is essential especially in regard to withdrawal periods prior to the birds being presented for shooting. To ensure both legal and welfare aspects are adequately covered, veterinary involvement is a necessity.

Drug administration. Drugs may be administered in the drinking water or in the feed when flock medication is necessary, or by intramuscular injection into the posterior aspect of the upper leg for the treatment of individual birds. In the earlier stages of rearing and before release, the birds are fairly easily handled and treated with medication administered in the drinking water or in the feed. However, fluid intake may vary due to weather conditions, unpalatability of the medicated drinking water, or if water is available from other sources such as streams or rainwater.

Feed medication may be impractical where the quantity of feed required is smaller than the usual minimum amount supplied by the mill as a single-mix batch. POM products for incorporation in feed must be prescribed under a Medicated Feeding Stuffs (MFS) prescription.

Antimicrobial therapy. Antimicrobial doses of drugs used in game birds are listed in Table 3. The normal antibacterial course should be 5 days. Infections caused by *E*.

coli, *Salmonella*, and *Staphylococcus* are commonly seen in game birds. *Salmonella* infection usually causes enteric disease, which under stress may lead to septicaemia and this condition has a high mortality rate especially in younger birds. Antibacterials should be given although they will only reduce the degree of infection rather than eliminate it. Neomycin is the drug of choice for enteric salmonellosis, while potentiated sulphonamides are effective for the systemic disease caused by *Salmonella* and colibacillosis. Apramycin, enrofloxacin, and lincomycin/spectinomycin combination can also be used in game birds for these conditions. Probiotics are commonly used in gamebirds to help reduce the incidence of disease and as an adjunct to antibacterial therapy.

Drugs used for the treatment of staphylococcal infections include chlortetracycline for infection within the joints and amoxicillin when the infection causes acute toxaemia. Infections caused by *Pasteurella* and *Erysipelothrix* are fairly common and may lead to high mortality. Acute disease should be treated with tetracycline or amoxicillin in the drinking water. A vaccine is available for pasteurellosis and erysipelas and may be used in pheasants. Vaccination is helpful on farms that have previously been affected by the disease.

Mycoplasma infection is endemic in game birds, particularly pheasants. Various treatment regimens are available. However, treament will control rather than eliminate the disease and therefore management practices, for example the formation of closed breeding flocks, need to be reviewed in order to reduce the incidence of the disease. *Mycoplasma* infection causes respiratory problems in all ages of bird and is characterised by excessive lacrimation and facial oedema. When complicated by secondary bacterial infection (usually *E. coli*) septicaemia is the sequel with subsequent mortality. Poultry respiratory viruses may play a role in the condition in game birds and should be considered by the veterinarian. Breeding birds carrying *Mycoplasma* suffer from poor egg production. The disease is egg transmitted and any suspect birds should be culled and all remaining birds treated before coming into lay to prevent disease and also improve chick quality. Treatment for *Mycoplasma* can be given via the drinking water or by injection; enrofloxacin, tiamulin, or tylosin are used for treatment. Tiamulin must not be given in combination with ionophore anticoccidials, such as monensin, narasin, or salinomycin, because concurrent administration may give rise to toxic effects. Ionophores are zootechnical feed additives and may only be prescribed for guinea fowl.

Coccidiosis is still commonly diagnosed in game birds but the availability of more efficacious coccidiostats has reduced its prevalence. Clopidol and lasalocid are authorised for use in pheasants and partridges.

Table 3 Antimicrobial doses of drugs for game birds[1]

Drug	By addition to drinking water	By addition to feed
Amoxicillin	17 g/100 L 20 mg/kg body-weight	—
Apramycin	25–50 g/100 L 40 mg/kg body-weight	—
Chlortetra-cycline	4–12 g/100 L 30 mg/kg body-weight	200–600 g/tonne
Clopidol	—	125 g/tonne[1] (guinea fowl, partridges, pheasants)
Dimetridazole 400 g/kg	20–40 g/30 litres[1]	200 g/tonne[1]
Enrofloxacin	5–10 g/100 L 10 mg/kg body-weight	—
Lasalocid	—	120 g/tonne[1] (partridges, pheasants)
Lincomycin/spectinomycin	50–150 mg of powder (Linco-Spectin)/kg body-weight	—
Metronidazole	100 g/kg body-weight	
Neomycin	12.6 g/100 L 11 mg/kg body-weight	220 g/tonne
Sulfadiazine with trimethoprim	10.7 g/100 L 30 mg/kg body-weight	—
Sulfaquinoxaline with trimethoprim	28 g/100 L 30 mg/kg body-weight	500 g/tonne
Tetracycline	4–12 g/100 L 30–60 mg/kg body-weight	200–600 g/tonne
Tiamulin	25–30 mg/kg body-weight	300–400 g/tonne
Tylosin	Treatment, 50 g/100 L, 50–200 mg/kg body-weight Prophylaxis.12.5 g/100 L	200 g/tonne

[1]drug doses for preparations that have a marketing authorisation for use in these species in the UK. Therefore unless marked [1], the drug or doses stated are not authorised for these species

A number of species of coccidia may be seen in game birds. They are host specific and no cross infection between the game bird species occurs. The disease tends to occur at about 3 weeks of age or in the release pen and it is often linked to a reduction in the intake of the anticoccidial due to intercurrent disease. Suitable reduction ('step down') anticoccial programmes should be employed to ensure that adequate immunity to infection develops. Toltrazuril or sulfaquinoxaline with trimethoprim administered in the drinking water may be used to treat clinical coccidiosis.

Infection with flagellate parasites such as *Hexamita meleagridis* and *Trichomonas phasioni* may lead to disease characterised by high mortality rate and chronic unthriftiness with severe weight loss. Clinical signs are often seen early in the rearing phase or in the release pen. The disease can be particularly debilitating in red-legged partridges. Dimetridazole in the feed or the water may be given as an aid in the prevention of the disease. Infections are treated with dimetridazole, tetracyclines, or a combination of both agents. Dimetridazole is given in the feed to guinea fowl for prophylaxis against histomoniosis.

The clinical effects of *Blastocystus* are debatable because no invasive forms have been observed. It is possibly a yeast or protozoan which depends on bacteria for its survival. The organism has been seen in birds which have lost weight and some authorities report that it causes earth-brown droppings and mortality. Medication of affected birds with oxytetracycline removes the organism while trimethoprim and dimetridazole may have some effect.

Parasiticidal therapy. The gapeworm, *Syngamus trachea*, affects game birds by causing an obstruction of the trachea characterised by 'gaping' respiration. Differential diagnosis for these clinical signs includes aspergillosis, which affects the air sacs.

Other helminths affecting game birds are the common intestinal roundworms (ascarids) and the much smaller *Capillaria* worm. *Capillaria* affects adult breeding stock causing a delay in onset of laying and reduced egg production. Treatment of helminth infection is based on the use of fenbendazole or flubendazole. Repeated doses may be given every 6 to 8 weeks for prevention of helminth infection. Breeding birds should be treated before commencement of lay to ensure maximum fertility and production. Growing birds are treated before entering the release pen and several weeks later.

Vaccines. Viral diseases seen in game birds include Newcastle disease, which can be a fatal condition in pheasants; authorised vaccines are available (see section 18.6.15). Vaccines for infectious bronchitis and avian rhinotracheitis are not authorised for game birds but may be used on veterinary advice. Rotavirus infection is a major disease in young pheasant chicks and increasingly in partridges; suitable vaccines are not yet available. Hygiene precautions and adequate nursing especially in relation to rehydration of the affected chicks are essential in overcoming and preventing the condition.

Table 4 Parasiticidal doses of drugs for game birds[1]

Drug	Dosage
Fenbendazole[1]	*By addition to feed.* **Partridges, pheasants**: *Syngamus, Heterakis, Ascaridia,* 12 mg/kg as a single dose *Capillaria,* 24 mg/kg in divided doses over 3 days **Grouse**: *Trichostrongylus,* 7–10 mg/kg in divided doses over 14 days
Flubendazole[1]	*By addition to feed.* **Partridges, pheasants**: 60 g/tonne feed for 7–14 days

[1]drug doses for preparations that have a marketing authorisation for use in these species in the UK. Therefore unless marked [1], the drug or doses stated are not authorised for these species

Pigeons

Many breeds and types of pigeons are kept solely for showing and others may be kept for meat production. Racing pigeons are kept for racing and showing. Other flying breeds such as tipplers, tumblers, and rollers, are kept for showing and display flying.

In the UK, few preparations are authorised for use in pigeons; in other European countries many preparations authorised for pigeons are available. Preparations available for other species, particularly poultry, are frequently used. Pigeon owners should be informed and consent obtained when prescribing preparations outwith the data sheet recommendations. It is important that withdrawal periods stated by the manufacturer are adhered to if the preparation is authorised for pigeons and the birds are intended for human consumption. If no withdrawal period is given or the preparation is not authorised for pigeons, standard withdrawal periods should be applied.

Drug administration. Pigeons may be medicated individually or as a group. While clinically ill birds are often treated individually, it is usually necessary to consider the group or the whole loft as a colony. For many infections only a few individuals may appear to be clinically affected but most of the birds in the group are likely to harbour the same infection. Treatment of the entire group is usually essential. Individual medication is therefore often given to sick birds with simultaneous mass medication to the group.

Individual treatment can be given by crop tubing, by injection, or by mouth with tablets, capsules, and liquids. Injections can be given subcutaneously on the back at the base of the neck, with the needle directed posteriorly and in the mid-line to avoid the plexus of vessels in the neck. Intramuscular injections may be given into the breast muscle close to the posterior end of the keel to avoid the major blood vessels in the anterior part of this muscle. Thigh muscle can also be used. However a proportion of the drug may be excreted via the renal portal system before reaching the systemic circulation. Some preparations may cause fibrosis at the site of injection and so could potentially adversely affect racing performance.

Most group medication is given via the drinking water. Drug dosages are commonly calculated on the assumption that a typical pigeon consumes about 50 mL per day but in practice this amount is variable and may range from 15 mL to 250 mL per day. Consumption will be low in cold dull weather, during illness and rest periods, and will increase considerably in hot dry conditions, racing, feeding nestlings, and some clinical conditions involving profuse diarrhoea. Intake may also be reduced by the unpalatability of some mdications. Many pigeons will drink less of any medicated water, particularly on the first day of treatment. Some individual birds appear to almost totally refuse medicated water with subsequent treatment 'failure' which may lead to re-infection of the group by some infections for example *Trichomonas* or *Hexamita* spp. Some drugs are particularly unpalatable and it may be necessary to withhold water for a few hours before offering medicated drinking water.

Pigeons are frequently offered much more water than they drink as the drinking vessels may be emptied and refilled several times each day to ensure water is fresh and not soiled. Pigeons normally drink mainly after feeding and therefore consume the bulk of their daily water intake within a fairly short period, following the main feed. It is therefore essential to accurately assess the amount of water being consumed (rather than the total amount being offered to the group of pigeons) and then use that volume to carry the appropriate amount of medication. In intensive poultry units, stable environmental conditions enable water consumption to be very accurately predicted, so that dosages for many poultry preparations may be given as mg or mL/litre of drinking water rather than mg/kg body-weight. Such dosages may therefore require adjustment when using these preparations for treating pigeons.

Preparations containing tylosin, citric acid, or copper sulphate should not be administered in galvanised water containers. Medicated water must not be disposed of into watercourses, ditches, or drains.

Absorption of many drugs from the digestive tract of pigeons is thought to be relatively poor. Calcium and magnesium contained in bird grit may further reduce the absorption of medicines. Some adjustment of dose may be required when treating systemic conditions.

Insoluble medication may be incorporated into the feed. Pigeons are often selective feeders so that unless medication is actually adherent to the feed grains, it is unlikely to be eaten. The estimated amount of food to be consumed daily is placed in a small container and sprinkled with vegetable oil. The oil is thoroughly mixed into the feed and the appropriate amount of drug in the form of oral powder added and likewise thoroughly mixed. Lemon juice and live unpasturised yoghurt are often used instead of vegetable oil.

The amount of medication consumed by any given individual following group medication is unpredictable. Therefore sick birds should be isolated and medicated individually. When birds are under mass medication via the feed or drinking water, they must be confined to prevent access to external sources, for example rainwater, garden ponds, and bird baths.

Drugs may also be administered topically either as localised treatment or with the intention that they may be absorbed through the skin and act systemically.

Although limited information is available on the toxic effects of drugs in pigeons, in general, drug administration should be avoided during the breeding season (mid-December to April) and periods of feather growth or moult.

Antimicrobial therapy. A variety of antibacterial and antiprotozoal preparations are in wide circulation and use in the pigeon fancy in the UK. Many antibacterial combination preparations are available in other European countries and are imported into the UK by visiting British fanciers. Pigeons treated with these products in their native country and imported into the UK may introduce resistant strains of bacteria and protozoa and also significantly increase the incidence of conditions such as hexamitosis. Consequently, when treating pigeons in the UK, the existence and usage of these products must be taken into account even though their use may not be admitted.

Suitable antibacterials for pigeons include amoxicillin, enrofloxacin, doxycycline, tetracyclines, tylosin, and erythromycin. Tiamulin is used but caution is recommended to avoid toxicity.

Coccidiosis is seen in pigeon flocks and anticoccidials such as amprolium, clazuril, and sulphonamides may be given prophylactically to control infection. Prolonged intermittent or continuous medication may be required for severe coccidiosis. For the treatment and prophylaxis of trichomoniosis (canker) caused by *Trichomonas gallinae* (*T. columbae*), carnidazole, dimetridazole, and metronidazole are used. Dimetridazole has a low safety margin and toxicity will result in CNS signs, incoordination, and death. These drugs are also used for the treatment of hexamitosis, a cause of severe debility and rapid death in young pigeons.

Antimicrobial drug doses for pigeons are given in Table 5. *For the purposes of this table, it is assumed that a cock racing pigeon weighs 500 g and a pigeon drinks 50 mL water per day.*

Parasiticidal therapy. Gastro-intestinal round-worms found in pigeons include *Ascaridia* and *Capillaria* spp. Drugs used for treatment include fenbendazole, febantel, ivermectin, levamisole, or piperazine. Oral levamisole may cause vomiting. Levamisole also gives a bitter taste when added to drinking water. Withholding drinking water for a time before feeding and offering medicated water is usually necessary. Benzimidazoles may cause feather abnormalities if used during feather development in young birds and during the moult. Ivermectin can be given by subcutaneous injection, individual oral dosing, or topically. In severely infected birds, oral levamisole may cause vomiting and medication is best given by injection. Gapeworm infection is rarely reported. Tapeworms may be treated with praziquantel.

Ivermectin is also used to control mites (skin, subcutaneous, quill, feather, nasal, and airsac mites) and lice. Permethrin or pyrethrins are commonly used on birds for control of lice and mites. Loft hygiene is important in the control of internal and external parasites and essential if red mite infestation occurs. Pesticides containing malathion and permethrins can be used on the loft and fittings.

Parasiticide doses for pigeons are listed in Table 6.

Other drugs. Betamethasone 500 micrograms by intramuscular injection as a single dose may be used for ana-phylactic reactions in pigeons. Ophthalmic preparations of chlortetracycline, cloxacillin, fusidic acid, and gentamicin can be used for ocular infections, applied twice daily for up to 7 days. Systemic treatment is recommended for unilateral conjunctivitis ('one-eyed cold'). Levothyroxine can be used to accelerate the moulting out and replacement of damaged feathers. Multivitamins, probiotics, and electrolyte preparations are widely used, particularly after medicinal treatments for prophylaxis and therapy during breeding and racing.

Anaesthetics. Ketamine is used for sedation and light anaesthesia of pigeons at a dose of 50 to 100 mg/kg by intramuscular injection. Recovery after ketamine anaesthesia may be characterised by excitation. Birds should be restrained by wrapping with a cloth and kept in the dark until recovery is complete. Ketamine is also used at 20 to 40 mg/kg in combination with diazepam 1 to 2 mg/kg. Isoflurane administered by mask is the anaesthetic of choice.

Vaccines. Under *The Diseases of Poultry Order 1994* (SI 1994/3141) as amended, all racing pigeons entered for races or shows must be vaccinated against pigeon paramyxovirus (see section 18.6.18). A vaccine against pigeon pox is also available (see section 18.6.19).

Table 5 Antimicrobial doses of drugs for pigeons[1]

Drug	By mouth	By addition to drinking water	By injection
Amoxicillin	40–80 mg/kg twice daily for 5 days	20 mg/kg daily for 3–5 days[1]	30 mg/kg i.m. twice daily for 5 days (formulation to use: long-acting preparation)
Amprolium	—	28 mL (Coxoid)/4.5 litres[1] for 7 days	—
Carnidazole	(adult birds) 10 mg/bird; (young birds) 5 mg/bird[1]	—	—
Cefalexin	50 mg/kg 4 times daily for 5 days (formulation to use: cefalexin 100 mg/mL oral suspension)	—	—
Clazuril	2.5 mg/bird[1]	—	—
Dimetridazole	—	1.2 g/4.5 litres[1] for 7 days	—
Doxycycline	10–20 mg/kg once daily for 3–5 days	15 mg/kg[1] daily for 3–5 days	—
Enrofloxacin	5–20 mg/kg 1–2 times daily for 5–10 days	5–20 mg/kg daily for 5 days *or* 100–200 mg/L for 5 days	10–20 mg/kg s.c. daily for 7–10 days
Erythromycin	—	[2]one 5-mL spoonful powder (Erythrocin Soluble, Ceva) in 2.27 L	—
Itraconazole	26 mg/kg twice daily		
Ketoconazole	30 mg/kg daily for 7 days (formulation to use: ketoconazole 200 mg tablets, crushed and suspended in water)	—	—
Lincomycin/spectinomycin	—	100 mg activity/kg *or* [2]one 5-mL spoonful powder (Linco-Spectin) in 3.4 L	—
Metronidazole	20 mg/kg once daily for 5 days *or* 50 mg/kg on alternate days for 3 treatments	—	—
Nystatin	20 000–100 000 units daily for 7 days	—	—

Table 5 Antimicrobial doses of drugs for pigeons[1] *(continued)*

Drug	By mouth	By addition to drinking water	By injection
Oxytetracycline	—	133–444 mg/L	100 mg/kg i.m. on alternate days
Sulfadimethoxine[1]		1 g/2 litres (40 birds) for 5 days	
Sulfadimidine	—	2 g/L for 3 days. Repeat dose 1–2 times at intervals of 2 days *or* 6 mL/L for 5 days. Repeat after 5 days (formulation to use: sulphadimidine injection 333 mg/mL)	—
Sulfatroxazole with trimethoprim	60 mg for 3 days (formulation to use: 480 mg dispersible tablets)	480 mg/L for 3–5 days	—
Tetracycline	—	[2]one 5-mL spoonful powder (tetracycline 500 mg/g) in 4.55 L	—
Tiamulin	—	250 mg/L for 3–5 days (formulation to use: Tiamutin 12.5% solution	—
Tylosin	100 mg/kg daily for 3 days	500 mg/L for 3–5 days	—

[1] drug doses for preparations that have a marketing authorisation for use in pigeons in the UK. Therefore unless marked [1], the drugs or doses stated are not authorised for this species

[2] 5-mL medical spoonful: a level spoonful is the amount of powder left in the spoon when the top of the heap has been gently scraped off with a straight edge but not packed down

Table 6 Parasiticidal doses of drugs for pigeons[1]

Drug	By mouth	By addition to drinking water	By injection	Topical application
Endoparasiticides				
Febantel	15 mg/bird[1]	—	—	—
Fenbendazole	8 mg/bird[1]	—	—	—
Ivermectin	200 micrograms/kg. May be repeated after 7–10 days	—	200 micrograms/kg s.c., i.m. May be repeated after 7–10 days	—
Levamisole	20 mg/bird, repeat after 3 weeks[1]	1 mL/420 mL (formulation to use: levamisole injection 75 mg/mL)	7.5 mg i.m.	—
Piperazine	—	1.9 g/litre for 30 birds[1]	—	—
Praziquantel	10–20 mg/kg. Repeat in 10–14 days (formulation to use: praziquantel 50 mg tablets, crushed and suspended in water)	0.1 mL/bird s.c. Repeat after 4 weeks (formulation to use: praziquantel injection 56.8 mg/mL)	—	—
Ectoparasiticides				
Benzyl benzoate	—	—	—	Apply benzyl benzoate 25% solution directly to lesions
Ivermectin	—	—	—	Apply one drop ivermectin 0.8% to skin weekly for 3 weeks
Permethrin	—	—	—	Dusting powder[1]
Pyrethrins	—	—	—	Dusting powder, spray[1]

[1] drug doses for preparations that have a marketing authorisation for use in pigeons in the UK. Therefore unless marked [1], the drugs or doses stated are not authorised for this species

Ostriches

Ostriches are farmed for meat, leather, and feathers. In the UK, ostriches are classified as dangerous wild animals under *The Dangerous Wild Animals Act 1976*. Ostriches can be easily stressed. Stock quality, diet, management procedures, and environmental conditions should be considered when investigating a disease problem. In all cases, specific therapy must be related to accurate diagnosis of the primary cause and any secondary (usually bacterial) sequelae.

There are no drugs authorised for ostriches in the UK. Preparations authorised for poultry are not always safe for use in ostriches.

Drug administration. Medication may be administered to ostriches by injection, or via the drinking water or feed. Care must be exercised when approaching a bird to administer treatment. However, in most cases, an adult caught and hooded with a dark hood will be a quiet patient. Intramuscular injection is usually given into the anterior or posterior aspect of the thigh muscles or rump area. Subcutaneous injection is best performed into the loose naked skin over the lower thorax cranial to the mass of the thigh, or at the base of the neck. Intravenous injection is given into the right jugular vein in the caudo-lateral aspect of the neck, or the radial or ulnar veins of the wing; a 19 gauge 2.5 cm angiocath is used for intravenous administration of anaesthetics and fluid therapy in adult birds.

Medication via the drinking water or feed may be unpredictable due to binding of drug to feed ingredients, reduced water or feed intake in sick birds, or apparent unpalatability of some preparations. In particular, young ostriches may not drink medicated water and may die of dehydration.

Routine vaccination, parasiticides, and vitamin therapy should be administered between breeding seasons in adult birds (for example, December in Northern Europe).

Antimicrobial therapy. Routine use of oral antibacterials in ostriches is not recommended because they are likely to lead to changes to intestinal flora especially the caecal bacteria which play a vital role in the reduction and digestion of vegetable matter. Following antibacterial therapy, probiotics are used to encourage normal flora development within the gut.

Infectious conditions involving *E. coli*, and other Gram-negative organisms can be treated with amoxicillin or potentiated amoxicillin. Amoxicillin with clavulanic acid administered by injection is the drug of choice if bacterial involvement in a disease process in any age of bird is suspected; usually a 5-day course is administered. Amoxicillin with clavulanic acid has been given by intramuscular injection to newly hatched ostriches where a significant bacterial challenge is expected. The use of other antimicrobials such as enrofloxacin is only justified on bacterial culture and sensitivity testing. Antibacterials are administered as an adjunct to treatment in birds that have aspergillosis and air sacculitis. In outbreaks of diarrhoea, samples should be taken and the causal agent determined. Cloacal swabs may be examined for the presence of *Cryptosporidia* spp. and other pathogenic protozoa for example *Ballantidium* spp. Virology may also be performed but as yet the role of enteric viruses in ostrich diseases is unclear.

Antibacterial over-usage may result in gastric and bowel mycoses. Certain antibacterials are recognised as toxic in ostriches and their use is not to be recommended. These include lincomycin, furazolidine and streptomycin.

Table 7 Antimicrobial doses of drugs for ostriches[1]

Drug	Dose
Amoxicillin	by addition to drinking water, 20 mg/kg daily
Amoxicillin with clavulanic acid	7–14 mg/kg i.m. daily
Copper sulphate	trichomoniosis, by addition to drinking water, 500–750 mg/L *or* by addition to feed, 1 g/kg feed
Dimetridazole	trichomoniosis, by addition to feed, 200–500 mg/kg feed (up to 3 months of age)
Enilconazole	by nebulisation, see notes above
Enrofloxacin	10–20 mg/kg i.m. daily
Ketoconazole	8 mg/kg p.o. twice daily for 30 days. 10–20 mg/kg p.o. once daily (May be crushed and reconstituted in orange or pineapple juice for smaller birds)
Nystatin	330 000 units/kg p.o. daily

[1] drug doses for preparations that have a marketing authorisation for use in ostriches in the UK. Therefore unless marked [1], the drugs or doses stated are not authorised for this species

Dimetridazole can be used for the control of trichomoniosis in ostrich chicks less then 3 months of age and copper sulphate can also be used. Some problems with palatability of the final ration have been observed. Sulfaquinoxaline has been successfully used in water to treat protozoal infections in 5 to 6 month old ostriches. Sulfadimethoxine have been used but is reported to be unpalatable. Coccidiosis is currently not a problem in ostriches in the UK. Ionophore coccidiostats can be toxic in ostriches.

Aspergillosis is a particular problem in ostriches kept in poorly ventilated or dusty environments. It can be differentiated from *E. coli* air sacculitis or *Pasturellosis* using serology. The site of the lesions of aspergillosis (air sac membranes) are often poorly vascularised and can extend into the femur bones and some of the spinal vertebrae. Treatment should be considered for high value birds. Therapy is intensive and involves oral and aerosol administration of antifungal agents. Ketoconazole is given orally. Enilconazole is administered by inhalation of an aerosol in a small sealed room such as sealed loose box. The drug solution is first diluted to 1:10 in sterile or potable water at 22 to 30°C. The fogging machine should produce a mist of fine particles of 5 to 20 microns to ensure efficient distribution of the drug into the airways. The bird should be placed in the room which is then completely filled with the mist and left closed for half an hour. The concentration of the mist should be maintained throughout this period. Fogging should be performed twice daily for five days then twice weekly for five weeks. The procedure is well tolerated but the birds should be constantly supervised and contingency plans made should release of the bird be necessary.

Candidiasis of the digestive tract is usually a result of antibacterial over-usage. Oral administration of nystatin or ketoconazole may be effective. Supportive therapy with vitamins is also indicated. Oxytetracycline spray is used for spraying navels of hatchlings and superficial wounds. Careful observation of the birds should be made to ensure the colour of the spray does not attract other birds to the treated site and encourage pecking.

Ostriches rely greatly on their eyesight. The eye is large and vulnerable to infections and traumatic damage. Eye infections are very painful and damaged eyes will affect the performance of the bird. Eyes must be thoroughly examined under local anaesthesia for corneal ulceration, conjunctivitis, and granuloma formation (for example in avian tuberculosis). Topical antimicrobial creams containing cefalonium or cloxacillin have been used for corneal ulceration and conjunctivitis and are applied daily.

Parasiticidal therapy. As intensification occurs within the European ostrich industry, ticks, lice, mites and endoparasites will probably become a major problem. These parasites may spread viral ostrich diseases for example, in South Africa, the zoonotic viral disease Crimean-Congo haemorrhagic fever is found in about 1% of ticks.

Infestations of the ostrich louse, *Struthiolipeurus struthionis* and the quill mite *Gabucinia* spp. are common. Cypermethrin or amitraz is used for treatment. **Lindane is extremely toxic in ostriches and should not be used**. All ectoparasitic treatment should be repeated after 10 days and the housing may need fumigation or the application of an environmental ectoparasiticide.

Currently endoparasites do not appear to be a problem in ostriches because the birds have not been established in Northern Europe for sufficient time. The ostrich tapeworm *Houttuynia struthionis* is abundant in South Africa where it causes unthriftiness in chicks. It has been seen in imported birds in Northern Europe but it is uncertain as to whether an intermediate host exists for the worm to complete its life cycle. It is treated effectively with fenbendazole, praziquantal, oxfendazole, or niclosamide.

The wireworm *Libostrongylus douglassi* is a strongyle worm of ostriches. The later larval stages and adults live in the glandular crypts of the proventriculus causing local inflammation and reduction of digestive secretions. This lack of secretions causes decay of food in the proventriculus and rotting of the stomach contents ('vrotmaag'). The eggs can survive in the faeces for one year and infective third stage larvae develop into adults in 29 days. Effective anthelmintics include levamisole, ivermectin, fenbendazole and oxfendazole.

Table 8 Parasiticidal doses of drugs for ostriches[1]

Drug	Dose
Endoparasiticides	
Fenbendazole	15–45 mg/kg p.o.
Ivermectin	200 micrograms/kg p.o. (formulation to use: ivermectin oral solution 800 micrograms/mL) 300 micrograms/kg s.c.
Levamisole	7.5 mg/kg p.o. (formulation to use: levamisole oral solution 15 mg/mL) 7.5 mg/kg s.c.
Niclosamide	100 mg/kg p.o.
Oxfendazole	5 mg/kg p.o.
Praziquantel	7.5 mg/kg p.o.
Ectoparasiticides	
Amitraz (12.5%)	by spraying, dilute 1 volume in 500 volumes water = 0.025% solution and use 2.5 L/bird
Cypermethrin (5%)	by spraying, dilute 1 volume in 100 volumes = 0.05% solution
Ivermectin	quill mites, 300 micrograms/kg s.c.

[1] drug doses for preparations that have a marketing authorisation for use in ostriches in the UK. Therefore unless marked [1], the drugs or doses stated are not authorised for this species

Other worms found in ratites include *Codiostromum struthionis*, a caecal strongyle that does not appear to have major clinical significance, and the large ostrich guinea worm *Dicheilonema specularum* which lives under the subperitoneal connective tissue and can grow up to 2.1 metres long and 12 cm diameter.

Syngamus trachea has been found causing haemorrhagic tracheitis in emus.

For worming prophylaxis in Northern Europe levamisole should be given at 6 months of age, followed by ivermectin by injection at 12 months, 24 months, and in adult breeders. If a significant worm burden exists, levamisole should be given at 3 and 6 months of age, followed by fenbendazole at 9 months of age. At 12 months of age ivermectin by injection is administered, followed by levamisole at 18 months. Then ivermectin by injection is given at 24 months and in adult breeders.

Birds should be vaccinated against clostridial diseases before treatment with praziquantel. **Morantel, tiabendazole and mebendazole have been reported as being toxic in ostriches**.

Other drugs. If nutritional deficiencies are suspected then a change of diet to that produced by a different manufacturer could be considered. Myopathies are a recognised problem in ostriches. A degenerative myopathy is seen in young birds less than 6 months old. Capture myopathy is seen commonly in stressed older stock and this may be an acute manifestation of a more chronic sub-clinical deficiency of selenium or vitamin E caused for example by a diet high in polyunsaturated fats that are undergoing oxidation. Injectable vitamin E and selenium preparations can be used to treat deficiencies, non-specific lameness conditions, and poor performance animals. Care should be taken because over dosage of selenium can result in intoxication.

Preparations containing B group vitamins, iron and other elements for parenteral injection are indicated for supportive therapy in birds with proventricular, gastric or gut stasis, anaemia, and parasitism. B group vitamins can also be used supportively to encourage appetite in sick birds. In breeders producing large numbers of eggs, problems of embryonic abnormalities from vitamin B deficiencies can occur. For example thiamine deficiency can cause polyneuritis, riboflavin deficiencies cause clubbed down, and folic acid deficiency can cause parrot beak and mandibular defects. B group vitamin deficiencies can also cause late embryonic death, low hatchability and weak chicks at hatch. Vitamin B therapy is indicated if deficiencies are diagnosed.

Pantothenic acid and biotin deficiency can occur if unbalanced high cereal diets are fed. Calcium pantothenate can be added to the feed at a rate of 5mg/kg. Alternatively parenteral products such as Haemo 15 (Arnolds) may be administered.

Multivitamin preparations have been used in the prevention and treatment of vitamin deficiencies during periods of illness, convalescence, stress, and ill thrift. Deficiencies of vitamins A, D and E can cause low egg production, low egg hatchability and embryonic death. The prophylactic use of a product such as Duphafral ADE Forte (Fort Dodge) is advised in breeding adults between the seasons and also in treatment of A, D and E deficiency.

Vitamin K has been used to treat rodenticide poisoning.

Corticosteriods are contra-indicated in ostriches because they damage the gonads. Flunixin is used in cases of shock, hyperthermic myopathy, 'downer ostrich', and in stressed birds. Ostriches appear to have a low pain threshold for joint or bowel pain for which flunixin is appropriate. Furosemide is used for the treatment of localised swelling and oedema of allergic, toxic, traumatic, or inflammatory conditions.

Levamisole can be used as an immunostimulant in debilitated birds.

Rehydration solutions are used in chicks from 4 days up to 28 days of age that are not gaining weight. Solutions are reconstituted as directed by the manufacturer and given by stomach tube at a rate of 5 to 10 mL/kg 2 to 4 times daily. Oral levothyroxine can be used in slow growing chicks less than 60 days of age.

Table 9 Doses of other drugs for ostriches[1]

Drug	Dose
Flunixin	1.5 mg/kg i.m. daily for 3 days
Furosemide	0.5–1.0 mg/kg i.m. 1–2 times daily
Levamisole	immunestimulation, 2.5 mg/kg s.c.
Levothyroxine	(<60 days of age), 100 micrograms/bird p.o. twice weekly
Multivitamins	Duphafral ADE Forte , 1 mL/40 kg i.m. Haemo 15 , 1 mL/15 kg i.m. weekly Multivitamin (Arnolds), 1 mL/6 kg i.m.
Vitamins and minerals	Dystosel, prophylaxis 1 mL/40 kg (outwith the breeding season); treatment 1 mL/25 kg i.m. Vitatrace 1mL/15 kg
Vitamin K	5 mg/kg i.m. daily for several days

[1] drug doses for preparations that have a marketing authorisation for use in ostriches in the UK. Therefore unless marked [1], the drugs or doses stated are not authorised for this species

Straw and vegetable matter proventricular impactions may be treated medically. Initially the degree of impaction should be assessed by abdominal palpation. A mixture of liquid paraffin (5 mL/kg) and vegetable oil (2.5 mL/kg) is given by stomach tube twice daily. In addition, a mixture of rumenal extract such as Vetrumex (Fort Dodge) at 1 g/kg and concentrate ration at 20 g/kg at body temperature is given twice daily. Vitatrace (Vétoquinol) is given on alternate days for up to 3 doses. Treatment is administered according to the patient's response and at each treatment the impacted mass should be massaged and broken up through the abdominal wall. Affected birds may be debilitated and require additional heat and light.

Non-organic impactions such as grit, sand, and foreign bodies may require surgical intervention. Small particulate foreign bodies may be removed by high pressure proventricular lavage. Bowel impactions occur in ostriches especially in birds less than 6 months of age. The aetiology of impaction is complex.

Anaesthetics. Ostriches appear to have a high pain threshold for skin and the amount of anaesthetic required is low for performing local anaesthesia.

Before sedating or anaesthetising an ostrich, consideration should be given to the provision of quiet surroundings, efficient dark hood, adequate manual assistance, and intravenous fluid therapy.

Injectable and inhalational anaesthetics have all been successfully used in ostriches. Ketamine should not be used as a sole anaesthetic agent. Azaperone is the drug of choice for sedation. If sedated birds are transported, they should be individually penned and be well supervised.

The method of choice for anaesthetising young handleable birds is to use an inhalational agent without premedication. A rapid response is seen with isoflurane but with halothane there is a lag phase of 2 to 5 minutes before changes in the gaseous anaesthetic concentration are reflected in the patient's response. Without premedication, some struggling is observed on induction with more objection to halothane than isoflurane being noted. Masking for induction is followed by intubation.

Larger birds are sedated with azaperone. As the azaperone takes effect, the bird may become unsteady on its feet at which point thiopental is administered according to the patient's response. Approximately 15 to 20 minutes of surgical anaesthesia time is obtained. Incremental doses of thiopental may be safely given but recovery will be protracted. For long procedures inhalational anaesthesia is preferred for maintenance.

Following anaesthesia, the patient should recover under constant supervision in a padded loose box with the bird hooded and the head and neck elevated.

Table 10 Sedative and anaesthetic doses of drugs for ostriches[1]

Drug	Dose
Sedatives and injectable anaesthetics	
Azaperone	sedation 1–4 mg/kg i.m. anaesthetic pre-medication, 1 mg/kg i.v.
Diazepam + Ketamine	250 micrograms/kg i.v. + 2–5 mg/kg i.v. according to the patient's response
Etorphine/ acepromazine	1 mL/50 kg i.m. Reversal: diprenorphine 2 mg/50 kg i.v.
Fentanyl/ droperidol	1 mL/9 kg i.m. Reversal: naloxone 400 micrograms/ 9 kg i.v.
Medetomidine	(< 15 kg body-weight) 15–20 mg/kg i.m.
Medetomidine + Azaperone	(< 15 kg body-weight)10–20 mg/kg i.m. + 3.3–6.6 mg/kg i.m.
Thiopental	0.5–1.0 g/90 kg i.v.
Tiletamine/ zolazepam	2–10 mg/kg i.m. 2–8 mg/kg i.v.
Xylazine + Ketamine	adults, 1 mg/kg i.m + 5 mg/kg i.m.
Xylazine + Ketamine	5–10 mg/kg i.m. + 2–3 mg/kg i.v. according to the patient's response
Xylazine + Ketamine	250 micrograms/kg i.v. + 2–5 mg/kg i.v. according to the patient's response
Inhalational anaesthetics	
Halothane	(with pre-anaesthetic medication) 1–4% (without pre-anaesthetic medication) 3–5%
Isoflurane	(with pre-anaesthetic medication) 0.5–4.0% (usually 1.5–2%) (without pre-anaesthetic medication) 3–5%

[1] drug doses for preparations that have a marketing authorisation for use in ostriches in the UK. Therefore unless marked [1], the drugs or doses stated are not authorised for this species

Vaccines. Ostriches are thought to have a poorly developed immune system and the protective response to vaccination has not been assessed. It is advisable that ostriches are vaccinated against Newcastle disease and clostridial diseases caused by *Clostridium perfringens* types A, B, and D. For protection against clostridial infections, 2 doses of 1 mL of vaccine effective against *Clostridium perfringens* types A, B, and D are given by subcutaneous injection at 7 and 28 days of age. Booster vaccinations are given every 3 months until 12 months of age. Then a twice yearly booster should be given.

Ostriches, especially those less than 6 months of age, are susceptible to Newcastle disease. Both living and inactivated Clone 30 vaccines are used. The live vaccine should be reconstituted to give *a dilution 5 times more concentrated than the poultry dilution*. One drop of this vaccine should be placed into each eye. Alternatively the vaccine should be reconstituted at the poultry dilution and 5 drops of the vaccine placed in each nostril. Birds over 5 months of age need to be hooded making the intranasal vaccination the method of choice. The inactivated vaccine is given by subcutaneous injection.

The vaccine protocol followed depends on the antibody status of the parent bird. If maternal antibody is present in chicks, birds are vaccinated with 3 mL inactivated Clone 30 at 45 days, 70 days, and 6 months of age, and 5 mL at 12 months and then annually. Living Clone 30 may also be given at 45 days of age. If no maternal antibody is present in chicks, birds are given additional vaccinations at 2 weeks of age (living Clone 30 and 0.5 mL inactivated Clone 30) and at 1 month of age (1 mL inactivated Clone 30). If a high risk situation exists, vaccination can be given to day-old chicks.

Prescribing for laboratory animals

Contributor:
P A Flecknell MA, VetMB, PhD, DLAS, DipECVA, MRCVS

Animals used in research include guinea pigs, mice, rats and other small rodents, rabbits, primates, dogs, cats, farm animals, and a range of less familiar species such as amphibians, reptiles, fish, and some invertebrates.

Vertebrates used in research are protected under the *Animals (Scientific Procedures) Act 1986* along with certain invertebrates such as the common octopus *Octopus vulgaris*. All premises registered under the Act must employ a 'named veterinary surgeon' to advise on the health and welfare of all laboratory animals. The animals are under the care of the named veterinary surgeon and it is appropriate that he or she should take responsibility for prescribing all required medication and formulating preventive health control programmes.

Before giving any medication, it is necessary to determine whether the animals are being or will be used for any experimental procedures. If so, the proposed therapy should be discussed with the Animal Care and Welfare Officer, the personal licensee, and the project licence holder. The personal licensee carries out the experiment described in the project licence and is the person immediately responsible for the welfare of the animals. The project licence holder is required to justify the use of the animals and to provide an assurance that no suitable *in vitro* techniques, which would avoid the need to use live animals, are available.

When determining a therapeutic regimen, the welfare of the animals concerned must be the most important consideration. In many instances it will be found that treatment cannot be undertaken, as it could influence the results of the proposed or current study, and in these circumstances it may be necessary to kill the animals humanely. Although treatment may interfere with an experiment, this should not be a total contra-indication for the use of medication. When withholding treatment would compromise the welfare of the animals, for example, when deciding whether to administer analgesics, special care must be taken to ensure that a specific scientific justification is provided if treatment is to be withheld. If the veterinary surgeon is still uncertain as to the correct action to be taken the Home Office Inspectorate may be consulted.

Treatment may require medication of an individual animal or mass medication. Drugs may be administered to groups of animals via the feed or drinking water. Antibacterials administered in the drinking water may be ineffective due to reduction in water consumption as a consequence of the disease process or unpalatability of medicated water. It is preferable, although very labour intensive, to administer preparations by injection or gavage to each individual animal.

Although the majority of preparations that have a veterinary marketing authorisation have not been approved for use in some of these species, most products authorised for human use will have been administered to laboratory animals previously in order to assess drug safety and efficacy. Therefore information may be obtained from scientific literature or pharmaceutical companies. In addition see Prescribing for fish, Prescribing for rabbits and rodents, Prescribing for invertebrates, Appendix 4 Dosage estimation, and chapters 1 to 17 for specific drug dosage regimens.

Prescribing for rabbits and rodents

Contributor:
P A Flecknell MA, VetMB, PhD, DLAS, DipECVA, MRCVS

In this section, prescribing for gerbils, guinea pigs, hamsters, mice, rabbits, and rats is discussed. These animals are kept as pets, exhibited, used for research, and rabbits may also be bred for meat or fur production. There is growing concern that pet rabbits are often kept in isolated conditions with poor housing and this may have an effect on the disorders seen in these animals.

Drug administration. Administration of medication to these species may be by mouth or by injection. Before treatment, animals should be accurately weighed in order to determine the correct dose of a drug. Many drug preparations will have to be diluted to obtain the required dose in a volume that can be administered accurately. Some drugs are not water soluble and may require dilution in other solvents. These species will often more readily accept oral medication if either palatable veterinary preparations or human paediatric sugar-based formulations are used. Medication may also be incorporated into highly palatable foods or cubes of fruit-flavoured jelly. The jelly should be reconstituted in half the recommended quantity of water, allowed to cool and the drug then added. Sucrose may be added to the drinking water to increase palatability (50 g/litre drinking water).

Antimicrobial therapy. The use of antimicrobial drugs in rabbits, guinea pigs, and hamsters is associated with a high incidence of undesirable side-effects. Clindamycin, lincomycin, erythromycin, and narrow-spectrum penicillins can produce fatal adverse reactions through an effect on gastro-intestinal micro-organisms. Cephalosporins can also be toxic in hamsters and guinea pigs, and oral tetracyclines may cause gastro-intestinal disturbance and death in guinea pigs. Alteration of the normal bacterial flora in the intestine results in proliferation of organisms such as *Clostridium* spp. and the production of an often fatal enterotoxaemia. When administering antibacterials to rabbits and guinea pigs, it may be advisable to provide a vitamin B and Vitamin K supplement (such as Ⓗ Abidec, Warner-Lambert) and lactobacilli (live yoghurt) and to continue this for five days after completion of therapy. If a rabbit develops diarrhoea during antibacterial therapy, or is presented with clinical signs of enterotoxaemia, treatment with colestyramine may be of value. In all species, if diarrhoea develops during antibacterial administration, drug treatment should be discontinued. Rats and mice appear much less susceptible to disturbances to the gastro-intestinal tract, but antibacterials such as streptomycin and dihydrostreptomycin have been reported to have a toxic effect in these species, causing flaccid paralysis, coma, respiratory arrest, and death. Griseofulvin should be used with caution in guinea pigs because the drug is derived from *Penicillium* cultures. The usual antibacterial course is 5 to 7 days.

The most common bacterial infections in rabbits and rodents are respiratory tract infections, gastro-intestinal tract disease, and subcutaneous abscesses caused by fight wounds or other injuries. Respiratory infection in rabbits is normally caused by *Pasteurella multocida*, and a remission of disease signs can usually be obtained using cefalexin or sulfadiazine with trimethoprim. Recurrence of infection is however common, even following prolonged periods of therapy of 10 to 21 days. Ocular involvement is frequently associated with naso-lacrimal blockage; flushing of the duct with either saline or antibacterial solutions may be beneficial. Pneumonia in guinea pigs caused by *Bordetella bronchiseptica* can be treated using enrofloxacin, provided therapy is commenced early in the course of the disease. Respiratory infection in rats and mice may involve infection by *Mycoplasma pulmonis*, and in the rat this may be treated using oxytetracycline or enrofloxacin, given by injection. Cephalosporins are also useful in treating respiratory diseases in rats and mice, but affected animals frequently develop chronic lung lesions, which can rarely be treated successfully.

Antibacterials are of limited value in the treatment of gastro-intestinal disturbances in rabbits and guinea pigs, and most emphasis should be given to maintaining fluid balance using both oral fluids (see section 16.1.1) and parenteral fluid therapy, for example, using Hartmann's solution, administered by intravenous, intraperitoneal, or subcutaneous injection. When treating diarrhoea in hamsters ('wet tail'), fluid therapy is of major importance, but neomycin given by mouth, may also be of value.

Subcutaneous abscesses are seen quite frequently, especially in rabbits and guinea pigs. These abscesses usually require surgical drainage and lavage with a wound cleansing preparation. Systemic antibacterial therapy should also be instituted. Treatment at an early stage of abscess development is usually successful, but if the lesion has become extensive, repeated drainage may be required.

Parasiticide therapy. Parenteral and topical ectoparasiticides may be used for the treatment of mites in rabbits and rodents. The safety and efficacy in rabbits and rodents of many products currently available is uncertain, and the most widely used therapy for ectoparasitic infection is ivermectin. Ear mites, *Psoroptes cuniculi*, in rabbits can be treated either with topical acaricides or by subcutaneous administration of ivermectin. Surface-living mites, for example, *Cheyletiella* and *Myobia* may be treated using permethrin-containing dusting powders. Treatment may need to be repeated on several occasions at 10 to 21 day intervals. Sarcoptic mange in guinea pigs is caused by *Trixacarus caviae* infection. The treatment of choice is ivermectin. Treatment of both affected and clinically normal in-contact animals may be required at 7 to 10 day intervals for six weeks. For all ectoparasitic infestations, the caging should be thoroughly cleaned.

Treatment of endoparasites, such as *Syphacia obvelata* the mouse pinworm, may be required. Ivermectin is effective and when treating large groups of animals it is most conveniently administered in the feed or drinking water. If necessary, treatment can be repeated after 2 to 3 weeks. Ivermectin has been reported to be effective in a range of small mammals, and the very wide range of dosages used suggests that this drug is generally safe for these species. Adverse reactions associated with high mortality have been noted in C57/BL6 mice and related strains, indicating the need for caution before treating large numbers of animals. For specific parasiticide doses and dosage regimens, see Table 12.

Anaesthetics. Many anaesthetics and analgesics are used in rabbits and rodents. A drug may be used alone or in combination, and specific drug regimens are given in Table 13. All of the commonly used volatile anaesthetics such as halothane, enflurane, and isoflurane can be used to provide safe and effective anaesthesia in rabbits and rodents. Ether is irritant to mucous membranes, inflammable, and explosive and should not be used. Volatile anaesthetics are generally recommended as the most suitable means of anaesthetising small rodents, because the depth of anaesthesia can be altered and both induction and recovery are generally rapid. Induction of anaesthesia with inhalational agents in rabbits is not recommended unless the animal has been heavily sedated. Safe inspired concentrations of volatile anaesthetics are similar to those used in dogs and cats. If injectable agents are used, then fentanyl/fluanisone + midazolam, or ketamine + medetomidine, or ketamine + xylazine are recommended. All of these combinations cause mild or moderate respiratory depression, and if possible, oxygen should be administered during anaesthesia. Respiratory depression can be reduced following surgery by partial reversal of fentanyl/fluanisone anaesthesia with butorphanol, buprenorphine or nalbuphine. Atipamezole should be administered to reverse medetomidine or xylazine if these have been used in combination with ketamine. If post-operative pain is present an analgesic such as buprenorphine or carprofen should be administered.

Rabbits and small rodents may be in poor clinical condition when presented for anaesthesia, especially those requiring dental treatment. These animals may be significantly dehydrated, and if a fluid deficit is considered likely, then replacement therapy before inducing anaesthesia may be of significant benefit. In small rodents, warmed fluid, (for example sodium chloride 0.18% + glucose 4% or Hartmann's solution) can be given by intraperitoneal or subcutaneous routes and this will be absorbed in 8 to 12 hours. In rabbits, fluid therapy may be administered intravenously via a catheter (20 to 22 gauge) placed in the ear vein. Placement of the catheter is facilitated by applying local anaesthetic cream (Ⓗ Emla, Astra) to the ear. The cream is covered with cling-film and an outer layer of self-adhesive bandage. After 45 to 60 minutes, the dressing is removed, the ear cleaned, and venepuncture undertaken.

Other drugs. Authorised preparations of buserelin are available for the induction of postpartum ovulation in rabbits (see section 8.1.2). A number of other drugs are reported to be of value in these species and dosages are listed in Table 14.

Vaccines. Rabbits may be vaccinated against infectious myxomatosis and viral haemorrhagic disease (see section 18.7).

Table 11 Antimicrobial doses of drugs for rabbits and rodents[1]

Drug	Gerbil	Guinea pig	Hamster	Mouse	Rabbit	Rat
Amoxicillin	—	—	—	100 mg/kg s.c. once daily	—	150 mg/kg i.m. once daily
Ampicillin	—	—	—	150 mg/kg s.c. twice daily		150 mg/kg s.c. twice daily
Benzyl-penicillin	—	—	—	60 mg/kg i.m. twice daily	—	12 mg/kg p.o. once daily (formulation to use: injection, powder for recon-stitution)
Cefalexin	25 mg/kg i.m. once daily	15 mg/kg i.m. twice daily	—	60 mg/kg p.o. daily in 3 divided doses 30 mg/kg i.m. once daily	15 mg/kg s.c. twice daily	60 mg/kg p.o. daily in 3 divided doses 15 mg/kg s.c. once daily
Chloram-phenicol	30 mg/kg i.m. once daily	50 mg/kg p.o. 3 times daily 20 mg/kg i.m. twice daily	30 mg/kg s.c. twice daily	200 mg/kg p.o. 3 times daily 50 mg/kg s.c. twice daily	50 mg/kg p.o. once daily 15 mg/kg i.m. twice daily	20–50 mg/kg p.o. twice daily 10 mg/kg i.m. twice daily
Chlortetra-cycline	—	—	—	—	1 g/L drinking water	—
Clopidol	—	—	—	—	200 g/tonne feed[1]	—
Enrofloxacin	50–100 mg/L drinking water 5 mg/kg p.o., s.c. twice daily[1]	50–100 mg/L drinking water 5 mg/kg p.o., s.c. twice daily[1]	50–100 mg/L drinking water 5 mg/kg p.o., s.c. twice daily[1]	50–100 mg/L drinking water 5 mg/kg p.o., s.c. twice daily[1]	50–100 mg/L drinking water 5 mg/kg p.o., s.c. twice daily[1]	50–100 mg/L drinking water 5 mg/kg p.o., s.c. twice daily[1]
Gentamicin	5 mg/kg i.m. once daily	5–8 mg/kg s.c. once daily	2–4 mg/kg s.c. twice daily	5 mg/kg i.m. once daily	4 mg/kg i.m. once daily	4.4 mg/kg i.m. twice daily
Griseofulvin	15–25 mg/kg p.o. once daily for 3 weeks	25 mg/kg p.o. once daily for 2 weeks 800 micro-grams/kg feed	25–30 mg/kg p.o. once daily for 3 weeks	25 mg/kg p.o. once daily for 2 weeks	25 mg/kg p.o. once daily for 4 weeks	25 mg/kg p.o. once daily for 2 weeks
Neomycin	100 mg/kg p.o. daily in divided doses	5 mg/kg p.o. twice daily	250 mg/kg p.o. daily in divided doses	2.5 g/L drinking water	200–800 mg/L drinking water	2 g/L drinking water
Oxytetracycline	5 g/L drinking water 20 mg/kg s.c. once daily	—	5 g/L drinking water 20 mg/kg s.c. once daily	400 mg/L drinking water 10 mg/kg s.c. twice daily	30 mg/kg p.o. twice daily 15 mg/kg i.m. twice daily	800 mg/L drinking water 10 mg/kg s.c. twice daily
Robenidine	—	—	—	—	50–66 g/tonne feed[1]	—
Streptomycin	—	—	25 mg/kg s.c. once daily	—	50 mg/kg i.m. once daily	—
Sulfadiazine with trimethoprim	—	120 mg/kg s.c. once daily	48 mg/kg s.c.once daily	—	48 mg/kg s.c. once daily	120 mg/kg s.c. once daily
Sulfadimidine	—	20 g/L drinking water	—	500 mg/L drinking water	100–233 mg/L drinking water	200 mg/L drinking water

Table 11 Antimicrobial doses of drugs for rabbits and rodents[1] *(continued)*

Drug	Gerbil	Guinea pig	Hamster	Mouse	Rabbit	Rat
Tetracycline	20 mg/kg p.o. twice daily	—	10 mg/kg p.o. once daily	500 mg/L drinking water	30 mg/kg p.o. twice daily	15–20 mg/kg p.o. twice daily
Tylosin	10 mg/kg s.c. once daily	—	500 mg/L drinking water 10 mg/kg s.c. once daily	10 mg/kg p.o., s.c.	—	10 mg/kg i.m. once daily

[1] drug doses for preparations that have a marketing authorisation for use in these species in the UK. Therefore, unless marked [1], the drug or doses stated are not authorised for these species

Table 12 Parasiticidal doses of drugs for rabbits and rodents[1]

Drug	Gerbil	Guinea pig	Hamster	Mouse	Rabbit	Rat
Endoparasiticides						
Ivermectin	200–400 micrograms/kg s.c.	200–500 micrograms/kg s.c. 500 micrograms p.o.	200–400 micrograms/kg s.c.	200–400 micrograms/kg s.c.	200–400 micrograms/kg s.c. 400 micrograms p.o.	200–400 micrograms/kg s.c.
Piperazine	5 g/L drinking water for 7 days	3 g/L drinking water for 7 days	10 g/L drinking water for 7 days	5 g/L drinking water for 7 days	500 micrograms/kg p.o., repeat after 10 days	2 g/L drinking water for 7 days
Ectoparasiticides						
Ivermectin			— as above for all species—			
Permethrin			— dusting powder —			

[1] drug doses for preparations that have a marketing authorisation for use in these species in the UK. Therefore, unless marked [1], the drug or doses stated are not authorised for these species

Table 13 Doses of analgesics and anaesthetics for rabbits and rodents[1]

Drug	Gerbil	Guinea pig	Hamster	Mouse	Rabbit	Rat
Acepromazine	2.5 mg/kg i.m., i.p.	2.5 mg/kg i.m.	2.5 mg/kg i.m., i.p.	2.5 mg/kg i.m.	1 mg/kg i.m.	2.5 mg/kg i.m., i.p.
Alfaxalone/ alfadolone	—	40 mg/kg i.p.	—	10 mg–15 mg/kg i.v.	6–9 mg/kg i.v.	10–12 mg/kg i.v.
Atipamezole	1 mg/kg s.c., i.m., i.p., i.v	1 mg/kg s.c., i.m., i.p., i.v	1 mg/kg s.c., i.m., i.p., i.v	1 mg/kg s.c., i.m., i.p., i.v	1 mg/kg s.c., i.m., i.p., i.v	1 mg/kg s.c., i.m., i.p., i.v
Atropine	40 micrograms/kg s.c., i.m.	50 micro-grams/kg s.c., i.m.	40 micrograms/ kg s.c., i.m.	40 micrograms/ kg s.c., i.m.	50 micrograms/ kg s.c., i.m.	40 micrograms/kg s.c., i.m.
Buprenorphine	100 micrograms/ kg s.c.	50 micro-grams/kg s.c.	100 micrograms/ kg s.c.	100 micrograms/ kg s.c.	50 micrograms/ kg s.c., i.v.	50 micrograms/kg s.c.
Butorphanol	—	2 mg/kg s.c.	—	1–5 mg/kg s.c.	100–500 micro-grams/kg s.c., i.v.	2 mg/kg s.c.
Carprofen	—	—	—	—	1.5 mg/kg p.o. twice daily	5 mg/kg s.c. twice daily
Diazepam	5 mg/kg i.p.	2.5 mg/kg i.m., i.p.	5 mg/kg i.p.	5 mg/kg i.m., i.p.	1–2 mg/kg i.m., i.v.	2.5 mg/kg i.p.
Doxapram	5–10 mg/kg i.v.	5–10 mg/kg i.v.	5–10 mg/kg i.v.	5–10 mg/kg i.v.	5–10 mg/kg i.v.	5–10 mg/kg i.v.
Fentanyl citrate/ fluanisone	0.5–1.0 mL/kg i.m.	0.5 mL/kg i.m.[1]	0.5 mL/kg i.m., i.p.	0.5 mL/kg i.m.[1]	0.5 mL/kg i.m.[1]	0.5 mL/kg i.m.[1]
Fentanyl citrate/ fluanisone + diazepam	0.3 mL/kg + 5 mg/kg i.p.	1 mL/kg i.m. + 2.5 mg/kg i.p.	1 mL/kg + 5 mg/kg i.p.	0.3 mL/kg i.p. + 5 mg/kg i.p.	0.3 mL/kg i.m. + 2 mg/kg i.p., i.v.	0.3 mL/kg i.m. + 2.5 mg/kg i.p.
Fentanyl citrate/ fluanisone + midazolam[2]	8 mL[2]/kg i.p.	8 mL[2]/kg i.p.	4 mL[2]/kg i.p.	10 mL[2]/kg i.p.	0.3 mL/kg i.m. + 2 mL/kg i.v. or i.p.	2.7 mL[2]/kg i.p.
Flunixin	—	—	—	2.5 mg/kg s.c. twice daily	1.1 mg/kg s.c. twice daily	2.5 mg/kg s.c. twice daily
Ketamine	200 mg/kg i.m., i.p.	100 mg/kg i.m., i.p.	200 mg/kg i.m., i.p.	150 mg/kg i.m., i.p.	50 mg/kg i.m.	100 mg/kg i.m., i.p.
Ketamine + medetomidine	—	40 mg/kg + 500 micrograms/ kg i.p.	100 mg/kg + 250 micrograms/ kg i.p.	75 mg/kg + 1 mg/kg i.p.	15 mg/kg + 250 micro-grams/kg s.c.	75 mg/kg + 500 micrograms/kg i.p.
Ketamine + xylazine	50 mg/kg + 2 mg/kg i.m.	40 mg/kg + 5 mg/kg i.m.	200 mg/kg + 10 mg/kg i.p.	100 mg/kg + 10 mg/kg i.p.	35 mg/kg + 5 mg/kg i.m.	90 mg/kg + 10 mg/kg i.p.
Ketoprofen	—	—	—	—	3 mg/kg i.m.	5 mg/kg i.m.
Methohexital	—	30 mg/kg i.p.	—	10 mg/kg i.v.	10 mg/kg i.v.	7–10 mg/kg i.v.
Morphine	—	5 mg/kg s.c.	—	5 mg/kg s.c.	5 mg/kg s.c.	5 mg/kg s.c.
Nalbuphine	—	—	—	4–8 mg/kg s.c.	1–2 mg/kg i.v.	1–2 mg/kg s.c.

Table 13 Doses of analgesics and anaesthetics for rabbits and rodents[1] *(continued)*

Drug	Gerbil	Guinea pig	Hamster	Mouse	Rabbit	Rat
Naloxone	10–100 micro-grams/kg i.m., i.p., i.v.	10–100 micro-grams/kg i.m., i.p., i.v.	10–100 micro-grams/kg i.m., i.p., i.v.	10–100 micro-grams/kg i.m., i.p., i.v.	10–100 micro-grams/kg i.m., i.p., i.v.	10–100 micro-grams/kg i.m., i.p., i.v.
Pentazocine	—	—	—	10 mg/kg s.c.	5 mg/kg i.v.	10 mg/kg s.c.
Pentobarbital	60–80 mg/kg i.p.	26 mg/kg i.v.[1]	50–90 mg/kg i.p.	40 mg/kg i.p.	26 mg/kg i.v.[1]	40 mg/kg i.p.
Pethidine	—	10 mg/kg s.c., i.m.	—	10 mg/kg s.c., i.m.	10 mg/kg s.c., i.m.	10 mg/kg s.c., i.m.
Propofol	—	—	—	26 mg/kg i.v.	10 mg/kg i.v.	10 mg/kg i.v.
Thiopental	—	—	—	30–40 mg/kg i.v.	30 mg/kg i.v.	30 mg/kg i.v.

[1] drug doses for preparations that have a marketing authorisation for use in these species in the UK. Therefore, unless marked [1], the drug or doses stated are not authorised for these species

[2] dose is in mL/kg of a mixture made up of 2 mL of Hypnorm (Janssen) plus 4 mL Water for injection plus 2 mL Hypnovel (Roche)

Table 14 Doses of other drugs for rabbits and rodents[1]

Drug	Gerbil	Guinea pig	Hamster	Mouse	Rabbit	Rat
Cisapride					500 micro-grams/kg p.o. three times daily	
Colestyramine	—	—	—	—	2 g/adult daily for 2 weeks	—
Dexamethasone	—	400 micrograms/kg s.c.	600 micrograms/kg s.c.	—	0.5–2.0 mg/kg s.c., i.m., i.v.	—
Metoclopramide	—	—	—	—	0.2–1.0 mg/kg p.o., s.c., i.m., i.v. twice daily	—
Oxytocin	—	1–3 units/kg i.m.	0.2–3.0 units/kg i.m.	—	—	—
Phenobarbital	10–20 mg/kg p.o.	—	—	—	—	—

[1] drug doses for preparations that have a marketing authorisation for use in these species in the UK. Therefore, unless marked [1], the drug or doses stated are not authorised for these species

Prescribing for ferrets

Contributors:
S W Cooke BVSc, MRCVS

In the UK, domesticated ferrets *Mustela putorius furo,* are now used for rabbit hunting, as pets, as show animals (including demonstrations such as ferret racing), and for biomedical research.

Ferrets are carnivorous and will take prey much larger than themselves killing it with their strong jaws and sharp canine teeth. They do not have a caecum and are unable to digest fibre. High concentration of carbohydrates in the diet may predispose to diabetes mellitus. The diet should contain a high concentration of good quality protein (26 to 36% wet matter weight) and fat (15 to 30% wet matter weight). Excess fat in the diet may cause obesity, lethargy, and poor reproductive performance. Hypovitaminosis E and excess polyunsaturated fats may cause a steatitis and is usually seen in young animals fed excessive amounts of fish or horsemeat. Fresh water should be provided *ad lib*. Thiamine deficiency may be caused by feeding young ferrets solely on whole chicks due to the thiaminase contained in day old chick yolk sacs.

The *Mustelinae* all possess anal glands and produce a strongly smelling 'musk'. However 90% of the animal's odour originates from the subaceous glands and is controlled by androgens. Neutering is effective at controlling odour and anal gland removal is not indicated for this purpose. In females, oestrus may last up to 6 months and ovulation is coitus induced. Sexual maturity is at 8 to 12 months but may be as early as 5 months.

Due to their inquisitive nature, varied diet, and ability to chew, gastro-intestinal foreign bodies are commonly diagnosed in ferrets.

Drug administration. Ferrets readily accept oral medication if the taste of the medicine is disguised in sweet or fatty foods, for example flavoured syrups (not real chocolate), cat laxatives, nutritional supplements, honey, fatty acid supplements, double cream, taramasalata, or couscous. Individuals may show a preference. Tablets may be given whole with a commercial tablet administrator, such as that used for cats, but ferrets are often not tolerant of tablet administration. Alternatively tablets may be crushed and mixed with a palatable substance.

Subcutaneous injections should be given in the neck and shoulder regions using small gauge needles (22 g to 27 g) to reduce discomfort. Up to 20 mL of fluid may be given at a single injection site. Intramuscular injections should be given in the semitendinous, semimembranous, biceps femoris, or lumbar muscles.

Intravenous injections may be given into the cephalic, jugular, or lateral saphenous veins; the jugular site is often poorly tolerated. Liberal application of spirit or alcohol to the fur often allows better visualisation of the vein than clipping. For long to medium term administration, 22 g to 24 g over-the-needle catheters should be used and may require chemical restraint to ease placement. Butterfly catheters (23 g to 25 g) are useful for short term fluid or chemotherapy administration. The animal should be prevented from chewing the catheter by covering the area with adhesive dressing.

Intra-osseous catheters are very useful in severely debilitated animals. The femur (most commonly used), humerus, or tibia are suitable bones. A 22 g to 20 g spinal needle or similar sized hypodermic using sterile orthopaedic wire as a stylet may be used. Anaesthesia is required for placement. Catheters may be left in place for several days for giving intravenous medication (except some chemotherapeutics); a syringe pump is necessary and antibiotic treatment is recommended during this time and for 3 days after removal.

Intraperitoneal injections should be restricted to euthanasia or fluid replacement in very debilitated animals due to the risk of organ damage if the animal struggles.

Blood transfusions may be performed in ferrets. They have no discernible blood types so a number of donors may be used for a single recipient. A maximum of 1% of bodyweight may be collected from the anaesthetised (preferably with isoflurane) donor with either heparin or ACD solution as anticoagulant and administered immediately to the recipient at a rate of 0.25 to 0.5 mL/minute.

Antimicrobial therapy. Abscesses caused by *Staphylococcus, Streptococcus, Pasteurella, Corynebacterium, Actinobacillus* and *E. coli* occur as opportunist infections secondary to penetrating wounds, for example bites from other ferrets or other animals, foreign bodies such as sharp bones in the diet, or skin injuries.

Bacterial pneumonia may be primary, or secondary to a viral infection for example influenza, or other illnesses such as hyperadrenocorticism or abscesses. Organisms implicated include *Streptococcus zooepidemicus, S. pneumoniae, E. coli, Klebsiella pneumoniae, Pseudomonas aeruginosa, Bordetella bronchiseptica* and *Listeria monocytogenes*.

Enteritis is commonly seen, especially in young ferrets, and may be husbandry related. Secondary opportunist infections with, for example *E. coli,* may cause sudden death. Proliferative bowel disease caused by *a Campylobacter (Desulfovibrio)* affects ferrets of less than 1 year of age and may require treatment with gentamicin or chloramphenicol. *Helicobacter mustelae* infection can be implicated in gastric ulceration and chronic atrophic gastritis. Treatment is with amoxicillin.

Ferrets are very susceptible to salmonellosis and tuberculosis caused by *Mycobacterium avium, M. bovis* and *M. tuberculosis*. They are not very susceptible to leptospirosis but may be exposed if used for rodent control. Infection due to *Listeria monocytogenes* has been reported.

Botulism (Types A, B, and especially the common C) may pose a risk to animals fed uncooked food or by soil exposure. Actimomycosis should be considered in the differential list for a 'lumpy jaw' presentation. Both *Mycoplasma* and *Chlamydia* have been isolated from ferrets but their clinical significance is not known.

Ferrets are extremely susceptible to canine distemper (usually from the dog) with mortality approaching 100%. Vaccination with an appropriate dog vaccine and prior advice from the manufacturer may be used. Ferrets are also very susceptible to rabies. Aleutian disease, which is usually a problem in mink farms, is caused by a parvovirus but often remains as an asymptomatic infection; morbidity and mortality is very variable. Human influenza virus infections are pathogenic for ferrets. In adults, infection is characterised by a short illness with spontaneous recovery and low mortality. Infection may cause high mortality in kits. Feline panleukopaenia, feline leukaemia virus, mink enteritis, and canine parvovirus are not thought to constitute a risk to ferrets.

Blastomycosis, cryptococcosis, histoplasmosis, coccidiomycosis, and mucormycosis are all reported (especially from the USA) and should be considered if other diseases are eliminated by appropriate diagnostic methods. Ringworm due to *Microsporum canis* and *Trichophyton mentagrophytes* are reported.

Coccidia (*Isospora* spp.), *Toxoplasma, Sarcocystis, Giardia* may occur in ferrets.

Antiparasiticidal therapy. Both internal and external parasites are common in ferrets and treatment is similar to that used for cats. Caution should be exercised with dosage of any preparation but particularly organophosphorus compounds because the animal's small body weight predisposes to overdose and toxic doses have not been established. It is recommended to treat several times with the minimal dose rather than attempt a single-dose medication.

Fleas (*Ctenocephalides spp*), ear mites (*Otodectes cynotis*), ticks (many species), and sarcoptes (*Sarcoptes scabiei*) affect ferrets. Sarcoptes infestation may be generalised or limited to the feet. *Toxascaris, Toxocara, Ancylostoma*, ces-todes, and (in the USA), heartworm (*Dirofilaria immitis*) are all reported as occuring in ferrets.

Other drugs. Insulinoma is commonly reported as is hyperadrenocorticism, diabetes mellitus, and oestrogen-induced anaemia due to persistent oestrus. Tumours such as lymphosarcoma, ovarian and other reproductive organ tumours (mammary tumours are uncommon), skin and subcutaneous tumours (mast cell tumours, squamous cell carcinomas and adenomas) occur in ferrets. Dilated and hypertrophic cardiomyopathies are commonly diagnosed and usually respond well to treatment initially. Gastric dilation (may be associated with *Clostridium welchii*), eosinophilic gastro-enteritis, periodontal disease, posterior paralysis/paresis and splenomegaly (the latter two may be caused by a number of other disease entities and are not pathognomic for any one) all are reported as being significant clinical entities. Zinc toxicosis is also reported as are cases of struvite urolithiasis and osteodystrophy. Treatment of conditions should be approached using conventional veterinary knowledge and techniques and modified where necessary by reference to known drug dosages and client/patient compliance.

Complete nutritional replacement therapy may be used in debilitated or convalesing animals. Hill's a/d may be given at a dose of 10 to 20 mL/kg 3 to 6 times daily. Pharyngostomy tubing (using 8 to 19 F paediatric feeding tube placed under general anaesthesia) is well tolerated if the protective dressings are light and not restrictive but are sufficient to prevent chewing of the cap or catheter end and subsequent gastro-intestinal foreign body problems. Calorific requirements are 200 to 300 kcal/kg/day.

For fluid administration in ferrets, maintenance replacement is approximately 60 to 70 mL/kg/24 hours. There is a high incidence of insulinoma in ferrets and glucose 2.5% or 5% + sodium chloride 0.9% solution should used rather than lactated Ringer's solution in animals over 3 years of age including during elective surgery if indicated.

Table 15 Antimicrobial doses of drugs for ferrets[1]

Drug	Dose
Amantadine	6 mg/kg p.o. or nebulisation twice daily
Amikacin	10–15 mg/kg s.c., i.m. twice daily
Amoxicillin	10–20 mg/kg p.o., s.c. 2–3 times daily for 7–10 days
Amoxicillin with clavulanic acid[2]	13–25 mg/kg p.o., s.c., i.m. twice daily
Amphotericin B	0.25–1.0 mg/kg i.v. daily or on alternate days until total dose of 7–25 mg given cryptococcosis, 150 micrograms/kg i.v. 3 times weekly for 2–4 months
Ampicillin	20 mg/kg p.o., s.c. twice daily 10 mg/kg i.m. twice daily
Cefadroxil	15–20 mg/kg p.o. twice daily
Cefalexin	15–30 mg/kg p.o. 2–3 times daily
Ciprofloxacin	10 mg/kg p.o. twice daily
Clindamycin	5.5–10.0 mg/kg p.o. twice daily
Enrofloxacin	5–10 mg/kg p.o. twice daily 3–5 mg/kg s.c., i.m. twice daily
Erythromycin	10 mg/kg p.o. 4 times daily
Gentamicin	5 mg/kg s.c., i.m. once daily
Griseofulvin	25 mg/kg p.o. once daily
Ketoconazole	10–30 mg/kg p.o. once daily for 60 days
Lincomycin	11 mg/kg p.o. 3 times daily
Metronidazole	20 mg/kg p.o. twice daily
Neomycin	10 mg/kg p.o. 4 times daily
Oxytetracycline	17–20 mg/kg p.o. 3 times daily 10 mg/kg i.m. twice daily
Sulfadiazine with trimethoprim	30 mg/kg p.o., s.c. twice daily
Sulfamethoxazole with trimethoprim	30 mg/kg p.o., s.c. twice daily
Tetracycline	20 mg/kg p.o. 3 times daily
Tylosin	10 mg/kg p.o. 3 times daily 5–10 mg/kg i.m., i.v. twice daily

[1] drug doses for preparations that have a marketing authorisation for use in these species in the UK. Therefore, unless marked [1], the drug or doses stated are not authorised for these species
[2] dose expressed as amoxicillin

Table 16 Parasiticidal doses of drugs for ferrets[1]

Drug	Dose
Endoparasiticides	
Fenbendazole	20 mg/kg p.o. daily for 5 days
Mebendazole	50 mg/kg p.o. twice daily for 2 days
Milbemycin oxime	1.15–2.30 mg/kg p.o. monthly
Praziquantel	5–10 mg/kg s.c.. Repeat after 2 weeks
Pyrantel	4.4 mg/kg p.o. as a single dose
Ectoparasiticides	
Carbaril	shampoo, once weekly for 3–5 weeks
Ivermectin	0.4–1.0 mg/kg s.c.. Repeat after one week
Pyrethrins	dusting powder, weekly for 3 weeks

[1] drug doses for preparations that have a marketing authorisation for use in these species in the UK. Therefore, unless marked [1], the drug or doses stated are not authorised for these species

Table 17 Doses of analgesics and anaesthetics for ferrets

Drug	Dose
Acepromazine	100–250 micrograms/kg s.c., i.m.
Alfadolone + Alfaxalone	10 mg/kg i.m.; 8-12 mg/kg i.v.
Atipamezole	0.4–1.0 mg/kg i.m.
Atropine	50 micrograms/kg s.c., i.m.
Buprenorphine	10–50 mg/kg s.c., i.m., i.v. 2–3 times daily
Butorphanol	10–50 mg/kg i.m. every 4–6 hours
Diazepam	1–2 mg/kg i.m.
Fentanyl + Droperidol	0.15 mL (Innovar-Vet)/kg i.m.
Fentanyl + Fluanisone	300 micrograms/kg i.m.
Glycopyrronium	10 micrograms/kg s.c.
Halothane	induction, 3.0–3.5%; maintenance, 0.5–2.5%
Isoflurane	induction, 3.0–5.0%; maintenance, 1.5–3.0%
Ketamine + Acepromazine	20–35 mg/kg s.c., i.m. 200–350 micrograms/kg for 30–35 minutes effect
Ketamine + Diazepam	25–35 mg/kg s.c., i.m. 2–3 mg/kg
Ketamine + Xylazine	10–25 mg/kg s.c., i.m. (**Use with caution**) 1–2 mg/kg i.m.
Medetomidine + Ketamine	80 micrograms/kg i.m. 5 mg/kg
Medetomidine + Ketamine + Butorphanol	80 micrograms/kg i.m. 5 mg/kg 100 micrograms/kg
Methoxyflurane	induction, 1–3 %; maintenance, 0.3–0.5%
Morphine	0.5–5.0 mg/kg s.c., i.m. every 2–6 hours
Nalbuphine	0.5–1.5 mg/kg i.m., i.v. every 2–3 hours
Naloxone	40 micrograms/kg s.c., i.m., i.v.
Oxymorphone	50–200 micrograms/kg s.c., i.m., i.v. 2–3 times daily
Pentazocine	5–10 mg/kg i.m. every 4 hours
Pentobarbital	25–35 mg/kg i.v.
Pethidine	5–10 mg/kg s.c., i.m., i.v. every 2–4 hours
Phencyclidine + Promazine	0.8–1.1 mg/kg i.m. 1 mg/kg i.m.
Propofol	2–10 mg/kg i.v.
Thiopental	8–12 mg/kg i.v.
Tiletamine + Zolazepam	8–22 mg/kg i.m.
Xylazine	4 mg/kg s.c.
Yohimbine	500 micrograms/kg i.m.

Table 18 Table of doses of other drugs for ferrets[1]

Drug	Dose
Aminophylline	4.4–6.6 mg/kg p.o., i.m. twice daily
Apomorphine	5 mg/kg s.c. as a single dose
Aspirin	0.5–20.0 mg/kg p.o. once daily or on alternate days
Atenolol	6.25 mg/kg p.o. once daily
Atropine	organophosphorus toxicity, 5–10 mg/kg s.c., i.m.
Barium sulphate	contrast radiography, 2–10 mL/kg p.o.
Betamethasone	100 micrograms/kg s.c.
Bismuth subsalicylate	0.25 mL (Pepto-Bismol)/kg p.o. every 4–6 hours
Buserelin	1 microgram i.m.
Chorionic gonadotrophin	20–100 units i.m.
Chlorphenamine	1–2 mg/kg p.o. 1–2 times daily
Cimetidine	5–10 mg/kg p.o., i.v. 3 times daily
Crisantaspase[2]	400 units i.p. total dose
Cyclophosphamide[2]	10 mg/kg s.c.
Dexamethasone	0.5–2.0 mg/kg s.c., i.m., i.v.
Diazepam	1.0 mg/kg i.v.
Diazoxide	2.5–30.0 mg/kg p.o. twice daily
Digitoxin	70–100 micrograms/kg p.o. once daily or on alternate days. Plasma-digitoxin concentration should be monitored
Diltiazem	3.75–7.5 mg/kg p.o. twice daily
Diphenhydramine	0.5–2.0 mg/kg p.o. 2–3 times daily
Doxapram	2 mg/kg i.m.
Doxorubicin[2]	1 mg/kg i.v.
Enalapril	500 micrograms/kg p.o. from 3 times daily to on alternate days
Famotidine	250–500 micrograms/kg p.o., i.v. once daily
Flunixin	inflammation, 1.1 mg/kg; analgesia, 0.3–2.0 mg/kg s.c., i.m. 1–2 times daily (on alternate days for long-term therapy)
Furosemide	1–2 mg/kg p.o., s.c., i.m., i.v. 2–3 times daily. may use up to 4 mg/kg i.m. for acute conditions
Hydrocortisone	25–40 mg/kg i.v. as a single dose
Immunoglobulins	0.2 mL (Maxaglobulin P)/kg s.c., i.m. for distemper prophylaxis
Insulin, protamine zinc	0.5–1.0 unit/kg s.c. once daily
Iohexol	contrast radiography, dilute 1 volume with 1 volume water, 10 mL/kg p.o.
Iron dextran	10 mg/kg i.m. weekly

Table 18 Table of doses of other drugs for ferrets[1]

Drug	Dose
Ketoconazole	hyperadrenocorticism, 15 mg/kg p.o. twice daily
Lactulose	150–750 mg/kg p.o. 2–3 times daily
Levothyroxine	200–400 micrograms/kg p.o. 2–3 times daily
Oxytocin	0.2–3.0 units/kg s.c., i.m.
Methotrexate[2]	500 micrograms/kg i.v.
Mitotane	50 mg/kg p.o. once daily. Reduce to every 3 days after 1 week
Nandrolone	1–5 mg/kg i.m. weekly
Prednisolone[2]	inflammation, 250–500 micrograms p.o. twice daily. May increase up to 2 mg/kg gradually; malignant disease, 1 mg/kg p.o. once daily
Proligestone[1]	50 mg/kg s.c. as a single dose
Propranolol	0.2–1.0 mg/kg p.o. 2–3 times daily
Sucralfate	25–30 mg p.o. 4 times daily
Theophylline	4.25 mg/kg p.o. 2–3 times daily
Vincristine[2]	70 micrograms/kg i.v.

[1] drug doses for preparations that have a marketing authorisation for use in these species in the UK. Therefore, unless marked [1], the drug or doses stated are not authorised for these species

[2] usually cyclophosphamide, prednisolone, and vincristine are given concurrently. Alternatively cyclophosphamide, prednisolone, and vincristine combination may be given with cristantaspase and methotrexate, or doxorubicin

Prescribing for fish

Contributors:
A E Wall, BVM&S, MSc, CertVOphthal, MRCVS
W H Wildgoose, BVMS, CertFHP, MRCVS

Fish are farmed as food-producing animals and also kept by enthusiasts as a hobby. In the UK, Atlantic salmon and rainbow trout are most commonly farmed. Species kept by enthusiasts may be divided into cold-water and tropical fish. Cold-water fish kept include goldfish in aquaria, Japanese koi carp in ponds, and occasionally temperate marine fish caught off the coast. Tropical fish may be freshwater or marine.

Preventive medicine is extremely important for fish health. Fish live in a 'bacterial soup' and poor water quality or frank infection may quickly lead to an acute cascade of disease within a cage, pond, or tank. Maintenance of good water quality, adequate feeding but not overfeeding, long quarantine, and low stocking densities will aid the production and maintenance of healthy fish.

Farmed fish

Antibacterial therapy. The majority of bacterial infections affecting fish are caused by Gram-negative organisms such as *Aeromonas*, *Vibrio*, and *Pseudomonas* spp., which cause furunculosis, septicaemia, and ulcer disease. *Yersinia ruckeri* infection causes enteric redmouth disease. The intracellular bacteria *Piscirikettsia salmonis* has been implicated in some disease outbreaks in salmon. Bacterial kidney disease (BKD) infection caused by the Gram-positive bacterium *Renibacterium salmoninarum* affects all salmonid stocks. This chronic disease causes highest mortality with changing water temperatures. Fish are lethargic, anorexic, and have darkened skin often with shallow ulcers on the flanks. Internally the kidney is very swollen and grey with a fibrinous peritonitis over the internal organs. Vertical transmission within the egg makes control of this disease difficult.

Bacterial resistance to antibacterials has been a problem in the fish industry. Good husbandry including single year classes, fallowing sites, and lower stocking densities and vaccination have significantly reduced the use of antibacterials in the UK.

Antibacterials are usually formulated as in-feed medications for farmed fish. The drug is surface coated on the prepared pellet and then oil is added to maintain adhesion. Rarely, the drug is mixed with oil and sprayed directly onto the pellet. Fish should be starved for 12 to 24 hours before treatment because in-feed medication may be unpalatable. Adequate oxygenation must always be maintained, particularly in treatment tanks.

Antibacterial preparations that are used in farmed fish include **amoxicillin, florfenicol, oxolinic acid, oxytetracycline, sarafloxacin, sulfadiazine with trimethoprim,** and **sulfadimethoxine with ormetoprim**. Further information on these antibacterials is given in section 1.1. The usual treatment course is 7 to 10 days, but readers should also refer to the manufacturer's data sheet. Sulfadiazine with trimethoprim administered at a dose of 30 mg/kg daily for 7 to 10 days has been found to cause lethargy and inappetance in Atlantic salmon. In practice, the usual dose administered is 15 mg/kg daily♦ or 30 mg/kg on alternate days♦. Concurrent treatment with dichlorvos, which can itself cause stress and panic in fish, has lead to large numbers of deaths on salmon farms.

When administering antibacterials to farmed fish, the appropriate withdrawal periods must be observed. Fish are ectothermic and their basal metabolic rate varies with water temperature. Therefore withdrawal periods, stated in degree days, vary with ambient water temperature. For example 400 degree days is 20 days at a water temperature of 20°C or 40 days at 10°C. The standard withdrawal period for fish of 500° days should be observed unless otherwise stated by the manufacturer.

In general, treatment with in-water antibacterials or methylthioninium chloride (methylene blue) should not be carried out in tanks with biological filters. Although some drugs are claimed not to disturb biological filters, many do so depending on the dose used. It is preferable to administer the treatment in a quarantine tank without filtration but with appropriate monitoring of water quality or water changes. Alternatively, with a commercial recirculation system, individual tanks may be isolated for treatment and then the water discharged to waste.

Vaccines are available for the control of some fish diseases caused by bacteria (see section 18.8).

AMOXICILLIN TRIHYDRATE
(Amoxycillin trihydrate)

UK
Indications. Amoxicillin-sensitive infections including furunculosis
Warnings. Penicillins and cephalosporins may cause hypersensitivity (allergy) following self-injection, inhalation, ingestion, or skin contact. Operators with known hypersensitivity should not handle these drugs. Clinical signs of allergic reaction in operators include skin rash, swelling of the face, lips, or eyes, or difficulty breathing. Operators should seek medical advice
Dose. *Fish*: *by addition to feed,* 40–80 mg/kg body-weight daily for 10 days

POM **Aquacil** (Vericore AP) *UK*
Powder, for addition to feed, amoxicillin trihydrate 800 g/kg, for *salmon*; 500 g, 1 kg, other sizes available
Withdrawal Periods. *Salmon*: slaughter 50° days (dose of amoxicillin 40 mg/kg), 80° days (dose of amoxicillin 80 mg/kg)

POM **Vetremox Fish** (Vetrepharm) *UK*
Powder, for addition to feed, amoxicillin trihydrate 100%, for **Atlantic salmon**
Withdrawal Periods. *Atlantic salmon*: slaughter 40° days

Eire

Indications. Amoxicillin-sensitive infections including furunculosis
Dose. *Fish*: *by addition to feed*, 80 mg/kg body-weight daily for 10 days

Aquacil (Cypharm) *Eire*
Oral powder, for addition to feed, amoxycillin trihydrate 500 g/kg, for *salmon*
Withdrawal Periods. Slaughter 50° days

FLORFENICOL

UK

Indications. Florfenicol-sensitive infections including furunculosis
Contra-indications. Brood stock
Warnings. Drug Interactions – anaesthetics
Dose. *Fish*: *by addition to feed*, 10 mg/kg body-weight daily for 10 days

MFS **Florocol** (Schering-Plough) *UK*
Powder, for addition to feed, florfenicol 500 mg/g, for *Atlantic salmon*
Withdrawal Periods. *Atlantic salmon*: slaughter 150° days

ORMETOPRIM WITH SULFADIMETHOXINE

USA

Indications. Ormetoprim/sulfadimethoxine-sensitive infections
Dose. Expressed as ormetoprim + sulphadiazine
Fish: 16.7 g/100 kg daily

Romet 30 (Roche Viamins) *USA*
Premix, ormetoprim 5%, sulfadimethoxine 25%, for *salmon, trout, catfish*
Withdrawal Periods. *Salmon, trout*: slaughter 42 days. *Catfish*: slaughter 3 days

OXOLINIC ACID

UK

Indications. Oxolinic acid-sensitive infections including furunculosis and enteric red mouth disease
Dose. *Fish*: *by addition to feed*, 10 mg/kg body-weight daily for 10 days; 30 mg/kg♦ body-weight (sea water)

POM **Aqualinic** (Vetrepharm) *UK*
Powder, for addition to feed, oxolinic acid 100%, for *Atlantic salmon, rainbow trout, brown trout*
Withdrawal Periods. *Atlantic salmon, rainbow trout, brown trout*: slaughter 500° days

POM **Aquinox** (Vericore AP) *UK*
Powder, for addition to feed, oxolinic acid 500 g/kg, for *salmon, trout, ornamental fish*; 1 kg, 2 kg, 20 kg
Withdrawal Periods. *Salmon, trout*: slaughter 500° days

Eire

Indications. Oxolinic acid-sensitive infections including furunculosis

Dose. *Fish*: *by addition to feed*, 10 mg/kg body-weight daily for 10 days

Aquinox (Cypharm) *Eire*
Oral powder, for addition to feed, oxolinic acid 50%, for *salmon*
Withdrawal Periods. Slaughter 500° days

OXYTETRACYCLINE

UK

Indications. Oxytetracycline-sensitive infections including furunculosis
Warnings. Chelated in hard water (not applicable for in-feed medication)
Dose. *Fish*: *by addition to feed*, 75 mg/kg body-weight daily for 4–10 days

POM **Aquatet** (Vetrepharm) *UK*
Powder, for addition to feed, oxytetracycline hydrochloride, for *Atlantic salmon, rainbow trout*; 1 kg, 2.5 kg
Withdrawal Periods. *Atlantic salmon, rainbow trout*: slaughter 400° days

POM **Tetraplex** (Vericore AP) *UK*
Powder, for addition to feed, oxytetracycline 500 g/kg, for *Atlantic salmon, ornamental fish*; 2 kg, 25 kg
Withdrawal Periods. *Atlantic salmon*: slaughter 500° days

Eire

Indications. Oxytetracycline-sensitive infections including furunculosis
Dose. *Fish*: *by addition to feed*, 75 mg/kg body-weight daily for 10 days

Maracycline 50% w/w Powder (Univet) *Eire*
Oral powder, for addition to feed, oxytetracycline 500 g/kg, for *salmon*
Withdrawal Periods. Slaughter 400° days

Maracycline Powder (Univet) *Eire*
Oral powder, for addition to feed, oxytetracycline hydrochloride, for *salmon*
Withdrawal Periods. Slaughter 400° days

Tetraplex (Cypharm) *Eire*
Oral powder, to mix with feed, oxytetracycline hydrochloride 500 g/kg, for *salmon*
Withdrawal Periods. Slaughter 400° days

USA

Indications. Oxytetracycline-sensitive infections
Dose. *Fish*: *by addition to feed*, 2.5–3.75 g/45.45 kg body-weight daily for 10 days

TM 100F (Pfizer) *USA*
Premix, oxytetracycline 220 g/kg premix, for *catfish*

SARAFLOXACIN HYDROCHLORIDE

UK

Indications. Sarafloxacin-sensitive infections including furunculosis
Dose. *Fish*: *by addition to feed*, 10 mg/kg body-weight daily for 5 days

POM **Sarafin** (Vetrepharm) *UK*
Powder, for addition to feed, sarafloxacin hydrochloride 100%, for *Atlantic salmon*
Withdrawal Periods. *Atlantic salmon*: slaughter 150° days

SULFADIAZINE WITH TRIMETHOPRIM

(Co-trimazine: preparations of trimethoprim and sulphadiazine in the proportions, by weight, 1 part to 5 parts

UK

Indications. Sulfadiazine/trimethoprim-sensitive infections including furunculosis
Side-effects. **Warnings**. High dosage may cause lethargy and inappetence, see notes above
Dose. Expressed as trimethoprim + sulphadiazine
Fish: *by addition to feed*, 30 mg/kg body-weight daily for 7–10 days but see dose♦ above

POM **Sulfatrim** (Vericore AP) *UK*
Powder, for addition to feed, sulphadiazine 416.7 g, trimethoprim 83.3 g/kg, for *salmon*; 2 kg
Withdrawal Periods. *Salmon*: slaughter 400° days

Eire

Indications. Sulfadiazine/trimethoprim-sensitive infections including furunculosis
Dose. Expressed as trimethoprim + sulphadiazine
Fish: *by addition to feed*, 30 mg/kg body-weight

Sulfatrim (Cypharm) *Eire*
Oral powder, to mix with feed, trimethoprim and sulphadiazine 50%, for *salmon*
Withdrawal Periods. Slaughter 400° days

Parasiticidal and antifungal therapy. The common protozoal infections affecting farmed fish include white spot caused by *Ichthyophthirius multifiliis*; slime disease due to *Chilodonella*, *Ichthyobodo* (*Costia*), and *Trichodina*; velvet disease caused by *Oodinium* spp.; and fin rot caused by traumatic injury, poor water quality, and protozoal and ectoparasitic infections. Other ectoparasites causing lesions include flukes such as *Gyrodactylus*, which attach onto the skin and *Dactylogyrus*, which affect the gills, and the anchor worm *Lernaea*. *Gyrodactylus salaris* causes widespread losses in Atlantic salmon in Norway due to skin damage. *Saprolegnia* is a common fungal infection of fish; it is usually a secondary infection.

Fish should be starved before any treatment because this reduces the metabolic rate of the fish and the organic loading of water from food and faeces, which increases the oxygen demand. Initially only a few fish in a group, as a representative sample, should be treated. After observing these fish for good recovery over a few hours, the remaining fish can be treated similarly. Adequate oxygenation should always be provided in treatment tanks.

Chemicals or drugs are added to the water, which is used as a bath, a flush, or a dip. To prepare a **bath**, a low concentration of drug is added to the water and the fish are placed in the solution for 30 to 60 minutes, or longer for prolonged immersion. When given as a **flush**, a higher concentration of drug is added to the water which is then flushed through with fresh incoming water. This usually means the fish remain in contact with the drug for 15 to 20 minutes. In a dip, a very concentrated solution of the drug is prepared and fish are netted into the solution for 30 to 60 seconds and then replaced in their original tank.

The organophosphorus compounds **azamethiphos** is used for the treatment of salmon infested by the sea lice, *Lepeophtheirus salmonis* and *Caligus* spp., before the stage at which serious skin damage is evident. Organophosphorus compounds affect mature sea lice (stages pre-adult 1 to adult); they do not affect juvenile stages. Therefore treatment may need to be repeated after 10 to 20 days and again after a further 14 days to ensure complete eradication of the infestation. Vigorous water aeration should be provided when using organophosphorus compounds. Gasping and rolling are signs of toxicity and asphyxiation of the fish.

Cypermethrin is a synthetic pyrethroid and is used for the treatment of sea lice and has largely superseded the organophosphorus compounds. Cypermethrin is used to treat and control all stages of sea lice. Treatment before the sea lice reach the reproductive stage should help to reduce the number of free-swimming infective stages released and fewer treatments will be required. Fish may be retreated when re-infestation occurs.

Goldsinney wrasse have been used, as an alternative to chemical treatment, to control sea louse infestation on salmon (the wrasse ingest the lice).

AZAMETHIPHOS

UK

Indications. Sea lice infestation
Warnings. Limit treatment to 30 minutes at water temperatures greater than 10°
Dose. *Fish*: *by bath*, 0.1 ppm for 30–60 minutes

POM **Salmosan** (Novartis) *UK*
Powder, azamethiphos 500 mg/g, for *salmon*; 20 g, 100 g
Withdrawal Periods. *Fish*: slaughter 1 day

CYPERMETHRIN

UK

Indications. Sea lice infestation
Warnings. Oxygen concentration should be maintained at greater than 7 mg/litre during treatment; safety in broodstock has not been established
Dose. *Fish*: *by seawater bath*, 0.005 ppm (5 micrograms/litre) for 60 minutes

POM **Excis** (Vericore) *UK*
Solution, for dilution with water, cypermethrin (cis:trans 40:60) 1%, for *Atlantic salmon*. Correct dose should be diluted with 40 litres of seawater before adding to the seacage
Withdrawal Periods. *Atlantic salmon*: slaughter 24 hours

EMAMECTIN

UK

Indications. Sea lice infestation
Contra-indications. Brood stock

Dose. *Fish*: *by addition to feed*, 50 micrograms/kg fish daily

POM **Slice** (Schering-Plough) *UK*
Premix, emamectin 2 g/kg, for Atlantic salmon
Withdrawal Periods. Slaughter withdrawal period nil. Do not treat more than once within 60 days before slaughter

---

Parasiticides may be toxic to animals and the operator. Care should be taken with dosage and handling of the product. The recommendations for storage, use, and disposal of unused materials and containers should be followed. For guidance and information, see:
- MAFF/HSE. *Code of practice for the safe use of pesticides on farms and holdings*. London: HMSO, 1998. PB3528
- *Animal medicines: A user's guide*. NOAH, 1995
- Control of Substances Hazardous to Health (COSHH) Regulations 1994.

Chemicals used in the treatment of fish diseases may be obtained in the UK from:
- AVL
- Dunwood
- James A Mackie (Agricultural)
- Vericore AP
- Vetark.

Addresses for these companies can be found in the Index of manufacturers and organisations.

There are many chemical treatments for ectoparasitic and fungal infections available. These chemicals may be used in fish destined for human consumption because they are considered as non-medicinal curative substances. Although reservations about their use have been expressed by consumer groups and fish farming organisations, any potential risks remain unproven . Malachite green residues persist in flesh and this component should only be used in rainbow trout eggs and fry less than 0.5 gram body-weight and Atlantic salmon in the fresh water phase.

In general, the ectoparasiticides of choice for farmed fish are formaldehyde, chloramine, Leteux-Meyer mixture, and sodium chloride. For fungal infections, malachite green or sodium chloride is employed.

Formaldehyde is a general ectoparasiticide and is also used for fluke infections due to *Gyrodactylus* and resistant *Chilodonella* infections. The dose of formaldehyde should be adjusted according to the water pH; low doses should be used at low pH and higher doses used at high pH. Toxic precipitates of paraformaldehyde form on storage which should be discarded before use. Formaldehyde actively depletes water oxygen and adequate aeration must therefore be provided.

Malachite green is primarily used for fungal infections and some ectoparasitic infections. Care should be taken with regard to the source of malachite green; some grades may be lethal to fish. Low doses should be used at low pH and higher doses used at high pH. Care must be taken when prescribing malachite green because residues of this chemical

have been found in rainbow trout at point of sale. Most freshwater trout farms grow their largest trout in water previously used by smaller fish and eggs. Therefore any treatment of eggs or young fish with malachite green may result in residues being found in market-sized fish. The use of this chemical is being increasingly discouraged by consumer groups and fish farming organisations. Malachite green and formaldehyde are often used in combination (**Leteux-Meyer mixture**) as an ectoparasiticide particularly for white spot and slime disease. It is effective against secondary fungal overgrowth.

Chloramine is effective against ectoparasites. It aids in the control of fin rot by decreasing the bacterial loading. Chloramine is more toxic in soft water with a low pH. **Sodium chloride** is used as a general antifungal and ectoparasiticide in freshwater fish and for supportive therapy.

Iodine compounds are used for disinfection of fish eggs and also for direct application to lesions. These compounds are toxic to newly hatched fish. **Benzalkonium chloride** is used as a general antibacterial. It acts as a surfactant, removing excess mucus and slime containing parasites and bacteria from the fish. It is also used as a disinfectant of rainbow trout eggs against *Flavobacterium psychrophilum*, which causes rainbow trout fry syndrome. Benzalkonium chloride tends to be more toxic in soft water and lower doses should then be used.

Copper sulphate is used for velvet disease but is potentially toxic in fresh water. It is inadvisable to use this compound where other treatments are available. The dose of copper sulphate in fresh water depends on the water hardness. It should be used with caution if the calcium carbonate level in the water is less than 50 mg/litre such as in soft water.

Potassium permanganate is toxic in water of high pH because manganese dioxide may precipitate onto the gills. Potassium permanganate acts by liberating oxygen and has been used in situations of intensive fish stocking in earth ponds where emergency aeration is needed. This oxidising effect is potentially dangerous and use of this chemical should be restricted to specialists. **Methylthioninium chloride** (methylene blue) is also used in cases of nitrite toxicity; it converts methaemoglobin to haemoglobin. Methylthioninium chloride is absorbed through the skin regardless of the condition of the gills. The agent is easily removed by charcoal filtration. However, it must not be used with biological filter systems.

---

1 ppm	= 1 mg/litre
	= 1 mL/1000 litres
	= 1 mL in 1 m³

After the use of any in-water medication, reliable water test kits should be used to monitor the water chemistry to ensure that appropriate water conditions are maintained. **With the exception of the combined use of formaldehyde and malachite green, water medications should not be used concurrently**. After medication to aquaria or ponds, water changes should be carried out before the use of other chemicals.

BENZALKONIUM CHLORIDE

UK

Indications. External bacterial infections, in particular bacterial gill disease; disinfection
Warnings. Toxicity is increased in soft water
Dose. *By bath*, as indicated in the following table: Where

Dose (ppm)	Duration of treatment
10	5–10 minutes
5	30 minutes
2	60 minutes
1	several hours

the water softness is unknown lower doses should be used and then increased as appropriate.

Ark Klens (Vetark) *UK*
Solution, benzalkonium chloride 12.5%; 250 mL, 1 litre

CHLORAMINE
(Chloramine-T)

There are many chloramines. Chloramine BP is synonymous with chloramine-T. Chloramine-B has similar uses. There are many other complex chloramines, some of which are toxic to fish and are contra-indicated for use in these species

UK

Indications. Ectoparasitic and external bacterial infections; disinfection; aid in control of fin rot
Warnings. Appropriate grade material (see definition above) must be used; avoid contact with metal
Dose. *By bath* (1 hour), dose dependent on pH and water hardness as indicated in the following table:

| pH of water | Dose (ppm) | |
	Soft water	Hard water
6.0	2.5	7.0
6.5	5.0	10.0
7.0	10.0	15.0
7.5	18.0	18.0
8.0	20.0	20.0

Chloramine-T (Vetark) *UK*
Powder, chloramine-T 100%; 50 g, 500 g

COPPER SULPHATE

UK

Indications. Ectoparasitic infections

Warnings. Specialist use only. Potentially toxic in low pH, soft water systems; kills marine invertebrates and elasmobranchs. (Copper can be removed from the system by water changes or activated charcoal 3 g/litre of water being treated)
Dose. Dissolve 400 mg in 1 litre water for stock solution.
By prolonged immersion, 1 mL stock solution/litre. Daily tests should be carried out to maintain a copper concentration of 100–200 micrograms/litre for at least 10 days. Water changes should be carried out if the copper-concentration rises. In fresh water, care needs to be taken because the dose depends on water hardness.

FORMALDEHYDE SOLUTION

Formaldehyde is available as formaldehyde solution (formalin) which is diluted before use, the percentage strength being expressed in terms of formaldehyde solution rather than formaldehyde (CH_2O). For example, in the UK, formaldehyde solution 3% consists of 3 volumes of Formaldehyde Solution BP diluted to 100 volumes with water and thus contains 1.02 to 1.14% w/w of formaldehyde (CH_2O).

UK

Indications. Ectoparasitic infections
Contra-indications. Should not be mixed with potassium permanganate; fish with gill disease
Warnings. Operators should avoid contact with skin and inhalation of formaldehyde fumes, see notes above. Oxygen depletion is rapid at high temperature. Therefore water-oxygen concentration should be monitored and emergency aeration employed if required.
Dose. Expressed in terms of formaldehyde solution 35–40%
By bath, 250 ppm (high pH) or 170 ppm (low pH), for 30 to 60 minutes
By prolonged immersion, 20 ppm for 12 hours

USA

Indications. Ectoparasitic infections
Dose. 170–250 ppm

Paracide-F (Argent) *USA*
Solution, formaldehyde 37%, for *salmon, trout, catfish, bass, bluegill*

FORMALDEHYDE and MALACHITE GREEN SOLUTION
(Leteux-Meyer mixture)

A stock solution containing malachite green 3.3 g/litre in formaldehyde solution 35–40%

UK

Indications. Fungal and ectoparasitic infections, particularly *Ichthyophthirius* infections
Contra-indications. Warnings. See under Malachite green and Formaldehyde solution
Dose. *By bath*, 25 ppm for 1 hour

By prolonged immersion, 15 ppm given as 3 treatments at 3–4 day intervals for *Ichthyophthirius* infections

IODINE COMPOUNDS

UK

Indications. Disinfection of fish eggs; cleaning wounds
Warnings. Toxic to unfertilised ova and live fish
Dose. See preparation details

Buffodine (Evans Vanodine) *UK*
Solution, iodine 1%; 1 litre
Dose. *Eggs*: *by bath*, 10 mL/litre for 10 minutes. Rinse ova thoroughly in clean water

Tamodine (Vetark) *UK*
Solution, povidone-iodine 0.75%; 250 mL, 1 litre
For topical application only

Tamodine-E (Vetark) *UK*
Solution, available iodine 1.6%; 250 mL, 1 litre
Dose. *Eggs*: *by bath*, 3 mL/litre for 10 minutes. Rinse ova thoroughly in clean water

Wescodyne (Novartis) *UK*
Solution, available iodine 1.6%; 25 litres
Dose. *Eggs*: *by bath*, 3 mL/litre for 10 minutes. Rinse ova thoroughly in clean water

MALACHITE GREEN (Zinc-free)

UK

Indications. Fungal and some ectoparasitic infections; fungal infections on eggs
Contra-indications. Toxic to Tetras and scaleless fish, may be toxic to small marine fish
Warnings. See notes above concerning residues. Toxicity resulting from blockage of cellular respiration occurs due to overdosage
Dose. *Fish*: *by dip*, 50–60 ppm for 10–30 seconds
By bath, 1–2 ppm for 30–60 minutes (the higher dose should only be used for large fish kept in hard water, see notes above)
By prolonged immersion, 0.1 ppm for 30–96 hours
Eggs: *by bath*, 0.5 ppm for 1 hour

METHYLTHIONINIUM CHLORIDE
(Methylene blue)

UK

Indications. Ectoparasitic and fungal infections
Contra-indications. Toxic to scaleless fish; should not be used in tanks with bacterial filters
Dose. Dissolve 10 g methylthioninium chloride in 1 litre water for stock solution.
By prolonged immersion, 0.2–0.4 mL stock solution/litre. Dose may be doubled with care

POTASSIUM PERMANGANATE

UK

Indications. Ectoparasitic infections, emergency oxygenation

Warnings. See notes above
Dose. Treatment.
By bath, 5 ppm for 1 hour
By dip, 10 ppm for 10–40 seconds. If organic load is high, repeat treatment after 24 hours
Emergency aeration.
By permanent bath, 2 ppm or 3–4 ppm if a high organic load is present

SODIUM CHLORIDE (Iodine-free)

UK

Indications. Fungal and ectoparasitic infections in freshwater fish; osmotic support for stressed or diseased freshwater fish
Contra-indications. Galvanised zinc containers
Dose. *By bath*, 10 000–15 000 ppm for 20 minutes
By dip, 20 000–30 000 ppm (2–3 kg/100 litres) until fish show signs of distress

Hormonal preparations authorised for fish are available. Buserelin (see section 8.1.2), a synthetic analogue of gonadotrophin-releasing hormone, is used to facilitate stripping in male and female rainbow trout and to reduce mortality due to egg binding.
Immunomodulators are available from various suppliers.
Anaesthetics should preferably be administered to fish after they have been starved for 12 to 14 hours. Constant aeration and a recovery tank of clean water should be available in case the fish become too deeply anaesthetised. If this occurs fish should be pushed through the water manually so that fresh water passes across their gills in an antero-posterior direction. Thumb/finger pressure ventrally between the operculae will usually open the fish's mouth and flare the operculae, therefore facilitating artificial ventilation. Excessive water flow in the wrong direction may severely damage the delicate structure of the gills.
A few fish are anaesthetised as a sample group. Sedation or anaesthesia should take 1 to 3 minutes to develop. Fish placed in a clean tank following anaesthesia usually recover within 2 to 3 minutes.
The anaesthetics most commonly used in fish are tricaine mesilate, benzocaine, and phenoxyethanol. They are used for tranquilisation of fish for transportation, weighing, examination or minor procedures such as treating a surface lesion, and for anaesthesia before drug administration by injection, for example vaccination. Sedative doses may be given by merely reducing the amount of anaesthetic which is placed in the bath to half the anaesthetic dose. For transportation one-fifth of the anaesthetic dose is used.
Tricaine mesilate may reduce the pH of soft water to about 3.8, which may cause stress to fish. The anaesthetic solution should be prepared using the type and composition of water normally needed for the fish species to be treated. **Benzocaine** should be dissolved in an organic solvent before use (see below).

BENZOCAINE

UK
Indications. Sedation and anaesthesia of fish
Warnings. Care should be taken when handling the organic solvent. Solutions should be stored protected from light
Dose. Dissolve 40 g benzocaine in 1 litre ethanol or acetone (benzocaine 40 mg/mL) stock solution.
By bath, 0.6–1.2 mL stock solution/litre

PHENOXYETHANOL

UK
Indications. Sedation and anaesthesia of fish
Warnings. May elute toxins from activated charcoal filters; solidifies below 5°C
Dose. *Fish*: *by bath*, 0.1–0.5 mL/litre
By prolonged immersion, 0.1 mL/litre for prolonged sedation

TRICAINE MESILATE
(Tricaine mesylate)

UK
Indications. Sedation and anaesthesia of fish
Contra-indications. Should not be used for certain tropical fish
Warnings. Solution should not be exposed to direct sunlight
Dose. *Fish*: *by bath*, 25–100 mg/litre

PML **MS-222** (Thomson & Joseph) *UK*
Powder, tricaine mesilate 100%, for *fish*; 25 g, 100 g
Withdrawal Periods. *Fish*: slaughter 10 days

USA
Indications. Sedation and anaesthesia of fish
Dose. *Fish*: *by bath*, 100–120 mg/litre

Finquel (Argent) *USA*
Powder, soluble, tricaine mesilate 100%, for *fish, frogs, salamanders*
Withdrawal Periods. *Fish*: slaughter 21 days

Viral conditions. Increased prevalence of many notifiable viral diseases is now seen. Infectious pancreatic necrosis (IPN) is classically a disease of first-feeding rainbow trout fry. The disease is often stress mediated and mortality can occur from overcrowding and transportation. This viral disease is characterised by skin darkening, inappetence, ascites, and exophthalmos. Although the virus has been isolated many times in Atlantic salmon, its involvement in clinical disease is unclear. Transmission is horizontal and, probably, vertical.

Infectious haemopoietic necrosis (IHN) is a viral disease affecting mainly very young fish with the highest losses occurring at temperatures over 10°C where morbidity can reach 100% of the population. Clinical signs include erratic swimming patterns, skin darkening, ascites, and exophthalmia. Haemorrhages may be seen on the fins and head with the fish appearing anaemic. Transmission is both horizontal and vertical.

Viral haemorrhagic septicaemia (VHS) is an acute to chronic disease occuring in rainbow trout but also seen in other species. The disease has been diagnosed in turbot in the UK. In the acute form, the fish are anaemic with extensive haemorrhages, exophthalmia, and skin darkening. The chronic form is characterised by very dark fish with pronounced ascites. Outbreaks are usually a continuum between the acute and chronic types. Transmission is only horizontal and so eradication can be achieved by using clean stocks.

Infectious salmon anaemia (ISA) caused by an orthomyxo-type (envelope) virus has been diagnosed on a number of marine salmon farms in Scotland. Anaemia, ascites, ocular haemorrhages and necrotic and haemorrhagic lesions in the liver are seen. Under UK law, large numbers of in-contact healthy fish must be slaughtered with the few affected fish.

Spring viraemia of carp (SVC) is a viral disease endemic in a number of European countries. The disease has occurred in the UK due to importation of infected stock. SVC is known to infect common carp and varieties such as koi as well as other ornamental species including goldfish. Strict importation controls are required for farmed and ornamental fish together with veterinary inspection and quarantine. Clinical signs of this disease are variable.

Ornamental fish

Management. Correct management is the most important aspect of maintaining ornamental fish health because the fish are kept in a confined body of water. Improving environmental conditions alone will often aid recovery without the need for drug therapy. Metabolic wastes and their products should be monitored regularly every two weeks (and more frequently if water conditions are poor). Simple and reliable test kits for ammonia, nitrite, nitrate, and pH are available from aquatic suppliers.

To limit the occurence of toxicity, the Ornamental Aquatic Trade Association (OATA) recommends the following concentrations:

ammonia (free)	< 0.01 mg/litre
nitrite	< 0.125 mg/litre
nitrate	< 40 mg/litre
oxygen (dissolved)	> 5.5 mg/litre.

Some fish species will have other minimum requirements for pH, water hardness, and salinity. Nitrifying bacteria in the environment and filter systems remove ammonia and nitrite but take several weeks to reach sufficient concentration in a new facility. These beneficial bacteria must be considered when adding any antibacterial medication to the water. High concentrations of ammonia and nitrite are toxic to fish while raised concentrations are physiologically stressful and may compromise the fish's natural resistance to infection and disease. Frequent water changes (30% every 2 to 3 days) may be required to improve water quality and reduce the chemical concentrations to acceptable levels. The addition of salt (2 g/litre) may benefit freshwater species in poor water conditions while water changes are taking place.

Many other chemicals are equally harmful to fish but may prove difficult to detect. Water changes should be performed if environmental poisoning is suspected, in which case, typically, all fish will be affected and the onset of clinical signs is sudden.

Raising the water temperature to 20°C with submersible electric heaters will benefit many cold-water species because their rate of metabolism and recovery from disease is related to ambient water temperature.

The clinical signs of many diseases that affect ornamental fish are similar and it is important to establish a cause where possible and identify disease agents. Parasites are always present on fish but stress often results in the parasites multiplying to a sufficient concentration so as to cause disease.

Attention to water quality and husbandry is the primary consideration in the management of diseases of ornamental fish

---

Drug administration. The operator should aim to use the least stressful method of treatment to achieve the therapeutic concentration of medication. Ornamental fish may be treated by the following methods: in-water medication (short dip or permanent bath), oral medication (in feed or by gavage), intramuscular injection, or topical application.

In-water medication is usually employed for the treatment of fungal infections and ectoparasites. This may involve short-timed dips in a strong chemical solution or a permanent bath of low-dose medication in a tank or pond. Where ultra-violet sterilizers are in use, these should be switched off when using some water treatments. Activated carbon or ozone should not be used in filters during medication.

There are several methods to make home-made in-feed medication for ornamental fish: gelatin solution may be mixed with the drug, then applied to the feed, and then allowed to solidify. Alternatively the feed may be dampened with a solution containing water-soluble drugs and then allowed to dry or the drug may be mixed with vegetable oil and then used to coat the feed.

Many fish are fastidious eaters and may prove difficult to treat orally. Commercial fish flake or pellet food medicated with oxolinic acid can be obtained from Sinclair (UK) on receipt of a MFS.

Antibacterials are more effective and commonly administered by intramuscular injection. The needle should be carefully angled so as not to damage or remove scales when injecting. Sites for injection vary according to personal preference but injections are usually given into the flank above the lateral line. Due to species differences in anatomy, it is not recommended that medication is administered by intraperitoneal injection in ornamental fish.

Topical preparations are often applied after debridement of skin wounds under general anaesthesia. Preparations used include skin disinfectants such as povidone-iodine, and topical antibacterials for example Panolog Ointment

(Novartis). This may be followed by application of a protective sealant for example, Ⓗ Orabase (ConvaTec)

Antibacterial therapy. The most common bacteria causing disease in ornamental fish are Gram-negative rods such as *Aeromonas*, *Pseudomonas*, *Vibrio*, *Flavobacterium*, and *Edwardsiella*. These bacteria are commonly associated with acute septicaemia and ulcerative skin lesions. *Nocardia* and *Mycobacteria* cause systemic chronic granulomata. The latter is a zoonotic disease. Ulcer disease is caused by atypical *Aeromonas salmonicida* and affects cyprinids such as carp and goldfish. The organism is a variant of the one that causes furunculosis in salmonids (see section 18.8.3).

Doses of antibacterials for ornamental fish are listed in Table 19. Because of increasing problems of bacterial resistance, it may be necessary to take samples for bacterial culture and sensitivity tests. Although results may not be available for 5 to 14 days, treatment should be instigated immediately to limit the severity and spread of the disease. Oral antibacterials are often administered for up to 3 weeks. Fish are given approximately 1 to 5% of their body-weight per day as medicated feed. Therapy is administered by injection to fish that are not feeding, are of suitable size and value, and to initiate treatment that is continued by oral medication. Injections may be repeated 3 to 4 times and may require anaesthesia. However, this is stressful and it may be preferable to attempt feeding oral antibacterials.

There are few antibacterial preparations authorised for use in ornamental fish in the UK. However, these species may be considered as 'minor or exotic species' under *The Medicines (Restrictions on the Administration of Veterinary Medicinal Products) Regulations 1994* (SI 1994/2987). Therefore, the final choice of drug usually depends on antibacterial resistance, availability of a suitable formulation, and palatability, where applicable.

The administration of antibacterials via the water is problematic. Small fish respond quite well and may be too small to inject. However in large fish, although treatment may appear to be clinically effective particularly where skin lesions are part of the condition, drugs may not be adequately absorbed and the condition may not be resolved. Concentrated or pure drugs should be used wherever possible to avoid potential water chemistry problems due to other agents in formulated preparations. Where pure preparations are not commercially available, it may be possible to obtain the drug directly from the manufacturer.

Attention to environmental conditions is important because correct treatment may prove ineffective unless water quality is adequate

---

In general, treatment with in-water antibacterials or methylthioninium chloride (methylene blue) should not be carried out in tanks with biological filters. Although some drugs are claimed not to disturb biological filters, many do so depending on the dose used. It is preferable to administer the treatment in a quarantine tank without filtration but with appropriate monitoring of water quality and water changes.

This will allow removal of the fish in case of accidental overdose.

Benzalkonium chloride, acriflavine, proflavine hemisulphate, and chloramine are used for external bacterial infections.

Parasiticidal and antifungal therapy. The common external protozoal infections of freshwater fish include white spot caused by *Ichthyophthirius multifiliis*; slime disease due to *Chilodonella*, *Ichthyobodo* (*Costia*), and Trichodinids; velvet disease caused by *Oodinium* spp.; and secondary infection of skin wounds with *Epistylis*. Other ectoparasites causing lesions include flukes such as *Gyrodactylus* (body fluke), which attach onto the skin and *Dactylogyrus* (gill fluke), which affect the gills. The crustacean parasites include the anchor worm *Lernaea* and the fish louse *Argulus*, which cause localised damage to the skin, and the gill maggot *Ergasilus*. The fish leech *Piscicola* is found in fresh and salt water. *Saprolegnia* (cotton wool fungus) is a common fungal infection in fish that usually develops from secondary invasion of lesions on the skin and gills. *Dermocystidium* is a fungal-like pathogen which affects the skin and gills.

The flagellate protozoan *Hexamita* infects the skin and the gut. Various microsporidia and myxosporidia are found internally in a wide variety of ornamental fish. The roundworms *Camallanus* and *Capillaria* may infect freshwater tropical fish. The tapeworm *Bothriocephalus* is occasionally found in the gastro-intestinal tract of carp. Doses of endoparasiticides for ornamental fish are listed in Table 20.

External parasitic and fungal infections affecting ornamental fish are usually treated by in-water medication. Fish should be starved before any treatment because this reduces their metabolic rate and the organic loading of water from food and faeces, which increases the oxygen demand. Initially only a few fish in a group, as a representative sample, should be treated. After observing these fish for good recovery over a few hours, the remaining fish can be treated similarly. Adequate aeration should always be provided in treatment tanks because some medications reduce dissolved oxygen, for example formaldehyde. Temporary treatment tanks may not be available for tropical fish and their capture and handling may be excessively stressful. Therefore medication is often administered directly into the tank. In general, when medicating ornamental fish, treatment should always begin at the lower end of a dose range, increasing as necessary. When treating fish in soft water or at low pH, low doses should be used because chemicals are more toxic under these conditions.

Many different chemical treatments are used for ectoparasitic and fungal infections (see Prescribing for farmed fish for information on individual chemicals). When treating ornamental fish the volume of diluted chemical required may be small and difficult to titrate correctly. Therefore it is preferable to advise the use of a proprietary preparation. There are many commercial preparations available which contain one or several ingredients and are recommended by the manufacturer for various conditions. **Proprietary preparations for ornamental fish should be the initial choice of treatment**. Complete eradication of the parasite may involve repeated treatments to kill resistant stages, for example eggs, and treatment of the environment to remove free-swimming parasites.

Proprietary preparations and the manufacturer's indications are listed below in alphabetical order. Although these preparations have been used for years by the aquarist, most of the products do not have a marketing authorisation. Manufacturer recommendations for conditions such as the treatment of viral infections, systemic bacterial infections, and lice infestation may not be able to be substantiated. Cases that fail to respond to these proprietary preparations for ornamental fish may be treated with chemicals such as listed in Prescribing for farmed fish.

After in-water medication, reliable water test kits should be used to monitor the water chemistry to ensure that appropriate water conditions are maintained. Following the addition of a medicament to aquaria or ponds, water changes should be carried out before the use of other chemicals.

Anaesthetics for fish are discussed under Prescribing for farmed fish. Great care must be taken to allow for species variation in tolerance to the anaesthetic agent. Efficacy and toxicity are also influenced by variations in water conditions and quality. Due to the anatomy of some species (for example some marine fish and eels which have a soft gill cover), assistance may be required during recovery and clean water should be flushed through the mouth.

Euthanasia of ornamental fish is carried out by using an overdose of anaesthetic followed by one of the following methods: severing the spinal cord just behind the gill covers, a sharp blow to the head using a blunt instrument, or administration of a lethal dose of pentobarbital into the heart or intravenously into the caudal vein found ventral to the vertebrae of the peduncle. In the absence of anaesthetics commonly used in fish, isoflurane at a dose of 5 mL/litre, or clove oil at a dose of 10 drops/litre have been used; their use has not been fully evaluated

Other drugs. Vitamin deficiencies are uncommon in species fed on commercial manufactured diets which have added vitamins and minerals. However, dietary deficiencies may arise in fish fed on a limited variety of natural foodstuffs. Compound multivitamin and mineral preparations for fish are available (see section 16.7).

Immuno-modulators are available from various suppliers. They may be given alone or in conjunction with antibacterials. Their main use has been in the fish farming industry but they are now incorporated into some commercial ornamental fish feeds.

Viral conditions. Carp pox and lymphocystis are viral diseases caused by Cyprinid herpesvirus (CHV) and an iridovirus, respectively. CHV causes smooth raised hyperplastic lesions, which resemble drops of candle wax on the skin of carp such as koi. It is not fatal, rarely causes secondary health problems, and occasionally resolves spontaneously. Usually only one or two fish are affected. There is no treatment. Lymphocystis causes similar discrete lesions due to hypertrophy of dermal fibroblasts, which swell to about 1 mm in diameter and frequently cluster to form larger masses up to 1 cm in size. Morbidity, clinical pattern, and lack of treatment is similar to carp pox but lymphocystis mainly affects tropical marine fish. Spring viraemia of carp is known to infect common carp and varieties such as koi as well as other ornamental species including goldfish; it is a notifiable disease (see Prescribing for farmed fish).

Proprietary preparations for ornamental fish

There are many preparations available. This is not a comprehensive list. This list contains preparations for which information on active ingredients is available from the manufacturer. It is preferable to use preparations for which the active ingredients are known in order to limit potential problems of toxicity in the operator, fish, and invertebrates.

UK

Indications. See preparation details
Contra-indications. Side-effects. Warnings. See monographs under Farmed fish, manufacturer's information, and preparation details
Dose. A measure is provided with many products, see manufacturer's instructions for dosage details

ACE-High (Vetark) *UK*
See section 16.7 for preparation details
Indications. Conditions requiring compound mineral and multivitamin supplement

Acriflavine (PPI, UK Pond Products) *UK*
Liquid, acriflavine, for *pond fish*; 250 mL, 500 mL, 1 litre
Indications. External bacterial, fungal, and protozoal infections

Aquarium Care Fungus (NT Labs.) *UK*
Liquid, malachite green, for *aquarium fish*
Indications. Fungal and ectoparasitic infections

Aquarium Care White Spot (NT Labs.) *UK*
Liquid, acetic acid, for *freshwater aquarium fish*
Indications. Protozoal infections (*Ichthyophthirius, Costia, Chilodonella, Oodinium*)

POM **Aquinox** (Vericore AP) *UK*
See Farmed fish for preparation details
Indications. Oxolinic acid-sentitive bacterial infections

Ark-Klens (Vetark) *UK*
Liquid, benzalkonium chloride, for *pond fish*; 250 mL, 1 litre
Indications. External bacterial infections
Comments. Harmful to filters; use half dosage in soft water

Bacterial Terminator (Sinclair) *UK*
Liquid, allantoin, formaldehyde, magnesium sulphate, sodium chloride, for *freshwater aquarium fish*; 150 mL, 1 litre
Indications. External bacterial and fungal infections

Bacta-pure (UK Pond Products) *UK*
Liquid, acriflavine, aminoacridine, formaldehyde, for *pond fish*; 250 mL, 1 litre, 5 litres
Indications. External bacterial and fluke infections
Comments. May cause skin sensitisation by skin contact, operators should avoid skin contact and inhalation of product

Bactocide (NT Lab.) *UK*
Liquid, acriflavine, aminoacridine hydrochloride, formaldehyde, for *freshwater and marine aquarium fish*; 125 mL, 500 mL
Indications. External bacterial, fluke, and *Oodinium* infections

Baktopur (Sera; distributed by John Allan) *UK*
Liquid, acriflavine, 1,3-butylglycol, methylthioninium chloride, for *freshwater aquarium fish*; 15 mL, 100 mL, 500 mL
Indications. External bacterial infections
Comments. Harmful to filters

Chloramine-T (Vetark) *UK*
Powder, chloramine-T, for *pond fish*; 50 g
Indications. External bacterial, protozoal (*Ichthyobodo, Ichthyophthirius*) and fluke (*Gyrodactylus*) infections
Comments. Use higher dosage in high pH and hard water

Costapur (Sera; distributed by John Allan) *UK*
Liquid, malachite green, potassium iodide, for *freshwater and marine aquarium fish*; 15 mL, 100 mL, 500 mL
Indications. Protozoal infections (*Ichthyophthirius, Costia, Chilodonella*)
Comments. Harmful to marine invertebrates

Cyprinopur (Sera; distributed by John Allan) *UK*
Liquid, 1,3 dihydroxybenzol, ethanol, phenol, for *pond fish*
Indications. Treatment of open wounds and ulcers

Diseasolve Aquarium Antiseptic (NT Lab.) *UK*
Liquid, acriflavine, methylthioninium chloride, for *aquarium fish and pond fish*; 150 mL, 1 litre
Indications. External bacterial and protozoal infections

Diseasolve for ponds (NT Lab.) *UK*
Liquid, acriflavine, methylthioninium chloride, for *ornamental pond fish*; 250 mL, 1 litre

Ectopur (Sera; distributed by John Allan) *UK*
Powder, sodium borate, sodium chloride, sodium perborate, for *freshwater and marine aquarium fish*; 100 g, 2.5 kg
Indications. Fungal and ectoparasitic infections

Fin-Rot (NT Lab.) *UK*
Liquid, acriflavine, aminoacridine hydrochloride, formaldehyde, for *freshwater aquarium fish*; 125 mL, 500 mL
Indications. External bacterial and fluke infections

Fin Rot Terminator (Sinclair) *UK*
Liquid, silver protein, mild, for *freshwater aquarium fish*; 150 mL, 1 litre
Indications. External bacterial infections
Comments. Harmful to marine fish; best at 10–30°C

Formaldehyde 30% Solution (UK Pond Products) *UK*
Liquid, formaldehyde, for *pond fish*; 250 mL, 1 litre, 5 litres
Indications. Ectoparasitic infections
Comments. May cause skin sensitisation by skin contact, causes burns

Formalachite (PPI) *UK*
Liquid, formaldehyde, malachite green, for *pond fish*; 250 mL, 500 mL, 1 litre
Indications. Protozoal (*Ichthyophthirius, Costia, Trichodina*) and fluke infections
Comments. May cause skin sensitisation by skin contact, operators should avoid skin contact and inhalation of product

Formalin (PPI) *UK*
Liquid, formaldehyde, for *pond fish*; 250 mL, 500 mL, 1 litre
Indications. Protozoal (*Ichthyophthirius, Costia, Trichodina*) and fluke infections

Fungal Terminator (Sinclair) *UK*
Liquid, 2-phenoxyethanol, for *freshwater aquarium fish*; 150 mL, 1 litre
Indications. Fungal infections
Comments. Harmful in salt water; best at 16–27°C

Fungicide (NT Lab.) *UK*
Liquid, 2-phenoxyethanol, for *aquarium fish*; 10 mL
Indications. Fungal infections
Comments. Harmful to filters

Gill-Pure (UK Pond Products) *UK*
Liquid, benzalkonium chloride, for *pond fish*; 250 mL, 1 litre, 5 litres
Indications. External bacterial and parasitic infections
Comments. Harmful to filters; use half dosage in soft water

Ichcide (NT Lab.) *UK*
Liquid, formaldehyde, malachite green, for *freshwater aquarium fish*; 125 mL, 500 mL
Indications. Fungal and protozoal (*Ichthyophthirius, Chilodonella*) infections
Comments. May cause skin sensitisation by skin contact, operators should avoid skin contact and inhalation of product

Koi Bath (PPI) *UK*
Liquid, benzalkonium chloride, stabiliser, aloe vera, witch hazel, for *pond fish*; 250 mL, 500 mL, 1 litre
Indications. External bacterial, and parasitic infections of the gills

Koi Care Acriflavin (NT Lab.) *UK*
Liquid, acriflavine, for *pond fish*; 250 mL, 500 mL, 1 litre
Indications. External bacterial infections

Koi Care Formaldehyde 30% Solution (NT Lab.) *UK*
Liquid, formaldehyde, for *pond fish*; 250 mL, 500 mL, 1 litre
Indications. Protozoal (*Ichthyophthirius, Trichodina, Costia*) and fluke infections

Koi Care F-M-G (NT Lab.) *UK*
Liquid, formaldehyde, malachite green, for *koi, goldfish*
Indications. Fungal or parasitic infections
Comments. Switch off ultraviolet light; harmful to orfe, rudd, tench, and sterlets; may cause skin sensitisation by skin contact, operators should avoid skin contact and inhalation of product

Koi Care Gill-Wash (NT Lab.) *UK*
Liquid, benzalkonium chloride, for *pond fish*; 250 mL, 500 mL, 1 litre
Indications. External bacterial infections of the gills
Comments. Harmful to filters; use half dosage in soft water

Koi Care Koi Calm (NT Lab.) *UK*
Liquid, clove oil; 30 mL
Indications. Use as a calmative
Comments. Harmful to skin

Koi Care Malachite Green Solution (NT Lab.) *UK*
Liquid, malachite green, for *pond fish*; 250 mL, 500 mL, 1 litre
Indications. Fungal and external parasitic infections
Comments. Irritant

Koi Care Ulcer Swab (NT Lab.) *UK*
Liquid, benzalkonium chloride, povidone, for *koi and other pond fish*; 30 mL, 125 mL
Indications. Cleanser and disinfectant for skin wounds
Comments. Topical use only; best used in conjunction with Koi Care Wound Seal (NT Lab.)

Koi Care Wound Seal (NT Lab.) *UK*
Liquid, zinc cream, for *koi and other pond fish*; 30 mL, 125 mL
Indications. Used to seal wounds and assist healing
Comments. Topical use only; best used in conjunction with Koi Care Ulcer Swab (NT Lab.)

Malachite (PPI) *UK*
Liquid, malachite green, for *pond fish*; 250 mL, 500 mL, 1 litre
Indications. Fungal, parasitic, and some bacterial infections

Malachite Green 2% Solution (UK Pond Products) *UK*
Liquid, malachite green, for *pond fish*; 250 mL, 1 litre, 5 litres
Indications. Fungal and some parasitic infections
Comments. May cause skin sensitisation by skin contact

Medifin (Tetra) *UK*
Liquid, formaldehyde, malachite green, for *pond fish*; 250 mL, 500 mL
Indications. External bacterial, fungal, fluke, and protozoal infections
Comments. May cause skin sensitisation by skin contact, operators should avoid skin contact and inhalation of product

Methylene Blue (Sinclair) *UK*
Liquid, methylthioninium chloride, for *freshwater aquarium fish*
Indications. Fungal, fluke and protozoal infections
Comments. Harmful to filters; harmful to marine fish and plants; best at 10–30°C

Mycopur (Sera; distributed by John Allan) *UK*
Liquid, acriflavine, copper chloride, copper sulphate, for *freshwater aquarium fish*; 15 mL, 100 mL, 500 mL
Indications. Fungal infections, fluke infestations

Myxocide (NT Lab.) *UK*
Liquid, benzalkonium chloride, for *aquarium fish*; 25 mL
Indications. External bacterial infections; disinfectant
Comments. Harmful to filters

Nishi-Cure Anti-Fin Rot (Nishikoi) *UK*
Liquid, acriflavine, aminoacridine hydrochloride, formaldehyde, for *pond fish*; 250 mL
Indications. External bacterial infections

Nishi-Cure Anti-Fungus (Nishikoi) *UK*
Liquid, malachite green, for *pond fish*; 250 mL
Indications. Fungal infections
Comments. Use above 6°C

Nishi-Cure Anti-White Spot (Nishikoi) *UK*
Liquid, formaldehyde, malachite green, for *pond fish*; 250 mL
Indications. Protozoal infections
Comments. May cause skin sensitisation by skin contact, operators should avoid skin contact and inhalation of product; use above 6°C

Oodinopur A (Sera; distributed by John Allan) *UK*
Liquid, copper chloride, copper sulphate, for *freshwater and marine aquarium fish*; 15 mL, 500 mL
Indications. Protozoal (*Oodinium*) infection
Comments. Harmful to marine invertebrates

Paracide (NT Lab.) *UK*
Liquid, citric acid, cupric sulphate, formaldehyde, for *freshwater and marine aquarium fish*; 125 mL, 500 mL
Indications. Protozoal infections including *Oodinium, Cryptocaryon*
Comments. Harmful to invertebrates

Para-Pure (UK Pond Products) *UK*
Liquid, formaldehyde, malachite green, for *pond fish*; 250 mL, 1 litre, 5 litres
Indications. Fungal and protozoal infections
Comments. May be applied topically for *Argulus, Lernaea*; may cause skin sensitisation by skin contact, operators should avoid skin contact and inhalation of product

Pond Care Bacterad (NT Lab.) *UK*
Liquid, acriflavine, aminoacridine hydrochloride, formaldehyde, for *pond fish*; 250 mL, 1 litre
Indications. External bacterial and fluke infections
Comments. May cause skin sensitisation by skin contact, operators should avoid skin contact and inhalation of product

Pond Care Clear Gills (NT Lab.) *UK*
Liquid, benzalkonium chloride, for *pond fish*; 125 mL, 500 mL
Indications. Decongestant bath for gill disease
Comments. Harmful to filters

Pond Care Erad-Ick (NT Lab.) *UK*
Liquid, formaldehyde, malachite green, for *pond fish*; 250 mL, 1 litre
Indications. Protozoal infections including *Ichthyophthirius, Chilodonella, Costia*
Comments. May cause skin sensitisation by skin contact, operators should avoid skin contact and inhalation of product

Pond Care Fin-Rot (NT Lab.) *UK*
Liquid, acriflavine, aminoacridine hydrochloride, formaldehyde, for *pond fish*; 125 mL, 500 mL
Indications. External bacterial and fluke infections
Comments. May cause skin sensitisation by skin contact, operators should avoid skin contact and inhalation of product

Pond Care Fungus (NT Lab.) *UK*
Liquid, malachite green, for *pond fish*; 125 mL, 500 mL
Indications. Fungal and ectoparasitic infections

Pond Care White Spot (NT Lab.) *UK*
Liquid, formaldehyde, malachite green, for *pond fish*; 125 mL, 500 mL
Indications. Protozoal infections including *Ichthyophthirius, Chilodonella, Costia, Oodinium*

Pond Pride No 3 – Parasite Control (Sinclair) *UK*
Liquid, acriflavine, malachite green, quinine sulphate, for *pond fish*
Indications. Protozoal infections
Comments. May cause sensitisation by skin contact

Pond Pride No 4 – Fungus Control (Sinclair) *UK*
Liquid, formaldehyde, malachite green, for *pond fish*; 250 mL, 500 mL
Indications. Fungal infections
Comments. May cause skin sensitisation by skin contact, operators should avoid skin contact and inhalation of product

Pond Pride No 5 – Fin and Tail Rot Control (Sinclair) *UK*
Liquid, silver protein, mild, for *pond fish*; 250 mL, 500 mL
Indications. External bacterial infections
Comments. May cause sensitisation by skin contact; may be used topically

Pond Pride No 8 – Open Wound Treatment (Sinclair) *UK*
Liquid, allantoin, formaldehyde, magnesium sulphate, sodium chloride, for *pond fish*; 250 mL, 500 mL
Indications. External bacterial infections
Comments. May cause skin sensitisation by skin contact, operators should avoid skin contact and inhalation of product

Potassium (PPI) *UK*
Liquid, potassium salts, for *pond fish*; 250 mL, 500 mL, 1 litre
Indications. Protozoal infections (*Ichthyophthirius, Trichodina*) anchor worm, fungal infections

Protoban (Vetark) *UK*
Liquid, formaldehyde, malachite green, for *pond fish*; 250 mL, 1 litre
Indications. External bacterial, fluke, and protozoal (*Costia, Trichodina, Chilodonella*) infections
Comments. May cause skin sensitisation by skin contact, operators should avoid skin contact and inhalation of product

Tamodine (Vetark) *UK*
Solution, povidone-iodine, for *all fish species*; 100 mL
Indications. Topical application to skin ulcers and wounds

Tamodine-E (Vetark) *UK*
Liquid, iodophor, for *all fish species*; 250 mL, 1 litre
Indications. Disinfection

TetraMedica ContraSpot (Tetra) *UK*
Liquid, formaldehyde, malachite green, for *freshwater aquarium fish*; 100 mL
Indications. Protozoal and fluke infections
Comments. May cause skin sensitisation by skin contact, operators should avoid skin contact and inhalation of product

TetraMedica FungiStop (Tetra) *UK*
Liquid, collidon, metanil yellow, silver in colloidal form, for *freshwater aquarium fish*; 100 mL
Indications. Fungal infections on fish and eggs
Comments. Not recommended for marine aquaria

TetraMedica General Tonic (Tetra) *UK*
Liquid, acriflavine, aminoacridine, ethacridine lactate, methylthioninium chloride, for *freshwater aquarium fish*; 100 mL
Indications. External bacterial infections

TetraMedica Goldmed-Goldfish Disease Aquarium Treatment (Tetra) *UK*
Liquid, formaldehyde, malachite green, for *aquarium goldfish*; 100 mL
Indications. External bacterial, fungal, fluke, and protozoal infections
Comments. May cause skin sensitisation by skin contact, operators should avoid skin contact and inhalation of product

POM **Tetraplex** (Vericore AP) *UK*
See Farmed fish for preparation details
Indications. Oxytetracycline-sensitive bacterial infections

Velvet Terminator (Sinclair) *UK*
Liquid, cupric sulphate, for *freshwater aquarium fish*; 150 mL, 1 litre
Indications. *Oodinium* infection
Comments. Use half dose for light scaled fish e.g. sharks, loaches; use at 20–30°C

White Spot Terminator (Sinclair) *UK*
Liquid, acriflavine, malachite green, quinine sulphate, for *freshwater aquarium fish*; 150 mL, 1 litre, 2 litres
Indications. Protozoal infections
Comments. Harmful to marine fish; best at 25–30°C

Table 19 Antimicrobial and ectoparasiticidal doses of drugs for ornamental fish[1]

Drug	Dose	Condition
Acriflavine (neutral)	by addition to water, 5–10 mg/L as prolonged bath *or* by addition to water, 500 mg/L daily as 30 minute bath	bacterial, fungal, and ectoparasitic infections
Amoxicillin	by addition to feed, 80 mg/kg body-weight 12.5 mg/kg i.m. as a single dose (formulation to use: long-acting preparation)	bacterial infections
Ampicillin	10 mg/kg i.m. daily	bacterial infections
Benzalkonium chloride	*see* Prescribing for farmed fish	external bacterial infections
Chloramine	*see* Prescribing for farmed fish	external bacterial and ectoparasitic infections
Chloramphenicol	40 mg/kg i.m. daily	bacterial infections
Copper sulfate	*see* Prescribing for farmed fish	ectoparasitic infections
Dimetridazole	by addition to feed, 28 mg/kg body-weight for 10 days by addition to water, 5 mg/litre	protozoal infections
Enrofloxacin	by addition to feed, 10 mg/kg body-weight for 10 days by addition to water, 2 mg/L for 5 days 5–10 mg/kg i.m. on alternate days for 15 days	bacterial infections
Formaldehyde	*see* Prescribing for farmed fish	ectoparasitic infections
Formaldehyde and malachite green mixture	*see* Prescribing for farmed fish	fungal and ectoparasitic infections
Gentamicin[3]	2.5 mg/kg i.m. on alternate days	bacterial infections
Griseofulvin	by addition to water, 10 mg/L as permanent bath by addition to feed, 50 mg/kg body-weight	fungal infections
Ivermectin	100–200 micrograms/kg i.m.	*Lernaea*
Malachite green	*see* Prescribing for farmed fish	fungal and protozoal infections
Mebendazole	1 mg/L as a 24 hour bath	ectoparasitic flukes
Methylthioninium chloride (Methylene blue)	*see* Prescribing for farmed fish	external bacterial, fungal, and ectoparasitic infections
Metronidazole	by addition to water, 7 mg/L (14 mg/L for *Oodinium*) by addition to feed, 10 mg/g feed for 5 days	protozoal infections
Miconazole	10–20 mg/kg i.m.	fungal infections
Neomycin	by addition to water, 50–75 mg/L (sea water) for 24–48 hours	bacterial infections
Oxolinic acid	by addition to feed, 10 mg/kg body-weight[1] (freshwater fish) by addition to feed, 30 mg/kg body-weight (marine fish)	bacterial infections
Oxytetracycline	by addition to water, 13–120 mg/L by addition to feed, 75 mg/kg body-weight[1] 10 mg/kg i.m. as a single dose (formulation to use: long-acting preparation)[2]	bacterial infections
Potassium permanganate	*see* Prescribing for farmed fish	external bacterial and ectoparasitic infections

Table 19 Antimicrobial and ectoparasiticidal doses of drugs for ornamental fish[1](continued)

Drug	Dose	Condition
Praziquantel	2 mg/L as a permanent bath *or* 10 mg/L as 4 hour bath	ectoparasitic flukes
Proflavine hemisulphate	by addition to water, 1 mg/L	mild bacterial infections
Sarafloxacin	10 mg/kg body-weight daily for 10 days	bacterial infections
Sodium chloride	by addition to fresh water, 20–30 g/L as a 15–30 minute bath	adult leeches only
Sulfadiazine + trimethoprim	by addition to feed, 30 mg/kg body-weight 30 mg/kg i.m. on alternate days	bacterial infections
Sulfadoxine + trimethoprim	75 mg/kg i.m. every 4 days (formulation to use: sulfadoxine 62.5 + trimethoprim 12.5 mg/mL)	bacterial infections
Water, fresh	(marine fish) 2–10 minute dip daily for 5 days. Add sufficient sodium bicarbonate to ensure pH equals that of tank water	protozoal infections

[1] drug doses for preparations that have a marketing authorisation for use in ornamental fish in the UK. Therefore, unless marked [1], the drug or doses stated are not authorised for ornamental fish
[2] may cause reaction at injection site with formation of sero-sanguineous fluid filled cavity; may also be immunosuppressive
[3] may cause renal toxicity in some species, for example *Opsanus* sp.

Table 20 Endoparasiticidal doses of drugs for ornamental fish[1]

Drug	Dose	Condition
Fenbendazole	by gavage or addition to feed, 50 mg/kg body-weight daily for 2 days, repeat after 14 days	roundworms
Ivermectin	100–200 micrograms/kg i.m.	roundworms
Levamisole	by addition to water, 5 mg/L as a single dose	roundworms
Mebendazole	by addition to feed, 25–50 mg/kg body-weight weekly for 3 weeks	roundworms
Piperazine	by addition to feed, 10 mg/kg body-weight for 3 days	roundworms
Praziquantel	by gavage, 50 mg/kg as a single dose by addition to feed, 35–125 mg/kg body-weight daily for 3 days 10–25 mg/kg i.m. as a single dose	tapeworms

[1] drug doses for preparations that have a marketing authorisation for use in ornamental fish in the UK. Therefore, unless marked [1], the drug or doses stated are not authorised for ornamental fish

Prescribing for invertebrates

Contributors:
L Jepson, MA, VetMB, CBiol, MIBiol, MRCVS
G F Rendall, BVSc, MRCVS
D L Williams, MA, VetMB, PhD, CertVOphthal, MRCVS

There are many species of invertebrates with diverse environmental, nutritional, and behavioural requirements. Species of economic importance include bees, crustaceans, snails, and silkworms. Others such as spiders and butterflies are kept as pets or for exhibition. Many are used in research, for example leeches and octopuses.

The majority of conditions affecting invertebrates kept in captivity are related to poor husbandry or nutritional deficiencies and thus conditions for which pharmacological intervention is appropriate are generally limited to infectious disease. With the increasing popularity of numerous invertebrates as pets, the growth of commercial snail farming, and the conservation importance of many endangered invertebrate species, further work on disease in these animals and the development of effective chemotherapeutic agents is important.

Many agents used for these animals are not authorised for the target species and are used under the responsibility of the veterinarian who has the animal 'under his care'. COSHH regulations should be adhered to when handling chemicals.

Terrestrial invertebrates

Although considerable work has been undertaken on the diseases of the honey bee *Apis mellifera* (see below) and the silkworm *Bombyx mori* because of their economic importance, little is known about the diseases of terrestrial invertebrates such as arachnids (spiders and scorpions), insects (cockroaches, mantids, and stick insects), myriapods (centipedes and millipedes), crustacea (land and tree crabs), or molluscs (snail species). Invertebrate pathology has concentrated on diseases in which invertebrates act merely as vectors, or on the use of diseases for biological control of pest species. Nevertheless even studies of disease agents used to control invertebrate pests can be useful when aiming to treat endangered species or those kept as pets.

Hygiene and quarantine measures for newly acquired invertebrates are important. Pathogenic viruses such as baculoviridae have been inadvertently introduced via food contamination leading to infection and a diseased animal introduced into a naive captive population can cause significant mortality and morbidity. Chemotherapeutic agents used in the control of insect virus diseases include unconventional treatments such as sub-lethal doses of arsenic sulphide 0.01% given in the feed to reduce the effects of viral disease in silkworms.

Problems occur with the diagnosis of bacterial disease in invertebrates. Firstly, little is known about the normal bacterial flora of many invertebrates and thus evaluation of a bacterial isolate from a lesion is difficult. An organism which is a normal commensal species in an external location can be pathogenic when introduced intracoelomically and as such interpretation of bacteriology should take into account the location of the sample. Many potentially pathogenic bacteria are common saprophytic species and therefore isolation of an organism does not necessarily indicate pathogenicity.

Bacteria such as *Bacillus thuringiensis* are recognised pathogens in some insect colonies. Control by the use of leaves soaked in chlortetracycline or streptomycin has been reported but the quantity of antibacterial ingested is highly variable. The use of antibacterial solutions in spray or preferably in nebulized formulations can be more useful. The inclusion of therapeutic agents in sugar solutions encourages oral uptake but the dose absorbed is unknown. Gram-negative species such as *Aeromonas hydrophila* have been considered important in die-offs of insects and have also been isolated from lesions in species as diverse as scorpions and banana slugs. Extrapolation between widely varying invertebrate species, however, is difficult.

Selection of an appropriate antibacterial for a bacterial infection should rely on bacteriological culture and sensitivity undertaken at the temperature of the environment inhabited by the host species. It may be necessary to ensure that the laboratory utilised can provide such a service. Oral or topical use of oxytetracycline and chlortetracycline has been reported in insects. However topical medicinal ointments designed for ocular or dermatological use, which may appear ideal for surface antibiosis, contain high drug concentrations, and may lead to toxicity if the compound is ingested or absorbed across mucous membranes. A potentiated sulphonamide, such as sulfatroxazole and trimethoprim, may be used in an oral paediatric elixir formulation or by intracoelomic injection of a diluted intravenous preparation. Sulphonamides have been reported as being safe and efficacious in grasshoppers, mealworms, and bees.

While it may appear advantageous to provide dosages for various drugs, unfortunately little work has been undertaken in this area and as such all treatment protocols are highly empirical. It may be assumed that dosage varies with the temperature at which the animals are kept as with other ectothermic species. However, limited data are available on dosage variation. At present, the only controllable factor is the selection of a suitable antibacterial by culture and sensitivity.

A number of fungi may be associated with disease in invertebrates, especially in species kept in humid conditions. Muscardine, caused by *Beauveria bassiana* has been a serious problem in silkworms, but has also been noted in other terrestrial invertebrate colonies. While control is a key feature limiting this disease, some antifungal drugs have been used in the past. Topical ketoconazole or enilconazole may be employed in a spray formulation or painted on, but again concentrations and frequencies of application are empirical.

Mermithid nematodes are seen as parasites in a number of invertebrate species. Trombiculid and erythrid mites parasitise arachnids and insects. In certain cases, such as the mite of the hissing cockroach *Gromphadorina potentosa* a commensal relationship exists and thus infestations with the mite should not be treated. The nematode *Nemihelix bakeri* is reported to cause reduced fecundity in snails such as *Achatina* and *Helix* but no treatment regimens have been suggested except hygiene measures.

For invertebrates infested with mites, treatment can be difficult without risking toxicity to the host species. Although flumethrin-containing acaricidal strips are used by the bee industry (see below) and may be appropriate, the laborious removal of individual mites with an alcohol-moistened cotton wool swab is the recommended treatment in most cases. Infestations of arachnids with acrocerid fly larvae and hymenopteran larval endoparasites are invariably fatal.

Anaesthesia of invertebrates to permit procedures ranging from full examination to invasive surgery is possible. Pain sensation and relief in invertebrates is a poorly researched area. Carbon dioxide 20% in air provides good immobilisation and is also used for artificial insemination in bees. Halothane 5% or preferably isoflurane 1% to 3% give good anaesthesia and are likely to be more humane than carbon dioxide. Hypothermia may be used to facilitate examination but should not be employed for invasive procedures because no analgesia is provided. Snails may be anaesthetised by placing the foot in appropriate solutions of benzocaine, phenoxyethanol, or tricaine mesilate.

Penetrating injuries or limb loss may result in a significant loss of haemolymph. In such cases tissue adhesive may be applied locally, although dysecdysis may occur later. Loss of limb is not necessarily fatal and many arachnids and insects will regenerate lost appendages during successive moults.

Bees

Honeybees, *Apis mellifera*, are kept for the production of honey, beeswax, pollen, royal jelly, venom, and propolis; for the propagation of queen bees and the preparation of new colonies; and for the purpose of pollination of agricultural and horticultural crops. Honeybees are also used in research into, for example the neural tract and giant neurons.

There is limited information available on the diseases and their treatment in bees. Some diseases have low economic value, have been incompletely researched, or the causative agent is unknown.

Bees are susceptible to a number of viral, bacterial, protozoal, fungal, and acarine infections, which affect either the adult bees or their brood. Diseases affecting adults include nosema caused by the microsporidian *Nosema apis*. The disease is spread in the faeces of infected bees. During the warmer period of the year the faeces are discharged away

from the hive and represent no risk to the colony, but in winter and early spring faecal contamination of the inside of the hive may occur if cleansing flights are limited by adverse weather. The young bees on 'house' duties are infected with the organism when cleaning soiled frames. The organism multiplies in the epithelial cells of the midgut producing huge numbers of spores.

'Amoeba disease' is caused by the protozoa *Malpighamoeba mellificae*. The organism encysts in the malpighian tubules, later moving into the ventriculus where it multiplies, becomes flagellated and then invades the malpighian tubules again to form cysts, some or which are discharged through the intestine.

Tracheal mites are acarine mites, *Acarapis woodi*, which live in the trachea behind the first thoracic spiracle. Eggs are laid in the trachea, which hatch, pass through a nymph stage, and when mature may emerge from the spiracle and transfer to other bees. It is believed that they can only enter the spiracle in young bees where the hairs guarding the entrance are still soft. Feeding on haemolymph through the tracheal wall, they have the potential of passing on infections to their host and their presence is usually associated with chronic bee paralysis virus, characterised by angled wings, fluttering, and bloated abdomen.

The larvae of the greater wax moths *Galleria mellonella* (honeybee moths) and the lesser wax moths *Achroia grisella* (*Meliphora grisella*) feed on larval skins and pupal remains together with some wax in the brood combs. Their tunnels are lined with silken threads and frass, which the bees dislike, causing the bees to abandon areas of comb. There may also be mechanical damage to any brood present resulting in the condition called 'bald brood'. In an empty hive, there is complete destruction of the combs, leaving a tangled mass of silk threads, frass, and debris, and probably erosions into the woodwork by the pupae.

Braula coeca ('bee louse') lives on the adult bees, rarely causing any problem. However its larval stages pass along the cappings of the stored honey, producing lines that disfigure the appearance of comb honey. (Subjecting the comb to freezing for a brief period will prevent development of the larvae.)

Chalkbrood is a widespread infection due to the fungus *Ascosphaera apis*. Most hives have a few cells of infected larvae but it can become more extensive if other factors, such as chilling, weaken the brood. The spores germinate in the ventriculus and invade the haemocoel. The larva die just after capping and when exposed by the bees are swollen and chalky white. They then shrink and are removed by the bees and dropped at the front of the hive (known as 'mummies' by beekeepers). Dead larvae are occasionally black due to the presence of fungal fruiting bodies. Stonebrood is a less frequent infection caused by *Aspergillus flavus* or *Aspergillus fumigatus* and is similar to the above.

Sac brood is fairly common and is caused by sac brood virus (SBV), which is able to cause clinical disease apparently without needing a triggering factor. The virus interferes with the production of a chitinase responsible for enabling the separation and sloughing of the skin at the final larval moult. The partially shed skin fills with fluid containing huge amounts of virus particles.

American foul brood (AFB) caused by *Paenibacillus larvae* infection and **European foul brood** (EFB) caused by *Melissococcus pluton* infection **are notifiable diseases in the UK**. The bacteria are passed to the newly hatched larvae by infected nurse bees and the concentration of bacteria increase at different stages dependent on the oxygen:carbon dioxide concentrations. The disease is characterised by death after capping (AFB) or usually before capping (EFB). Dried remnants of the AFB infected larvae are difficult to remove from the comb and the contained spores provide a very durable source of further infections, hence the requirement to destroy by burning any infected material such as frames and combs. EFB is not so persistent and does not form spores but does appear unexpectedly in colonies; current thought is tending to the view that it may persist as a subclinical or latent infection in an otherwise normal colony. Biological control of EFB is being investigated.

Varroosis caused by infestation by the acarine mite, *Varroa jacobsoni* is also a notifiable disease in the UK. A high concentration of varroa mites on the bee brood will result in developmental damage such as deformed wings and abdomens, also abnormal salivary glands so that the emerging bee is unable to carry out normal duties in the hive and the lifespan is shortened. Recent developments for the control of varroosis include pheromones, fungi, and bees resistant to *Varroa* infection.

For many years it has been known that several honeybee viruses persist as inapparent infections, difficult to detect by normal techniques. It has been found that in combination with infections, such as *Varroa jacobsoni* or *Nosema apis*, these viruses can increase to lethal levels. Slow paralysis (SPV) in the UK, acute paralysis virus (APV) in other parts of Europe, deformed wing virus, and cloudy wing virus are associated with varroosis. Kashmir bee virus, a virulent and highly infective bee virus, previously found in *Apis cerana* in Asia and in *A. mellifera* in Australia has been recovered in Canada and the USA and recently in Spain in conjunction with *Varroa* infection. Similarly *Nosema* infections can be associated with black queen cell virus, bee virus Y, and filamentous virus. The latter is common in the UK, fortunately showing little pathogenicity.

Drug administration. Drugs can be administered to bees as powder, in syrup, in gel, by aerosol, in smoke, or by contact with a medicated strip. Fumigation is used to treat combs. Great care should be taken to ensure that the bees utilise the drug immediately rather than store it because the drug may contaminate the honey. This is achieved in the case of medicated sugar syrup by using a slow feeder from which the drug is taken over 2 to 3 days, rather than a rapid feeder which allows the bees to take litres of syrup overnight, which is then likely to be put into the honey super. However, medication should not normally be administered with honey supers still on the hive. There is a risk that certain drugs may accumulate in the wax of the comb and remain potent for a considerable period with little break-down even if the wax is heat processed. This has occured with some varroacidal preparations. Therefore the manufacturer recommends that bee products other than honey, for example comb honey, is not taken for human consumption until the spring following treatment. Transfer to extracted honey is negligible. The duration of treatment specified in the data sheet should not be exceeded.

The formulation of the preparation may affect its stability within the hive, for example oxytetracycline degrades rapidly in aqueous solution but retains potency for several months in sugar syrup. The ambient temperature has a significant effect on the activity of the bees and also affects the vaporisation of chemicals such as formic acid; ambient temperature should be monitored to ensure adequate, but not toxic, concentration of medication.

Few preparations for bees have a UK marketing authorisation; preparations for bees available in other countries may be obtained by veterinarians under a Special Treatment Authorisation from the VMD. The *Medicines (Restrictions on the Administration of Veterinary Medicinal Products) Amendment Regulations 1997* prohibits personal imports of products not authorised in the UK.

Under the *Animal and Animal Products (Examination for Residues and Maximum Residue Limits) Regulations 1997*, bees are considered as food-producing animals. The VMD have indicated that non-medicinal curative substances such as industrial talc, lactic acid, oxalic acid, thymol, other essential oils, homoeopathic treatments, oil of wintergreen, liquid paraffin, and formic acid may be used for bees if such agents are unlikely to be harmful to human health, if transmitted to honey. Frow mixture (containing ligroin, methyl salicylate, nitrobenzene, petrol, and safrol) should not be used.

In the UK, preparations for bees are available from drug manufacturers and also bee equipment suppliers including:

- Maisemore Apiaries
- Exeter Bee Supplies
- Thorne (beehives)
- Vita
- Kemlea Bee Supplies
- Beesy
- Loveridge.

ACETIC ACID

UK

Indications. Eggs and larvae of wax moths, *Nosema apis*, *Malpighamoeba mellificae*

Warnings. Concentrated solutions are irritant to skin; operators should take care not to inhale fumes; corrosive to metal hive parts

Dose. *As fumigant*, soak pads of cotton wool in 150 mL acetic acid 80% and place between hive bodies full of combs in winter storage. Ventilate the combs before offering them to the bees

BACILLUS THURINGIENSIS

UK

Indications. Infestation of comb by the larvae of the greater wax moth *Galleria mellonella*

Warnings. Not effective against the lesser waxmoth. Store the suspension at <20°C, do not freeze

Dose. Dilute 1 volume in 19 volumes water. *By spraying*, 10 mL of diluted solution on each comb surface, ensuring penetration of the open cells. Apply in autumn before storing the combs, or in spring prior to placing on the hive.

Certan (Swarm, distributed by Thorne) *UK*

ESSENTIAL OILS

Essential oils such as oil of citronella and oil of sandalwood act by repelling the mites from beeswax that has oil incorporated. Other oils, especially oil of cinnamon, are toxic to mites.

FORMIC ACID

Formic acid is a liquid at less than 50°C, is soluble in water and honey, is a small molecule, and penetrates porous wax cappings. Therefore it may be used in the treatment of sealed brood.

UK

Indications. Control of mites *Acarapis woodii* and *Varroa jacobsoni*, bee louse *Braula coeca*, wax moth larvae

Side-effects. A few bees may be killed and bees emerging from sealed cells and queens appear to be at greatest risk

Warnings. Corrosive, causes severe burns to skin and dangerous if inhaled; reported to be cytotoxic. Operator should take adequate precautions; remove honey spurs before treatment

Dose. By vaporiser, formic acid 60% or 85%. Treatment can be applied at any time of year if ambient temperature is high enough to achieve adequate vaporisation and the bees are not clustered

FLUMETHRIN

UK, Eire

Indications. Diagnosis and control of mites *Varroa jacobsoni*

Warnings. Avoid use during periods of honey flow except for diagnosis, or treatment if necessary for survival of the colony; avoid contact of preparation and honey to be harvested for human consumption

Dose. Treatment, suspend 2–4 impregnated strips between the combs in the brood chamber. Leave in place for a maximum of 6 weeks

Diagnosis, leave in place for 24 hours. Dead mites seen on floor tray, which must be protected by a mesh or screen to prevent removal by the bees. The level of infestation can be estimated by the number of mites. Interpretation of the result must relate the number of mites to the size and condition of the colony, previous treatment, time of year, the breeding activity of bees at the time.

GSL **Bayvarol** (Bayer) *UK, Eire*
Impregnated strip, flumethrin 3.6 mg/strip, for *honey bees*; 20
Withdrawal Periods. *Bees*: honey withdrawal period nil; other bee produce intended for human consumption should not be taken until the spring following treatment

FLUVALINATE

UK

Indications. Diagnosis and control of mites *Varroa jacobsoni*

Contra-indications. Leaving strips in the hive for more than 8 weeks

Warnings. Keep in original packing until ready for use; operator should take adequate precautions such as wearing gloves, avoiding contact with skin, mouth, or eyes

Dose. Treatment, suspend 2 strips between the combs in the brood chamber; leave for 6–8 weeks. May be used throughout the period of honeyflow if required.

GSL **Apistan** (Vita) *UK*
Impregnated strip, fluvalinate 10%, for *honey bees*
Withdrawal Periods. *Bees*: honey withdrawal period nil

FORMALDEHYDE SOLUTION

UK

Indications. *Nosema apis*, *Malpighamoeba mellificae*, European Foul Brood, wax moths

Warnings. Use only on empty combs or hive bodies; operators should take care not to inhale fumes

Dose. *As fumigant*, add 500 mL Formaldehyde Solution BP to 240 g potassium permanganate (sufficient for 30 m³). Leave in contact with combs or hive bodies for 14 to 17 days

FUMAGILLIN

UK

Indications. Control of *Nosema apis*

Dose. *By addition to sugar syrup*, 166 mg (8 g of powder)/colony. Feed in autumn or spring

Fumidil B (distributed by Thorne) *UK*
Powder, fumagillin 20 mg/g, for *bees*

LACTIC ACID

UK

Indications. Treatment of mites *Varroa jacobsoni*

Contra-indications. Brood cappings are not penetrated by the acid, therefore should not be used in presence of brood

Warnings. Chilling of bees by the spray is stressful and treatment at low temperatures should be avoided. Lactic acid is corrosive and likely to cause skin burns. Operator should wear protective clothing

Dose. *By spray*, 5 mL lactic acid 15% solution each side of combs directly onto the bees, ensuring that they are thoroughly wetted. Repeat 4 times at weekly intervals. Ambient temperature should be between 5°C and 10°C (late autumn) when minimal flying is taking place so that most bees are treated and there is little brood to conceal mites. May be used in summer on broodless stocks such as natural or artificial swarms.

METHYL SALICYLATE

UK

Indications. Prevention of migration of mites *Acarapis woodi* from infested bee to healthy bee. Mites are not killed
Warnings. May taint honey if used when honey supers are present
Dose. *As fumigant*, moisten a gauze pad with 2.5 mL and apply over frames daily for 6 days *or* fill a small bottle fitted with a wick and place it at the back of the hive, allowing natural evaporation

OXALIC ACID

UK

Indications. Control of mites *Varroa jacobsoni*
Warnings. Care must be taken not to contaminate honey (if applied as directed accumulation in wax does not occur and no residues remain); operators should wear face mask with filter, goggles or protective glasses, and rubber gloves
Dose. Reconstitute 30 g oxalic acid dihydrate in 1 litre water (= oxalic acid 2.1% solution)
By hand spray or pressure pump with a very fine nozzle, apply 3–4 mL oxalic acid 2.1% solution to the bees on each side of combs. May be repeated 2–3 times. Time of treatment depends on level of infestation, but likely to be July to December. Ambient temperature should be more than 5°C

OXYTETRACYCLINE

UK

Indications. Oxytetracycline-sensitive infections
Dose. *By addition to sugar syrup*, 250–400 mg/5 litres sugar syrup
By addition to patty, 250–500 mg mixed with yeast, pollen, and honey and placed on top of frames *or* up to 1 g mixed with sugar and vegetable fat and placed on top of frames
By dusting, 250–500 mg mixed with powdered sugar and dusted on frames

POM **Terramycin** (Pfizer) *UK*
See section 1.1.2 for preparation details
Note. In the UK, use is only permitted under the supervision of MAFF and issued for the treatment of European Foul Brood

Australia

Indications. European foul brood
Contra-indications. American foul brood; placement in honey supers
Warnings. Do not move hives for 4 weeks after treatment
Dose. Pour over top bars of the frames in the brood nest.
By addition to sugar syrup, 10 g/500 mL sugar syrup (sugar 340 g in water 300 mL) *or* 5 g/250 mL sugar syrup *or* 2.5 g/125 mL sugar syrup

Oxymav 100 (Mavlab) *Austral.*
Powder, oxytetracycline 100 g/kg, for *calves* (see section 1.1.2), *pigs* (see section 1.1.2), *poultry* (see section 1.1.2), *honey bees*
Withdrawal Periods. *Bees*: honey 8 weeks

USA

Indications. American foul brood and European foul brood
Warnings. Use so that medication consumed before period of main honey flow
Dose. *By addition to sugar syrup*, 1 5-mL spoonful/2 L sugar syrup
By dusting, 121 g mixed with 900 g powdered sugar. Per colony, 28 g of mixture dusted on outer parts or end of frames

Terramycin Soluble Powder (Pfizer) *USA*
Powder, oxytetracycline 10 g/181 g, for *cattle* (see section 1.1.2), *pigs* (see section 1.1.2), *sheep* (see section 1.1.2), *mink*, *poultry* (see section 1.1.2), *honey bees*
Withdrawal Periods. *Bees*: honey 8 weeks

PARADICHLORBENZENE
(PDB crystals)

UK

Indications. Adults and larvae of wax moths
Warnings. Wax moth eggs may not be killed. Air combs before replacing on the hive. May be carcinogenic
Dose. Sprinkle crystals throughout stored stacks of comb

POWDER

Inert dust or powder such as glucose powder, talcum, chalk, flour, corn starch, milk powder, cellulose, icing sugar, finely ground pollen, diatomaceous earth. Minimal drug residues or drug resistance occur because powder such as sugars, pollen, and milk powder are utilised by the bees and other powders are removed by grooming

UK

Indications. Control of mites *Varroa jacobsoni*
Contra-indications. Do not apply near the honey super
Warnings. Excessive amounts of powder should be avoided because of risk of damage to uncapped brood; very fine powder may cause blockage of the spiracles of bees
Dose. *By sprinkling* (using container with fine holes such as flour dredger), lightly cover all bees on each side of combs in the brood box. Close the hive entrance for 20–30 minutes. Collect mites on floor tray (mites are not killed but lose their grip on bees because of the effect of the powder on the sticky tarsal pads). Repeat as necessary at 4-day intervals

THYMOL

UK

Indications. Control of mites *Acarapis woodi, Varroa jacobsoni*, and chalkbrood
Contra-indications. Use at temperatures <15°C; use for longer than 6 weeks
Side-effects. Strong odour persistant in the hive after treatment, which can adhere to the honey
Dose. *As fumigant and by contact*, place one tray with lid removed on top of brood frames. Allow sufficient space overtop of tray to allow access by bees and circulation of

air. After 14 days, place another tray alongside and leave for 4 weeks or until supers are required

Apiguard (Vita) *UK*
Gel, thymol 25%, for bees

VEGETABLE OILS/LIGHT PARAFFIN OILS

UK

Indications. Control of mites *Acarapis woodi, Varroa jacobsoni*
Warnings. Care must be taken not to contaminate honey; use at temperature > 12°C
Dose. *By addition to sugar patty,* vegetable oils. Mites are not killed directly but attractiveness of host bee diminished
By spray (fine nozzle), apply an emulsion to bees on each side of the comb; repeat twice after 1-week interval

Aquatic invertebrates

Aquatic invertebrates, for example bivalve molluscs and crustaceans such as lobsters (*Homarus*), shrimps, and prawns are farmed for food. They are also used in research, for example *Daphnia* have been used in pollution studies. Aquatic invertebrates are exhibited in private, public, and educational establishments. These animals are important in medicine, for example leeches *Hirudo medicinalis* are used in skin graft management and also for the isolation, characterisation, and production of their beneficial salivary components such as hirudin, a very potent anticoagulant.

When administering drugs to aquatic invertebrates used for human consumption, withdrawal periods should be considered. Where no withdrawal period for invertebrates is given, it is advisable to apply the withdrawal period for fish. The health and welfare of aquatic invertebrates, like all aquatic animals, is closely dependent upon their immediate environment. Each species has its own environmental parameters within which it is able to survive, grow, and multiply. Therefore consideration must be given to the substrate and water temperature, composition, pH, and hardness. In some species, provision of light of the correct wavelength is required. Unfortunately, information about the physiology and habitat requirements of many species, particularly tropical marine invertebrates, is incomplete and therefore there may be unknown factors influencing captive success. Furthermore, marine organisms have evolved in a stable environment and may lack the range of physiological and behavioural responses to cope with any alteration in their habitat.

Generally, invertebrates appear to be relatively resistant to infections providing water quality and environmental considerations are met. Detectable levels of ammonia, nitrites, and other pollutants, as well as overstocking can readily predispose to viral, bacterial, and fungal disease. Most of the diseases recognised in aquatic invertebrates are those encountered in commercially important species, but some are known from studies in the wild.

Antimicrobial therapy. Although there are many bacterial infections to which aquatic invertebrates are susceptible the commonest are caused by *Aeromonas* and *Pseudomonas* spp., and in marine invertebrates, *Vibrio* spp. Bacteria associated with marine invertebrates are mainly Gram-negative while those affecting freshwater invertebrates are both Gram-positive and Gram-negative. An important bacterial disease of the lobster is gaffkaemia ('red tail') caused by *Aerococcus viridans*. This is a natural commensal of lobsters with 5 to 7% of individuals in a population being carriers of the bacteria. Treatment is with antibacterials (see Table 19). In the past, commercial vaccines against gaffkaemia have been available and therefore autogenous vaccination delivered by injection to individual animals may be considered.

Antibacterials have an optimal pH for maximal activity. Marine systems usually have a pH greater than 8.0 and this will limit the effectiveness of, for example the tetracyclines, which have optimal activity at pH 6.0 to 6.6. Chloramphenicol or streptomycin may be preferred because their optimal activity is at pH 7.4 to 8.0. Antibacterials in solution are constantly being deactivated due to reducing substances, chelation (for example tetracyclines), and high pH. Streptomycin, chloramphenicol, kanamycin, and neomycin have a long half-life in solution. Penicillin and erythromycin have a short half-life and therefore medication will need to be repeated. Neomycin, kanamycin, and chloramphenicol are considered potentially toxic to invertebrates. Attempts should be made to determine the toxicity for each new drug used with a different invertebrate species. One cannot safely extrapolate from one species to another, for example in the marine crustacean *Artemia,* benzylpenicillin is toxic at 200 mg/litre whereas 40 mg/litre is toxic to the freshwater crustacean *Daphnia*. See Table 19 for dosage regimens for antimicrobials for aquatic invertebrates. In general, treatment with antibacterials should not be carried out in tanks with biological filters.

Probiotics may aid prevention of bacterial diseases. Epicin (Pharm-X) has been shown to significantly reduce the incidence of *Vibrio* spp. in pond cultures both directly by production of natural bacteriostatic products (bactocillins) and indirectly by competition at substrate sites. For lobsters the dose is 30 g/455 litres for 4 weeks, then every 2 weeks. For shrimp, the dose is 0.5 to 1 ppm for vibriosis.

Rickettsial and chlamydial infections have been recorded in scallops, cockles, mussels, crayfish, and clams.

Fungal infections such as freshwater *Saprolegnia* are also of major importance. Other fungal diseases seen include *Aphanomyces asataci* infection ('crayfish plague') and *Fusarium* spp. infection of lobsters (fungus disease, 'burn spot disease').

For protozoan diseases such as thelohaniosis ('porcelain disease') of crayfish or microsporidiosis of oyster eggs (one of the causes of oyster egg disease) there is no practical treatment in open systems. Some promising *in vitro* studies with the protozoan affecting lobsters *Anophryoides haemophila* suggests that formaldehyde, pyrimethamine combined with sulphaquinoxaline, and monensin are possible treatments but amprolium is not effective. Alternative methods of disease control include the production of resistant stock;

this has been used for *Haplosporidium nelsoni* infection (MSX disease) in oysters.

Viral conditions. Many viral infections have been recognised in invertebrates including herpes-type virus disease of oysters, baculovirus penaei (BP virus disease) of shrimps and prawns, hepatopancreatic parvovirus (HPV) disease of shrimps and prawns, and baculovirus of blue crayfish. The management of viral diseases involves regular health monitoring, the correction of predisposing factors, and the disposal of affected stock.

Parasiticidal therapy. Parasitic diseases are common and problematic to control. Drugs that are toxic to the parasite may also be toxic to the host. The red worm parasite of oysters, mussels, clams, and cockles is a copepod (Crustacea) and there is no known method of prevention or control. Various insecticides for terrestrial species have been used in the control of aquatic parasites. For example carbaryl has been used in the USA for the control of oyster parasites including pea crabs, boring gastropods, and ghost shrimps.

However, there are concerns about persistant drug residues in marine sediments and drug action on non-target species and use is not recommended.

Anaesthetics. Anaesthetics for aquatic invertebrates are usually added to the water, the depth of anaesthesia being controlled by a combination of the concentration and time of exposure. Recovery from anaesthesia is achieved by returning the animal to fresh, well aerated water and can be accelerated, where practical, by manually moving the animal forwards and backwards in an attempt to increase the water flow over the gills. In octopuses, flushing fresh sea water through the mantle cavity and massaging the musculature will aid recovery. The use of hypothermia to induce 'anaesthesia' must be approached with caution. Many of the criteria for assessing the depth of anaesthesia such as cessation of respiration and loss of chromatophore tone have a temperature dependence in these ectotherms and so may not be a reflection of the degree of analgesia experienced by the animal.

Table 21 Antimicrobial doses of drugs for aquatic invertebrates[1]

Drug	Dose	Condition	Species
Amphotericin B	1–25 mg/L for 2–7 days (formulation to use: amphotericin, powder for reconstitution)	fungal infections	crustacea
Benzylpenicillin	80 mg/kg body-weight i.co.	gaffkaemia	lobsters
Chloramine	5.5–100 mg/L for 2 days	protozoal and fungal infections	paenid prawns
Chloramphenicol	20 mg/L (formulation to use: chloramphenicol (as sodium succinate), powder for reconstitution)	bacterial infections	tropical marine invertebrates
Chlortetracycline	1 mg/L	bacterial infections	tropical marine invertebrates
	30 mg/L	bacterial infections	oyster and clam larvae
Erythromycin	0.65–1.3 mg/L	bacterial necrosis	crustacea
Griseofulvin	100 mg/L for 2 days (formulation to use: griseofulvin 75 mg/g, oral powder)	fungal infections	*Penaeus*
Methylthioninium chloride (Methylene blue)	8–10 mg/L	protozoal and fungal infections	crustacea
Neomycin	100 mg/L for 2 days	fungal infections	*Penaeus*
Nystatin	1 mg/L (formulation to use: nystatin 100 000 units/mL, oral suspension)	fungal infections	*Penaeus*
Oxytetracycline	450 mg/kg biomass	*Vibrio* infection	paenid prawn larvae
	75 mg/kg p.o. or injection into abdominal sinus	gaffkaemia	lobsters
Streptomycin	10–100 mg/L	bacterial infections	variety of invertebrates
	100 mg/L	bacterial infections	oyster and clam larvae
Tetracycline	1.2 mg/L	bacterial necrosis	paenid prawn larvae
Vancomycin	25 mg/kg injection into abdominal sinus	gaffkaemia	lobsters

[1] drug doses for preparations that have a marketing authorisation for use in these species in the UK. Therefore, unless marked [1], the drug or doses stated are not authorised for these species

Table 22 Anaesthetic doses of drugs for aquatic invertebrates

Drug	Dose	Species
Benzocaine	Dissolve 100 g in 1 litre ethanol for stock solution. Add stock solution to water dropwise according to the animal's response	univalve molluscs
Carbon dioxide	Bubble gas through water *or* Dilute 1 volume soda water in 1 volume water	*Hirudo medicinalis*
Ethanol 96%	2.0–2.5 mL/100 mL sea water 8 mL/100 mL water	cephalopods (may be irritant to octopuses) *Hirudo medicinalis*, univalve molluscs
Isobutanol	1–2 mL/10 g body-weight, by injection into the abdominal sinus	*Homarus americanus*
Tricaine mesilate	Add in incremental doses until desired effect achieved	various aquatic invertebrates (**not** *Homarus americanus, Actinosphaerum, Hydra, Planaria*)

[1] drug doses for preparations that have a marketing authorisation for use in these species in the UK. Therefore, unless marked [1], the drug or doses stated are not authorised for these species

Prescribing for amphibians

Contributors:
S J Divers BSc (Hons), BVetMed, CertZooMed, CBiol, MIBiol, MRCVS
M Lafortune DMV

Most commonly kept amphibia are of the orders Urodela (the salamanders including the neotenic axolotl) and Anura. The Anura includes about 4000 species of frogs and toads such as the common frog (*Rana temporaria*) and common toad (*Bufo bufo*), neotropical animals for example White's tree frog (*Litoria caerulea*) and the green tree frog (*Hyla cinerea*), and more exotic species such as poison arrow frogs (*Dendrobates* spp.) and horned toads (*Ceratophrys* spp., *Pyxicephalus* spp.). Laboratory species include the African clawed toad (*Xenopus laevis*) and the leopard frog (*Rana pipiens*).

Successful care of the captive amphibians is based on an understanding of the basic biology of these animals in general and also on a knowledge of the environment normally inhabited by the particular species in question; texts on amphibian husbandry should be consulted. Environmental factors are important in the vast majority of amphibian disease and water quality is paramount in maintaining amphibian health.

Amphibians are ectothermic. They have a preferred body temperature, or more correctly, a preferred optimal temperature zone (POTZ), within which their body functions operate at maximal efficiency (see Table 21). This reliance on heat from the surrounding environment has important ramifications for captive animals. Suboptimal temperatures will result in delayed neurological reactions and abnormal behaviour, reduced digestion and absorption of food, and impaired immunological defences. The absorption, metabolism, and excretion of drugs will be markedly slower than if the animal was kept at the correct temperature range.

Amphibians have an unusually fragile and permeable skin. The *stratum corneum*, although having some effective barrier functions, is only a few cell layers thick since it acts, in adults, as the prime respiratory organ. While epidermal and dermal glands secrete mucus and wax, passage of water through the skin allows substantial cutaneous water loss, and absorption of electrolytes and toxins occurs even through undamaged skin. Trauma leads to infection with organisms normally occuring in the environment, as does toxic damage. Therefore amphibians should be restrained with care and the operator's hands should be kept moist or ideally disposable plastic gloves should be worn.

The difference between the tadpole stage of all amphibia and the adult form is very marked, which results not so much in different diseases in tadpole and adult but different methods of diagnosis and treatment. In general, it is the adult animal that is seen in veterinary practice and mainly pet frogs and toads.

Amphibians produce urea as a nitrogenous waste product and excrete ammonia when in water.

Drug administration. The use of drugs such as antibacterials given by addition to the water is to be discouraged. Although uptake is generally good because of the nature of amphibian skin, it is impossible to judge exact dosages received by the animal via this route. Also, antibacterials in tank water can predispose to fungal overgrowth, and compromise bacterial filters in many water purification systems.

If a topical route is to be used, the animal should be placed in a treatment tank for a defined period each day; doses and exposure times being empirically defined.

The subcutaneous injectable route is preferred. Although each animal must be handled, this allows brief clinical inspection of the patient. Hands should be washed or gloves changed between individuals where infectious disease is suspected.

Drug dosage. Limited data are available on the pharmacokinetics and pharmacodynamics of drugs in amphibians and most dosages have to be extrapolated from other groups. However, significant variation occurs between species and at different temperatures. Determination of dosages of parenterally or orally administered drugs could use allometric scaling whereby the dose is defined as $mg/kg^{0.75}$ rather than mg/kg. This, together with the variation at different body temperatures, renders the calculation of doses complicated. Doses are given in the standard mg/kg assuming that the drug will be given within the POTZ of the animal. In general, at higher temperatures, the required dose will be increased from that at lower temperatures. The metabolism of the drug actually varies with the log of the temperature but such considerations become somewhat academic when variations from the optimum temperature zone are small.

Antimicrobial therapy. While several viral diseases have been reported in amphibians, bacterial conditions lead to most significant morbidity and mortality. 'Red leg' is the main cause of death in captive amphibians. The petechial epidermal lesions are a clinical sign of Gram-negative septicaemia caused by several bacteria but predominantly by *Aeromonas hydrophilia*. Other epidermal lesions include ulceration and subcutaneous oedema. Poor water quality and nutrition, and suboptimal environmental temperatures may be predisposing factors. In these cases culling or at least isolation of affected animals and prophylactic treatment of in-contact individuals is important; tetracycline is the treatment of choice.

Chlamydiosis is characterised by similar dermatological lesions and postmortem histopathological diagnosis is required.

Mycobacterial disease is seen sporadically. The condition may be characterised by dermal lesions such as pale nodules and occasionally ulceration, or cause systemic disease with visceral involvement and subsequent non-specific clinical signs such as weight loss. Non-specific antibacterial agents are used in addition to antibiotics, and may be useful for prophylaxis in in-contact or at risk animals. These atypical mycobacteria are zoonoses, causing aquarists nodule; operators should wear gloves.

Fungal diseases in amphibians are variable. Saprolegniasis is seen in aquatic species and is characterised by cotton wool-like growths on skin and gills. Systemic infections include chromomycosis caused by pigmented fungi for example *Cladosporium* and phycomycosis caused by the non-pigmented *Mucor* and *Basidiobolus.* All these conditions present as similar dermal lesions and diagnosis must be by culture and biopsy rather than clinical presentation alone.

Some fungal diseases in aquatic species may be ameliorated by physical removal and topical treatment with dilute chlorhexidine or merbromin (mercurochrome). Deep cutaneous or systemic infections require either concerted topical treatment or parenteral therapy. Amphotericin B should not be given by intramuscular injection; severe muscle necrosis may occur. Caution is required when applying topical agents to amphibians because relatively 'harmless' substances, for example dilute povidone-iodine, can induce severe dermatitis and toxicity.

Protozoa are mainly non-pathogenic in amphibians. However, *Entamoeba ranarum* causes amoebiosis characterised by enteritis and hepatic abscesses. Aquatic protozoa such as *Oodinium, Trichodina,* and *Voticella* may cause skin irritation and lesions in tadpoles but rarely affect adults.

Parasiticidal therapy. Parasitic infections include nematodiosis with strongyle infection either of the gastro-intestinal tract or lungs. *Capillaria* infection of the skin is commonly found in *Xenopus* and large numbers of filarid roundworms in tissues and blood vessels may be significant.

Anthelmintic treatment should be administered when parasitic ova are present in a faecal sample on a routine health check even in the absence of physical clinical signs. Non-specific parasiticidal agents are used in addition to anthelmintics. For visceral roundworm infections, ivermectin is particularly useful. However, the death of large numbers of roundworm larvae or microfilaria *in situ* may give rise to a severe inflammatory reaction, compromising the patient. Fenbendazole and tiabendazole do not appear to produce such a reaction. A levamisole bath is reported to be as efficacious as parenteral treatment.

Trombiculid mite larvae may be found subcutaneously with minute vesicles containing the parasite and the fish louse *Argulus* may be found on aquatic adults and tadpoles.

Other drugs. Nutritional deficiencies seen in amphibians include inadequate calcium intake resulting in metabolic bone disease in meat eating species, thiamine deficiency causing flaccid paralysis, or amino acid deficiency resulting in nutritional myopathy. Gout has been reported in amphibia fed a high protein diet. Dropsy or anasarca may be a clinical sign of osmotic dysfunction or may occur in otherwise healthy animals.

Hormonal drugs are used increasingly to manipulate captive breeding in various amphibian species. Although these techniques were originally employed in biomedical research, they are proving useful for the captive breeding of endangered species and mass propagation of pet stock.

Intracoelomic injection is the normal route for fluid administration in a dehydrated amphibian. The preferred solution is sodium chloride 0.18% + glucose 4%. Other solutions used are 1:2 sodium chloride 0.9%:glucose 5% or 1:2 Hartmann's solution:glucose 5%.

Anaesthetics. Anaesthetics can be administered by injection, gaseous induction, or transcutaneously using an anaesthetic bath. Reversal of anaesthesia is facilitated by transferring the animal to a bath of clean oxygenated water. Dopram also aids recovery by stimulating respiration.

Tricaine mesilate, isoflurane, and propofol are the anaesthetic agents of choice.

Table 23 Husbandry requirements for amphibians

Species	Habitat/ Vivarium type	POTZ (°C)[1]	Lighting[2]	Diet
European common frog (*Rana temporaria*)	best kept outdoors in garden enclosure, pond for breeding	0–25	broad spectrum, sunlight recommended	various invertebrates including flies, worms, crickets, maggots. Vitamin/ mineral supplementation recommended
Common toad (*Bufo bufo*)	garden enclosures, well drained site, pond for breeding	5–20	broad spectrum, sunlight recommended	various invertebrates including insects, worms, slugs, crickets. Vitamin/mineral supplementation recommended
White's tree frog (*Litoria caerulea*)	well ventilated vivarium with land and water partition for breeding, leaf-litter of bark chips as substrate, stout branches for climbing	5–25	broad spectrum	larger insects and other invertebrates, dead neonate mice. Vitamin/mineral supplementation recommended
European tree frog (*Hyla arborea*)	outside enclosure with high humidity and protection from frost, or large unheated indoor vivaria	5–25	broad spectrum	various invertebrates including flies, waxworms, mealworms, moths. Vitamin/ mineral supplementation recommended
Poison arrow frog (*Dendrobates* spp.)	large tropical vivarium with good ventilation, frequent spraying essential	22–28	bright, broad spectrum	small invertebrates including fruit flies (*Drosophilia*) and small crickets. Vitamin/mineral supplementation recommended
African clawed toads (*Xenopus* spp.)	aquatic species, 10 to 20 cm freshwater depth	18–22	broad spectrum	small fish, earthworms, aquatic insects. Vitamin/mineral supplementation recommended
Horned toads (*Ceratophrys* spp.)	large tropical vivarium with spacious shallow water area (depth of water approximately half height of frog)	25–28	broad spectrum	various insects and small pre-killed rodents. Vitamin/mineral supplementation recommended if feeding invertebrate prey, unnecessary if feeding whole dead rodents
European fire salamander (*Salamandra salamandra*)	large vivarium with shallow water dish and substrate of peat, leaf-litter, and moss	5–20	broad spectrum, subdued	small invertebrates including worms, crickets, waxworms, mealworms, and slugs. Vitamin/mineral supplementation recommended
Japanese fire bellied newt (*Cynops pyrrhogaster*)	aquatic species (but may leave water at end of breeding season), large aquarium, 20 cm freshwater depth	10–20	broad spectrum	*Daphnia*, *Tubifex*, and various invertebrates including worms. Vitamin/ mineral supplementation recommended
Axolotl (*Ambystoma mexicanum*)	large aquarium, 45 cm freshwater depth	16–22	broad spectrum	small invertebrates including worms, crickets, waxworms, mealworms, and slugs; small whole fish. Vitamin/mineral supplementation recommended

[1] temperature requirements are air temperature gradients
[2] broad-spectrum lighting includes ultra-violet B light

Table 24 Antimicrobial doses of drugs for amphibians[1]

Drug	Dose	Comments
Acriflavine	0.025% in water for 5 days *or* 500 mg/L as 30 minute bath once daily	
Amikacin	5 mg/kg i.m. on alternate days	
Ampicillin	6 mg/L as bath	
Amphotericin B	1 mg/kg i.co daily for 15–20 days	
Benzalkonium chloride	2 mg/L as 60 minute bath once daily *or* 0.25 mg/L water as 2 hour bath	fungal infections
Chloramphenicol	50 mg/kg i.m. twice daily *or* 20 mg/L as bath	
Doxycycline	10–50 mg/kg p.o. once daily	chlamydiosis in African clawed frogs
Enrofloxacin	5–10 mg/kg s.c., i.m. once daily	
Gentamicin	2.5–5.0 mg/kg s.c., i.m., i.co. once daily at 22°C *or* 10 mg/L as bath (poor efficacy) *or* 1.3 mg/L as soak 1 hour daily	caution: may be toxic
Isoniazid	12.5 mg/L as bath	
Ketoconazole	10 mg/kg p.o. daily	
Malachite green	150 micrograms/L as soak daily	fungal infections
Merbromin (Mercurochrome)	3 mg/L as 72 hour bath	
Methylthioninium chloride (Methylene blue)	2–4 mg/L	decreases mortality in tadpoles
Metronidazole	100–150 mg/kg p.o. weekly *or* 50 mg/kg p.o. daily for 3 days *or* 5 mg/kg food *or* 50 mg/L as 24 hour bath	protozoal infections
Miconazole	5 mg/kg i.co. daily	
Nalidixic acid	10 mg/L	
Oxytetracycline	25 mg/kg i.m., s.c. daily *or* 50 mg/kg p.o. twice daily *or* 1 g/kg food daily for 7 days	
Paromomycin	55 mg/kg p.o., repeat after 14 days *or* 25 mg/kg p.o., repeat after 7 days	
Piperacillin	100 mg/kg s.c., i.m. once daily	anaerobic infections
Rifampicin	25 mg/L as bath	
Sodium chloride	4–6 g/L as 72 hour bath *or* 10–25 g/L as 5–10 minute bath	protozoal infections; osmotic complications may occur depending on the species
Sulfadimidine	1 g/L as bath	
Sulphonamide + Trimethoprim	3 mg/kg p.o., s.c. once daily	
Tetracycline	50 mg/kg p.o. twice daily	
Water, distilled	2–3 hours bath	

[1] drug doses for preparations that have a marketing authorisation for use in these species in the UK; unless marked [1], the drug or doses stated are not authorised for these species

Table 25 Parasiticidal doses of drugs for amphibians[1]

Drug	Dose	Indications
Copper sulphate	500 mg/L bath for 2 minutes daily	parasites
Fenbendazole	50–100 mg/kg p.o. every 14 days	roundworms
Formaldehyde (10%)	1.5 mL/L as 10 minute dip every 48 hours	ectoparasites
Ivermectin	200–400 micrograms p.o. every 14 days *or* 200 micrograms/kg i.m. as a single dose *or* 400 micrograms/kg i.m. as a single dose *or* 2 mg/kg by topical application on thorax (*Rana* spp.)	roundworms rhabdiosis
Levamisole	300 mg/L as 24-hour bath *or* 8–10 mg/kg i.co. every 14–21 days *or* 50–75 mg in 4.0–6.5 L tank water/frog	
Mebendazole	20 mg/kg p.o., repeat after 14 days	
Niclosamide	150 mg/kg p.o., repeat after 14 days	tapeworms
Oxfendazole	5 mg/kg p.o. as a single dose	
Praziquantel	10 mg/L bath for 3 hours as a single dose *or* 8–24 mg/kg p.o., s.c. daily for 14 days	
Tiabendazole	50–100 mg/kg p.o., repeat after 14 days	

[1] drug doses for preparations that have a marketing authorisation for use in these species in the UK; unless marked [1], the drug or doses stated are not authorised for these species

Table 26 Doses of other drugs for amphibians[1]

Drug	Dose	Indications
Chorionic gonadotrophin (hCG)	2000–5000 units/kg s.c., i.m. *Xenopus* spp., 300–400 units s.c., i.m. *Ambystoma* spp., (female) 250 units s.c., i.m., (male) 300 units i.m.	breeding
Dopram	5–10 mg/kg i.m., i.v.	respiratory stimulation
Serum gonadotrophin	*Xenopus* spp., 50 units s.c., i.m., then 600 units after 72 hours	breeding
Thiamine	25 mg/kg of fish	
Vitamin E	200 units/kg food	

[1] drug doses for preparations that have a marketing authorisation for use in these species in the UK. Therefore, unless marked [1], the drug or doses stated are not authorised for these species

Table 27 Anaesthetic doses of drugs for amphibians[1]

Drug	Dose	Comments
Benzocaine	(Dissolve in ethanol) 50 mg/L water 200–300 mg/L water	larvae frogs, salamanders
Isoflurane	4–5% bubbled into water administered according to animal's response or place animal on damp towels in induction chamber	all species
Ketamine	50–100 mg/kg s.c., i.m.	long recovery period
Pentobarbital	60 mg/kg by injection into dorsal lymph sacs	frogs
Phenoxyethanol	0.1–0.5 mL/L	
Propofol	10 mg/kg i.v.	all large species; for salamanders use ventral tail vein, for frogs and toads use abdominal vein or heart
Tiletamine/zolazepam	10–15 mg/kg i.m.	variable response
Tricaine mesilate (MS-222)	200–500 mg/L 0.5–2.0 g/L 1–3 g/L 50–150 mg/kg s.c., i.m., i.co.	tadpoles, newts; administered according to animal's response frogs, salamanders; buffer with sodium bicarbonate toads; buffer with sodium bicarbonate

[1] drug doses for preparations that have a marketing authorisation for use in these species in the UK; unless marked [1], the drug or doses stated are not authorised for these species

Prescribing for exotic birds

Contributor:
B H Coles BVSc, DipECAMS, RCVS Specialist in Zoo and Wildlife Medicine (Avian), FRCVS

Exotic birds include passerines, psittacines, and raptors. Drug preparations authorised for use in exotic birds are not generally available. Preparations authorised for use in other species or authorised human preparations may be administered under the responsibility of the veterinarian who has the animal 'under his care'.

When prescribing for exotic birds, it is important to ascertain the normal feeding and husbandry of the birds; additional texts should be consulted. For some species it may be preferable to refer to the section on Prescribing for birds, which contains information on poultry, game birds, pigeons, and ostriches.

Disease in exotic birds may be influenced by nutrition, housing, and stress. It is often advisable to treat them under hospital care where an ambient temperature of 29°C to 32°C and supportive therapy, such as fluids, can be provided. An initial volume of lactated Ringer's solution (Hartmann's solution) or sodium chloride 0.9% and glucose 5% solution given by intravenous injection or into the cloaca often produces considerable clinical improvement. For guidance, the volume of fluid that may be administered by intravenous injection into the jugular vein is 5% of the body-weight, given in 4 divided doses over 12 hours. The volume of fluid for cloacal administration into the rectum is usually 0.5 mL (budgerigars), 1 mL (cockatiels), 4 mL (amazons), or 6 to 7 mL (macaws). Thereafter, the minimal daily fluid requirement of 50 mL/kg may be met by oral administration, subcutaneous or slow intravenous injection, or by administration into the medullary cavity of the ulna or tibiotarsal bone using a 20 to 22 gauge needle with an indwelling stylet. In avian patients with hypovolaemic shock, a plasma substitute such as Dextran 70 (see section 16.2), may be used at a dose of 10 to 20 mL/kg

Drug administration. Drugs may be administered to exotic birds by addition to drinking water or feed. The drug dose is mixed in half the daily ration of feed, which should be consumed before offering any further food. This method is non-stressful and convenient for groups of birds on either a therapeutic or prophylactic basis. However, often the correct dose may not be consumed because sick birds may be anorexic or polydipsic leading to under or overdosage. Palatability of drugs, such as chlortetracycline or ivermectin, may be improved by mixing with honey, syrup, or fruit juice or, alternatively, a sweetened paediatric preparation may be used where available.

Oral medication may also be given by gavage using a metal tube for parrots, or plastic catheters for other birds. This direct method of medication is more reliable but requires frequent handling, which may cause stress. It is important that the fluid is placed directly into the crop and not into the upper oesophagus. The volume of fluid administered will depend on the individual bird. For guidance: 0.5 mL (budgerigars), 2 mL (cockatiels), 5 mL (amazons), or 10 mL (macaws). Capsules or tablets can be given to birds of pigeon size and larger.

Therapy may also be administered by parenteral injection but frequent handling of the patient is necessary. Subcutaneous injection may be given in the inguinal region and over the breast muscle, but is most readily given at the back of the base of the neck. Care should be taken not to puncture the crop or the cervical-cephalic air sac, both of which may extend into this area. For critically ill birds, intramuscular or intravenous injection is preferred. Intramuscular injection is given in the posterior part of the pectoral muscles or the quadriceps muscle. Certain preparations given by intramuscular injection may cause pain and muscular damage. Birds have a renal-portal system and a proportion of a medicament may therefore be excreted before reaching the systemic circulation when the drug is given into the leg muscles. Intravenous injection is given into the right jugular, the brachial vein, or the superficial medial metatarsal vein in some larger species. In larger birds, medication may be injected directly into the infra-orbital sinus to treat localised infections.

Nebulisation may be used for treatment of disease of the respiratory tract or the skin. This requires specialised equipment which produces a droplet size of 0.5 to 5.0 microns. Equipment for human use, such as the ⒽPorta-Neb 50 nebuliser (Medic-Aid), may be employed with a small air compressor, or with oxygen flow provided by an anaesthetic machine delivering not less than 6 litres oxygen per minute. Drugs administered by nebulisation include amphotericin B, chloramphenicol, erythromycin, spectinomycin, and tylosin (see 28 for dilution details).

Drugs may also be applied topically although preparations should be used sparingly. Ointments and creams used in excess are easily spread through preening and may damage plumage, which can lead to loss of body heat. Some drugs, such as ivermectin, are absorbed percutaneously.

Antimicrobial therapy. Many antimicrobial drugs are used in avian medicine and suggested doses are listed in Table 28. Therapy may be required before results of bacterial sensitivity are available. In these circumstances the following antibacterials are the drugs of choice: amoxicillin with clavulanic acid for respiratory-tract infections; aminoglycosides in combination with sulfadiazine with trimethoprim for gastro-intestinal or urinary-tract infections; and amoxicillin with clavulanic acid or sulfadiazine with trimethoprim for skin infections.

Probenecid reduces the renal tubular excretion of particular antibacterials and was used to reduce dose frequency. However it also decreases active secretion of uric acid and may result in gout; probenecid is no longer recommended.

Many adverse reactions to antimicrobials have been reported in exotic birds particularly in smaller birds such as finches, canaries, and soft bills. The aminoglycoside antibacterials are potentially nephrotoxic. Sulphonamides may cause tissue haemorrhage and anaemia. Sulfadiazine with trimethoprim may cause gastro-intestinal disturbances such as crop stasis or emesis. Enrofloxacin may cause vomiting in raptors.

> All birds should be weighed before being medicated because the estimation of weight by sight alone may be grossly inaccurate

Calcium and magnesium found in bird grit may affect the absorption of tetracyclines, although this effect may be reduced by adding citric acid 500 mg/100 mL of drinking water. Ideally, tetracyclines, and in particular oxytetracycline, should only be used after bacterial sensitivity has been established because resistance to these antibacterials is now widespread.

Psittacosis is a zoonotic disease caused by *Chlamydia psittaci*. Tetracyclines (in particular chlortetracycline or doxycycline) are the drugs of choice for the treatment of the disease in birds. Fluoroquinolones may also be used but only after bacterial sensitivity tests. A minimum 45-day course of treatment is recommended, after which the bird should be retested for presence of *Chlamydia* and therapy continued if necessary.

Candida albicans is a normal component of the gastrointestinal microflora. Overgrowth of *C. albicans* in the gastro-intestinal tract may occur with prolonged antibacterial therapy, retinol (vitamin A) deficiency, crop impaction, or feeding of infected grain. Nystatin is effective against candidiasis. Alternatively, flucytosine may be given in combination with amphotericin B, itraconazole, or ketoconazole.

Treatment of aspergillosis includes amphotericin B in combination with ketoconazole or itraconazole, and fluid therapy, and immunostimulants such as levamisole. Amphotericin B and imidazoles are hepatotoxic and should not be used in birds that are dehydrated or have renal impairment. However, the side-effect of hepatotoxicity should not prohibit the use of these drugs for the treatment of aspergillosis, a severe and life-threatening disease. The drinking water should be acidified with citric acid or apple cider vinegar during treatment with amphotericin B.

Metronidazole, dimetronidazole, carnidazole, and ronidazole are used for *Giardia, Trichomonas, Cochlosoma,* and *Hexamita* infections. Coccidiosis may occasionally be a problem, particularly in finches, budgerigars, and parrots. Sulphadimidine is an effective treatment for coccidiosis; the dosage must be adequate (see Table 28).

Parasiticidal therapy. General control measures include the following: to avoid contact with invertebrates birds should be kept in free-standing cages with wire mesh flooring or aviaries with solid concrete flooring, birds should be isolated to avoid indirect contact with wild birds, and regular faecal examination should be carried out every 4 to 6 months.

Endoparasiticides such as fenbendazole or levamisole may be used regularly (every 4 to 6 months) for prophylaxis in groups of birds. The parasiticide group used should be alternated to avoid problems of drug resistance. The benzimidazole endoparasiticides may cause feather abnormalities in some birds during the moult, and may lead to vomiting and death in nestlings if used during the breeding season. Levamisole gives a bitter taste when added to drinking water and the addition of sweeteners may improve palatability. The margin of safety with levamisole is relatively narrow and some species are particularly sensitive to this drug. Levamisole should not be administered parenterally to birds. Parenterally administered ivermectin may be toxic to finches and budgerigars but is relatively safe when applied to the skin and subsequently absorbed and distributed throughout the body.

Ectoparasiticides such as pyrethrins, coumafos, fipronil, and carbaril are used in birds to control *Cnemidocoptes*, feather mites, and lice infestations. A dichlorvos-impregnated strip such as Vapona (Sara Lee; distributed by Chemist Brokers) may be placed in the bird room for up to 3 days, with removal at night. Birds should not come into direct contact with the strip. The strip should be removed immediately and the room ventilated if signs of toxicity such as ruffled feathers occur.

Other drugs are used for the treatment of a variety of disorders in exotic birds (see Table 30).

Medroxyprogesterone acetate may be given to stop persistent egg laying due to ovarian cysts. Chronic use of medroxyprogesterone acetate may lead to obesity and polydipsia. Medical treatment for egg binding includes oxytocin in combination with calcium gluconate 10% solution, or the prostaglandin dinoprost; 50% of cases requiring medical treatment also need surgery.

Birds normally excrete uric acid but renal impairment or incorrect diet may lead to retention and hence gout. Allopurinol administered orally may aid recovery. However it is not effective in reducing uric acid tophi already present in joints and other tissues. In addition, the use of allopurinol in high dosage may lead to the deposition of both xanthine and hypoxanthine in the renal tubules.

The NSAIDs ketoprofen and carprofen have been used in exotic birds for treatment of shock, inflammatory conditions, and trauma. NSAIDs are contra-indicated in patients with renal impairment. These drugs may occasionally cause vomiting.

In general, the routine use of corticorticoids is not recommended in birds because these drugs have severe effects on the immune system and organ function. Short-acting glucocorticoids may be used in acutely ill patients.

Respiratory system and epidermal disorders in birds are often caused by an underlying vitamin A deficiency. Bird seed often does not provide adequate vitamin A, which may need to be provided as a supplement (see section 16.7). Treatment is given daily by injection for 2 weeks followed by maintenance with an oral supplement. The diet should be changed to include sources high in vitamin A such as car-

Table 28 Antimicrobial doses of drugs for exotic birds[1]

Drug	By mouth	By addition to drinking water	By addition to feed	By injection	Other methods of administration
Amikacin	—	—	—	15–20 mg/kg 2–3 times daily i.m. (psittacines)	
Amoxicillin	150–175 mg/kg 2 times daily (formulation to use: tablets or oral suspension)	1.5–4.5g/L	600 mg/kg soft feed	150 mg/kg i.m. daily (formulation to use: long-acting preparation)	—
Amoxicillin with clavulanic acid[2]	125 mg/kg 4 times daily	—	—	100 mg/kg i.m.	—
Amphotericin B	treatment of megabacteriosis in budgerigars, 0.2 mL/bird twice daily for 10 days (formulation to use: intravenous infusion 5 mg/mL)	—	—	1.5 mg/kg i.v. daily for 7 days	By oral topical application, 10 % solution By nebulisation, 100 mg diluted in 15 mL of sodium chloride 0.9% solution By intratracheal administration, 1 mg/kg daily for 12 days then on alternate days for 5 weeks
Carnidazole	10 mg (adults); 5 mg (young birds)				
Cefalexin	35–50 mg/kg, repeat 4 times daily (>500 g body-weight); 35–50 mg/ kg repeat 8 times daily (<500 g body-weight)	—	—	25–50 mg/kg i.m.	—
Chlortetra-cycline	100 mg/kg 4 times daily	Treatment. 5 g/ L for 45 days Prophylaxis. 1 g/L for 45 days	Treatment. 5 g/kg soft feed for 45 days Prophylaxis. 1 g/ kg soft feed for 45 days	—	—
Dimetridazole	40 mg/kg daily	100 mg/L (finches); 100–250 mg/L (other species)	—	—	—
Doxycycline	25 mg/kg twice daily♦ 15 mg/kg[1]	500 mg/L♦ 260 mg/2 litres[1]. Birds with low daily water intake, 260 mg/500 mL[1]	—	75–100 mg/kg i.m. every 5–7 days	—
Enrofloxacin	10 mg/kg twice daily[1]	100–200 mg/L for 5–10 days	—	10 mg/kg i.m. twice daily[1]	—
Erythromycin	10–20 mg/kg	250–500 mg/L for 3–5 days	200 mg/kg soft feed	—	By nebulisation, 200 mg diluted in 15 mL sodium chloride 0.9% soln.
Flucytosine	50 mg/kg twice daily for 2–4 weeks	—	80–300 mg/kg feed (psittacines, mynahs)	—	—

Table 28 Antimicrobial doses of drugs for exotic birds[1] *(continued)*

Drug	By mouth	By addition to drinking water	By addition to feed	By injection	Other methods of administration
Itraconazole	10 mg/kg twice daily for 30–60 days (formulation to use: itraconazole 100 mg capsules)	—	10 mg/kg twice daily for 30–60 days (formulation to use: itraconazole 100 mg capsules)	—	—
Ketoconazole	20 mg/kg daily for 2 weeks		40–100 mg/kg soft feed	—	—
Lincomycin/ spectinomycin	—	1 g (Linco-Spectin (Pharmacia & Upjohn)/L	—	—	—
Metronidazole	20–50 mg/kg once daily for 7 days	100 mg/L	—	5 mg/kg i.m. twice daily	—
Nystatin	300 000–600 000 units/kg 2–3 times daily for 1–2 weeks	100 000 units/L for 3–6 weeks	200 000 units/kg soft feed for 3–6 weeks	—	—
Oxytetracycline	25–50 mg/kg	Treatment. 0.65–2.0 g/L for 5–14 days	Treatment. 300 mg/kg soft feed for 5–14 days 4.5 mg/bird (as medicated seed[1])	50 mg/kg i.m. daily (> 400 g body-weight); 100 mg/kg i.m. daily (< 400 g body-weight)	—
Sulfadiazine with trimethoprim	75 mg/kg for up to 7 days	—	—	20 mg/kg s.c., i.m. twice daily	—
Sulphadimidine	50 mg/kg	220 mg/L for 3 days, repeat after 2 days	—	30 mg/kg s.c., i.m.	—
Toltrazuril	—	2 mg/L, give on 2 consecutive days per week	—	—	—
Tobramycin	—	—	—	2.5 mg/kg i.m. 3 times daily for 14 days (raptors); 5 mg/kg i.m. 2–3 times daily for 14 days (other species)	—
Tylosin	20 mg/kg daily for 3 days	500 mg/L	—	20–40 mg/kg i.m. 3 times daily (use higher dose for smaller birds)	By nebulisation, 100 mg diluted in 5 mL DMSO and 10 mL sodium chloride 0.9% solution

[1] drug doses for preparations that have a marketing authorisation for use in these species in the UK. Therefore, unless marked [1], the drug or doses stated are not authorised for these species

[2] dose expressed as amoxicillin

Table 29 Parasiticidal doses of drugs for exotic birds[1]

Drug	By mouth	By addition to drinking water	By injection	Other methods of administration
Endoparasiticides				
Fenbendazole	50–100 mg/kg once, repeat after 10 days (nematodes); 33 mg/kg, repeat daily for 3 days (microfilaria, trematodes); 20 mg/kg, repeat daily for 5 days (*Capillaria*)	10 mg/L (finches)	—	—
Ivermectin	200 micrograms/kg. Repeat after 2–3 weeks	—	200 micrograms/kg i.m. Repeat after 2–3 weeks (not finches, budgerigars)	By topical application, one drop of 1% solution
Levamisole	10–20 mg/kg, repeat after 2 weeks	80 mg/L (finches); 100–200 mg/L daily for 3 days (other species)	—	—
Praziquantel	5–10 mg/kg, repeat after 2–4 weeks	—	7.5 mg/kg s.c., i.m., repeat after 2–4 weeks (not finches)	—
Ectoparasiticides				
Carbaril				Dusting powder, spray
Coumafos, propoxur, and sulfanilamide (Negasunt, Bayer)				Dusting powder; use sparingly
Dichlorvos-impregnated strips (bird room)	—	—	—	Minimum air space 30 m^3 per strip, use for up to 3 days, see notes above
Fipronil				Spay on to *skin* one, repeat after 14 days if required
Pyrethrins[1]	—	—	—	Dusting powder, spray

[1] drug doses for preparations that have a marketing authorisation for use in these species in the UK. Therefore, unless marked [1], the drug or doses stated are not authorised for these species

Table 30 Doses of other drugs for exotic birds[1]

Drug	Dose	Indications
Allopurinol (**but see text**)	10–15 mg/kg p.o.	gout
Bromhexine	3–6 mg/kg i.m. 6.5 mg/L drinking water	respiratory disorders
Butorphanol	2 mg/kg i.m. daily. May be used for up to 28 days	analgesia
Calcium gluconate 10%	1–2 mL/kg i.m. + oxytocin	egg binding
Carprofen	2–10 mg/kg i.m.	inflammatory disorders
Clomipramine	1–2 mg/kg daily by addition to drinking water (formulation to use: clomipramine syrup 5 mL diluted in 50 mL drinking water)	behaviour modification
Diazepam	0.5–1.5 mg/kg p.o., i.m., i.v. 3 times daily	seizures
Digoxin	10–20 micrograms/kg p.o. twice daily *or* 4 micrograms/30 mL drinking water (formulation to use: Lanoxin PG elixir 50 micrograms/mL)	congestive cardiac failure
Dinoprost	20–100 micrograms/kg i.m. as a single dose	egg binding
Doxapram	(<2 kg body-weight) one drop p.o.; (>2 kg body-weight) 7 mg/kg i.m.	respiratory stimulation in apnoea and newly hatched chicks
Doxepin	initial dose, 1 mg/kg daily in 2 divided doses (formulation to use: contents of doxepin capsule as an oral solution or by addition to drinking water)	behaviour modification
Haloperidol	by addition to drinking water, initial dose 200 micrograms/kg (<1 kg body-weight); initial dose 170 micrograms/kg (>1 kg body-weight) (formulation to use: haloperidol oral liquid). Gradually increase dose to 900 micrograms/kg over a 9 week period. Maintenance doses of 400 micrograms/kg may be required if a relapse occurs and may be given for more than 12 months	behaviour modification
Hydrocortisone	10 mg/kg i.v.	see text
Iodine	Dilute 1 volume Aqueous Iodine Oral Solution with 14 volumes water. Add 1 drop of this solution to 30 mL drinking water daily for 3 weeks	hypothyroidism
Ketoprofen	2 mg/kg i.m.	inflammatory disorders
Levamisole	2 mg/kg s.c. every 4 days for a total of 3 doses	immunostimulant
Lactulose	0.3 mL/kg p.o.	
Medroxyprogesterone acetate	30 mg/kg s.c., i.m. Repeat dose once every 4 weeks	persistant egg laying
Metoclopramide	500 micrograms/kg p.o., i.m.	anti-emetic, to increase motility of upper gastro-intestinal tract
Naltrexone	1.5 mg/kg by addition to drinking water (formulation to use: naltrexone 50 mg tablet, dissolved in 10 mL water)	behaviour modification
Oxytocin	3–5 units/kg i.m. + calcium gluconate	egg binding
Penicillamine	50–55 mg/kg p.o. daily for 7–14 days	copper, zinc, mercury, and lead poisoning
Potassium bromide	75 mg/kg p.o. (parrots)	idiopathic epilepsy
Sodium calciumedetate (**but see text**)	10–40 mg/kg i.m., slow i.v.	lead and zinc poisoning
Succimer	30 mg/kg p.o. daily for 10 days	lead and zinc poisoning
Vitamin A	5000 units/kg i.m. daily for 2 weeks, then 250–1000 units/kg daily p.o.	respiratory and epithelial disorders

Table 30 Doses of other drugs for exotic birds[1] *(continued)*

Drug	Dose	Indications
Vitamin E /selenium	68 micrograms/kg i.m. every 7–14 days (formulation to use: 0.01 mL (Vitesel, Norbrook)/kg)	cockatiel paralysis, paresis syndrome and similar neuropathies in other psittacines
Vitamin K	0.2–2.5 mg/kg i.m.	coagulopathies

[1] drug doses for preparations that have a marketing authorisation for use in these species in the UK. Therefore, unless marked [1], the drug or doses stated are not authorised for these species

rots and spinach. Bromhexine with concurrent Vitamin A therapy, may also aid recovery.

Hypothyroidism is a common condition in budgerigars fed loose-bought seed. Treatment consists of iodine supplementation.

Antiepileptics such as diazepam and potassium bromide are used in exotic birds to aid in the treatment of seizures due to various disorders including lead poisoning. Succimer and sodium calciumedetate are used for treatment of lead and zinc poisoning. There is decreased occurrence of renal toxicity with succimer.

Some neuroleptics (antipsychotic) and antidepressant drugs have undergone limited trials in exotic birds for behavioural problems, in particular feather picking in parrots. Before using these drugs it is essential that all other possible causes of feather picking have been eliminated. Owner compliance may be a problem with the use of these drugs because they may need to be administered continuously for 3 to 4 months before they can be shown to be effective and cost may preclude their use in some patients. Many of the drugs are administered by addition to the drinking water. To ensure that the bird receives the full dose, the average daily water intake should be calculated and the dose added to this volume of drinking water. Birds drink on average 50 to 150 mL water/kg body-weight daily, depending on diet and basal metabolic weight.

Doxepin is administered at a dose which may be progressively increased at 14-day intervals. Doxepin should not be used in birds with cardiac, hepatic, or renal impairment, or recent infectious disease.

Clomipramine has been found to be effective in 50% of patients. Side-effects of overdosage include drowsiness and incoordination, which are reversible with cessation of treatment or reduction of dosage.

Haloperidol has been found to be effective in a broad range of psittacine species and is considered to have a wide margin of safety. Regrowth of feathers may be seen in about 3 months. Side-effects of haloperidol include depression, inappetance, and occasionally hyperactivity or excitability, which are resolved when treatment is discontinued and recommenced at a lower dosage after an interval of 2 to 3 days.

Naltrexone has also been used successfully to treat feather picking.

Anaesthetics. Ketamine given in combination with sedatives is the injectable drug of choice. When ketamine is combined with medetomidine or xylazine, side-effects of the alpha$_2$-adrenoceptor stimulant can be antagonised by administration of atipamezole at the same volume as that previously administered for medetomidine. Isoflurane is the preferred inhalational anaesthetic. Administration of butorphanol 1 mg/kg by intramuscular injection 10 minutes before isoflurane anaesthesia is found to reduce the amount of anaesthetic required.

Table 31 Anaesthetic doses of drugs for exotic birds[1]

Drug	Dose
Injectable anaesthetics	
Ketamine	50 mg/kg i.m.
Ketamine + acepromazine	25–50 mg/kg i.m. 0.5–1.0 mg/kg i.m.
Ketamine + diazepam	10–40 mg/kg i.m. 0.5–1.5 mg i.m.
Ketamine + medetomidine	5–10 mg/kg i.m. 100 micrograms/kg i.m.
Ketamine + midazolam	20 mg/kg i.m. 4 mg/kg i.m.
Ketamine + xylazine	20 mg/kg i.m. 4 mg/kg i.m.
Inhalational anaesthetics	
Halothane	Induction, 0.5–4.0% (increase concentration slowly) Maintenance, 1.5–3.0%
Isoflurane[1]	Induction, 5% Maintenance, 2.5–3.5%

[1] drug doses for preparations that have a marketing authorisation for use in these species in the UK. Therefore, unless marked [1], the drug or doses stated are not authorised for these species

Prescribing for reptiles

Contributors:
S J Divers BSc (Hons), BVetMed, CertZooMed, CBiol, MIBiol, MRCVS
M Lafortune DMV

The class Reptilia consists of more than 6500 species. However reptiles most likely to be seen in practice are snakes (order Squamata, suborder Serpentes), lizards (order Squamata, suborder Sauria), and tortoises, terrapins, and turtles (order Chelonia). The large number of species necessitates a knowledge of specific nutritional and husbandry systems, including that of desert dwelling insectivores, rain forest herbivores, and carnivorous snakes. Texts on basic husbandry and nutrition of pet reptiles should be consulted.

> All reptiles should be weighed before being medicated to avoid overdosage and during treatment to monitor response

All reptiles are ectothermic and rely on environmental heat and behaviour to maintain their preferred body temperature (PBT). The PBT varies with species, age, season, and time of day, and is the temperature at which metabolism is optimal. The PBT for specific metabolic processes is variable, so that the PBT for gametogenesis and reproduction is likely to be different from the PBT for immunocompetence and fighting infection. The preferred optimum temperature zone (POTZ) is the temperature range that permits the reptile to achieve the PBT, and should therefore be provided by a thermal gradient within the home, in the hospital vivarium, on the operating table, or in recovery from anaesthesia (see Table 32). A change in temperature may have profound influences on drug distribution, metabolism, excretion, and hence elimination half-life. Some therapeutic regimens state a fixed temperature at which the reptile should be held during treatment. The advantage of this approach is that where pharmacokinetic evidence exists the elimination of the drug will be known and constant. However, if this stated temperature is below or above the POTZ for the species being treated then stress and debilitation may ensue. In addition, where the stated therapeutic temperature is within the POTZ for the species being treated, constant exposure to a fixed temperature is likely to cause stress and maladaptation over a period of time.

Reptiles have a well developed renal portal system where blood from the caudal half of the body passes through the kidneys before reaching the systemic venous circulation. Therefore drugs that are injected into the caudal half of the body may have a significantly reduced half-life if excreted via the kidneys, while nephrotoxic drugs may reach renal tissue in high concentration. However, studies have demonstrated that this effect does not always occur. There appears to be a valve mechanism capable of shunting blood through or around the kidneys, but the precise hormonal and neural control has yet to be described. It is recommended that in most cases, medication should be injected into the cranial half of the reptile.

Another anatomical consideration is the large voluminous bladder of chelonians which may act as a drug reservoir and lead to a second therapeutic peak many hours after drug administration.

The shell of tortoises, turtles, and terrapins is largely living tissue and therefore all chelonian medication should be based on total body-weight.

Drug administration. There are few drug preparations authorised for use in reptiles. Drugs authorised for use in other species or for humans may be administered under the responsibility of the veterinarian who has the animal 'under his care'. A limited number of pharmacokinetic studies for reptiles have been published and where possible these should always be used. Where species specific information is not available, it is sometimes possible to extrapolate to closely related species. For example, data for Hermann's tortoise (*Testudo hermanni*) could be used for the Spurthigh tortoise (*Testudo graeca*).

Medication may be administered to reptiles by mouth or stomach tube or by subcutaneous, intramuscular, intravenous, intracoelomic, intraosseous, intrasynovial, or intratracheal injection. Some drugs may be applied topically, given per cloaca, or administered by inhalation (nebulisation).

Antimicrobial therapy. The majority of bacterial infections in reptiles are caused by Gram-negative bacteria, particularly *Pseudomonas*, *Aeromonas*, *Citrobacter*, *Klebsiella*, and *Proteus* spp. Bacterial resistance to many commonly used antibacterials is seen and many Gram-negative bacteria can have unexpected sensitivity to particular antibacterials. Therefore sampling for microbial culture and sensitivity testing should be carried out before commencing therapy. Antibacterial therapy must usually be given while awaiting the results of sensitivity tests. In these circumstances, amikacin, ceftazidime, and enrofloxacin or ciprofloxacin are the drugs of choice. In severe infections, amikacin may be combined with ampicillin or amoxicillin for respiratory tract infections, or ceftazidime for generalised or systemic infections. Chloramphenicol in combination with neomycin may be given for gastro-intestinal infections. Anaerobic infections are also seen and metronidazole, lincomycin, or clindamycin are used.

Fungal and yeast infections may occur in reptiles. Gastro-intestinal mycoses are particularly common in reptiles that have been maintained on inappropriately long-term broad-spectrum antibacterials. Cutaneous mycoses can often be treated by debridement and the topical application of malachite green or povidone-iodine, although griseofulvin can be employed. Gastro-intestinal infections can be treated with nystatin while systemic infections may require ketoconazole, amphotericin B, or polymixin B. In cases of pul-

Table 32 Husbandry requirements for reptiles

Species	Habitat/ Vivarium type	POTZ (°C)[1]	Humidity (%)	Lighting[2]	Diet
Bearded dragon (*Pogona vitticeps*)	terrestrial/ desert	20–32	20–30[3]	broad-spectrum	mainly insectivorous, also carnivorous, herbivorous
Boa constrictor (*Boa constrictor*)	terrestrial/ rain forest (semi-arboreal, aquatic)	28–32	50–80	special requirements not known	carnivorous
Box tortoise (*Terrapene carolina*)	terrestrial/ semi-aquatic, temperate	24–30	50–80	broad-spectrum	mainly herbivorous and insectivorous, also carnivorous
Burmese python (*Python molurus*)	terrestrial/ rain forest, scrub land	26–30	50–80	special requirements not known	carnivorous
Corn/Rat snake (*Elaphe guttata*)	terrestrial/ scrub land	25–30	30–70	special requirements not known	carnivorous
Garter snake (*Thamnophis sirtalis*)	terrestrial/ temperate	21–28	50–80	special requirements not known	carnivorous
Green anole (*Anolis carolinensis*)	arboreal/ rain-forest	23–29	70–80	broad-spectrum	mainly insectivorous
Green iguana (*Iguana iguana*)	arboreal/ rain-forest	29–34	60–85	broad-spectrum	herbivorous
Leopard gecko (*Eublepharus macularius*)	terrestrial/ desert	25–30	20–30[3]	special requirements not known	mainly insectivorous, also carnivorous
King snake (*Lampropeltis* spp.)	terrestrial/ scrub land	25–30	30–70	special requirements not known	carnivorous
Plumed basilisk (*Basiliscus plumifrons*)	arboreal/ rain-forest	24–32	70–85	broad-spectrum	mainly insectivorous, also carnivorous
Red-eared terrapin (*Trachemys scripta elegans*)	aquatic/ subtropical	20–26	60–90	broad-spectrum	mainly carnivorous, also herbivorous
Royal python (*Python regius*)	terrestrial/ scrub land	26–30	50–80	special requirements not known	carnivorous
Sand boa (*Eryx* spp.)	burrowing/ desert	25–30	20–30[2]	special requirements not known	carnivorous
Mediterranean tortoise (*Testudo* spp.)	terrestrial/ subtropical, temperate	20–28	30–50	broad-spectrum	mainly herbivorous
Water dragon (*Physignathus cocincinus*)	arboreal (semi-aquatic)/ rain-forest	25–32	80–90	broad-spectrum	mainly insectivorous, also herbivorous

[1] temperature requirements are air temperature gradients. In general, basking temperature should be 5°C greater and night temperature should be 5°C less

[2] broad-spectrum lighting includes ultra-violet B light

[3] humidity requirements will be significantly greater during ecdysis

monary mycoses, antifungal medication may be given by nebulisation, or intratracheal or intrapulmonary injection.

Viral diseases including ophidian paramyxovirus, boid inclusion body disease virus, and herpesviruses are identified in reptiles; aciclovir has been used with some success against herpesviruses.

Entamoeba invadens is a fatal protozoan disease of snakes that can penetrate the gastro-intestinal mucosa causing severe gastro-enteritis and invade other organs including the liver. Protozoa are not necessarily restricted to the alimentary tract and some, notably *Hexamita*, can cause kidney and bladder disease in tortoises. Metronidazole is the drug of choice for treatment. However, neurological signs have been reported with repeated use of metronidazole and, in general, a single dose of 250 mg/kg (maximum 400 mg/animal) is recommended. Adverse effects have been reported in indigo snakes, king snakes, and uracoan rattlers and a maximum dose of metronidazole 40 mg/kg is recommended for these species. Cryptosporidiosis can cause hypertrophy of the gastric mucosa and chronic regurgitation in snakes and treatment is largely ineffective. Many other protozoa are commonly seen in the faeces of healthy reptiles; these are usually part of the normal gut flora and indiscriminate treatment may be counterproductive.

Parasiticidal therapy. Helminth parasites that require an intermediate host and ticks are more commonly associated with wild caught imports while mites and helminths with a direct life cycle are usually seen in captive bred reptiles.

Individual ticks can be removed while heavy tick infestations are treated with the localised application of a topical spray or the use of systemic ivermectin (not Chelonia). Mites, particularly the snake mite *Ophionyssus natricis*, can be difficult to eradicate due to their motile nature and environmental contamination. Mite infested reptiles should be placed in a temporary vivarium and treated with ivermectin (given by injection or spray) or fipronil. Meanwhile the main vivarium is treated with an organophosphorus compound such as a dichlorvos-impregnated strip (Vapona, Sara Lee: distributed by Chemist Brokers) for at least 4 weeks. The main enclosure should be thoroughly cleaned before the reptile is returned. If it is not possible to remove the snake then Vapona can be used repeatedly for 2 to 3 days every week; alternatively fipronil or ivermectin may be used on a weekly basis. Avoid contamination of food and water by environmental parasiticides.

Occasionally large ascarids may be passed in the faeces of tortoises. The faeces or a cloacal wash should be examined for eggs and larvae to identify the parasite(s) present. In general, worming should be repeated until faecal examinations are negative. For certain species, particularly Mediterranean tortoises kept on contaminated ground, regular worming during spring and late summer is recommended. Oxfendazole is the benzimidazole of choice for the treatment of roundworms.

Most endoparasites affect the gastro-intestinal tract. However, *Kalicephalus* (hookworm) can penetrate the skin and cause extensive damage by tissue migration. *Rhabdias* (lungworm) and Pentastomids (arthropods) are parasites of

the respiratory tract of snakes and examination of a lung wash and lung endoscopy are recommended.

Parasiticide overdosage may lead to drug toxicity, which may manifest as neurological signs including seizures. **Ivermectin is contra-indicated in Chelonia**, and adverse reactions have been reported in iguanid lizards, skinks, and indigo snakes. Milbemycin has been used successfully in box tortoises and terrapins but it is recommended that avermectins and milbemycins are avoided in Chelonia.

Other drugs. Nutritional disease in reptiles is still very common. Ocular problems in terrapins due to hypovitaminosis A can be treated with vitamin A supplementation, although a change in diet is essential to produce a permanent cure. Hypovitaminosis B causes neurological signs in garter and ribbon snakes fed fish that contain thiaminase. Thiamine produces a rapid recovery but a change of diet is needed. Hypovitaminosis C is implicated in cases of stomatitis, iron deficiency is associated with anaemia in alligators, and iodine supplementation is required in cases of goitre in tortoises. Nutritional metabolic bone disease (NMBD) remains the primary nutritional disease of captive reptiles fed an inappropriate diet (high protein, low Ca:P ratio) and/or kept in an unsuitable environment (lack of UVB light). High calcium and phosphorus concentrations may cause soft tissue mineralisation. Oral calcium therapy should always be used in preference to injectable calcium (unless serum hypocalcaemia has been confirmed) in order to avoid resultant soft tissue mineralisation. Nutrobal (Vetark) is a multivitamin and high calcium supplement given at a maintenance rate of 0.1 mg/kg daily. This supplement has been used orally at 1 to 2 mg/kg daily ♦ to treat NMBD without inducing hypercalcaemia or any side-effects. The use of calcitonin has been advocated to improve bone density more rapidly, but should only be used once serum-calcium concentrations are within the normal range. Commercial reptile diets (for example Pretty Pets available from Pretty Bird International) may help in preventing nutritional disease in the pet reptiles.

Most sick reptiles present in a state of dehydration and because of their uricotelic nitrogenous metabolism (uric acid rather than urea), gout is of important clinical concern and may necessitate the use of allopurinol to reduce further uric acid production. For reptiles receiving potentially nephrotoxic drugs such as potentiated sulphonamides or aminoglycosides, oral or subcutaneous fluid therapy at 20 mL/kg daily is sufficient. In cases of severe dehydration, parenteral hypotonic fluids are recommended. Historically this has been achieved by the intracoelomic administration of warm fluids. More recently the use of syringe drivers, either electrical or spring action, has enabled the more effective administration of intravenous or intraosseous fluids to reptiles as small as 75 g body-weight. The intraosseous route is used for lizards (proximal tibia) and chelonia (cancellous bone of the lateral bridge that connects the plastron and carapace or proximal tibia). For larger iguanas and monitor lizards, the cephalic vein may be catheterised. In snakes, the right jugular vein may be catheterised using a cut-down technique. In emergencies, an intracardiac cathe-

Table 33 Antimicrobial doses of drugs for reptiles[1]

Drug	Dose[2]	Comments
Aciclovir	80 mg/kg p.o. daily topical cream 1–2 times daily	
Amikacin	gopher snakes, initial dose 5 mg/kg i.m., then 2.5 mg/kg i.m. every 3 days gopher tortoises, 5 mg/kg i.m. on alternate days at 30°C American alligators (juvenile), 2.25 mg/kg i.m. every 3–4 days at 22°C royal python, 3.5 mg/kg i.m. every 4–5 days	
Amoxicillin	22 mg/kg p.o. 1–2 times daily 10 mg/kg i.m. daily	often ineffective unless given in combination with aminoglycosides
Amphotericin B	0.5–1.0 mg/kg i.co, i.v every 1–3 days for 14–28 days	aspergillosis; fluid therapy recommended
Ampicillin	Hermann's tortoises, 50 mg/kg i.m. on alternate days 20 mg/kg i.m. daily at 26°C for 7–14 days	
Cefalexin	20–40 mg/kg p.o. twice daily	
Ceftazidime	20–40 mg/kg i.m. every 3 days snakes, 20 mg/kg i.m. every 3 days at 30°C	
Ceftiofur	tortoises, 20 mg/kg i.m. daily; 4 mg/kg i.m. daily (upper respiratory tract infection) snakes, 2.2 mg/kg i.m. on alternate days turtles, 2.2 mg/kg i.m. daily	
Cefuroxime	100 mg/kg i.m. daily for 10 days at 30°C	
Ciprofloxacin	10 mg/kg p.o. on alternate days	
Clarithromycin	desert tortoises, 15 mg/kg p.o. every 2–3 days	mycoplasmal infection
Clindamycin	5 mg/kg p.o. daily	
Chloramphenicol	indigo snakes, 50 mg/kg i.m. twice daily Midland water snakes, 50 mg/kg i.m. every 4 days bull snakes, 40 mg/kg i.m. daily	
Dimetridazole	40 mg/kg p.o. daily for 5 days	
Doxycycline	2.5–10.0 mg/kg p.o. 1–2 times for 10 days Hermann's tortoises, initial dose 50 mg/kg i.m., then 25 mg/kg i.m. every 3 days	
Enrofloxacin	5 mg/kg p.o., i.m. every 1–2 days[1] upper respiratory tract infection in tortoises, 15 mg/kg i.m. every 3 days; nasal flush, 1–3 mL every 1–2 days (using solution of enrofloxacin 200 mg/L water) Burmese pythons (juvenile), initial dose 10 mg/kg i.m., then 5 mg/kg i.m. on alternate days; *Pseudomonas* infection, 10 mg/kg i.m. on alternate days Hermann's tortoises, 10 mg/kg i.m. daily gopher tortoises, snakes, 5 mg/kg i.m. every 1–2 days Indian star tortoises, 5 mg/kg 1–2 times daily box tortoises, 5 mg/kg i.m. every 4–5 days	

Table 33 Antimicrobial doses of drugs for reptiles[1] *(continued)*

Drug	Dose[2]	Comments
Gentamicin	American alligators, 1.75 mg/kg i.m. every 3–4 days at 22°C painted turtles, 10 mg/kg i.m. on alternate days at 26°C red-eared terrapins, 6 mg/kg i.m. every 2–5 days gopher snakes, 2.5 mg/kg i.m. every 3 days at 24°C	
Griseofulvin	20–40 mg/kg p.o. every 3 days	fungal dermatitis
Itraconazole	spiny lizard, 23.5 mg/kg p.o. daily for 3 days	
Kanamycin	10 mg/kg i.m. daily at 24°C	fluid therapy recommended
Ketoconazole	crocodilians, 50 mg/kg p.o. daily turtles, 25 mg/kg p.o. daily for 14–28 days tortoises, 15 mg/kg p.o. daily	
Lincomycin	10 mg/kg p.o. daily 5 mg/kg i.m. 1–2 times daily	
Malachite green	150 micrograms/L water, 1 hour dip daily for 14 days	
Metronidazole	bacterial infections, 150 mg/kg p.o. every 7 days *or* 50 mg/kg p.o. daily for 5–7 days protozoal infections, 250 mg/kg p.o. as a single dose (may be repeated after 14 days) *or* 100 mg/kg p.o., repeat after 14 days and 28 days *or* 25–40 mg/kg p.o., repeat after 3–4 days	maximum dose 400 mg maximum dose for tricolour snakes, king snakes, indigo snakes, or Uracoan rattles is 40 mg/kg. Repeat after 14 days and 28 days for protozoal infections
Neomycin	10 mg/kg p.o. daily	should not be given systemically
Nystatin	turtles, 100 000 units/kg p.o. daily for 10 days	enteric fungal conditions
Oxytetracycline	5–10 mg/kg p.o., i.m. daily for 7 days American alligators, upper respiratory tract infection, 10 mg/kg i.v. every 4–10 days	pain, irritation, and inflammation at i.m. injection site
Piperacillin	50–100 mg/kg i.m. every 1–2 days	fluid therapy recommended
Polymixin B	1–2 mg/kg i.m. daily	
Sulfadoxine + trimethoprim	15–25 mg/kg p.o., i.m. daily 30 mg/kg i.m. on alternate days	fluid therapy recommended
Sulfamethoxy-pyridazine	initial dose 80 mg/kg s.c., then 40 mg/kg s.c. daily for 4 days *or* 50 mg/kg p.o. daily for 3 days, repeat after an interval of 3 days	coccidial infections
Tobramycin	turtles, 10 mg/kg i.m. daily tortoises and terrapins, 10 mg/kg i.m. every 1–2 days Chelonia, snakes, and lizards, 2 mg/kg i.m. daily	fluid therapy recommended
Tylosin	5 mg/kg i.m. daily	

[1] drug doses for preparations that have a marketing authorisation for use in these species in the UK; unless marked [1], the drug or doses stated are not authorised for these species

[2] where a particular temperature is not stated, the reptile should be maintained at the species-specific PBT

[3] species-specific data should be used wherever possible

Table 34 Parasiticidal doses of drugs for reptiles[1]

Drug	Dose	Parasite	Comments
Endoparasiticides			
Albendazole (25 mg/mL)	50 mg/kg p.o. as a single dose	ascarids	
Fenbendazole	50–100 mg/kg p.o. every 5–7 days	roundworms	
Ivermectin	200 micrograms/kg s.c., i.m., repeat after 28 days		should not be used in Chelonia; care in skinks and indigo snakes
Levamisole	5–10 mg/kg i.m., repeat after 14 days 400 mg/kg p.o. as a single dose	roundworms in snakes, lizards	care in tortoises
Mebendazole	20–25 mg/kg p.o., repeat after 14 days	strongyles and ascarids	
Oxfendazole	66 mg/kg p.o. as a single dose	roundworms	
Praziquantel	8 mg/kg p.o., i.m., repeat after 14 days and 28 days *or* 30 mg/kg p.o. as a single dose	tapeworms, flukes	
Ectoparasiticides			
Dichlorvos-impregnated strip	1 cm^2 of strip/30 cm^3 vivarium for 28 days *or* 2.5 cm^2 of strip/25 cm^3 vivarium for 2–3 days every week		toxic, vivarium should be emptied, keep out of direct contact of animals
Fipronil	by spraying, every 7–10 days	mites and ticks	
Ivermectin (10 mg/mL)	by spraying, 1–2 mL/L water every 7–10 days 200 micrograms/kg i.m. every 7 days	mites and ticks	should not be used in Chelonia, care in skinks and indigo snakes

[1] drug doses for preparations that have a marketing authorisation for use in these species in the UK; unless marked [1], the drug or doses stated are not authorised for these species

ter may be safely left in place for 24 hours. For parenteral fluid therapy sodium chloride 0.18% + glucose 4% solution or lactated Ringer's (Hartmann's) solution is effective. In cases of shock or severe dehydration, fluids may be given at a dose of 50 to 100 mL/kg/24 hours by intravenous or intra-osseous infusion for 2 to 3 hours before reducing the infusion rate to 20 to 30 mL/kg/24 hours. For oral therapy, warm (30°C) electrolyte mixtures (see section 16.1.1) may be employed but the solution should be diluted an additional 10% beyond that stated for mammals.

Egg-bound reptiles should initially be radiographed to provide a good quality dorsoventral radiograph. In cases of post-ovulatory egg stasis the eggs may occupy most of the coelomic cavity, often appear oval in shape and possess a thin, sometimes barely perceptible, shell. In cases of pre-ovulatory stasis, the ova can also occupy most of the coelomic cavity and often appear as more rounded without any shell. Injecting a small volume of air into the coelomic cavity can improve contrast and visualisation of the individual ova. Many egg-bound reptiles are dehydrated on presentation and parenteral fluid therapy is usually indicated. Parenteral calcium should not be administered unless hypocalcaemia has been confirmed. In most cases provision of a suitable nesting environment will stimulate most reptiles to lay or give birth. Oxytocin may be given by slow intravenous or intraosseous administration. Chelonia respond well to oxytocin, lizards and snakes less so. In snakes, the concurrent use of prostaglandins E and $F_{2\alpha}$ has been successful. Any evidence of abnormality such as large or deformed eggs or oviductal or cloacal obstruction precludes medical therapy and the reptile should be stabilised for surgery.

Respiratory disease is common in reptiles kept constantly below their POTZ, exposed to draughts, inappropriate humidity, poor ventilation, and kept in squalid conditions. Diagnosis relies on good quality horizontal beam radiographs (lateral views in Squamata; lateral and cranio-caudal views in Chelonia), endoscopy, and lung washing (using up to 1 mL fluid/100 g body-weight) for microscopy (parasites), cytology (inflammatory cells), and aerobic and anaerobic bacterial and fungal culture and sensitivity. Treatment options include husbandry improvements (temperature, humidity and ventilation), surgical removal of caseous lung material, coopage, bronchodilators, and antimicrobial drugs. Antimicrobial drugs can be given by intratracheal or intrapulmonary injection, or by nebulisation. In cases of partial tracheal blockage or lung surgery the air sac can be cannulated in the mid-caudal third of many snakes to provide an airway through which oxygen and isoflurane can be delivered. The cannula may be safely left in place for up to 5 days.

Ulcerative stomatitis in snakes is a multifactorial disorder which may arise from mouth trauma from cage furnishings or prey items, secondary to pneumonia or systemic infection, parasites (for example *Kalicephalus* spp), persistent hypothermia, squalid conditions, stress, maladaptation, or following hibernation. Most cases are seen in snakes and tortoises although certain lizards, such as water dragons, are also frequently affected. Most serpentine cases are due to Gram-negative bacteria while tortoises can often have fungal and yeast involvement. Untreated cases may progress to maxillary/mandibular osteomyelitis, aspiration pneumonia, ear abscesses, septicaemia and death. Treatment involves the correction of underlying husbandry factors, surgical debridement, and antimicrobial therapy based on culture and sensitivity. Daily debridement using dilute povidone-iodine is usually necessary and in severe cases fluid and nutritional support (including vitamin C) may be required.

'Runny nose syndrome' in Mediterranean tortoises (*Testudo* spp) is a common presentation of a multifactorial disease. The nasal discharge may be clear and serous, haemorrhagic, or purulent in nature. Various environmental, bacterial, and viral aetiologies have been advocated but none appear to be universally applicable. It appears that this syndrome is more common in the Spur-thighed tortoise (*Testudo graeca*) than in the Hermann's tortoise (*Testudo hermanni*) and outbreaks have often followed the mixing of these two species. Diagnostic investigation includes haematology, nasal flushing for cytological examination, bacterial and fungal culture and an accurate assessment of husbandry is essential. Treatment includes isolation of affected individuals and improvements in husbandry, particulary temperature, humidity, and ventilation. Antimicrobial drugs can be given by mouth, by injection ,or by nasal flushing. In refractory cases, scanning electron microscopy for viruses (for example herpesviruses) can be considered. Ideally, affected animals should not be allowed to hibernate.

Anaesthetics. Propofol is the injectable anaesthetic of choice because of its rapid smooth induction and recovery, minimal accumulation on repeated injections, and limited excitatory side-effects; the drug is administered by intravenous or intraosseous injection.

Ketamine may be given by intramuscular injection and its effect is dose dependent. At higher doses apnoea and recovery may be prolonged, taking up to 72 hours in certain circumstances. Ketamine should be used with care in debilitated reptiles.

Once anaesthesia has been induced, the reptile should be intubated and anaesthesia mantained with an inhalational agent. Many species such as iguanid and monitor lizards may be induced using a face mask. Conscious intubation and intermittent positive pressure ventilation (IPPV) is advised only for snakes.

Many reptiles have sub-clinical liver disease and isoflurane is the inhalational anaesthetic of choice because it is less hepatotoxic than halothane. The respiratory drive in most reptiles is governed by hypoxia and not hypercapnia. Therefore, it is not uncommon for reptiles to be apnoeic for much of the anaesthetic period and part of the recovery phase if the inhalational agent is delivered with pure oxygen, necessitating IPPV every 5 to 30 seconds. Maintaining anaesthetised reptiles using air (20% oxygen) seems to induce most species to breathe spontaneously, but in such circumstances it is important to monitor peripheral blood oxygen using an oesophageal or cloacal (ventral aspect) pulse oximeter.

Table 35 Doses of other drugs for reptiles[1]

Drug	Dose[2]	Indications
Allopurinol	10–20 mg/kg p.o. daily	gout, reduction of uric acid production
Aminophylline	2–4 mg/kg i.m.	respiratory disease where bronchodilation required
Argipressin	0.01–1.0 micrograms/kg	egg binding (more potent than oxytocin)
Ascorbic acid	10–200 mg/kg i.m. as required	ulcerative stomatitis
Calcitonin	1.5 units/kg s.c. 3 times daily 50 units/kg i.m., repeat after 2 weeks	hypercalcaemia (fluid therapy also recommended) secondary hyperparathyroidism
Calcium gluconate (10 mg/mL)	100 mg/kg i.m. 4 times daily or 400 mg/kg i.v., i.o. given over 24 hours	hypocalcaemia in iguanas
Cimetidine	4 mg/kg p.o. 3–4 times daily	regurgitation, vomiting, gastritis, gastro-intestinal ulceration
Cisapride	0.5–2.0 mg/kg p.o. daily	gastro-intestinal motility modification. (Concurrent use with clarithromycin in tortoises not recommended)
Colecalciferol	100–1000 units/kg i.m. as a single dose	hypocalcaemia, fibrous osteodystrophy in iguanas
Cyanocobalamin	50 micrograms/kg s.c., i.m.	appetite stimulation
Dexamethasone	30–150 micrograms/kg i.m., i.v., i.o.	inflammation, shock
Dinoprost	500 micrograms/kg i.m. as a single dose	egg binding in snakes
Doxapram	5–10 mg/kg i.v., i.o.	respiratory stimulation
Flunixin	100–500 micrograms/kg i.m., i.v. 1–2 times daily	inflammation, pain
Furosemide	2–5 mg/kg i.m., i.v. 1–2 times daily	diuresis
Iodine	2–4 mg/kg p.o. every 7 days	prophylaxis for goitrogenic diets
Iron	12 mg/kg i.m. every 7 days (alligators)	anaemia in alligators
Levothyroxine	20 micrograms/kg p.o. on alternate days	hypothyroidism in tortoises
Metoclopramide	60 micrograms/kg p.o. daily for 7 days	stimulation of gastric emptying in tortoises
Prednisolone	1–2 mg/kg p.o.	anti-inflammatory, reduction of nephrocalcinosis
Selenium	25–500 micrograms/kg i.m.	deficiency in lizards
Sucralfate	0.5–1.0 g/kg p.o. 3–4 times daily	gastric irritation
Thiamine	50–100 mg/kg i.m.	thiamine deficiency
Vitamin A	10 000 units/kg p.o., i.m. every 7 days	hypovitaminosis A (iatrogenic hypervitaminosis A may result from repeated treatment)
Vitamin B Complex	0.2 mL (Combivit, Norbrook)/kg	
Vitamin E	50–100 mg/kg i.m.	vitamin E deficiency

[1] drug doses for preparations that have a marketing authorisation for use in these species in the UK; unless marked [1], the drug or doses stated are not authorised for these species

[2] where a particular temperature is not stated, the reptile should be maintained at the species-specific PBT

Table 36 Doses of pre-medicants, sedatives, and anaesthetics for reptiles[1]

Drug	Dose	Anaesthetic times	Comments
Alfadolone/ alfaxalone	9–15 mg/kg i.m. 6–9 mg/kg i.v.	induction: <1 min (i.v.), 15–20 mins (i.m.) duration: 10–20 mins (i.v.), 20–30 mins (i.m.) recovery: 30–45 mins	incremental doses may be given every 30 minutes
Atropine	10–20 micrograms/kg i.m.		
Diazepam	220–620 micrograms/kg i.m.		administered to alligators before suxamethonium
Etorphine	crocodilians, 0.05–5.0 mg/kg i.m. sedation and analgesia in turtles, 0.5–2.75 mg/kg i.m.		
Gallamine	crocodilians, 0.4–1.0 mg/kg i.m.	induction: 15–30 mins recovery: 1.5–15 hours	may cause respiratory arrest; no analgesia; can be reversed with neostigmine
Isoflurane[1]	induction, 3–5% maintenance, 1–3%	induction: 2–10 mins recovery: 2–10 mins	less hepatotoxic than halothane
Ketamine	sedation, 10–50 mg/kg i.m. anaesthesia, 50–100 mg/kg i.m.	induction: 10–30 mins duration: 10–60 mins recovery: 12–72 hours	should not be used in debilitated animals; prolonged apnoea at high doses
Propofol	Squamata, 10–14 mg/kg i.v. Chelonia, 12–15 mg/kg i.v.	induction: <1 min duration: 15–25 mins recovery: 20–40 mins	must be given i.v. or i.o.
Suxameth- onium	Crocodilians, tortoises, 0.25–5.0 mg/kg i.m.	induction: < 4 mins duration: 1–9 hours recovery: 1–9 hours	may cause respiratory arrest; no analgesia
Tiletamine/ zolazepam	4–5 mg/kg i.m.	induction: 9–15 mins recovery: 1–12 hours	more sedation than anaesthesia; not suitable as sole agent

[1] drug doses for preparations that have a marketing authorisation for use in these species in the UK; unless marked [1], the drug or doses stated are not authorised for these species

Prescribing in hepatic impairment

Contributor:
P-J M Noble BVM&S, BSc, MRCVS

Hepatic disease can alter the bioavailability and disposition of a drug and influence the pharmacological effects produced by the drug; these effects are dependent on the nature and severity of the disease. The liver is the principal organ for metabolism of lipid-soluble drugs and for the production of plasma proteins.

The enhanced effect of drugs in patients with hepatic disease is mainly due to *decreased drug metabolism* and therefore increased duration of drug action. Glucuronide conjugation of drugs appears to be relatively unaffected by hepatic disease. Other reasons for augmented effect, particularly of those drugs that act on the CNS, could be attributed to *decreased drug-protein binding* due to hypoalbuminaemia, or increased permeability of the blood-brain barrier due to release of substances from the damaged liver, or a combination of both.

The occurrence of *drug-induced hepatotoxicity* is more commonly associated with chronic medication or overdosage of certain drugs than with short courses of therapy. The halogenated anaesthetic agents, paracetamol, antiepileptics, and corticosteroids are among the most significant causes of drug-related hepatotoxicity encountered in veterinary practice. Drugs that should be avoided in patients with hepatic disease are listed in the table.

Diagnosis of hepatic impairment. Routine hep-atic function tests poorly correlate with liver dysfunction, drug metabolising activity, or both. Serum-albumin concentration might serve as a prognostic indicator of hepatic drug-metabolising activity. Increases in activity of serum enzymes such as alanine aminotransferase (ALT) while indicative of hepatic damage in dogs, cats, and primates, do not relate to the degree of loss of liver function, which may be reduced by 100% before values reflect the dysfunction. In chronic hepatic disease, clearance of sulphobromoph-thalein (bromsulphthalein, BSP, sulfobromophthalein), which evaluates the functional capacity of the liver, may be decreased but in severely hypoalbuminaemic conditions, more efficient BSP clearance occurs which may underestimate the severity of hepatic disease. For practical reasons the BSP clearance test has largely been replaced by the measurement of serum-bile acid concentration, which gives a sensitive but variably specific test of hepatocellular function and the integrity of the enterohepatic portal circulation, and is not affected by hypoalbuminaemia. Although elevation of bile acid indicates liver dysfunction, correlation with the degree of functional loss is poor.

Ultrasonographic examination may show focal or diffuse changes in liver size and texture but specific diagnosis of chronic hepatic failure usually requires a liver biopsy.

Drug dosage in hepatic impairment. Although the effect of hepatic disease on the bioavailability and disposition of drugs is highly variable and difficult to predict, there are well-recognised principles for modifying dosage. The dose of drugs administered parenterally, or low clearance drugs given orally, should be reduced by 50%. Drugs with high hepatic clearance for example propranolol, and the opioid analgesics pentazocine and pethidine, should be given orally at 10 to 50% of the usual dose. In general, when administering drugs that depend on hepatic metabolism to animals with liver disease, the dosage interval should be increased.

Drugs to be avoided or used with caution in animals with hepatic disease. This list is not comprehensive; absence from the table does not imply safety.

Anabolic steroids
Anaesthetics, halogenated
Antiepileptics
Beta-adrenoceptor blocking drugs
Butorphanol
Chloramphenicol
Chlorpromazine
Copper salts
Corticosteroids
Diazepam
Doxapram
Doxorubicin
Fentanyl citrate + fluanisone (Hypnorm™)
Flucytosine
Griseofulvin
Halothane
Heparin
Ketamine
Ketoconazole
Lidocaine
Lincosamides
Megestrol acetate
Methoxyflurane
NSAIDs
Pancuronium
Paracetamol
Pentobarbital
Pentosan polysulphate sodium
Phenylbutazone
Polysulphated glycosaminoglycan
Propofol
Quinidine
Sulphonamides
Suxamethonium
Thiacetarsamide
Tubocurarine
Vecuronium

Prescribing in renal impairment

Contributor:
Professor A S Nash BVMS, PhD, CBiol, FIBiol, DipECVIM, MRCVS

Renal excretion is the principal process of elimination for drugs that are predominantly ionised at physiological pH and for polar drugs and drug metabolites with low lipid solubility. Renal excretion is dependent on renal blood flow, urinary pH, drug polarity, and lipid solubility. While the same basic mechanisms of renal excretion apply to mammalian species, the glomerular filtration rate, activity of tubular secretion, and contribution of pH-dependent passive reabsorption vary among species.

The degree to which impaired renal function affects drug elimination is determined by the fraction of the dose that is excreted unchanged by the kidneys. In severe renal disease, decreased drug excretion and changes in drug distribution occur, thereby enhancing the pharmacological effect of the drug. In uraemic patients and patients with nephrotic syndrome, plasma-protein binding of many drugs, notably furosemide, phenylbutazone, and phenytoin is decreased. Permeability of the blood-brain barrier may be increased in renal disease and therefore the anaesthetic effect of, for example, thiopental is enhanced. Decreased renal function affects not only the excretion of drugs that are eliminated by the kidneys, but may also alter the distribution and metabolism of drugs that are eliminated by the liver.

Nephrotoxic renal failure is most commonly associated with injury to the proximal tubules. It may be caused by antimicrobial drugs such as aminoglycosides, amphotericin B, cefaloridine, and polymyxins, and by heavy metals including mercuric salts, arsenic salts, bismuth, and copper. Nephrotoxic drugs should, if possible, be avoided in patients with pre-existing renal disease because consequences of nephrotoxicity are likely to be more serious when the renal reserve is already reduced. Nephrotoxicity caused by aminoglycosides is dose-related; the total amount of drug administered is probably more important than the daily dose in determining toxicity. Dehydration due to reduced water intake and increased loss due to vomiting in animals in renal failure, sodium deprivation, or administration of diuretics in particular furosemide, increases the nephrotoxic potential of aminoglycosides. Diuretic-induced potassium loss may be a contributing factor. Neonates are more susceptible than adult animals to aminoglycoside nephrotoxicity.

Drugs that should be avoided or used with caution in patients with renal impairment are listed in the tables.

Diagnosis of renal impairment. Reduced renal function is commonly assessed from the plasma (or serum) concentrations of urea or creatinine. Increased urea and creatinine concentrations result from moderate to severe renal dysfunction but plasma-urea concentration may be complicated by diet and protein metabolism. It is important to rule out pre-renal causes of azotaemia, such as dehydration from any cause, circulatory disorders, hypotension, and hypovolaemia. Glomerular filtration rate (GFR) will be reduced by 75% before plasma-urea and creatinine concentrations rise and signs of clinical disease are readily evident. This is because of the large functional reserve of the kidney. In adult animals, creatinine clearance provides a better quantitative indication of the degree of renal impairment and is the parameter on which calculation of dosage adjustment should be based. A limitation associated with the use of plasma creatinine as an indicator of renal function impairment is that patients with the same plasma-creatinine concentration may have widely varying renal function; hence the justification for using creatinine clearance. More recently, measurement of iohexol clearance has become possible. It is easier to measure than creatinine clearance and gives an accurate measurement of glomerular filtration but specialist equipment is required.

Drug dosage in renal impairment. There are several approaches which can be applied to dose adjustment in renal disease. Most of the methods assume that the required plasma therapeutic concentration of the drug in patients with renal dysfunction is similar to that required in those with no renal impairment. The objective is therefore to maintain uraemic patients at the same average steady state concentration after multiple doses or the same steady state concentration for infusions as those for normal individuals.

The design of dosage regimens is based on the pharmacokinetic changes that have occurred. In general pharmacokinetic approaches to dosage adjustment in renal failure can be based either on drug clearance or the GFR as an estimate of elimination rate constant. The latter is the more commonly used and requires assessment of the patient's renal function. It might be thought that active excretion or reabsorption of drug by the nephron might invalidate this approach. However, although occasional significant discrepancies can arise, in most circumstances, GFR is an adequate measure. For example, although procainamide and penicillins are actively secreted their renal elimination is in each case proportional to measured GFR, regardless of the nature of the renal dysfunction. The simplest reliable assessment of GFR is by measurement of plasma-creatinine concentration.

Creatinine is a obligatory by-product of muscle metabolism and is produced at constant rate and eliminated by renal clearance. Thus, under steady state conditions, the plateau principle applies to creatinine and, since its production rate is invariant and equals its whole-body clearance, the plasma concentration is inversely related to GFR. It should be noted, however, that reduced muscle mass will reduce creatinine production and thus steady-state plasma concentrations. Uraemic animals often have significant muscle wasting and the degree of renal function impairment will therefore be underestimated and GFR overestimated. Nonetheless plasma-creatinine concentration gives a simple measure on which to base alterations in dosing regimen which are sufficiently accurate for most purposes in chronic renal failure. It can therefore be used as a substitute for measurement of creatinine clearance although the latter is preferable, if practical. Plasma-creatinine concentration will lag several hours to days behind changing renal function in acute renal failure.

The dosage regimen can be adjusted by reducing the dose, increasing the dosage interval, or altering both. Changing the dosing interval alone may result in very large fluctuations in plasma concentration between doses. Altering the maintenance dose alone minimises fluctuations. However, since toxicity may be related both to the peak and trough concentrations for some drugs, and since peak concentrations may be important for therapeutic effect, there is merit in adjusting both variables so as to match the variations in concentration in the normal as closely as possible in the compromised patient.

If the plasma-creatinine concentration were found to be increased fourfold, the maintenance dose could be quartered and the dosage interval increased fourfold, but a better option is to halve the dose and double the dosage interval.

To find the most satisfactory dosage regimen to use in the uraemic patient, use the following equations:

U = uraemic patient
N = normal patient
Dose rate = average hourly rate
C = proportion increase in plasma-creatinine concentration

$$\text{Dose (U)} = \text{Dose (N)} \times \frac{1}{\sqrt{C}}$$

$$\text{Dose interval (U)} = \text{Dose interval (N)} \times \sqrt{C}$$

$$\text{Dose rate (U)} = \frac{\text{Dose rate (N)}}{C}$$

If a significant proportion of the drug (greater than 20%) is eliminated by non-renal routes the correction should be applied for that proportion of the dose eliminated by renal excretion. Basing the adjustment of dosage on plasma creatinine is an imperfect approach; in particular the reduction in dose required may be overestimated at low GFR. However, since caution in drug usage is required at very low GFR this may be an acceptable failing. It is certainly preferable to use this approach rather than to avoid dosage adjustment at all simply because creatinine clearance or drug clearance can not easily be measured in practice.

One or more loading doses may be required if a prompt therapeutic effect is sought because the desired steady-state plasma concentration will not be reached until after five times the half-life, and this will be greatly prolonged if the half-life is significantly lengthened as a consequence of reduced elimination.

Drug prescribing should be kept to a minimum in all patients with severe renal disease. If renal impairment is considered on clinical grounds, renal function should be assessed before prescribing *any* drug which requires dose modification even when renal impairment is mild.

Drugs that are nephrotoxic. This list is not comprehensive; absence from the table does not imply safety.

Amphotericin B
Aminoglycosides
Cisplatin
Doxorubicin
Methotrexate
Methoxyflurane

Drugs to be avoided or used with caution in animals with renal impairment. This list is not comprehensive; absence from the table does not imply safety.

Acepromazine
Alcuronium
Allopurinol
Captopril
Cardiac glycosides
Cephalosporins
Chloramphenicol
Chlorpromazine
Clindamycin
Doxapram
Fentanyl citrate + fluanisone (Hypnorm)
Flucytosine
Fluorouracil
Furosemide
Gallamine
Glucocorticoids
Hydroxycarbamide
Ketamine
Metronidazole
NSAIDs
Pancuronium
Pentosan polysulphate sodium
Pethidine
Piperazine
Polysulphated glycosaminoglycan
Procainamide
Propofol
Spironolactone
Sulphonamides
Tetracyclines (except doxycycline)
Thiazides
Tubocurarine

Prescribing for pregnant animals

Contributor:
R J Evans MA, PhD, VetMB, MRCVS

Effect of drugs used during pregnancy.

Important physiological changes occur during pregnancy that may alter the processes of drug absorption, distribution, and elimination. Changes occur in the cardiovascular, pulmonary, renal, and gastro-intestinal systems, and in body water compartments. The placenta, amniotic fluid, and fetus constitute additional distribution compartments for drugs. Drug exposure of offspring during pregnancy is determined by transplacental transfer. The rate and degree of transplacental transfer is influenced by the same principles and factors which affect transfer across other cellular barriers. These are: the concentration of free drug on each side of the barrier, the degree of ionisation, and the lipid solubility of the unionised drug. As a general rule, if a drug can be absorbed from the gut it will usually cross the placenta and enter the fetus. The fetus is susceptible to damage during implantation, when embryonic death is the outcome; during the embryonic and fetogenic stages when teratogenesis may result, and at birth when CNS, cardiovascular and respiratory depression are the most serious effects.

Some drugs may cause abortion, congenital malformations or neonatal disease if administered during pregnancy. Drugs that are known to cause teratogenesis in animals include some benzimidazoles such as albendazole and oxfendazole (particularly at high doses), corticosteroids, griseofulvin, ketoconazole, and methotrexate. Drugs that may affect the fetus or neonate, include opioids and barbiturates, which may alter respiration. Diethylstilbestrol administered for misalliance, may cause aplastic anaemia in offspring. Chlorpropamide and tolbutamide may cause hypoglycaemia. Salicylates (including aspirin) are teratogenic and prolonged use may also increase the risk of haemorrhage. Tetracyclines may cause dental discoloration and malformation in the offspring. Corticosteroids may cause teratogenesis and also affect skeletal calcification. Steroid hormones including androgens, anabolic steroids, and progestogens may affect the sexual development of the offspring. Drugs may induce abortion or premature parturition and these are are discussed below.

This does not mean that the use of drugs is contra-indicated in pregnant animals, but drug selection and manufacturer's warnings on the data sheets and package inserts must be considered. The need for therapy of the dam must be weighed against the generally uncertain risk to the fetus. It is important that the balance of risks is fully discussed with the client. Sometimes, administration during a certain period of pregnancy is not recommended. In many cases, safety has not been established and limited data are available on the consequences of administering drugs to the dam during pregnancy; manufacturer's information on the effect of drugs in laboratory animals may be helpful when assessing drug safety in other species. The pharmacological class of drug, the physicochemical properties that influence its passage by passive non-ionic diffusion across the placental barrier, and the mechanisms of elimination of the drug must also be taken into account. Modification in dosage, if required, should be based on changes in pharmacokinetic parameters, such as bioavailablity, systemic clearance, apparent volume of distribution, and half-life. It must be remembered that the dam's cardiovascular, respiratory, renal and metabolic physiology are changing throughout pregnancy, as are those of the fetus.

Drugs to be avoided or used with caution in pregnant animals. Care should also be taken by operators such as women of child-bearing age and pregnant women. This list is not comprehensive; absence from the table does not imply safety.

Barbiturates
Beta-adrenoceptor blocking drugs
Some benzimidazoles
Corticosteroids
Cytotoxic drugs
Diethylstilbestrol
Fluoroquinolones
Gentamicin
Griseofulvin
Some inhalational anaesthetics
Ketoconazole
Netobimin
Pethidine
Phenothiazines
Polysulphated glycosaminoglycan
Primidone
Prostaglandins
Salicylates
Sex hormones
Tetracyclines
Vaccines, live (but refer to individual vaccine information)
Warfarin

Unfortunately, too few studies of the absorption, distribution, and disposition kinetics of drugs have been performed in pregnant animals to allow even general recommendations to be made on dosage modifications.

Effect of drugs used at parturition.

Drugs may cause pregnancy termination or premature parturition. Abortion may be induced by corticosteroids, some prostaglandins, and $alpha_2$-adrenoceptor stimulants such as xylazine. Prostaglandins are used therapeutically to terminate early pregnancy in cattle, and to induce parturition in cattle and pigs. When drugs are used to induce early parturition, the length of gestation should be calculated to minimise the risk of non-viable offspring.

Drugs may also prolong normal delivery. Clenbuterol is used as a bronchodilator and also to reduce uterine motility. When used to treat a respiratory condition, therapy should be discontinued before the expected date of parturition. Progestogens may delay parturition. NSAIDs may delay or prolong parturition.

Drugs to be avoided or used with caution at parturition. This list is not comprehensive; absence from the table does not imply safety.

Barbiturates
Chlorpropamide
Clenbuterol
NSAIDs
Opioid analgesics
Progestogens
Tolbutamide
Xylazine

Prescribing for lactating animals

Contributor:
P E Edmondson MVB, CertCHP, FRCVS

Drug therapy in lactating animals should preferably only be instituted with a knowledge of the possible effects of that drug on lactation, the amount of drug likely to pass into the milk, whether the presence of the drug in milk is likely to be harmful to a neonate feeding from the dam, and, for food-producing animals, a knowledge of the withdrawal period for both meat and milk. When no authorised product for a particular situation exists, the choice of product and withdrawal period applied must take into account provisions of European and UK law including whether a drug is included in Annex IV of Regulation 2377/90/EEC and *The Medicines (Restrictions on the Administration of Veterinary Medicinal Products) Regulations 1994.*

During lactation lipid-soluble drugs pass from the systemic circulation into milk. The concentration of drug attained in the milk is influenced by the extent of plasma protein-binding, its lipid solubility, and degree of ionisation. Milk is separated from the general circulation by an intact membrane through which only the non-ionised lipophilic form of a drug may pass. When the non-ionised form of a basic drug such as a macrolide enters the relatively acid milk it dissociates and so becomes trapped resulting in high concentrations in milk - the so called 'ion-trap'. Therefore erythromycin, novobiocin, and trimethoprim achieve high concentrations in milk and diffuse well throughout the udder. Polar organic bases, such as the aminoglycosides streptomycin and neomycin, and organic acids are less concentrated in milk than in plasma. The pH difference between blood (pH 7.4) and normal milk (pH 6.7) is reduced in patients with mastitis, when milk pH may rise to pH 7.3. Increased blood flow and increased capillary permeability contribute to the transfer of antibacterials and other drugs into mastitic milk. The presence of milk has an inhibitory effect on some antibacterials when tested *in vitro*. This effect is most pronounced with oxytetracycline, dihydrostreptomycin, erythromycin, and trimethoprim-containing preparations.

Drugs achieving high concentrations in milk include: erythromycin, metronidazole, quinidine, trimethoprim and verapamil (metronidazole is included in Annex IV of Regulation 2377/90 and its use is effectively banned in food-producing animals).

Limited data are available on the effect of drugs on the offspring being suckled. Chloramphenicol may be found in milk but safety to neonates has not been established (chloramphenicol is included in Annex IV of Regulation 2377/90 and its use is effectively banned in food-producing animals). Dantron preparations, for example, should not be administered to lactating mares because the drug may affect the nursing foal. Barbiturates could also theoretically pass into milk to affect the neonate. Phenobarbital may inhibit the sucking reflex. Many topical ectoparasiticides should not be used on nursing bitches or queens. In general, any treatment given to the dam during lactation should be used with caution.

Drugs such as atropine, bromocriptine, cabergoline, and furosemide may inhibit lactation and cause agalactia. Repeated glucocorticoid therapy may also depress appetite and milk yield.

There may be potential problems for humans arising from drug residues in milk. For example, iodides are concentrated in milk. Milk iodine is primarily affected by dietary intake, but pre- and post-milking teat dipping, if not performed correctly, has a significant effect on milk-iodine concentration. Also antibacterial residues in milk can be sufficient to trigger an anaphylactic reaction in a sensitive individual.

Prescribing for neonates

Contributor:
R J Evans MA, PhD, VetMB, MRCVS

The neonatal period varies between species: from one week in foals to 6 to 8 weeks in calves and puppies. Physiological systems that affect drug absorption and disposition differ during the neonatal period and undergo rapid development particularly during the first 24 hours after birth. Characteristics of the neonatal period include more efficient absorption from the gastro-intestinal tract compared to older animals, lower binding to plasma proteins, increased volume of distribution of drugs that are distributed in extracellular fluid or total body water, increased permeability of the blood-brain barrier, and slower elimination of many drugs. These differences largely account for the clinical observation that neonates are often more sensitive to the effects of some drugs. Enhanced effect or toxicity may be seen with a number of drugs including chloramphenicol, nitrofurantoin, sulphonamides, and tetracyclines. There is generally, however, a reduced risk of immunological hypersensitivity.

Some antimicrobial agents that are poorly absorbed after oral administration to adult animals, particularly aminoglycosides, may attain effective systemic concentrations in neonates.

The gastro-intestinal absorption pattern of drugs in young ruminants is similar to that in monogastric species, depending on dietary composition, until the functional rumen has developed. The high incidence of diarrhoea in this period of life is a common cause of unpredictable alterations in oral bioavailability.

There is wide variation among species in the rate of development of hepatic microsomal oxidative reactions and glucuronide conjugation, which constitute the principal pathways of metabolism for various lipid-soluble drugs. Until the pathways are fully developed at between 1 and 8 weeks of age, depending on the species, drugs are metabolised at a slower rate. Most other hepatic metabolic pathways develop rapidly within the first 1 to 2 weeks after birth. For kittens and puppies it is often assumed that the hepatic drug metabolising system is mature by 4 to 6 weeks of age. This may, however, be too optimistic, because maturity for some substrates may require 6 months. Slow clearance and prolonged half-life of chloramphenicol, sulphonamides, tetracyclines, macrolides and lincosamides persist beyond 6 weeks of age.

Renal excretion mechanisms are poorly developed in neonates, particularly in puppies, kittens, and piglets. In calves and foals, glomerular filtration reaches functional maturity 24 to 48 hours after birth, whereas in puppies it may take 2 weeks. Tubular secretion develops more slowly and at a rate which is also species-specific.

Neonates of all species produce acidic urine, which promotes tubular reabsorption of lipid-soluble organic acids prolonging the duration of action of these drugs. The combined effect of slow hepatic metabolic reactions and inefficient renal excretion in very young animals may considerably decrease the elimination of lipid-soluble drugs and their metabolites. Therefore care must be exercised in the calculation of drug dose and dose frequency.

Limited data is available on the side-effects of drugs in neonates and young animals. Tetracyclines may cause staining of the teeth and fluoroquinolones may adversely affect the articular cartilage during periods of rapid growth.

Precise recommendations cannot be made on dosage adjustment of drugs for neonates. In *The Veterinary Formulary* the dose for young animals, in mg/kg, is the same as that given for adults, unless otherwise stated. In general, the dose frequency should be reduced to allow for the decreased rate of elimination of the drug. It is clearly important to select drugs with a wide therapeutic dose range and therapeutic index whenever possible, given the uncertainties over absorption and elimination. It is essential whenever possible to weigh the patient.

The oral route is generally preferable to parenteral administration, for convenience and relative safety, but when the parenteral route is required it may be best to administer the drug by intravenous infusion, which should be given slowly to avoid circulatory overload and to ensure complete systemic availability of the dose, although difficulties can arise because of small fragile veins and the difficulty of immobilising the patient. Low muscle mass and poor muscle blood supply can cause irregular and unpredictable absorption from intramuscular administration sites. Haematoma formation and discomfort are more common than in adult animals. It is wise to avoid topical or aerosol insecticides, although fipronil is an exception to this generalisation, and to exercise care with topical glucocorticoids, medicated shampoos, ointments, creams, and occlusive dressings because of the risk of high drug absorption rates. The intraperitoneal route has little to recommend it, being hazardous, due to risks of infection and of hyperosmolarity, and giving slow absorption. For particularly small patients insulin syringes are useful for dosing because measurement of volumes to 0.01mL are facilitated.

Due to the immunodeficient condition of the neonatal animal combined with the decreased ability to eliminate drugs, antimicrobial drugs that have a bactericidal action and wide margin of safety should be used in the treatment of systemic infections. Such drugs include penicillins (for example amoxicillin or ticarcillin combined with clavulanic acid), potentiated sulphonamides, and most of the cephalosporins.

Gut colonisation by micro-organisms is an important process in the neonate. This is susceptible to disturbance, particularly by antibiotics. Studies in humans and experimental animals, particularly in respect of colonisation by anaerobes, show marked inhibition of colonisation following administration of metronidazole, furazolidone, or oral ampicillin or cloxacillin. Moderate inhibition is produced by amoxicillin, tetracycline and chloramphenicol, whilst aminoglycosides, trimethoprim, sulphonamides, erythromycin, and parenteral penicillins are without effect. Some agents may be beneficial in this period in increasing resistance to colonisation by pathogens and these include potentiated sulphonamides, polymyxin B and neomycin. The extent to which these findings can be extrapolated to veterinary clinical circumstances is unknown.

When normal nourishment of offspring is not possible for any reason, it may be necessary to feed neonates with a milk substitute. **Colostrum replacers** should be administered within 12 hours of birth. These primarily provide a source of immunoglobulins.

Milk replacers do not contain immunoglobulins but are an important source of nutrition when for example the dam is unable to feed the offspring due to eclampsia or other causes.

Prescribing for geriatric animals

Contributor:
R J Evans MA, PhD, VetMB, MRCVS

Advances in nutrition, husbandry, welfare and veterinary practice are leading to increased longevity in animals. A greater proportion of elderly dogs and cats will be seen by veterinarians, and, as the horse population is anticipated to continue increasing, more elderly horses are likely to be encountered. Elderly farm animals are least likely to be presented but this too is changing with the increasing popularity of organic and extensive systems and of hobby farming or small-holding.

Ageing is a process of progressive degeneration of tissues, organs and body systems coupled with reduced regenerative capacity and an associated decline in functional reserve capacity. This leads to discernible anatomical changes and to an impaired ability to adapt to environmental variables and to respond to and survive stress. The animal can be considered geriatric once these deficiencies come to have a detectable impact on the animal's lifestyle and/or its veterinary care and maintenance. This reduced response capacity may not be apparent until the animal is stressed by disease, kennelling, hospitalisation, anaesthesia, or surgery. In humans, elderly (60 to 75 years) and aged (beyond 75 years) categories are distinguished but it is currently impracticable to attempt such discrimination in veterinary work. The age at which the changes become clinically significant vary with species and, within species, with breed, size, individual, and the use to which the animal is put. It is therefore difficult to generalise but the threshold is in the range 10 to 13 years for cats; 9 to 13 years for small to medium dogs, 7 to 10 years for most large breeds of dog and as early as 6 years for some giant breeds.

Ageing affects all body systems and the consequences are wide-ranging. Those most likely to be noticed by the dog or cat owner include changes in coat quality and pigmentation, thinning and loss of pliability of the skin, increased sensitivity to cold, obesity, reduced mobility, reduced alertness, cataract development, and loss of fastidiousness in urination, defecation and grooming. These are not necessarily of diagnostic significance or amenable to treatment.

Cattle, sheep and goats can survive, breed and lactate well into their second decade and some individuals have lived much longer, however by 8 to 10 years of age many will be requiring special attention in terms of husbandry and possibly veterinary intervention. Degenerative joint disease, foot problems and tooth loss all of which may contribute to difficulty in feeding are most likely to be encountered. The consequent inability to graze sufficiently or to compete with younger animals may lead to the need for separate feeding and require the use of compound feeds. It is important in dealing with these older animals that full clinical investigation is pursued otherwise false assumptions may be made, for example loss of condition may be due to overlooked parasitism rather than poor feed intake.

With horses, particularly competition animals, as with farm livestock, there is strong pressure to eliminate animals with compromised performance early in life. This must result in marked selection of the animals surviving into old-age and thus may account for the lower incidence of problems encountered than for other species. Nevertheless a significant proportion of horses and numerous ponies are roughed-off and kept into old age without particular problem. Old age can be considered to begin at 15 years, and at 20 years of age many horses will be distinctly geriatric, but animals can survive to twice this. Many owners will be neither working nor breeding from animals over 20 years of age. Renal and hepatic dysfunction is rare in old horses and when liver disease occurs it is usually characterised by fibrosis and decreased hepatic mass associated with ragwort ingestion or unknown causes, as in younger animals. The commonest problems of older horses are pituitary adenoma and the associated endocrine problems, degenerative joint disease, and dental problems. Joint disease involves a range of joints but most commonly the hock and distal limb joints. The dental problems encountered include overgrowth, spontaneous tooth decay, and infundibular abscesses. There is no particular evidence for important pharmacokinetic changes in older horses and generally clinicians use the range of drugs and dosage regimens employed in younger horses.

Prescribing for older dogs and cats requires complex judgements. Because of the increased prevalence of many diseases (see Tables below), older animals are more likely to be affected by several concurrent conditions. The need for polypharmacy is thus more common than in younger animals. Conditions needing long-term treatment are also more prevalent in older animals. There is thus greater likelihood of drug interactions and adverse reactions and also contraindications to treatment. In some cases, there can be considerable difficulty in selecting safe and effective treatments, particularly when several conditions exist concurrently. Because of the increased risk of adverse effects and drug interactions, it is prudent to minimise drug therapy as far as practicable. It may be necessary to leave conditions untreated if they interfere with the therapy of a more significant disorder, to tolerate adverse effects which may be less acceptable in younger animals, to accept limited therapeutic responses, or to elect for euthanasia. Which of these is more appropriate will depend not only upon the clinical circumstance but on the welfare implications for the animal and the perceptions, philosophy, and financial resources of the owner. It is important that there is discussion of the available options. Elderly owners are likely to have older companion animals, limited financial resources but to be greatly dependent on the companionship afforded by the human-animal bond and such circumstances will require particularly delicate consideration.

Factors influencing pharmacokinetics in older animals include renal insufficiency, with reduced GRF, leading to reduced renal clearance; hepatic insufficiency with reduced drug metabolism, conjugation or biliary clearance; reduced first pass effect; and reduced body water proportion.

There is no evidence that age-related changes influence drug absorption, whether following oral or parenteral administration. There is reduced plasma-albumin concentration, but the magnitude of the change is small and has not been shown to have a significant influence on bound to free ratio.

Reduction in body water proportion can be of greater significance. For hydrophilic drugs, the volume of distribution is generally reduced by this, whereas, for lipophilic drugs, the distribution volume is increased.

The dose regimen adjustment appropriate for the animal's GFR can be estimated using the method outlined in the section Prescribing in renal impairment. However this formula is unreliable for animals with muscle wasting and thus for many older patients. Reduced muscle mass (and thus creatinine production) means that plasma-creatinine concentration will be inappropriately low for a given GFR. In consequence, adjusted dose rates will be overestimated when using the formula based on plasma-creatinine concentration. In such circumstances creatinine clearance is a more reliable estimate of drug clearance and therefore adjusted dose rate.

Even in animals without clinically detectable hepatic dysfunction, drug uptake and clearance may be reduced because with ageing, hepatic blood flow decreases and the activity of the microsomal oxidative enzymes and of conjugating systems declines. Unfortunately there is no clinically applicable method of estimating the degree of impairment of hepatic drug handling. Thus empirical reduction in dose rate, coupled with close clinical monitoring of therapeutic and adverse effects in order to titrate the dose, must be employed.

When administering fluid therapy it is important to remember that reduced renal functional reserve, decreased ability to concentrate urine and less facile cardiovascular compensatory responses together render the animal less tolerant of fluid eletrolyte and pH disturbances and to volume and electrolyte overload. Renal ability to excrete H^+ ions is also reduced and influences the clearance of drugs by ion-trapping.

Discomfort associated with oral lesions and greater risk of aspiration associated with sluggish laryngeal reflex responses may render oral adminstration problematical.

Other miscellaneous effects can be significant. Myelin loss results in enhancement of the effect of local anaesthetics. Decreased immunocompetence may lead to greater susceptibility to disease, reduced ability to eliminate infections, and require prompt, more aggresive antibiotic therapy preferably with bactericidal agents. Infected teeth may lead to a higher incidence of bacteraemic episodes and bacterial seeding to other organs. Chronic airway disease and reduced mucociliary clearance increase susceptibility to bronchopulmonary infection and the difficulty of attaining bacteriological cure, so that longer-term and more aggressive antimicrobial therapy may be required.

Agents to be employed with caution in aged animals

Acepromazine (may result in prolonged recovery time)
Aminoglycosides
Antidysrhythmic agents
Barbiturates (and repeat dosing should be avoided)
Cholinergic agonists and antagonists (may lead to exaggerated cardiac rate changes)
Digoxin
Ketamine
Tiletamine
Xylazine

It is those conditions for which long-term or aggressive treatment are needed which will present greatest difficulty. Drugs with a narrow therapeutic index will need careful individualisation of dosage regimen, particularly if affected by one of the pharmacokinetic variables.

Common conditions seen in older dogs and cats

	Dogs	Cats
Anaemia	+	+
Cardiovascular disease	+	+
Cataracts	+	
Cystitis	+	+
Degenerative joint disease[1]	+	+
Dental calculus	+	
Diabetes mellitus[1]	+	+
Endocardiosis	+	
Endocrine disease	+	
Gingivitis	+	+
Hepatic insufficiency[2]	+	+
Hepatic lipidosis	+	+
Hyperadrenocorticism	+	
Hyperthyroidism	+	+
Hypothyroidism[2]	+	
Myocardial insufficiency	+	
Mitral insufficiency	+	
Neoplasms[1]	+	
Obesity[2]	+	+
Oral disease	+	+
Periodontitis	+	+
Prostatic disease[1] (abscessation, hypertrophy)	+	
Prostatitis	+	
Renal insufficency[2]	+	+
Tooth decay	+	+
Urinary incontinence	+	
Urinary tract disease	+	+
Urolithiasis	+	+

[1] Conditions likely to require long-term therapy
[2] Conditions where dosage regimen individualisation is essential

Treatment of poisoning

Contributor:
R J Evans MA, PhD, VetMB, MRCVS

Poisoned patients commonly present as emergencies, and often without definitive evidence of poisoning. General supportive therapy, essentially as for any other emergency, is outlined in the plan below. Useful specific antidotes are rare. It is important to collect diagnostic specimens before initiating therapy and to keep detailed contemporary records in case of possible litigation.

Veterinary Poisons Information Service

The Veterinary Poisons Information Service (VPIS) centres in London and Leeds offer an information and advice service to veterinary surgeons and animal welfare organisations who have registered and have paid an annual subscription fee. The registration fee is scaled according to the number of veterinarians in the practice. Subscribers are issued with a membership number that should be quoted when an enquiry is made.

VPIS (London)
Telephone: 020 7635 9195
Facsimile: 020 7771 5309
E-mail: vpis@gstt.sthames.nhs.uk

VPIS (Leeds)
Telephone: 0113 243 0530
Facsimile: 0113 244 5849

Treatment of poisoning

- **Remove the animal(s) from the source of intoxicant** or any suspected material such as partly eaten food. Any vomitus should be kept, together with a sample of the suspected poison and its packaging, for subsequent examination, identification, and possible analysis.
- **Decontaminate the patient, minimise and prevent further absorption, and enhance elimination.** Wash any contaminants from the skin, fur, or fleece with running water. Oily materials, paint, or tar should be removed with rags or paper towels and then the area cleaned using cooking oil or margarine. Commercial grease solvents or hand cleaners may be used sparingly following the application of oil or margarine, provided they are washed off with plenty of water, and the animal then washed using soap or liquid detergent. It may be necessary to clip the coat to remove contamination. If the animal has been in contact with strong alkalis, wash with copious amounts of water, and vinegar or lemon juice. If acids are implicated, wash with water and a weak solution of sodium bicarbonate. The owner should be advised to be careful of self-exposure to the toxicant and to wear protective clothing, particularly gloves, if necessary. In dogs and cats, ingested materials may be removed by inducing vomiting.

Vomiting should not be induced if the poison has been ingested for more than 2 hours or if the ingesta are thought to contain paraffin, petroleum products, or other oily or volatile organic materials due to the risk of inhalation. The risk of inhalation is also great and vomiting should not be induced if the animal is unconscious, convulsing, or has a reduced or absent cough reflex. In such cases, endotracheal intubation followed by gastric lavage is indicated in small animals and, in ruminants, rumenotomy may be performed. Ingesta containing strong acids or alkalis may cause further oesophageal damage if emesis is attempted. Ingested alkalis can be partly neutralised using lemon juice or vinegar diluted 1 volume with 4 volumes of water. Ingested acids should not be neutralised with sodium bicarbonate because of gas formation; *magnesium hydroxide mixture is preferable*.

Gastric lavage with **water, sodium chloride 0.9% (saline) solution**, or a slurry of **activated charcoal** may be carried out; isotonic saline is the treatment of choice. Some activated charcoal should be left in the stomach after lavage. Activated charcoal is the residue from destructive distillation of vegetable material. Adsorption of intoxicants is due to surface binding and activity is therefore greatest with small particle sizes. Saline or laxatives may also aid elimination of the toxin.

Paediatric Ipecacuanha Emetic Mixture may be used to induce emesis. In cases of poisoning, ipecacuanha syrup should not be used in association with activated charcoal because the effectiveness of the charcoal is reduced. **Apomorphine** is also a useful emetic and if employed with care produces self-limiting emesis within a few minutes. It is more effective as an emetic after subcutaneous administration than by other routes; a dose at the lower end of the dosage range is less likely to induce hyperemesis. Apomorphine is not recommended for use in cats.

Although **not** generally recommended, in an emergency information on emesis may be given to the owner. Crystalline **washing soda** (sodium carbonate), **salt** (sodium chloride), or **mustard** deposited at the back of the tongue and swallowed can cause vomiting.

In large animal practice, emesis and gastric lavage are not used. Laxatives may be used to eliminate toxin from the gastro-intestinal tract. In ruminants, gastric emptying may be performed only by rumenotomy. If the ruminal contents are removed, they should be replaced by suitable fluids and roughage, and the bacterial microflora re-established.

APOMORPHINE

UK
Indications. Induction of emesis
Contra-indications. General contra-indications to emesis, see notes above; CNS depression; cats

Side-effects. Hyperemesis, respiratory depression, sedation

Dose. *Dogs*: *by subcutaneous or intramuscular injection*, 40–100 micrograms/kg

by intravenous injection, 20–40 micrograms/kg

POM Ⓗ **Britaject** (Britannia) *UK*
Injection, apomorphine 10 mg/mL; 2 mL, 3 mL, 5 mL

IPECACUANHA

UK

Indications. Induction of emesis

Contra-indications. Poisoning with corrosive compounds or petroleum products (risk of aspiration); shock; see notes above

Side-effects. Cardiac effects if absorbed

Dose. *Dogs, cats*: 1–2 mL/kg. Maximum dose 15 mL for dogs

P Ⓗ **Paediatric Ipecacuanha Emetic Mixture** (Non-proprietary) *UK*
Ipecacuanha liquid extract 0.7 mL, hydrochloric acid 0.025 mL, glycerol 1 mL, syrup to 10 mL

CHARCOAL, ACTIVATED

UK

Indications. See notes above

Dose. Administer as an aqueous slurry of 2 g charcoal in 10 mL water

Horses: 1–3 g/kg

Ruminants: 2–8 g/kg

Pigs: 2 g/kg. Administer saline purge 30 minutes after charcoal

Dogs, cats: 0.5–2.0 g/kg by oesophageal tube following gastric lavage. Administer saline purge 30 minutes after charcoal

GSL **BCK** (Fort Dodge) *UK*
See section 3.1.1 for preparation details

P Ⓗ **Carbomix** (Penn) *UK*
Oral powder, activated charcoal; 25 g, 50 g

Liqui-Char-Vet (Arnolds) *UK*
Mixture, activated charcoal USP 50 g/240 mL

GSL Ⓗ **Medicoal** (Concord) *UK*
Oral granules, effervescent, activated charcoal 5 g/sachet

● **Collect samples for diagnosis**: (a) blood for haematological and biochemical examinations including fluid and electrolyte balance; (b) vomitus, lavage washings, urine, blood, faeces, plus other defined samples for particular intoxicants (after seeking laboratory advice) for possible toxicological examination.

● **Ensure that the airway is clear** of vomitus, tongue, and debris. Intubate and ventilate if required. Avoid the use of analeptics to stimulate respiration.

● **Regularly monitor and record** body temperature, respiration, pulse and peripheral perfusion, hydration, electrolyte balance, and urine output.

● **Institute fluid therapy** to correct any detected imbalances.

● **Correct and maintain body temperature** as appropriate using heat sources or cooling.

● **Ensure urine output**. If the animal is oliguric or anuric indicating renal shutdown administer, by intravenous injection, mannitol (see section 4.2.5) or sodium chloride 0.18% and glucose 4% solution (see section 16.1.2) with furosemide (see section 4.2.2) to re-establish renal function and induce diuresis.

For weak acid intoxicants, excretion may be enhanced by alkalinisation of the urine with 7 mL/kg of sodium bicarbonate 1.26% solution given intravenously every 3 to 4 hours in rotation with glucose saline solution.

For weak bases, acidification may be achieved with 7 mL/kg glucose 5% solution, to which has been added 1 g ammonium chloride per 100 mL of glucose 5% solution, given intravenously every 3 to 4 hours in rotation with glucose saline solution. Ammonium chloride may be administered by mouth at a dosage of 66 mg/kg 3 times daily for dogs, and for cats the dosage is 20 mg/kg twice daily.

Urinary output and pH should be monitored and the regimen adjusted on this basis whenever diuresis with urinary acidification or alkalinisation is employed to enhance elimination of intoxicants.

● **Treat convulsions, cardiac dysfunction, gastrointestinal irritation, and pain appropriately**. Treatment of convulsions should include diazepam (see section 6.9.2) or pentobarbital sodium (see section 6.6.2.1), administered by intravenous injection. The dose is dependent on the degree of CNS depression required and each animal should be treated according to response. *Acepromazine lowers the seizure threshold and should not be administered to animals with, or at risk of, seizures*.

● **Administer antidote** if the intoxicant has been identified and a suitable antidotal treatment is available. Other supportive therapy should be maintained until the toxicant has been metabolised or eliminated.

● **Keep detailed contemporary records**. This is particularly important where there is the possibility of litigation. Ideally, all samples for analysis should be labelled, dated, and sealed in the presence of a witness. If possible, samples should be divided so that they may be analysed by more than one laboratory.

Antidotes and other specific therapy

Antidotes act in a variety of ways. They may antagonise the toxin, react with it to form less active or inactive complexes, or interfere with the metabolism of the poison. For the purpose of this section intoxicants are considered under the following classification: household products; medicinal preparations intended for humans; pesticides; minerals and inorganic substances; miscellaneous chemicals; food, feed additives, and food toxins; poisonous plants; and poisonous animals. The toxicity of veterinary drugs is dealt with under the relevant monographs in Chapters 1 to 19.

Household products

Detergents, *bleaches*, and *disinfectants* commonly contain hypochlorite, phenols, or pine oils and are widely used in the home, veterinary practices, and boarding establishments. Dilute bleach is a mild to moderate irritant but ingestion of concentrated solutions causes severe erosion of the gastro-intestinal mucosa. Surface-active agents such as detergents and soaps damage membranes and remove mucus thus enhancing damage to mucosal surfaces. Alkalis also produce damage to membranes and epithelia causing severe burns with little or no initial pain so that the injury may be overlooked. The marked alkalinity of many dishwasher powders, particularly older high bulk products, can result in stomatitis and pharyngitis with oesophageal ulceration and perforation; neutralisation with a weak acid such as lemon juice or vinegar is indicated.

Phenols and *coal tar* products are corrosive, may cause local coagulative necrosis, and are absorbed from the gastro-intestinal tract and percutaneously. Hepatic and renal damage may result. Cats are particularly susceptible to phenols. *Pine oil* is a gastro-intestinal irritant and is also absorbed causing CNS depression and renal damage.

Carbon monoxide is generated by the incomplete combustion of hydrocarbon fuels and thus by gas heaters and solid fuel stoves which are improperly adjusted or have an inadequate air supply. Poisoning in the domestic situation is not uncommon and poultry and pig houses are also particularly at risk. The gas is intensely toxic and is absorbed by inhalation. It reacts with the iron atom of haemoglobin to form carboxyhaemoglobin which is incapable of oxygen transport. The clinical consequences depend upon carbon monoxide concentration. Up to approximately 200 ppm is without discernible clinical effect. Above this level and up to around 2000 ppm ataxia, muscle weakness, dyspnoea, and cardiac dysrhythmias may be noted. Above 2000 ppm death occurs in 2 to 4 hours or less as the concentration rises. Affected animals have cherry red mucous membranes and blood. Treatment is symptomatic and supportive. Affected animals should be removed from the carbon monoxide atmosphere (with due regard for human safety in doing so) and allowed to breath fresh air or an oxygen 95% and carbon dioxide 5% gas mixture.

Smoke injury is relatively common as a consequence of fires. The effects are complex. There is direct thermal injury of upper airways. In addition, chemical and particle injury of lower airways and lung parenchyma occurs due to low oxygen tension in the fire atmosphere and carbon monoxide and other combustion products. The pathology and clinical signs are progressive. Acute pulmonary insufficiency with upper airway obstruction and lower airway oedema occur over the first 36 hours. Pulmonary parenchymal oedema with alveolar proteinosis may develop over one to three days and secondary bacterial bronchopneumonia may occur up to a week following smoke exposure. Initial clinical signs include tachypnoea, dyspnoea, marked increase in expiratory effort, paroxysmal coughing, nasal discharge, and cyanosis. Auscultation reveals decreased air movement,

crackles, and wheezes. Radiology indicates pulmonary oedema with diffuse or patchy densities early in the progress, with bronchial interstitial and alveolar patterns developing later. Treatment includes administration of oxygen 95% and carbon dioxide 5% gas mixture, preferably humidified. Cautious fluid therapy with crystalloids may be needed initially. Plasma and colloids should not be administered for at least the first 12 to 24 hours. Bronchodilators are helpful and aminophylline may be administered at a dosage of 4 to 10 mg/kg 3 times daily in dogs and cats. The use of glucocorticoids is controversial but brief use may have some benefit if there is severe pulmonary oedema. Antibacterials should be used only in the face of documented infection and not for prophylaxis.

Acrolein is an unsaturated aldehyde generated by the decomposition of hot fats, notably overheated chip pans. It is a severe corneal irritant, lachrimatory agent, and causes dyspnoea. Hepatotoxicity, tonsillar enlargement, airway constriction and oedema, epistaxis, pulmonary haemorrhage, and cyanosis can also result. Most cases encountered involve dogs and prolonged exposure can be fatal.

Polytetrafluoroethylene (PTFE, Teflon) degradation products are formed when the material decomposes and vapourises when overheated. The products cause pulmonary oedema, acute haemorrhagic peritonitis, and cardiac and hepatic degeneration. Birds are particularly susceptible and in these species exposure is often fatal.

There are no specific antidotes for these household materials and supportive and symptomatic treatment should be instigated.

Medicinal preparations intended for humans

P and GSL medicines for humans that may be sold over the counter, such as paracetamol and the NSAIDs aspirin and ibuprofen, are not infrequently administered by pet owners to dogs and cats.

Aspirin and other *salicylates* have a longer half-life in dogs (9 to 13 hours) compared to man (3 to 4 hours) and a markedly longer half life in cats (22 to 45 hours). In both dogs and cats, the half life is dose dependent such that it is increased at higher doses. Intoxication may result from a single ingestion of an excessive quantity, from over frequent administration, or from the repeated administration of small or moderate overdose.

Intoxication usually presents as gastro-enteritis, which may be haemorrhagic. Steps should be taken to minimise absorption and enhance elimination. Treatment is symptomatic: **H₂-receptor antagonists,** such as cimetidine (see section 3.8.2), and **sucralfate** (see section 3.8.2) may be of value to minimise gastritis and ulceration. **Misoprostol** (see section 3.8.2), an analogue of prostaglandin E₁ is cytoprotective to the mucosa and may be used in the treatment of gastritis. Severe intoxication may result in initial respiratory acidosis followed by metabolic acidosis or by fluctuating acid-base status. The acidosis should be ameliorated by administration of intravenous fluid therapy and the judicious use of sodium bicarbonate (see section 16.1.2).

Ibuprofen has a narrow margin of safety in dogs and cats such that repeated doses of more than 5 mg/kg daily can result in intoxication in dogs. Overdose or intoxication gives rise to gastro-intestinal irritation with enteritis, haemorrhage and possible perforation, in addition to renal failure and metabolic acidosis. Treatment for this, and intoxication with most other NSAIDs, is as for the gastro-intestinal disturbances due to salicylates.

Paracetamol (acetaminophen) intoxication is most common in cats due to the deficiency of hepatic glucuronidation in this species. Also, feline haemoglobin is particularly susceptible to oxidative damage. The resulting methaemoglobinaemia is the major clinical sign of paracetamol poisoning in cats rather than hepatic necrosis as in other species. Paracetamol poisoning occurs in cats at doses greater than 45 mg/kg. Large overdoses (of more than 250 mg/kg) can cause clinical signs of hepatic failure and nephropathy in dogs. The reactive metabolite of paracetamol, *N*-acetyl-*p*-benzoquinoneimine (NABQI) is inactivated by conjugation with glutathione leading to preferential depletion of glutathione. Free NABQI then accumulates leading to damage. **Acetylcysteine** is a precursor for replenishment of glutathione. Acetylcysteine reduces free NABQI concentrations, decreases toxicity, and is the major element of treatment. In cats, in addition to acetylcysteine, administration of **ascorbic acid** (see section 16.6.3) 30 mg/kg every 6 hours by intravenous injection or orally, is also of value in order to reduce methaemoglobin to haemoglobin.

Palatable laxatives, for example *phenolphthalein* in a chocolate basis, are potential sources of poisoning. Ferrous sulphate may be toxic when ingested in the form of iron tablets, iron-supplemented vitamin preparations, or moss killer for lawns. Ferrous sulphate (iron) poisoning presents as severe gastro-enteritis and cardiovascular shock followed by pulmonary oedema and pallor or grey cyanosis. Haematemesis or black-stained vomitus may be noted and the faeces may be black and offensive. Acute liver necrosis may also develop, as may anuria or oliguria. After recent ingestion, gastric lavage is essential. The use of **desferrioxamine** as a chelating antidote may be useful in severe cases. Ointments containing the vitamin D derivative calcipotriol (Ⓗ Dovonex, Leo) are prescribed for the management of psoriasis in humans. Ingestion of ointment by animals by chewing of the tube or licking of the area to which application has been made can result in toxicity with acute and severe hypercalcaemia, hypercalciuria, bone resorption, nephrocalcinosis, and respiratory and cardiovascular dysfunction. Treatment should be as for intoxication with ergocalciferol (see Pesticides below).

Direct-acting *beta2-adrenoceptor stimulants* are used in aerosol or nebulised form for the symptomatic managment of asthma in humans. Cases of toxicosis in dogs have been reported following the ingestion or inhalation of orciprenaline (metaproterenol) or terbutaline when the animal has chewed into the owner's inhaler. Animals may present with anxious demeanour, weakness, rapid shallow respiration, cardiac tachydysrhythmia, premature contractions, pulse deficit and vomiting. Pulse strength may be increased or

decreased. Fluid therapy and beta-adrenoceptor blocking drugs are indicated. Propranolol (100 to 300 micrograms/kg, by slow intravenous injection repeated if necessary within one hour and after a further 2 to 3 hours) alone, or followed by oral propranolol (0.3 to 1.0 mg/kg 3 times daily) or atenolol (700 micrograms/kg twice daily) for up to five days, are suggested on the basis of reported cases.

Poisoning with *caffeine* or 'doping' may be seen in horses or dogs used in competitions. In dogs, pentobarbital sodium (see section 6.6.2.1) is used to control the clinical symptoms of excitement, incoordination, and convulsions.

ACETYLCYSTEINE

UK
Indications. Paracetamol poisoning
Dose. *Dogs*: *by intravenous injection,* 140 mg/kg as soon as possible after ingestion. Then 70 mg/kg 30 minutes and 1 hour after the initial dose.
Cats: *by intravenous injection,* 140 mg/kg then *by mouth,* 70 mg/kg every 6 hours for 5 days

POM Ⓗ **Parvolex** (Medeva) *UK*
Injection, acetylcysteine 200 mg/mL; 10 mL

DESFERRIOXAMINE MESILATE
(Deferoxamine mesilate, Deferoxamine mesylate)

UK
Indications. Ferrous sulphate (iron) poisoning
Side-effects. Hypotension, when given by rapid intravenous injection
Dose. *Dogs, cats*: *by intramuscular injection,* 20 mg/kg
By intravenous infusion, 10–15 mg/kg per hour (max. dose 75 mg/kg over 24 hours)

POM Ⓗ **Desferal** (Novartis) *UK*
Injection, powder for reconstitution, desferrioxamine mesilate 500 mg

Pesticides

Pesticides include insecticides, molluscicides, rodenticides, and herbicides.

The *organochlorine* insecticides, for example lindane and dieldrin, have largely been phased out of use. Cases of poisoning are, however, still encountered and present with CNS stimulation and seizures. Convulsions may be controlled with diazepam (see section 6.9.2) or pentobarbital sodium (see section 6.6.2.1).

The *organophosphorus* and *carbamate* insecticides are inhibitors of cholinesterase and poisoning results in severe muscarinic stimulation. **Atropine** (see section 6.6.1) at a dose of 25 to 200 micrograms/kg is used to control muscarinic signs; it is usually recommended that one-quarter to one-half of the dose is administered according to response by intravenous injection and the remainder by subcutaneous injection. Atropine administration should be repeated as required. **Pralidoxime** may also be used to reactivate cholinesterase in cases of organophosphorus poisoning presented within 24 hours of exposure. It has generally been thought that pralidoxime is contra-indicated in poisoning by carbamate anticholinesterases. Recent findings suggest that *pralidoxime may be of benefit in toxicity due to many carbamate insecticides but not that due to carbaril.*

Pyrethrum and *pyrethroid* insecticide poisonings are frequently reported in dogs and cats. Hypersalivation is a common sign after ingestion of pyrethrum-containing powder. In more severe cases vomiting, diarrhoea, CNS disturbances including hyperexcitability, tremors, or fasciculations are seen. Diazepam may be used to control the CNS signs.

Metaldehyde is a widely used molluscicide and many older preparations were highly palatable to dogs and cats. The resulting CNS stimulation, with hyperexcitability or convulsions, should be controlled with diazepam or pentobarbital sodium.

Many rodenticides contain *warfarin* or related *coumarin* anticoagulants, sometimes in combination with *ergocalciferol*. The coumarins inhibit the synthesis of vitamin K dependent coagulation factors. Treatment is by administration of **phytomenadione** (vitamin K₁). In large animals each dose should be divided between a number of injection sites. In severe cases, the drug may be given initially by *slow* intravenous injection. *Menadione is ineffective and should not be used.* Treatment should be continued for 7 days in cases of warfarin intoxication. Second generation coumarins, for example bromadiolone, brodifacoum, and difenacoum, have a very long half-life and treatment for 4 to 8 weeks is required. The one stage prothrombin time should be checked 3 to 4 days after the cessation of treatment. In severe cases blood transfusion may be indicated to replenish coagulation factors immediately because there is a 6 to 8 hour delay before the action of phytomenadione is evident.

Ergocalciferol causes hypercalcaemia, hyperphosphataemia, and renal failure. To reduce the hypercalcaemia, saline diuresis and furosemide (see section 4.2.2) at a dose♦ of 2.5 to 4 mg/kg 3 times daily by mouth may be employed. A low calcium diet, prednisolone (see section 7.2.1) at a dose♦ of 2 to 4 mg/kg daily by mouth and, if necessary, treatment of renal failure are indicated. Exposure to sunlight should be avoided. In severe cases, the use of **calcitonin** (see section 7.7.1) by subcutaneous or intramuscular injection at a dose of 8 to 18 units/kg daily in divided doses for up to 28 days may help to reduce bone resorption, although vomiting may be an unacceptable adverse effect. Aluminium hydroxide (see section 3.8.1) at a dose of 10 to 30 mg/kg by mouth 2 to 3 times daily has also been recommended to limit intestinal phosphate absorption.

Alphachloralose induces hypothermia, which may be fatal in small animals including mice, hedgehogs, and birds. Cats are more susceptible to poisoning than dogs. Maintenance of body temperature is essential. *Strychnine* is used under rigorous control for killing moles and rodents. Blockade of spinal inhibitory transmission results in rigidity and seizures. There is no antidote; symptoms may be controlled with diazepam or pentobarbital sodium.

While most herbicides, and particularly those for garden use, are of low toxicity, the bipyridylium agents *paraquat* and *diquat* are extremely dangerous. They are inactivated on contact with soil. Paraquat and diquat poisoning is characterised by severe oral and pharyngeal ulceration, vomiting, diarrhoea, and marked abdominal pain followed by renal function impairment, pulmonary oedema, and progressive pulmonary fibrosis. In cases presented within 4 hours of ingestion, **fuller's earth** (available from home winemaking shops and pharmaceutical suppliers), **bentonite**, **activated charcoal**, or clay soil (as a last resort) should be administered by stomach tube or orally. Forced diuresis to enhance clearance is also of value in the first 12 to 24 hours after ingestion. Administration of oxygen enhances pulmonary damage and should be avoided. Massive doses of glucocorticoids and cytotoxics have been employed with inconsistent results.

Poisoning with *sodium chlorate*, which is used as weedkiller, causes conversion of haemoglobin to methaemoglobin. **Methylthioninium chloride** (methylene blue) (see under Poisonous plants) is administered as the antidote.

PHYTOMENADIONE
(Vitamin K₁)

UK
Indications. Warfarin and coumarin poisoning
Dose. *Horses, ruminants, pigs*: by intramuscular injection, 0.5–1.0 mg/kg daily in divided doses. For second generation coumarins, continue treatment after the first week with *by subcutaneous or intramuscular injection*, 1 mg/kg daily as a single dose in ruminants
Dogs, cats: by intramuscular injection, 3–5 mg/kg daily in divided doses for 1–3 days followed by oral administration. In severe cases, initial treatment may be given by slow intravenous injection. For second generation coumarins, continue treatment after the first week with *by mouth*, 1 mg/kg daily in 3 divided doses

Ⓗ **Konakion** (Roche) *UK*
P *Tablets*, s/c, phytomenadione 10 mg; 25
POM *Injection*, phytomenadione 2 mg/mL; 0.5 mL
Note. Contains polyethoxylated castor oil which has been associated with anaphylaxis; should not be diluted therefore **not** for intravenous infusion

POM Ⓗ **Konakion MM** (Roche) *UK*
Injection, phytomenadione 10 mg/mL; 1 mL
Note. May be administered by slow intravenous injection or intravenous infusion in glucose 5%; **not** for intramuscular injection

PRALIDOXIME MESILATE
(Pralidoxime mesylate)

UK
Indications. Adjunct to atropine in organophosphorus and carbamate (see notes above) poisoning
Dose. Administer within 24 hours of exposure and repeat after 12 hours if required
Horses, ruminants: by slow intravenous injection, 10–40 mg/kg
Dogs: by slow intravenous injection, 20–50 mg/kg

Cats: *by slow intravenous injection*, 20 mg/kg

POM Ⓗ **Pralidoxime Mesilate** (Non-proprietary) *UK*
Injection, pralidoxime mesilate 200 mg/mL; 5 mL
Information on availability from the Veterinary Poisons Information Service

Minerals and inorganic substances

Lead is still a common intoxicant, especially of calves, dogs, and birds. Sources include old paint, lead accumulators (especially car batteries), curtain weights, lead toys, golf balls, linoleum, putty and, for water fowl, fishermen's lead weights. Growing awareness of the risks arising from lead is leading to reduction of its use in such products. Lead poisoning is characterised by severe abdominal pain, variable gastro-intestinal motility disturbances, and neurological signs, which may include convulsions, hyperexcitability, hysteria, depression, and blindness. In horses, pharyngeal and laryngeal paralysis may be seen. Treatment includes removing any solid lead from the gastro-intestinal tract together with the use of chelating agents to enhance urinary elimination.

Magnesium sulphate (Epsom salts) (see section 3.6.3) precipitates lead in the gastro-intestinal tract as lead sulphate and has a mild cathartic action hastening elimination. **Sodium calciumedetate** is the chelating agent of choice. It mobilises lead from bone and tissues and enhances removal of lead from the body by forming a stable, water-soluble lead complex that is readily excreted by the kidneys. Sodium calciumedetate should not be administered orally because solubilisation of the lead in the gastro-intestinal tract may enhance absorption. **Penicillamine** is a chelating agent, which may be used in the treatment of lead poisoning. It may also be of benefit in copper poisoning in dogs. It is administered orally and may therefore enhance lead absorption from the gastro-intestinal tract. It is often poorly tolerated especially at higher doses. Both sodium calciumedetate and penicillamine may induce renal and gastro-intestinal adverse effects. **Succimer** is an alternative agent which appears, on limited evidence currently available from dogs, to offer advantages.

It is advisable to measure blood-lead concentration to confirm the diagnosis and blood- and urine-lead concentration to monitor effectiveness of therapy.

Lead shot in the tissues usually becomes encapsulated in fibrous tissue and has generally been thought to be biologically inert. Recently, a number of cases of lead poisoning resulting from retained lead shot have been described in humans. In cases of doubt in animals with retained pellets and compatible clinical signs, blood-lead concentrations should be measured.

Arsenic, cyanide, copper, mercury, and *nitrite* and *nitrate* are inorganic compounds contained in pesticides, plants, and therapeutic preparations.

Sodium thiosulphate in conjunction with **sodium nitrite** is given in the treatment of cyanide poisoning. In the body sodium nitrite converts some haemoglobin to methaemoglobin. The lethal cyanide ion binds with methaemoglobin forming cyanmethaemoglobin. This is converted to the readily eliminated thiocyanate following sodium thiosulphate administration. Sodium thiosulphate is also used in the treatment of poisoning by *arsenic* and *mercury*.

Sodium thiosulphate in combination with **ammonium molybdate** is used for *copper* poisoning in sheep. An alternative treatment is ammonium tetrathiomolybdate 3 to 4 mg/kg given by subcutanous injection and repeated after 2 days. Molybdenum (7 mg/kg daily by addition to feed) has been used to prevent copper poisoning in lambs exposed to high copper intake.

Penicillamine may be of benefit in copper poisoning in dogs.

Animals may exhibit signs of *molybdenum* poisoning when grazing on pastures deficient in copper and having high sulphate levels. Copper supplements (see section 16.5.6) are used in the treatment of molybdenosis.

AMMONIUM MOLYBDATE

UK

Indications. Copper poisoning
Dose. *Sheep*: *by mouth*, 100 mg ammonium molybdate with 1 g sodium thiosulphate daily

Ammonium molybdate is available from chemical suppliers

PENICILLAMINE

UK

Indications. Lead and copper poisoning in dogs; cystine calculi (see section 9.4); copper hepatotoxicosis (see section 3.10)
Side-effects. Anorexia, vomiting, pyrexia, nephrotic syndrome
Warnings. May enhance the absorption of lead from the gastro-intestinal tract
Dose. *Dogs*: lead poisoning, *by mouth,* 110 mg/kg daily in 3–4 divided doses for 2 weeks given on an empty stomach. Antiemetics (see section 3.4.1) administered 30 minutes before penicillamine may help to reduce vomiting. Lower doses of 33–55 mg/kg daily may be better tolerated and as efficacious. Repeat with either regimen after 1 week if required
Copper poisoning, *by mouth,* 10–15 mg/kg twice daily

See section 9.4 for preparation details

SODIUM CALCIUMEDETATE
(Sodium calciumedetate)

UK

Indications. Lead poisoning
Warnings. Urine-lead concentrations should be monitored. Excessive lead mobilisation may enhance intoxication and result in renal tubular damage
Dose. *Horses* ♦: *by slow intravenous injection*, 100 mg/kg twice daily for 5 days. Repeat after 2–5 days if required
Cattle, dogs, cats ♦: *by subcutaneous* ♦ *or slow intravenous injection or infusion*, 75 mg/kg daily in 4 divided doses for 2–5 days. Repeat after 2–3 days if required. (Maximum dose for dogs 2 g)

Birds ♦: *by intramuscular or slow intravenous injection*, 35-50 mg/kg 1–3 times daily for 5 days. Repeat after 5 days if required

POM **Sodium Calciumedetate (Strong)** (Animalcare) *UK*
Injection, sodium calciumedetate 250 mg/mL, for *cattle, dogs*; 100 mL. To be diluted before use
Dilute 1 mL in 4 mL glucose 5% or sodium chloride 0.9%
Withdrawal Periods. *Cattle*: slaughter dependent on 2 successive blood-lead concentrations below 150 micrograms/litre. Blood-lead concentration should be measured at intervals of at least 7 days commencing after 28 days of clinical recovery. Milk dependent on 2 successive milk-lead concentrations below 20 micrograms/litre. *Other food-producing animals*: produce from treated animals should not be used for human consumption

SODIUM NITRITE

UK
Indications. Cyanide poisoning (in combination with sodium thiosulphate)
Dose. *Cattle, sheep*: *by intravenous injection*, sodium nitrite 1% injection, 22 mg/kg, followed by sodium thiosulphate 25% injection, 660 mg/kg. Then sodium thiosulphate 30 g *by mouth* every hour to prevent further absorption of cyanide
Dogs, cats: *by intravenous injection*, sodium nitrite 1% injection, 25 mg/kg, followed by sodium thiosulphate 25% injection, 1.25 g/kg

POM (H) **Sodium Nitrite** *UK*
Injection, sodium nitrite 30 mg/mL (3%). To be diluted before use
Available by 'Special Order' from Martindale

SODIUM THIOSULPHATE

UK
Indications. Arsenic, mercury, cyanide poisoning (in combination with sodium nitrite); copper poisoning (in combination with ammonium molybdate)
Dose. Cyanide poisoning, see under Sodium nitrite. Copper poisoning, see under Ammonium molybdate
Horses, cattle: arsenic poisoning, mercury poisoning, *by intravenous injection*, 8-10 g and *by mouth*, 20-30 g diluted in 300 mL water
Sheep, goats: arsenic poisoning, mercury poisoning, *by intravenous injection*, 2.0–2.5 g and *by mouth*, 5–7 g

POM (H) **Sodium Thiosulphate** *UK*
Injection, sodium thiosulphate 500 mg/mL
Available as a 'Special Order' from Martindale

Crystalline sodium thiosulphate is available from Loveridge and other wholesalers

SUCCIMER

UK
Indications. Lead poisoning
Dose. *Dogs*: *by mouth*, 10 mg/kg 3 times daily for 10 days

Preparations of succimer are not generally available. (H) Chemet (Bock, *USA*) may be obtained under a Special Treatment Authorisation from the VMD

Miscellaneous chemicals

Ethylene glycol is used as an antifreeze, industrial solvent, and in some photographic solutions. The initial signs of poisoning are similar to those produced by ethanol: incoordination and 'drunkenness'. Ethylene glycol is metabolised by alcohol dehydrogenase to oxalate and precipitation of calcium oxalate crystals in the kidney produces renal failure and, in the CNS, convulsions. Treatment involves saturating the enzyme, alcohol dehydrogenase, with **ethanol** thus preventing the formation of oxalate. Ideally alcohol BP should be used but vodka is a readily available source of ethanol containing approximately 40% by volume. The dose of ethanol 25%, by intravenous injection, is initially 4 mL/kg followed by 2 mL/kg every 4 hours for 4 days. **Fomepizole**, an inhibitor of alcohol dehydrogenase has also been recommended for use in the dog but cost may prohibit routine use. Fluid therapy, and, in cases of acidosis, sodium bicarbonate must be given (see section 16.1.2).
Turpentine, white spirit, kerosene, and *petrol* (light-weight hydrocarbons) and *tar* and *creosote* (phenols) usually present as topical contamination. The toxin should be removed with rags or paper towels or, for tarry substances, by clipping. Vegetable oils and hand degreasers are then applied. Emesis is generally contra-indicated for ingested light-weight hydrocarbons due to the risk of aspiration. In the UK, the Creosote Council publishes information on safe use of creosote including *Livestock & Creosote* Fact Sheet no. X02/1/95 and *Creosote: the facts and fiction* Fact sheet no. X01/2.

FOMEPIZOLE

UK
Indications. Ethylene glycol poisoning
Dose. *Dogs*: *by intravenous injection*, initial dose 20 mg/kg, then 15 mg/kg 12 and 24 hours later, then 5 mg/kg every 12 hours until blood-ethylene glycol concentration neglible or animal has visibly recovered

POM (H) **Antizol** (Cambridge) *UK*
Concentrate for intravenous infusion, fomepizole 1 g/mL

Foods, feed additives, and food toxins

Chocolate and cocoa (drinking chocolate) contain theobromine, a methylxanthine, which like caffeine, is not an uncommon cause of poisoning in dogs. Dark chocolate is more dangerous than milk or white chocolate. Doses of theobromine as low as 115 mg/kg (10 g of cooking chocolate/kg body-weight) have been reported to be fatal. Poisoning is characterised by hyperexcitability, tachycardia, dysrhythmias, and, in severe cases, convulsions and death. The cardiac signs may be controlled with anti-arrhythmic drugs such as **propranolol** (see section 4.4.2) and the CNS stimulation with diazepam (see section 6.9.2) or pentobarbital sodium (see section 6.6.2.1).
Feed additives may be toxic when feedstuffs are incorrectly compounded or when cross contamination occurs, for example, copper supplements for pig foods contaminate

sheep rations. Copper poisoning in sheep is treated with ammonium molybdate and sodium sulphate.

Aflatoxins are fungal toxins. The source is contaminated seeds and nuts such as mouldy peanuts. Aflatoxins are hepatotoxic causing marked bile duct hyperplasia and hepatic fibrosis and cirrhosis.

Botulism is the clinical manifestation of poisoning by pre-formed neurotoxins of the obligate anaerobic spore-forming bacterium *Clostridium botulinum*. Some neurotoxins are known and differing strains may produce different spectra of toxins. Toxin production is also influenced by substrate type and availability. Disease may result from the ingestion of feedstuffs, carrion, garbage, soil, or mud containing the toxins. All species are susceptible but dogs are commonly affected, as are water birds in hot dry summers. Botulinum toxins block acetylcholine release from motor nerve terminals resulting in flaccid paralysis which is symmetrical and commonly sufficiently severe that the animal becomes quadriplegic. Gastro-intestinal disturbance, hyposalivation, and pupillary dilation may be present. The animal remains conscious and aware. Death usually results from respiratory paralysis. Definitive diagnosis depends on the demonstration of toxin(s) in the source material, serum, or both. Although mixed (A, B and E) botulinum antitoxin is available from hospitals, it is of little use once a significant amount of toxin is bound to receptors. Antitoxin is therefore not generally employed in veterinary practice but has been used in treatment of botulism in foals and horses at a dose of approximately 1 mL/kg body-weight. Supportive therapy is given, with intermittent positive pressure ventilation, if practicable, should respiratory failure supervene. Clearance of residual toxin from the gastro-intestinal tract by emesis and enema may be of some value. Since the toxin is generally preformed, antimicrobial drugs are not indicated.

Poisonous plants

Poisonous plants may be ingested from roadsides, neglected pastures, dried in hay, or in preserved forage. Plants infected with fungi such as ergot may also cause poisoning. Before treatment, potentially poisonous plants should be identified. Identification systems are available on CD-ROM: *Poisonous Plants and Fungi in Britain and Ireland* produced by Nightshade (Royal Botanic Gardens, Kew and Medical Toxicology Unit, Guy's & St Thomas' Hospital Trust). This includes information on plants that are toxic in humans and some of signifance for animals.

Sweet vernal grass *Anthoxanthum odoratum* contains *coumarin*, which may cause clinical signs in cattle similar to warfarin poisoning. **Phytomenadione** (vitamin K₁) is given intramuscularly at a dose of 1 to 3 mg/kg body-weight.

Cyanogenetic glycosides found in plants such as cherry laurel, bird cherry, linseed, and some grasses and clovers are toxic and may affect cattle and sheep. Treatment includes sodium nitrite injection followed by sodium thiosulphate injection.

The *nitrite* and *nitrate* content of various plants such as grasses, kale, rape, turnips and swedes is influenced by climate and use of nitrogenous fertilisers. Poisoning results in conversion of haemoglobin to methaemoglobin within the body and also vasodilation with consequent hypotension. Oxygen delivery is compromised resulting in tissue anoxia with dyspnoea, with muddy brown cyanosis and weakness being prominent clinical signs. **Methylthioninium chloride** (methylene blue) is used as an antidote because it converts methaemoglobin to haemoglobin. A wide range of dosages has been suggested (for ruminants 1 mg/kg up to 20 mg/kg). Methylthioninium chloride in excess may itself cause methaemoglobinaemia and caution is advised.

Beet tops should be wilted before feeding to stock and introduced into the diet slowly because these and other plants such as *Oxalis* species may be toxic due to their *oxalate* content. *Rhubarb* leaves commonly cause oxalate poisoning in goats kept in gardens. Clinical signs are those of hypocalcaemia and treatment is by subcutaneous or intravenous injection of **calcium borogluconate** (see section 16.5.1).

Bracken and *Equisetum* species contain thiaminases, which may cause thiamine deficiency. **Thiamine** (see section 16.6.2) at a dose of 0.25 to 1.25 mg/kg twice daily for up to 7 days by intramuscular or slow intravenous injection is used for the treatment of thiaminase poisoning in horses and pigs. In cattle, bracken poisoning is unrelated to thiaminase and causes aplastic anaemia with thrombocytopenia and bladder neoplasia.

Oak and acorn poisoning due to the leaves and fruit of trees of the genus *Quercus* may affect ruminants, horses, and pigs and is relatively common. Toxicity results from high concentrations of tannins in the plant and is manifested as gastro-enteritis, which is often haemorrhagic, and hepatic and renal damage with consequent jaundice and haematuria. The mortality rate is very high and there is no specific treatment. If ingestion is known to have occurred, oral administration of calcium hydroxide may have a protective effect.

European yew *Taxus baccata* and Japanese yew *Taxus cuspidata* contain a highly poisonous alkaloid taxine. The main action is on the heart and toxicity is generally characterised by sudden death. All species are susceptible but poisoning is most commonly seen in cattle, sheep, and horses. There is no specific antidote and the extreme rapidity of effect generally precludes any attempt at treatment. In ruminants, rumenotomy to remove any ingested material may be of value.

Laburnum *Laburnum anagyroides* is the most toxic tree in Britain after the yew. All parts of the plant are poisonous, containing the alkaloid cytisine, but the fallen seeds and seed pods represent a particular hazard. Cases of poisoning are severe but infrequent and have been recorded in cattle, horses, pigs, and dogs. Vomiting, excitement, incoordination, and convulsions progress to coma, asphyxia, and death. There is no specific therapy but control of convulsions and general supportive therapy are indicated.

The abuse of cannabis (Indian hemp, hashish, marijuana, *Cannabis sativa*) by humans means that opportunities for intoxication of animals arise with considerable frequency. The main pharmacologically active and toxic compound is tetrahydrocannabinol. The dried plant is of low toxicity and even after ingestion of large amounts the prognosis is good with fatalities being rare. The intoxication presents as inco-ordination, depression and stupor, slow strong pulse, and reduced respiratory rate. Sometimes there are intervening periods of wakefulness and hyperaesthesia and occasionally collapse supervenes. Clinical signs seen in animals are not necessarily similar to the effects observed in humans. Supportive therapy is indicated but recovery is usually spontaneous after a few hours and uneventful. There is no specific treatment.

In periods of intense algal bloom, ingestion of water containing high densities of blue-green algae *Cyanophyceae* may result in poisoning. A number of syndromes are seen depending on the algal species involved. A severe syndrome characterised by hypotension, tachycardia, hyperglycaemia, and marked liver damage resulting in jaundice and photosensitisation due to ingestion of *Anacystis cyanea* (*Microcystis aeruginosa*) is probably most common. Death may occur within hours in the worst affected cases. There is no specific treatment.

Plants of the genus *Senecio*, notably various ragworts, contain pyrrolizidine alkaloids. They cause poisoning as a result of ingestion directly from pasture or by contamination in hay, silage, or other preserved forage. Ragwort poisoning occurs in horses and cattle. The alkaloids may induce acute or, more commonly, chronic liver disease with consequent hepatic function impairment. Jaundice, photosensitisation, and hepatic encephalopathy may ensue. There is no specific treatment and euthanasia is normally indicated once clinical signs are apparent although there have been reports of full recovery of mild cases in horses.

A variety of species and hybrids of daffodil and narcissus (*Narcissus* spp.) occur in the UK as native plants as naturalised introductions or are grown as ornamental plants. A mixture of alkaloids is present throughout the plants but in highest concentration in the bulbs. Calcium oxalate crystals are also present and may act as mechanical irritants. The alkaloids are emetic, purgative and irritant, thus inducing a marked gastro-enteritis. Dogs are most commonly affected and ingestion of as little as 15 g of bulbs can be fatal. In addition to the gastro-enteritis, severe cases may develop hyperglycaemia, ataxia, cardiovascular collapse and or coma. Rehydration and symptomatic treatment are indicated.

Aesculus hippocastanum the familiar white-flowered horse chestnut is a common introduced tree now with many naturalised specimens. A pink-flowered hybrid (*Aesculus carnea*) is also grown in the UK but is not naturalised. A number of glycosides, alkaloids and saponins are present in *Aesculus* spp. The hydroxycoumarin saponin glycoside aesculin is probably the most significant toxic principle. Although the bark reputedly has a high aesculin content and young leaves and flowers are the most toxic parts of the tree, poisoning is commonly due to the ingestion of the seeds ('conkers'). Poisoning is reported for a variety of species including horses, cattle, pigs, and dogs. The clinical signs include gastro-enteritis and abdominal discomfort,

depression, , incoordination with muscle tremor and weakness or paralysis. There is no specific treatment. Decontaminative and supportive measures should be instituted.

Many garden and house plants are poisonous and represent a potential hazard to dogs, cats, and other domestic pets. *Dieffenbachia* spp. (dumbcane), *Philodendron* spp. (for example sweetheart vine), and *Monstera* spp. (Swiss cheese plant) contain numerous fine oxalate crystals and, when ingested, these penetrate the gastro-intestinal mucosa causing marked stomatitis, pharyngitis, oesophagitis, and intestinal irritation. *Euphorbia* spp. (for example poinsettia) contain chemical irritants and cause severe vomiting, diarrhoea, anorexia, and depression.

METHYLTHIONINIUM CHLORIDE
(Methylene blue)

UK

Indications. Nitrite and nitrate poisoning; sodium chlorate poisoning

Dose. Administer according to the patient's response, *by slow intravenous injection*. Treatment may be repeated after 4 to 6 hours if required.

Cattle: initially 1–2 mg/kg, may be given up to 10–15 mg/kg

Sheep: initially 1–2 mg/kg, may be given up to 20 mg/kg

Dogs, cats: 5-10 mg/kg

POM Ⓗ **Methylthioninium chloride** *UK*
Injection, methylthioninium chloride 10 mg/mL; 10 mL
Available as a 'Special Order' from Martindale

Poisonous animals

The only venomous snake indigenous to the UK is the common adder *Vipera berus*. Dogs are the main species affected and are usually bitten on the head or neck. **Snake venom antiserum (Europe)**, available from P & D Pharmaceuticals, is the antidote. The small size of dogs and cats means that the venom load per unit body weight is high. This has two consequences: the risk of fatality is greater and a large dose of antivenin relative to body-weight is required. A dose of 15 to 100 mL of antivenin may be required for the treatment of a moderately sized dog bitten by an adder. Glucocorticoids, antihistamines, and antibacterials may be of some benefit.

Localised swelling occurs after bee, hornet, or wasp stings. Insect stings around the larynx may cause respiratory distress. **Glucocorticoids** (see section 7.2.1) and **antihistamines** (see section 5.2.1) are used as systemic therapy. Topical treatment such as weak acids for wasp stings or sodium bicarbonate for bee stings may be applied to the affected area.

The common toad *Bufo vulgaris* secretes venom from glands within the skin. Dogs and cats may be poisoned when they 'mouth' the amphibian and will show clinical symptoms of profuse salivation. Mouth-washes containing **sodium bicarbonate** and administration of **atropine** (see section 6.6.1) are used as therapy.

1 Drugs used in the treatment of
BACTERIAL, FUNGAL, VIRAL, and PROTOZOAL INFECTIONS

Contributors:
M Bennett BVSc, PhD, MRCVS
J Elliott MA, VetMB, PhD, CertSAC, DipECVPT, MRCVS
L M Sommerville BVMS, MRCVS
Professor M A Taylor BVMS, PhD, CBiol, MIBiol, MRCVS

1.1 Antibacterial drugs
1.2 Antifungal drugs
1.3 Antiviral drugs
1.4 Antiprotozoal drugs

1.1 Antibacterial drugs

1.1.1 Beta-lactam antibacterials
1.1.2 Tetracyclines
1.1.3 Aminoglycosides
1.1.4 Macrolides and lincosamides
1.1.5 Chloramphenicols
1.1.6 Sulphonamides and potentiated sulphonamides
1.1.7 Nitrofurans
1.1.8 Nitroimidazoles
1.1.9 Quinolones
1.1.10 Pleuromutilins
1.1.11 Other antibacterial drugs
1.1.12 Compound antibacterial preparations
1.1.13 Compound preparations for bacterial enteritis

Selection of a suitable drug

Bacterial sensitivity. Antibacterial drugs are often used unnecessarily and sometimes (as in uncomplicated diarrhoea) when they are clearly contra-indicated. However, when antibacterial therapy is essential, there is a rational basis for deciding which antibacterial drug to use in a specific case. For time-dependent bactericidal drugs and bacteriostatic drugs, the aim of therapy is to maintain an effective concentration of the drug at the site of infection for as long as necessary. An effective concentration may be defined as that which is sufficiently in excess of the minimum inhibitory concentration (MIC) of the drug for an adequate period of time appropriate for the causal micro-organisms. Effective therapy is thus dependent on the susceptibility of the micro-organisms to the drug and the pharmacokinetics which determine its ability to attain and maintain effective concentrations at the infection site.

Except in the rare cases where sensitivity data are available, assessment of the potential sensitivity of the micro-organisms concerned depends firstly upon accurate clinical diagnosis and secondly upon the knowledge that these are the micro-organisms likely to be implicated and of their susceptibility to antibacterial drugs. Fortunately, detailed knowledge of MIC values is not required because microbial sensitivity to a drug can be expressed in terms of the concentrations attained in body tissues. In this chapter, a micro-organism will be deemed 'sensitive' to a drug if, following administration according to the recommended dosage regimen, tissue concentrations are likely to be in excess of the MIC for that micro-organism for a major part of the time between doses. The spectrum of activity for antimicrobial drugs is given in Table 1.1. Having narrowed the list of possible drugs to those likely to be active against the micro-organism or micro-organisms concerned, the final choice is based on the following criteria.

Species, breed, and age differences affect an animal's ability to eliminate antibacterial drugs; the following of which are examples. Cats are less able than other species to metabolise chloramphenicol, which may accumulate following prolonged administration in this species. The young of all species are similarly deficient in their ability to metabolise drugs. Antibacterial action can disrupt bacterial fermentation and therefore animals with a functional rumen should not be given broad-spectrum antibacterials by mouth. Many antibacterials and particularly tetracyclines by any route may be associated with a fatal enterocolitis in horses subjected to stress. Penicillins, macrolides, and lincosamides should not be administered to gerbils, guinea pigs, hamsters, or rabbits in which they are likely to cause a fatal enterotoxaemia. See also Prescribing for equines, ruminants, pigs, dogs, cats, and neonates.

Predisposition to toxicity. Certain conditions may exacerbate the toxicity of antibacterial drugs; the following are examples. Renal disease may predispose animals, especially cats, to the toxic effects of aminoglycosides because they are eliminated solely by renal excretion and so may accumulate in renal failure. Tetracyclines are contra-indicated in bitches and queens in late pregnancy when they may cause enamel defects and discoloration in the offsprings' milk teeth. In growing dogs and cats, fluoroquinolones may cause an arthropathy.

Site of infection. Special considerations apply to the treatment of infections at particular sites. For example, antibacterials such as chloramphenicol and the macrolides are extensively metabolised and so are not used to treat urinary-tract infections for which drugs undergoing renal excretion and which are therefore concentrated in the urine are preferred. In addition, in the treatment of urinary-tract infections it is important to choose a drug with actions that are favoured by the prevailing urinary pH to maximise efficacy. In particular, aminoglycosides are much more active in alkaline urine.

Some body compartments, notably the brain and the internal structures of the eye, are penetrated only by lipophilic drugs that are able to cross intact cell membranes. Permeability is increased by inflammation. Although chloramphenicol and sulphonamides normally enter the brain, ampicillin and doxycycline do so only in the presence of inflammation. Similarly, milk is separated from the general circulation by an intact membrane through which only the non-ionised lipophilic form of a drug may pass. When the non-ionised form of a basic drug such as a macrolide enters the relatively acid milk it dissociates and so becomes trapped resulting in high concentrations in milk – the so called 'ion-trap'. Conversely, acidic drugs such as benzylpenicillin are largely excluded from the healthy udder. Both factors cease to operate in the presence of inflammation so that drugs penetrate the acutely inflamed mammary gland to the same extent as any other inflamed tissue. The physicochemical properties of antimicrobial drugs is given in Table 1.2.

Mode of antibacterial action. As noted in the sections dealing with individual groups of drugs, some are bactericidal, that is they are able to kill bacteria, whereas others are bacteriostatic, only inhibiting multiplication and hence relying upon host defences to clear the infection. Although the advantages of bactericidal drugs have probably been exaggerated in the past, there are certain situations in which their use is essential. These include the treatment of endocarditis, and in cases of immunosuppression occurring either naturally or due to administration of corticosteroids.

Antibacterial policy. It is essential that antibacterials are given according to a predetermined policy in order that efficacy may be monitored. Changes in resistance patterns in a particular area should be noted and therapy altered accordingly. The BVA have published *General Guidelines on Prudent use of Antimicrobials* and also species-specific guidelines on prudent antimicrobial usage in horses, cattle, sheep, dogs, cats, poultry, and fish; these are included in *The Veterinary Formulary*.

Before commencing therapy

The **dose** of an antibacterial drug expressed as weight of drug per kg body-weight will vary with a number of factors including intercurrent disease, severity of the infection, and size of the animal. In serious infections high doses are administered more frequently. Depot preparations are long-acting but attain relatively low plasma-drug concentrations; they are not suitable for the treatment of severe acute infections. In general, the larger the animal the smaller the dosage per unit body-weight.

The dosing regimen used should also reflect the mode of action of the antibacterial drug. For bactericidal drugs, such as beta-lactams, and bacteriostatic drugs which operate time-dependent killing mechanisms it is important to maintain tissue concentration of the drug above the MIC for as long as possible during the inter-dosing interval. For bactericidal drugs, such as aminoglycosides and fluoroquinolones, which operate concentration-dependent killing mechanisms, the most successful dosing regimen is one

which produces a peak tissue concentration of the drug which greatly exceeds the MIC value for the bacterium and the time the concentration of the drug is above the MIC is much less significant.

The **duration of therapy** depends upon the nature of the infection and the response to treatment. In general, therapy should continue for 2 to 3 days beyond the clinical cure for acute infections and for 1 to 2 weeks beyond the clinical cure for chronic infections. However, this guidance does not apply in all instances. For example, acute cystitis in the bitch often responds very quickly to antibacterial drugs (24 to 48 hours) but if treatment is not continued for 7 to 10 days, relapses may well occur. This more extended period of treatment allows the important mucosal defence mechanisms within the bladder to heal fully and therefore be effective in preventing re-infection when the treatment stops. Clinical experience has shown that some chronic infections may require more prolonged duration of therapy (for example, deep pyodermas, chronic prostatitis and osteomyelitis in dogs). Empirically, therapy for 4 to 6 weeks may be required in these cases.

The **route of administration** depends upon the severity of the disease and ease of administration. In the treatment of severe infections it is advantageous to give the initial dose by the intravenous route in appropriate cases. In companion animals subcutaneous injection may be preferred to the more painful intramuscular route. In order to attain effective concentrations in the cerebrospinal fluid, an initial intrathecal injection may be administered. However, **penicillins should not be administered by the intrathecal route because seizures may result**.

Although oral medication given with food is often convenient, it may considerably reduce the amount of drug absorbed. For example, ampicillin (unlike amoxicillin) is poorly absorbed in dogs if administered following a meal. Milk, iron salts, and antacids all interfere with the absorption of tetracyclines from the gastro-intestinal tract. However, in some cases, for example ketoconazole, administration with food will reduce side-effects such as nausea. In other cases, giving the drug with food is important to aid in its absorption, for example, griseofulvin is highly lipid soluble and requires biliary secretion to allow optimal absorption from the gastro-intestinal tract.

1.1.1 Beta-lactam antibacterials

1.1.1.1 Narrow-spectrum penicillins
1.1.1.2 Beta-lactamase resistant penicillins
1.1.1.3 Broad-spectrum penicillins
1.1.1.4 Antipseudomonal penicillins
1.1.1.5 Cephalosporins

This group comprises the penicillins and the cephalosporins. They are bactericidal by interfering with cell wall synthesis. Beta-lactam antibacterials are not metabolised in the body, but are rapidly excreted unchanged in the urine. Relatively insoluble depot preparations are often used to prolong action, albeit at the expense of concentrations

Table 1.1 Summary of spectrum of activity for antimicrobial drugs[1]

Bacteria	Antimicrobials	Additional information
Narrow spectrum antimicrobials for aerobes and facultative anaerobes		
Mainly Gram-positive	lincosamides	also very active against many obligate anaerobes
	glycopeptides:vancomycin	
Gram-positive and fastidious Gram-negative organisms (for example *Haemophilus*)	benzylpenicillin, phenoxymethylpenicillin	poor activity against beta-lactamase producing *Staphylococcus*
	cloxacillin, flucloxacillin	active against beta-lactamase producing *Staphylococcus*
	macrolides	also active against *Chlamydia* and mycoplasmas
	rifampicin	also active against pox viruses, *Chlamydia*, some protozoa and fungi (**but** antiviral and anti-fungal activity not used clinically)
Mainly Gram-negative	aminoglycosides: kanamycin, neo-mycin, streptomycin	neomycin is active against *Pseudomonas aeruginosa*; aminoglycosides should usually be reserved for treatment of infections caused by particularly resistant Gram-negative organisms
	nalidixic acid	
	polymixins	active against *Pseudomonas aeruginosa*; should usually be reserved for treatment of infections caused by particularly resistant Gram-negative organisms
Broad spectrum antimicrobials for aerobes and facultative anaerobes		
Many Gram-positive and Gram-negative bacteria	aminoglycosides: amikacin, gentamicin, tobramycin	sometimes active against *Pseudomonas aeruginosa*; should usually be reserved for treatment of infections caused by particularly resistant Gram-negative organisms
	aminopenicillins	poor activity against beta-lactamase producing *Staphylococcus*
	carboxypenicillins: ticarcillin	active against *Pseudomonas aeruginosa*; should usually be reserved for treatment of infections caused by particularly resistant Gram-negative organisms
	cephalosporins	third generation cephalosporins active against *Pseudomonas aeruginosa*; should usually be reserved for treatment of infections caused by particularly resistant Gram-negative organisms
Many Gram-positive and Gram-negative bacteria	baquiloprim, trimethoprim, ormetoprim	

Table 1.1 Summary of spectrum of activity for antimicrobial drugs[1]

Bacteria	Antimicrobials	Additional information
Broad spectrum antimicrobials for aerobes and facultative anaerobes		
Many Gram-positive and Gram-negative bacteria, also some protozoa, rickettsiae, *Chlamydia*	chloramphenicol	also active against rickettsiae and *Chlamydia*
	fluoroquinolones	also active against rickettsiae
	nitrofurans	also active against protozoa
	sulphonamides	also active against protozoa and *Chlamydia*
	tetracyclines	also active against protozoa, rickettsiae, and *Chlamydia*
Antimicrobials for special organisms		
Obligate anaerobic bacteria	cephalosporins	*Bacteroides fragilis* is resistant to all cephalosporins except cefoxitin
	clindamycin, chloramphenicol, nitroimidazoles	
	penicillins	*Bacteroides fragilis* is resistant to all penicillins except piperacillin
Mycobacteria	rifampicin, streptomycin, azithromycin, clarithromycin, fluroquinolones	
Mycoplasma	fluroquinolones	active against *Pseudomonas aeruginosa*; should usually be reserved for treatment of infections caused by particularly resistant Gram-negative organisms
	lincosamides, macrolides, nitrofurans, tetracyclines	

[1] The information given is for guidance. Antimicrobial sensitivity testing will be necessary in the clinical situation, particularly for coagulase positive staphylococci, many Gram-negative enterobacteriaceae, and *Pseudomonas aeruginosa*, whose sensitivities are unpredictable and change due to plasmid-mediated resistance

Table 1.2 Physicochemical properties of antimicrobial drugs and effect on tissue distribution

Polar (hydrophilic) drugs of low lipophilicity

These drugs do not readily penetrate 'natural body barriers' so that effective concentrations in CSF, milk, and other transcellular fluids will not always be achieved. Adequate concentrations may be achieved in joints, and pleural and peritoneal fluids where the barrier to penetration is less. (Penetration may be assisted by acute inflammation.)

Acids	*Bases*
Beta-lactams	Polymixins: polymixin B, colistin
Penicillins: aminopenicillins, carbenicillin, isoxazolypenicillins[1], benzylpenicllin, phenoxymethylpenicllin, piperacillin, ticarcillin	Aminoglycosides: amikacin, dihydrostreptomycin, gentamicin, kanamycin, neomycin, streptomycin, tobramycin
Cephalosporins (all)	Spectinomycin
Beta-lactamase inhibitors: clavulanate	

Drugs of moderate to high lipophilicity

These drugs cross cellular barriers more readily than polar molecules so enter transcellular fluids to a greater extent. Weak bases will be ion trapped (concentrated) in fluids which are more acidic than plasma, for example prostatic fluid, milk, or intracellular fluid (for example macrolides, which are sufficiently lipophilic to penetrate). Penetration into CSF and ocular fluids (in absence of acute inflammation) is affected by plasma protein binding and also lipophilicity. Sulphonamides and diaminopyrimidines penetrate effectively whereas insufficient penetration is achieved with macrolides, lincosamides, and tetracyclines.

Weak acids	*Weak bases*	*Amphoteric substances*
Sulphonamides: sulfadiazine, sulfadimethoxine, sulfadoxine, sulfafurazole, sulfamethazine, sulfamethoxazole, sulfathiazole	Diaminopyrimidines: baquiloprim, ormetoprim, trimethoprim	Tetracyclines: chlortetracycline, oxytetracycline, tetracycline
	Lincosamides: clindamycin, lincomycin, pirlimycin	
	Macrolides: azithromycin, clarithromycin, erythromycin, spiramycin, tilmicosin, tylosin	

Highly lipophilic molecules with low ionisation

These drugs cross cellular barriers very readily. They penetrate into transcellular fluids such as prostatic fluid and bronchial secretions. All these drugs penetrate into intracellular fluids. All these drugs, except tetracyclines and rifampicin, penetrate into CSF.

Fluroquinolones: danofloxacin, difloxacin, enrofloxacin, orbifloxacin, marbofloxacin

Tetracyclines (lipophilic): doxycycline, minocycline

Other antimicrobials: chloramphenicol, florphenicol, metronidazole, rifampicin, thiamphenicol

---

[1] cloxacillin, flucloxacillin, and oxacillin are highly plasma protein bound (> 95%) in dogs

achieved in body fluids. An initial high concentration of drug in body fluids combined with prolonged activity may be achieved by simultaneous administration of a soluble and a less soluble penicillin salt.

1.1.1.1 Narrow-spectrum penicillins

Benzylpenicillin, also known as penicillin G, was the first of the penicillins, and remains an important and useful antibacterial. It is particularly active against Gram-positive bacteria. Sensitive micro-organisms include Gram-positive aerobes such as *Staphylococcus aureus*, streptococci, most *Actinomyces* spp., *Erysipelothrix*, and *Bacillus* spp. Most anaerobic bacteria including *Clostridium* and some *Bacteroides* spp., although not *B. fragilis*, are also sensitive. Benzylpenicillin has activity against the more fastidious Gram-negative aerobes such as *Haemophilus*, *Pasteurella*, *Leptospira*, and some *Actinobacillus* spp. Benzylpenicillin is broken down by the beta-lactamase enzymes produced by staphylococci and *Bacteroides* spp. A high proportion of strains of these micro-organisms are now resistant to benzylpenicillin. Other organisms mentioned retain their sensitivity to benzylpenicillin because of their inability to produce beta-lactamase.

Benzylpenicillin is inactivated by gastric acid and so is not administered by mouth. It is available as a range of salts that differ in their solubility and hence their duration of action. The sodium salt is very soluble and therefore rapidly absorbed following injection, but gives effective concentrations for no more than 4 hours.

Procaine benzylpenicillin is slightly soluble. Following parenteral administration, it forms a 'depot' which slowly releases free benzylpenicillin into the circulation, maintaining effective concentrations against the more susceptible micro-organisms for up to 24 hours. It is thought that the procaine component of procaine benzylpenicillin may give rise to a febrile reaction and abortions in sows infected with *Erysipelothrix*. **Benzathine benzylpenicillin** is a very slightly soluble ester, which has a prolonged action after intramuscular injection although plasma concentrations produced are low. It is available in combination with procaine benzylpenicillin.

Phenoxymethylpenicillin, or penicillin V, has a similar antibacterial spectrum to benzylpenicillin but is less active. It is gastric acid-stable and thus suitable for oral administration (not horses). It should not be used for severe infections because absorption can be unpredictable and plasma-drug concentrations variable.

BENZYLPENICILLIN
(Penicillin G, Penethamate hydriodide)

UK
Indications. Penicillin-sensitive infections
Contra-indications. Penicillin or cephalosporin hypersensitivity; should not be administered to gerbils, guinea pigs, hamsters, rabbits; should not be administered by intrathecal injection

Side-effects. Allergic reactions; diarrhoea
Warnings. Penicillins and cephalosporins may cause hypersensitivity (allergy) following self-injection, inhalation, ingestion, or skin contact. Operators with known hypersensitivity should not handle these drugs. Clinical signs of allergic reaction in operators include skin rash, swelling of the face, lips, or eyes, or difficulty breathing. Operators should seek medical advice
Dose. *Horses*: *by intravenous injection*, 10 mg/kg twice daily for 1 day

POM **Crystapen 5 Mega for Injection (Veterinary)** (Schering-Plough) *UK*
Injection, powder for reconstitution, benzylpenicillin (as sodium salt) 3 g, for *horses*
Withdrawal Periods. Should not be used in *horses* intended for human consumption

Australia
Indications. Penicillin-sensitive infections
Contra-indications. Penicillin or cephalosporin hypersensitivity; should not be administered to gerbils, guinea pigs, hamsters, rabbits
Side-effects. Allergic reactions; diarrhoea
Warnings. Penicillins and cephalosporins may cause hypersensitivity (allergy) following self-injection, inhalation, ingestion, or skin contact. Operators with known hypersensitivity should not handle these drugs. Clinical signs of allergic reaction in operators include skin rash, swelling of the face, lips, or eyes, or difficulty breathing. Operators should seek medical advice

Leocillin (Boehringer Ingelheim) *Austral.*
Injection, powder for reconstitution, penethamate hydiodide 5 g (= benzylpenicillin 5 g), for *horses, cattle, pigs, sheep*
Withdrawal Periods. *Cattle*: slaughter 5 days, milk 36 hours (single dose) or 72 hours (multiple dose). *Horses, pigs, sheep*: slaughter 5 days

Eire
Indications. Penicillin-sensitive infections
Contra-indications. Penicillin or cephalosporin hypersensitivity; should not be administered to gerbils, guinea pigs, hamsters, rabbits
Side-effects. Allergic reactions; diarrhoea
Warnings. Penicillins and cephalosporins may cause hypersensitivity (allergy) following self-injection, inhalation, ingestion, or skin contact. Operators with known hypersensitivity should not handle these drugs. Clinical signs of allergic reaction in operators include skin rash, swelling of the face, lips, or eyes, or difficulty breathing. Operators should seek medical advice

POM **Crystapen** (Schering-Plough) *Eire*
Injection, powder for reconstitution, benzylpenicillin (as sodium salt) 3 g, for *horses*
Withdrawal Periods. Should not be used in *horses* intended for human consumption

New Zealand
Indications. Penicillin-sensitive infections
Contra-indications. Penicillin or cephalosporin hypersensitivity; should not be administered to gerbils, guinea pigs, hamsters, rabbits
Side-effects. Allergic reactions; diarrhoea

Warnings. Penicillins and cephalosporins may cause hypersensitivity (allergy) following self-injection, inhalation, ingestion, or skin contact. Operators with known hypersensitivity should not handle these drugs. Clinical signs of allergic reaction in operators include skin rash, swelling of the face, lips, or eyes, or difficulty breathing. Operators should seek medical advice

Procillin (Boehringer Ingelheim) *NZ*
Injection, benzylpenicillin (as potassium salt), for *horses, cattle, pigs*
Withdrawal Periods. *Horses, pigs*: slaughter 6 days. *Cattle*: slaughter 6 days, milk 48 hours

Leocillin (Boehringer Ingelheim) *NZ*
Injection, penethamate hydriodide 5 g, for *horses, cattle, sheep, pigs*
Withdrawal Periods. Horses, pigs: slaughter 7 days. Cattle, sheep: slaughter 7 days, milk 48 hours

USA

Indications. Penicillin-sensitive infections,
Contra-indications. Hypersensitivity to the drug
Warnings. Penicillins and cephalosporins may cause hypersensitivity (allergy) following self-injection, inhalation, ingestion, or skin contact. Operators with known hypersensitivity should not handle these drugs. Clinical signs of allergic reaction in operators include skin rash, swelling of the face, lips, or eyes, or difficulty breathing. Operators should seek medical advice

Penicillin G Potassium USP (AgriLabs, DurVet, Osborn, RXV) *USA*
Oral powder, for addition to drinking water, benzylpenicillin potassium, for *turkeys*
Withdrawal Periods. Slaughter 1 day, should not be used in turkeys producing eggs for human consumption

R-Pen (ID Russell) *USA*
Oral solution, for addition to drinking water, benzylpenicillin (as potassium salt), for *turkeys*
Withdrawal Periods. Slaughter 1 day, should not be used in turkeys producing eggs for human consumption

Solu-Pen (Wade Jones) *USA*
Oral powder, for addition to drinking water, benzylpenicillin (as potassium salt), for *turkeys*
Withdrawal Periods. Slaughter 1 day, should not be used in turkeys producing eggs for human consumption

PHENOXYMETHYLPENICILLIN
(Penicillin V)

UK

Indications. Penicillin-sensitive infections,
Contra-indications. Side-effects. Warnings. See notes above and under Benzylpenicillin; should not be used in horses
Dose. *Pigs: by addition to feed,* 200 g/tonne feed
Dogs, cats: by mouth, 10 mg/kg 3 times daily

POM Ⓗ **Phenoxymethylpenicillin** (Non-proprietary) *UK*
Tablets, phenoxymethylpenicillin (as potassium salt) 250 mg
Oral solution, powder for reconstitution, phenoxymethylpenicillin (as potassium salt) 25 mg/mL, 50 mg/mL; 100 mL

POM **Potencil** (Vericore LP) *UK*
Oral powder, for addition to feed, phenoxymethylpenicillin potassium 100 g/kg, for *pigs*
Withdrawal Periods. Slaughter 1 day

Eire

Indications. Penicillin-sensitive infections,
Contra-indications. Hypersensitivity to the drug
Warnings. Penicillins and cephalosporins may cause hypersensitivity (allergy) following self-injection, inhalation, ingestion, or skin contact. Operators with known hypersensitivity should not handle these drugs. Clinical signs of allergic reaction in operators include skin rash, swelling of the face, lips, or eyes, or difficulty breathing. Operators should seek medical advice
Dose. *Pigs*: 10 mg/kg

Potencil (Cypharm) *Eire*
Oral powder, for addition to feed, phenoxymethylpenicillin 10%, for *pigs*
Withdrawal Periods. Slaughter 24 hours

PROCAINE BENZYLPENICILLIN
(Procaine penicillin)

UK

Indications. Penicillin-sensitive infections
Contra-indications. Side-effects. Warnings. See under Benzylpenicillin; see also notes above
Dose. Dosages vary, for guidance.
Horses: by intramuscular injection, 10 mg/kg once daily
Cattle: by intramuscular injection, 10 mg/kg once daily
cattle, non lactating: by depot subcutaneous or intramuscular injection, 20 mg/kg. Repeat after 3 days if required
cattle, lactating: by depot intramuscular injection, 20 mg/kg. Repeat after 3 days if required
Sheep: by intramuscular injection, 10 mg/kg once daily
Pigs: by intramuscular injection, 10 mg/kg once daily
by depot intramuscular injection, 20 mg/kg. Repeat after 3 days if required
Dogs, cats: by subcutaneous injection, 30 mg/kg once daily

POM **Depocillin** (Intervet) *UK*
Injection, procaine benzylpenicillin 300 mg/mL, for *horses, cattle, sheep, pigs, dogs, cats*; 100 mL
Withdrawal Periods. Should not be used in *horses* intended for human consumption. *Cattle*: slaughter 4 days, milk 3 days. *Sheep*: slaughter 4 days, should not be used in sheep producing milk for human consumption. *Pigs*: slaughter 5 days

POM **Duphapen** (Fort Dodge) *UK*
Injection, procaine benzylpenicillin 300 mg/mL, for *cattle, sheep, pigs*; 40 mL, 100 mL
Withdrawal Periods. *Cattle*: slaughter 5 days, milk 2 days. *Sheep*: slaughter 5 days, should not be used in sheep producing milk for human consumption. *Pigs*: slaughter 5 days

POM **Econopen Injection** (Vericore VP) *UK*
Injection, procaine benzylpenicillin 300 mg/mL, for *horses, cattle, sheep, pigs*; 100 mL
Withdrawal Periods. *Cattle*: slaughter 5 days, milk 2.5 days. *Sheep*: slaughter 5 days, should not be used in sheep producing milk for human consumption. *Pigs*: slaughter 5 days

POM **Lenticillin** (Merial) *UK*
Injection, procaine benzylpenicillin 300 mg/mL, for *cattle, sheep, pigs*; 100 mL
Withdrawal Periods. *Cattle*: slaughter 5 days, milk 60 hours. *Sheep*: slaughter 5 days, should not be used in sheep producing milk for human consumption. *Pigs*: slaughter 5 days

POM **Norocillin** (Norbrook) *UK*
Injection, procaine benzylpenicillin 300 mg/mL, for *cattle, sheep, pigs*; 50 mL, 100 mL
Withdrawal Periods. *Cattle*: slaughter 5 days, milk 2 days. *Sheep*: slaughter 5 days, should not be used in sheep producing milk for human consumption. *Pigs*: slaughter 5 days

POM **Penacare** (Animalcare) *UK*
Injection, procaine benzylpenicillin 300 mg/mL, for *cattle, sheep, pigs*
Withdrawal Periods. *Cattle*: slaughter 5 days, milk 60 hours. *Sheep*: slaughter 5 days, should not be used in sheep producing milk for human consumption. *Pigs*: slaughter 5 days

POM **Ultrapen LA** (Norbrook) *UK*
Depot injection, procaine benzylpenicillin 300 mg/mL, for *cattle, pigs*
Withdrawal Periods. *Cattle*: slaughter 10 days (subcutaneous administration), 21 days (intramuscular administration), milk 5 days. *Pigs*: slaughter 7 days

Australia

Indications. Penicillin-sensitive infections
Dose. Dosages vary, consult manufacturer's information

Aquacaine G Injectable Suspension (Boehringer Ingelheim) *Austral..*
Injection, procaine benzylpenicillin 300 mg/mL, for *horses, cattle, sheep, cats, dogs*
Withdrawal Periods. *Cattle*: slaughter 5 days, milk 36 hours (single dose) or 72 hours (multiple dose). *Horses, sheep*: slaughter 5 days

Bomacillin (Pharmtech) *Austral..*
Injection, procaine benzylpenicillin 300 mg/mL, for *horses, cattle, sheep, pigs, dogs, cats*
Withdrawal Periods. *Cattle*: slaughter 5 days, milk 36 hours (single dose) or 72 hours (multiple dose). *Horses, sheep, pigs*: slaughter 5 days

Depocillin (Intervet) *Austral..*
Injection, procaine benzylpenicillin 300 mg/mL, for *horses, cattle, sheep, pigs, dogs, cats*
Withdrawal Periods. Cattle: slaughter 5 days, milk 36 hours (single dose) or 72 hours (multiple dose). Horses, sheep, pigs: slaughter 5 days

Norocillin SA Injection (Novartis) *Austral..*
Injection, procaine benzylpenicillin 300 mg/mL, for *cattle, horses, sheep, pigs, dogs, cats*
Withdrawal Periods. *Horses, pigs, sheep*: slaughter 5 days. *Cattle*: slaughter 5 days, milk 36 hours

Propen (Ilium) *Austral..*
Injection, procaine benzylpenicillin 300 mg/mL, for *horses, cattle, sheep, pigs, dogs, cats*
Withdrawal Periods. *Cattle*: slaughter 5 days, milk 36 hours (single dose) or 72 hours (multiple dose). *Horses, sheep, pigs*: slaughter 5 days

Eire

Indications. Penicillin-sensitive infections
Dose. Dosages vary, consult manufacturer's information

Depocillin (Intervet) *Eire*
Injection, procaine benzylpenicillin 300 mg/mL, for *horses, cattle, sheep, pigs, dogs, cats*
Withdrawal Periods. Should not be used in *horses* intended for human consumption. *Cattle*: slaughter 4 days, milk 72 hours. *Sheep*: slaughter 4 days, should not be used in sheep producing milk for human consumption. Pigs: slaughter 5 days

Duphapen (Interchem) *Eire*
Injection, procaine benzylpenicillin 300,000 i.u./mL, for *horses, cattle, sheep, goats, pigs*
Withdrawal Periods. *Horses*: slaughter 28 days. *Cattle*: slaughter 5 days, milk 72 hours. *Sheep*: slaughter 5 days, should not be used in sheep producing milk for human consumption. *Goats, pigs*: slaughter 5 days

Norocillin (Norbrook) *Eire*
Injection, procaine benzylpenicillin 300 mg/mL, for *horses, cattle, sheep, pigs*
Withdrawal Periods. Should not be used in *horses* intended for human consumption, in emergency, slaughter 28 days. *Cattle*: slaughter 5 days, milk 72 hours. *Sheep*: slaughter 5 days, should not be used in sheep producing milk for human consumption. *Pigs*: slaughter 5 days

Pharmacillin Injection (Interpharm) *Eire*
Injection, procaine benzylpenicillin 300 mg/mL, for *cattle, sheep, pigs*
Withdrawal Periods. *Cattle*: slaughter 5 days, milk 3 days. *Sheep*: slaughter 5 days, should not be used in sheep producing milk for human consumption. *Pigs*: slaughter 5 days

Unicillin (Univet) *Eire*
Injection, procaine benzylpenicillin 300 mg/mL, for *cattle, sheep, pigs*
Withdrawal Periods. *Cattle*: slaughter 7 days, milk 72 hours. *Sheep*: slaughter 7 days, should not be used in sheep producing milk for human consumption. *Pigs*: slaughter 7 days

Ultrapen LA (Norbrook) *Eire*
Injection, procaine benzylpenicillin 300 mg/mL, for *cattle, pigs*
Withdrawal Periods. *Cattle*: slaughter 21 days (after im) or 10 days (after sc), milk 5 days. *Pigs*: slaughter 7 days

New Zealand

Indications. Penicillin-sensitive infections
Dose. Dosages vary, consult manufacturer's information

Bomacillin (Bomac) *NZ*
Injection, procaine benzylpenicillin 300 mg/mL, for *horses, cattle, sheep, goats, pigs, dogs, cats*
Withdrawal Periods. *Horses*: slaughter 28 days. *Cattle, sheep*: slaughter 5 days, milk 48 hours (1 dose), 60 hours (2 doses), 72 hours (3 or more doses). *Goats*: slaughter 30 days, milk 48 hours (1 dose), 60 hours (2 doses), 72 hours (3 or more doses). *Pigs*: slaughter 5 days

Bovipen (Stockguard) *NZ*
Injection, procaine benzylpenicillin 300 mg/mL, for *cattle*
Withdrawal Periods. Slaughter 30 days, milk 48 hours (1 dose), 60 hours (2 doses), 72 hours (3 or more doses)

Cowpen 5000 (Bomac) *NZ*
Injection, procaine benzylpenicillin 300 mg/mL, for *cattle*
Withdrawal Periods. Slaughter 5 days, milk 48 hours (1 dose), 60 hours (2 doses), 72 hours (3 or more doses)

Depocillin (Chemavet) *NZ*
Injection, procaine benzylpenicillin 300 mg/mL, for *large and small animals*
Withdrawal Periods. *Horses*: slaughter 28 days. *Cattle, sheep*: slaughter 4 days, milk 48 hours (1 dose), 60 hours (2 doses), 72 hours (3 or more doses). *Pigs*: slaughter 5 days

Intracillin (Stockguard) *NZ*
Injection, procaine benzylpenicillin 300 mg/mL, for *horses, cattle, sheep, pigs, dogs, cats*
Withdrawal Periods. *Horses, pigs*: slaughter 30 days. *Cattle, sheep*: slaughter 30 days, milk 48 hours (1 dose), 60 hours (2 doses), 72 hours (3 or more doses)

Intracillin High Potency 500 (Stockguard) *NZ*
Injection, procaine benzylpenicillin 500 mg/mL, for *horses, cattle, sheep, pigs, dogs, cats*
Withdrawal Periods. *Horses, pigs*: slaughter 30 days. *Cattle, sheep*: slaughter 30 days, milk 48 hours (1 dose), 60 hours (2 doses), 72 hours (3 or more doses)

Mylipen (Schering-Plough) *NZ*
Injection, procaine benzylpenicillin 300 mg/mL, for *horses, cattle, sheep, pigs, dogs, cats*
Withdrawal Periods. *Horses, pigs*: slaughter 30 days. *Cattle, sheep*: slaughter 30 days, milk 72 hours

Penicillin-300 (Ethical) *NZ*
Injection, procaine benzylpenicillin 300 mg/mL, for *horses, cattle, sheep, pigs, dogs, cats*
Withdrawal Periods. *Horses*: slaughter 28 days. *Cattle, sheep*: slaughter 5 days, milk 48 hours (1 dose), 60 hours (2 doses), 72 hours (3 or more doses). *Pigs*: slaughter 5 days

Penovet (Boehringer Ingelheim) *NZ*
Injection, procaine benzylpenicillin 300 mg/mL, for *horses, cattle, sheep, pigs, dogs, cats*
Withdrawal Periods. *Horses, pigs*: slaughter 30 days. *Cattle, sheep*: slaughter 30 days, milk 48 hours (1 dose), 60 hours (2 doses), 72 hours (3 or more doses)

Pharmacillin 300 (Phoenix) *NZ*
Injection, procaine benzylpenicillin 300 mg/mL, for *horses, cattle, sheep, pigs, dogs, cats*
Withdrawal Periods. *Horses, pigs*: slaughter 30 days. *Cattle, sheep*: slaughter 30 days, milk 48 hours (1 dose), 60 hours (2 doses), 72 hours (3 or more doses)

Procal 5000 (Stockguard) *NZ*
Injection, procaine benzylpenicillin 5 g/vial, for *cattle*
Withdrawal Periods. Slaughter 30 days, milk 48 hours (1 dose), 60 hours (2 doses), 72 hours (3 or more doses)

USA

Indications. Penicillin-sensitive infections
Dose. *By intramuscular injection.*
Horses, cattle, sheep, pigs: 6.6 mg/kg

Agri-Cillin (AgriLabs) *USA*
Injection, procaine benzylpenicillin 300mg/ml, for *cattle*
Withdrawal Periods. Milk 48 hours

Aquacillin Injection (Vedco) *USA*
Injection, procaine benzylpenicillin 300 mg/ml, for *horses, cattle, sheep, pigs*
Withdrawal Periods. Milk 48 hours

Crysticillin (Fort Dodge) *USA*
Injection, procaine benzylpenicillin 300 mg/mL, for *cattle, sheep, pigs, horses*
Withdrawal Periods. Should not be used in *horses* intended for human consumption. *Cattle* (calves): slaughter 7 days. Cattle: slaughter 4 days. *Sheep*: slaughter 8 days. *Pigs*: slaughter 6 days. Should not be used in animals producing milk for human consumption

Microcillin (Anthony) *USA*
Injection, procaine benzylpenicillin 300 mg/mL, for *cattle, sheep, pigs, horses*
Withdrawal Periods. Should not be used in *horses* intended for human consumption. *Cattle*: slaughter 4 days (pre-ruminating calves 7 days), milk 48 hours. *Sheep*: slaughter 8 days. *Pigs*: slaughter 6 days

Pen-Aqueous (AgriPharm) *USA*
Injection, procaine benzylpenicillin 300 mg/mL, for *horses, cattle, sheep, pigs,*
Withdrawal Periods. Should not be used in horses intended for human consumption. *Cattle*: slaughter 4 days, milk 48 hours. *Calves (non-ruminating)*: slaughter 7 days. *Sheep*: slaughter 8 days. *Pigs*: slaughter 6 days.

Pen-Aqueous (DurVet) *USA*
Injection, procaine benzylpenicillin 300 mg/mL, for *cattle, sheep, pigs, horses*
Withdrawal Periods. Horses: should not be used in horses intended for human consumption. Cattle: slaughter 10 days, milk 48 hours, should not be used in calves intended for veal production. Sheep: slaughter 9 days. Pigs: slaughter 7 days

Pen-Aqueous (RXV, Western Veterinary Supply) *USA*
Injection, procaine benzylpenicillin 300 mg/mL, for *horses, cattle, sheep, pigs*
Withdrawal Periods. Should not be used in *horses* intended for human consumption. *Cattle*: slaughter 10 days, milk 48 hours. *Sheep*: slaughter 9 days. *Pigs*: slaughter 7 days

Pen-G (Phoenix) *USA*
Injection, procaine benzylpenicillin 300 mg/mL, for *cattle, sheep, pigs, horses*
Withdrawal Periods. Should not be used in *horses* intended for human consumption. *Cattle*: slaughter 10 days, milk 48 hours, should not be used in calves intended for veal production. *Sheep*: slaughter 9 days. *Pigs*: slaughter 7 days

Pen-G Procaine (VetTek) *USA*
Injection, procaine benzylpenicillin 300 mg/mL, for *horses, cattle, sheep, pigs,*
Withdrawal Periods. Should not be used in *horses* intended for human consumption. *Cattle*: slaughter 10 days, milk 48 hours, should not be used in calves intended for veal production. *Sheep*: slaughter 9 days. *Pigs*: slaughter 7 days

Penicillin G Procaine (Aspen, GC Hanford) *USA*
Injection, procaine benzylpenicillin 300 mg/mL, for *horses, cattle, sheep, pigs*
Withdrawal Periods. *Horses*: should not be used in horses intended for human consumption. *Cattle*: slaughter 10 days, milk 48 hours, should not be used in calves intended for veal production. *Sheep*: slaughter 9 days. *Pigs*: slaughter 7 days

Penicillin G Procaine Suspension (Butler) *USA*
Injection, procaine benzylpenicillin 300 mg/mL, for *horses, cattle, sheep, pigs*
Withdrawal Periods. Should not be used in *horses* intended for human consumption. *Cattle*: slaughter 10 days, milk 48 hours. *Sheep*: slaughter 9 days. *Pigs*: slaughter 7 days

Penject (Vetus) *USA*
Injection, procaine benzylpenicillin 300 mg/mL, for *horses, cattle, sheep, pigs*
Withdrawal Periods. Should not be used in *horses* intended for human consumption. *Cattle*: 4 days, milk 48 hours. *Sheep*: slaughter 8 days. *Pigs*: slaughter 6 days. *Calves (non ruminating)*: slaughter 7 days.

PFI-Pen G (Pfizer) *USA*
Injection, procaine benzylpenicillin 300 mg/mL, for *horses, cattle, sheep, pigs*
Withdrawal Periods. Should not be used in *horses* intended for human consumption. *Cattle*: slaughter 10 days, milk 48 hours, should not be used in calves intended for veal production. *Sheep*: slaughter 9 days. *Pigs*: slaughter 7 days

BENZATHINE BENZYLPENICILLIN and PROCAINE BENZYLPENICILLIN
(Benzathine Penicillin and Procaine Penicillin)

UK

Indications. Penicillin-sensitive infections
Contra-indications. Side-effects. Warnings. See under Benzylpenicillin
Dose. Expressed for a suspension containing benzathine benzylpenicillin 112.5 mg + procaine benzylpenicillin 150 mg/mL
Horses, cattle, sheep, pigs: *by intramuscular injection,* 1 mL/25 kg body-weight, repeat after 3–4 days if required
Dogs, cats: *by intramuscular injection,* 1 mL/10 kg body-weight, repeat after 3–4 days if required

POM **Duphapen LA** (Fort Dodge) *UK*
Depot injection, benzathine benzylpenicillin 112.5 mg, procaine benzylpenicillin 150 mg/mL, for *horses, cattle, sheep, pigs, dogs, cats*; 40 mL, 100 mL
Withdrawal Periods. Should not be used in *horses* intended for human consumption. *Cattle*: slaughter 60 days, milk 3 days. *Sheep*: slaughter 60 days, should not be used in sheep producing milk for human consumption. *Pigs*: slaughter 60 days

POM **Duplocillin LA** (Intervet) *UK*
Depot injection, benzathine benzylpenicillin 112.5 mg, procaine benzylpenicillin 150 mg/mL, for *horses, cattle, sheep, pigs, dogs, cats*; 50 mL, 100 mL
Withdrawal Periods. Should not be used in *horses* intended for human consumption. *Cattle*: slaughter 60 days, milk 3 days. *Sheep*: slaughter 60 days, should not be used in sheep producing milk for human consumption. *Pigs*: slaughter 60 days

POM **Lentrax 100** (Merial)
Depot injection, benzathine benzylpenicillin 112.5 mg, procaine benzylpenicillin 150 mg/mL, for *horses, cattle, sheep, pigs, dogs, cats*; 100 mL
Withdrawal Periods. Should not be used in *horses* intended for human consumption. *Cattle*: slaughter 60 days, milk 3 days. *Sheep*: slaughter 60 days, should not be used in sheep producing milk for human consumption. *Pigs*: slaughter 60 days

POM **Norocillin LA** (Norbrook) *UK*
Depot injection, benzathine benzylpenicillin 112.5 mg, procaine benzylpenicillin 150 mg/mL, for *horses, cattle, sheep, pigs, dogs, cats*; 50 mL, 100 mL
Withdrawal Periods. Should not be used in *horses* intended for human consumption. *Cattle*: slaughter 60 days, milk 3 days. *Sheep*: slaughter 60 days, should not be used in sheep producing milk for human consumption. *Pigs*: slaughter 60 days

Australia

Indications. Penicillin-sensitive infections
Dose. Dosages vary, consult manufacturer's information

Aquacaine L/A Injectable Suspension (Boehringer Ingelheim) *Austral.*.
Injection, benzathine benzylpenicillin 112.5 mg/mL and procaine benzylpenicillin 150 mg/mL, for *horses, cattle, sheep, cats, dogs*
Withdrawal Periods. *Horses, sheep*: slaughter 30 days. *Cattle*: slaughter 30 days, milk 13 days

Benacillin (Ilium) *Austral.*.
Injection, procaine benzylpenicillin 150 mg/mL, benzathine benzylpenicillin 150 mg/mL and procaine hydrochloride 20 mg/mL, for *horses, cattle, pigs dogs, cats*
Withdrawal Periods. *Horses, pigs*: slaughter 30 days. *Cattle*: slaughter 30 days, milk 13 days

Bomacillin LA (Pharmtech) *Austral.*.
Injection, procaine benzylpenicillin 150 mg/mL and benzathine benzylpenicillin 112.5 mg/mL, for *horses, cattle, sheep, pigs, dogs, cats*
Withdrawal Periods. *Horses, sheep*: slaughter 30 days.*Cattle*: slaughter 30 days, milk 13 days.

Duplocillin (Intervet) *Austral.*.
Injection, procaine benzylpenicillin 150 mg/mL, benzathine benzylpenicillin 115 mg/mL, for *horses, cattle, sheep, pigs, dogs, cats*
Withdrawal Periods. *Horses, sheep*: slaughter 30 days.*Cattle*: slaughter 30 days, milk 13 days

Norocillin LA (Novartis) *Austral.*.
Injection, procaine benzylpenicillin 150 mg/mL, benzathine benzylpenicillin 112.5 mg/mL, for *cattle, horses, sheep, pigs, dogs, cats*
Withdrawal Periods. *Horses, sheep, pigs*: slaughter 30 days. *Cattle*: slaughter 30 days, milk 13 days

Eire

Indications. Penicillin-sensitive infections
Dose. Expressed for a suspension containing benzathine benzylpenicillin 112.5 mg + procaine benzylpenicillin 150 mg/mL
Horses, cattle, sheep, pigs: by intramuscular injection, 1 mL/25 kg body-weight
Dogs, cats: by intramuscular injection, 1 mL/10 kg body-weight

Duphapen LA (Interchem) *Eire*
Injection, procaine benzylpenicillin 150 mg/mL, benzathine penicillin 112.5 mg/mL, for *horses, cattle, sheep, pigs, dogs, cats*

Withdrawal Periods. Should not be used in *horses* intended for human consumption. *Cattle*: slaughter 14 days, milk 5 days. *Sheep*: slaughter 14 days, should not be used in sheep producing milk for human consumption. *Pigs*: slaughter 14 days

Duplocillin LA (Intervet) *Eire*
Injection, procaine benzylpenicillin 150 mg/mL, benzathine penicillin 112.5 mg/mL, for *horses, cattle, sheep, pigs, dogs, cats*
Withdrawal Periods. *Horses*: slaughter 70 days. *Cattle*: slaughter 14 days, milk 108 hours. *Sheep*: slaughter 14 days, should not be used in sheep producing milk for human consumption. *Pigs*: slaughter 14 days

Norocillin LA (Norbrook) *Eire*
Injection, benzathine benzylpenicillin 112.5 mg/mL, procaine benzylpenicillin 150.0 mg/mL, for *horses, cattle, sheep, pigs*
Withdrawal Periods. Should not be used in *horses* intended for human consumption, in emergency slaughter 28 days. *Cattle*: slaughter 14 days, milk 5 days. *Sheep*: slaughter 14 days, should not be used in sheep producing milk for human consumption. *Pigs*: slaughter 14 days

Pharmacillin LA (Interpharm) *Eire*
Injection, benzathine benzylpenicillin 112.5 mg/mL, procaine benzylpenicillin 150.0 mg/mL, for *horses, cattle, sheep, pigs*
Withdrawal Periods. Should not be used in *horses* intended for human consumption. *Cattle*: slaughter 14 days, milk 5 days. *Sheep*: slaughter 14 days, should not be used in sheep producing milk for human consumption. *Pigs*: slaughter 14 days

New Zealand

Indications. Penicillin-sensitive infections
Dose. Dosages vary, consult manufacturer's information

Bomacillin LA (Bomac) *NZ*
Depot injection, benzathine benzylpenicillin 112.5 mg/mL, procaine benzylpenicillin 150 mg/mL, for *horses, cattle, sheep, pigs, dogs, cats*
Withdrawal Periods. *Horses*: slaughter 28 days. *Cattle, sheep*: slaughter 14 days, milk 128 hours. *Pigs*: slaughter 10 days

Bomacillin LA for Sheep (Bomac) *NZ*
Depot injection, benzathine benzylpenicillin 112.5 mg/mL, procaine benzylpenicillin 150 mg/mL, for *sheep*
Withdrawal Periods. Slaughter 30 days, should not be used in sheep producing milk for human consumption

Duplocillin LA (Chemavet) *NZ*
Depot injection, benzathine benzylpenicillin 112.5 mg/mL, procaine benzylpenicillin 150 mg/mL, for *horses, cattle, sheep, pigs, dogs, cats*
Withdrawal Periods. *Horses, pigs*: slaughter 30 days. *Cattle, sheep*: slaughter 30 days, milk 120 hours

Intracillin L.A. (Stockguard) *NZ*
Depot injection, benzathine benzylpenicillin 112.5 mg/mL, procaine benzylpenicillin 150 000 units/mL, for *horses, cattle, sheep, pigs, dogs, cats*
Withdrawal Periods. *Horses, pigs*: slaughter 30 days. *Cattle, sheep*: slaughter 30 days, milk 108 hours

Ovipen (Stockguard) *NZ*
Depot injection, benzathine benzylpenicillin 112.5 mg/mL, procaine benzylpenicillin 150 mg/mL, for *sheep*
Withdrawal Periods. Slaughter 30 days

Penodure LA (Boehringer Ingelheim) *NZ*
Depot injection, benzathine benzylpenicillin 112.5 mg/mL, procaine benzylpenicillin 150 mg /mL, for *horses, cattle, sheep, pigs, dogs, cats*
Withdrawal Periods. *Horses, pigs*: slaughter 30 days. *Cattle, sheep*: slaughter 30 days, milk 108 hours

Pharmacillin L.A. (Phoenix) *NZ*
Depot injection, benzathine benzylpenicillin 112.5mg/mL, procaine benzylpenicillin 150 mg/mL, for *horses, cattle, sheep, pigs, dogs, cats*
Withdrawal Periods. *Horses, pigs*: slaughter 30 days. *Cattle, sheep*: slaughter 30 days, milk 108 hours

Procal 500 (Stockguard) *NZ*
Injection, per single-dose tube: benzylpenicillin 125 000 units, procaine benzylpenicillin 375 000 units, for *sheep, pigs*
Withdrawal Periods. *Sheep*: slaughter 30 days, milk 96 hours. *Pigs*: slaughter 30 days

Propen LA (Schering-Plough) *NZ*
Injection, benzathine benzylpenicillin 141.5 mg/mL, procaine benzylpenicillin 150 mg/mL, for *horses, cattle, sheep, pigs, dogs, cats*
Withdrawal Periods. *Horses, pigs*: slaughter 30 days. *Cattle, sheep*: slaughter 30 days, milk 132 hours

Tripen L A (Ethical) *NZ*
Depot injection, benzathine benzylpenicillin 112.5 mg/mL, procaine benzylpenicillin 150 mg/mL, for *horses, cattle, sheep, pigs, dogs, cats*
Withdrawal Periods. *Horses*: slaughter 180 days. *Cattle*: slaughter 30 days, milk 120 hours. *Sheep*: slaughter 30 days, should not be used in sheep producing milk for human consumption. *Pigs*: slaughter 30 days

USA

Indications. Penicillin-sensitive infections
Dose. *Horses, cattle*: *by subcutaneous injection*, 1 mL/34 kg body-weight

Ambi-Pen (Butler) *USA*
Injection, benzathine benzylpenicillin 112.5 mg/mL, procaine benzylpenicillin 150 mg/ml, for *horses, cattle, dogs*
Withdrawal Periods. Should not be used in *horses* intended for human consumption. *Cattle*: slaughter 30 days

Combicillin (Anthony) *USA*
Injection, benzathine benzylpenicillin 112.5 mg/mL, procaine benzylpenicillin 150 mg/mL, for *horses, cattle, dogs*
Withdrawal Periods. Should not be used in *horses* intended for human consumption. *Cattle*: slaughter 30 days

Crystiben (Fort Dodge) *USA*
Injection, benzathine benzylpenicillin 112.5 mg/mL, procaine benzylpenicillin 150 mg/mL, for *horses, cattle, dogs*
Withdrawal Periods. Should not be used in *horses* intended for human consumption. *Cattle*: slaughter 30 days

Benza-Pen (Western Veterinary Supply) *USA*
Injection, benzathine benzylpenicillin 112.5 mg/mL, procaine benzylpenicillin 150 mg/ml, for *horses, cattle*
Withdrawal Periods. Should not be used in *horses* intended for human consumption. *Cattle*: slaughter 30 days, should not be used in calves intended for veal production

Dual-Cillin (Phoenix) *USA*
Injection, benzathine benzylpenicillin 112.5 mg/mL, procaine benzylpenicillin 150 mg/mL, for *cattle*
Withdrawal Periods. Slaughter 30 days, should not be used in cattle producing milk for human consumption

Dura-Pen (DurVet) *USA*
Injection, benzathine benzylpenicillin 112.5 mg/mL, procaine benzylpenicillin 150 mg/mL, for *cattle*
Withdrawal Periods. Slaughter 30 days, should not be used in cattle producing milk for human consumption, should not be used in calves intended for veal production

Durapen Injection (Vedco) *USA*
Injection, benzathine benzylpenicillin 112.5 mg/mL, procaine benzylpenicillin 150 mg/mL, for *cattle, horses, dogs*
Withdrawal Periods. Should not be used in *horses* intended for human consumption. *Cattle*: slaughter 30 days, should not be used in cattle producing milk for human consumption

Duo-Pen (AgriPharm, RXV, VetTek) *USA*
Injection, benzathine benzylpenicillin 112.5 mg/mL, procaine benzylpenicillin 150 mg/mL, for *cattle*
Withdrawal Periods. Slaughter 30 days, should not be used in cattle producing milk for human consumption

Pen BP-48 (Pfizer) *USA*
Injection, benzathine benzylpenicillin 112.5 mg/mL, procaine benzylpenicillin 150 mg/mL, for *cattle*
Withdrawal Periods. Slaughter 30 days, should not be used in calves intended for veal production

Penicillin G Benzathine And Penicillin G Procaine (Aspen) *USA*
Injection, benzathine benzylpenicillin 112.5 mg/mL, procaine benzylpenicillin 150 mg/mL, for *cattle*
Withdrawal Periods. Slaughter 30 days, should not be used in calves intended for veal production

Sterile Penicillin G Benzathine And Penicillin G Procaine (GC Hanford) *USA*
Injection, benzathine benzylpenicillin 112.5 mg/mL, procaine benzylpenicillin 150 mg/mL, for *cattle*
Withdrawal Periods. Slaughter 30 days, should not be used in calves intended for veal production

Twin-Pen (AgriLabs) *USA*
Injection, benzathine benzylpenicillin 112.5 mg and procaine benzylpenicillin 150 mg/mL, for *cattle*
Withdrawal Periods. Slaughter 30 days

1.1.1.2 Beta-lactamase resistant penicillins

Isoxazolylpenicillins have the antibacterial spectrum of benzylpenicillin but in addition are stable in the presence of staphylococcal beta-lactamases. They are effective in infections caused by penicillin-resistant staphylococci, the sole indication for their use. **Cloxacillin** and **oxacillin** are incorporated into intramammary or ophthalmic preparations. **Flucloxacillin** is absorbed from the gastro-intestinal tract and is available for oral administration. Its bioavailability is significantly reduced by the presence of food thus this drug should be given before feeding.

FLUCLOXACILLIN

UK

Indications. Infections caused by beta-lactamase-producing staphylococci
Contra-indications. Side-effects. See under Benzylpenicillin (see section 1.1.1.1)
Dose. *Dogs, cats*: *by mouth*, 15 mg/kg 4 times daily

POM Ⓗ **Flucloxacillin** (Non-proprietary) *UK*
Capsules, flucloxacillin (as sodium salt) 250 mg, 500 mg
Oral solution, powder for reconstitution, flucloxacillin (as sodium salt) 25 mg/mL; 100 mL

1.1.1.3 Broad-spectrum penicillins

Ampicillin and **amoxicillin** have slightly less activity than benzylpenicillin against Gram-positive bacteria and anaerobes but considerably greater activity against Gram-negative bacteria, although their action is poor against *Klebsiella*, some *Proteus* spp., and *Pseudomonas* spp. In addition, they are broken down by beta-lactamases, both the staphylococcal enzymes and those produced by Gram-negative organisms such as *E. coli* and *Haemophilus* spp. Acquired resistance in such organisms has limited the usefulness of these antibiotics.

Amoxicillin is better absorbed following administration by mouth than ampicillin, giving higher plasma and tissue concentrations. Its absorption is less affected by the presence of food in the stomach. Ampicillin should be given to fasted animals and at least an hour should then elapse before food is provided. Ampicillin and amoxicillin are excreted into both bile and urine.

Depot preparations of both amoxicillin and ampicillin are available. The drug is incorporated into an oily vehicle to prolong the action of the antibacterial. Depot oil-based ampicillin preparations include aluminium monostearate in the formulation.

Pivampicillin is the pivaloyloxymethyl ester of ampicillin and as such is a prodrug. It is hydrolysed by non-specific esterases in the mucosal wall of the gastro-intestinal tract and in plasma to release ampicillin (75% by weight is converted to ampicillin).

Clavulanic acid has no significant antibacterial activity, but is a potent beta-lactamase inhibitor. Therefore, its inclusion in preparations of amoxicillin (co-amoxiclav) renders the combination active against most strains of *Staph. aureus*, some *E. coli* spp., in addition to *Bacteroides* and *Klebsiella* spp.

AMOXICILLIN
(Amoxycillin)

UK

Indications. Amoxicillin-sensitive infections; hepatic encephalopathy (see section 3.10)
Contra-indications. Oral administration to horses or calves with a functional rumen; see under Benzylpenicillin (see section 1.1.1.1)
Side-effects. Warnings. See under Benzylpenicillin (see section 1.1.1.1)
Dose. Dosages vary. For guidance.
Cattle: by *intramuscular injection*, 7 mg/kg daily
by *depot intramuscular injection*, 15 mg/kg, repeat after 2 days
calves: by *mouth*, 8 mg/kg twice daily
Sheep: by *intramuscular injection*, 7 mg/kg daily
by *depot intramuscular injection*, 15 mg/kg, repeat after 2 days
Pigs: by *addition to drinking water*, 20 mg/kg daily
by *intramuscular injection*, 7 mg/kg daily
by *depot intramuscular injection*, 15 mg/kg, repeat after 2 days
piglets: by *addition to feed*, 15mg/kg bodyweight daily for 14 days
Dogs, cats: by *mouth*, 10 mg/kg twice daily
by *subcutaneous or intramuscular injection*, 7 mg/kg daily
by *depot subcutaneous or intramuscular injection*, 15 mg/kg, repeat after 2 days
Poultry: by *addition to drinking water*, 15–20 mg/kg
Pigeons, ducks: by *addition to drinking water*, 20 mg/kg
Fish: see Prescribing for fish for preparation details and dosage

Note. Amoxicillin 1 g = amoxicillin trihydrate 1.15 g

POM **Amoxinsol 50** (Vétoquinol) *UK*
Oral powder, for addition to drinking water, amoxicillin trihydrate 500 mg/g, for *pigs, chickens, turkeys, ducks*; 150 g, 750 g, 2.5 kg
Withdrawal Periods. *Pigs, chickens*: slaughter 1 day. *Turkeys*: slaughter 5 days. *Ducks*: slaughter 7 days. Should not be used in *birds* producing eggs for human consumption

POM **Amoxinsol Tablets** (Vétoquinol) *UK*
Tablets, scored, amoxicillin (as trihydrate) 40 mg, for *dogs, cats*; 100, 500
Tablets, scored, amoxicillin (as trihydrate) 200 mg, for *dogs*; 100, 250

POM **Amoxycare Capsules** (Animalcare) *UK*
Capsules, amoxicillin (as trihydrate) 250 mg, for *dogs*; 500

POM **Amoxycare Injection** (Animalcare) *UK*
Injection, amoxicillin (as trihydrate) 150 mg/mL, for *cattle, sheep, pigs, dogs, cats*; 50 mL, 100 mL
Withdrawal Periods. *Cattle*: slaughter 18 days, milk 1 day. *Sheep*: slaughter 18 days, should not be used in sheep producing milk for human consumption. *Pigs*: slaughter 18 days

POM **Amoxycare LA Injection** (Animalcare) *UK*
Depot injection, amoxicillin (as trihydrate) 150 mg/mL, for *cattle, sheep, pigs, dogs, cats*; 50 mL, 100 mL
Withdrawal Periods. *Cattle*: slaughter 21 days, milk 2.5 days. *Sheep*: slaughter 21 days, should not be used in sheep producing milk for human consumption. *Pigs*: slaughter 21 days

POM **Amoxycare Palatable Drops** (Animalcare) *UK*
Oral suspension, powder for reconstitution, amoxicillin (as trihydrate) 50 mg/mL, for *dogs, cats*; 15-mL dropper bottle. Life of reconstituted suspension 7 days

POM **Amoxycare Tablets** (Animalcare) *UK*
Tablets, scored, amoxicillin (as trihydrate) 40 mg, for *dogs, cats*; 100, 500
Tablets, scored, amoxicillin (as trihydrate) 200 mg, for *dogs*; 100, 250

POM **Amoxypen** (Intervet) *UK*
Tablets, scored, amoxicillin (as trihydrate) 40 mg, for *dogs, cats*; 500
Tablets, scored, amoxicillin (as trihydrate) 200 mg, for *dogs*; 250

POM **Amoxypen Injection** (Intervet) *UK*
Injection (oily), amoxicillin (as trihydrate) 150 mg/mL, for *cattle, sheep, pigs, dogs, cats*; 100 mL
Withdrawal Periods. *Cattle*: slaughter 18 days, milk 1 day. *Sheep*: slaughter 10 days, should not be used in sheep producing milk for human consumption. *Pigs*: slaughter 16 days

POM **Amoxypen LA** (Intervet) *UK*
Depot injection (oily), amoxicillin (as trihydrate) 150 mg/mL, for *cattle, sheep, pigs, dogs, cats*; 100 mL
Withdrawal Periods. *Cattle*: slaughter 21 days, milk 2.5 days. *Sheep*: slaughter 21 days, should not be used in sheep producing milk for human consumption. *Pigs*: slaughter 21 days

POM **Amoxypen Oral Suspension** (Intervet) *UK*
Oral suspension, powder for reconstitution, amoxicillin (as trihydrate) 50 mg/mL, for *dogs, cats*; 15-mL dropper bottle. Life of reconstituted suspension 7 days

POM **Amoxypen SP** (Intervet) *UK*
Oral powder, for addition to drinking water, amoxicillin (as trihydrate) 697 mg/g, for *chickens*; 100 g, 250 g
Withdrawal Periods. *Chickens*: slaughter 1 day, should not be used in laying birds

POM **Betamox** (Norbrook) *UK*
Tablets, scored, amoxicillin (as trihydrate) 40 mg, for *dogs, cats*; 100, 500
Tablets, scored, amoxicillin (as trihydrate) 200 mg, for *dogs*; 100, 250
Tablets, scored, amoxicillin (as trihydrate) 400 mg, for *calves*; 20, 50
Withdrawal Periods. *Calves*: slaughter 10 days
Dose. *Calves*: by *mouth*, 1 tablet/50 kg body-weight twice daily

POM **Betamox** (Norbrook) *UK*
Injection, amoxicillin (as trihydrate) 150 mg/mL, for *cattle, sheep, pigs, dogs, cats*; 50 mL, 100 mL

Withdrawal Periods. *Cattle*: slaughter 18 days, milk 1 day. *Sheep*: slaughter 10 days, should not be used in sheep producing milk for human consumption. *Pigs*: slaughter 16 days

POM **Betamox LA** (Norbrook) *UK*
Depot injection, amoxicillin (as trihydrate) 150 mg/mL, for *cattle, sheep, pigs, dogs, cats*; 50 mL, 100 mL
Withdrawal Periods. *Cattle*: slaughter 21 days, milk 2.5 days. *Sheep*: slaughter 16 days, should not be used in sheep producing milk for human consumption. *Pigs*: slaughter 16 days

POM **Bimoxyl** (Bimeda) *UK*
Capsules, amoxicillin 250 mg, for *dogs*; 100, 500, 1000

POM **Bimoxyl LA** (Bimeda) *UK*
Depot injection (oily), amoxicillin (as trihydrate) 150 mg/mL, for *cattle, sheep, pigs, dogs*; 100 mL
Withdrawal Periods. *Cattle*: slaughter 21 days, milk 3 days. *Sheep*: slaughter 21 days, should not be used in sheep producing milk for human consumption. *Pigs*: slaughter 11 days

POM **Clamoxyl** (Pfizer) *UK*
Tablets, scored, amoxicillin (as trihydrate) 40 mg, for *dogs, cats*; 100, 500
Tablets, scored, amoxicillin (as trihydrate) 200 mg, for *dogs*; 250

POM **Clamoxyl Oral Multidoser** (Pfizer) *UK*
Mixture, amoxicillin (as trihydrate) 40 mg/dose, for *piglets*; 100-dose applicator
Withdrawal Periods. *Piglets*: slaughter 7 days
Dose. *Piglets*: *by mouth,* (up to 7 kg body-weight) 1 dose twice daily, (7–15 kg body-weight) 2 doses twice daily

POM **Clamoxyl LA** (Pfizer) *UK*
Depot injection (oily), amoxicillin (as trihydrate) 150 mg/mL, for *cattle, sheep, pigs, dogs, cats*; 100 mL, 250 mL
Withdrawal Periods. *Cattle*: slaughter 21 days, milk 96 hours. *Sheep*: slaughter 21 days, should not be used in sheep producing milk for human consumption. *Pigs*: slaughter 21 days

POM **Clamoxyl Ready to Use Injection** (Pfizer) *UK*
Injection, amoxicillin (as trihydrate) 150 mg/mL, for *cattle, sheep, pigs, dogs, cats*; 100 mL, 250 mL
Withdrawal Periods. *Cattle*: slaughter 21 days, milk 2 days. *Sheep*: slaughter 35 days, milk from treated sheep should not be used for human consumption. *Pigs*: slaughter 14 days

POM **Duphamox** (Fort Dodge) *UK*
Tablets, scored, amoxicillin (as trihydrate) 40 mg, for *dogs, cats*; 500
Tablets, scored, amoxicillin (as trihydrate) 200 mg, for *dogs*; 100, 250

POM **Duphamox** (Fort Dodge) *UK*
Injection, amoxicillin (as trihydrate) 150 mg/mL, for *cattle, sheep, pigs, dogs, cats*; 100 mL
Withdrawal Periods. *Cattle*: slaughter 18 days, milk 1 day. *Sheep*: slaughter 18 days, should not be used in sheep producing milk for human consumption. *Pigs*: slaughter 18 days

POM **Duphamox LA** (Fort Dodge) *UK*
Depot injection, amoxicillin (as trihydrate) 150 mg/mL, for *cattle, sheep, pigs, dogs, cats*; 100 mL
Withdrawal Periods. *Cattle*: slaughter 21 days, milk 2.5 days. *Sheep*: slaughter 21 days, should not be used in sheep producing milk for human consumption. *Pigs*: slaughter 21 days

POM **Duphamox Palatable Drops** (Fort Dodge)
Oral suspension, powder for reconstitution, amoxicillin (as trihydrate) 50 mg/mL, for *dogs, cats*; 15-mL dropper bottle. Life of reconstituted suspension 7 days

POM **Qualamox 15** (Merial) *UK*
Injection, amoxicillin (as trihydrate) 150 mg/mL, for *cattle, sheep, pigs, dogs, cats*; 100 mL
Withdrawal Periods. *Cattle*: slaughter 18 days, milk 1 day. *Sheep*: slaughter 18 days, should not be used in sheep producing milk for human consumption. *Pigs*: slaughter 18 days

POM **Qualamox LA** (Merial) *UK*
Depot injection, amoxicillin (as trihydrate) 150 mg/mL, for *cattle, sheep, pigs, dogs, cats*; 100 mL
Withdrawal Periods. *Cattle*: slaughter 21 days, milk 2.5 days. *Sheep*: slaughter 21 days, should not be used in sheep producing milk for human consumption. *Pigs*: slaughter 21 days

POM **Stabox 5% Premix** (Virbac) *UK*
Premix, amoxicillin 5%, for *weaned piglets*; 25 kg
Withdrawal Periods. *Pigs*: slaughter 3 days

POM **Trioxyl LA** (Tulivin) *UK*
Depot injection (oily), amoxicillin (as trihydrate) 150 mg/mL, for *cattle, sheep, pigs*; 100 mL
Withdrawal Periods. *Cattle*: slaughter 21 days, milk 5 days. *Sheep*: slaughter 21 days, should not be used in sheep producing milk for human consumption. *Pigs*: slaughter 21 days

POM **Ultramox LA** (Schering-Plough) *UK*
Depot injection, amoxicillin (as trihydrate) 150 mg/mL, for *cattle, sheep, pigs*; 100 mL
Withdrawal Periods. *Cattle*: slaughter 21 days, milk 3 days. *Sheep*: slaughter 21 days, should not be used in sheep producing milk for human consumption. *Pigs*: slaughter 11 days

POM **Vetremox** (Vetrepharm) *UK*
Oral powder, for addition to drinking water, amoxicillin trihydrate 100%, for *chickens, turkeys*; 25 g, 75 g
Withdrawal Periods. *Chickens*: slaughter 24 hours. *Turkeys*: slaughter 5 days. Should not be used in chickens or turkeys laying eggs for human consumption

POM **Vetremox Pigeon** (Vetrepharm) *UK*
Oral powder, for addition to drinking water, amoxicillin trihydrate 100%, for *pigeons*; 25 g, 75 g
Withdrawal Periods. Should not be used in *pigeons* intended for human consumption

POM **Vetrimoxin Tablets** (Ceva) *UK*
Tablets, or to prepare an oral solution, scored, amoxicillin (as trihydrate) 150 mg, for *dogs*; 10

POM **Vetrimoxin Paste** (Ceva) *UK*
Oral paste, amoxicillin (as trihydrate) 20 mg/mL, for *small dogs, cats*; 15-mL metered dose applicator

POM **Vidamox Tablets** (Vericore VP) *UK*
Tablets, scored, amoxicillin (as trihydrate) 40 mg, for *dogs, cats*; 200, 1000
Tablets, scored, amoxicillin (as trihydrate) 200 mg, for *dogs*; 100, 500

POM **Vidamox Injection** (Vericore VP) *UK*
Injection, amoxicillin (as trihydrate) 150 mg/mL, for *cattle, sheep, pigs, dogs, cats*; 100 mL
Withdrawal Periods. *Cattle*: slaughter 18 days, milk 1 day. *Sheep*: slaughter 10 days, should not be used in sheep producing milk for human consumption. *Pigs*: slaughter 16 days

POM **Vidamox LA Injection** (Vericore VP) *UK*
Depot injection, amoxicillin (as trihydrate) 150 mg/mL, for *cattle, sheep, pigs, dogs, cats*; 100 mL
Withdrawal Periods. *Cattle*: slaughter 21 days, milk 2.5 days. *Sheep*: slaughter 21 days, should not be used in sheep producing milk for human consumption. *Pigs*: slaughter 21 days

Australia

Indications. Amoxicillin-sensitive infections
Contra-indications. Penicillin hypersensitivity; should not be administered to gerbils, guinea pigs, hamsters, rabbits
Side-effects. Local irritation at site of injection
Dose. Dosages vary, consult manufacturer's information

A.F.S. Amoxcillin Soluble (Controlled Medications) *Austral..*
Powder, for addition to drinking water, amoxicillin trihydrate 840 mg/g, for *poultry*

Withdrawal Periods. Slaughter 1 day, should not be used in poultry producing eggs for human consumption

Amoxil Aqueous Drops (Jurox) *Austral..*
Drops (powder for reconstitution), amoxicillin (as trihydrate) 50 mg/mL, for *dogs*

Amoxil LA Injectable Suspension (Jurox) *Austral..*
Injection, amoxicillin (as trihydrate) 150 mg/mL in aluminium stearate/fractionated coconut oil base, for *cattle, sheep, pigs, dogs, cats*
Withdrawal Periods. *Cattle, sheep*: slaughter 28 days, milk 72 hours. *Pigs*: slaughter 28 days

Amoxil Palatable Tablets (Jurox) *Austral..*
Tablets, amoxicillin (as trihydrate) 50 mg, 200 mg, for *dog, cats*

Amoxil Ready-To-Use Injectable (Jurox) *Austral..*
Injection, amoxicillin (as trihydrate) 150 mg/mL in aluminium stearate/ethyloleate gel, for *cattle, pigs, sheep, dogs, cats*
Withdrawal Periods. *Cattle*: slaughter 14 days, milk 48 hours. *Pigs*: slaughter 14 days

Amoxycillin 200 (Apex) *Austral..*
Tablets, amoxicillin (as trihydrate) 200 mg, 400, for *dogs, cats*

Amoxycillin Soluble Powder (Agrotech) *Austral..*
Powder, for addition to drinking water, amoxicillin (as trihydrate) 865 mg/g powder, for *poultry*
Withdrawal Periods. Slaughter 2 days, should not be used in poultry producing eggs for human consumption.

Amoxycillin Trihydrate for Poultry (CCD) *Austral..*
Powder, for addition to drinking water, amoxicillin as trihydrate 870 mg/g powder, for *poultry*
Withdrawal Periods. Slaughter 2 days, should not be used in poultry producing eggs for human consumption.

Betamox (Novartis) *Austral..*
Oral drops (powder for reconstitution), amoxicillin (as trihydrate) 50 mg/mL, for *dogs, cats*

Betamox (Novartis) *Austral..*
Injection, amoxicillin (as trihydrate) 150 mg/mL, for *horses, cattle, sheep, pigs, dogs, cats*
Withdrawal Periods. *Horses, pigs, sheep*: slaughter 28 days. *Cattle*: slaughter 28 days, milk 72 hours.

Betamox Long-Acting Injection (Novartis) *Austral.*
Injection, amoxicillin (as trihydrate) 150 mg/mL, for *dogs, cats*

Betamox Palatable Tablets (Novartis) *Austral..*
Tablets, amoxicillin (as trihydrate) 40 mg and 200 mg, for *dogs, cats*

Bimoxyl LA (Bimeda) *Austral.*
Injection, amoxicillin (as trihydrate) 150 mg/mL (oil base), for *cattle, sheep, pigs, dogs, cats*
Withdrawal Periods. *Pigs, sheep*: slaughter 30 days. *Cattle*: slaughter 30 days, milk 72 hours

Deltamox '200' Tablets (Delvet) *Austral.*
Tablets, amoxicillin 200 mg, for *dogs, cats*

Paracillin SP (Intervet) *Austral.*
Powder, for addition to drinking water, amoxicillin trihydrate 800 mg/g, for *poultry*
Withdrawal Periods. Slaughter 2 days, should not be used in poultry producing eggs for human consumption

Eire

Indications. Amoxicillin-sensitive infections
Contra-indications. Penicillin hypersensitivity; should not be administered to gerbils, guinea pigs, hamsters, rabbits
Dose. Dosages vary, consult manufacturer's information. For guidance:
Cattle, sheep, pigs: *by intramuscular injection*, 7 mg/kg
by depot intramuscular injection, 15 mg/kg

calves: *by mouth*, 8 mg/kg
Dogs, cats: *by mouth*, 10 mg/kg
by subcutaneous or intramuscular injection, 7 mg/kg
by depot subcutaneous or intramuscular injection, 15 mg/ kg

Amoxinsol 50 (Vetoquinol) *Eire*
Oral powder, for addition to drinking water, amoxicillin trihydrate 75 g (50%), for *chickens, turkeys, ducks, pigs*
Withdrawal Periods. *Pigs*: slaughter 1 day. *Chickens*: slaughter 1 day. *Turkeys*: slaughter 5 days. *Ducks*: slaughter 7 days

Amoxypen Bolus (Intervet) *Eire*
Oral bolus, amoxicillin (as trihydrate) 400, for *calves*
Withdrawal Periods. Slaughter 10 days

Amoxypen Injection (Intervet) *Eire*
Injection, amoxicillin (as trihydrate) 150 mg/mL, for *cattle, sheep, pigs, dogs, cats*
Withdrawal Periods. *Cattle*: slaughter 18 days, milk 48 hours. *Sheep*: slaughter 18 days, should not be used in sheep producing milk for human consumption. *Pigs*: slaughter 18 days

Amoxypen LA (Intervet) *Eire*
Depot injection, amoxicillin (as trihydrate) 150 mg/mL, for *cattle, sheep, pigs, dogs, cats*
Withdrawal Periods. *Cattle*: slaughter 21 days, milk 48 hours. *Sheep*: slaughter 21 days, should not be used in sheep producing milk for human consumption. *Pigs*: slaughter 21 days

Amoxypen Tablets (Intervet) *Eire*
Tablets, amoxicillin (as trihydrate) 40, 200 mg, for *dogs, cats*

Betamox (Norbrook) *Eire*
Injection, amoxicillin (as trihydrate) 150 mg/mL, for *cattle, sheep, pigs, dogs, cats*
Withdrawal Periods. *Cattle*: slaughter 18 days, milk 48 hours. *Sheep*: slaughter 7 days, should not be used in sheep producing milk for human consumption. *Pigs*: slaughter 14 days

Betamox 400 mg Tablets (Norbrook) *Eire*
Tablets, amoxicillin (as trihydrate) 400 mg, for *calves*
Withdrawal Periods. Slaughter 10 days, should not be given to cattle producing milk for human consumption

Betamox LA (Norbrook) *Eire*
Depot injection, amoxicillin (as trihydrate) 150 mg/mL, for *cattle, sheep, pigs, dogs, cats*
Withdrawal Periods. *Cattle*: slaughter 21 days, milk 48 hours. *Sheep*: slaughter 14 days, should not be used in sheep producing milk for human consumption. *Pigs*: slaughter 14 days

Betamox Palatable Drops (Norbrook) *Eire*
Oral drops, powder for reconstitution, amoxicillin (as trihydrate) 750 mg (50 mg/ml when reconstituted), for *dogs, cats*

Betamox Palatable Tablets (Norbrook) *Eire*
Tablets, amoxicillin (as trihydrate) 40 mg, 200 mg, for *dogs, cats*

Clamoxyl LA Injection (Pfizer) *Eire*
Injection, amoxicillin (as trihydrate) 150 mg/mL, for *cattle, sheep, pigs, dogs, cats*
Withdrawal Periods. *Cattle, sheep, pigs*: slaughter 21 days. *Cattle*: milk 4 days

Clamoxyl Oral Multidoser (Pfizer) *Eire*
Cream, amoxicillin (as trihydrate) 40 mg/dose, for *pigs*
Withdrawal Periods. Slaughter 7 days

Clamoxyl Palatable Tablets (Pfizer) *Eire*
Tablets, amoxicillin (as trihydrate) 40 mg, for *dogs, cats*

Clamoxyl Ready-to-Use Injection (Pfizer) *Eire*
Injection, amoxicillin (as trihydrate) 150 mg/mL, for *cattle, sheep, pigs, dogs, cats*

Withdrawal Periods. *Cattle, sheep, pigs*: slaughter 28 days. *Cattle, sheep*: milk 3 days

Duphamox LA (Interchem) *Eire*
Depot injection, amoxicillin (as trihydrate) 150 mg/mL, for *cattle, sheep, pigs, dogs, cats*
Withdrawal Periods. *Cattle*: slaughter 21 days, milk 48 hours. *Sheep*: slaughter 21 days, should not be used in sheep producing milk for human consumption. *Pigs*: slaughter 21 days

Duphamox RTU (Interchem) *Eire*
Injection, amoxicillin (as trihydrate) 150 mg/mL, for *cattle, sheep, pigs, dogs, cats*
Withdrawal Periods. *Cattle*: slaughter 18 days, milk 48 hours. *Sheep*: slaughter 18 days, should not be used in sheep producing milk for human consumption. *Pigs*: slaughter 18 days

Hostamox LA (Hoechst Roussel Vet) *Eire*
Depot injection, amoxicillin (as trihydrate) 150 mg/mL, for *cattle, sheep, pigs*
Withdrawal Periods. *Cattle*: slaughter 18 days, milk 72 hours. *Sheep*: slaughter 21 days, should not be used in sheep producing milk for human consumption. *Pigs*: slaughter 11 days

Trioxyl LA (Univet) *Eire*
Depot injection (oily), amoxicillin (as trihydrate) 150 mg/mL, for *cattle, sheep, pigs*
Withdrawal Periods. *Cattle, sheep, pigs*: slaughter 21 days. *Cattle, sheep*: milk 5 days

New Zealand
Indications. Amoxicillin-sensitive infections
Contra-indications. Penicillin hypersensitivity; should not be administered to gerbils, guinea pigs, hamsters, rabbits
Side-effects. Local irritation at site of injection
Dose. Dosages vary, consult manufacturer's information

Amoxil (Jurox) *NZ*
Injection, amoxicillin (as trihydrate) 150 mg/mL, for *cattle, sheep, pigs, dogs, cats*
Withdrawal Periods. *Cattle*: slaughter 28 days, milk 36 hours. *Sheep*: slaughter 28 days, should not be used in sheep producing milk for human consumption. *Pigs*: slaughter 7 days

Amoxil Palatable Drops (Jurox) *NZ*
Oral suspension, amoxicillin 50 mg/mL, for *dogs, cats*

Amoxil Palatable Tablets (Jurox) *NZ*
Tablets, amoxicillin 50 mg, 200 mg, for *dogs, cats*

Amoxycillin-400 (Ethical) *NZ*
Tablets, amoxicillin (as trihydrate) 400 mg, for *dogs, cats*

Betamox LA (Bomac) *NZ*
Injection, amoxicillin (as trihydrate) 150 mg/mL, for *horses, cattle, sheep, pigs, dogs, cats*
Withdrawal Periods. *Horses*: slaughter 28 days. *Cattle, sheep*: slaughter 14 days, milk 60 hours. *Pigs*: slaughter 14 days

Bimoxyl LA (Reamor) *NZ*
Injection, amoxicillin trihydrate 150 mg/mL, for *cattle, sheep, pigs*
Withdrawal Periods. *Cattle, sheep*: slaughter 14 days, milk 60 hours after first dose plus 12 hours for each additional dose. *Pigs*: slaughter 10 days

Deltamox-200 (Ethical) *NZ*
Tablets, amoxicillin (as trihydrate) 200 mg, for *dogs, cats*

Longamox (Ethical) *NZ*
Injection, amoxicillin trihydrate 150 mg/mL, for *cattle, sheep, pigs*
Withdrawal Periods. *Cattle*: slaughter 36 days, milk 60 hours. *Sheep*: slaughter 21 days, milk 60 hours. *Pigs*: slaughter 21 days

Moxylan Aqueous Drops (Jurox) *NZ*
Oral solution, amoxicillin 50 mg/mL, for *dogs, cats*

Moxylan Ready-to-use (Jurox) *NZ*
Injection, amoxicillin 150 mg/mL, for *cattle, sheep, pigs, dogs, cats*
Withdrawal Periods. *Cattle*: slaughter 28 days, milk 36 hours. *Sheep*: slaughter 28 days, should not be used in sheep producing milk for human consumption. *Pigs*: slaughter 7 days

Moxylan Tablets (Jurox) *NZ*
Tablets, amoxicillin 50 mg, 200 mg, for *dogs, cats*

Tecamox L.A. (Virbac) *NZ*
Injection, amoxicillin (as trihydrate) 150 mg/mL, for *cattle*
Withdrawal Periods. Slaughter 14 days, milk 60 hours

USA
Indications. Amoxicillin-sensitive infections
Contra-indications. Penicillin hypersensitivity; should not be administered to gerbils, guinea pigs, hamsters, rabbits
Dose. Dosages vary, consult manufacturer's information. For guidance
Cattle: *by subcutaneous or intramuscular injection*, 6.6–11.0 mg/kg
Dogs, cats: by mouth 11 mg/kg twice daily
by subcutaneous or intramuscular injection, 11 mg/kg

Amoxi-Drop (Pfizer) *USA*
Oral suspension, amoxicillin (as trihydrate) 50 mg/mL, for *dogs, cats*

Amoxi-Inject (Pfizer) *USA*
Injection, amoxicillin (as trihydrate) 3 g, for *dogs, cats*

Amoxi-Inject (Pfizer) *USA*
Injection, amoxicillin (as trihydrate) 25 g, for *cattle*
Withdrawal Periods. Slaughter 25 days, milk 96 hours

Biomox (Delmarva) *USA*
Oral suspension, amoxicillin (as trihydrate) 50 mg/mL (after reconstitution), for *dogs*

Biomox (Delmarva) *USA*
Tablets, amoxicillin 50 mg, 100 mg, 200 mg, 400mg, for *dogs*

Robamox-V (Fort Dodge) *USA*
Oral powder, for preparation of suspension, amoxycillin (as trihydrate) 50 mg/mL after reconstitution, for *dogs*

Robamox-V (Fort Dodge) *USA*
Tablets, amoxycillin 50 mg, 100 mg, 200 mg, 400 mg, for *dogs*

AMOXICILLIN with CLAVULANIC ACID
(Co-amoxiclav: preparations of amoxicillin (as trihydrate or the sodium salt) and clavulanic acid (as potassium clavulanate); the proportions are expressed in the form x/y, where x and y are the strengths in milligrams of amoxicillin and clavulanic acid respectively)

UK
Indications. Amoxicillin-sensitive infections including beta-lactamase-producing micro-organisms
Contra-indications. Side-effects. See under Benzylpenicillin (see section 1.1.1.1)
Dose. Expressed as amoxicillin
Cattle: *by intramuscular injection*, 7 mg/kg once daily
calves: *by mouth*, 5–10 mg/kg twice daily
Pigs: *by intramuscular injection*, 7 mg/kg once daily
Dogs, cats: *by mouth*, 10–20 mg/kg twice daily
by subcutaneous or intramuscular injection, 7 mg/kg once daily

POM **Synulox 500 mg Bolus** (Pfizer) *UK*
Tablets, f/c, scored, amoxicillin (as trihydrate) 400 mg, clavulanic acid (as potassium salt) 100 mg, for *calves*; 20, 100
Withdrawal Periods. *Calves*: slaughter 4 days

POM **Synulox Palatable Drops** (Pfizer) *UK*
Oral suspension, powder for reconstitution, amoxicillin (as trihydrate) 40 mg, clavulanic acid (as potassium salt) 10 mg/mL, for *dogs, cats*; 15-mL dropper bottle. Life of reconstituted suspension 7 days (1 drop = amoxicillin 2.3 mg)

POM **Synulox Palatable Tablets** (Pfizer) *UK*
Tablets, scored, amoxicillin (as trihydrate) 40 mg, clavulanic acid (as potassium salt) 10 mg, for *dogs, cats*; 10, 100, 500
Tablets, scored, amoxicillin (as trihydrate) 200 mg, clavulanic acid (as potassium salt) 50 mg, for *dogs*; 100, 250
Tablets, scored, amoxicillin (as trihydrate) 400 mg, clavulanic acid (as potassium salt) 100 mg, for *dogs*; 10, 20, other sizes available

POM **Synulox Ready to Use Injection** (Pfizer) *UK*
Injection, amoxicillin (as trihydrate) 140 mg, clavulanic acid (as potassium salt),35 mg/mL, for *cattle, pigs, dogs, cats*; 40 mL, 100 mL
Withdrawal Periods. *Cattle*: slaughter 14 days, milk 60 hours. *Pigs*: slaughter 14 days

Australia

Indications. Amoxicillin-sensitive infections including beta-lactamase-producing micro-organisms
Dose. Expressed as amoxicillin
Cattle: *by subcutaneous or intramuscular injection*, 7 mg/kg once daily
calves: *by mouth*, 5–10 mg/kg twice daily
Dogs, cats: *by mouth*, 10–20 mg/kg twice daily
by subcutaneous or intramuscular injection, 7 mg/kg once daily

Clavulox Palatable Drops (Pfizer) *Austral.*
Oral drops (powder for reconstitution), clavulanic acid (as potassium salt) 12.5 mg/mL and amoxicillin (as trihydrate) 50 mg/mL, for *dogs, cats*

Clavulox Palatable Tablets (Pfizer) *Austral.*
Tablets, clavulanic acid (as potassium salt)/amoxicillin (as trihydrate) 10 mg/40 mg, 50 mg/200 mg, for *dogs, cats*

Clavulox 500 mg Tablets (Pfizer) *Austral.*
Tablets, clavulanic acid (as potassium salt)/amoxicillin (as trihydrate) 100 mg/400 mg, for *calves, dogs*
Withdrawal Periods. *Calves*: slaughter 4 days

Clavulox Injectable (Pfizer) *Austral.*
Injection, amoxicillin (as trihydrate) 140 mg/mL, clavulanic acid (as potassium salt) 35 mg/mL in oil base, for *dogs, cats*

Eire

Indications. Amoxicillin-sensitive infections including beta-lactamase-producing micro-organisms
Dose. Expressed as amoxicillin
Cattle: *by subcutaneous or intramuscular injection*, 7 mg/kg once daily
calves: *by mouth*, 5–10 mg/kg twice daily
Dogs, cats: *by mouth*, 10–20 mg/kg twice daily
by subcutaneous or intramuscular injection, 7 mg/kg once daily

Synulox 500 mg Bolus (Pfizer) *Eire*
Tablets, amoxicillin (as trihydrate) 400 mg, clavulanic acid (as potassium clavulanate) 100 mg, for *calves*
Withdrawal Periods. Slaughter 4 days

Synulox Palatable Tablets (Pfizer) *Eire*
Tablets, 50 mg: clavulanic acid (as potassium clavulanate) 10 mg, amoxicillin (as trihydrate) 40 mg; 250 mg: clavulanic acid (as potassium clavulanate) 50 mg, amoxicillin (as trihydrate) 200 mg, for *dogs, cats*

Synulox Ready-to-Use Injection (Pfizer) *Eire*
Injection (oily), clavulanic acid (as potassium clavulanate) 35 mg/mL, amoxicillin (as trihydrate) 200 mg, prednisolone 140 mg/mL, for *cattle, sheep, pigs, dogs, cats*
Withdrawal Periods. *Cattle*: slaughter 14 days, milk 80 hours. *Sheep*: slaughter 28 days, milk 48 hours. *Pigs*: slaughter 14 days

New Zealand

Indications. Amoxicillin-sensitive infections including beta-lactamase-producing micro-organisms
Dose. Expressed as amoxicillin
Cattle, sheep, pigs: *by subcutaneous or intramuscular injection*, 7 mg/kg once daily
calves: *by mouth*, 5–10 mg/kg twice daily
Dogs, cats: *by mouth*, 10–20 mg/kg twice daily
by subcutaneous or intramuscular injection, 7 mg/kg once daily

Clavulox Palatable Drops (Pfizer) *NZ*
Oral solution, amoxicillin (as trihydrate) 50 mg/mL, clavulanic acid (as potassium salt) 12.5 mg/mL, for *dogs, cats*

Clavulox Palatable Tablets 50 mg (Pfizer) *NZ*
Tablets, amoxicillin (as trihydrate) 40mg, clavulanic acid (as potassium salt) 10 mg, for *dogs, cats*

Clavulox Palatable Tablets 250 mg (Pfizer) *NZ*
Tablets, amoxicillin (as trihydrate) 200 mg, clavulanic acid (as potassium salt) 50 mg, for *dogs, cats*

Clavulox Palatable Tablets 500 mg (Pfizer) *NZ*
Tablets, amoxicillin (as trihydrate) 400 mg, clavulanic acid (as potassium salt) 100 mg, for *cattle, dogs*
Withdrawal Periods. *Cattle*: slaughter 4 days

Clavulox RTU (Pfizer) *NZ*
Injection, amoxicillin (as trihydrate) 140 mg/mL, clavulanic acid (as potassium salt) 35 mg/mL, for *cattle, dogs, cats*
Withdrawal Periods. *Cattle*: slaughter 28 days, milk 36 hours

USA

Indications. Amoxicillin-sensitive infections including beta-lactamase-producing micro-organisms
Dose. Expressed as amoxicillin
Dogs, cats: *by mouth*, 10–20 mg/kg twice daily

Clavamox Drops (Pfizer) *USA*
Oral solution, amoxicillin (as trihydrate) 50 mg/mL, clavulanic acid 12.5 mg/mL, for *dogs, cats*

Clavamox Tablets (Pfizer) *USA*
Tablets, amoxicillin (as trihydrate)/clavulanic acid; 50 mg/12.5 mg, 100 mg/25mg, 200 mg/50 mg, 300mg/75 mg, for *dogs, cats*

AMPICILLIN

UK

Indications. Ampicillin-sensitive infections
Contra-indications. Side-effects. See under Benzylpenicillin (see section 1.1.1.1); occasional irritation at siteof injection
Dose.
Horses: *by intramuscular injection*, 7.5 mg/kg once daily

Cattle, sheep: *by intramuscular injection*, 7.5 mg/kg once daily

by depot intramuscular injection, 15 mg/kg, repeat after 2 days

calves: *by mouth*, 10–15 mg/kg twice daily dissolved and given in milk replacer

Pigs: *by intramuscular injection*, 7.5 mg/kg once daily

by depot intramuscular injection, 25 mg/kg, repeat after 2 days

Dogs: *by mouth*, 10–20 mg/kg twice daily given on an empty stomach

by subcutaneous or intramuscular injection, 7.5 mg/kg once daily

by depot subcutaneous injection, 15 mg/kg, repeat after 2 days

Cats: *by mouth*, 10–20 mg/kg twice daily given on an empty stomach

by subcutaneous or intramuscular injection, 7.5 mg/kg once daily

by depot subcutaneous injection, 20 mg/kg, repeat after 2 days

POM **Amfipen** (Intervet) *UK*
Tablets, ampicillin 50 mg, 125 mg, for *dogs, cats*; 100, 400
Tablets, ampicillin 500 mg, for *calves, dogs*; 30
Withdrawal Periods. *Calves*: slaughter 14 days
Capsules, ampicillin 250 mg, for *calves, dogs*; 250, 1000
Withdrawal Periods. *Calves*: slaughter 14 days

POM **Amfipen 15%** (Intervet) *UK*
Injection (oily), ampicillin 150 mg/mL, for *horses, dogs, cats*; 100 mL
Withdrawal Periods. Should not be used in *horses* intended for human consumption

POM **Amfipen 30%** (Intervet) *UK*
Injection (oily), ampicillin 300 mg/mL, for *cattle, sheep, pigs*; 100 mL
Withdrawal Periods. *Cattle*: slaughter 21 days, milk 1 day. *Sheep*: slaughter 21 days, should not be used in sheep producing milk for human consumption. *Pigs*: slaughter 28 days

---

Accidental self-injection with oil-based formulations can cause severe pain and intense swelling, which may result in ischaemic necrosis and loss of a digit. Prompt medical attention is essential.

POM **Amfipen LA** (Intervet)
Depot injection (oily), ampicillin 100 mg/mL with aluminium monostearate, for *cattle, sheep, pigs, dogs, cats*; 80 mL
Withdrawal Periods. *Cattle*: slaughter 60 days, milk 7 days. *Sheep*: slaughter 60 days, should not be used in sheep producing milk for human consumption. *Pigs*: slaughter 60 days

POM **Ampicaps** (Bimeda) *UK*
Capsules, ampicillin (as trihydrate) 250 mg, for *dogs more than 10 kg body-weight*; 100, 250, 500

POM **Ampicare** (Animalcare) *UK*
Capsules, ampicillin (as trihydrate), for *dogs more than 10 kg body-weight*; 500

POM **Ampicare 15% Injection** (Animalcare) *UK*
Injection (oily), ampicillin 150 mg/mL, for *cattle, sheep, pigs*; 100 mL
Withdrawal Periods. *Cattle*: slaughter 18 days, milk 1 day. *Sheep*: slaughter 18 days, should not be used in sheep producing milk for human consumption. *Pigs*: slaughter18 days

POM **Duphacillin** (Fort Dodge) *UK*
Injection (oily), ampicillin (as trihydrate) 150 mg/mL, for *cattle, sheep, pigs*
Withdrawal Periods. *Cattle*: slaughter 18 days, milk 1 day. *Sheep*: slaughter 18 days, should not be used in sheep producing milk for human consumption. *Pigs*: slaughter18 days

POM **Embacillin** (Merial) *UK*
Injection, ampicillin (as trihydrate) 150 mg/mL, for *cattle, sheep, pigs*
Withdrawal Periods. *Cattle*: slaughter 18 days, milk 1 day. *Sheep*: slaughter 18 days, should not be used in sheep producing milk for human consumption. *Pigs*: slaughter 18 days

POM **Norobrittin** (Norbrook) *UK*
Injection, ampicillin (as trihydrate) 150 mg/mL, for *cattle, sheep, pigs*
Withdrawal Periods. *Cattle*: slaughter 18 days, milk 1 day. *Sheep*: slaughter 18 days, should not be used in sheep producing milk for human consumption. *Pigs*: slaughter 18 days

POM **Vidocillin Injection** (Vericore VP) *UK*
Injection, ampicillin (as trihydrate) 150 mg/mL, for *horses, cattle, sheep, pigs*; 100 mL
Withdrawal Periods. *Cattle*: slaughter 18 days, milk 1 day. *Sheep*: slaughter 18 days, should not be used in sheep producing milk for human consumption. *Pigs*: slaughter 18 days

Eire

Indications. Ampicillin-sensitive infections
Dose. Dosages vary, consult manufacturer's information

Amfipen 15% (Intervet) *Eire*
Injection, ampicillin 150 mg/mL, for *horses, dogs, cats*
Withdrawal Periods. Should not be used in *horses* intended for human consumption

Amfipen LA (Intervet) *Eire*
Depot injection (oily), ampicillin (anhydrous) 100 mg/mL, for *cattle, sheep, pigs, dogs, cats*
Withdrawal Periods. *Cattle*: slaughter 28 days, milk 4 days. *Sheep*: slaughter 28 days, should not be used in sheep producing milk for human consumption. *Pigs*: slaughter 28 days

Amfipen Soluble Powder (Intervet) *Eire*
Oral powder, for addition to drinking water, ampicillin trihydrate 10 g/200 g, for *calves*
Withdrawal Periods. Slaughter 48 hours

Amfipen Tablets (Intervet) *Eire*
Tablets, ampicillin (anhydrous) 50, 125, 500 mg, for *calves, dogs, cats*

Norobrittin (Norbrook) *Eire*
Injection (oily), ampicillin (as trihydrate) 150 mg/mL, for *cattle, sheep, pigs*
Withdrawal Periods. *Cattle*: slaughter 18 day, milk 24 hours. *Sheep*: slaughter 18 days, should not be used in sheep producing milk for human consumption. *Pigs*: slaughter 18 days

Penbritin Injectable Suspension (Pfizer) *Eire*
Injection, ampicillin (as trihydrate) 15%, for *cattle, dogs, cats*
Withdrawal Periods. *Cattle*: slaughter 28 days, 48 hours

Penbritin Veterinary Injectable (Pfizer) *Eire*
Injection, ampicillin (as sodium salt), for *horses, dogs, cats*
Withdrawal Periods. Should not be used in *horses* intended for human consumption

New Zealand

Indications. Ampicillin-sensitive infections
Dose. Dosages vary, consult manufacturer's information

Albipen (Chemavet) *NZ*
Tablets, ampicillin 50 mg, 125 mg, 500 mg, for *horses, cattle, pigs, dogs, cats*
Withdrawal Periods. *Horses*: slaughter 28 days. *Cattle*: slaughter 2 days, milk 72 hours. *Pigs*: slaughter 2 days

Albipen L.A. (Chemavet) *NZ*
Depot injection, ampicillin 100 mg/mL, for *cattle, sheep, pigs, dogs, cats*
Withdrawal Periods. *Cattle, sheep*: slaughter 28 days, milk 72 hours. *Pigs*: slaughter 28 days

Ampitras 20% (Phoenix) *NZ*
Injection, ampicillin trihydrate 200 mg/mL, for *large animals, dogs, cats*
Withdrawal Periods. *Horses*: slaughter 28 days. *Cattle*: slaughter 6 days, milk 72 hours. *Pigs*: slaughter 6 days

USA

Indications. Ampicillin-sensitive infections
Dose. Consult manufacturer's information

Polyflex (Fort Dodge) *USA*
Injection, ampicillin (as trihydrate) 10 g, 25 g, for *cattle, dogs, cats*
Withdrawal Periods. *Cattle*: slaughter 6 days, milk 48 hours

Polyflex (Fort Dodge) *USA*
Injection, ampicillin (as trihydrate) 10 g, 25 g, for *cattle, dogs, cats*
Withdrawal Periods. *Cattle*: slaughter 6 days, milk 48 hours

1.1.1.4 Antipseudomonal penicillins

The carboxypenicillin **ticarcillin** is principally indicated for the treatment of *Pseudomonas aeruginosa* infections although it is also active against a number of other Gram-negative organisms including *Proteus* and *Bacteroides* spp. Ticarcillin is broken down by the beta-lactamase produced by some strains of *Ps. aeruginosa* and is available in preparations to which clavulanic acid has been added to inhibit beta-lactamase. The ureidopenicillin, **piperacillin** is broad spectrum and is more active than ticarcillin against *Pseudomonas aeruginosa*.

PIPERACILLIN

UK

Indications. Dose. See Prescribing for reptiles and Prescribing for amphibians

POM Ⓗ **Pipril** (Lederle) *UK*
Injection, powder for reconstitution, piperacillin (as sodium salt) 1 g, 2 g

TICARCILLIN with CLAVULANIC ACID

UK

Indications. See notes above
Contra-indications. Side-effects. See under Benzylpenicillin (see section 1.1.1.1)
Dose. Expressed as ticarcillin + clavulanic acid
Foals: *by intravenous injection*, 50 mg/kg 4 times daily
Dogs, cats: *by intravenous infusion*, 15–25 mg/kg 3 times daily

POM Ⓗ **Timentin** (SmithKline Beecham) *UK*
Injection, powder for reconstitution, ticarcillin (as sodium salt) 3 g, clavulanic acid (as potassium salt) 200 mg; 3.2 g

1.1.1.5 Cephalosporins

The cephalosporins comprise a large group of antibacterials containing the beta-lactam ring. They are closely related to the penicillins. Like the penicillins they are bactericidal (operating time-dependent killing), are relatively non-toxic, and less likely to cause allergic reactions. Cephalosporins are suitable for use in rabbits and rodents.

It is difficult to generalise about the spectrum of activity of cephalosporins and each individual drug can be different. The tradition of classifying these drugs as first, second and third generation can cause confusion particularly as newer drugs are developed. The first generation drugs are active against a range of both Gram-positive and Gram-negative organisms comprising staphylococci (including beta-lactamase-producing strains), *Pasteurella, E. coli, Actinobacillus, Actinomyces, Haemophilus, Erysipelothrix, Clostridium*, and *Salmonella* spp. However *Pseudomonas* and many *Proteus* spp. are resistant.

Successive generations of cephalosporins are characterised by being less well absorbed following oral administration (so that only first generation cephalosporins are available as oral preparations and most other cephalosporins are not suitable for oral administration), have increased stability to Gram-negative beta-lactamases, and generally increased activity against Gram-negative organisms, but reduced activity against Gram-positive organisms particularly staphylococci.

As a general rule, the second generation cephalosporins have good activity against Gram-positive organisms and the enterobacteriaceae but are not effective against the most intractable Gram-negative organisms such as *Klebsiella* spp. or *Pseudomonas aeruginosa*. Further developments amongst the cephalosporins have been made to produce drugs which are effective against *Klebsiella* spp. or *Pseudomonas aeruginosa* or to produce drugs which are effective against the refractory anaerobes, such as *Bacteroides fragilis*. These developments have been made sometimes at the expense of the Gram-positive spectrum, such that potency against *Staphylococcus* spp, in particular, may be reduced. Cefoperazone is an example of a cephalosporin (third generation) with activity against *Pseudomonas aeruginosa*. Cefoxitin is a cephalosporin which is noted for its activity against *Bacteroides fragilis*. Cefquinome is a recently developed cephalosporin (sometimes termed fourth generation). It is extremely broad-spectrum being highly active against enterobacteriaceae, staphylococci (including methicillin resistant strains), and enterococci. In addition, it is not destroyed by the most common plasmid or chromosomal beta lactamases of *Klebsiella* spp. and *Pseudomonas aeruginosa*.

CEFADROXIL

UK

Indications. Cefadroxil-sensitive infections
Contra-indications. Hypersensitivity to cephalosporins or penicillins
Side-effects. Occasional vomiting, diarrhoea; lethargy
Warnings. See under Benzylpenicillin (see section 1.1.1.1)
Dose. *By mouth.*
Dogs: 10 mg/kg twice daily. May be administered with food if vomiting occurs

Cats: 20 mg/kg once daily. May be given twice daily for acute or severe infections. May be administered with food if vomiting occurs

POM Cefa-Tabs (Fort Dodge) *UK*
Tablets, f/c, cefadroxil 50 mg, 100 mg, for *dogs, cats*; 100, 500
Tablets, f/c, cefadroxil 200 mg, for *dogs*; 100, 250

Australia
Indications. Cefadroxil-sensitive infections
Contra-indications. Hypersensitivity to cephalosporins or penicillins
Dose. *Dogs, cats*: *by mouth*, 20 mg/kg

Cefa-Cure (Intervet) *Austral.*
Tablets, cefadroxil 50 mg, 200 mg, 1000 mg, for *dogs, cats*

New Zealand
Indications. Cefadroxil-sensitive infections
Contra-indications. Hypersensitivity to cephalosporins or penicillins
Dose. *Dogs, cats*: *by mouth*, 20 mg/kg

Cefa-Cure (Chemavet) *NZ*
Tablets, cefadroxil 50 mg, 200 mg , 1000 mg, for *dogs, cats*

USA
Indications. Cefadroxil-sensitive infections
Contra-indications. Hypersensitivity to cephalosporins or penicillins
Dose. *Dogs, cats*: *by mouth*, 22 mg/kg

Cefa-Drops (Fort Dodge) *USA*
Oral suspension, powder for reconstitution, cefadroxil 50 mg/mL (reconstituted), for *dogs, cats*

Cefa-Tabs (Fort Dodge) *USA*
Tablets, cefadroxil 50mg, 100mg, 200mg, 1 g, for *dogs, cats*

CEFALEXIN
(Cephalexin)

UK
Indications. Cefalexin-sensitive infections
Contra-indications. Hypersensitivity to cephalosporins or penicillins
Side-effects. Local tissue reaction
Warnings. Reduce dose in renal impairment; see under Benzylpenicillin (see section 1.1.1.1)
Dose. Dosages vary. For guidance.
Cattle: *by intramuscular injection*, 7 mg/kg once daily
Sheep, pigs: *by intramuscular injection*, 10 mg/kg once daily
Dogs, cats: *by mouth*, 10–15 mg/kg twice daily. May be increased to 20–30 mg/kg twice daily for severe infections
by subcutaneous or intramuscular injection, 10 mg/kg once daily

POM Ceporex Injection (Schering-Plough) *UK*
Injection (oily), cefalexin (as sodium salt) 180 mg/mL, for *cattle, sheep, pigs, dogs, cats*; 100 mL
Withdrawal Periods. *Cattle*: slaughter 4 days, milk withdrawal period nil.
Sheep: slaughter 3 days, should not be used in sheep producing milk for human consumption. *Pigs*: slaughter 2 days

POM Ceporex Veterinary Tablets (Schering-Plough) *UK*
Tablets, f/c, cefalexin 50 mg, for *dogs 6–9 kg body-weight, cats*; 100, 500
Tablets, f/c, cefalexin 250 mg, for *dogs more than 10 kg body-weight*; 100, 250

POM Ceporex Oral Drops (Schering-Plough) *UK*
Oral suspension, granules for reconstitution, cefalexin 100 mg/mL, for *dogs up to 20 kg body-weight, cats*; 10-mL dropper bottle. Life of reconstituted suspension 10 days

POM Rilexine Tablets (Virbac) *UK*
Tablets, cefalexin 75 mg, for *dogs, cats*
Tablets, cefalexin 300 mg, 600 mg, for *dogs*

Australia
Indications. Cefalexin-sensitive infections
Contra-indications. Hypersensitivity to cephalosporins or penicillins
Dose. *Dogs, cats*: *by mouth or by intramuscular injection*, 10–15 mg/kg

Cephalexin 200 (Apex) *Austral.*
Tablets, cefalexin 200 mg, 600 mg, for *dogs, cats*

Kefvet Granules for Oral Suspension (Elanco) *Austral.*
Oral granules, for preparation of suspension, cefalexin (as monohydrate) 78.7 mg/g granules, for *dogs, cats*

Kefvet Tablets (Elanco) *Austral.*
Tablets, cefalexin (as monohydrate) 500 mg and 1000 mg, for *dogs, cats*

Rilexine Paste (Virbac) *Austral.*
Oral paste, cefalexin (as monohydrate) 600 mg/5 mL, for *dogs, cats*

Rilexine Tablets (Virbac) *Austral.*
Tablets, cefalexin (as monohydrate) 75 mg, 300 mg, 600 mg, for *dogs, cats*

Rilexine 150 Suspension (Virbac) *Austral.*
Injection, cefalexin (as monohydrate) 15 g/100 mL, for *dogs, cats*

Eire
Indications. Cefalexin-sensitive infections
Contra-indications. Hypersensitivity to cephalosporins or penicillins
Side-effects. Local tissue reaction
Warnings. Reduce dose in renal impairment; see under Benzylpenicillin (see section 1.1.1.1)
Dose.
Cattle: *by intramuscular injection*, 7 mg/kg
Sheep, pigs: *by intramuscular injection*, 10 mg/kg
Dogs, cats: *by subcutaneous or intramuscular injection*, 10 mg/kg

Ceporex Injection (Schering-Plough) *Eire*
Injection (oily), cephalexin (as sodium) 18%, for *cattle, sheep, pigs, dogs, cats*
Withdrawal Periods. *Cattle*: slaughter 4 days, milk withdrawal period nil.
Sheep: slaughter 3 days, should not be used in sheep producing milk for human consumption. *Pigs*: slaughter 2 days

New Zealand
Indications. Cefalexin-sensitive infections
Contra-indications. Hypersensitivity to cephalosporins or penicillins
Dose. *Cattle, sheep, pigs*: *by intramuscular injection*, 7 mg/kg
Dogs, cats: *by mouth*, 10–15 mg/kg
by subcutaneous or intramuscular injection, 10 mg/kg

Ceporex (Schering-Plough) *NZ*
Injection, cefalexin (as sodium salt) 180 mg/mL, for *horses, cattle, sheep, pigs, dogs, cats*
Withdrawal Periods. *Horses*: slaughter 28 days. *Cattle*: slaughter 4 days, milk withdrawal period nil. *Sheep*: slaughter 10 days, milk withdrawal period nil. *Pigs*: slaughter 10 days

Ceporex Oral Drops (Schering-Plough) *NZ*
Oral suspension, cefalexin 100 mg/mL, for *dogs, cats*

Ceporex Tablets (Schering-Plough) *NZ*
Tablets, cefalexin 50 mg, 250 mg, for *dogs, cats*

Rilexine 150 (Virbac) *NZ*
Injection, cefalexin 150 mg/mL, for *dogs, cats*

Rilexine Paste (Virbac) *NZ*
Oral paste, cefalexin 120 mg/mL, for *dogs, cats*

Rilexine Tablets (Virbac) *NZ*
Tablets, cefalexin 75 mg, 300 mg, 600 mg, for *dogs, cats*

CEFQUINOME

UK
Indications. Cefquinome-sensitive infections
Contra-indications. Hypersensitivity to cephalosporins or penicillins
Warnings. See under Benzylpenicillin (see section 1.1.1.1)
Dose. *By intramuscular injection.*
Cattle: 1 mg/kg daily; *calves*: 2 mg/kg daily
Pigs: by intramuscular injection, 1–2 mg/kg

POM **Cephaguard** (Intervet) *UK*
Injection (oily), cefquinome 25 mg/mL, for *cattle*, *pigs*
Withdrawal Periods. *Cattle*: slaughter 5 days, milk not less than 12 hours. *Calves*: slaughter 4 days. *Pigs*: slaughter 3 days

Eire
Indications. Cefquinome-sensitive infections
Contra-indications. Hypersensitivity to cephalosporins or penicillins
Warnings. See under Benzylpenicillin (see section 1.1.1.1)
Dose. *By intramuscular injection.*
Cattle: 1 mg/kg

Cephaguard (Hoechst Roussel Vet) *Eire*
Injection (oily), cefquinome (as sulphate) 25 mg/mL, for *cattle*
Withdrawal Periods. Slaughter 5 days, not for use in lactating animals

CEFTAZIDIME

UK
Indications. Ceftazidime-sensitive infections
Dose. See Prescribing for reptiles

POM Ⓗ **Fortum** (GlaxoWellcome) *UK*
Injection, powder for reconstitution, ceftazidime (as pentahydrate) 250 mg, 500 mg, other sizes available

POM Ⓗ **Kefadim** (Lilly) *UK*
Injection, powder for reconstitution, ceftazidime (as pentahydrate) 500 mg, 1 g, 2 g

CEFTIOFUR

UK
Indications. Ceftiofur-sensitive infections
Contra-indications. Hypersensitivity to cephalosporins or penicillins
Side-effects. Transient occasional pain on injection
Warnings. Safety in pregnant or breeding animals not established
Dose.
Horses: by intramuscular injection, 2 mg/kg once daily
Cattle: by intramuscular injection, 1 mg/kg once daily
Pigs: by intramuscular injection, 3 mg/kg once daily
Poultry: (day-old chicks) by subcutaneous injection, 80–200 micrograms

POM **Excenel Sterile Powder** (Pharmacia & Upjohn) *UK*
Injection, powder for reconstitution, ceftiofur (as sodium salt) 1 g, 4 g, for *horses, cattle, pigs, day-old chicks*
Withdrawal Periods. Should not be used in *horses* intended for human consumption. *Cattle*: slaughter 8 hours, milk withdrawal period nil. *Pigs*: slaughter 12 hours. *Chicks*: slaughter 21 days

POM **Excenel RTU** (Pharmacia & Upjohn) *UK*
Injection, ceftiofur (as hydrochloride) 50 mg/mL, for *pigs*; 100 mL
Withdrawal Periods. *Pigs*: slaughter 5 days

Australia
Indications. Ceftiofur-sensitive infections
Contra-indications. Hypersensitivity to cephalosporins or penicillins
Dose.
Horses: by intramuscular injection, 2 mg/kg once daily
Cattle: by intramuscular injection, 1 mg/kg once daily
Dogs: by subcutaneous injection, 2 mg/kg once daily

Excenel Injectable (Pharmacia & Upjohn) *Austral.*
Injection, ceftiofur (as sodium salt) 50 mg/mL (when reconstituted), for *cattle, horses, dogs*
Withdrawal Periods. Horses: slaughter 28 days. *Cattle*: slaughter 1 day, milk withdrawal period nil

Eire
Indications. Ceftiofur-sensitive infections
Contra-indications. Hypersensitivity to cephalosporins or penicillins
Dose. *Cattle*: by intramuscular injection, 1 mg/kg
Pigs: by intramuscular injection, 3 mg/kg

Excenel RTU (Pharmacia & Upjohn) *Eire*
Injection, ceftiofur (as hydrochloride) 50 mg/mL, for *pigs*
Withdrawal Periods. Slaughter 5 days

Excenel Sterile Powder (Pharmacia & Upjohn) *Eire*
Injection, powder for reconstitution, ceftiofur (as sodium) 1 g, 4 g vials (50 mg/mL when reconstituted), for *cattle, pigs*
Withdrawal Periods. *Cattle*: slaughter 24 hours, milk withdrawal period nil. *Pigs*: slaughter 12 hours

New Zealand
Indications. Ceftiofur-sensitive infections
Contra-indications. Hypersensitivity to cephalosporins or penicillins

Dose. *Horses*: *by intramuscular injection*, 2 mg/kg once daily
Cattle: *by intramuscular injection*, 1 mg/kg once daily
Pigs: *by intramuscular injection*, 3 mg/kg once daily

Excenel (Pharmacia & Upjohn) *NZ*
Injection, ceftiofur (as sodium salt) 50 mg/mL, for *horses, cattle, pigs*
Withdrawal Periods. *Horses, pigs*: slaughter withdrawal period nil. *Cattle*: slaughter withdrawal period nil, milk withdrawal period nil

USA

Indications. Ceftiofur-sensitive infections
Contra-indications. Hypersensitivity to cephalosporins or penicillins
Dose.

Horses: *by intramuscular injection*, 2.2 mg/kg
Cattle, sheep: *by intramuscular injection*, 1.1–2.2 mg/kg
Pigs: *by intramuscular injection*, 3–5 mg/kg once daily
Dogs: *by subcutaneous injection*, 2.2 mg/kg
Poultry: (day-old chicks) *by subcutaneous injection*, 80–200 micrograms

Excenel (Pharmacia & Upjohn) *USA*
Injection, ceftiofur 50 mg/mL, for *pigs*
Withdrawal Periods. Slaughter withdrawal period nil

Naxel (Pharmacia & Upjohn) *USA*
Injection, powder for reconstitution, ceftiofur 50 mg/mL of reconstituted solution, for *horses, cattle, sheep, pigs, dogs, chickens, turkeys*
Withdrawal Periods. Should not be used in *horses* intended for human consumption. *Cattle*: slaughter withdrawal period nil, milk withdrawal period nil. *Sheep*: slaughter withdrawal period nil. *Chickens, turkeys*: slaughter withdrawal period nil

CEFUROXIME

UK

Indications. Cefuroxime-sensitive infections
Dose. See Prescribing for reptiles

POM Ⓗ **Zinacef** (GlaxoWellcome) *UK*
Injection, powder for reconstitution, cefuroxime (as sodium salt) 250 mg, 750 mg, 1.5 g

1.1.2 Tetracyclines

The tetracyclines are broad-spectrum antibacterials active against *Mycoplasma*, *Chlamydia*, and *Rickettsia* in addition to bacteria. They are active against a range of Gram-positive and Gram-negative bacteria but have little useful activity against *E. coli*, *Salmonella*, *Proteus*, or *Pseudomonas* spp. Tetracyclines are bacteriostatic and acquired resistance is now widespread among bacteria.

The widely-used **oxytetracycline** and the less often-used **tetracycline** and **chlortetracycline** have similar properties. When given by intramuscular injection they may be irritant, depending on the vehicle used. For this reason some preparations incorporate a local anaesthetic. Depot preparations will maintain effective plasma concentrations for 72 to 96 hours. Some preparations may be given intravenously, but rapid injection by this route in cattle may cause cardiovascular collapse, apparently due to chelation of calcium. Oral administration may cause diarrhoea. Absorption of tetracy-

clines from the gastro-intestinal tract is variable and is reduced by milk (not doxycycline), antacids, and by calcium, iron, magnesium, and zinc salts.

Tetracyclines are deposited in developing teeth by binding to calcium and if given to puppies, kittens, or bitches or queens in late pregnancy they may cause discoloration and defects of the enamel of the puppies' temporary dentition. Horses that are given parenteral or enteral tetracyclines and also exposed to stress may suffer a severe enterocolitis, which can prove fatal. Photodermatitis has occurred following treatment with tetracyclines after exposure to intense sunlight or ultraviolet light. There are reports of nephrotoxicity being associated with use of tetracyclines. These may have been due to degradation products which accumulate in preparations which are used beyond the expiry date.

The main excretory routes for tetracyclines are the urinary system and the gastro-intestinal tract via the biliary system. **Doxycycline** and **minocycline** are more lipophilic than the older tetracyclines and have a number of advantages. Absorption of orally administered doxycycline and minocycline are better and are less affected by milk and calcium salts. These drugs also penetrate better into several body compartments and fluids, notably bronchial secretions and prostatic fluid. Doxycycline enters the gastro-intestinal tract through the bile and is particularly liable to produce enterocolitis in the horse. Minocycline is metabolised prior to excretion in the bile. These lipid soluble tetracyclines are safer to use in animals with renal impairment.

CHLORTETRACYCLINE

UK

Indications. Chlortetracycline-sensitive infections; theileriosis (see section 1.4.8)
Contra-indications. Oral administration to ruminants with a functional rumen is not recommended; renal impairment; last 2–3 weeks of gestation in pregnant animals and up to 4 weeks of age in neonates, see notes above; avoid use in patients with dysphagia or diseases accompanied by vomiting
Side-effects. May cause vomiting, diarrhoea
Dose. *By mouth*.
Calves: 10–20 mg/kg body-weight daily
Pigs: 10–20 mg/kg body-weight daily
by addition to feed, 400–600 g/tonne feed
Chickens: 20–50 mg/kg body-weight
by addition to feed, 300–400 g/tonne feed
Turkeys, ducks: 10–30 mg/kg body-weight; 300–400 g/tonne feed

POM **Aureomycin Soluble Oblets** (Fort Dodge) *UK*
Tablets, or to prepare an oral solution, scored, chlortetracycline hydrochloride 500 mg, for *calves*; 48
Withdrawal Periods. *Calves*: slaughter 25 days

POM **Aureomycin Soluble Powder** (Fort Dodge) *UK*
Oral powder, for addition to drinking water or to prepare an oral solution, chlortetracycline hydrochloride 55 g/kg, for *calves, pigs, chickens, turkeys*; 225 g, 5 kg
Withdrawal Periods. *Calves*: slaughter 25 days. *Pigs*: slaughter 10 days. *Chickens, turkeys*: slaughter 1 day, egg withdrawal period nil

MFS Aurofac 100 Granular (Alpharma) *UK*
Premix, chlortetracycline hydrochloride 100 g/kg, for *pigs, chickens, turkeys, ducks*; 3 kg, 24 kg
Withdrawal Periods. *Pigs*: slaughter 10 days. *Chickens, turkeys*: slaughter 1 day, egg withdrawal period nil. *Ducks*: slaughter 2 days

MFS Aurofac 200 MA (Fort Dodge) *UK*
Oral powder, for addition to milk, milk replacer, or to prepare an oral solution, chlortetracycline hydrochloride 200 g/kg, for *calves*; 500 g, 10 kg
Withdrawal Periods. *Calves*: slaughter 15 days

POM Aurogran (Vericore LP) *UK*
Premix, chlortetracycline 100 g/kg, for *pigs, chickens, turkeys*
Withdrawal Periods. *Pigs*: slaughter 7 days. *Chickens, turkeys*: slaughter 3 days, egg withdrawal period nil

POM Aurogran 150 (Vericore LP) *UK*
Premix, chlortetracycline 150 g/kg, for *pigs, broiler chickens*
Withdrawal Periods. *Pigs*: slaughter 7 days. *Chickens*: slaughter 3 days, egg withdrawal period nil

MFS Auromix 100 (Pharmacia & Upjohn) *UK*
Premix, chlortetracycline hydrochloride 100 g/kg, for *pigs 5–90 kg body-weight, non-laying chickens*; 2 kg, 3 kg, 25 kg
Withdrawal Periods. *Pigs*: slaughter 5 days. *Chickens*: slaughter 12 hours
Contra-indications. Laying hens

POM Chlorsol 50 (Vétoquinol) *UK*
Oral powder, for addition to drinking water, chlortetracycline hydrochloride 500 g/kg, for *pigs, broiler chickens*; 200 g, 300 g
Withdrawal Periods. *Pigs*: slaughter 6 days. *Chickens*: slaughter 3 days
Contra-indications. Pregnant sows; laying hens

MFS Chlortet FG 100 (ECO) *UK*
Premix, chlortetracycline 100 g/kg, for *pigs*
Withdrawal Periods. *Pigs*: slaughter 7 days

Australia

Indications. Chlortetracycline-sensitive infections
Dose. Dosages vary, consult manufacturer's information
For guidance. *By mouth.*
Cattle: 10–20 mg/kg body-weight daily
Pigs: 20 mg/kg body-weight daily
Chickens: 20–30 mg/kg body-weight

Aureomycin 950 Soluble Concentrate (Fort Dodge) *Austral.*
Premix, chlortetracycline hydrochloride 950 mg/g premix, for *cattle, sheep, pigs, poultry*
Withdrawal Periods. *Cattle, sheep*: slaughter 5 days. *Pigs*: slaughter 4 days. *Poultry*: slaughter 7 days, should not be used in poultry producing eggs for human consumption

Aureomycin Soluble Powder (Whelehan) *Eire*
Oral powder, for addition to drinking water, chlortetracycline hydrochloride 55 g/kg, for *calves, pigs, chickens, turkeys*
Withdrawal Periods. *Calves*: slaughter 25 days. *Pigs*: slaughter 10 days. *Chickens, turkeys*: 1 day

Aureomycin Water Soluble Powder (CCD) *Austral.*
Powder, for addition to drinking water, chlortetracycline hydrochloride 950 mg/g powder, for *poultry*
Withdrawal Periods. *Poultry*: slaughter 7 days (therapeutic dose) or 5 days (prophylactic dose), should not be used in poultry producing eggs for human consumption

Aurofac 200 Antibiotic Feed Supplement (Roche) *Austral.*
Premix, chlortetracycline hydrochloride 200 g/kg premix, for *poultry, pigs*
Withdrawal Periods. *Pigs*: slaughter 5 days (100 ppm) or 7 days (400 ppm). *Poultry*: slaughter 2 days (100 ppm dose) or 7 days (400 ppm), egg withdrawal period nil

Tricon Powder (Apex) *Austral.*
Powder, for addition to drinking water, chlortetracycline hydrochloride 55 mg/g powder, for *poultry, pigs, dogs, cats, caged birds*

Withdrawal Periods. *Pigs*: slaughter 7 days. *Poultry*: slaughter 7 days, should not be used in poultry producing eggs for human consumption

Eire

Indications. Chlortetracycline-sensitive infections
Dose. Dosages vary, consult manufacturer's information
For guidance. *By mouth.*
Cattle: 10–20 mg/kg body-weight daily
Pigs: 20 mg/kg body-weight daily
Chickens: 20 mg/kg body-weight

Aureosup on Crystakon (Cypharm) *Eire*
Oral powder, to mix with feed, chlortetracycline hydrochloride 100 g/kg, for *pigs, chickens*
Withdrawal Periods. *Pigs*: slaughter 7 days. *Chickens*: 3 days

Aurogran (Cypharm) *Eire*
Oral granules, to mix with feed, chlortetracycline hydrochloride 10%, for *pigs, chickens*
Withdrawal Periods. *Pigs*: slaughter 7 days. *Chickens*: 3 days

Auromix 100 (Pharmacia & Upjohn) *Eire*
Oral powder, chlortetracycline hydrochloride 100 g/kg, for *pigs, chickens*
Withdrawal Periods. *Pigs*: slaughter 5 days. *Chickens*: slaughter 12 hours, should not be used in chickens producing eggs for human consumption

CTC 10% Premix (Univet) *Eire*
Premix, chlortetracycline hydrochloride 100 g/kg, for *calves, pigs*
Withdrawal Periods. *Calves*: slaughter 28 days. *Pigs*: slaughter 5 days

CTC 15% Premix (Univet) *Eire*
Premix, chlortetracycline hydrochloride 150 g/kg, for *cattle, pigs*
Withdrawal Periods. *Calves*: slaughter 28 days, should not be used in cattle producing milk for human consumption. *Pigs*: slaughter 5 days

Intercrison 100 (Intervet) *Eire*
Oral powder, to mix with feed, chlortetracycline hydrochloride 100 mg/g
Withdrawal Periods. Slaughter 5 days

New Zealand

Indications. Chlortetracycline-sensitive infections
Dose. Consult manufacturer's information

Aurofac D (Bomac) *NZ*
Oral powder, chlortetracycline hydrochloride 10 g/kg, for *cattle, pigs*
Withdrawal Periods. Slaughter 28 days

USA

Indications. Chlortetracycline-sensitive infections
Dose. Dosages vary, consult manufacturer's information
For guidance. *By mouth.*
Cattle: 11–22 mg/kg body-weight daily
Pigs: 22 mg/kg body-weight daily

Aureomycin (Roche Vitamins) *USA*
Premix, chlortetracycline hydrochloride (as calcium complex) 110 g, 198 g, 220 g/kg, for *cattle, sheep, pigs, chickens, turkeys, ducks*
Withdrawal Periods. *Cattle*: slaughter withdrawal period nil, should not to be used in calves processed for veal. *Sheep*: slaughter withdrawal period nil. *Pigs*: slaughter withdrawal period nil

Aureomycin Soluble Calf Oblets (Fort Dodge) *USA*
Tablets, chlortetracycline 500mg, for *cattle*
Withdrawal Periods. Slaughter 24 hours

Aureomycin Soluble Powder (Fort Dodge) *USA*
Oral powder, for addition to drinking water, chlortetracycline hydrochloride 55 g/kg, for *pigs, calves, chickens, turkeys*
Withdrawal Periods. *Chickens (high dose),pigs, calves, turkeys*: slaughter 24 hours, should not be used in chickens producing eggs for human consumption

Aureomycin Soluble Powder Concentrate (Fort Dodge) *USA*
Oral powder, for addition to drinking water, chlortetracycline hydrochloride 145.2 g/kg, for *pigs, calves, chickens, turkeys*
Withdrawal Periods. *Chickens (high dose) pigs, calves, turkeys*: slaughter 24 hours, should not be used in chickens producing eggs for human consumption

Aureomycin Tablets (Fort Dodge) *USA*
Tablets, chlortetracycline 25 mg, for *calves*
Withdrawal Periods. Slaughter 24 hours

Calf Scour Bolus Antibiotic (DurVet) *USA*
Tablets, chlortetracycline hydrochloride 500 mg, for *calves*
Withdrawal Periods. Slaughter 3 days, should not be used in calves intended for veal production

Chlora-Cycline (RXV) *USA*
Oral powder, to add to drinking water, chlortetracycline hydrochloride 181.4 g/measuring cup (225 mL), for *chickens, turkeys, pigs*
Withdrawal Periods. *Pigs*: slaughter 5 days. *Chickens, turkeys*: slaughter 1 day, should not be used in chickens producing eggs for human consumption

Chlormax 50 (Alpharma) *USA*
Premix, chlortetracycline 110 g/kg premix, for *cattle, pigs, tukeys, chickens, sheep*
Withdrawal Periods. Should not be used in *chickens or turkeys* producing eggs for human consumption. Should not be used in *calves* intended for veal production

CLTC 100 MR (Pfizer) *USA*
Premix, chlortetracycline 220 mg/g, for *calves*

CTC 50 (DurVet) *USA*
Premix, chlortetracycline (as hydrochloride) 110 g/kg premix, for *chickens, turkeys, pigs, sheep*
Withdrawal Periods. *Cattle*: slaughter 2 days. *Pigs*: slaughter withdrawal period nil. *Chickens*: slaughter 24 hours

CTC Soluble Powder (AgriLabs) *USA*
Oral powder, to add to drinking water, chlortetracycline (as hydrochloride) 141 g/kg powder, for *chickens, turkeys, pigs*
Withdrawal Periods. *Pigs*: slaughter 5 days. *Chickens, turkeys*: slaughter 1 day, should not be used in chickens producing eggs for human consumption

Purina Chek-R-Mycin 10X (Purina Mills) *USA*
Oral powder, for addition to drinking water, chlortetracycline hydrochloride 140.8 g/kg powder, for *pigs, chickens, turkeys, cattle, pigs*
Withdrawal Periods. *Pigs, calves*: slaughter 1 day. *Chickens*: slaughter 1 day (but depends on dose used), should not be used in chickens producing eggs for human consumption

DOXYCYCLINE

UK
Indications. Doxycycline-sensitive infections
Contra-indications. Side-effects. Use in pregnant animals is contra-indicated. See under Chlortetracycline. May be used in renal impairment
Warnings. Avoid use during reproductive period of birds. Manufacturer advises that birds do not participate in races during treatment. Deionised or distilled water should be used. Drug Interactions – see Appendix 1
Dose.
Dogs: *by mouth,* 10 mg/kg daily
Cats: *by mouth,* 10 mg/kg daily
Feline chlamydial infections♦, *by mouth,* 5 mg/kg 1–2 times daily
Birds: *by addition to drinking water,* 15 mg/kg *or* 260 mg/2 litres drinking water. For birds with low daily water intake, 260 mg/500 mL drinking water

POM **Ornicure** (Vetrepharm) *UK*
Oral powder, for addition to drinking water, doxycycline (as hyclate) 260 mg/sachet, for *pigeons, cage birds*; 4-g sachets
Withdrawal Periods. Should not be used in *pigeons, cage birds* intended for human consumption

POM **Ronaxan** (Merial) *UK*
Tablets, doxycycline 20 mg, for *dogs, cats*; 100
Tablets, doxycycline 100 mg, for *dogs*; 100

Australia
Indications. Doxycycline-sensitive infections
Dose. *Dogs, cats*: *by mouth,* 5 mg/kg, then 2.5 mg/kg
Birds: consult manufacturer's information

Psittavet (Vetafarm) *Austral.*
Powder, for addition to drinking water, doxycycline hydrochloride 40 mg/g powder, for *parrots, pigeons*
Withdrawal Periods. Should not be used in animals intended for human consumption

VibraVet (Pfizer) *Austral.*
Paste, doxycycline (as monohydrate) 100 mg/g, for *dogs, cats*
Tablets, doxycycline (as monohydrate) 50 mg, 100 mg, for *dogs, cats*

Eire
Indications. Doxycycline-sensitive infections
Dose. *Dogs, cats*: *by mouth,* 10 mg/kg daily

Ronaxan (Merial) *Eire*
Tablets, doxycycline 20 mg, for *dogs, cats*
Tablets, doxycycline 100 mg, for *dogs*

New Zealand
Indications. Doxycycline-sensitive infections
Dose. *Cattle*: *by mouth or by intravenous injection,* 10 mg/kg
Dogs, cats: *by mouth,* 5 mg/kg, then 2.5 mg/kg

Doxycycline 5% Powder (Phoenix) *NZ*
Oral powder, doxycycline (as hyclate) 50 mg/g, for *cattle*
Withdrawal Periods. Slaughter 14 days, should not be used in cattle producing milk for human consumption

Doxycycline 10% Injection (Phoenix) *NZ*
Injection, doxycycline (as hyclate) 100 mg/mL, for *cattle*
Withdrawal Periods. Slaughter 14 days, should not be used in cattle producing milk for human consumption

Vibravet 100 Paste for Cats and Dogs (Pfizer) *NZ*
Oral paste, doxycycline 100 mg/g, for *dogs, cats*

Vibravet Tablets (Pfizer) *NZ*
Tablets, doxycycline 50 mg, for *dogs, cats*
Tablets, doxycycline 100 mg, for *dogs*

USA
Indications. Doxycycline-sensitive infections
Dose. Consult manufacturer's information

Heska Periodontal Disease Therapeutic (Heska) *USA*
Periodontal mixture, doxycycline 88 mg/mL, for *dogs*

OXYTETRACYCLINE

UK
Indications. Oxytetracycline-sensitive infections; theileriosis (see section 1.4.8)

Contra-indications. Side-effects. See under Chlortetracy-cline. Avoid subcutaneous injection in horses. Some manufacturers recommend that intravenous injection in dogs should be avoided; avoid oral administration in calves with a functional rumen; photodermatitis may be observed after treatment with oxytetracycline

Warnings. Caution with use in animals with renal or hepatic impairment; Drug Interactions – see Appendix 1

Dose. Dosages vary. For guidance.

Horses: *by intramuscular or intravenous injection*, 2–10 mg/kg daily

Cattle, sheep, goats, pigs: *by intramuscular or intravenous injection*, 2–10 mg/kg daily

by depot intramuscular injection, 20 mg/kg, repeat after 2–4 days *or*

30 mg/kg (preparations containing oxytetracycline 300 mg/mL), repeat after 6 days

calves, pigs: *by mouth*, dosage varies, for guidance 10–30 mg/kg 1–2 times daily but see also manufacturer's information

Red deer: *by depot intramuscular injection*, 20 mg/kg, repeat after 2–4 days

Dogs: *by mouth*, 25 mg/kg twice daily

by subcutaneous or intramuscular injection, 2–10 mg/kg daily

Cats: *by subcutaneous or intramuscular injection*, 2–10 mg/kg daily

Poultry: *by addition to drinking water*, 7–27 g/100 litres

Cage birds: see preparation details

Fish: see Prescribing for fish

POM **Alamycin 10** (Norbrook) *UK*
Injection, oxytetracycline hydrochloride 100 mg/mL, for *cattle, pigs*
Withdrawal Periods. *Cattle*: slaughter 15 days, milk 2.5 days. *Pigs*: slaughter 15 days

POM **Alamycin LA** (Norbrook) *UK*
Depot injection, oxytetracycline (as dihydrate) 200 mg/mL, for *cattle, sheep, pigs*; 50 mL, 100 mL
Withdrawal Periods. *Cattle*: slaughter 28 days, milk 7 days. *Sheep*: slaughter 21 days, should not be used in sheep producing milk for human consumption. *Pigs*: slaughter 14 days

POM **Alamycin LA 300** (Norbrook) *UK*
Depot injection, oxytetracycline (as dihydrate) 300 mg/mL, for *cattle, sheep, pigs*; 100 mL
Withdrawal Periods. (20 mg/kg dose) *Cattle*: slaughter 28 days, milk 7 days. *Sheep*: slaughter 28 days, milk 8 days. *Pigs*: slaughter 14 days. (30 mg/kg dose) *Cattle*: slaughter 35 days, milk 7 days. *Sheep*: slaughter 28 days, milk 8 days. *Pigs*: slaughter 28 days

POM **Duphacycline 50** (Fort Dodge) *UK*
Injection, oxytetracycline hydrochloride 50 mg/mL, for *cattle, pigs, dogs*
Withdrawal Periods. *Cattle*: slaughter 15 days, milk 2 days. *Pigs*: slaughter 15 days

POM **Duphacycline 100** (Fort Dodge) *UK*
Injection, oxytetracycline hydrochloride 100 mg/mL, for *cattle, pigs*;
Withdrawal Periods. *Cattle*: slaughter 15 days, milk 2.5 days. *Pigs*: slaughter 15 days

POM **Duphacycline LA** (Fort Dodge) *UK*
Depot injection, oxytetracycline dihydrate 200 mg/mL, for *cattle, sheep, pigs*; 100 mL
Withdrawal Periods. *Cattle*: slaughter 14 days, milk 7 days. *Sheep*: slaughter 14 days, should not be used in sheep producing milk for human consumption. *Pigs*: slaughter 14 days

POM **Duphacycline XL** (Fort Dodge) *UK*
Depot injection, oxytetracycline (as dihydrate) 300 mg/mL, for *cattle, pigs*
Withdrawal Periods. (20 mg/kg dose) *Cattle*: slaughter 28 days, milk 7 days. *Pigs*: slaughter 14 days. (30 mg/kg dose) *Cattle*: slaughter 35 days, milk 7 days. *Pigs*: slaughter 28 days

POM **Embacycline 5** (Merial) *UK*
Injection, oxytetracycline hydrochloride 50 mg/mL, for *cattle, pigs, dogs*;
Withdrawal Periods. *Cattle*: slaughter 15 days, milk 2 days. *Pigs*: slaughter 15 days

POM **Embacycline LA** (Merial) *UK*
Depot injection, oxytetracycline (as dihydrate) 200 mg/mL, for *cattle, sheep, pigs*; 50 mL, 100 mL
Withdrawal Periods. *Cattle*: slaughter 14 days, milk 7 days. *Sheep*: slaughter 14 days, should not be used in sheep producing milk for human consumption. *Pigs*: slaughter 14 days

POM **Engemycin 10% (DD)** (Intervet) *UK*
Depot injection, oxytetracycline (as hydrochloride) 100 mg/mL, for *cattle, sheep, pigs*; 100 mL
Withdrawal Periods (Prolonged-action dosage). *Cattle*: slaughter 10 days, milk 3 days. *Sheep*: slaughter 10 days, milk 2 days. *Pigs*: slaughter 10 days

POM **Engemycin LA** (Intervet) *UK*
Depot injection, oxytetracycline 200 mg/mL, for *cattle, sheep, pigs*; 50 mL, 100 mL
Withdrawal Periods. *Cattle*: slaughter 28 days, milk 7 days. *Sheep*: slaughter 14 days, milk 8 days. *Pigs*: slaughter 14 days

POM **Engemycin 5%** (Intervet) *UK*
Injection, oxytetracycline (as hydrochloride) 50 mg/mL, for *horses, cattle, sheep, pigs, dogs, cats*; 100 mL
Withdrawal Periods. Should not be used in *horses* intended for human consumption. *Cattle, sheep*: slaughter 8 days, milk 2 days. *Pigs*: slaughter 8 days

POM **Engemycin 10% (DD)** (Intervet) *UK*
Injection, oxytetracycline (as hydrochloride) 100 mg/mL, for *horses, cattle, sheep, pigs, dogs, cats*; 100 mL
Withdrawal Periods (Daily dosage). Should not be used in *horses* intended for human consumption. *Cattle, sheep*: slaughter 8 days, milk 2 days. *Pigs*: slaughter 8 days
Note. May also be given as a Depot intramuscular injection

POM **Finabiotic** (Schering-Plough) *UK*
Injection, oxytetracycline (as hydrochloride) 100 mg, flunixin (as meglumine) 20 mg/mL, for *cattle*; 100 mL
Withdrawal Periods. *Cattle*: slaughter 21 days, milk 5 days
Dose. *Cattle*: respiratory disease, *by intramuscular or intravenous injection*, 0.1 mL/kg daily for 3–5 days
Acute mastitis, *by intravenous injection*, 0.1 mL/kg daily

POM **Hexasol HB** (Norbrook) *UK*
Injection, oxytetracycline 300 mg, flunixin 20 mg/mL, for *cattle*
Withdrawal Periods. Slaughter 21 days, should not be used in pregnant cattle or cattle producing milk for human consumption
Dose. *Cattle*: 0.1 mL/kg

POM **Mycen 5** (Vericore VP) *UK*
Injection, oxytetracycline hydrochloride 50 mg/mL, for *cattle, pigs, dogs*
Withdrawal Periods. *Cattle*: slaughter 15 days, milk 2 days. *Pigs*: slaughter 15 days

POM **Mycen 10** (Vericore VP) *UK*
Injection, oxytetracycline hydrochloride 100 mg/mL, for *cattle, pigs*
Withdrawal Periods. *Cattle*: slaughter 15 days, milk 2.5 days. *Pigs*: slaughter 15 days

POM **Mycen 20 LA** (Vericore VP)
Depot injection, oxytetracycline 200 mg/mL, for *cattle, sheep, pigs*
Withdrawal Periods. *Cattle*: slaughter 28 days, milk 7 days. *Sheep*: slaughter 21 days, should not be used in sheep producing milk for human consumption. *Pigs*: slaughter 14 days

POM **Occrycetin Bolus** (Fort Dodge) *UK*
Tablets, scored, oxytetracycline hydrochloride 500 mg, for *calves*; 20
Withdrawal Periods. *Calves*: slaughter 10 days

POM **Ornimed Oxytetracycline** (LAB; distributed by Millpledge) *UK*
Medicated seed, oxytetracycline 3 mg/g, for *budgerigars*; 20 g
Side-effects. May cause fungal infections and soft shelled eggs with prolonged treatment
Dose.*Birds*: 1.5 g of seed twice daily

POM **Oxycare 5%** (Animalcare) *UK*
njection, oxytetracycline hydrochloride 50 mg/mL, for *cattle, pigs, dogs*
Withdrawal Periods. *Cattle*: slaughter 15 days, milk 2 days. *Pigs*: slaughter 15 days

POM **Oxycare 10%** (Animalcare) *UK*
njection, oxytetracycline hydrochloride 50 mg/mL, for *cattle, pigs*
Withdrawal Periods. *Cattle*: slaughter 15 days, milk 2.5 days. *Pigs*: slaughter 15 days

POM **Oxycare 20/LA** (Animalcare) *UK*
Depot injection, oxytetracycline (as dihydrate) 200 mg/mL, for *cattle, sheep, pigs*; 50 mL, 100 mL
Withdrawal Periods. *Cattle*: slaughter 14 days, milk 7 days. *Sheep*: slaughter 14 days, should not be used in sheep producing milk for human consumption. *Pigs*: slaughter 14 days

POM **Oxycare Tablets** (Animalcare) *UK*
Tablets, s/c, oxytetracycline dihydrate 50 mg, 100 mg, 250 mg, for *dogs*; 500, 1000

POM **Oxycomplex NS** (Bimeda) *UK*
Injection, oxytetracycline (as hydrochloride) 100 mg, flunixin (as meglumine) 20 mg/mL, for *cattle*; 100 mL
Withdrawal Periods. *Cattle*: slaughter 28 days, milk 7 days
Dose. *Cattle*: initially *by intravenous injection*, then *by intramuscular injection*, 0.1 mL/kg daily for up to 5 days

POM **Oxytetrin 5** (Schering-Plough) *UK*
Injection, oxytetracycline hydrochloride 50 mg/mL, for *cattle, sheep, pigs*
Withdrawal Periods. *Cattle*: slaughter 7 days, milk 3 days. *Sheep*: slaughter 5 days, should not be used in sheep producing milk for human consumption. *Pigs*: slaughter 11 days

POM **Oxytetrin 10 DD** (Schering-Plough) *UK*
Injection, oxytetracycline hydrochloride 100 mg/mL, for *cattle, sheep, pigs*; 100 mL
Withdrawal Periods. *Cattle*: slaughter 10 days, milk 80 hours. *Sheep*: slaughter 5 days, should not be used in sheep producing milk for human consumption. *Pigs*: slaughter 11 days
Note. May also be given as a Depot intramuscular injection in cattle

POM **Oxytetrin 10 DD** (Schering-Plough) *UK*
Depot injection, oxytetracycline hydrochloride 100 mg/mL, for *cattle*; 100 mL
Withdrawal Periods. *Cattle*: slaughter 10 days, milk 80 hours

POM **Oxytetrin 20 LA** (Schering-Plough) *UK*
Depot injection, oxytetracycline dihydrate 200 mg/mL, for *cattle, sheep, pigs*; 100 mL
Withdrawal Periods. *Cattle*: slaughter 14 days, milk 7 days. *Sheep*: slaughter 21 days, should not be used in sheep producing milk for human consumption. *Pigs*: slaughter 35 days

POM **Terramycin LA Injectable Solution** (Pfizer)
Depot injection, oxytetracycline (as dihydrate) 200 mg/mL, for *cattle, sheep, red deer, pigs*; 100 mL
Withdrawal Periods. *Cattle*: slaughter 21 days, milk 7 days. *Sheep*: slaughter 21 days, should not be used in sheep producing milk for human consumption. *Pigs*: slaughter 21 days. *Red deer*: slaughter 30 days
Note. Administered by intravenous injection in cattle for short-acting effect

POM **Terramycin Q-50 Injectable Solution** (Pfizer) *UK*
Injection, oxytetracycline hydrochloride (as magnesium complex) 50 mg/mL, for *cattle, sheep, pigs*; 40 mL, 100 mL
Withdrawal Periods. *Cattle*: slaughter 14 days, milk 4 days. *Sheep*: slaughter 14 days, should not be used in sheep producing milk for human consumption. *Pigs*: slaughter 14 days
Note. May also be given by subconjunctival injection in cattle

POM **Terramycin Q-100 Injectable Solution** (Pfizer) *UK*
Injection, oxytetracycline hydrochloride (as magnesium complex) 100 mg/mL, for *cattle, sheep, pigs*; 100 mL
Withdrawal Periods. *Cattle*: slaughter 14 days, milk 5 days. *Sheep*: slaughter 28 days, should not be used in sheep producing milk for human consumption. *Pigs*: slaughter 21 days

POM **Terramycin Soluble Powder 5.5%** (Pfizer) *UK*
Oral powder, for addition to drinking water or feed, or to prepare an oral solution, oxytetracycline hydrochloride 55 g/kg, for *cattle, pigs, chickens, turkeys*; 225 g, 2 kg (measure provided = oxytetracycline 200 mg)
Withdrawal Periods. *Cattle*: slaughter 10 days, milk withdrawal period nil. *Pigs*: slaughter 7 days. *Chickens, turkeys*: slaughter 7 days, eggs 1 day

POM **Terramycin Soluble Powder Concentrate 20%** (Pfizer) *UK*
Oral powder, for addition to drinking water or feed or to prepare an oral solution, oxytetracycline hydrochloride 200 g/kg, for *cattle, pigs, chickens, turkeys*; 225 g, 2 kg (measure provided = oxytetracycline 1 g)
Withdrawal Periods. *Cattle*: slaughter 10 days, milk withdrawal period nil. *Pigs*: slaughter 7 days. *Chickens, turkeys*: slaughter 7 days, eggs 1 day

POM **Tetcin 5** (Vétoquinol)
Injection, oxytetracycline hydrochloride 50 mg/mL, for *cattle, sheep, pigs*; 100 mL
Withdrawal Periods. *Cattle*: slaughter 7 days, milk 3 days. *Sheep*: slaughter 5 days, should not be used in sheep producing milk for human consumption. *Pigs*: slaughter 11 days

MFS **Tetramin 100, 200** (Pharmacia & Upjohn) *UK*
Premix, oxytetracycline dihydrate 100 g/kg, 200 g/kg, for *pigs 5–90 kg body-weight*; 2 kg, 25 kg
Withdrawal Periods. *Pigs*: slaughter 5 days

POM **Tetroxy 5%** (Bimeda) *UK*
Injection, oxytetracycline hydrochloride (as magnesium complex) 50 mg/mL, for *cattle less than 150 kg body-weight, sheep, pigs*; 100 mL
Withdrawal Periods. *Cattle*: slaughter 7 days, milk 3 days. *Sheep*: slaughter 5 days, should not be used in sheep producing milk for human consumption. *Pigs*: slaughter 11 days

POM **Tetroxy 10% DD** (Bimeda) *UK*
Injection, oxytetracycline hydrochloride (as magnesium complex) 100 mg/mL, for *cattle, sheep, pigs*; 100 mL
Withdrawal Periods. *Cattle*: slaughter 10 days, milk 80 hours. *Sheep*: slaughter 5 days, should not be used in sheep producing milk for human consumption. *Pigs*: slaughter 11 days
Note. May also be given as a Depot intramuscular injection

POM **Tetroxy LA** (Bimeda) *UK*
Depot injection, oxytetracycline (as magnesium complex) 200 mg/mL, for *cattle, sheep, pigs*; 100 mL
Withdrawal Periods. *Cattle*: slaughter 14 days, milk 7 days. *Sheep*: slaughter 21 days, should not be used in sheep producing milk for human consumption. *Pigs*: slaughter 35 days

Australia
Indications. Oxytetracycline-sensitive infections
Dose. Dosages vary, consult manufactuer's information

A.F.S. Oxytet Soluble (Controlled Medications) *Austral.*
Powder, for addition to drinking water, oxytetracycline hydrochloride 980 mg/g, for *poultry, pigeons*
Withdrawal Periods. Slaughter 7 days, should not be given to poultry producing eggs for human consumption

Alamycin 10 Injection (Novartis) *Austral.*
Injection, oxytetracycline 100 mg/mL, for *cattle, sheep, pigs*
Withdrawal Periods. *Cattle*: slaughter 42 days, milk 60 hours. *Pigs, sheep*: slaughter 42 days

Alamycin LA Injection (Novartis) *Austral.*
Injection, oxytetracycline 200 mg/mL, for *cattle, sheep, pigs*
Withdrawal Periods. *Cattle:* slaughter 42 days, milk 7 days. *Pigs, sheep:* slaughter, 42 days

Bivatop 200 Long Acting Injectable for Cattle and Pigs (Boehringer Ingelheim) *Austral.*
Injection, oxytetracycline 200 mg/mL, for *cattle, pigs*
Withdrawal Periods. *Cattle*: slaughter 28 days, milk 7 days. *Pigs*: slaughter 42 days

Delcycline 200 LA (Delvet) *Austral.*
Injection, oxytetracycline 200 mg/mL, for *cattle, sheep, pigs*
Withdrawal Periods. *Cattle*: slaughter 42 days, milk 7 days. *Sheep, pigs*: slaughter 42 days

Engemycin 100 (Intervet) *Austral.*
Injection, oxytetracycline (as hydrochloride)100 mg/mL, for *horses, cattle, pigs, sheep, dogs, cats*
Withdrawal Periods. *Cattle*: slaughter 10 days, milk 3 days. *Horses, sheep, pigs*: slaughter 10 days

OTC-200 for Feed Medication (Rhône-Poulenc) *Austral.*
Powder, oxytetracycline 9as hydrochloride) 200 g/kg powder, for *cattle, pigs, poultry*
Withdrawal Periods. *Cattle*: slaughter 5 days, milk 72 hours. *Pigs*: slaughter 5 days. *Poultry*: slaughter 7 days, should not be used in poultry producing eggs for human consumption

Oxymav 100 (Mavlab) *Austral.*
Powder, for addition to drinking water, oxytetracycline hydrochloride 100 g/kg powder, for *cattle, poultry, pigs, bees*
Withdrawal Periods. *Calves*: slaughter 21 days, milk 7 days. *Pigs*: slaughter 21 days. *Poultry*: slaughter 21 days, should not be used in poultry producing eggs for human consumption

Oxymav B (Mavlab) *Austral.*
Powder, for addition to drinking water, oxytetracycline hydrochloride 10 g/kg, for *parrots, cockatoos, canaries, finches, budgerigars*

Oxytet-200 LA (Ilium) *Austral.*
Injection, oxytetracycline (as base) 200 mg/mL, for *cattle, sheep, pigs*
Withdrawal Periods. *Cattle*: slaughter 42 days, milk 7 days. *Sheep, pigs*: slaughter 42 days

Oxytetracycline 100 Premix (CCD) *Austral.*
Premix, oxytetracycline hydrochloride 100 g/kg, for *pigs, poultry, cattle*
Withdrawal Periods. *Pigs*: slaughter 4 days. *Calves*: slaughter 5 days. *Poultry*: slaughter 7 days, should not be used in poultry producing eggs for human consumption

Oxytetracycline Hydrochloride Water Soluble Powder (CCD) *Austral.*
Powder, for addition to drinking water, oxytetracycline hydrochloride 980 mg/g powder, for *poultry*
Withdrawal Periods. Slaughter 7 days, should not be used in poultry producing eggs for human consumption

Roscocycline-5 (Apex) *Austral.*
Injection, oxytetracycline hydrochloride 50 mg/mL, for *horses, cattle, pigs, poultry, dogs, cats*
Withdrawal Periods. *Cattle*: slaughter 22 days, milk 36 hours (single dose) or 72 hours (multiple dose). *Horses, pigs, poultry*: slaughter 22 days

Roscocycline-10 (Apex) *Austral.*
Injection, oxytetracycline hydrochloride 100 mg/mL, for *horses, cattle, pigs, sheep, goats,*
Withdrawal Periods. *Cattle*: slaughter 22 days, milk 36 hours (single dose) or 72 hours (multiple dose). *Horses, pigs, sheep, goats*: slaughter 22 days

Terramycin 100 Injectable (Pfizer) *Austral.*
Injection, oxytetracycline hydrochloride (as magnesium complex) 100 mg/mL in a PVP base, for *horses, cattle, pigs, deer*
Withdrawal Periods. *Horses*: slaughter 28 days. *Cattle*: slaughter 14 days, milk 7 days. *Sheep, pigs, deer*: slaughter 14 days

Terramycin 200 Feed Supplement (Pfizer) *Austral.*
Powder, for addition to feeds, oxytetracycline hydrochloride (as arquad salt) 200 g/kg powder, for *cattle, sheep, pigs, poultry*

Withdrawal Periods. *Cattle*: slaughter 5 days, milk 72 hours. *Sheep*: slaughter 5 days. *Pigs*: slaughter 4 days. *Poultry*: slaughter 7 days, should not be used in poultry producing eggs for human consumption

Terramycin 400 Feed Supplement (Pfizer) *Austral.*
Powder, for addition to feeds, oxytetracycline hydrochloride 400 g/kg, for *pigs, cattle, poultry*
Withdrawal Periods. *Cattle*: slaughter 5 days, milk 72 hours. *Pigs*: slaughter 4 days. *Poultry*: slaughter 7 days, should not be used in poultry producing eggs for human consumption

Terramycin 550 Feed Supplement (Pfizer) *Austral.*
Powder, for addition to feeds, oxytetracycline hydrochloride 550 g/kg, for *cattle, pigs, poultry*
Withdrawal Periods. *Cattle*: slaughter 5 days, milk 72 hours. *Pigs*: slaughter 4 days. *Poultry*: slaughter 7 days, should not be used in poultry producing eggs for human consumption

Terramycin 880 Soluble Powder (Pfizer) *Austral.*
Powder, for addition to drinking water, oxytetracycline hydrochloride 880 g/kg powder, for *cattle, pigs, poultry*
Withdrawal Periods. *Cattle*: slaughter 5 days, milk 72 hours. *Pigs*: slaughter 4 days. *Poultry*: slaughter 7 days, should not be used in poultry producing eggs for human consumption

Terramycin L/A (Pfizer) *Austral.*
Injection, oxytetracycline 200 mg/mL, for *cattle, sheep, pigs*
Withdrawal Periods. *Cattle*: slaughter 42 days, milk 7 days. *Sheep, pigs*: slaughter 42 days

Tetravet 100 Injection (Pharmtech) *Austral.*
Injection, oxytetracycline hydrochloride 100 mg/mL, for *horses, cattle, sheep, pigs*
Withdrawal Periods. *Horses*: slaughter 28 days. *Cattle*: slaughter 18 days, milk 96 hours. *Sheep*: slaughter 14 days. *Pigs*: slaughter 10 days

Tetravet 100 Soluble Antibiotic Powder (Pharmtech) *Austral.*
Powder, for addition to drinking water, oxytetracycline hydrochloride 10 g/100 g powder, for *cattle, pigs, poultry, caged birds, pigeons*
Withdrawal Periods. *Calves*: slaughter 5 days. *Pigs*: slaughter 4 days. *Poultry*: 7 days, should not be used in poultry producing eggs for human consumption

Tetravet 200 LA (Pharmtech) *Austral.*
Injection, oxytetracycline (as dihydrate in stable magnesium complex) 200 mg/mL, for *cattle, sheep, pigs*
Withdrawal Periods. *Cattle*: slaughter 42 days, milk 7 days. *Sheep, pigs*: slaughter 42 days

Tetroxy LA (Bimeda, Jurox) *Austral.*
Injection, oxytetracycline 200 mg/mL, for *cattle, sheep, pigs*
Withdrawal Periods. *Cattle*: slaughter 42 days, milk 7 days. *Sheep, pigs*: slaughter 42 days

Eire

Indications. Oxytetracycline-sensitive infections
Dose. Dosages vary, consult manufactuer's information

Alamycin 10% (Norbrook) *Eire*
Injection, oxytetracycline hydrochloride 100 mg/mL, for *cattle, sheep, pigs*
Withdrawal Periods. *Cattle, sheep, pigs*: slaughter 15 days. *Cattle*: milk 60 hours. Should not be used in sheep producing milk for human consumption

Alamycin Injection (Norbrook) *Eire*
Injection, oxytetracycline hydrochloride 50 mg/mL, for *cattle, pigs*
Withdrawal Periods. *Cattle*: slaughter 15 days, milk 48 hours. *Pigs*: slaughter 15 days

Alamycin LA (Norbrook) *Eire*
Injection, oxytetracycline (as dihyrate) 200 mg/mL, for *cattle, sheep, pigs*
Withdrawal Periods. *Cattle*: slaughter 14 days, milk 7 days. *Sheep*: slaughter 28 days, should not be used in sheep producing milk for human consumption. *Pigs*: slaughter 14 days

Alamycin LA 300 (Norbrook) *Eire*
Injection, oxytetracycline (as dihyrate) 300 mg/mL, for *cattle, pigs*

Withdrawal Periods. (20 mg/kg): *Cattle*: slaughter 28 days, milk 7 days. *Sheep*: slaughter 28 days, milk 8 days. *Pigs*: slaughter 14 days. (30 mg/kg): *Cattle*: slaughter 35 days, milk 7 days. *Sheep*: slaughter 28 days, milk 8 days. *Pigs*: slaughter 28 days

Bisolvomycin (Boehringer Ingelheim) *Eire*
Injection, bromhexine hydrochloride 3 mg/mL, oxytetracycline hydrochloride 50 mg/mL, lignocaine 20 mg/mL, for *cattle*
Withdrawal Periods. Slaughter 21 days, should not be used in cattle producing milk for human consumption

Bivatop (Boehringer Ingelheim) *Eire*
Injection, oxytetracycline (as dihydrate) 200 mg/mL, for *cattle, pigs*
Withdrawal Periods. *Cattle*: slaughter 21 days, should not be used in cattle producing milk for human consumption. *Pigs*: slaughter 14 days

Chanacycline 5% (Chanelle) *Eire*
Injection, oxytetracycline hydrochloride 50 mg/mL, for *cattle, sheep, pigs*
Withdrawal Periods. *Cattle*: slaughter 28 days, milk 96 hours. *Sheep*: slaughter 28 days, should not be used in sheep producing milk for human consumption. *Pigs*: slaughter 28 days

Chanacycline 10% (Chanelle) *Eire*
Injection, oxytetracycline hydrochloride 100 mg/mL, for *cattle, sheep, pigs*
Withdrawal Periods. *Cattle*: slaughter 28 days, milk 96 hours. *Sheep*: slaughter 28 days, should not be used in sheep producing milk for human consumption. *Pigs*: slaughter 28 days

Chanacycline LA (Chanelle) *Eire*
Injection, oxytetracycline hydrochloride 200 mg/mL, for *cattle, sheep, pigs*
Withdrawal Periods. *Cattle*: slaughter 28 days, milk 8 days. *Sheep*: slaughter 28 days, should not be used in sheep producing milk for human consumption. *Pigs*: slaughter 28 days

Duocycline 5 (Univet) *Eire*
Injection, oxytetracycline hydrochloride 50 mg/mL, for *cattle, sheep, pigs*
Withdrawal Periods. *Cattle*: slaughter 28 days, milk 96 hours. *Sheep*: slaughter 28 days, should not be used in sheep producing milk for human consumption. *Pigs*: slaughter 28 days

Duocycline 10 (Univet) *Eire*
Injection, oxytetracycline hydrochloride 100 mg/mL, for *cattle, sheep, pigs*
Withdrawal Periods. *Cattle*: slaughter 28 days, milk 96 hours. *Sheep*: slaughter 28 days, should not be used in sheep producing milk for human consumption. *Pigs*: slaughter 28 days

Duocycline LA (Univet) *Eire*
Injection, oxytetracycline dihydrate 200 mg/mL, for *cattle, sheep, pigs*
Withdrawal Periods. *Cattle*: slaughter 28 days, milk 8 days. *Sheep*: slaughter 28 days, should not be used in sheep producing milk for human consumption. *Pigs*: slaughter 28 days

Duphacycline 10% (Interchem) *Eire*
Injection, oxytetracycline hydrochloride 100 mg/mL, for *cattle, sheep, pigs*
Withdrawal Periods. *Cattle*: slaughter 15 days, milk 60 hours. *Sheep*: slaughter 15 days, should not be used in sheep producing milk for human consumption. *Pigs*: slaughter 15 days

Duphacycline 20% LA (Interchem) *Eire*
Injection, oxytetracyline hydrochloride 200 mg/mL, for *cattle, sheep, pigs*
Withdrawal Periods. *Cattle*: slaughter 14 days, milk 7 days. *Sheep*: slaughter 28 days, should not be used in sheep producing milk for human consumption. *Pigs*: slaughter 14 days

Engemycin 5% (Intervet) *Eire*
Injection, oxytetracyline (as hydrochloride) 50 mg/mL, for *horses, cattle, sheep, pigs, dogs, cats*
Withdrawal Periods. Should not be used in *horses* intended for human consumption. *Cattle*: slaughter 8 days, milk 60 hours. *Sheep*: slaughter 8 days, milk 48 hours. *Pigs*: slaughter 8 days

Engemycin 10% (DD) (Intervet) *Eire*
Injection, oxytetracycline (as hydrochloride) 100 mg/mL, for *horses, cattle, sheep, pigs, dogs, cats*
Withdrawal Periods. (24-hour dosage): *Horses*: slaughter 8 days. *Cattle*: slaughter 8 days, milk 60 hours. *Sheep*: slaughter 8 days, milk 48 hours. *Pigs*: slaughter 8 days. (Prolonged action): Should not be used in *horses*

intended for human consumption. *Cattle*: slaughter 10 days, milk 72 hours. *Sheep*: slaughter 10 days, milk 48 hours. *Pigs*: slaughter 14 days

Engemycin Soluble Powder 5% (Intervet) *Eire*
Oral powder, for addition to drinking water, oxytetracycline hydrochloride 50 g/kg, for *cattle, pigs*
Withdrawal Periods. *Cattle*: slaughter 10 days, milk withdrawal period nil. *Pigs*: slaughter 7 days

Finabiotic Injection (Schering-Plough) *Eire*
Injection, oxytetracycline (as hydrochloride) 100 mg/mL, flunixin (as meglumine) 20 mg, for *cattle*
Withdrawal Periods. Slaughter 21 days, milk 120 hours

Hostacycline LA (Hoechst Roussel Vet) *Eire*
Injection, oxytetracyclin (as dihydrate) 200 mg/mL, for *cattle, sheep, pigs*
Withdrawal Periods. *Cattle*: slaughter 21 days, milk 7 days. *Sheep*: slaughter 21 days, should not be used in sheep producing milk for human consumption. *Pigs*: slaughter 21 days

Maxoject 10 Injection (Interpharm) *Eire*
Injection, oxytetracycline hydrochloride 100 mg/mL, for *cattle, sheep, pigs*
Withdrawal Periods. *Cattle*: slaughter 15 days, milk 60 hours. *Sheep*: slaughter 15 days, should not be used in sheep producing milk for human consumption. *Pigs*: slaughter 15 days

Maxoject LA Injection (Interpharm) *Eire*
Injection, oxytetracycline (as dihydrate) 200 mg/mL, for *cattle, sheep, pigs*
Withdrawal Periods. *Cattle*: slaughter 14 days, milk 7 days. *Sheep*: slaughter 28 days, should not be used in sheep producing milk for human consumption. *Pigs*: slaughter 14 days

Occrycetin Bolus (Fort Dodge) *Eire*
Tablets, oxytetracyline hydrochloride 500 mg/tablet, for *calves*
Withdrawal Periods. Slaughter 10 days

Oxytetrasol 10% Injectable Solution (Virbac) *Eire*
Injection, oxytetracycline hydrochloride 100 mg/mL, for *cattle*
Withdrawal Periods. Slaughter 14 days, milk 60 hours

Terrafungine 20% LA Injectable Solution (Virbac) *Eire*
Injection, oxytetracycline (as hydrochloride) 200 mg/mL, for *cattle, pigs*
Withdrawal Periods. *Cattle*: slaughter 21 days, milk 7 days. *Pigs*: slaughter 21 days

Terramycin/LA Injectable Solution (Pfizer) *Eire*
Injection, oxytetracycline (as dihydrate) 200 mg/mL, for *cattle, sheep, deer, pigs*
Withdrawal Periods. *Cattle*: slaughter 21 days, milk 7 days. *Sheep*: slaughter 21 days, should not be used in sheep producing milk for human consumption. *Deer*: slaughter 30 days. *Pigs*: slaughter 21 days

Terramycin Q-50 Injectable Solution (Pfizer) *Eire*
Injection, oxytetracycline hydrochloride 50 mg/mL (as magnesium complex), for *cattle, sheep, pigs*
Withdrawal Periods. *Cattle*: slaughter 13 days or 5 days (after single iv dose), milk 96 hours. *Sheep*: slaughter 7 days, should not be used in sheep producing milk for human consumption. *Pigs*: slaughter 14 days or 7 days (after single im dose)

Terramycin Q-100 Injectable Solution (Pfizer) *Eire*
Injection, oxytetracycline hydrochloride 100 mg/mL (as magnesium complex), for *cattle, sheep, pigs*
Withdrawal Periods. *Cattle*: slaughter 14 days, milk 108 hours. *Sheep*: slaughter 28 days, should not be used in sheep producing milk for human consumption. *Pigs*: slaughter 21 days

Terramycin Soluble Powder 5.5% (Pfizer) *Eire*
Oral powder, oxytetracycline hydrochloride 55 g/kg, for *cattle, pigs, chickens, turkeys*
Withdrawal Periods. *Cattle*: slaughter 10 days, milk withdrawal period nil. *Pigs*: slaughter 7 days. *Chickens, turkeys*: slaughter 7 days, eggs 1 day

Terramycin Soluble Powder Concentrate 20% (Pfizer) *Eire*
Oral powder, oxytetracycline hydrochloride 200 g/kg, for *cattle, pigs, chickens, turkeys*
Withdrawal Periods. *Cattle*: slaughter 10 days, milk withdrawal period nil. *Pigs*: slaughter 7 days. *Chickens, turkeys*: slaughter 7 days, eggs 1 day

New Zealand

Indications. Oxytetracycline-sensitive infections
Dose. Dosages vary, consult manufactuer's information

Alphamycin (PCL) *NZ*
Premix, oxytetracycline 100 g/kg, for *cattle, pigs, poultry*
Withdrawal Periods. *Cattle*: slaughter 10 days, milk 96 hours. *Pigs*: slaughter 10 days. *Poultry*: slaughter 10 days, should not be used in birds producing eggs for human consumption

Bisolvomycin Vet (Boehringer Ingelheim) *NZ*
Injection, bromhexine hydrochloride 3 mg/mL, lidocaine 20 mg/mL, oxytetracycline hydrochloride 50 mg/mL, for *horses, cattle, pigs, dogs, cats*
Withdrawal Periods. *Horses*: slaughter 28 days. *Cattle*: slaughter 19 days, milk 144 hours. *Pigs*: slaughter 19 days

Bivatop 200 (Boehringer Ingelheim) *NZ*
Injection, oxytetracycline dihydrate 200 mg/mL, for *cattle, sheep, goats, deer, pigs*
Withdrawal Periods. *Cattle, sheep, goats*: slaughter 28 days, milk 168 hours. *Deer, pigs*: slaughter 28 days

Engemycin 10% (DD) (Chemavet) *NZ*
Injection, oxytetracycline 100 mg/mL, for *horses, cattle*
Withdrawal Periods. *Horses, pigs*: slaughter 10 days (short-acting regimen) or 14 days (long-acting regimen). *Cattle, sheep*: slaughter 10 days (short-acting regimen) or 14 days (long-acting regimen), milk 96 hours (short-acting regimen) or 120 hours (long-acting regimen)

Oxycomplex NS (Reamor) *NZ*
Injection, flunixin (as meglumine) 20 mg/mL, oxytetracycline (as hydrochloride) 100 mg/mL, for *cattle*
Withdrawal Periods. Slaughter 28 days, milk 144 hours

Oxytetra MA 10% (Phoenix) *NZ*
Injection, oxytetracycline (as hydrochloride) 100 mg/mL, for *cattle, pigs*
Withdrawal Periods. *Cattle*: slaughter 14 days, milk 120 hours. *Pigs*: slaughter 14 days

Oxytetra LA (Phoenix) *NZ*
Injection, oxytetracycline (as hydrochloride) 200 mg/mL, for *cattle, sheep, pigs*
Withdrawal Periods. *Cattle*: slaughter 21 days, milk 168 hours. *Sheep*: slaughter 28 days, milk 168 hours. *Pigs*: slaughter 28 days

Oxytetrin LA (Schering-Plough) *NZ*
Injection, oxytetracycline (as dihydrate) 200 mg/mL, for *cattle, sheep, pigs*
Withdrawal Periods. *Cattle, sheep*: slaughter 28 days, milk 168 hours. *Pigs*: slaughter 28 days

Oxyvet LA (Ethical) *NZ*
Injection, oxytetracycline dihydrate 200 mg/mL, for *cattle, sheep, pigs*
Withdrawal Periods. *Cattle, sheep*: slaughter 28 days, milk 168 hours. *Pigs*: slaughter 28 days

Tecoxy LA (Virbac) *NZ*
Injection, oxytetracycline (as magnesium complex) 200 mg/mL, for *cattle, sheep, pigs*
Withdrawal Periods. *Cattle, sheep*: slaughter 28 days, milk 168 hours. *Pigs*: slaughter 28 days

Terasol (PCL) *NZ*
Oral powder, oxytetracycline 100 g/kg, for *cattle, pigs, poultry*
Withdrawal Periods. Slaughter 10 days. Should not be used in birds producing eggs for human consumption

Terramycin 200 Feed Supplement (Pfizer) *NZ*
Premix, oxytetracycline hydrochloride 200 mg/g, for *cattle, pigs, poultry*
Withdrawal Periods. *Cattle*: slaughter 10 days, milk 96 hours. *Pigs, poultry*: slaughter 10 days

Terramycin/LA (Pfizer) *NZ*
Injection, oxytetracycline 200 mg/mL, for *cattle, sheep, goats, deer, pigs*
Withdrawal Periods. *Cattle, sheep, goats*: slaughter 21 days, milk 7 days. *Deer, pigs*: slaughter 21 days

Tetravet 100 (Bomac) *NZ*
Oral powder, oxytetracycline hydrochloride 100 g/kg, for *horses, cattle, sheep, pigs, dogs, cats, poultry*
Withdrawal Periods. *Horses*: slaughter 28 days. *Cattle, sheep*: slaughter 10 days, milk 96 hours. *Pigs*: slaughter 10 days. *Poultry*: slaughter 10 days, should not be used in birds producing eggs for human consumption

Tetravet 100 (Bomac) *NZ*
Injection, oxytetracycline hydrochloride (as magnesium complex) 100 mg/mL, for *horses, cattle, sheep, pigs*
Withdrawal Periods. Horses: slaughter 28 days. Cattle: slaughter 21 days, milk 96 hours. Sheep: slaughter 14 days, milk 96 hours. Pigs: slaughter 10 days

Tetravet 200 (Bomac) *NZ*
Oral powder, oxytetracycline hydrochloride 200 g/kg, for *cattle, pigs, poultry*
Withdrawal Periods. Slaughter 10 days. Should not be used in birds producing eggs for human consumption

Tetravet 200 LA (Bomac) *NZ*
Injection, oxytetracycline (as dihydrate) 200 mg/mL, for *cattle, sheep, pigs*
Withdrawal Periods. *Cattle, sheep*: slaughter 28 days, milk 7 days. *Pigs*: slaughter 28 days

Tetroxy LA (Reamor) *NZ*
Injection, oxytetracycline (as dihydrate complex with magnesium) 200 mg/mL, for *cattle, sheep, pigs*
Withdrawal Periods. *Cattle, sheep*: slaughter 21 days, milk 6 days. *Pigs*: slaughter 21 days

USA

Indications. Oxytetracycline-sensitive infections
Dose. Dosages vary, consult manufactuer's information

Agrimycin 200 (AgriLabs) *USA*
Injection, oxytetracycline 200mg/mL (as amphoteric), for *cattle, pigs*
Withdrawal Periods. *Cattle*: slaughter 28 days; should not be used in cattle producing milk for human consumption. *Pigs*: slaughter 42 days

Agrimycin-343 (AgriLabs) *USA*
Oral powder, for addition to drinking water, oxytetracycline hydrochloride 102.4g/135.5g powder, for *pigs, chickens, turkeys*
Withdrawal Periods. *Pigs*: slaughter 13 days. *Chickens*; should not be used in chickens producing eggs for human consumption. *Turkeys*: slaughter 5 days

Agrimycin Injection (AgriLabs) *USA*
Injection, oxytetracycline (as hydrochloride) 100mg/500mL, for *cattle*
Withdrawal Periods. Slaughter 19 days

Biocyl-50 (Anthony) *USA*
Injection, oxytetracycline 50 mg/mL, for *cattle*
Withdrawal Periods. Slaughter 19 days, should not be used in cattle producing milk for human consumption, should not be used in calves intended for veal production

Biocyl-100 (Anthony) *USA*
Injection, oxytetracycline 100 mg/mL, for *cattle*
Withdrawal Periods. Slaughter 19 days, should not be used in cattle producing milk for human consumption, should not be used in calves intended for veal production

Bio-Mycin 200 (Boehringer Ingelheim Vetmedica) *USA*
Injection, oxytetracycline 200 mg/mL, for *cattle, pigs*
Withdrawal Periods. *Cattle*: slaughter 28 days (after im or iv) and 36 days (after sc), should not be used in cattle producing milk for human consumption. *Pigs*: slaughter 42 days

Bio-Mycin C (Bio-Ceutic) *USA*
Injection, oxytetracycline (as hydrochloride) 100 mg/mL, for *cattle, pigs*
Withdrawal Periods. *Cattle*: slaughter 18 days, should not be used in cattle producing milk for human consumption. *Pigs*: slaughter 26 days

Duramycin 50 (DurVet) *USA*
Injection, oxytetracycline hydrochloride 50 mg/mL, for *cattle*

Withdrawal Periods. Slaughter 19 days, should not be used in cattle producing milk for human consumption

Duramycin 72-200 (DurVet) *USA*
Injection, oxytetracycline (as amphoteric) 200 mg/mL, for *cattle, pigs*
Withdrawal Periods. *Cattle*: slaughter 28 days, should not be used in cattle producing milk for human consumption. *Pigs*: slaughter 28 days.

Duramycin-100 (DurVet) *USA*
Injection, oxytetracycline hydrochloride 100 mg/mL, for *cattle*
Withdrawal Periods. Slaughter 19 days, should not be used in cattle producing milk for human consumption, should not be used in calves intended for veal production

Liquamycin LA-200 (Pfizer) *USA*
Injection, oxytetracycline 200 mg/mL, for *cattle, pigs*
Withdrawal Periods. Slaughter 28 days, should not be used in cattle producing milk for human consumption

Maxim-200 (Phoenix) *USA*
Injection, oxytetracycline (as amphoteric) 200 mg/mL, for *cattle, pigs*
Withdrawal Periods. Slaughter 28 days, should not be used in cattle producing milk for human consumption

Medamycin-100 (Boehringer Ingelheim Vetmedica) *USA*
Injection, oxytetracycline hydrochloride 100 mg/mL, for *cattle*
Withdrawal Periods. Slaughter 22 days, should not be used in cattle producing milk for human consumption, should not be used in calves intended for veal production

OT 200 (Vetus) *USA*
Injection, oxytetracycline (as amphoteric) 200 mg/mL, for *cattle, pigs*
Withdrawal Periods. *Cattle*: slaughter 28 days, should not be used in cattle producing milk for human consumption. *Pigs*: slaughter 28 days

OTC 50 (DurVet) *USA*
Premix, oxytetracycline 110 g/kg, for *cattle, pigs, chickens, turkeys*
Withdrawal Periods. *Chickens*: slaughter 24 hours, should not be used in chickens producing eggs for human consumption.

OXTC 50 (Pfizer) *USA*
Premix, oxytetracycline 11%, for *chickens, turkeys, pigs, cattle*
Withdrawal Periods. *Cattle*: slaughter 5 days. *Pigs*: slaughter 5 days. *Chickens, turkeys*: slaughter 3 days

OXTC 100 (Pfizer) *USA*
Premix, oxytetracycline 22%, for *chickens, turkeys, pigs, cattle*
Withdrawal Periods. *Cattle*: slaughter 5 days. *Pigs*: slaughter 5 days. *Chickens, turkeys*: slaughter 3 days

Oxybiotic-100 (Butler) *USA*
Injection, oxytetracycline (as hydrochloride) 100 mg/mL, for *cattle*
Withdrawal Periods. Slaughter 19 days, should not be used in cattle producing milk for human consumption

Oxybiotic 200 (Vedco) *USA*
Injection, oxytetracycline 200 mg/mL, for *cattle, pigs*
Withdrawal Periods. *Cattle*: slaughter 28 days, should not be used in cattle producing milk for human consumption. *Pigs*: slaughter 28 days

Oxy-Mycin (AgriPharm) *USA*
Injection, oxytetracycline (as amphoteric) 200 mg/mL, for *cattle, pigs*
Withdrawal Periods. *Cattle*: slaughter 28 days, should not be used in cattle producing milk for human consumption. *Pigs*: slaughter 28 days

Oxy-Mycin 100 (RXV) *USA*
Injection, oxytetracycline hydrochloride 100 mg/mL, for *cattle*
Withdrawal Periods. Slaughter 22 days, should not be used in cattle producing milk for human consumption, should not be used in calves intended for veal production

Oxy-Mycin 100P (AgriPharm) *USA*
Injection, oxytetracycline (as hydrochloride) 100 mg/mL, for *cattle, pigs*
Withdrawal Periods. *Cattle*: slaughter 18 days,should not be used in cattle producing milk for human consumption. *Pigs*: slaughter 26 days

Oxy-Mycin 200 (RXV) *USA*
Injection, oxytetracycline (as hydrochloride) 200 mg/mL, for *cattle, pigs*

Withdrawal Periods. Slaughter 28 days, should not be used in cattle producing milk for human consumption

Oxyshot LA (Osborn) *USA*
Injection, oxytetracycline (as amphoteric) 200 mg/mL, for *cattle, pigs*
Withdrawal Periods. *Cattle*: slaughter 28 days, should not be used in cattle producing milk for human consumption. *Pigs*: slaughter 28 days

Oxy-Tet 100 (Anchor) *USA*
Injection, oxytetracycline (as hydrochloride) 100 mg/mL, for *cattle, pigs*
Withdrawal Periods. *Cattle*: slaughter 18 days,should not be used in cattle producing milk for human consumption. *Pigs*: slaughter 26 days

Oxytet HCL Injection (Vedco) *USA*
Injection, oxytetracycline (as hydrochloride) 100 mg/mL, for *cattle*
Withdrawal Periods. Slaughter 19 days, should not be used in cattle producing milk for human consumption

Oxytet Soluble (ID Russell) *USA*
Oral powder, for addition to drinking water, oxytetracycline 102.4 g/280 gpowder, for *chickens, turkeys, pigs*
Withdrawal Periods. *Pigs*: slaughter 13 days. *Chickens, turkeys*: slaughter 5 days, should not be used in chickens or turkeys producing eggs for human consumption

Oxytetracycline-343 (DurVet) *USA*
Oral powder, for addition to drinking water, oxytetracycline 34 g/scoop, for *chickens, turkeys, pigs*
Withdrawal Periods. *Pigs*: slaughter 13 days. *Chickens, turkeys*: slaughter 5 days, should not be used in chickens or turkeys producing eggs for human consumption

Oxy-Vet 100 (Western Veterinary Supply) *USA*
Injection, oxytetracycline (as hydrochloride) 100 mg/mL, for *cattle*
Withdrawal Periods. Slaughter 22 days, should not be used in cattle producing milk for human consumption

Oxy-Vet 200 (Western Veterinary Supply) *USA*
Injection, oxytetracycline 200 mg/mL, for *cattle, pigs*
Withdrawal Periods. *Cattle*: slaughter 28 days, should not be used in cattle producing milk for human consumption. *Pigs*: slaughter 28 days

Promycin (Phoenix) *USA*
Injection, oxytetracycline (as hydrochloride) 50 mg/mL, for *cattle*
Withdrawal Periods. Slaughter 19 days, should not be used in cattle producing milk for human consumption

Promycin (Phoenix) *USA*
Injection, oxytetracycline (as hydrochloride) 100 mg/mL, for *cattle*
Withdrawal Periods. Slaughter 22 days, should not be used in cattle producing milk for human consumption, should not be used in calves intended for veal production

Status SQ (Boehringer Ingelheim Vetmedica) *USA*
Injection, oxytetracycline (as hydrochloride) 100 mg/mL, for *cattle, pigs*
Withdrawal Periods. *Cattle*: slaughter 2 days (after sc), 13 days (after iv). *Pigs*: slaughter 20 days

Terramycin TM-50D (Pfizer) *USA*
Premix, oxytetracycline 110 g/kg premix, for *cattle*
Withdrawal Periods. Slaughter 5 days

Terra-Vet 100 (Aspen) *USA*
Injection, oxytetracycline hydrochloride 100 mg/mL, for *cattle*
Withdrawal Periods. *Cattle*: slaughter 22 days, should not be used in cattle producing milk for human consumption, should not be used in calves intended for veal production.

Terramycin (Pfizer) *USA*
Premix, oxytetracycline hydrochloride (as quaternary salt) 110g and 220 g/kg , for *pigs*
Withdrawal Periods. *Pigs*: slaughter 5 days

Terramycin-343 Soluble Powder (Pfizer) *USA*
Oral powder, for addition to drinking water, oxytetracycline 754.6 g/ kg powder, for *chickens, turkeys, pigs, cattle, sheep*
Withdrawal Periods. *Cattle, pigs, sheep, turkeys*: slaughter 5 days. *Chickens, turkeys*: should not be used in chickens or turkeys producing eggs for human consumption

Terramycin Scours Tablets (Pfizer) *USA*
Tablets, oxytetracycline hydrochloride 250 mg, for *cattle*
Withdrawal Periods. Slaughter 7 days, should not be used in cattle producing milk for human consumption

Terramycin Soluble Powder (Pfizer) *USA*
Oral powder, for addition to drinking water, oxytetracycline hydrochloride 10 g/181 g pack, for *cattle, pigs, sheep, turkeys, chickens, mink, bees*
Withdrawal Periods. *Cattle*: slaughter 5 days, milk 60 hours. *Bees*: use in early spring or autumn before main honey flow begins

Terramycin TM-50 (Pfizer) *USA*
Premix, oxytetracycline hydrochloride (as quaternary salt) 110 g/kg, for *cattle, pigs, chickens, sheep, turkeys, mink*

TETRACYCLINE HYDROCHLORIDE

UK

Indications. Tetracycline-sensitive infections
Contra-indications. Side-effects. See under Chlortetracycline
Dose. *By addition to drinking water.*
Pigs: 40 mg/kg daily
Poultry: 60 mg/kg

POM **Tetsol 800** (Vericore LP) *UK*
Oral powder, for addition to drinking water, tetracycline hydrochloride 800 g/kg, for *pigs, poultry*; 125 g, 2 kg
Withdrawal Periods. *Pigs*: slaughter 5 days. *Poultry*: slaughter 2 days, egg withdrawal period nil

New Zealand

Indications. Tetracycline-sensitive infections
Dose. *Dogs, cats*: *by mouth*, 50 mg/kg daily

Panmycin Aquadrops (Pharmacia & Upjohn) *NZ*
Oral suspension, tetracycline hydrochloride 100 mg/mL, for *dogs, cats*

USA

Indications. Tetracycline-sensitive infections
Dose. Consult manufacturer's information

Duramycin 10 (DurVet) *USA*
Oral powder, to add to drinking water, tetracycline hydrochloride 55 g/kg, for *pigs, chickens, turkeys*

Duramycin-324 (DurVet) *USA*
Oral powder, to add to drinking water, tetracycline hydrochloride 713 g/ kg powder, for *pigs, calves, turkeys*
Withdrawal Periods. *Calves*: slaughter 5 days. *Pigs*: slaughter 4 days. *Chickens, turkeys*: slaughter 24 days, should not be used in chickens or turkeys producing eggs for human consumption

Panmycin 500 Bolus (Pharmacia & Upjohn) *USA*
Tablets, tetracycline hydrochloride 500 mg, for *cattle*
Withdrawal Periods. Slaughter 12 days

Panmycin Aquadrops (Pharmacia & Upjohn) *USA*
Oral solution, tetracycline hydrochloride (as base) 100 mg/mL, for *dogs, cats*

Polyotic Concentrate Soluble Powder (Fort Dodge) *USA*
Oral powder, for solution, tetracycline hydrochloride 25.6 g/packet, for *cattle, pigs*
Withdrawal Periods. *Calves*: slaughter 4 days. *Pigs*: slaughter 7 days

Polyotic Oblets (Fort Dodge) *USA*
Tablets, tetracycline hydrochloride 500 mg, for *cattle*
Withdrawal Periods. Slaughter 14 days

Solutet Soluble Powder (Vedco) *USA*
Oral powder, for addition to drinking water, tetracycline hydrochloride 55 g/kg (22 g/packet), for *pigs, cattle, chickens, turkeys*
Withdrawal Periods. *Chickens, turkeys*: slaughter 4 days, should not be used in chickens or turkeys producing eggs for human consumption

Tet-324 (Phoenix) *USA*
Oral powder, for addition to drinking water, tetracycline hydrochloride 713 g/kg powder, for *pigs, cattle, chickens, turkeys*
Withdrawal Periods. *Cattle*: slaughter 5 days. *Pigs*: slaughter 4 days. *Chickens, turkeys*: should not be used in chickens and turkeys producing eggs for human consumption

Tet-Sol 10 (Wade Jones) *USA*
Oral powder, for addition to drinking water, tetracycline hydrochloride 55 g/kg powder, for *pigs, cattle, chickens, turkeys*
Withdrawal Periods. *Calves*: slaughter 5 days. *Pigs, chickens, turkeys*: slaughter 4 days, should not be used in chickens or turkeys producing eggs for human consumption

Tet-Sol 324 (Wade Jones) *USA*
Oral powder, for addition to drinking water, tetracycline hydrochloride 712.8 g/kg powder, for *pigs, cattle, chickens, turkeys*
Withdrawal Periods. *Calves*: slaughter 5 days. *Pigs, chickens, turkeys*: slaughter 4 days, should not be used in chickens and turkeys producing eggs for human consumption.

Tetracycline Hydrochloride Capsules (Global) *USA*
Capsules, tetracycline hydrochloride 50 mg, 100 mg, 250 mg and 500 mg, for *dogs*

Tetracycline Hydrochloride Soluble Powder (Butler) *USA*
Oral powder, for addition to drinking water, tetracycline hydrochloride 55g/ kg powder, for *cattle, pigs, chickens, turkeys*
Withdrawal Periods. *Pigs, chickens, turkeys*: slaughter 4 days, should not be used in chickens or turkeys producing eggs for human consumption. *Calves*: slaughter 5 days.

Tetracycline Hydrochloride Soluble Powder-324 (Butler) *USA*
Oral powder, for addition to drinking water, tetracycline hydrochloride 712.8 g/kg powder, for *cattle, pigs, chickens, turkeys*
Withdrawal Periods. *Pigs, chickens, turkeys*: slaughter 4 days, should not be used in chickens or turkeys producing eggs for human consumption. *Calves*: slaughter 5 days

Tetracycline Hydrochloride Soluble Powder 324 (Boehringer Ingelheim Vetmedica) *USA*
Oral powder, for addition to drinking water, tetracycline hydrochloride 21.45 g/30 g powder, for *cattle, pigs, chickens, turkeys*
Withdrawal Periods. *Pigs, chickens, turkeys*: slaughter 4 days, should not be used in chickens or turkeys producing eggs for human consumption. *Calves*: slaughter 5 days, should not be used in calves intended for veal production.

Tetracycline HCL Soluble Powder-324 (Vedco) *USA*
Oral powder, for addition to drinking water, tetracycline hydrochloride 712.8 g/kg powder, for *cattle, pigs, chickens, turkeys*
Withdrawal Periods. *Pigs, chickens, turkeys*: slaughter 4 days, should not be used in chickens or turkeys producing eggs for human consumption. *Calves*: slaughter 5 days

Tetracycline Soluble Powder (AgriPharm) *USA*
Oral powder, for addition to drinking water, tetracycline hydrochloride 712.8 g/kg powder, for *cattle, pigs, chickens, turkeys*
Withdrawal Periods. *Pigs, chickens, turkeys*: slaughter 4 days, should not be used in chickens or turkeys producing eggs for human consumption. *Calves*: slaughter 5 days

Tetracycline Soluble Powder 324 (RXV, Western Veterinary Supplies) *USA*
Oral powder, for addition to drinking water, tetracycline hydrochloride 712.45 g/kg powder, for *cattle, pigs, chickens, turkeys*

Withdrawal Periods. *Pigs, chickens, turkeys*: slaughter 4 days, should not be used in chickens or turkeys producing eggs for human consumption. *Calves*: slaughter 5 days

Tetrasol Soluble Powder (Med-Pharmex) *USA*
Oral powder, for addition to drinking water, tetracycline hydrochloride 712.45 g/kg powder, for *cattle, pigs, chickens, turkeys*
Withdrawal Periods. *Pigs, calves, turkeys*: slaughter 4 days, should not be used in chickens or turkeys producing eggs for human consumption. *Calves*: slaughter 5 days, should not be used in calves intended for veal production

Polyotic Soluble powder (Fort Dodge) *USA*
Oral powder, for addition to drinking water, tetracycline 10 g/packet, for *cattle, pigs*
Withdrawal Periods. *Calves*: slaughter 4 days. *Pigs*: slaughter 7 days

Solu-Tet 324 (Wade Jones) *USA*
Oral powder, for addition to drinking water, tetracycline hydrochloride 712.8 g/kg powder, for *chickens*
Withdrawal Periods. *Chickens*: slaughter 4 days, should not be used in chickens producing eggs for human consumption)

1.1.3 Aminoglycosides

This group includes **streptomycin, dihydrostreptomycin, neomycin, framycetin, gentamicin, paromomycin, amikacin, kanamycin, tobramycin,** and **apramycin**. All are bactericidal and active against Gram-negative organisms and some Gram-positive organisms, but not streptococci. Amikacin, gentamicin, and tobramycin are active against *Pseudomonas aeruginosa*. Aminoglycosides are taken up into bacteria by an oxygen-dependent process and are therefore inactive against anaerobic bacteria. They are more active in alkaline media, which is of particular importance when treating urinary infections. Aminoglycosides show synergism with beta-lactam antibacterials.

Bacteria may rapidly acquire resistance to these antibiotics. Enteric bacteria may gain the ability to produce a range of aminoglycoside-inactivating enzymes particularly if a sub-therapeutic dose is given. The different members of the group vary in their susceptibility to these inactivating enzymes.

The aminoglycosides are not absorbed from the gastro-intestinal tract following oral administration; therefore this route is used for the treatment of gastro-intestinal infections and hepatic encephalopathy. The treatment of systemic infections, including invasive enteric organisms, requires that the drug is administered by injection. Aminoglycosides are poorly distributed into body compartments such as the brain, cerebrospinal fluid, and the eye. Elimination is solely by renal excretion.

The important side-effects of aminoglycosides are vestibular or auditory ototoxicity, and nephrotoxicity. Risk of toxicity following systemic administration varies with different members of the group. Neomycin is particularly toxic to the auditory and renal systems. Streptomycin and dihydrostreptomycin are ototoxic and gentamicin is ototoxic and nephrotoxic. Due to their potential nephrotoxic effect, they should be used with care and for short periods of time. The toxic effects on the kidney vary with the individual drugs but dosing regimens that have short interdosing intervals are more likely to cause damage to the kidneys than dosing regimens where long interdosing intervals are used. As these drugs kill by a concentration-dependent mechanism, giving the daily dose once rather than dividing and giving it every 8 hours is also more likely to be successful since higher peak concentrations of the drug will be achieved by the former method. If there is renal impairment, an alternative drug should be chosen. If this is not possible, the inter-dosing interval should be increased on the basis of the animal's plasma-creatinine concentration (see Prescribing in renal impairment) and the plasma levels of the drug should be monitored. The trough drug concentration should be measured just before the next dose is given to ensure that, in the case of gentamicin, it has fallen below 1 microgram/mL to avoid toxicity.

Simultaneous administration with other potentially ototoxic drugs such as loop diuretics should be avoided (see Drug Interactions – Appendix 1). Aminoglycosides may impair neuromuscular transmission and so are not given to animals with myasthenia gravis. These drugs are well absorbed from the peritoneal cavity and instillation during surgery may result in drug overdose and transient respiratory paralysis.

AMIKACIN

UK
Indications. Amikacin-sensitive infections
Dose. See Prescribing for reptiles

POM Ⓗ **Amikacin** (Non-proprietary)
Injection, amikacin (as sulphate) 250 mg/mL; 2 mL

POM Ⓗ **Amikin** (Bristol-Myers)
Injection, amikacin (as sulphate) 50 mg/mL, 250 mg/mL; 2 mL

USA
Indications. Amikacin-sensitive infections
Dose. *Dogs: by subcutaneous or intramuscular injection,* 10 mg/kg

Amiglyde-V (Fort Dodge) *USA*
Injection, amikacin sulphate 50 mg/mL, for *dogs*

Amiject D (Vetus) *USA*
Injection, amikacin sulphate 50 mg/mL, for *dogs*

Amikacin C Injection (Phoenix) *USA*
Injection, amikacin (as sulphate) 50 mg/mL, for *dogs*

Amikacin Sulfate Injection (VetTek) *USA*
Injection, amikacin (as sulphate) 50 mg/mL, for *dogs*

APRAMYCIN

UK
Indications. Apramycin-sensitive infections
Contra-indications. Cats, myasthenia gravis, see notes above
Side-effects. Ototoxicity, nephrotoxicity, see notes above
Warnings. Caution in renal impairment; Drugs Interactions – see Appendix 1 (aminoglycosides); aminoglycosides may cause hypersensitivity reactions in operators following injection, inhalation, ingestion, or skin contact

Dose. *Calves*: by addition to drinking water, milk, or milk replacer, 20–40 mg/kg daily
by intramuscular injection, 20 mg/kg daily
Lambs: by mouth, 10 mg/kg daily
Pigs: by addition to drinking water, 7.5–12.5 mg/kg daily or 5 g/100 litres drinking water
by addition to feed, 100 g/tonne feed
piglets: by mouth, 10–20 mg/kg daily
Poultry: by addition to drinking water, 25–50 g/100 litres

POM **Apralan 200 Injection** (Elanco) *UK*
Injection, apramycin (as sulphate) 200 mg/mL, for *calves up to 6 months of age*; 100 mL
Withdrawal Periods. *Calves*: slaughter 6 months

POM **Apralan Bolus** (Elanco) *UK*
Tablets, f/c, apramycin (as sulphate) 800 micrograms, for *calves less than 120 kg body-weight*; 20
Withdrawal Periods. *Calves*: slaughter 28 days
Dose. Calves: (<40 kg body-weight) 1 tablet daily, (40–80 kg body-weight) 2 tablets daily, (80–120 kg body-weight) 3 tablets daily

MFS **Apralan G200** (Elanco) *UK*
Premix, apramycin (as sulphate) 200 g/kg, for *pigs*; 5 kg
Withdrawal Periods. *Pigs*: slaughter 14 days

POM **Apralan Oral Doser** (Elanco) *UK*
Mixture, apramycin (as sulphate) 20 mg/unit dose, for *lambs, piglets*; 150-mL dose applicator (1 unit dose = 1.1 mL)
Withdrawal Periods. *Lambs*: slaughter 35 days. *Piglets*: slaughter 28 days
Dose. *Piglets*: 1–2 unit doses daily
Lambs: 1 unit dose/2 kg body-weight

POM **Apralan Soluble Powder** (Elanco) *UK*
Oral powder, for addition to drinking water, milk, or milk replacer, apramycin (as sulphate) 1 g, 50 g, 1 kg, for *calves, pigs, poultry* (measure provided = apramycin 5 g with 50-g bottle, apramycin 25 g with 1-kg bag)
Withdrawal Periods. *Calves*: slaughter 28 days. *Pigs*: slaughter 14 days. *Poultry*: slaughter 7 days, should not be used in birds producing eggs for human consumption

Australia
Indications. Apramycin-sensitive infections
Dose. Consult manufacturer's information

Apralan 100 Premix (Elanco) *Austral.*
Premix, apramycin 100g/kg premix, for *pigs*
Withdrawal Periods. Slaughter 28 days

Apralan Soluble (Elanco) *Austral.*
Powder, for addition to drinking water, apramycin sulphate 50 g, for *cattle, pigs, poultry*
Withdrawal Periods. Slaughter 14 days

Eire
Indications. Apramycin-sensitive infections
Dose.
Calves: by addition to drinking water, milk, or milk replacer, 20–40 mg/kg daily
by intramuscular injection, 20 mg/kg daily
Lambs: by mouth, 10 mg/kg daily
Pigs: by addition to drinking water, 7.5–12.5 mg/kg daily
by addition to feed, 100 g/tonne feed
piglets: by mouth, 10–20 mg/kg daily

Apralan 200 mg Injection (Elanco) *Eire*
Injection, apramycin (as sulphate) 200 mg/mL, for *calves*
Withdrawal Periods. Slaughter 35 days

Apralan G 100 Premix (Elanco) *Eire*
Premix, apramycin (as sulphate) 100 g/kg, for *pigs*
Withdrawal Periods. Slaughter 14 days

Apralan Oral Doser (Elanco) *Eire*
Liquid, apramycin (as sulphate) 20 mg/1.1 mL, for *lambs, piglets*
Withdrawal Periods. *Lambs*: slaughter 35 days. *Piglets*: slaughter 28 days

Apralan Soluble Powder (Elanco) *Eire*
Oral powder, for addition to drinking water or milk, apramycin (as sulphate) 50 g/150 cm3, for *calves, pigs, poultry*
Withdrawal Periods. *Calves*: slaughter 28 days. *Pigs*: slaughter 14 days. *Poultry*: slaughter 7 days

New Zealand
Indications. Apramycin-sensitive infections
Dose. Consult manufacturer's information

Apralan 100 (Elanco) *NZ*
Premix, apramycin (as sulphate) 100 g/kg, for *pigs*
Withdrawal Periods. Slaughter 21 days

Apralan Soluble (Elanco) *NZ*
Oral powder, apramycin 50 g/container, for *pigs, poultry*
Withdrawal Periods. *Pigs*: slaughter 28 days. *Poultry*: slaughter withdrawal period nil

USA
Indications. Apramycin-sensitive infections
Dose. Consult manufacturer's information

Apralan 75 (Elanco) *USA*
Premix, apramycin (as sulphate) 165 g/ kg , for *pigs*
Withdrawal Periods. Slaughter 28 days

Apralan Soluble Powder (Elanco) *USA*
Oral powder, for addition to drinking water, apramycin (as sulphate) 48 g, for *pigs*
Withdrawal Periods. Slaughter 28 days

DIHYDROSTREPTOMYCIN

Australia
Indications. Dihydrostreptomycin-sensitive infections
Dose. Consult manufacturer's information

Vibrostrep (Jurox) *Austral.*
Injection, dihyrostreptomycin (as sulphate) 500 mg/mL, for *cattle*
Withdrawal Periods. Slaughter 30 days, milk 1 day (single treatment); 3 days (multiple dose)

FRAMYCETIN SULPHATE

UK
Indications. Framycetin-sensitive infections, in particular acute bovine mastitis with systemic involvement
Contra-indications. Side-effects. Warnings. See under Apramycin; concomitant use of calcium borogluconate at parturition advised because aminoglycosides may cause hypocalcaemia; hypersensitivity to framycetin; concurrent cephalosporins
Dose. *Dairy cattle*: by intramuscular injection, 5 mg/kg twice daily for up to 3 days

POM **Framomycin Injection 15%** (Vericore VP) *UK*
Injection, framycetin sulphate 150 mg/mL, for *dairy cattle*; 100 mL
Withdrawal Periods. *Cattle*: slaughter 49 days, milk 56 hours

Eire
Indications. Apramycin-sensitive infections
Dose. *Cattle*: *by intramuscular injection*, 5 mg/kg
calves: *by mouth*, 10 mg/kg
Pigs: *by mouth*, 10 mg/kg

Framomycin Injection 15% (Cypharm) *Eire*
Injection, framycetin sulphate 150 mg/mL, for *cattle*
Withdrawal Periods. Slaughter 49 days, milk 56 hours

Framomycin Sachets (Cypharm) *Eire*
Oral powder, to mix with water, framycetin sulphate 250 mg/g, for *calves*
Withdrawal Periods. Slaughter 7 days

Framomycin Soluble Powder (Cypharm) *Eire*
Oral powder, to mix with water, framycetin sulphate 250 mg/g, for *pigs*
Withdrawal Periods. Slaughter 14 days

GENTAMICIN

UK
Indications. Gentamicin-sensitive infections
Contra-indications. Pregnant animals, concurrent use of other drugs that may induce ototoxicity
Warnings. Care in renal impairment
Dose. *Horses*: *by intravenous injection*, 6.6 mg/kg once daily
Dogs, cats: *by subcutaneous or intramuscular injection*, 5 mg/kg twice daily for 24 hours then once daily

POM Pangram 5% (Bimeda)
Injection, gentamicin 50 mg/mL, for *dogs, cats*

Australia
Indications. Gentamicin-sensitive infections
Dose.
Horses♦: *by intramuscular or intravenous injection*, 1.5 mg/kg
Dogs, cats: *by subcutaneous, intramuscular, or intravenous*, 4.4 mg/kg

Gentam (Ilium) *Austral.*
Injection, gentamicin (as sulphate) 50 mg/mL, for *horses, dogs, cats*
Withdrawal Periods. Should not be used in *horses* intended for human consumption

Gentamicin (Parnell) *Austral.*
Injection, gentamicin (as sulphate) 50 mg/mL, for *horses, dogs, cats*
Withdrawal Periods. Should not be used in *horses* intended for human consumption.

Gentamicin 50 (RWR) *Austral.*
Injection, gentamicin (as sulphate) 50 mg/mL, for *horses, dogs, cats*
Withdrawal Periods. *Horses*: slaughter 28 days

Gentapex-50 (Apex) *Austral.*
Injection, gentamicin (as sulphate) 50 mg/mL, for *dogs, cats*

New Zealand
Indications. Gentamicin-sensitive infections
Dose. Dosages vary, consult manufacturer's information. For guidance:
Horses: *by intramuscular or intravenous injection*, 1.5 mg/kg
Dogs, cats: *by subcutaneous, intramuscular, or intravenous*, 5 mg/kg

Genta 50 (Phoenix) *NZ*
Injection, gentamicin 50 mg/mL, for *horses, dogs, cats*
Withdrawal Periods. *Horses*: slaughter 28 days

Gentamicin 50 (Vetpharm) *NZ*
Injection, gentamicin (as sulphate) 50 mg/mL, for *horses, dogs, cats*

Gentamicin Injection (Parnell) *NZ*
Injection, gentamicin (as sulphate) 50 mg/mL, for *horses, dogs, cats*
Withdrawal Periods. *Horses*: slaughter 28 days

Gentavet (Bomac) *NZ*
Injection, gentamicin (as sulphate) 50 mg/mL, for *horses, dogs, cats*
Withdrawal Periods. *Horses*: slaughter 28 days

USA
Indications. Gentamicin-sensitive infections
Dose. Dosages vary, consult manufacturer's information. For guidance:
Pigs: *by mouth or by intramuscular injection*, 5 mg
by addition to drinking water, 1.1–2.2 mg/kg body-weight
Dogs, cats: by intramuscular or intravenous injection, 4.4 mg/kg

Garacin (DurVet) *USA*
Injection, gentamicin (as sulphate) 5 mg/mL, for *pigs*
Withdrawal Periods. Slaughter 40 days

Garacin (Schering-Plough) *USA*
Oral solution, for addition to drinking water , gentamicin (as sulphate) 50 mg/mL , for *pigs*
Withdrawal Periods. Slaughter 3 days

Garacin (DurVet) *USA*
Oral solution , gentamicin (as sulphate) 4.35 mg/mL, for *pigs*
Withdrawal Periods. Slaughter 14 days

Garacin (Schering-Plough) *USA*
Oral solution, gentamicin (as sulphate) 4.35 mg/mL, for *pigs*
Withdrawal Periods. Slaughter 14 days

Garacin (Schering-Plough) *USA*
Injection, gentamicin (as sulphate) 5 mg/mL, for *pigs*
Withdrawal Periods. Slaughter 40 days

Garacin (Schering-Plough) *USA*
Oral powder, to add to drinking water, gentamicin 66.7 mg/g powder, for *pigs*
Withdrawal Periods. Slaughter 10 days

Garacin (Schering-Plough) *USA*
Oral powder, to add to drinking water, gentamicin 333.33 mg/g powder, for *pigs*
Withdrawal Periods. Slaughter 10 days

Garasol (Schering-Plough) *USA*
Injection, gentamicin (as sulphate) 50 mg/mL , for *chickens, turkeys*
Withdrawal Periods. *Chickens*: slaughter 5 weeks. *Turkeys*: slaughter 9 weeks.

Garasol (Schering-Plough) *USA*
Injection, gentamicin (as sulphate) 100 mg/mL, for *chickens, turkeys*
Withdrawal Periods. Chickens: slaughter 5 weeks. Turkeys: slaughter 9 weeks.

Gen-Gard (AgriLabs) *USA*
Oral powder, to add to drinking water, gentamicin (as sulphate) 333.33 mg/g powder, for *pigs*
Withdrawal Periods. Slaughter 10 days

Gentaject (Vetus) *USA*
Injection, gentamicin (as sulphate) 50 mg/mL , for *dogs*

Gentamicin Sulfate Injection (Boehringer Ingelheim Vetmedica) *USA*
Injection, gentamicin (as sulphate) 50 mg/mL , for *dogs*

Gentaved 50 (Vedco) *USA*
Injection, gentamicin (as sulphate) 50 mg/mL , for *dogs*

Gentocin (Schering-Plough) *USA*
Injection/Intra-uterine solution, gentamicin (as sulphate) 50 mg/mL , for *horses, dogs, cats*
Withdrawal Periods. Should not be used in *horses* intended for human consumption.

KANAMYCIN

UK

Indications. Kanamycin-sensitive infections
Dose. See Prescribing for reptiles

POM Ⓗ **Kannasyn** (Sanofi-Synthelabo) *UK*
Injection, powder for reconstitution, kanamycin (as acid sulphate) 1 g

USA

Indications. Kanamycin-sensitive infections
Dose. *Dogs, cats*: by intramuscular or intravenous injection, 11 mg/kg

Kantrim (Fort Dodge) *USA*
Injection, kanamycin sulphate 200 mg/mL, for *dogs, cats*

NEOMYCIN SULPHATE

UK

Indications. Neomycin-sensitive   infections;   hepatic encephalopathy♦ (see section 3.10)
Contra-indications. Side-effects. Warnings. See   under Apramycin; caution in animals with urinary obstruction; do not use in foals manifesting signs of toxaemia
Dose.
Horses: hepatic encephalopathy♦, see section 3.6.3
foals: bacterial infections, see preparation details
Calves, lambs: see preparation details
Pigs: see also preparation details
by addition to drinking water, 12.5 g/100 litres
by addition to feed, 230 g/tonne feed
Dogs, cats: bacterial infections, 11 mg/kg daily in divided doses
Hepatic encephalopathy♦, see section 3.6.3
Poultry: 11 mg/kg
by addition to feed, 230 g/tonne feed

POM **Neobiotic Pump** (Pharmacia & Upjohn) *UK*
Oral solution, neomycin sulphate 60 mg/unit dose, for *foals, lambs, pigs*; 120-mL dose applicator (1 unit dose = 1.2 mL)
Withdrawal Periods. Should not be used in *foals* intended for human consumption. *Lambs*: slaughter 8 days. *Pigs*: slaughter 14 days
Dose. *Foals, lambs, piglets*: 1 unit dose/5.5 kg body-weight

POM **Neobiotic Soluble Powder 70%** (Pharmacia & Upjohn) *UK*
Oral powder, for addition to drinking water or feed, neomycin sulphate 700 mg/g, for *pigs, broiler chickens*; 500 g
Withdrawal Periods. *Pigs*: slaughter 14 days. *Chickens*: slaughter withdrawal period nil

POM **Neomycin Premix** (Pharmacia & Upjohn) *UK*
Premix, neomycin sulphate 100%, for *pigs, broiler chickens*; 466 g, 699 g
Withdrawal Periods. *Pigs*: slaughter 14 days. *Chickens*: slaughter withdrawal period nil

POM Ⓗ **Nivemycin** (Sovereign) *UK*
Tablets, neomycin sulphate 500 mg

POM **Orojet N** (Fort Dodge) *UK*
Oral liquid, neomycin sulphate 70 mg/unit dose, for *lambs, piglets*; 210-mL dose applicator (1 unit dose = 1 mL)
Withdrawal Periods. Slaughter 6 days
Dose. *Lambs, piglets*: 1 unit dose/5 kg body-weight

Australia

Indications. Neomycin-sensitive infections
Dose. *Horses, cattle, sheep, pigs*: by intramuscular or intravenous injection, 2–4 mg/kg
Dogs, cats: by intramuscular or intravenous injection,10 mg/kg

Neoject '200' Injection (Delvet) *Austral.*
Injection, neomycin sulphate 200 mg/mL, for *cattle, horses, sheep, pigs*
Withdrawal Periods. *Cattle*: slaughter 30 days, milk 36 hours (single dose) , 72 hours (multiple dose). *Sheep*: slaughter 30 days. *Pigs*: slaughter 7 days

Neomycin Sulfate Sterile Injection (Jurox) *Austral.*
Injection, neomycin sulphate 200 mg/mL, for *cattle, sheep, pigs, horses, dogs, cats*
Withdrawal Periods. *Horses*: slaughter 28 days.*Cattle*: slaughter 10 days, milk 36 hours (single dose), 72 hours (multiple dose). *Sheep*: slaughter 10 days. *Pigs*: slaughter 15 days

Neomycin Water Soluble Powder (CCD) *Austral.*
Powder, for addition to drinking water, neomycin sulphate 600 mg/g powder, for *poultry*
Withdrawal Periods. Slaughter 5 days

Eire

Indications. Neomycin-sensitive infections
Dose. Dosages vary, consult manufacturer's information

CNF Scour-diet (Chanelle) *Eire*
Oral powder, to mix with water, neomycin sulphate 40mg/g, for *calves*
Withdrawal Periods. Slaughter 30 days

Edomycin Soluble Powder (Norbrook) *Eire*
Oral powder, for addition to drinking water, neomycin sulphate 35,000 units/g, for *calves*
Withdrawal Periods. Slaughter 28 days

Hyspan (Rice Steele) *Eire*
Oral powder, neomycin sulphate 400 mg/sachet, for *calves*
Withdrawal Periods. Slaughter 28 days

Neobiotic Soluble Powder 70% (Pharmacia & Upjohn) *Eire*
Oral powder, for addition to drinking water, neomycin sulphate 700 mg/g, for *pigs, chickens*
Withdrawal Periods. Pigs: slaughter 14 days. Chickens: slaughter withdrawal period nil

New Zealand

Indications. Neomycin-sensitive infections
Dose. *Cattle, pigs, poultry*: by addition to drinking water or feed, 11 mg/kg

Neomix Concentrate (Pharmacia & Upjohn) *NZ*
Oral powder, neomycin sulphate 700 mg/g, for *cattle,pigs, poultry*
Withdrawal Periods. *Cattle*: slaughter 30 days. *Pigs*: slaughter 20 days. *Poultry, turkeys*: slaughter 14 days, broilers slaughter 5 days, should not be used in birds within 14 days of commencement of laying

USA

Indications. Neomycin-sensitive infections
Dose. *Cattle, sheep, sheep, goats, pigs*: by mouth, 22 mg/ kg

Biosol Liquid (Pharmacia & Upjohn) *USA*
Oral solution, neomycin sulphate 200 mg/mL, for *cattle, sheep, pigs, goats*
Withdrawal Periods. *Cattle, goats*: slaughter 30 days, should not be used in calves intended for veal production. *Pigs, sheep*: slaughter 20 days

Neomix 325 (Pharmacia & Upjohn) *USA*
Oral powder, for addition to drinking water, neomycin sulphate 71.5 g/100 g powder, for *cattle, sheep, goats, pigs*
Withdrawal Periods. *Cattle*: slaughter 1 day, should not be used in calves intended for veal production. *Sheep*: slaughter 2 days. *Pigs, goats*: slaughter 3 days

Neomix AG 325 (Pharmacia & Upjohn) *USA*
Oral powder, for addition to drinking water, neomycin sulphate 715 g/kg powder, for *cattle, sheep, goats, pigs*
Withdrawal Periods. *Cattle*: slaughter 1 day, should not be used in calves intended for veal production. *Sheep*: slaughter 2 days. *Pigs, goats*: slaughter 3 days

Neo-Sol 50 (Wade Jones) *USA*
Oral powder, for addition to drinking water, neomycin sulphate 71.5 g/100 g powder, for *cattle, sheep, goats, pigs*
Withdrawal Periods. *Cattle*: slaughter 1 day, should not be used in calves intended for veal production. *Sheep*: slaughter 2 days. *Pigs, goats*: slaughter 3 days

Neomycin 200 (Aspen) *USA*
Oral solution, neomycin sulphate 200 mg/mL, for *cattle, sheep, goats, pigs*
Withdrawal Periods. *Cattle, goats*: slaughter 30 days, should not be used in calves intended for veal production. *Pigs, sheep*: 20 days

Neomycin 325 (AgriLabs) *USA*
Oral powder, for addition to drinking water, neomycin sulphate 71.5 g/100g powder, for *cattle, sheep, goats, pigs*
Withdrawal Periods. *Cattle, goats*: slaughter 30 days, should not be used in calves intended for veal production. *Pigs, sheep*: 20 days

Neomycin 325 Soluble Powder (DurVet, Osborn) *USA*
Oral powder, for addition to drinking water, neomycin sulphate 71.5 g/100 g powder, for *cattle, sheep, goats, pigs*
Withdrawal Periods. *Cattle*: slaughter 1 day, should not be used in calves intended for veal production. *Sheep*: slaughter 2 days. *Pigs, goats*: slaughter 3 days

Neomycin Oral Solution (AgriLabs, DurVet, Phoenix) *USA*
Oral solution, neomycin sulphate 200 mg/mL, for *cattle, sheep, goats, pigs*
Withdrawal Periods. *Cattle, goats*: slaughter 30 days, should not be used in calves intended for veal production. *Pigs, sheep*: 20 days

Neosol Soluble Powder (Med-Pharmex) *USA*
Oral powder, for addition to drinking water, neomycin (as sulphate) 500g/kg, for *cattle, sheep, goats, pigs*
Withdrawal Periods. *Cattle, goats*: slaughter 30 days, should not be used in calves intended for veal production. *Pigs, sheep*: 20 days

Neovet Neomycin Oral Solution (RXV) *USA*
Oral solution, neomycin sulphate 200 mg/mL, for *cattle, pigs, sheep, goats*
Withdrawal Periods. *Cattle, goats*: slaughter 30 days, should not be used in calves intended for veal production. *Pigs, sheep*: 20 days

PAROMOMYCIN

Indications. Paromomycin-sensitive infections
Dose. See Prescribing for amphibians

Preparations containing paromomycin are not generally available in the UK. Preparations may be obtained on a named-patient basis from IDIS

STREPTOMYCIN SULPHATE

UK
Indications. Streptomycin-sensitive infections

Contra-indications. Side-effects. Warnings. See under Apramycin
Dose. *By intramuscular injection.*
Horses, cattle, sheep, goats: 10 mg/kg daily
Dogs, cats: 25 mg/kg daily

POM **Devomycin** (Norbrook) *UK*
Injection, streptomycin sulphate 250 mg/mL, for *horses, cattle, sheep, goats, dogs, cats*; 100 mL
Withdrawal Periods. Should not be used in *horses* intended for human consumption. *Cattle*: slaughter 14 days, milk 2 days. *Sheep, goats*: slaughter 14 days, should not be used in sheep, goats producing milk for human consumption

Eire
Indications. Streptomycin-sensitive infections
Dose. *By intramuscular injection.*
Cattle, sheep, goats: 12 mg/kg daily

Devomycin Injection (Norbrook) *Eire*
Injection, streptomycin (as sulphate) 250 mg/mL, for *cattle, sheep, pigs*
Withdrawal Periods. *Cattle, sheep, pigs*: slaughter 14 days. *Cattle*: milk 48 hours. Should not be used in sheep producing milk for human consumption

Dulphar Streptomycin (Interchem) *Eire*
Injection, streptomycin (as sulphate) 250 mg/mL, for *cattle, sheep, pigs*
Withdrawal Periods. Cattle: slaughter 14 days, milk 48 hours. Sheep: slaughter 14 days, should not be used in sheep producing milk for human consumption. Pigs: slaughter 14 days

Streptomycin Injection (Interpharm) *Eire*
Injection, streptomycin (as sulphate) 250 mg/mL, for *cattle, sheep, pigs*
Withdrawal Periods. *Cattle*: slaughter 14 days, milk 48 hours. *Sheep*: slaughter 14 days, should not be used in sheep producing milk for human consumption. *Pigs*: slaughter 14 days

DIHYDROSTREPTOMYCIN and STREPTOMYCIN

The antibacterial activity of these drugs is similar, but they differ in their toxic effects, dihydrostreptomycin being more likely to cause auditory damage while streptomycin is more likely to produce vestibular damage. Hence, it is claimed that a mixture of the two may have the same activity as, but may be less toxic than, either alone. See under apramycin for contra-indications, side-effects, warnings.

UK
POM **Devomycin-D** (Norbrook) *UK*
Injection, dihydrostreptomycin sulphate 150 mg, streptomycin sulphate 150 mg/mL, for *horses, cattle, sheep, goats, dogs, cats*; 100 mL
Withdrawal Periods. Should not be used in *horses* intended for human consumption. *Cattle*: slaughter 21 days, milk 2 days. *Sheep, goats*: slaughter 21 days, should not be used in sheep, goats producing milk for human consumption
Dose. *By intramuscular injection.*
Horses, cattle, sheep, goats: 0.03 mL/kg daily (1 mL/30 kg body-weight)
Dogs, cats: 0.08 mL/kg daily (1 mL/12 kg body-weight)

Eire
Devomycin D Injection (Norbrook) *Eire*
Injection, streptomycin (as sulphate) 150 mg/mL, dihyrdrostreptomycin (as sulphate) 150 mg/mL, for *cattle, sheep, pigs*
Withdrawal Periods. Cattle, sheep, pigs: slaughter 21 days. Cattle: milk 48 hours. Should not be used in sheep producing milk for human consumption

New Zealand

Bomastrep (Bomac) *NZ*
Injection, dihydrostreptomycin sulphate 150 mg/mL, streptomycin sulphate 150 mg/mL, for *cattle, sheep, pigs*
Withdrawal Periods. *Cattle*: slaughter 30 days, milk 72 hours. *Sheep*: slaughter 30 days, should not be used in sheep producing milk for human consumption. *Pigs*: slaughter 30 days

Strepolin (Schering-Plough) *NZ*
Injection, dihydrostreptomycin (as sulphate) 500 mg/mL, streptomycin (as sulphate) 500 mg/mL, for *horses, cattle, sheep, pigs, dogs, cats, poultry*
Withdrawal Periods. *Horses, pigs, poultry*: slaughter 30 days. *Cattle, sheep*: slaughter 30 days, milk 72 hours

Strepto 50 (Ethical) *NZ*
Injection, dihydrostreptomycin (as sulphate) 250 mg/mL, streptomycin (as sulphate) 250 mg/mL, for *cattle*
Withdrawal Periods. Slaughter 30 days, milk 72 hours

Streptovet 500 (Phoenix) *NZ*
Injection, dihydrostreptomycin (as sulphate) 250 mg/mL, streptomycin (as sulphate) 250 mg/mL, for *cattle, sheep, pigs*
Withdrawal Periods. *Cattle, sheep*: slaughter 30 days, milk 72 hours. *Pigs*: slaughter 30 days

Vibrostrep (Stockguard) *NZ*
Injection, dihydrostreptomycin (as sulphate) 250 mg/mL, streptomycin (as sulphate) 250 mg/mL, for *cattle, sheep, pigs*
Withdrawal Periods. *Cattle, sheep*: slaughter 30 days, milk 72 hours. *Pigs*: slaughter 30 days

TOBRAMYCIN

UK

Indications. Tobramycin-sensitive infections
Dose. See Prescribing for reptiles and Prescribing for exotic birds

POM Ⓗ **Tobramycin** (Non-proprietary) *UK*
Injection, tobramycin (as sulphate) 40 mg/mL; 1 mL, 2 mL

POM Ⓗ **Nebcin** (Lilly) *UK*
Injection, tobramycin (as sulphate) 10 mg/mL, 40 mg/mL

1.1.4 Macrolides and lincosamides

The macrolides include erythromycin, josamycin, spiramycin, tilmicosin, and tylosin, while clindamycin, pirlimycin and lincomycin belong to the related lincosamide group. They are usually bacteriostatic in action. All are basic compounds that are well absorbed following oral administration and inactivated by hepatic metabolism. Due to their basic nature they are concentrated by the 'ion-trap' in acidic fluids such as milk and prostatic fluid. Ion trapping also occurs within cells and macrolides, in particular, will attain high concentrations inside cells, including macrophages which may target the drug to sites of infection. They can be effective against intracellular pathogens (for example *Mycobacteria* spp.).

Tylosin has good activity against *Mycoplasma* spp. and *Serpulina hyodysenteriae (Treponema hyodysenteriae)* and a number of Gram-positive aerobes, but little activity against Gram-negative organisms or anaerobes.

Erythromycin is active against streptococci, *Staph. aureus* including penicillin-resistant strains, the more fastidious Gram-negative bacteria, and anaerobes. It is likely to be the drug of choice for *Campylobacter* and also *Rhodococcus*

equi in foals. Erythromycin has less activity than tylosin against *Mycoplasma* spp. or *Serpulina hyodysenteriae*. Vomiting is a common side-effect of erythromycin due to a gastric irritant effect. Fatal enterocolitis has been reported in horses following ingestion of erythromycin. In addition, this drug also inhibits the metabolism of other drugs by the liver and, in humans, has given rise to serious drug interactions. These interactions have not been studied in veterinary species but care should be taken when administering erythromycin with theophylline, cyclosporin, oral anticoagulants, methylprednisolone, and antihistamines such as terfenidine.

Azithromycin and **clarithromycin** are structural analogues of erythromycin produced for human medicine. They have longer half lives and less frequent dosing is required. In addition, the gastro-intestinal side-effects are less of a problem in humans and azithromycin does not inactivate the cytochrome P450 enzymes inhibited by erythromycin so the potential for serious drug interactions is much less. In addition, both azithromycin and clarithromycin have greater activity than erythromycin against *Mycobacterium avium* complex (and can be used in treating atypical mycobacterial infections) and against *Toxoplasma gondii*. Azithromycin is also highly active against *Chlamydia* and clarithromycin is active against *M. leprae*. Little work has been done on these drugs in domestic animals and much data in the literature is extrapolated from human studies. Azithromycin appears to have a long half-life of 35 hours in cats.

Spiramycin is a macrolide which achieves very high tissue concentrations (in excess of those found in plasma) and penetrates well into milk, lacrimal fluids, respiratory secretions and other body fluids partly because of ion trapping of this weak base in fluids which are more acidic than plasma. The high tissue levels found are partly due to binding of the drug to tissue proteins, a feature which prolongs the residence time of spiramycin within tissue compartments. Its spectrum of activity is similar to that of erythromycin. It has greater acid stability than erythromycin and good oral bioavailability in monogastric animals. There is some evidence of a synergistic action with metronidazole against anaerobic bacteria. Spiramycin also has activity against *Toxoplasma gondii* and *Isospora* spp.

Tilmicosin is indicated for the treatment of pneumonia associated with *Pasteurella* spp. in cattle and sheep and *Actinobacillus pleuropneumoniae, Mycoplasma hyopneumoniae*, and *Pasteurella multocida* in pigs. It is also effective against ovine mastitis associated with *Staphylococcus aureus* and *Mycoplasma agalactiae*.

Lincomycin is effective against Gram-positive bacteria, anaerobes, and *Mycoplasma* but has little activity against Gram-negative organisms. **Clindamycin** has more potent antibacterial activity than lincomycin. It is particularly indicated in staphylococcal osteomyelitis. Lincosamides may cause a fatal enterocolitis in horses, rabbits, and rodents. Accidental administration of feedstuffs contaminated with trace amounts of lincomycin to cattle may cause a drop in milk production, inappetence, diarrhoea, and in some cases ketosis.

CLARITHROMYCIN

UK

Indications. Clarithromycin-sensitive infections
Dose. See Prescribing for reptiles

POM ⒣ **Klaricid** (Abbott) *UK*
Oral suspension, clarithromycin 25 mg/mL when reconstituted with water

CLINDAMYCIN

UK

Indications. See notes above
Contra-indications. Clindamycin or lincomycin hypersensitivity; horses, ruminants, rabbits, hamsters, guinea pigs, chinchillas
Side-effects. Occasional vomiting and diarrhoea
Warnings. Drug Interactions – see Appendix 1. Safety in breeding animals has not been established, care in patients with renal or hepatic impairment; renal and hepatic function and blood parameters should be monitored during prolonged treatment
Dose.
Dogs: infected wounds, dental infections, superficial pyoderma, *by mouth*, 5 mg/kg twice daily *or* 11 mg/kg once daily for 5–7 days
Osteomyelitis, *by mouth*, 11 mg/kg twice daily for minimum 28 days
by intramuscular injection, 10 mg/kg twice daily
Cats: infected wounds, dental infections, *by mouth*, 5 mg/kg twice daily *or* 11 mg/kg once daily for 5–7 days
by intramuscular injection, 10 mg/kg twice daily
Toxoplasmosis♦, *by mouth*, 25 mg/kg daily in divided doses for at least 2 weeks

POM **Antirobe Capsules** (Pharmacia & Upjohn) *UK*
Capsules, clindamycin (as hydrochloride) 25 mg, for *dogs, cats*; 150
Capsules, clindamycin (as hydrochloride) 75 mg, 150 mg, for *dogs*; 150

POM ⒣ **Dalacin C** (Pharmacia & Upjohn) *UK*
Injection, clindamycin (as phosphate) 150 mg/mL; 2 mL, 4 mL

Australia
Indications. Clindamycin-sensitive infections
Dose. *Dogs, cats*: *by mouth*, 5.5 mg/kg *or* 11 mg/kg (depending on the condition)

Antirobe Capsules (Pharmacia & Upjohn) *Austral.*
Capsules, clindamycin (as hydrochloride) 25 mg, 75 mg,and 150 mg, for *dogs, cats*

Antirobe Aquadrops (Pharmacia & Upjohn) *Austral.*
Oral drops, clindamycin (as hydrochloride) 25 mg/mL, for *dogs, cats*

Eire
Indications. Clindamycin-sensitive infections
Dose. *Dogs, cats*: *by mouth*, 5.5 mg/kg *or* 11 mg/kg (depending on the condition)

Antirobe Capsules (Pharmacia & Upjohn) *Eire*
Oral capsules, clindamycin (as hydrochloride) 25 mg, 75 mg, 150 mg, for *dogs, cats*

New Zealand
Indications. Clindamycin-sensitive infections
Dose. *Dogs, cats*: *by mouth*, 5.5 mg/kg *or* 11 mg/kg (depending on the condition)

Antirobe Aquadrops (Pharmacia & Upjohn) *NZ*
Oral solution, clindamycin hydrochloride 25 mg/mL, for *dogs, cats*

Antirobe Capsules (Pharmacia & Upjohn) *NZ*
Capsules, clindamycin hydrochloride 25 mg or 75 mg, for *dogs, cats*

USA
Indications. Clindamycin-sensitive infections
Dose. *Dogs, cats*: *by mouth*, 5.5 mg/kg *or* 11 mg/kg (depending on the condition)
Cats: *by mouth*, 11–22 mg/kg (depending on the condition)

Antirobe Capsules (Pharmacia & Upjohn) *USA*
Capsules, clindamycin (as hydrochloride) 25 mg, 75 mg, 150 mg, for *dogs, cats*

Antirobe Aquadrops (Pharmacia & Upjohn) *USA*
Oral solution, clindamycin (as hydrochloride) 25 mg/ML, for *dogs, cats*

Clindadrops (Phoenix) *USA*
Oral solution, clindamycin (as hydrochloride) 25 mg/mL, for *dogs*

Clindamycin Hydrochloride Oral Liquid (Butler) *USA*
Oral solution, clindamycin (as hydrochloride) 25 mg/mL, for *dogs*

Clindrops (Vetus) *USA*
Oral solution, clindamycin (as hydrochloride) 25 mg/mL, for *dogs*

ERYTHROMYCIN

UK

Indications. Erythromycin-sensitive infections, especially those caused by *Campylobacter* spp.; reduction of gastric motility (see section 3.7)
Dose.
Foals: *by mouth*, 25 mg/kg 3 times daily
Dogs, cats: *by mouth*, 2–10 mg/kg daily
Poultry: *by addition to drinking water*, 25 g/100 litres

POM ⒣ **Erythromycin** (Non-proprietary) *UK*
Tablets, e/c, erythromycin 250 mg

POM ⒣ **Erythromycin Ethyl Succinate** (Non-proprietary) *UK*
Oral suspension, powder for reconstitution, erythromycin (as ethyl succinate) 25 mg/mL, 50 mg/mL, 100 mg/mL; 100 mL

POM **Erythrocin Proportioner** (Ceva) *UK*
Oral powder, for reconstitution and then addition to drinking water, erythromycin activity (as phosphate) 300 mg/g, for *chickens*; 78 g
Reconstitute erythromycin 23.12 g (78 g powder) in 1.1 litres water then add to drinking water at a rate of 13 mL/litre drinking water
Withdrawal Periods. *Chickens*: slaughter 3 days, eggs 6 days

POM **Erythrocin Soluble** (Ceva) *UK*
Oral powder, for reconstitution and then addition to drinking water, erythromycin activity (as thiocyanate) 165 mg/g, for *chickens*; 70 g
Reconstitute erythromycin 11.56 g (70 g powder) in 2.5 litres water then add to drinking water to make a total volume of 45 litres
Withdrawal Periods. *Chickens*: slaughter 3 days, eggs 6 days

Australia
Indications. Erythromycin-sensitive infections
Dose. Consult manufacturer's information

Erythromycin Water Soluble Powder (CCD) *Austral.*
Powder, for addition to drinking water, erythromycin thiocyanate 750 mg/g
powder, for *poultry*
Withdrawal Periods. Slaughter 7 days

Gallimycin-200 (Merial) *Austral.*
Injection, erythromycin 200 mg/mL, for *cattle, sheep, pigs*
Withdrawal Periods. *Cattle*: slaughter 14 days, milk 72 hours. *Sheep*: slaughter 3 days. *Pigs*: slaughter 7 days.

Eire

Indications. Erythromycin-sensitive infections
Dose. Consult manufacturer's information

Erythrocin Soluble (Interpharm) *Eire*
Oral powder, for addition to drinking water, erythromycin (as thiocyanate)
11.56 g/70 g sachet, for *chickens*
Withdrawal Periods. Slaughter 3 days, eggs 6 days

New Zealand

Indications. Erythromycin-sensitive infections
Dose. Consult manufacturer's information

Erythrosol (Bomac) *NZ*
Oral powder, erythromycin 100 g/200 g, for *poultry*
Withdrawal Periods. Slaughter 3 days

Gallimycin 200 (Virbac) *NZ*
Injection, erythromycin 200 mg/mL, for *cattle, pigs*
Withdrawal Periods. *Cattle*: slaughter 3 days, milk 108 hours. *Pigs*: slaughter 3 days

USA

Indications. Erythromycin-sensitive infections
Dose. Consult manufacturer's information

Gallimycin-100 (Osborn) *USA*
Injection, erythromycin 100 mg/mL, for *pigs, cattle, sheep*
Withdrawal Periods. *Cattle*: slaughter 14 days, milk 72 hours. *Sheep*: slaughter 3 days. *Pigs*: slaughter 7 days

LINCOMYCIN

UK
Indications. See notes above
Contra-indications. Lincomycin hypersensitivity; horses, rabbits, and rodents; concurrent treatment with erythromycin
Side-effects. Transient soft stools, mild swelling of the anus, skin erythema, mild irritable behaviour
Dose. *Pigs*:
Swine dysentery
treatment, *by addition to drinking water,* 3.3 g/100 litres
by addition to feed, 110 g/tonne feed
by intramuscular injection, 10 mg/kg once daily for up to 2 days
prophylaxis, *by addition to feed,* 44 g/tonne feed
Swine mycoplasmal pneumonia
treatment and prophylaxis, *by addition to feed,* 220 g/tonne feed
by intramuscular injection, 10 mg/kg daily

Other bacterial infections, *by intramuscular injection*, 4.5–11.0 mg/kg daily
Dogs, cats: *by mouth*, 22 mg/kg twice daily *or* 15 mg/kg 3 times daily
by intramuscular injection, 22 mg/kg once daily *or* 11 mg/kg twice daily
by slow intravenous injection, 11–22 mg/kg 1–2 times daily

MFS **Lincocin Premix** (Pharmacia & Upjohn) *UK*
Premix, lincomycin (as hydrochloride) 44 g/kg, for *pigs*; 2.5 kg, 25 kg
Withdrawal Periods. *Pigs*: slaughter 1 day

POM **Lincocin Soluble Powder** (Pharmacia & Upjohn) *UK*
Oral powder, for addition to drinking water, lincomycin (as hydrochloride)
400 mg/g, for *pigs*; 7.5 g, 150 g
Withdrawal Periods. *Pigs*: slaughter 1 day

POM **Lincocin Sterile Solution** (Pharmacia & Upjohn) *UK*
Injection, lincomycin (as hydrochloride) 100 mg/mL, for *pigs, dogs, cats*; 50
mL, 100 mL
Withdrawal Periods. *Pigs*: slaughter 2 days

POM **Lincocin Tablets** (Pharmacia & Upjohn) *UK*
Tablets, scored, lincomycin (as hydrochloride) 100 mg, 500 mg, for *dogs, cats*; 100-mg tablets 100; 500-mg tablets 50

Australia

Indications. Erythromycin-sensitive infections
Dose. Consult manufacturer's information

Lincocin Solution (Pharmacia & Upjohn) *Austral.*
Injection, lincomycin (as hydrochloride monohydrate) 100 mg/mL, for *pigs, dogs, cats*
Withdrawal Periods. Slaughter 2 days

Lincocin Tablets (Pharmacia & Upjohn) *Austral.*
Tablets, lincomycin (as hydrochloride monohydrate) 200 mg, 500 mg, for *dogs, cats*

Lincomix 600 Concentrate (Pharmacia & Upjohn) *Austral.*
Premix, lincomycin (as hydrochloride monohydrate) 600 g/kg powder, for *pigs*
Withdrawal Periods. Slaughter 1 day (at less than 110 ppm) or 2 days (at 110- 220 ppm)

Lincomix Antibiotic Premix (Pharmacia & Upjohn) *Austral.*
Premix, lincomycin (as hydrochloride monohydrate) 44 g/kg premix, for *pigs*
Withdrawal Periods. Slaughter 1 day (at 110 ppm) or 2 days (at 220 ppm)

Lincomix Antibiotic Soluble Powder (Pharmacia & Upjohn) *Austral.*
Powder, for addition to drinking water, lincomycin (as hydrochloride monohydrate) 400 g/kg powder, for *pigs*
Withdrawal Periods. Slaughter 2 days

Lincomix Antibiotic Solution (Pharmacia & Upjohn) *Austral.*
Injection, lincomycin (as hydrochloride monohydrate) 300 mg/mL, for *pigs*
Withdrawal Periods. Slaughter 2 days

Lincomycin 500 mg Tablets (Apex) *Austral.*
Tablets, lincomycin (as hydrochloride) 500 mg, for *dogs, cats*

Eire

Indications. Erythromycin-sensitive infections
Dose. Consult manufacturer's information

Lincocin Premix (Pharmacia & Upjohn) *Eire*
Premix, lincomycin (as hydrochloride) 44 g/kg, for *pigs*
Withdrawal Periods. Slaughter 24 hours

Lincocin Soluble Powder (Pharmacia & Upjohn) *Eire*
Oral powder, for addition to drinking water, lincomycin (as hydrochloride) 400 mg/g, for *pigs*
Withdrawal Periods. Slaughter 24 hours

Lincocin Sterile Solution (Pharmacia & Upjohn) *Eire*
Injection, lincomycin (as hydrochloride) 100 mg/mL, for *pigs, dogs, cats*
Withdrawal Periods. Slaughter 48 hour

Lincocin Tablets (Pharmacia & Upjohn) *Eire*
Tablets, lincomycin (as hydrochloride) 100 mg, 500 mg, for *dogs, cats*

New Zealand
Indications. Erythromycin-sensitive infections
Dose. Consult manufacturer's information

Lincocin (Pharmacia & Upjohn) *NZ*
Tablets, lincomycin (as hydrochloride) 100 mg, 200 mg, 500 mg, for *dogs, cats*

Lincocin (Pharmacia & Upjohn) *NZ*
Injection, lincomycin (as hydrochloride) 100 mg/mL, for *dogs, cats*

Lincocin Aquadrops (Pharmacia & Upjohn) *NZ*
Oral solution, lincomycin (as hydrochloride) 50 mg/mL, for *dogs, cats*

Lincomix Premix (Pharmacia & Upjohn) *NZ*
Premix, lincomycin 110 g/kg, for *pigs, poultry*
Withdrawal Periods. *Pigs*: slaughter 24 hours

USA
Indications. Erythromycin-sensitive infections
Dose. Consult manufacturer's information

Lincocin (Pharmacia & Upjohn) *USA*
Injection, lincomycin hydrochloride, for *dogs, cats*

Lincocin (Pharmacia & Upjohn) *USA*
Tablets, lincomycin (as hydrochloride) 100mg, 200 mg or 500 mg, for *dogs, cats*

Lincomix (Pharmacia & Upjohn) *USA*
Injection, lincomycin 25 mg/mL. 100 mg/mL and 300 mg/mL, for *pigs*
Withdrawal Periods. Slaughter 2 days

Lincomix (Pharmacia & Upjohn) *USA*
Oral powder, for addition to drinking water, lincomycin (as hydrochloride) 32 g/ packet, for *chickens, pigs*
Withdrawal Periods. *Pigs*: slaughter 6 days. *Chickens*: slaughter withdrawal period nil

Lincomix 10 (Pharmacia & Upjohn) *USA*
Premix, lincomycin 22 g/kg premix, for *chickens, pigs*
Withdrawal Periods. Pigs: slaughter 6 days. *Chickens*: slaughter withdrawal period nil (at recommended doses), should not be used in chickens producing eggs for human consumption

Lincomix 20 Feed Medication (Pharmacia & Upjohn) *USA*
Premix, lincomycin 44 g/kg premix, for *chickens, pigs*
Withdrawal Periods. *Pigs*: slaughter 6 days. *Chickens*: slaughter withdrawal period nil (at recommended doses), should not be used in chickens producing eggs for human consumption

Lincomix 50 Feed Medication (Pharmacia & Upjohn) *USA*
Premix, lincomycin 110 g/kg premix, for *chickens, pigs*
Withdrawal Periods. *Pigs*: slaughter 6 days. *Chickens*: slaughter withdrawal period nil (at recommended doses), should not be used in chickens producing eggs for human consumption

Lincomycin Soluble (ID Russell) *USA*
Oral powder, for addition to drinking water, lincomycin (as hydrochloride) 32 g/ packet, for *chickens, pigs*
Withdrawal Periods. *Pigs*: slaughter 6 days. *Chickens*: slaughter withdrawal period nil

TILMICOSIN

UK
Indications. Tilmicosin-sensitive organisms
Contra-indications. Intravenous injection, goats, horses; incorporation into pig feeds containing bentonite
Side-effects. Occasional swelling at injection site
Warnings. Self-injection may cause cardiovascular system toxicity, operators should use extreme caution; safety of premix in pregnant sows and animals used for breeding purposes has not been established. Drug Interactions – see Appendix 1
Dose.
Cattle, sheep: by subcutaneous injection, 10 mg/kg
Pigs: by addition to feed, 400 g/tonne feed

POM **Micotil** (Elanco) *UK*
Injection, tilmicosin 300 mg/mL, for *young cattle, sheep more than 15 kg body-weight*; 50 mL
Withdrawal Periods. *Cattle*: slaughter 60 days, should not be used in cattle producing milk for human consumption. *Sheep*: slaughter 42 days, milk 15 days

POM **Pulmotil G100** (Elanco) *UK*
Premix, tilmicosin (as phosphate) 100 g/kg, for *growing fattening pigs*; 2 kg, 5 kg, 10 kg
Withdrawal Periods. *Pigs*: slaughter 14 days

MFS **Pulmotil G200** (Elanco) *UK*
Premix, tilmicosin (as phosphate) 200 g/kg, for *growing fattening pigs*
Withdrawal Periods. *Pigs*: slaughter 14 days

Australia
Indications. Tilmicosin-sensitive infections
Dose.
Cattle: by subcutaneous injection, 10 mg/kg
Pigs: by addition to feed, 200–400 g/tonne feed

Micotil 300 Injection (Elanco) *Austral.*
Injection, tilmicosin (as phosphate) 300 mg/mL, for *cattle*
Withdrawal Periods. Slaughter 28 days, should not be used in cattle producing milk for human consumption

Pulmotil 200 Premix (Elanco) *Austral.*
Premix, tilmicosin 200 g/kg, for *pigs*
Withdrawal Periods. Slaughter 14 days

Eire
Indications. Tilmicosin-sensitive infections
Dose.
Cattle, sheep: by subcutaneous injection, 10 mg/kg
Pigs: by addition to feed, 200–400 g/tonne feed; 8–16 mg/kg body-weight

Micotil (Elanco) *Eire*
Injection, tilmicosin 300 mg/mL, for *cattle, sheep*
Withdrawal Periods. *Cattle*: slaughter 42 days, should not be used in cattle producing milk for human consumption. *Sheep*: slaughter 42 days, milk 15 days

Pulmotil G40 Premix (Elanco) *Eire*
Premix, tilmicosin (as phosphate) 40 g/kg, for *pigs*
Withdrawal Periods. Slaughter 14 days

Pulmotil G100 Premix (Elanco) *Eire*
Premix, tilmicosin (as phosphate) 100 g/kg, for *pigs*
Withdrawal Periods. Slaughter 14 days

Pulmotil G140 Premix (Elanco) *Eire*
Premix, tilmicosin (as phosphate) 200 g/kg, for *pigs*
Withdrawal Periods. Slaughter 14 days

New Zealand
Indications. Tilmicosin-sensitive infections
Dose.
Cattle: *by subcutaneous injection*, 10 mg/kg
Pigs: *by addition to feed*, 200–400 g/tonne feed;

Micotil 300 (Elanco) *NZ*
Injection, tilmicosin 300 mg/mL, for *cattle*
Withdrawal Periods. Slaughter 28 days

Pulmotil 200 (Elanco) *NZ*
Premix, tilmicosin phosphate, for *pigs*
Withdrawal Periods. Slaughter 21 days

USA
Indications. Tilmicosin-sensitive infections
Dose.
Cattle: *by subcutaneous injection*, 10 mg/kg
Pigs: *by addition to feed*, 200–400 g/tonne feed;

Micotil 300 Injection (Elanco) *USA*
Injection, tilmicosin (as phosphate) 300 mg/mL, for *cattle*
Withdrawal Periods. Slaughter 28 days, should not be used in cattle producing milk for human consumption

Pulmotil 90 (Elanco) *USA*
Premix, tilmicosin 200 g/kg premix, for *pigs*
Withdrawal Periods. Slaughter 7 days

TYLOSIN

UK
Indications. Tylosin-sensitive organisms; to improve growth-rate and feed conversion efficiency in pigs (see section 17.1)
Side-effects. Transient swelling at injection site with depot injection
Dose.
Cattle: *by addition to milk or milk replacer*, 1 g/calf twice daily
by intramuscular injection, 2–10 mg/kg daily
Pigs: *by addition to drinking water,* 25 g/100 litres
prophylaxis of swine dysentery, enzootic pneumonia, *by addition to feed,* 100 g/tonne feed for 21 days, then 40 g/tonne feed during period of risk
treatment and prophylaxis *Lawsonia intracellularis, by addition to feed,* 100 g/tonne feed for 21 days
by intramuscular injection, 2–10 mg/kg daily
by depot intramuscular injection, 20 mg/kg as a single dose
Dogs: *by mouth*, 40 mg/kg daily in divided doses
Poultry: *by addition to drinking water,* 50 g/100 litres

POM Bilosin 200 (Bimeda) *UK*
Injection, tylosin 200 mg/mL, for *pigs*; 50 mL, 100 mL
Withdrawal Periods. *Pigs*: slaughter 28 days

POM Norotyl LA (Norbrook) *UK*
Depot injection, tylosin 150 mg/mL, for *pigs*; 50 mL, 100 mL
Withdrawal Periods. Slaughter 7 days

POM Tylacare (Animalcare) *UK*
Tablets, scored, tylosin 200 mg, for *dogs*; 50

POM Tylan 50 (Elanco) *UK*
Injection, tylosin 50 mg/mL, for *cattle, pigs*; 50 mL
Withdrawal Periods. *Cattle*: slaughter 28 days, milk 3.5 days. *Pigs*: slaughter 3 weeks

POM Tylan 200 (Elanco) *UK*
Injection, tylosin 200 mg/mL, for *cattle, pigs*; 100 mL
Withdrawal Periods. *Cattle*: slaughter 28 days, milk 3.5 days. *Pigs*: slaughter 3 weeks

MFS Tylan G20 (Elanco) *UK*
Premix, tylosin (as phosphate) 20 g/kg, for *pigs*
Withdrawal Periods. *Pigs*: slaughter withdrawal period nil

MFS Tylan G50 (Elanco) *UK*
Premix, tylosin (as phosphate) 50 g/kg, for *pigs*
Withdrawal Periods. *Pigs*: slaughter withdrawal period nil

MFS Tylan G250 (Elanco) *UK*
Premix, tylosin (as phosphate) 250 g/kg, for *pigs*
Withdrawal Periods. *Pigs*: slaughter withdrawal period nil

POM Tylan Soluble (Elanco) *UK*
Oral powder, for addition to drinking water, milk, or milk replacer, tylosin (as tartrate) 100 g, for *calves, pigs, broiler chickens, turkeys*
Withdrawal Periods. *Calves*: slaughter 14 days. *Pigs*: slaughter withdrawal period nil. *Chickens, turkeys*: slaughter withdrawal period nil, should not be used in birds producing eggs for human consumption

POM Tyluvet-20 (Vétoquinol) *UK*
Injection, tylosin 200 mg/mL, for *pigs*; 100 mL
Withdrawal Periods. *Pigs*: slaughter 28 days

Australia
Indications. Tylosin-sensitive infections
Dose. Consult manufacturer's information

A.F.S. Tylan Soluble (Controlled Medications) *Austral.*
Powder, for addition to drinking water, tylosin tartrate 850 mg/g powder, for *chickens, turkeys*
Withdrawal Periods. *Chickens*: slaughter 2 days, should not be used in chickens producing eggs for human consumption. *Turkeys*: slaughter 5 days, should not be used in turkeys producing eggs for human consumption

Tylan 200 Tablets (Elanco) *Austral.*
Tablets, tylosin 200 mg, for *dogs, cats*

Tylan Injection 200 (Elanco) *Austral.*
Injection, tylosin 200 mg/mL, for *cattle, pigs*
Withdrawal Periods. *Cattle*: slaughter 21 days, milk 3 days. *Pigs*: slaughter 3 days

Tylan Soluble (Elanco) *Austral.*
Powder, for addition to drinking water, tylosin 100 g, for *chickens, turkeys, pigs*
Withdrawal Periods. *Pigs, chickens, turkeys*: slaughter withdrawal period nil, should not be used in poultry producing eggs for human consumption

Tylan Soluble (Elanco) *Austral.*
Powder, for addition to drinking water, tylosin tartrate 850 mg/g powder, for *chickens, turkeys*
Withdrawal Periods. Slaughter withdrawal period nil.

Eire
Indications. Tylosin-sensitive infections
Dose. *Cattle, pigs*: *by intramuscular injection*, 10 mg/kg
Pigs: *by intramuscular injection*, 10 mg/kg
by addition to feed, 100 g/tonne feed, then 40 g/tonne feed

Tylan 50 (Elanco) *Eire*
Injection, tylosin 50 mg/mL, for *cattle, pigs*

Withdrawal Periods. *Cattle*: slaughter 7 days, milk 96 hours. *Pigs*: slaughter 3 weeks

Tylan 200 (Elanco) *Eire*
Injection, tylosin 200 mg/mL, for *cattle, pigs*
Withdrawal Periods. *Cattle*: slaughter 7 days, milk 96 hours. *Pigs*: slaughter 3 weeks

Tylan 20 (Elanco) *Eire*
Premix, tylosin (as phosphate) 20 g/kg, for *pigs*
Withdrawal Periods. Slaughter withdrawal period nil

Tylan G100 Premix (Elanco) *Eire*
Premix, tylosin (as phosphate) 100 g/kg, for *pigs*
Withdrawal Periods. Slaughter withdrawal period nil

Tylan Soluble (Elanco) *Eire*
Oral powder, to add to drinking water, tylosin (as tartrate) 100 g/bottle, for *cattle, pigs, chickens, turkeys*
Withdrawal Periods. *Calves*: slaughter 14 days. *Pigs, broiler chickens, turkeys*: slaughter withdrawal period nil

New Zealand
Indications. Tylosin-sensitive infections
Dose. Consult manufacturer's information

Tylan 100 (Elanco) *NZ*
Premix, tylosin (as phosphate) 100 g/kg, for *cattle, pigs, chickens*
Withdrawal Periods. *Cattle*: slaughter withdrawal period nil, should not be used in cattle producing milk for human consumption. *Pigs, chickens*: slaughter withdrawal period nil

Tylan 200 (Bomac) *NZ*
Injection, tylosin 200 mg/mL, for *cattle, sheep, goats, pigs*
Withdrawal Periods. *Cattle, sheep, goats*: slaughter 21 days, milk 72 hours. *Pigs*: slaughter 21 days

Tylan Soluble (Elanco) *NZ*
Oral powder, per container: tylosin (as tartrate) 100 g, for *poultry*
Withdrawal Periods. Slaughter withdrawal period nil

Tylasul-G (Elanco) *NZ*
Premix, tylosin (as phosphate) 20 g/kg, for *pigs*
Withdrawal Periods. Slaughter 15 days

Tylo 200 (Phoenix) *NZ*
Injection, tylosin (as tartrate) 200 mg/mL, for *cattle, sheep, goats, pigs*
Withdrawal Periods. *Cattle, sheep, goats*: slaughter 21 days, milk 72 hours. *Pigs*: slaughter 21 days

Tylomix (Bomac) *NZ*
Premix, tylosin (as tartrate) 100 g/kg, for *pigs, chickens*
Withdrawal Periods. Slaughter withdrawal period nil

USA
Indications. Tylosin-sensitive infections
Dose. Consult manufacturer's information

Tylan 40 (Elanco) *USA*
Premix, tylosin 88 g/kg premix, for *pigs, cattle, chickens*
Withdrawal Periods. *Chickens*: slaughter 5 days (depends on dose level)

Tylan 100 (Elanco) *USA*
Premix, tylosin (as phosphate) 220 g/kg premix, for *pigs, cattle, chickens*
Withdrawal Periods. *Chickens*: slaughter 5 days (depends on dose level)

Tylan 200 Injection (Elanco) *USA*
Injection, tylosin 200 mg/mL, for *cattle, pigs*
Withdrawal Periods. *Cattle*: slaughter 21 days, should not be used in cattle producing milk for human consumption, should not be used in calves intended for veal production. *Pigs*: slaughter 14 days

Tylan Soluble (Elanco) *USA*
Oral powder, for addition to drinking water, tylosin (as tartrate) 100 g, for *chickens, turkeys, pigs, cattle, sheep*

Withdrawal Periods. *Pigs*: slaughter 2 days. *Chickens*: slaughter 1 day, should not be used in chickens producing eggs for human consumption. *Turkeys*: slaughter 5 days, should not be used in turkeys producing eggs for human consumption

Tylosin Injection (Aspen, Boehringer Ingelheim Vetmedica) *USA*
Injection, tylosin 50 mg/mL, 200 mg/mL, for *cattle, pigs*
Withdrawal Periods. *Cattle*: slaughter 21 days, should not be used in cattle producing milk for human consumption, should not be used in calves intended for veal production. *Pigs*: slaughter 14 days

Tylosin Injection (AgriLabs) *USA*
Injection, tylosin 200 mg/mL, for *cattle, pigs*
Withdrawal Periods. *Cattle*: slaughter 21 days, should not be used in cattle producing milk for human consumption, should not be used in calves intended for veal production. *Pigs*: slaughter 14 days

1.1.5 Chloramphenicols

Chloramphenicol is a broad-spectrum bacteriostatic antibacterial. It is active against rickettsial and chlamydial infections, the majority of anaerobes, most Gram-positive aerobes, and non-enteric aerobes including *Actinobacillus*, *Bordetella*, *Haemophilus*, and *Pasteurella* spp. Enterobacteriaceae including *Escherichia* and *Salmonella* spp. are intrinsically susceptible but plasmid-mediated resistance is widespread. Chloramphenicol has activity against *Mycoplasma* and *Proteus* spp. but is unreliable. It is inactive against *Pseudomonas* spp.

Chloramphenicol is used in the treatment of human *Salmonella typhi* infection (typhoid). In veterinary medicine, the use of chloramphenicol is restricted to non-food producing animals; the drug is included in Annex IV of Regulation 2377/90/EEC which effectively prohibits its use in food-producing animals. Chloramphenicol should be used to treat individual animals rather than a group. Operators must wear impervious gloves and avoid drug-skin contact.

Chloramphenicol is a simple uncharged lipid-soluble compound which readily crosses cellular barriers. Chloramphenicol diffuses throughout the body and reaches sites of infection inaccessible to many other antibacterial drugs including cerebrospinal fluid, brain, and internal structures of the eye. It is inactivated in the liver by conjugation and then excreted in urine and bile.

Drug metabolism is particularly rapid in horses and chloramphenicol is therefore of limited use in this species. Due to limited drug metabolism in the cat, chloramphenicol may accumulate giving rise to reversible bone-marrow suppression. Treatment should be restricted to one week in cats.

The bacteriostatic action of chloramphenicol may inhibit the bactericidal action of beta-lactam antibacterials and these drugs should not therefore be used concurrently. Chloramphenicol is an irreversible inhibitor of the cytochrome P450 enzymes involved in the metabolism of barbiturates and will affect the metabolism of these drugs by dogs for up to 3 weeks following a single dose of 50 mg/kg of chloramphenicol.

Thiamphenicol has a broad spectrum of activity similar to chloramphenicol. **Florfenicol**, a fluorinated analogue of chloramphenicol, shares the general properties of the parent substance but is less liable to produce blood dyscrasias. It is a less satisfactory substrate for bacterial chloramphenicol acetyl-transferase and may be active against some strains resistant to chloramphenicol. Both florfenicol and thiamphenicol lack the nitrobenzene component of chloramphenicol which is thought to be responsible for the idiosyncratic reaction to chloramphenicol seen in humans.

CHLORAMPHENICOL

UK

Indications. See notes above
Contra-indications. Hepatic impairment, see notes above
Side-effects. Bone marrow suppression, diarrhoea, vomiting
Warnings. Administer with caution to cats, safety in pregnant or lactating animals and neonates not established; Drug Interactions – see Appendix 1
Dose.
Dogs: *by mouth or by slow intravenous injection*, 50 mg/kg 1–2 times daily. See also preparation details
Cats: *by mouth or by slow intravenous injection*, 25 mg/kg 1–2 times daily. See also preparation details

POM **Chloramphenicol '100' Tablets** (Fort Dodge) *UK*
Tablets, s/c, chloramphenicol 100 mg, for *dogs, cats*; 250
Dose. *Dogs, cats*: *by mouth*, 1 tablet/2 kg body-weight daily in 2–3 divided doses

POM Ⓗ **Kemicetine** (Pharmacia & Upjohn) *UK*
Injection, powder for reconstitution, chloramphenicol (as sodium succinate) 1 g
For intravenous injection

Australia

Indications. Chloramphenicol-sensitive infections
Contra-indications. Horses
Dose. *Dogs, cats*: *by mouth*, 50 mg/kg
by intramuscular injection, 10–30 mg/kg

Chlor-B Tablets (Delvet) *Austral.*
Tablets, chloramphenicol 125 mg, 250 mg, 500 mg, for *dogs, cats*

Chloramphenicol '150' 100 mL (Delvet) *Austral.*
Injection, chloramphenicol 150 mg/mL, for *dogs, cats*
Withdrawal Periods. Should not be used in animals intended for human consumption

Eire

Indications. Chloramphenicol-sensitive infections
Contra-indications. Renal or hepatic impairment
Warnings. Blood dyscrasia with prolonged treatment; Drug Interactions – barbiturate anaesthesia
Dose. *Dogs, cats*: *by mouth*, 50 mg/kg

Chloramphenicol 100 Tablets (Fort Dodge) *Eire*
Tablets, chloramphenicol 100 mg, for *dogs, cats*

USA

Indications. Chloramphenicol-sensitive infections
Contra-indications. Concurrent use of penicillin or streptomycin, with or2 hours before pentobarbital anaesthesia
Warnings. Care in animals with hepatic or renal impairment or haematopoietic dysfunction
Dose. *Dogs*: *by mouth*, 55 mg/kg

Duricol (Nylos) *USA*
Capsules, chloramphenicol 50 mg, 100 mg, 250 mg, 500 mg, for *dogs*

FLORFENICOL

UK

Indications. Florfenicol-sensitive infections
Side-effects. Transient decrease in appetite and softening of stools; inflammatory lesions at site of injection
Warnings. Manufacturer does not recommend use in adult bulls intended for breeding purposes because the effect on bovine reproductive performance has not been established
Dose. *Cattle*: *by subcutaneous injection*, 40 mg/kg as a single dose
by intramuscular injection, 20 mg/kg. Repeat after 2 days

POM **Nuflor** (Schering-Plough) *UK*
Injection, florfenicol 300 mg/mL, for *cattle*
Withdrawal Periods. *Cattle*: slaughter 30 days (20 mg/kg), 44 days (40 mg/kg), should not be used in cattle producing milk for human consumption

Eire

Indications. Florfenicol-sensitive infections
Dose. *Cattle*: *by intramuscular injection*, 20 mg/kg

Nuflor Injectable Solution (Schering-Plough) *Eire*
Injection, florfenicol 300 mg/mL, for *cattle*
Withdrawal Periods. Slaughter 30 days, should not be used in cattle producing milk for human consumption

USA

Indications. Florfenicol-sensitive infections
Dose. *Cattle*: *by intramuscular injection*, 20 mg/kg

Nuflor (Schering-Plough) *USA*
Injection, florfenicol 300 mg/mL, for *cattle*
Withdrawal Periods. Slaughter 28 days, should not be used in cattle producing milk for human consumption, should not be used in calves intended for veal production

1.1.6 Sulphonamides and potentiated sulphonamides

1.1.6.1 Sulphonamides
1.1.6.2 Potentiated sulphonamides

1.1.6.1 Sulphonamides

The sulphonamides form an extensive series of drugs that differ more in their physicochemical characteristics, and hence in mode of administration and pharmacokinetics, than they do in their antibacterial activity. They act by competing with tissue factors, notably *p*-aminobenzoic acid, and are therefore inactive in the presence of necrotic tissue. They are bacteriostatic to a range of Gram-positive and Gram-negative bacteria. They are active against aerobic Gram-positive cocci and some rods and many Gram-negative rods including Enterobacteriaceae. *Leptospira* and *Pseudomonas* spp. are resistant. Sulphonamides are also active against *Chlamydia*, *Toxoplasma*, and coccidia (see section 1.4). Acquired resistance to sulphonamides is widespread in the UK.

The sodium salts are alkaline and hence irritant by intramuscular injection and so are often given intravenously. Sulphonamides are well absorbed following oral administration. They diffuse well into body tissues and are partly inactivated in the liver, mainly by acetylation. The acetylated derivatives are relatively insoluble in acidic urine and so may precipitate in the renal tubules of carnivores leading to crystalluria and renal failure. This problem may be reduced by increasing the urine volume or by increasing the urine pH.

Prolonged administration of certain sulphonamides may cause keratoconjunctivitis sicca (dry eye) in dogs, and sulfadiazine-containing preparations may promote a reversible immune-mediated sterile polyarthritis in dogs. Sulphonamides may cause petechial haemorrhages in poultry as a result of vitamin K antagonism. Prolonged treatment with sulphonamides may lead to vitamin K deficiency causing agranulocytosis and haemolytic anaemia. Sulphonamides may inhibit thyroid hormone synthesis and, in some dogs can cause sub-clinical hypothyroidism with subnormal T_4 concentrations and high concentrations of TSH detected in plasma in these cases. This effect is reversible when the therapy is stopped. Concurrent administration of sulphonamides and sedatives or anaesthetics is contra-indicated in horses because severe cardiac arrhythmias and collapse may result. Intravenous administration of sulphonamides to cattle and horses can result in sudden collapse.

SULFACHLORPYRIDAZINE

USA

Indications. Sulfachlorpyridazine-sensitive infections
Dose. *Cattle*: *by mouth or intravenous injection*, 66–99 mg/kg
Pigs: *by mouth*, 44–77 mg/kg

Vetisulid Boluses (Fort Dodge) *USA*
Tablets, sulfachlorpyridazine (as sodium salt) 2 g, for *cattle*
Withdrawal Periods. Slaughter 7 days

Vetisulid Injection (Fort Dodge) *USA*
Injection, sulfachlorpyridazine (as sodium salt) 200 mg/mL, for *cattle*
Withdrawal Periods. Slaughter 5 days

Vetisulid Powder (Fort Dodge) *USA*
Oral powder, sulfachlorpyridazine (as sodium salt) 50 g, for *cattle, pigs*
Withdrawal Periods. *Calves*: slaughter 7 days. *Pigs*: slaughter 4 days

SULFADIMETHOXINE

USA

Indications. Sulfadimethoxine-sensitive infections; coccidiosis in poultry
Dose. Dosages vary, consult manufactuer's information

Albon (Pfizer) *USA*
Solution, for addition to drinking water, sulfadimethoxine 125 mg/mL, for *cattle, chickens, turkeys*
Withdrawal Periods. *Cattle*: slaughter 7 days. *Chickens, turkeys*: slaughter 5 days

Albon (Pfizer) *USA*
Tablets, sulfadimethoxine 5 g, 15 g, for *cattle*
Withdrawal Periods. Slaughter 7 days, milk 60 hours, should not be used in calves intended for veal production

Albon (Pfizer) *USA*
Injection, sulfadimethoxine 400 mg/mL, for *horses, cattle, dogs, cats*
Withdrawal Periods. Should not be used in *horses* intended for human consumption. *Cattle*: slaughter 5 days, milk 60 hours, should not be used in calves intended for veal production

Albon (Pfizer) *USA*
Tablets, sulfadimethoxine 125 mg, 250 mg, 500 mg, for *dogs, cats*

Albon (Pfizer) *USA*
Oral suspension, sulfadimethoxine 50 mg/mL, for *dogs, cats*

Albon SR (Pfizer) *USA*
Tablets, sulfadimethoxine 12.5 g, for *cattle*
Withdrawal Periods. Slaughter 21 days; should not be used in cattle producing milk for human consumption, should not be used in calves intended for veal production

Di-Methox (AgriLabs) *USA*
Injection, sulfadimethoxine 400 mg/mL, for *cattle*
Withdrawal Periods. Slaughter 5 days, milk 60 hours, should not be used in calves intended for veal production

Di-Methox (AgriLabs) *USA*
Oral solution, for addition to drinking water , sulfadimethoxine 12.5% (concentrated soln), for *cattlechickens, turkeys*
Withdrawal Periods. *Cattle*: slaughter 7 days.*Chickens, turkeys*: slaughter 5 days, should not be given to chickens over 16 weeks of age or turkeys over 24 weeks old

Di-Methox (AgriLabs) *USA*
Oral powder, to add to drinking water, sulfadimethoxine (as sodium salt), for *cattle, chickens, turkeys*
Withdrawal Periods. *Cattle*: slaughter 7 days. *Chickens, turkeys*: slaughter 5 days, should not be given to chickens over 16 weeks of age or turkeys over 24 weeks old

SDM Injection (Phoenix) *USA*
Injection, sulfadimethoxine 400 mg/mL, for *cattle*
Withdrawal Periods. Slaughter 5 days, milk 60 hours

SDM Solution (Phoenix) *USA*
Oral solution, for addition to drinking water, sulfadimethoxine 125 mg/mL, for *cattle, chickens, turkeys*
Withdrawal Periods. *Cattle*: slaughter 7 days, should not be used in calves intended for veal production. *Chickens, turkeys*: slaughter 5 days (not for chickens over 16 weeks old or turkeys over 24 weeks)

Sulfadimethoxine Injection-40 % (Aspen, DurVet, RXV,Vedco) *USA*
Injection, sulfadimethoxine 400 mg/mL, for *cattle*
Withdrawal Periods. Slaughter 5 days, milk 60 hours, should not be used in calves intended for veal production

Sulfadimethoxine Oral Solution (Aspen, Butler, DurVet, Vedco) *USA*
Oral solution, sulfadimethoxine 125 mg/mL, for *cattle, chickens, turkeys*
Withdrawal Periods. *Cattle*: slaughter 7 days, should not be used in calves intended for veal production. *Chickens, turkeys*: slaughter 5 days

Sulfadimethoxine Soluble Powder (DurVet, RXV,Vedco) *USA*
Oral powder, for addition to drinking water, sulfadimethoxine (as sodium salt) 94.6 g/107 g packet, for *cattle, chickens, turkeys*
Withdrawal Periods. *Cattle:* slaughter 7 days. *Chickens, turkeys:* slaughter 5 days

SULFADIMIDINE
(Sulphadimidine)

UK

Indications. Sulfadimidine-sensitive infections; coccidiosis (see section 1.1.4)
Contra-indications. Renal or hepatic impairment, sulphonamide hypersensitivity, blood dyscrasias
Side-effects. Transient irritation at injection site, occasional crystalluria (ensure patient has adequate water intake); see notes above
Warnings. Drug Interactions – see Appendix 1
Dose. Bacterial infections.
Cattle: by subcutaneous or intravenous (preferred) injection, initial dose 200 mg/kg then 100 mg/kg daily
calves: by mouth or by subcutaneous injection, initial dose 200 mg/kg then 100 mg/kg daily
Sheep, pigs: by subcutaneous or intravenous (preferred) injection, initial dose 200 mg/kg then 100 mg/kg daily

POM **Bimadine Tablets** (Bimeda) *UK*
Tablets, scored, sulfadimidine 5 g, for *cattle with a functional rumen up to 250 kg body-weight*; 200
Withdrawal Periods. *Cattle:* slaughter 8 days, should not be used in cattle producing milk for human consumption
Dose.
Cattle: by mouth, initial dose 2 tablets/50 kg body-weight, then 1 tablet/50 kg body-weight daily for 2 days

POM **Bimadine 33 1/3** (Bimeda) *UK*
Injection, sulfadimidine sodium 333 mg/mL, for *dairy cows, calves up to 12 months of age, sheep*; 500 mL, 2.5 litres
Withdrawal Periods. Should not be used in *adult cattle* intended for human consumption. *Cattle:* milk 3 days. *Calves:* slaughter 7 days. *Sheep:* slaughter 7 days, should not be used in sheep producing milk for human consumption

POM **Intradine** (Norbrook) *UK*
Injection, sulfadimidine sodium 333 mg/mL, for *cattle, sheep, pigs*; 500 mL
Withdrawal Periods. *Cattle:* slaughter 7 days, milk 3 days. *Sheep:* slaughter 7 days, should not be used in sheep producing milk for human consumption. *Pigs:* slaughter 7 days

POM **Sulfoxine 333 Injection** (Vétoquinol) *UK*
Injection, sulfadimidine sodium 333 mg/mL, for *cattle, sheep, pigs*; 500 mL
Withdrawal Periods. *Cattle:* slaughter 7 days, milk 3 days. *Sheep:* slaughter 7 days, should not be used in sheep producing milk for human consumption. *Pigs:* slaughter 7 days

POM **Vesadin** (Merial) *UK*
Injection, sulfadimidine sodium 333 mg/mL, for *cattle, sheep, pigs*; 500 mL
Withdrawal Periods. *Cattle:* slaughter 7 days, milk 3 days. *Sheep:* slaughter 7 days, should not be used in sheep producing milk for human consumption. *Pigs:* slaughter 7 days

Australia

Indications. Sulfadimethoxine-sensitive infections
Dose. Dosages vary, consult manufactuer's information

Cliftons Coccee Solution (Virbac) *Austral.*
Oral liquid, sulfadimidine sodium 220 mg/mL, for *cattle, sheep*
Withdrawal Periods. Slaughter 15 days, milk 36 hours (single dose) or 72 hours (multiple dose)

Suldim (David) *Austral.*
Liquid, for addition to drinking water, sulfadimidine sodium 70 g/L liquid, for *caged birds*

Sulfa 3 (Inca) *Austral.*
Liquid, sulfathiazole 120 g, sulfadimidine 40 g, sulfamerazine 40 g/ L, for *caged birds*

Sulfadimidine Feed Additive Premix (CCD) *Austral.*
Premix, sulfadimidine 1000g/kg, for *cattle,sheep, pigs, poultry*
Withdrawal Periods. *Cattle:* slaughter 15 days, milk 72 hours. *Pigs:* slaughter 15 days. *Sheep:* slaughter 15 days. *Poultry:* slaughter 15 days, should not be used in poultry producing eggs for human consumption

Sulfadimidine Sodium Soluble (CCD) *Austral.*
Oral powder, for addition to drinking water, sulfadimidine sodium 1000 g/kg, for *cattle, sheep, pigs, poultry*
Withdrawal Periods. *Cattle:* slaughter 15 days, milk 15 days. *Pigs, sheep:* slaughter 15 days. *Poultry:* slaughter 15 days, should not be used in poultry producing eggs for human consumption

Eire

Indications. Sulfadimethoxine-sensitive infections
Dose. *Cattle, sheep, pigs*: by subcutaneous or intravenous injection, 200 mg/kg, then 100 mg/kg

Intradine (Norbrook) *Eire*
Injection, sulfadimidine sodium 33 1/3%, for *cattle, sheep, pigs*
Withdrawal Periods. *Cattle, sheep, pigs:* slaughter 7 days. *Cattle:* milk 72 hours. Should not be used in sheep producing milk for human consumption

Sulpha No. 2 Powder (Chanelle) *Eire*
Oral powder, sulfadimidine 99%, for *calves*
Withdrawal Periods. Slaughter 28 days

Sulphadimidine 33 1/3 % Injection (Interpharm) *Eire*
Injection, sulfadimide 333 mg/mL, for *cattle, sheep, pigs*
Withdrawal Periods. *Cattle:* slaughter 7 days, milk 72 hours. *Sheep, pigs:* slaughter 7 days

USA

Indications. Sulfadimethoxine-sensitive infections
Dose. Consult manufacturer's information

Bovazine SR Calf Bolus (Vedco) *USA*
Tablets, sulfadimidine 8.25 g, for *cattle*
Withdrawal Periods. Slaughter 8 days, should not be used in cattle producing milk for human comsumption

Bovazine SR Cattle Bolus (Vedco) *USA*
Tablets, sulfadimidine 30 g, for *cattle*
Withdrawal Periods. Slaughter 8 days, should not be used in cattle producing milk for human comsumption

Sodium Sulfamethazine Antibacterial Soluble Powder (DurVet) *USA*
Oral powder, for addition to drinking water, sulfadimidine (contents of 1 pack in 3.785 L water = 125 mg/mL solution), for *cattle, pigs, chickens, turkeys*
Withdrawal Periods. *Cattle:* slaughter 5 days, should not be used in calves under 1 month old and those on all-milk diet,or in dairy cattle under 20 months old. *Pigs:* slaughter 15 days. *Chickens, turkeys:* slaughter 10 days, should not be used in chickens or turkeys producing e

Sulfa-Max III Calf Bolus (AgriLabs) *USA*
Tablets, sulfadimidine 8.25 g, for *cattle*
Withdrawal Periods. Slaughter 8 days, should not be used in cattle producing milk for human consumption

Sulfa-Max III Cattle Bolus (AgriLabs) *USA*
Tablets, sulfadimidine 30 g, for *cattle*
Withdrawal Periods. Slaughter 8 days, should not be used in cattle producing milk for human consumption

Sulfasure SR Calf Bolus (Aspen, Boehringer Ingelheim Vetmedica, Butler, DurVet) *USA*
Tablets, sulfadimidine 8.25 g, for *cattle*
Withdrawal Periods. Slaughter 8 days, should not be used in cattle producing milk for human consumption

Sulfasure SR (Butler, DurVet) *USA*
Tablets, sulfadimidine 30 g, for *cattle*
Withdrawal Periods. Slaughter 8 days, should not be used in cattle producing milk for human consumption

Sulfasure SR Cattle Bolus (Boehringer Ingelheim Vetmedica) *USA*
Tablets, sulfadimidine 30 g, for *cattle*
Withdrawal Periods. Slaughter 8 days, should not be used in cattle producing milk for human consumption

Sulmet Drinking Water Solution 12.5% (Fort Dodge) *USA*
Oral solution, sulfadimidine (as sodium salt) 12.5 %, for *cattle, pigs, chickens, turkeys*
Withdrawal Periods. *Cattle*: slaughter 10 days, should not be used in cattle producing milk for human consumption. *Pigs*: slaughter 15 days. *Chickens, turkeys*: slaughter 10 days, should not be used in chickens and turkeys producing eggs for human consumption

Sulmet Oblets (Fort Dodge) *USA*
Tablets, sulfadimidine 2.5 or 5 g/ tablet, for *horses, cattle*
Withdrawal Periods. Should not be used in *horses* intended for human consumption. *Cattle*: slaughter 10 days

Sulmet Soluble Powder (Fort Dodge) *USA*
Oral powder, for solution, sulfadimidine sodium 100%, for *cattle, pigs, chickens, turkeys*
Withdrawal Periods. *Cattle*: slaughter 10 days, should not be used in cattle producing milk for human consumption. *Pigs*: slaughter 15 days. *Chickens, turkeys*: slaughter 10 days, should not be used in chickens and turkeys producing eggs for human consumption

Suprasulfa III Calf Bolus (RXV) *USA*
Tablets, sulfadimidine 8.02 g, for *cattle*
Withdrawal Periods. Slaughter 12 days, should not be used in cattle producing milk for humanconsumption

Suprasulfa III Calf Bolus (Western Veterinary Supplies) *USA*
Tablets, sulfadimidine 8.25 g, for *cattle*
Withdrawal Periods. Slaughter 8 days, should not be used in cattle producing milk for human consumption

Suprasulfa III Cattle Bolus (Western Veterinary Supplies) *USA*
Tablets, sulfadimidine 30 g, for *cattle*
Withdrawal Periods. Slaughter 8 days, should not be used in cattle producing milk for human consumption

Suprasulfa SR (RXV) *USA*
Tablets, sulfadimidine 30 g, for *cattle*
Withdrawal Periods. Slaughter 8 days, should not be used in cattle producing milk for human consumption

Sustain III (AgriLabs, AgriPharm, DurVet) *USA*
Tablets, sulfadimidine 32.1 g, for *cattle*
Withdrawal Periods. Slaughter 12 days, should not be used in cattle producing milk for humanconsumption

Sustain III Calf Bolus (AgriLabs, AgriPharm, Osborn, Vedco) *USA*
Tablets, sulfadimidine 8.02 g, for *cattle*
Withdrawal Periods. Slaughter 12 days, should not be used in cattle producing milk for humanconsumption

Sustain III Cattle Bolus (Osborn, Vedco) *USA*
Tablets, sulfadimidine 32.1 g, for *cattle*
Withdrawal Periods. Slaughter 12 days, should not be used in cattle producing milk for humanconsumption

SULFAMETHOXYPYRIDAZINE
(Sulphamethoxypyridazine)

UK

Indications. Sulfamethoxypyridazine-sensitive infections; coccidiosis in sheep (see section 1.4.1)
Contra-indications. Side-effects. Warnings. See under Sulfadimidine
Dose. Dosages vary. For guidance.
Cattle, sheep: bacterial infections, *by subcutaneous, intramuscular, or intravenous injection*, 20 mg/kg daily

POM **Bimalong** (Bimeda) *UK*
Injection, sulfamethoxypyridazine (as sodium salt) 250 mg/mL, for *cattle, sheep*; 100 mL, 250 mL
Withdrawal Periods. *Cattle*: slaughter 21 days, milk 2 days. *Sheep*: slaughter 7 days, should not be used in sheep producing milk for human consumption
For intravenous injection in cattle, subcutaneous injection in sheep

POM **Midicel Parenteral** (Pharmacia & Upjohn) *UK*
Injection, sulfamethoxypyridazine 250 mg/mL, for *cattle, sheep*
Withdrawal Periods. *Cattle*: slaughter 7 days, milk 2 days. *Sheep*: slaughter 7 days, should not be used in sheep producing milk for human consumption
For subcutaneous or intramuscular injection

POM **Sulfapyrine LA** (Vétoquinol) *UK*
Injection, sulfamethoxypyridazine 250 mg/mL, for *cattle, sheep*
Withdrawal Periods. *Cattle*: slaughter 21 days, milk 2 days. *Sheep*: slaughter 7 days, should not be used in sheep producing milk for human consumption
For intravenous injection in cattle, subcutaneous injection in sheep

Eire

Indications. Sulfamethoxypyridazine-sensitive infections; coccidiosis in sheep (see section 1.4.1)
Dose. *Cattle, sheep*: *by subcutaneous, intramuscular, or intravenous injection*, 22 mg/kg daily

Midicel Parenteral (Pharmacia & Upjohn) *Eire*
Injection, sulfamethoxypyridazine 250 mg/mL, for *sheep, cattle*
Withdrawal Periods. Sheep: slaughter 7 days, should not be used in sheep producing milk for human consumption. Cattle; slaughter 7 days, milk 48 hours

SULFAMONOMETHOXINE

Eire

Indications. Sulfamonomethoxine-sensitive infections
Dose. *Horses*: *by intravenous injection*, 20 mg/kg
Cattle: *by intramuscular or intravenous injection*, 20 mg/kg

Duphadin S20 (Interchem) *Eire*
Injection, sulfamonomethoxine 20%, for *horses, cattle*
Withdrawal Periods. *Horses*: 7 days. *Cattle*: slaughter 7 days (by iv injection), 14 days (by im injection), milk 48 hours

SULFAQUINOXALINE

USA

Indications. Sulfaquinoxaline-sensitive infections; coccidiosis
Dose. Consult manufactuer's information

Purina Liquid Sulfa-Nox (Purina Mills) *USA*
Solution, for addition to drinking water, sulfaquinoxaline 34.4 mg/mL, for *cattle, sheep, rabbits, poultry*

Withdrawal Periods. *Cattle*: slaughter 10 days, should not be used in cattle producing milk for human consumption. *Sheep, rabbits, chickens, turkeys, pheasant, quail*: slaughter 10 days.

Sulfa-Q 20% Concentrate (RXV) *USA*
Oral solution, for addition to drinking water, sulfaquinoxaline 20 g/100 mL, for *cattle, chickens, turkeys*
Withdrawal Periods. *Cattle*: slaughter 10 days, should not be used in cattle producing milk for human consumption. *Chickens, turkeys*: slaughter 10 days, should not be used in chickens or turkeys producing eggs for human consumption

Sul-Q-Nox (Russell) *USA*
Oral solution, for addition to drinking water, sulfaquinoxaline (as sodium and potassium salts) 319.2 mg/mL, for *cattle, chickens, turkeys*
Withdrawal Periods. *Cattle*: slaughter 10 days, should not be used in cattle producing milk for human consumption, should not be used in calves intended for val production. *Chickens, turkeys*: slaughter 10 days, should not be used in chickens or turkeys producing eggs for human consumption

1.1.6.2 Potentiated sulphonamides

Sulphonamides may be combined with the dihydrofolate reductase inhibitors **baquiloprim**, **ormetoprim**, or **trimethoprim**. They inhibit the conversion of bacterial dihydrofolic acid to tetrahydrofolic acid which is necessary for the synthesis of certain amino acids, purines, and DNA synthesis. Potentiated sulphonamides block sequential stages in the synthesis of tetrahydrofolate and thus have a synergistic antibacterial action. This combination may be bactericidal and allows a smaller dose of sulphonamide to be used. The antibacterial spectrum of the combination is broad and includes a high proportion of anaerobic bacteria, *Nocardia*, *Chlamydia*, and *Toxoplasma* spp. Plasmid-mediated resistance to trimethoprim occurs. Side-effects seen with sulphonamides also occur with potentiated sulphonamide administration.

Compound preparations usually contain 5 parts sulphonamide and one part trimethoprim, baquiloprim, or ormetoprim. The sulphonamides most commonly used in conjunction with trimethoprim are sulfadiazine (co-trimazine) and sulfadoxine, the latter acting for a longer period. Sulfadimidine or sulfadimethoxine are combined with baquiloprim, and sulfadimethoxine with ormetoprim.

Trimethoprim, like the sulphonamides, diffuses well into body tissues and so the combination is the treatment of choice for disorders such as coliform meningitis. Unfortunately, in domesticated animals, trimethoprim is more rapidly inactivated than the sulphonamide component so that useful ratios are present in the body for a short time only. Trimethoprim is active against Gram-negative and Gram-positive bacteria. Trimethoprim is used alone in human medicine in the treatment of urinary tract infections and prostatic infections. The rapid clearance of trimethoprim from the plasma of domestic species makes its use as a sole agent less likely to be successful.

Baquiloprim is however more slowly inactivated and its prolonged half-life more closely matches the half-life of sulfadimidine in cattle and pigs or sulfadimethoxine in dogs and cats.

Ormetoprim has been less well studied in domestic animals but appears to have similar pharmacokinetic properties to trimethoprim in those species in which it has been studied

(horses and cattle) such that the drug is more rapidly cleared from the plasma than the sulphonamides with which it is combined.

Trimethoprim (and possibly baquiloprim) retain some slight activity on mammalian dihydrofolate reductase and so may predispose to a folate deficiency and hence to a reduction in bone marrow function. Intravenous administration of potentiated sulphonamides may precipitate collapse in horses and cattle.

BAQUILOPRIM with SULFADIMETHOXINE

UK
Indications. Baquiloprim/sulfadimethoxine-sens-itive infections
Contra-indications. Sulphonamide hypersensitivity, severe hepatic impairment, blood dyscrasias
Side-effects. Transient pain at injection site
Warnings. Ensure free access to water, coated tablets should not be divided or crushed
Dose. Expressed as baquiloprim + sulfadimethoxine
Dogs: *by mouth*, 30 mg/kg on alternate days
by subcutaneous injection, 12 mg/kg daily *or* 30 mg/kg at 3-day intervals
Cats: *by mouth*, 20–40 mg/kg once daily
by subcutaneous injection, 20 mg/kg as a single dose. Further oral treatment may be given after 12 hours

POM **Zaquilan** (Schering-Plough) *UK*
Tablets, coated, baquiloprim 10 mg, sulfadimethoxine 50 mg, for *dogs, cats more than 1.5 kg body-weight*; 96
Tablets, scored, baquiloprim 100 mg, sulfadimethoxine 500 mg, for *dogs*; 48

Eire
Indications. Baquiloprim/sulfadimethoxine-sens-itive infections
Dose. Expressed as baquiloprim + sulfadimethoxine
Dogs: *by mouth*, 30 mg/kg

Zaquilan 60 mg Tablets for Dogs (Schering-Plough) *Eire*
Tablets, baquiloprim 10 mg, sulfadimethoxine 50 mg, for *dogs*

Zaquilan 600 mg Tablets for Dogs (Schering-Plough) *Eire*
Tablets, baquiloprim 100 mg, sulfadimethoxine 500 mg, for *dogs*

BAQUILOPRIM with SULFADIMIDINE

UK
Indications.   Baquiloprim/sulfadimidine-sensitive infections
Contra-indications. Sulphonamide hypersensitivity, severe hepatic impairment, renal impairment, blood dyscrasias
Warnings. Coated tablets should not be divided or crushed
Dose. Expressed as baquiloprim + sulfadimidine
Cattle: *by mouth*, 40–80 mg/kg

POM **Zaquilan 15 g 2 day** (Schering-Plough)
Tablets, scored, baquiloprim 800 mg, sulfadimidine 7.2 g, for *cattle*; 30
Withdrawal Periods. *Cattle*: slaughter 28 days, should not be used in cattle producing milk for human consumption

Eire

Indications. Baquiloprim/sulfadimidine-sensitive infections
Dose. Consult manufacturer's information

Zaquilan 15 g 2 Day Bolus for Cattle (Schering-Plough) *Eire*
Tablets, baquiloprim 0.8 g, sulfadimidine 7.2 g, for *cattle*
Withdrawal Periods. Slaughter 28 days, should not be used in cattle producing milk for human consumption

Zaquilan 20% Injection for Cattle (Schering-Plough) *Eire*
Injection, baquiloprim 33.3 mg/mL, sulfadimidine 166.7 mg/mL, for *cattle*
Withdrawal Periods. Slaughter 28 days, milk 4 days

New Zealand

Indications. Baquiloprim/sulfadimidine-sensitive infections
Dose. Consult manufacturer's information

Zaquilan (Schering-Plough) *NZ*
Tablets, baquiloprim 0.8 g, sulfadimidine 7.2 g, for *cattle*
Withdrawal Periods. Slaughter 28 days, should not be used in cattle producing milk for human consumption

Zaquilan 20% (Schering-Plough) *NZ*
Injection, baquiloprim 33.3 mg/mL, sulfadimidine 41.7 mg/mL, sulfadimidine sodium 134.9 mg/mL, for *cattle*
Withdrawal Periods. Slaughter 35 days, milk 108 hours

ORMETOPRIM WITH SULFADIMETHOXINE

USA

Indications. Ormetoprim/sulfadimethoxine-sensitive infections; coccidiosis
Dose. Consult manufacturer's information

Primor (Pfizer) *USA*
Tablets, ormetoprim 40 mg, sulphadimethoxine 200 mg; ormetoprim 100 mg, , sulphadimethoxine 500 mg; ormetoprim 200 mg, , sulphadimethoxine 1000 mg, for *dogs*

Rofenaid 40 (Roche Vitamins) *USA*
Premix, ormetoprim 150 mg/g, sulfadimethoxine 250 mg/g, for *chickens, turkeys, ducks*
Withdrawal Periods. Slaughter 5 days, should not be used in chickens, turkeys, ducks producing eggs for human consumption

SULFADIAZINE with TRIMETHOPRIM

(Co-trimazine: preparations of trimethoprim and sulfadiazine in the proportions, by weight, of 1 part to 5 parts)

UK

Indications. Sulfadiazine/trimethoprim-sensitive infections
Contra-indications. Sulphonamide hypersensitivity, severe hepatic impairment, blood dyscrasias, horses with drug-induced cardiac arrhythmias, dogs with keratoconjunctivitis sicca, oral administration to calves with a functional rumen
Side-effects. Occasional transient polyarthritis and keratoconjunctivitis sicca in dogs, drowsiness in cats
Warnings. Drug Interactions – see Appendix 1; the drug may cause salivation in cats and coated tablets should be fed whole, should not be halved, crushed, or chipped; ensure sufficient water intake to avoid crystalluria
Dose. Dosages vary. For guidance.
Expressed as trimethoprim + sulfadiazine
Horses, cattle: *by mouth*, 30 mg/kg daily
by intramuscular or slow intravenous injection, 15–24 mg/kg daily
Sheep: *by intramuscular or slow intravenous injection*, 15–24 mg/kg daily
Pigs: *by mouth*, 30 mg/kg body-weight daily
by addition to feed, 300–450 g/tonne feed
by intramuscular or slow intravenous injection, 15–24 mg/kg daily
Dogs, cats: *by mouth or by subcutaneous injection*, 30 mg/kg daily
Poultry: *by addition to drinking water*, 15 mg/kg body-weight daily
by addition to feed, 300 g/tonne feed
Fish: see Prescribing for fish for preparation details and dosage

POM Delvoprim Coject (Intervet) *UK*
Injection, sulfadiazine 200 mg, trimethoprim 40 mg/mL, for *horses, cattle, sheep, pigs, dogs, cats*; 100 mL
Withdrawal Periods. Should not be used in *horses* intended for human consumption. *Cattle*: slaughter 10 days, milk 2.5 days. *Sheep*: slaughter 18 days. *Pigs*: slaughter 10 days

POM Delvoprim Horse Paste (Intervet) *UK*
Oral paste, sulfadiazine 1.25 g, trimethoprim 250 mg /division, for *horses*; 45-g metered-dose applicator
Withdrawal Periods. Should not be used in *horses* intended for human consumption

POM Delvoprim Piglet Suspension (Intervet) *UK*
Oral suspension, sulfadiazine 50 mg, trimethoprim 10 mg/unit dose, for *piglets*; 250-mL dose applicator (1 unit dose = 1.1 mL)
Withdrawal Periods. *Piglets*: slaughter 28 days

POM Delvoprim Tablets (Intervet) *UK*
Tablets, s/c, sulfadiazine 100 mg, trimethoprim 20 mg, for *dogs, cats*
Tablets, scored, sulfadiazine 400 mg, trimethoprim 80 mg, for *dogs*

POM Duphatrim (Fort Dodge) *UK*
Tablets, s/c, sulfadiazine 100 mg, trimethoprim 20 mg, for *dogs, cats*; 100
Tablets, scored, sulfadiazine 400 mg, trimethoprim 80 mg, for *dogs*; 100, 500
Tablets, or to prepare an oral solution, scored, sulfadiazine 1 g, trimethoprim 200 mg, for *calves*; 20
Withdrawal Periods. *Calves*: slaughter 28 days

POM Duphatrim Equine Formula (Fort Dodge) *UK*
Oral paste, sulfadiazine 1.3 g, trimethoprim 260 mg/division, for *horses*; 45-g metered-dose applicator
Withdrawal Periods. Should not be used in *horses* intended for human consumption

POM Duphatrim Granules for Horses (Fort Dodge) *UK*
Oral granules, for addition to feed, sulfadiazine 12.5 g, trimethoprim 2.5 g/sachet, for *horses*; 37.5-g sachets
Withdrawal Periods. Should not be used in *horses* intended for human consumption

POM Duphatrim IS (Fort Dodge) *UK*
Injection, sulfadiazine 200 mg, trimethoprim 40 mg/mL, for *horses, cattle, sheep, pigs, dogs, cats*; 100 mL
Withdrawal Periods. Should not be used in *horses* intended for human consumption. *Cattle*: slaughter 10 days, milk 2.5 days. *Sheep*: slaughter 18 days, should not be used in sheep producing milk for human consumption. *Pigs*: slaughter 10 days

POM **Duphatrim Piglet Suspension** (Fort Dodge)
Oral suspension, sulfadiazine 50 mg, trimethoprim 10 mg/unit dose, for *piglets*; 250-mL dose applicator (1 unit dose = 1.1 mL)
Withdrawal Periods. *Piglets*: slaughter 28 days

POM **Equitrim Granules** (Boehringer Ingelheim) *UK*
Oral granules, sulfadiazine 12.5 g, trimethoprim 2.5 g/sachet, for *horses*; 37.5-g sachet
Withdrawal Periods. Should not be used in *horses* intended for human consumption

POM **Equitrim Equine Paste** (Boehringer Ingelheim) *UK*
Oral paste, sulfadiazine 1.25 g, trimethoprim 250 mg /division, for *horses*; 45-g metered-dose applicator
Withdrawal Periods. Should not be used in *horses* intended for human consumption

POM **Norodine** (Norbrook) *UK*
Tablets, s/c, sulfadiazine 100 mg, trimethoprim 20 mg, for *dogs, cats*; 100
Tablets, scored, sulfadiazine 400 mg, trimethoprim 80 mg, for *dogs*; 100, 500
Tablets, or to prepare an oral solution, scored, sulfadiazine 1 g, trimethoprim 200 mg, for *calves*; 20, 50
Withdrawal Periods. *Calves*: slaughter 28 days

POM **Norodine 24** (Norbrook) *UK*
Injection, sulfadiazine 200 mg, trimethoprim 40 mg/mL, for *horses, cattle, sheep, pigs, dogs, cats*; 50 mL, 100 mL
Withdrawal Periods. Should not be used in *horses* intended for human consumption. *Cattle*: slaughter 10 days, milk 2.5 days. *Sheep*: slaughter 18 days, should not be used in sheep producing milk for human consumption. *Pigs*: slaughter 10 days

POM **Norodine Granules** (Norbrook) *UK*
Oral granules, for addition to feed, sulfadiazine 12.5 g, trimethoprim 2.5 g/ sachet, for horses; 37.5-g sachet
Withdrawal Periods. Should not be used in *horses* intended for human consumption

POM **Norodine Equine Paste** (Norbrook) *UK*
Oral paste, sulfadiazine 1.25 g, trimethoprim 250 mg /division, for *horses*; 45-g metered-dose applicator
Withdrawal Periods. Should not be used in *horses* intended for human consumption

POM **Norodine Oral Piglet Suspension** (Norbrook) *UK*
Oral suspension, sulfadiazine 50 mg, trimethoprim 10 mg/unit dose, for *piglets*; 250-mL dose applicator (1 unit dose = 1.1 mL)
Withdrawal Periods. *Piglets*: slaughter 28 days

POM **Scorprin Bolus** (Fort Dodge) *UK*
Tablets, scored, sulfadiazine 1 g, trimethoprim 200 mg, for *calves*; 20
Withdrawal Periods. *Calves*: slaughter 5 days

POM **Strinacin II** (Merial) *UK*
Tablets, or to prepare an oral solution, scored, sulfadiazine 1 g, trimethoprim 200 mg, for *calves*; 20
Withdrawal Periods. *Calves*: slaughter 28 days

POM **Synutrim-300** (Vericore LP) *UK*
Oral powder, for addition to feed, sulfadiazine 250 g, trimethoprim 50 g/kg, for *chickens*; 2 kg, 3 kg, other sizes available
Withdrawal Periods. *Chickens*: slaughter 5 days, should not be used in laying hens

POM **Synutrim Fortesol** (Vericore LP) *UK*
Oral powder, for addition to drinking water, sulfadiazine (as sodium salt) 625 g, trimethoprim 125 g/kg, for *pigs, chickens*; 150 g, 2 kg
Withdrawal Periods. *Pigs*: slaughter 5 days. *Chickens*: slaughter 5 days, eggs from treated birds should not be used for human consumption

POM **Synutrim Granular** (Vericore LP) *UK*
Oral granules, for addition to feed, sulfadiazine 250 g, trimethoprim 50 g/kg, for *pigs, chickens, turkeys*
Withdrawal Periods. *Pigs*: slaughter 10 days. *Chickens*: slaughter 5 days, should not be used in birds producing eggs for human consumption. *Turkeys*: slaughter 2 days

POM **Tribrissen** (Schering-Plough) *UK*
Tablets, s/c, sulfadiazine 100 mg, trimethoprim 20 mg, for *dogs, cats more than 1 kg body-weight*; 100
Tablets, scored, sulfadiazine 400 mg, trimethoprim 80 mg, for *dogs*

POM **Tribrissen 24%/48%** (Schering-Plough) *UK*
Injection, sulfadiazine 200 mg, trimethoprim 40 mg/mL, for *dogs, cats*; 50 mL
Injection, sulfadiazine 400 mg, trimethoprim 80 mg/mL, for *horses, cattle, pigs*; 100 mL
Withdrawal Periods. Should not be used in *horses* intended for human consumption. *Cattle*: slaughter 28 days, milk 2 days. *Pigs*: slaughter 28 days

POM **Tribrissen Boluses** (Schering-Plough) *UK*
Tablets, or to prepare an oral solution, scored, sulfadiazine 1 g, trimethoprim 200 mg, for *horses, calves*; 10
Withdrawal Periods. Should not be used in *horses* intended for human consumption. *Calves*: slaughter 8 days, should not be used in lactating cattle

POM **Tribrissen Oral Paste** (Schering-Plough) *UK*
Oral paste, sulfadiazine 1.25 g, trimethoprim 250 mg/division, for *horses*; 37.5-g metered-dose applicator
Withdrawal Periods. Should not be used in *horses* intended for human consumption

POM **Tribrissen Piglet Suspension** (Schering-Plough) *UK*
Oral suspension, sulfadiazine 50 mg, trimethoprim 10 mg/unit dose, for *piglets*; 200-mL dose applicator (1 unit dose = 1.1 mL)
Withdrawal Periods. *Piglets*: slaughter 5 days

POM **Trimabac** (Vericore VP) *UK*
Tablets, s/c, sulfadiazine 100 mg, trimethoprim 20 mg, for *dogs, cats*; 100, 1000
Tablets, scored, sulfadiazine 400 mg, trimethoprim 80 mg, for *dogs*; 500
Tablets, or to prepare an oral solution, scored, sulfadiazine 1 g, trimethoprim 200 mg,for *calves*; 20
Withdrawal Periods. *Calves*: slaughter 28 days

POM **Trimabac Injection 24%** (Vericore VP) *UK*
Injection, sulfadiazine 200 mg, trimethoprim 40 mg/mL, for *horses, cattle, sheep, pigs, dogs, cats*; 100 mL
Withdrawal Periods. Should not be used in *horses* intended for human consumption. *Cattle*: slaughter 10 days, milk 2.5 days. *Sheep*: slaughter 18 days. *Pigs*: slaughter 10 days

POM **Trimacare** (Animalcare) *UK*
Tablets, sulfadiazine 100 mg, trimethoprim 20 mg, for *dogs, cats*
Tablets, scored, sulfadiazine 400 mg, trimethoprim 80 mg, for *dogs*
Tablets, or to prepare an oral solution, scored, sulfadiazine 1 g, trimethoprim 200 mg,for *calves*
Withdrawal Periods. *Calves*: slaughter 28 days

POM**Trimacare 24%** (Animalcare) *UK*
Injection, sulfadiazine 200 mg, trimethoprim 40 mg/mL, for *horses, cattle, sheep, pigs, dogs, cats*
Withdrawal Periods. Should not be used in *horses* intended for human consumption. *Cattle*: slaughter 10 days, milk 2.5 days. *Sheep*: slaughter 18 days, should not be used in sheep producing milk for human consumption. *Pigs*: slaughter 10 days

POM **Trimediazine 15** (Vétoquinol) *UK*
Oral powder, sulfadiazine 125 g, trimethoprim 25 g/kg, for *pigs, chickens, turkeys*; 2 kg, 6 kg, other sizes available
Withdrawal Periods. *Pigs*: slaughter 7 days. *Chickens*: slaughter 1 day, should not be used in birds producing eggs for human consumption. *Turkeys*: slaughter 3 days

POM **Trimediazine BMP** (Vétoquinol) *UK*
Oral powder, for addition to feed, sulfadiazine 125 g, trimethoprim 25 g/kg, for *pigs, chickens, turkeys*; 2 kg, 6 kg, other sizes available
Withdrawal Periods. *Pigs*: slaughter 7 days. *Chickens*: slaughter 1 day, should not be used in birds producing eggs for human consumption. *Turkeys*: slaughter 3 days

POM **Trimediazine Paste** (Vétoquinol) *UK*
Oral paste, sulfadiazine 1.3 g, trimethoprim 260 mg/division, for *horses*; 45-g metered-dose applicator

Withdrawal Periods. Should not be used in *horses* intended for human consumption

POM Trimediazine Piglet Suspension (Vétoquinol) *UK*
Oral suspension, sulfadiazine 50.05 mg, trimethoprim 10.01 mg/unit dose, for *piglets*; 250-mL dose applicator (1 unit dose = 1.1 mL)
Withdrawal Periods. *Pigs*: slaughter 28 days

POM Trimediazine Plain (Vétoquinol) *UK*
Oral powder, for addition to feed, sulfadiazine 250 mg, trimethoprim 50 mg/g, for *horses*; 50 g
Withdrawal Periods. Should not be used in *horses* intended for human consumption

POM Trimedoxine 4S (Vétoquinol) *UK*
Tablets, or to prepare an oral solution, sulfadiazine, trimethoprim, for *calves*; 20
Withdrawal Periods. *Calves*: slaughter 28 days
Dose. *Calves*: by mouth, 1 tablet/40 kg body-weight

POM Trimedoxine Injection (Vétoquinol) *UK*
Injection, sulfadiazine 200 mg, trimethoprim 40 mg/mL, for *horses, cattle, sheep, pigs, dogs, cats*; 50 mL, 100 mL
Withdrawal Periods. Should not be used in *horses* intended for human consumption. *Cattle*: slaughter 10 days, milk 2.5 days. *Sheep*: slaughter 18 days. *Pigs*: slaughter 10 days

POM Trimedoxine Tablets (Vétoquinol) *UK*
Tablets, s/c, sulfadiazine 100 mg, trimethoprim 20 mg, for *dogs, cats*; 100
Tablets, scored, sulfadiazine 400 mg, trimethoprim 80 mg, for *dogs*; 100, 500

POM Trinacol (Boehringer Ingelheim) *UK*
Injection, sulfadiazine 200 mg, trimethoprim 40 mg/mL, for *cattle, sheep, pigs, dogs*; 100 mL
Withdrawal Periods. *Cattle*: slaughter 10 days, milk 2.5 days. *Sheep*: slaughter 18 days, should not be used in sheep producing milk for human consumption. *Pigs*: slaughter 10 days

MFS Uniprim 150S (Pharmacia & Upjohn) *UK*
Oral powder, for addition to feed, sulfadiazine 125 g, trimethoprim 25 g/kg, for *pigs, non-laying chickens, turkeys*
Withdrawal Periods. *Pigs*: slaughter 5 days. *Chickens*: slaughter 1 day. *Turkeys*: slaughter 10 days. Should not be used in birds producing eggs for human consumption

POM Uniprim for Horses (Pharmacia & Upjohn) *UK*
Oral powder, for addition to feed, sulfadiazine 12.5 g, trimethoprim 2.5 g/sachet, for *horses*; 37.5-g sachet
Withdrawal Periods. Should not be used in *horses* intended for human consumption

POM Ventipulmin TMP/S (Boehringer Ingelheim) *UK*
Oral powder, for addition to feed, clenbuterol 21.44 micrograms, sulfadiazine 335 mg, trimethoprim 67 mg/g, for *horses*; 190 g
Withdrawal Periods. Should not be used in *horses* intended for human consumption
Dose. *Horses*: 9 g (measure provided) of powder/250 kg body-weight twice daily

Australia

Indications. Sulfadiazine/trimethoprim-sensitive infections
Dose. Consult manufacturer's information

A.F.S. Trimsul (Controlled Medications) *Austral.*
Oral solution, for dilution, sulfadiazine 400 g/kL and trimethoprim 80 g/kL solution, for *poultry, pigeons*
Withdrawal Periods. *Chicken, turkeys, pigeons*: slaughter 14 days, should not be used in poultry producing eggs for human consumption

Tribrissen Bolus/Pessary (Jurox) *Austral.*
Pessary/Tablet, sulfadiazine 1000 mg, trimethoprim 200 mg, for *cattle, horses, sheep, pigs*

Withdrawal Periods. *Cattle*: slaughter 14 days, milk 36 hours (single dose) or 72 hours (multiple dose). *Horses, sheep, pigs*: slaughter 14 days

Tribrissen Piglet Suspension (Jurox) *Austral.*
Oral suspension, trimethoprim 10 mg/mL, sulfadiazine 50 mg/mL, for *pigs, dogs*
Withdrawal Periods. Slaughter 14 days

Trimethosol Powder (Agrotech) *Austral.*
Powder, for addition to drinking water, sulfadiazine sodium 440 g/kg and trimethoprim 80 g/kg powder, for *chickens, turkeys, pigs*
Withdrawal Periods. *Pigs*: slaughter 14 days. *Poultry*: slaughter 14 days, should not be used in poultry producing eggs for human consumption

Tribrissen Injection (Jurox) *Austral.*
Injection, sulfadiazine 400 mg/mL, trimethoprim 80 mg/mL, for *cattle, sheep, pigs, horses*
Withdrawal Periods. *Cattle*: slaughter 14 days, milk 36 hours (single dose) or 72 hours (multiple dose). *Sheep, pigs, horses*: slaughter 14 days.

Tribrissen Tablets (Jurox) *Austral.*
Tablets, sulfadiazine/ trimethoprim, 100 mg/20 mg and 400 mg/80 mg, for *dogs, cats*

Tribrissen Water Medication (Jurox) *Austral.*
Liquid, for addition to drinking water, sulfadiazine 400 g/L, trimethoprim 80 g/L, for *pigs, chickens, turkeys*
Withdrawal Periods. *Pigs*: slaughter 14 days. *Poultry*: slaughter 14 days, should not be used in poultry producing eggs for human consumption

Tridexine-S (Bioceuticals) *Austral.*
Oral powder, sulfadiazine 650 mg/g, trimethoprim 130 mg/g, bromhexine hydrochloride 5.5 mg/g powder, for *horses*
Withdrawal Periods. Slaughter 28 days

Trimethotab 120 (Pharmtech) *Austral.*
Tablets, sulfadiazine 100 mg, trimethoprim 20 mg, for *dogs, cats*

Trimethotab 480 (Pharmtech) *Austral.*
Tablets, sulfadiazine 400 mg, trimethoprim 80 mg, for *dogs*

Tridiazine Oral Paste (Jurox) *Austral.*
Oral paste, sulfadiazine 333 mg/g, trimethoprim 67 mg/g, for *horses*
Withdrawal Periods. Slaughter 28 days

Trimazine Boluses (Apex) *Austral.*
Tablets, sulfadiazine 1000 mg, trimethoprim 200 mg/ pessary/tablet, for *cattle, horses, sheep, pigs*
Withdrawal Periods. *Cattle*: slaughter 14 days, milk 36 hours (single dose) or 72 hours (multiple dose). *Sheep, pigs, horses*: slaughter 14 days

Trimethosol Suspension (Agrotech) *Austral.*
Oral suspension, for addition to drinking water, sulfadiazine sodium 440 g/L and trimethoprim 80 g/L, for *chickens, turkeys, pigs*
Withdrawal Periods. *Pigs*: slaughter 14 days. *Poultry*: slaughter 14 days, should not be used in poultry producing eggs for human consumption

Trizine Oral Powder For Horses (Delvet) *Austral.*
Oral granules, sulfadiazine 650 mg/g and trimethoprim 130 mg/g granules, for *horses*
Withdrawal Periods. Horses: slaughter 28 days

Norodine 24 Injection (Novartis) *Austral.*
Injection, sulfadiazine 200 mg/mL, trimethoprim 40 mg/mL, for *horses, cattle, sheep, pigs, dogs, cats*
Withdrawal Periods. *Cattle*: slaughter 10 days, milk 72 hours. *Sheep*: slaughter 10 days. *Pigs*: slaughter 15 days

Sulphatrim (International Animal Health Products) *Austral.*
Powder, for addition to drinking water, sulfadiazine 400 g/kg, trimethoprim 80 g/kg powder, for *horses, cattle, sheep, pigs, chickens, turkeys*
Withdrawal Periods. *Cattle*: slaughter 14 days, milk 7 days. *Pigs*: slaughter 15 days. *Horses, sheep*: slaughter 14 days. *Poultry*: slaughter 14 days, should not be used in poultry producing eggs for human consumption

Tribactral Duals (Jurox) *Austral.*
Pessary/Tablet, sulfadiazine 1000 mg, trimethoprim 200 mg, for *horses, cattle, sheep*

Withdrawal Periods. *Cattle*: slaughter 14 days, milk 36 hour (single dose) or 72 hours (multiple dose). *Horses, sheep*: slaughter 14 days

Tribactral Injection (Jurox) *Austral.*
Injection, sulfadiazine 400 mg/mL, trimethoprim 80 mg/mL, for *horses, cattle, sheep, pigs*
Withdrawal Periods. *Cattle*: slaughter 14 days, milk 36 hours (single dose) or 72 hours (multiple dose). *Horses, sheep, pigs*: slaughter 14 days

Trimazine L/S Tablets (Apex) *Austral.*
Tablets, sulfadiazine 100 mg, trimethoprim 20 mg, for *dogs, cats*

Trimazine Tablets (Apex) *Austral.*
Tablets, sulfadiazine 400 mg, trimethoprim 80 mg, for *dogs*

Trisoprim (Ilium) *Austral.*
Tablets, sulfadiazine 400 mg, trimethoprim 80 mg, for *dogs*

Trisoprim-480 (Ilium) *Austral.*
Injection, sulfadiazine 400 mg/mL, trimethoprim 80 mg/mL, for *horses, cattle, sheep, pigs*
Withdrawal Periods. *Cattle*: slaughter 14 days, milk 36 hours (single dose) or 72 hours (multiple dose). *Horses, sheep, pigs*: slaughter 14 days

Trizine 120 Tablets (Delvet) *Austral.*
Tablets, sulfadiazine 100 mg, trimethoprim 20 mg, for *dogs, cats*

Trizine 480 Caplets (Delvet) *Austral.*
Tablets, sulfadiazine 400 mg, trimethoprim 80 mg, for *dogs*

Ventipulmin + TMPS (Boehringer Ingelheim) *Austral.*
Oral powder, sulfadiazine 33.5 g, trimethoprim 6.7 g, clenbuterol/100 g powder, for *horses*
Withdrawal Periods. Should not be used in *horses* intended for human consumption

Eire

Indications. Sulfadiazine/trimethoprim-sensitive infections

Aprimazine (Bioceuticals) *Austral.*
Oral powder, sulfadiazine 650 mg/g, trimethoprim 130 mg/g powder, for *horses*
Withdrawal Periods. Slaughter 28 days

Aquaprim Injection (Univet) *Eire*
Injection, sulfadiazine 200 mg/mL, trimethroprim 40 mg/mL, for *cattle, pigs*
Withdrawal Periods. *Cattle*: slaughter 25 days, milk 72 hours. *Pigs*: slaughter 25 days

Chanoprim Bolus (Chanelle) *Eire*
Oral bolus, trimethoprim 200 mg, sulfadiazine 1 g, for *horses, calves, sheep*
Withdrawal Periods. Should not be used in *horses* intended for human consumption. *Cattle*: slaughter 21 days. *Sheep*: slaughter 21 days, should not be used in sheep producing milk for human consumption

Chanoprim Injection (Chanelle) *Eire*
Injection, trimethoprim 40 mg/mL, sulfadiazine 200 mg/mL, for *cattle, pigs*
Withdrawal Periods. *Cattle*: slaughter 25 days, milk 72 hours. *Pigs*: slaughter 25 days

Delvoprim Bolus (Intervet) *Eire*
Oral bolus, trimethoprim 200 mg, sulfadiazine 1 g, for *calves*
Withdrawal Periods. Slaughter 30 days

Delvoprim Coject (Intervet) *Eire*
Injection, trimethoprim 40 mg/mL, sulfadiazine 200 mg/mL, for *horses, cattle, sheep, pigs, dogs, cats*
Withdrawal Periods. Should not be used in *horses* intended for human consumption. *Cattle*: slaughter 10 days, milk 48 hours. *Sheep*: slaughter 18 days, should not be used in sheep producing milk for human consumption. *Pigs*: slaughter 10 days

Delvoprim Tablets (Intervet) *Eire*
Tablets, 120: trimethoprim 20 mg, sulfadiazine 100 mg; 480: trimethoprim 80 mg, sulfadiazine 400 mg, for *dogs, cats*

Equitrim Equine Paste (Boehringer Ingelheim) *Eire*
Oral paste, per 45 g syringe: trimethoprim 2.6 g, sulfadiazine 13.0 g, for *horses*
Withdrawal Periods. Slaughter 28 days

Equitrim Granules (Boehringer Ingelheim) *Eire*
Oral granules, sulfadiazine 333.3 mg/g, trimethoprim 66.7 mg/g, for *horses*
Withdrawal Periods. Slaughter 28 days

InterTrim Bolus (Interpharm) *Eire*
Tablets, trimethoprim 200 mg, sulphadiazine 1 g, for *calves*
Withdrawal Periods. Slaughter 30 days, should not be used in cattle producing milk for human consumption

InterTrim Injection (Interpharm) *Eire*
Injection, trimethoprim 40 mg/mL, sulphadiazine, for *horses, cattle, sheep, pigs, dogs, cats*
Withdrawal Periods. Should not be used in *horses* intended for human consumption. *Cattle*: slaughter 18 days, milk 48 hours. *Sheep, pigs*: slaughter 18 days

Norodine 120 mg Tablets (Norbrook) *Eire*
Tablets, sulfadiazine 100 mg, trimethoprim 20 mg, for *dogs, cats*

Norodine 480 mg Tablets (Norbrook) *Eire*
Tablets, sulfadiazine 400 mg, trimethoprim 80 mg, for *dogs*

Norodine 24% (Norbrook) *Eire*
Injection, sulfadiazine 200 mg/mL, trimethoprim 40 mg/mL, for *horses, cattle, sheep, pigs, dogs, cats*
Withdrawal Periods. Should not be used in *horses* intended for human consumption. *Cattle*: slaughter 10 days, milk 48 hours. *Sheep*: slaughter 18 days, should not be used in sheep producing milk for human consumption. *Pigs*: slaughter 10 days

Norodine Bolus (Norbrook) *Eire*
Tablets, sulfadiazine 1 g, trimethoprim 200 mg, for *calves*
Withdrawal Periods. Slaughter 30 days

Norodine Equine Paste (Norbrook) *Eire*
Oral paste, sulfadiazine 13 g, trimethoprim 2.6 g, for *horses*
Withdrawal Periods. Slaughter 28 days

Noroprim Granules (Norbrook) *Eire*
Oral granules, to mix with feed, per 37.5-g sachet: sulfadiazine 12.5 g, trimethoprim 2.5 g, for *horses*
Withdrawal Periods. Slaughter 28 days

Norodine Oral Piglet Suspension (Norbrook) *Eire*
Oral suspension, sulfadiazine 45.5 mg, trimethoprim 9.10 mg, for *piglets*
Withdrawal Periods. Slaughter 28 days

Olab Sultrim 21% Premix (Oldcastle) *Eire*
Premix, sulphadiazine 178.4 g/kg, trimethoprim 35.6 g/kg, for *pigs*
Withdrawal Periods. Slaughter 7 days

Septotryl II (Vetoquinol) *Eire*
Injection, sulfadiazine 200 mg/mL, trimethroprim 40 mg/mL, for *horses, cattle, sheep, pigs, dogs, cats*
Withdrawal Periods. Should not be used in *horses* intended for human consumption. *Cattle*: slaughter 10 days, milk 48 hours. *Sheep*: slaughter 18 days, should not be used in sheep producing milk for human consumption. *Pigs*: slaughter 10 days

Strinaxin Tablets (Merial) *Eire*
Tablets, sulfadiazine 1.0 g, trimethroprim 200 mg, for *calves*
Withdrawal Periods. Slaughter 30 days

Sulfoprim 15% Meal Mix (Univet) *Eire*
Premix, sulfadiazine 125 g/kg, trimethoprim 25 g/kg, for *pigs*
Withdrawal Periods. Pigs: slaughter 10 days

Sulfoprim 21% Meal Mix (Univet) *Eire*
Premix, sulfadiazine 178.4 g/kg, trimethoprim 35.6 g/kg, for *pigs*
Withdrawal Periods. Slaughter 7 days

Synutrim Bolus (Cypharm) *Eire*
Bolus, trimethoprim 200 mg, sulphadiazine 1 g, for *horses, cattle, sheep*

Withdrawal Periods. Should not be used in *horses* intended for human consumption. *Cattle*: slaughter 21 days. *Sheep*: slaughter 21 days, should not be used in sheep producing milk for human consumption

Synutrim 300 (Cypharm) *Eire*
Oral powder, to mix with feed, trimethoprim, sulphadiazine, for *poultry*
Withdrawal Periods. Slaughter 5 days

Synutrim 30% Soluble (Cypharm) *Eire*
Oral powder, for addition to drinking water or milk, trimethoprim, sodium sulphadiazine, for *calves*
Withdrawal Periods. Slaughter 10 days

Tribrissen Boluses (Schering-Plough) *Eire*
Tablets, sulfadiazine 1.0 g, trimethoprim 0.2 g, for *calves*
Withdrawal Periods. Slaughter 8 days, should not be used in cattle producing milk for human consumption

Tribrissen Oral Paste (Schering-Plough) *Eire*
Oral paste, per 37.5-g syringe: sulfadiazine 12.5 g, trimethoprim 2.5 g, for *horses*
Withdrawal Periods. Slaughter 6 days

Trimediazine 30 (Vetoquinol) *Eire*
Oral powder, for addition to feed, sulfadiazine 250 mg/g, trimethoprim 50 mg/g, for *horses*
Withdrawal Periods. Should not be used in *horses* intended for human consumption

Trinacol Injection (Boehringer Ingelheim) *Eire*
Injection, sulfadiazine 200 mg/mL, trimethoprim 40 mg/mL, for *cattle, sheep, pigs, dogs*
Withdrawal Periods. *Cattle*: slaughter 10 days, milk 60 hours. *Sheep*: slaughter 18 days, should not be used in sheep producing milk for human consumption. *Pigs*: slaughter 10 days

Uniprim 150 (Pharmacia & Upjohn) *Eire*
Premix, sulfadiazine 125 g/kg, trimethoprim 25 g/kg, for *pigs, chickens*
Withdrawal Periods. *Pigs*: slaughter 5 days. *Chickens*: slaughter 24 hours, should not be used in chickens producing eggs for human consumption

Uniprim for Horses (Pharmacia & Upjohn) *Eire*
Oral powder, per 37.5-g sachet: sulfadiazine 12.5 g, trimethoprim 2.5 g, for *horses*
Withdrawal Periods. Should not be used in horses intended for human consumption

Ventipulmin TMP/S (Boehringer Ingelheim) *Eire*
Oral powder, clenbuterol hydrochloride 21.44 micrograms/g, sulfadiazine 335 mg/g, trimethoprim 67 mg/g, for *horses*
Withdrawal Periods. Slaughter 28 days

New Zealand
Indications. Sulfadiazine/trimethoprim-sensitive infections
Dose. Consult manufacturer's information

Aquaprim (Ethical) *NZ*
Injection, sulfadiazine 200 mg/mL, trimethoprim 40 mg/mL, for *cattle, pigs*
Withdrawal Periods. *Cattle*: slaughter 35 days, milk 72 hours. *Pigs*: slaughter 35 days

Norodine 24 (Bomac) *NZ*
Injection, sulfadiazine 200 mg/mL, trimethoprim 40 mg/mL, for *horses, cattle, sheep, pigs, dogs, cats*
Withdrawal Periods. *Horses, pigs*: slaughter 18 days. *Cattle*: slaughter 18 days, milk 48 hours. *Sheep*: slaughter 18 days, should not be used in sheep producing milk for human consumption

Tribactral (Jurox) *NZ*
Tablets, sulfadiazine 400 mg, trimethoprim 80 mg, for *all species, except cats, fish*

Tribrissen (Jurox) *NZ*
Oral paste, sulfadiazine 333 mg/g, trimethoprim 67 mg/g, for *horses, cattle*
Withdrawal Periods. *Horses*: slaughter 28 days. *Cattle*: slaughter 8 days

Tribrissen 48% (Schering-Plough) *NZ*
Injection, sulfadiazine 400 mg/mL, trimethoprim 80 mg/mL, for *horses, cattle, sheep, goats, pigs*
Withdrawal Periods. *Horses, pigs*: slaughter 28 days. *Cattle, sheep, goats*: slaughter 28 days, milk 48 hours

Tribrissen 80 mg (Schering-Plough) *NZ*
Tablets, sulfadiazine 400 mg, trimethoprim 80 mg, for *dogs*

Trimethotab 120 (Bomac) *NZ*
Tablets, sulfadiazine 100 mg, trimethoprim 20 mg, for *dogs, cats*

Trimethotab 480 (Bomac) *NZ*
Tablets, sulfadiazine 400 mg, trimethoprim 80 mg, for *dogs*

Trizine Plus (Ethical) *NZ*
Oral granules, bromhexine hydrochloride 112.5 mg, sulfadiazine 13.5 g, trimethoprim 2.7 g/sachet, for *horses*
Withdrawal Periods. Slaughter 28 days

Ventipulmin TMP/S (Boehringer Ingelheim) *NZ*
Oral powder, clenbuterol hydrochloride 21.44 micrograms/g, sulfadiazine 335 mg/g, trimethoprim 67 mg/g, for *horses*
Withdrawal Periods. Slaughter 28 days

USA
Indications. Sulfadiazine/trimethoprim-sensitive infections
Dose. Consult manufacturer's information

Tribrissen 400 Oral Paste (Schering-Plough) *USA*
Oral paste, sulfadiazine 333 mg/g and trimethoprim 67 mg/g (37.5 g/ Dial-A-Dose syringe, for *horses*
Withdrawal Periods. Should not be used in *horses* intended for human consumption

Tribrissen Tablets (Schering-Plough) *USA*
Tablets, sulfadiazine/trimethoprim /tablet; 20 mg/5 mg, 100 mg/20 mg, 400mg/80 mg, and 800 mg/160 mg per tablet, for *dogs*
Withdrawal Periods. n/a

Uniprim Powder for Horses (Macleod) *USA*
Oral Powder, sulfadiazine 333 mg/g and trimethoprim 67 mg/g, for *horses*
Withdrawal Periods. Should not be used in *horses* intended for human consumption

SULFADIMIDINE with TRIMETHOPRIM

Australia
Indications. Sulfadimidine/trimethoprim-sensitive infections
Dose. Consult manufacturer's information

Amphoprim S (Virbac) *Austral.*
Injection, sulfadimidine 20 g, trimethoprim 4 g/ 100 mL, for *cattle, horses, sheep, pigs, dogs, cats*
Withdrawal Periods. *Cattle*: slaughter 15 days, milk 72 hours. *Horses, sheep, pigs*: slaughter 15 days

Bromotrimidine (Parnell) *Austral.*
Oral paste, sulfadimidine 450 mg/g, trimethoprim 90 mg/g, bromhexine hydrochloride 9 mg/g powder, for *horses*
Withdrawal Periods. Slaughter 28 days

Bromotrimidine (Parnell) *Austral.*
Oral powder, sulfadimidine 430 mg/g, trimethoprim 86 mg/g, bromhexine hydrochloride 8.6 mg/g, for *horses*
Withdrawal Periods. *Horses*: slaughter 28 days

Trimidine Powder (Parnell) *Austral.*
Oral powder, sulfadimidine 430 mg/g, trimethoprim 86 mg/g, for *horses, cattle, pigs, poultry*

Withdrawal Periods. Horses: slaughter 28 days. *Calves, pigs, poultry:* 15 days, should not be used in poultry producing eggs for human consumption

Triprim (Ausrichter) *Austral.*
Injection, sulfadimidine 200mg/mL, trimethoprim 40 mg/mL, for *cattle, sheep, pigs, horses, dogs, cats*
Withdrawal Periods. *Cattle:* slaughter 15 days, milk 72 hours. *Horses, sheep, pigs:* slaughter 15 days.

Eire
Indications. Sulfadimidine/trimethoprim-sensitive infections
Dose. Consult manufacturer's information

Amphoprim Injectable Aqueous Solution (Virbac) *Eire*
Injection, sulfadimidine (as sodium ethane sulphonate) 200 mg/mL, trimethoprim 40 mg/mL, for *horses, cattle, pigs, dogs*
Withdrawal Periods. Should not be used in *horses* intended for human consumption. *Cattle:* slaughter 21 days, milk 4 days. *Pigs:* slaughter 21 days

New Zealand
Indications. Sulfadimidine/trimethoprim-sensitive infections
Dose. Consult manufacturer's information

Amphoprim (Virbac) *NZ*
Injection, sulfadimidine 200 mg/mL, trimethoprim 40 mg/mL, for *horses, cattle, sheep, pigs, dogs, cats*
Withdrawal Periods. *Horses, pigs:* slaughter 5 days. *Cattle, sheep:* slaughter 5 days, milk 48 hours

Bromotrimidine Powder (Parnell) *NZ*
Oral powder, bromhexine hydrochloride 8.6 mg/g, sulfadimidine 430 mg/g, trimethoprim 86 mg/g, for *horses*
Withdrawal Periods. Slaughter 28 days

Bromtrimsulp (Phoenix) *NZ*
Oral powder, bromhexine hydrochloride 8.6 mg/g, sulfadimidine 430 mg/g, trimethoprim 86 mg/g, for *horses*
Withdrawal Periods. Slaughter 28 days

Trimidine Paste (Parnell) *NZ*
Oral paste, sulfadimidine 450 mg/g, trimethoprim 90 mg/g, for *horses*
Withdrawal Periods. Slaughter 28 days

Trimidine Powder (Parnell) *NZ*
Oral powder, sulfadimidine 430 mg/g, trimethoprim 86 mg/g, for *horses*
Withdrawal Periods. Slaughter 28 days

Trimsulp (Phoenix) *NZ*
Oral powder, sulfadimidine 430 mg/g, trimethoprim 86 mg/g, for *horses*
Withdrawal Periods. Slaughter 28 days

SULFADOXINE with TRIMETHOPRIM

UK
Indications. Sulfadoxine/trimethoprim-sensitive infections
Contra-indications. Side-effects. See under Sulfadimidine
Warnings. Drug Interactions – see Appendix 1
Dose. Dosages vary. For guidance.
Expressed as sulfadoxine + trimethoprim
Horses: by intramuscular or slow intravenous (preferred) injection, 15 mg/kg
Cattle, pigs: by subcutaneous, intramuscular (preferred), or intravenous injection, 15 mg/kg daily
Dogs: by mouth, 15–20 mg/kg daily

by subcutaneous, intramuscular, or slow intravenous (preferred) injection, 15 mg/kg daily or on alternate days
Cats: by subcutaneous or intramuscular injection, 15 mg/kg daily

POM **Bimotrim Co** (Bimeda) *UK*
Injection, sulfadoxine 200 mg, trimethoprim 40 mg/mL, for *horses, cattle;* 100 mL
Withdrawal Periods. Should not be used in *horses* intended for human consumption. *Cattle:* slaughter 10 days, milk 2 days

POM **Borgal** (Intervet) *UK*
Tablets, or to prepare an oral solution, sulfadoxine 250 mg, trimethoprim 50 mg, for *dogs;* 50

POM **Borgal 7.5%** (Intervet) *UK*
Injection, sulfadoxine 62.5 mg, trimethoprim 12.5 mg, lidocaine hydrochloride 1 mg/mL, for *dogs, cats;* 50 mL

POM **Borgal 24%** (Intervet) *UK*
Injection, sulfadoxine 200 mg, trimethoprim 40 mg/mL, for *horses, cattle, pigs;* 100 mL
Withdrawal Periods. *Horses:* slaughter 8 days. *Cattle:* slaughter 8 days, milk 2 days. *Pigs:* slaughter 8 days

POM **Trivetrin** (Schering-Plough) *UK*
Injection, sulfadoxine 200 mg, trimethoprim 40 mg/mL, for *horses, cattle, pigs, dogs;* 100 mL
Withdrawal Periods. Should not be used in *horses* intended for human consumption. *Cattle:* slaughter 5 days, milk 2 days. *Pigs:* slaughter 5 days

Australia
Indications. Sulfadoxine/trimethoprim-sensitive infections
Dose. Consult manufacturer's information

Bimotrim CO (Bimeda) *Austral.*
Injection, sulfadoxine 200 mg/mL, trimethoprim 40 mg/mL, for *cattle, sheep, goats, pigs, dogs, horses*
Withdrawal Periods. *Horses:* slaughter 28 days. *Cattle:* slaughter 10 days, milk 36 hours (single dose) or 72 hours (multiple dose). *Sheep:* slaughter 10 days. *Pigs:* slaughter 15 days

Tribactral S (Jurox) *Austral.*
Injection, sulfadoxine 200 mg/mL, trimethoprim 40 mg/mL, for *cattle, horses, sheep, pigs, dogs, cats*
Withdrawal Periods. *Cattle:* slaughter 14 days, milk 36 hours (single dose) or 72 hours (multiple dose). *Horses, sheep, pigs:* slaughter 14 days

Tridox Injection (Delvet) *Austral.*
Injection, sulfadoxine 200 mg/mL, trimethoprim 40 mg/mL, for *cattle, horses, sheep, pigs, dogs, cats*
Withdrawal Periods. *Cattle:* slaughter 14 days, milk 36 hours (single dose) or 72 hours (multiple dose). *Horses, sheep, pigs:* slaughter 14 days

Trivetrin (Jurox) *Austral.*
Injection, sulfadoxine 200 mg/mL, trimethoprim 40 mg/mL, for *cattle, horses, sheep, pigs, cats, dogs*
Withdrawal Periods. *Cattle:* slaughter 14 days, milk 36 hours (single dose) or 72 hours (multiple dose). *Horses, sheep, pigs:* slaughter 14 days

Eire
Indications. Sulfadoxine/trimethoprim-sensitive infections
Dose. Consult manufacturer's information

Borgal 24% Solution (Hoechst Roussel Vet) *Eire*
Injection, sulfadoxine 200 mg/mL, triemethroprim 40 mg/mL, for *horses, cattle, pigs*
Withdrawal Periods. *Horses, cattle, pigs:* slaughter 10 days. *Cattle:* milk 96 hours

Primidoxine Injection (Norbrook) *Eire*
Injection, sulfadoxine 200 mg/mL, trimethoprim 40 mg/mL, for *horses, cattle, pigs, dogs, cats*
Withdrawal Periods. Should not be used in *horses* intended for human consumption. *Cattle*: slaughter 10 days, milk 36 hours. *Pigs*: slaughter 10 days

Tribrissen Oral Suspension Sulphadiazine and Trimethoprim Mixture BP (Vet) (Schering-Plough) *Eire*
Oral suspension, sulfadiazine 400 mg/mL, trimethoprim 80 mg/mL, for *chickens*
Withdrawal Periods. Slaughter 5 days

Trivetrin Injection (Schering-Plough) *Eire*
Injection, sulfadoxine 200 mg/mL, trimethoprim 40 mg/mL, for *horses, cattle, pigs, dogs*
Withdrawal Periods. *Horses*: slaughter 28 days. *Cattle*: slaughter 5 days, milk 48 hours. *Pigs*: slaughter 5 days

New Zealand
Indications. Sulfadoxine/trimethoprim-sensitive infections
Dose. Consult manufacturer's information

Dofatrim-ject (Technipharm) *NZ*
Injection, sulfadoxine 200 mg/mL, trimethoprim 40 mg/mL, for *horses, cattle, sheep, goats, pigs, dogs, cats*
Withdrawal Periods. *Horses, goats, pigs*: slaughter 14 days. *Cattle*: slaughter 14 days, milk 24 hours. *Sheep*: slaughter 14 days, milk 48 hours

SULFAFURAZOLE WITH TRIMETHOPRIM

Australia
Indications. Sulfafurazole/trimethoprim-sensitive infections
Dose. Consult manufacturer's information

Trimazol (Apex) *Austral.*
Injection, sulfafurazole 200 mg/mL, trimethoprim 40 mg/mL, for *horses, dogs, cats*
Withdrawal Periods. *Horses*: should not be used in horses intended for human consumption.

New Zealand
Indications. Sulfafurazole/trimethoprim-sensitive infections
Dose. Consult manufacturer's information

Trimazol (Bomac) *NZ*
Injection, sulfafurazole 200 mg/mL, trimethoprim 40 mg/mL, for *horses, cattle, sheep, pigs, dogs, cats*
Withdrawal Periods. *Horses, pigs*: slaughter 28 days. *Cattle, sheep*: slaughter 28 days, milk 24 hours

SULFAMETHOXAZOLE with TRIMETHOPRIM
(Co-trimoxazole: preparations of trimethoprim and sulfamethoxazole in the proportions, by weight, of 1 part to 5 parts)

UK
Indications. Sulfamethoxazole/trimethoprim-sensitive infections
Contra-indications. See under Sulfadimidine
Side-effects. Occasionally erythema and petechiae of the skin, internal haemorrhage, haematuria, keratoconjunctivitis sicca
Warnings. Drug Interactions – see Appendix 1

Dose. Expressed as sulfamethoxazole + trimethoprim
Dogs, cats: *by mouth,* 30 mg/kg daily

POM Ⓗ **Co-trimoxazole** (Non-proprietary) *UK*
Tablets, sulfamethoxazole 400 mg, trimethoprim 80 mg,
Paediatric oral suspension, sulfamethoxazole 40 mg, trimethoprim 8 mg/mL; 100 mL
Oral suspension, sulfamethoxazole 80 mg, trimethoprim 16 mg/mL; 100 mL
Strong sterile solution, sulfamethoxazole 80 mg, trimethoprim 16 mg/mL; 5 mL, 10 mL. For dilution and use as an intravenous infusion

New Zealand
Indications. Sulfamethoxazole/trimethoprim-sensitive infections
Dose. Consult manufacturer's information

Amphoprim T-600 (Virbac) *NZ*
Tablets, sulfamethoxazole 400 mg, trimethoprim 80 mg, for *dogs, cats*

Sulphatrim (Ethical) *NZ*
Tablets, sulfamethoxazole 400 mg, trimethoprim 80 mg, for *dogs, cats*

SULFAMETHOXYPYRIDAZINE with TRIMETHOPRIM

Eire
Indications. Sulfamethoxypyridazine/trimethoprim-sensitive infections
Dose. Consult manufacturer's information

Amphoprim Bolus (Virbac) *Eire*
Tablets, sulfamethoxypyridazine 1 g, trimethoprim 0.2 g, for *calves*

New Zealand
Indications. Sulfamethoxypyridazine/trimethoprim-sensitive infections
Dose. Consult manufacturer's information

Amphoprim Bolus (Virbac) *NZ*
Tablets, sulfamethoxypyridazine 1000 mg, trimethoprim 200 mg, for *horses, cattle, sheep, goats*
Withdrawal Periods. *Horses*: slaughter 21 days. *Cattle, sheep, goats*: slaughter 21 days, milk 120 hours

SULFAQUINOXALINE with TRIMETHOPRIM

UK
Indications. Sulfadimidine/trimethoprim-sensitive infections; treatment of coccidiosis in chickens (see section 1.4)
Dose. Expressed as sulfaquinoxaline + trimethoprim
Chickens, turkeys: bacterial infections, *by addition to drinking water or feed*, 30 mg/kg body-weight

POM **Tribrissen (SQX) Poultry Formula** (Schering-Plough) *UK*
Granules, for addition to feed or drinking water, sulfaquinoxaline (as sodium) 500 mg/g, trimethoprim 165 mg/g, for *chickens, turkeys more than 21 days of age*
Withdrawal Periods. *Broiler chickens*: slaughter 7 days. *Turkeys*: slaughter 9 days. Should not be used in layer or breeder flocks when birds are in lay

SULFATROXAZOLE with TRIMETHOPRIM

Australia
Indications. Sulfatroxazole/trimethoprim-sensitive infections

Leotrox Injection (Boehringer Ingelheim) *Austral.*
Injection, sulfatroxazole 200 mg/mL, trimethoprim 40 mg/mL, for *horses, cattle, sheep, pigs, dogs, cats*
Withdrawal Periods. *Horses*: slaughter 28 days. *Cattle*: slaughter 16 days (im) or 10 days (iv), milk 60 hours. *Sheep*: slaughter 16 days (im) or 10 days (iv), should not be used in sheep producing milk for human consumption or within 16 days of lambing. *Pigs*: slaughter 9 days

Eire

Indications.   Sulfatroxazole/trimethoprim-sensitive infections
Dose. Consult manufacturer's information

Leotrox 24% Injection (Leo) *Eire*
Injection, sulfatroxazole 200 mg/mL, trimethoprim 40 mg/mL, for *cattle, sheep, pigs*
Withdrawal Periods. *Cattle*: slaughter 10 days (by iv injection), 16 days (by im injection), milk 60 hours. *Sheep*: slaughter 16 days. *Pigs*: slaughter 9 days

1.1.7 Nitrofurans

The nitrofurans, which include **furazolidone** and **nitrofurantoin**, are relatively broad-spectrum bactericidal drugs. They are active against *Salmonella* spp., coliforms, *Mycoplasma* spp., *Coccidia* spp., and some other protozoa. Resistance is by chromosomal mutation. Plasmid-mediated transmissible resistance is rare.

Furazolidone and nitrofurantoin are included in Annex IV of Regulation 2377/90/EEC, which effectively prohibits their use in medicinal products for food-producing species. Nitrofurantoin is well absorbed following oral administration and rapidly excreted in the urine. Blood and tissue concentrations are too low for the treatment of systemic infection and it is mainly used for urinary tract infections in dogs and cats.

FURALTADONE

New Zealand

Indications. Furaltadone-sensitive infections
Dose. *Poultry*: 111 mg/800 litres drinking water

Furactosol (PCL) *NZ*
Oral powder, furaltadone 222 g/kg, for *poultry*
Withdrawal Periods. Should not be used in laying birds

FURAZOLIDONE

New Zealand

Indications. Furazolidone-sensitive infections
Dose. *Pigs, poultry*: 100–400 g/tonne feed

Furamycin (PCL) *NZ*
Premix, furazolidone 200 g/kg, for *pigs, poultry*

NITROFURANTOIN

UK

Indications. Urinary-tract infections
Dose. *By mouth.*
Dogs, cats: 4 mg/kg 3 times daily

POM Ⓗ **Nitrofurantoin** (Non-proprietary) *UK*
Tablets, nitrofurantoin 50 mg, 100 mg

POM Ⓗ **Furadantin** (Goldshield) *UK*
Tablets, scored, nitrofurantoin 50 mg, 100 mg; 100

1.1.8 Nitroimidazoles

The nitroimidazoles include dimetridazole and metronidazole, which are bactericidal to most obligate anaerobic bacteria. They have negligble activity against aerobic bacteria. They are active against *Serpulina hyodysenteriae* (*Treponema hyodysenteriae*) and a variety of protozoa. Acquired resistance among susceptible organisms is rare.

Dimetridazole is included in Annex IV of Regulation 2377/90/EEC which effectively prohibits its use in food-producing species in Europe. However it is available in the UK as an authorised veterinary medicine (see sections 1.4.2, 1.4.3, and 1.4.6) for use in pheasants and partridges for health and welfare reasons; it may not be prescribed for any other food-producing species under the 'cascade'. Dimetridazole may be used as a zootechnical feed additive but only in accordance with Annex I of Directive 70/524/EEC; it is used for the prevention of blackhead (see section 1.4.2) in turkeys and guinea fowl.

Metronidazole is well absorbed by mouth and penetrates tissues throughout the body including the brain and cerebrospinal fluid. It is administered for a variety of anaerobic infections including gingivitis and empyema. The injectable solution may also be used for local irrigation of wounds. The action of metronidazole is restricted to obligate anaerobic organisms but infections are often mixed. Therefore, it may be necessary to concurrently administer a drug which is active against aerobic organisms. One such drug, whose spectrum of activity is complementary to metronidazole, is spiramycin which is effective against Gram-positive aerobes and appears to be synergistic with metronidazole against the obligate anaerobes.

DIMETRIDAZOLE

Australia

Indications. Bacterial infections in pigs; histomoniosis in turkeys; trichomoniosis in caged birds
Dose. Consult manufacturer's information

Dimetridazole 225 Premix (CCD) *Austral.*
Premix, dimetridazole 225 g/kg premix, for *pigs, turkeys, chickens*
Withdrawal Periods. *Pigs*: slaughter 5 days. *Turkeys, chickens*: slaughter 5 days, should not be used in poultry producing eggs for human consumption

Dimetridazole Water Soluble Powder (CCD) *Austral.*
Powder, for addition to drinking water, dimetridazole 980 mg/g powder, for *pigs, turkeys, cage birds*
Withdrawal Periods. *Pigs*: slaughter 5 days. *Turkeys*: slaughter 5 day, should not be used in turkeys producing eggs for human consumption

Emtryl Premix (Rhône-Poulenc) *Austral.*
Premix, dimetridazole 200 g/kg premix, for *poultry, pigs*
Withdrawal Periods. *Pigs*: slaughter 5 days. *Turkeys, chickens*: slaughter 5 days, should not be used in poultry producing eggs for human consumption

Emtryl Soluble (Rhône-Poulenc) *Austral.*
Powder, for addition to drinking water, dimetridazole 400 g/kg powder, for *poultry, pigs, pigeons*

Withdrawal Periods. *Pigs*: slaughter 5 days. *Turkeys, chickens, pigeons*: slaughter 5 days, should not be used in poultry producing eggs for human consumption

New Zealand
Indications. Bacterial infections in pigs; trichomoniosis in pigeons; histomoniosis in turkeys and game birds
Dose. Consult manufacturer's information

Dimetrasol (PCL) *NZ*
Oral powder, dimetridazole 400 mg/g, for *pigs, poultry, game birds, pigeons*
Withdrawal Periods. Slaughter 5 days. Should not be used in birds producing eggs for human consumption

METRONIDAZOLE

UK
Indications. Infections caused by anaerobic bacteria; treatment of giardiosis (see section 1.4.5); hepatic encephalopathy♦ (see section 310)
Contra-indications. Very small birds such as zebra finches
Warnings. Care in patients with renal or hepatic impairment; overdosage may cause reversible neurological depression, ataxia, hepatic impairment; operators should wear impervious gloves when applying topical treatment.
Drug Interactions – see Appendix 1
Dose.
Horses: by mouth, 20 mg/kg twice daily
by intramuscular or slow intravenous injection or intravenous infusion, 20 mg/kg daily
Dogs, cats: by mouth or by subcutaneous or intramuscular injection or intravenous infusion, 20 mg/kg daily
Birds, rodents: by addition to drinking water, 20 mg/kg

POM (H) **Metronidazole** (Non-proprietary) *UK*
Tablets, metronidazole 200 mg, 400 mg, 500 mg

POM **Metronex for Horses** (Pharmacia & Upjohn) *UK*
Oral paste, metronidazole 500 mg/g, for *horses*; 20-g metered dose applicator
Withdrawal Periods. Should not be used in *horses* intended for human consumption

POM **Torgyl** (Merial) *UK*
Injection, intravenous infusion, oral solution, or topical application, metronidazole 5 mg/mL, for *horses, dogs, cats, birds, rodents*; 50 mL
Withdrawal Periods. Should not be used in *horses, birds* intended for human consumption. Should not be used in *birds* producing eggs for human consumption
For subcutaneous or intravenous injection. Use undiluted for irrigations or wound dressings

POM **Torgyl Forte** (Merial) *UK*
Injection, powder for reconstitution, metronidazole 450 mg/mL, for *horses, dogs, cats*; 80 mL
Withdrawal Periods. Should not be used in *horses* intended for human consumption
For intramuscular injection. May be given by subcutaneous injection in dogs and cats

Australia
Indications. Infections caused by anaerobic bacteria; protozoal infections
Dose. *Horses, dogs, cats*: by mouth or by subcutaneous or intravenous injection, 20 mg/kg

Metrin Solution (Parnell) *Austral.*
Solution, metronidazole 5 mg/mL, for *horses, dogs, cats, birds*
Withdrawal Periods. *Horses*: slaughter 28 days

Eire
Indications. Infections caused by anaerobic bacteria
Dose. *Horses, dogs, cats*: by intramuscular injection, 22.5 mg/kg

Torgyl Forte (Merial) *Eire*
Injection, powder for reconstitution, metronidazole 450 mg/mL when reconstituted, for *horses, dogs, cats*
Withdrawal Periods. Should not be used in horses intended for human consumption

1.1.9 Quinolones

Oxolinic acid, pipemidic acid, and **nalidixic acid** are 4-quinolone antibacterial agents. They are active against Gram-negative bacteria. However Gram-positive bacteria, *Pseudomonas aeruginosa*, and obligate anaerobes are not susceptible.

Fluoroquinolone derivatives such as **difloxacin, danofloxacin, enrofloxacin, flumequine, marbofloxacin, orbifloxacin,** and **sarafloxacin** have a broader spectrum of activity than the parent compounds and are well distributed to tissues. They are bactericidal by inhibiting microbial DNA gyrase and are active against a wide range of Gram-negative bacteria, including *Pseudomonas aeruginosa* and *Klebsiella* spp., and also against some Gram-positive micro-organisms and *Mycoplasma* spp. They are not active against obligate anaerobes. Fluoroquinolones are not particularly effective against streptococcal and enterococcal infections. For this reason they tend to spare the normal gut flora of animals under treatment and are therefore the treatment of choice for neutropeanic patients undergoing cancer chemotherapy.

Fluoroquinolones operate by a concentration-dependent killing mechanism and the most successful dosing regimens are those which produce high peak plasma concentrations.

Fluoroquinolones may inhibit the growth of load-bearing articular cartilage and therefore should not be administered to growing dogs or cats. There is some evidence to suggest that fluoroquinolones may pre-dispose to seizure activity in patients suffering from epilepsy. These drugs should therefore be used with caution in epileptic patients.

There is concern about the increasing resistance of certain bacteria to fluoroquinolones. These include some zoonotic organisms such as *Salmonella* spp., *Campylobacter* spp. and *E. coli*. The resistance is often due to chromosomal mutations either in the Gyr A gene or in proteins in the bacterial cell membrane which allow the drug to enter the bacterial cell. Resistance within a population of bacteria becomes evident whenever antibacterial drugs are heavily used due to selection pressure. **It is recommended to perform antimicrobial sensitivity tests before using fluoroquinolones or to limit the use of this group of drugs to the treatment of intractable Gram-negative infections.** Examples of such infections are those that are potentially life-threatening or resistant infections where other antibacterial drugs do not penetrate well enough to the site of infection and are therefore not likely to be successful in treating the problem (for example, chronic prostatic infections in dogs or recurrent and resistant urinary tract infections).

DANOFLOXACIN

UK

Indications. Danofloxacin-sensitive infections
Dose. *Cattle*: *by intramuscular or intravenous injection*, 1.25 mg/kg daily
Pigs: *by intramuscular injection*, 1.25 mg/kg daily for 3 days

POM **Advocin** (Pfizer) *UK*
Injection, danofloxacin (as danofloxacin mesilate) 25 mg/mL, for *cattle, pigs*
Withdrawal Periods. *Cattle*: slaughter 5 days, milk 48 hours. *Pigs*: slaughter 3 days

Eire

Indications. Danofloxacin-sensitive infections
Dose. *Cattle*: *by intramuscular or intravenous injection*, 1.25 mg/kg daily

Advocin Injectable Solution (Pfizer) *Eire*
Injection, danofloxacin 25 mg/mL, for *cattle*
Withdrawal Periods. Slaughter 5 days, should not be used in cattle producing milk for human consumption

DIFLOXACIN

UK

Indications. Difloxacin-sensitive infections
Contra-indications. Dogs under 8 to 18 months of age (depending on the breed), see notes above
Side-effects. Occasional vomiting; inappetance, diarrhoea, anal irritation rarely
Warnings. Concurrent use of NSAIDs may cause seizures in epileptic patients, Drug Interactions - see Appendix 1. Manufacturer does not recommend use in pregnant or lactating bitches, male stud dogs, or birds with existing leg weakness or osteoporosis because safety has not been established
Dose.
Dogs: *by mouth*, 5 mg/kg once daily for 5–10 days
Poultry: *by addition to drinking water*, 10 mg/kg for 5 days

POM **Dicural** (Fort Dodge) *UK*
Tablets, difloxacin (as hydrochloride) 15 mg, 50 mg, 100 mg, for *dogs*; 10
Oral solution, difloxacin (as hydrochloride) 100 mg/mL, for *broiler chickens, future breeder chickens, turkeys up to 2 kg body-weight*; 250 mL, 1 litre
Withdrawal Periods. *Poultry*: slaughter 1 day, should not be used in laying hens

USA

Indications. Difloxacin-sensitive infections
Dose. *Dogs*: *by mouth*, 5–10 mg/kg

Dicural Tablets RX (Fort Dodge) *USA*
Tablets, difloxacin (as hydrochloride) 11.4 mg, 45.5 mg, 136 mg, for *dogs*

ENROFLOXACIN

UK

Indications. Enrofloxacin-sensitive infections
Contra-indications. Dogs under 12 to 18 months of age and cats under 8 weeks of age, see notes above
Side-effects. Occasional skin reactions in kennelled Greyhounds, occasional muscle bruising in reptiles and birds after injection
Warnings. Care in pregnant or lactating exotic animals because safety has not been established
Dose. *Cattle*: *by subcutaneous injection*, 2.5 mg/kg daily for 3 days. Dose may be increased to 5 mg/kg for 5 days for salmonellosis or complicated respiratory disease
by depot subcutaneous injection, 7.5 mg/kg as a single dose
calves: *by mouth*, 2.5 mg/kg daily for 3 days. Dose may be increased to 5 mg/kg for 5 days for salmonellosis and complicated respiratory disease
Pigs: *by intramuscular injection*, 2.5 mg/kg daily for 3 days. Dose may be increased to 5 mg/kg for 5 days for salmonellosis or complicated respiratory disease
piglets: *by mouth*, (up to 3 kg body-weight) 5 mg; (up to 10 kg body-weight) 15 mg
Dogs, cats: *by mouth*, 5 mg/kg once daily *or* as a divided dose given twice daily
by subcutaneous injection, 5 mg/kg daily
Poultry: *by addition to drinking water*, 10 mg/kg daily for 3-10 days
Exotic animals: see Prescribing for rabbits and rodents, Prescribing for reptiles, and Prescribing for exotic birds. Contact the manufacturer for specific case information

POM **Baytril 2.5% Injection** (Bayer) *UK*
Injection, enrofloxacin 25 mg/mL, for *dogs, cats, exotic animals such as small mammals, reptiles, birds*; 50 mL
Withdrawal Periods. Should not be used in *exotic animals and birds* intended for human consumption

POM **Baytril 5% Injection** (Bayer) *UK*
Injection, enrofloxacin 50 mg/mL, for *cattle, pigs, dogs, cats*; 100 mL
Withdrawal Periods. *Cattle*: slaughter 14 days, should not be used in cattle producing milk for human consumption. *Pigs*: slaughter 10 days

POM **Baytril 10% Injection** (Bayer) *UK*
Injection, enrofloxacin 100 mg/mL, for *cattle, pigs*; 50 mL, 100 mL
Withdrawal Periods. *Cattle*: slaughter 14 days, milk 84 hours. *Pigs*: slaughter 10 days

POM **Baytril 2.5% Oral Solution** (Bayer) *UK*
Oral solution, for addition to milk, milk replacer, oral electrolyte solution, or water, enrofloxacin 25 mg/mL, for *calves, exotic animals such as small mammals, reptiles, birds*; 100 mL
Withdrawal Periods. *Calves*: slaughter 8 days. Should not be used in *exotic animals and birds* intended for human consumption
Dilute 1 volume in 4 volumes water for oral administration by gavage in exotic animals
Contra-indications. Chickens, turkeys

POM **Baytril 10% Oral Solution** (Bayer) *UK*
Oral solution, for addition to drinking water, enrofloxacin 100 mg/mL, for *broiler chickens, broiler breeders, replacement chickens, turkeys*; 100 mL, 1 litre
Withdrawal Periods. *Chickens, turkeys*: slaughter 8 days, should not be used in birds producing eggs for human consumption
Note. Should not be given to replacement birds within 14 days of commencement of laying

POM **Baytril Piglet Doser** (Bayer) *UK*
Oral solution, enrofloxacin 5 mg/mL, for *piglets up to 10 kg body-weight*;
100-mL dose applicator (1 unit dose = 1 mL)
Withdrawal Periods. *Piglets*: slaughter 10 days

POM **Baytril Max** (Bayer) *UK*
Depot injection, enrofloxacin 100 mg/mL, for *cattle*; 100 mL
Withdrawal Periods. *Cattle*: slaughter 14 days, milk 84 hours

POM **Baytril Tablets** (Bayer) *UK*
Tablets, enrofloxacin 15 mg, for *dogs, cats*; 100
Tablets, enrofloxacin 50 mg, 150 mg, for *dogs*; 100

Australia
Indications. Enrofloxacin-sensitive infections
Dose. *Dogs, cats*: *by mouth or by subcutaneous injection*,
5 mg/kg

Baytril Oral Solution (Bayer) *Austral.*
Oral solution, enrofloxacin 25 mg/mL, for *dogs, cats*

Baytril Tablets (Bayer) *Austral.*
Tablets, enrofloxacin 50 mg, 150 mg, for *dogs, cats*

Baytril Injection (Bayer) *Austral.*
Injection, enrofloxacin 50 mg/mL, for *dogs, cats*

Eire
Indications. Enrofloxacin-sensitive infections
Dose.
Cattle: *by subcutaneous injection*, 2.5 mg/kg
by depot subcutaneous injection, 7.5 mg/kg
calves: *by mouth*, 2.5 mg/kg
Pigs: *by subcutaneous injection*, 2.5 mg/kg
piglets: *by mouth*, (up to 3 kg body-weight) 5 mg; (up to 10
kg body-weight) 15 mg
Dogs, cats: *by mouth*, 5 mg/kg
by subcutaneous injection, 5 mg/kg daily

Baytril 2.5% Oral Solution (Bayer) *Eire*
Oral solution, enrofloxacin 25 mg/mL, for *calves, exotic animals (small
mammals, reptiles, birds)*
Withdrawal Periods. Slaughter 7 days

Baytril 10% Oral Solution (Bayer) *Eire*
Solution, for addition to drinking water, enrofloxacin 100 mg/mL, for *poultry*
Withdrawal Periods. *Chickens*: slaughter 9 days. *Turkeys*: slaughter 11 days

Baytril 2.5% Injection (Bayer) *Eire*
Injection, enrofloxacin 25 mg/mL, for *dogs, cats, exotic animals (small
mammals, reptiles, birds)*

Baytril 5% Injection (Bayer) *Eire*
Injection, enrofloxacin 50 mg/mL, for *dogs, cats*

Baytril 5% Injection (Bayer) *Eire*
Injection, enrofloxacin 50 mg/mL, for *cattle, pigs*
Withdrawal Periods. *Cattle*: slaughter 14 days, should not be used in cattle
producing milk for human consumption. *Pigs*: slaughter 10 days

Baytril 0.5% Oral Solution (Bayer) *Eire*
Oral solution, enrofloxacin 5 mg/mL, for *piglets*
Withdrawal Periods. Slaughter 10 days

Baytril Tablets (Bayer) *Eire*
Tablets, enrofloxacin 15 mg, 50 mg, 150 mg, for *dogs, cats*

Baytril 10% Injection (Bayer) *Eire*
Injection, enrofloxacin 100 mg/mL, for *cattle, pigs*
Withdrawal Periods. *Cattle*: slaughter 14 days, should not be used in cattle
producing milk for human consumption. *Pigs*: slaughter 10 days

Baytril Max Injection (Bayer) *Eire*
Injection, enrofloxacin 100 mg/mL, for *cattle*
Withdrawal Periods. Slaughter 14 days, should not be used in cattle producing milk for human consumption.

New Zealand
Indications. Enrofloxacin-sensitive infections
Dose. *Cattle, pigs*: *by subcutaneous injection*, 2 mg/kg
Dogs, cats: *by mouth or by subcutaneous injection*, 5 mg/kg

Baytril (Bayer) *NZ*
Tablets, enrofloxacin 15 mg, 50 mg , 150 mg, for *dogs, cats*

Baytril 2.5% (Bayer) *NZ*
Injection, enrofloxacin 25 mg/mL, for *dogs, cats*

Baytril 10% (Bayer) *NZ*
Injection, enrofloxacin 100 mg/mL, for *cattle, pigs*
Withdrawal Periods. *Cattle*: slaughter 7 days, milk 168 hours. *Pigs*: slaughter 7 days

USA
Indications. Enrofloxacin-sensitive infections
Dose.
Cattle: *by subcutaneous injection*, 2.5–5.0 mg/kg
Dogs: *by mouth*, 5–20 mg/kg
by intramuscular injection, 2.5 mg/kg daily
Cats: *by mouth*, 5–20 mg/kg

Baytril 3.23% Concentrate Antimicrobial Solution (Bayer) *USA*
Solution, for addition to drinking water, 32.3 mg/mL, for *chickens, turkeys*
Withdrawal Periods. Slaughter 2 days, should not be used in hens producing eggs for human consumption

Baytril 100 (Bayer) *USA*
Injection, 100 mg/mL, for *cattle*
Withdrawal Periods. Slaughter 28 days, should not be used in cattle producing milk or calves intended for veal production

Baytril Injectable Solution (Bayer) *USA*
Injection, 22.7 mg/mL, for *dogs*

Baytril Taste Tabs (Bayer) *USA*
Tablets, 22.7 mg, 68 mg, for *dogs, cats*

MARBOFLOXACIN

UK
Indications. Marbofloxacin-sensitive infections
Contra-indications. Dogs less than 12 months of age or to 18 months of age for large breeds such as Great Danes or Mastiffs, cats less than 16 weeks of age, see notes above
Side-effects. Occasional vomiting, loose faeces, modification of thirst, transient increase in activity in dogs and cats; occasional transient inflammatory reaction at injection site
Warnings. Safety in pregnant animals has not been established. Caution in young animals and epileptics; overdosage may cause neurological symptoms. Possible reduced drug activity in patients with low urinary pH. Drug Interactions – see Appendix 1
Dose.
Cattle: *by mouth*, 1–2 mg/kg daily for up to 3 days
by subcutaneous or intravenous injection, 2 mg/kg daily
Pigs: *by intramuscular injection*, 2 mg/kg daily
Dogs, cats: *by mouth*, 2 mg/kg once daily
by subcutaneous or intravenous injection, 2 mg/kg

POM **Marbocyl 2%** (Vétoquinol) *UK*
Injection, marbofloxacin 20 mg/mL, for *pre-ruminant cattle up to 100 kg body-weight, pigs*
Withdrawal Periods. *Cattle*: slaughter 6 days. *Pigs*: slaughter 2 days
Note. For subcutaneous or intravenous injection in cattle

POM **Marbocyl 10%** (Vétoquinol) *UK*
Injection, marbofloxacin 100 mg/mL, for *cattle, pigs*
Withdrawal Periods. *Cattle*: slaughter 6 days, milk 1.5 days. *Pigs*: slaughter 2 days

POM **Marbocyl Bolus** (Vétoquinol) *UK*
Tablets, marbofloxacin 50 mg, for *calves 25–50 kg body-weight*
Withdrawal Periods. *Cattle*: slaughter 6 days

POM **Marbocyl SA** (Vétoquinol) *UK*
Injection, powder for reconstitution, marbofloxacin 10 mg/mL, 20 mg/mL, for *dogs, cats*

POM **Marbocyl Tablets** (Vétoquinol) *UK*
Tablets, scored, marbofloxacin 5 mg, for *dogs, cats*; 100
Tablets, scored, marbofloxacin 20 mg, for *dogs*; 100
Tablets, scored, marbofloxacin 80 mg, for *dogs*; 72

Eire
Indications. Marbofloxacin-sensitive infections
Dose.
Cattle: *by subcutaneous, intramuscular, or intravenous injection*, 2 mg/kg daily
Pigs: *by intramuscular injection*, 2 mg/kg daily
Dogs, cats: *by mouth*, 2 mg/kg once daily

Marbocyl 2% (Vetoquinol) *Eire*
Injection, marbofloxacin 2%, for *cattle, pigs*
Withdrawal Periods. *Calves*: slaughter 4 days. *Pigs*: slaughter 2 days

Marbocyl 10% (Vetoquinol) *Eire*
Injection, marbofloxacin 10%, for *cattle, pigs*
Withdrawal Periods. *Cattle*: slaughter 4 days, milk 24 hours. *Pigs*: slaughter 2 days

Marbocyl 5 mg, 20 mg, 80 mg (Vetoquinol) *Eire*
Tablets, marbofloxacin 5 mg, 20 mg, 80 mg, for *dogs, cats*

NALIDIXIC ACID

UK
Indications. Nalidixic acid-sensitive infections
Dose. See Prescribing for amphibians

POM (H) **Negram** (Sanofi Synthelabo) *UK*
Oral suspension, nalidixic acid 60 mg/mL

POM (H) **Uriben** (Rosemont) *UK*
Oral suspension, nalidixic acid 60 mg/mL

ORBIFLOXACIN

UK
Indications. Orbifloxacin-sensitive infections, in particular cystitis in dogs
Contra-indications. Dogs less than 8 months of age in small and medium sized breeds, up to 12 months of age in large breeds, or to 18 months of age for giant breeds, see notes above
Warnings. Safety in pregnant and lactating animals or animals intended for breeding has not been established; Drug Interactions – see Appendix 1

Dose. *Dogs*: *by mouth*, 2.5 mg/kg once daily for at least 10 days

POM **Orbax** (Schering-Plough) *UK*
Tablets, orbifloxacin 6.25 mg, 25 mg, 75 mg, for *dogs*

USA
Indications. Orbifloxacin-sensitive infections
Dose. *Dogs*: *by mouth*, 2.5–7.5 mg/kg

Orbax Tablets (Schering-Plough) *USA*
Tablets, orbifloxacin 5.7 mg, 22.7 mg, 68 mg, for *dogs*

SARAFLOXACIN

UK
See Prescribing for fish

USA
Indications. Orbifloxacin-sensitive infections
Dose. *Chickens*: *by addition to drinking water*, 20–40 g/1000 litres
(day-old chicks): *by subcutaneous injection*, 100 micrograms
Turkeys: *by addition to drinking water*, 30–50 g/1000 litres

Saraflox Injection (Abbott) *USA*
Injection, sarafloxacin (as hydrochloride) 50 mg/mL, for *chickens*
Withdrawal Periods. Slaughter withdrawal period nil, should not be used in chickens producing eggs for human consumption

Saraflox WSP (Abbott) *USA*
Oral powder, for addition to drinking water, sarafloxacin 14.5 g/145 g powder, for *chickens, turkeys*
Withdrawal Periods. *Chickens*: slaughter withdrawal period nil, should not be used in chickens producing eggs for human consumption. *Turkeys*: slaughter withdrawal period nil

1.1.10 Pleuromutilins

Tiamulin and **valnemulin** are antibiotics belonging to the pleuromutilin group, which act by the inhibition of the initiation of protein synthesis at the level of the bacterial ribosome. They have a broad spectrum of action, which includes more fastidious Gram-negative organisms such as *Haemophilus*, *Bordetella*, *Pasteurella*, and *Actinobacillus* spp., and also a number of anaerobic organisms.
Concurrent administration of pleuromutilins and ionophore antibiotics may result in severe growth depression, ataxia, paralysis, or death.

TIAMULIN FUMARATE

UK
Indications. Tiamulin-sensitive organisms
Side-effects. Rarely, skin erythema
Warnings. Should not be given at tiamulin 100 g/tonne feed or 5 mg/kg body-weight within 7 days of administration of monensin, narasin, or salinomycin (Drug Interactions – see Appendix 1)
Dose. *Pigs*:
Swine dysentery

treatment, *by addition to drinking water*, 8.8 mg/kg body-weight *or* 60 g/100 litres for 3–5 days

by addition to feed, 5 mg/kg body-weight *or* 100 g/tonne feed for 7–10 days

by intramuscular injection, 10 mg/kg as a single dose prophylaxis, *by addition to feed*, 1.5–2.0 mg/kg body-weight *or* 30–40 g/tonne feed and given during period of risk

Enzootic pneumonia complex

treatment, *by intramuscular injection*, 15 mg/kg daily for 3 days

prophylaxis, *by addition to feed*, 1.5–2.0 mg/kg body-weight *or* 30–40 g/tonne feed and given for up to 2 months during period of risk

Mycoplasmal arthritis, treatment, *by intramuscular injection*, 15 mg/kg daily for 3 days

MFS Tiamutin 2% Premix (Leo) *UK*
Premix, tiamulin fumarate 20 g/kg, for *pigs*; 1 kg, 5 kg
Withdrawal Periods. *Pigs*: slaughter 1 day

MFS Tiamutin 25% Premix (Leo) *UK*
Premix, tiamulin fumarate 250 g/kg, for *pigs*; 1.2 kg, 24 kg
Withdrawal Periods. *Pigs*: slaughter 1 day

POM Tiamutin 12.5% Oral Solution (Leo) *UK*
Oral solution, for addition to drinking water, tiamulin fumarate 125 mg/mL, for *pigs*; 250 mL, 1 litre
Withdrawal Periods. *Pigs*: slaughter 1 day

POM Tiamutin 200 Injection (Leo) *UK*
Injection (oily), tiamulin fumarate 200 mg/mL, for *pigs*; 100 mL
Withdrawal Periods. *Pigs*: slaughter 10 day

Australia
Indications. Tiamulin-sensitive organisms
Dose. *Pigs, chickens*: treatment, 200 mg/kg; prophylaxis, 25 mg/kg

Dynamutalin 25 Feed Premix (Rhône-Poulenc) *Austral.*
Premix, tiamulin hydrogen fumarate 25 g/kg powder, for *pigs, chickens*
Withdrawal Periods. *Pigs*: slaughter 5 days. *Chickens*: slaughter 5 days, should not be used in chickens producing eggs for human consumption

Eire
Indications. Tiamulin-sensitive organisms
Dose. Consult manufacturer's information

Tiamutin 2% Premix (Leo) *Eire*
Premix, tiamulin hydrogen fumarate 20 g/kg, for *pigs*
Withdrawal Periods. Slaughter 24 hours

Tiamutin 12.5% Solution (Leo) *Eire*
Oral solution, for addition to drinking water, tiamulin hydrogen fumarate 125 mg/mL, for *pigs*
Withdrawal Periods. Slaughter 24 hours

Tiamutin 25% Premix (Leo) *Eire*
Premix, tiamulin hydrogen fumarate 250 g/kg, for *pigs*
Withdrawal Periods. Slaughter 24 hours

Tiamutin 80% Granulate (Leo) *Eire*
Premix, tiamulin hydrogen fumarate 800 mg/g, for *pigs*
Withdrawal Periods. Slaughter 24 hours

Tiamutin 200 Injection (Leo) *Eire*
Injection (oily), tiamulin hydrogen fumarate 200 mg/mL, for *pigs*
Withdrawal Periods. Slaughter 10 days

USA
Indications. Tiamulin-sensitive organisms
Dose. Consult manufacturer's information

Denagard (Boehringer Ingelheim NOBL) *USA*
Oral liquid, to add to drinking water, tiamulin fumarate 123 mg/kg, for *pigs*
Withdrawal Periods. Slaughter 3 or 7 days depending on dose

Denagard (Boehringer Ingelheim NOBL) *USA*
Oral powder, to add to drinking water, tiamulin fumarate 450 g/kg, for *pigs*
Withdrawal Periods. Slaughter 3 or 7 days depending on dose

Denagard 10 (Boehringer Ingelheim NOBL) *USA*
Premix, tiamulin (as fumarate) 22 g/kg premix, for *pigs*
Withdrawal Periods. Slaughter 2 days

VALNEMULIN HYDROCHLORIDE

UK
Indications. Tiamulin-sensitive organisms
Contra-indications. Rabbits
Side-effects. Rarely, perianal erythema or mild dermal oedema; transient inappetance at concentrations above 200 ppm
Warnings. Should not be given within 5 days of administration of monensin, narasin, or salinomycin (Drug Interactions – see Appendix 1). Safety in pregnant and lactating sows has not been established
Dose. *Pigs*:
Swine dysentery

treatment, *by addition to feed*, 3–4 mg/kg body-weight daily
prophylaxis, *by addition to feed*, 1.0–1.5 mg/kg body-weight daily

Swine enzootic pneumonia (Econor 10%), treatment and prevention, *by addition to feed*, 10–12 mg/kg body-weight daily

POM Econor 1% (Novartis)
Premix, valnemulin (as hydrochloride) 10 g/kg, for *pigs*
Withdrawal Periods. *Pigs*: slaughter 1 day

POM Econor 10% (Novartis)
Premix, valnemulin (as hydrochloride) 100 g/kg, for *pigs*
Withdrawal Periods. *Pigs*: slaughter 1 day

1.1.11 Other antibacterial drugs

Rifampicin is bactericidal against a wide range of micro-organisms and interferes with their synthesis of nucleic acids by inhibiting DNA-dependent RNA polymerase. The ability of rifampin to penetrate into cells makes it an ideal drug for treating intracellular infections. Rifampin is used in the treatment of tuberculosis in humans and has been suggested for use in treating atypical mycobacterial infections in cats. Rifampicin is frequently used in combination with erythromycin for the treatment of some pneumonic conditions in foals, particularly those caused by *Rhodococcus equi* infection. Rifampicin is an inducer of cytochrome P450 enzymes in the liver and enhances the metabolism of many other drugs including anticonvulsants and anticoagulants.

Polymixin B and other polymixin antibiotics such as **colistin** are active against Gram-negative bacteria. They act primarily by binding to membrane phospholipids and disrupting the bacterial cytoplasmic membrane. Polymixins are highly charged basic (cationic) molecules which cross biological membranes very poorly and are not absorbed from the gastro-intestinal tract. They are used in oral preparations for the treatment of gastro-intestinal disturbances and also in topical formulations (ear preparations) for the treatment of Gram-negative infections including *Pseudomonas aeruginosa*. If given systemically, they cause pain at the site of injection and have a narrow therapeutic index being both nephrotoxic and neurotoxic. These drugs are renally excreted and should never be given systemically to patients with renal insufficiency. They do have a capacity to bind endotoxins and some authorities advocate their use for this purpose.

Fusidic acid is a steroidal antibiotic with bacteriostatic or bacteriocidal activity mainly against Gram-positive bacteria. It selectively inhibits bacterial protein synthesis; there is poor penetration of the host cell.

Novobiocin acts by inhibiting DNA gyrase. It is active against many Gram-positive bacteria. Novobiocin is mainly used topically in intramammary preparations. This drug is highly potent against *Staphylococcus* spp. and *Streptococcus* spp. and may have a synergistic action with benzylpenicillin hence it is often co-formulated with this drug.

Vancomycin is a glycopeptide antibiotic and is active against Gram-positive bacteria. It exerts its action by inhibiting the formation of the peptidoglycan polymers of the bacterial cell wall. Vancomycin is not absorbed if given by the oral route and has a narrow therapeutic index when given parenterally. In human medicine, vancomycin is used to treat life threatening resistant staphylococcal infections. Oral administration can be used to treat pseudomembranous colitis in humans which is caused by overgrowth of *Clostridium difficile*.

Spectinomycin is an aminocyclitol antibiotic which acts by binding to the 30S subunit of the bacterial ribosome and inhibiting protein synthesis. It is active against some Gram-positive and Gram-negative bacteria; anaerobic microorganisms are mostly resistant. Spectinomycin is similar to steptomycin but it is not an aminoglycoside.

BACITRACIN

USA

Indications. Bacitracin-sensitive infections

Solu-Tracin 200 (Alpharma) *USA*
Oral powder, for addition to drinking water, bacitracin (as methylene disalicylate), for *pigs, chickens, turkeys*

FUMAGILLIN

UK

See Prescribing for bees

ISONIAZID

UK

Indications. Isoniazid-sensitive infections
Dose. *Horses*: *by mouth*, 5–20 mg/kg once daily

POM Ⓗ **Isoniazid** (Non-proprietary) *UK*
Injection, isoniazid 25 mg/mL
Available from Cambridge

NOVOBIOCIN

USA

Indications. Bacitracin-sensitive infections

Albamix Feed Medication (Pharmacia & Upjohn) *USA*
Premix, novobiocin 55g/kg, for *turkeys, chickens, mink, ducks*
Withdrawal Periods. *Turkeys, chickens*: slaughter 4 days; should not be used in laying turkeys or chickens. *Ducks*: slaughter 3 days; should not be used in laying ducks

RIFAMPICIN

UK

Indications. Rifampicin-sensitive infections
Dose. *Foals*: *by mouth*, 5 mg/kg twice daily

POM Ⓗ **Rifampicin** (Non-proprietary) *UK*
Capsules, rifampicin 150 mg, 300 mg

SPECTINOMYCIN

UK

Indications. Spectinomycin-sensitive infections
Contra-indications. Side-effects. Warnings. See under Apramycin
Dose.

Calves: *by intramuscular injection*, 20–30 mg/kg once daily for up to 5 days
Lambs: *by mouth*, 50 mg once only
Piglets: *by mouth*, (<4.5 kg body-weight) 50 mg twice daily; (4.5–7 kg body-weight) 100 mg twice daily

POM **Spectam Injectable** (Ceva) *UK*
Injection, spectinomycin activity (as dihydrochloride) 100 mg/mL, for *calves*; 100 mL
Withdrawal Periods. *Calves*: slaughter 10 days

POM **Spectam Scour Halt** (Ceva) *UK*
Mixture, spectinomycin activity (as dihydrochloride pentahydrate) 50 mg/unit dose, for *lambs, piglets up to 7 kg body-weight or 4 weeks of age*; 100-mL dose applicator (1 unit dose = 1 mL)
Withdrawal Periods. *Lambs, piglets*: slaughter 10 days
Dose. *Lambs*: 1 unit dose once only as soon as possible after birth
Piglets: (<4.5 kg body-weight) 1 unit dose twice daily, (4.5–7.0 kg body-weight) 2 unit doses twice daily

Eire

Indications. Spectinomycin-sensitive infections
Dose. Consult manufacturer's information

Spectam Scour Halt (Interpharm) *Eire*
Oral liquid, spectinomycin (as dihydrochloride pentahydrate) 50 mg/mL, for *piglets*
Withdrawal Periods. Slaughter 21 days

Spectam Injection (Interpharm) *Eire*
Injection, spectinomycin (as dihydrochloride) 100 mg/mL, for *cattle, sheep, pigs, dogs, cats, poultry, turkeys*
Withdrawal Periods. *Cattle, sheep, pigs, poultry*: slaughter 5 days. *Cattle*: milk 48 hours

Spectam Soluble (Interpharm) *Eire*
Oral powder, for addition to drinking water, spectinamycin (as dihydrochloride) 500 g/kg, for *calves, lambs, piglets, poultry, turkeys*
Withdrawal Periods. Slaughter 5 days

USA
Indications. Spectinomycin-sensitive infections
Dose. Consult manufacturer's information

Adspec (Pharmacia & Upjohn) *USA*
Injection, spectinomycin 100mg/mL (as sulphate tetrahydrate), for *cattle*
Withdrawal Periods. Slaughter 11 days

Prospec (Valdar) *USA*
Injection, spectinomycin 100 mg/mL, for *chickens, turkeys*

Spectam Injectable (Osborn) *USA*
Injection, spectinomycin (as dihydrochloride pentahydrate) 100 mg/mL, for *turkeys, chickens*

Spectam Scour-Halt (AgriLabs, AgriPharm, DurVet, Osborn, RXV) *USA*
Oral solution, spectinomycin (as dihydrochloride pentahydrate) 50 mg/mL, for *pigs*
Withdrawal Periods. Slaughter 21 days

Spectam Water Soluble (Osborn) *USA*
Oral solution, for addition to drinking water, spectinomycin (as dihydrochloride pentahydrate) 50 g/100g bottle, for *chickens*
Withdrawal Periods. Slaughter 5 days, should not be used in chickens producing eggs for human consumption

Spectinomycin Hydrochloride Injectable (Aspen, DurVet) *USA*
Injection, spectinomycin (as dihydrochloride pentahydrate) 100 mg/mL, for *turkeys, chickens*

VANCOMYCIN

UK
Indications. Vancomycin-sensitive infections
Dose. Prescribing for aquatic invertebrates

POM Ⓗ **Vancomycin** (Non-proprietary) *UK*
Injection, powder for reconstitution, vancomycin (as hydrochloride) 500 mg, 1 g

POM Ⓗ **Vancocin** (Lilly) *UK*
Injection, powder for reconstitution, vancomycin (as hydrochloride) 250 mg, 500 mg, 1 g

1.1.12 Compound antibacterial preparations

Although in principle the use of antibacterial mixtures is **not** recommended, in some cases two antibacterials may be used in combination for their activity against two specific and co-existing infections, for example, a mixture of a macrolide and a sulphonamide for enteric or respiratory disease in pigs.

The main components of combination parenteral preparations are procaine benzylpenicillin and a streptomycin which are complementary, having bactericidal activity against Gram-positive and Gram-negative organisms respectively and may be synergistic. Unfortunately, while the procaine benzylpenicillin component may remain effective for up to 24 hours, the streptomycin component is only effective for up to 12 hours.

UK
MFS **Cyfac HS Granular** (Alpharma) *UK*
Premix, chlortetracycline hydrochloride 73.2 g, procaine benzylpenicillin 36.6 g, sulfadimidine 73.2 g/kg, for *pigs*; 2.25 kg, 22.5 kg
Withdrawal Periods. *Pigs*: slaughter 15 days
Dose. *Pigs*: 2.25 kg of premix/tonne feed

POM **Depomycin Forte** (Intervet) *UK*
Injection, dihydrostreptomycin (as sulphate) 250 mg, procaine benzylpenicillin 200 mg/mL, for *horses, cattle, sheep, pigs, dogs, cats*; 100 mL
Withdrawal Periods. Should not be used in *horses* intended for human consumption. *Cattle*: slaughter 21 days, milk 2.5 days. *Sheep*: slaughter 35 days, should not be used in sheep producing milk for human consumption. *Pigs*: slaughter 21 days
Dose. *Horses, cattle*: *by intramuscular injection*, 0.04 mL/kg
Sheep, pigs: *by intramuscular injection*, 0.05 mL/kg
Dogs, cats: *by subcutaneous injection*, 0.1 mL/kg

POM **Dipen Forte** (Bimeda) *UK*
Injection, dihydrostreptomycin (as sulphate) 250 mg, procaine benzylpenicillin 200 mg/mL, for *cattle, sheep, pigs*; 100 mL
Withdrawal Periods. *Cattle*: slaughter 28 days, milk 72 hours. *Sheep*: slaughter 28 days, should not be used in sheep producing milk for human consumption. *Pigs*: slaughter 35 days
Dose. *Cattle, sheep, pigs*: *by intramuscular injection*, 0.04 mL/kg

POM **Duphapen + Strep** (Fort Dodge) *UK*
Injection, dihydrostreptomycin sulphate 250 mg, procaine benzylpenicillin 200 mg/mL, for *horses, cattle, sheep, pigs*; 50 mL, 100 mL
Withdrawal Periods. Should not be used in *horses* intended for human consumption. *Cattle*: slaughter 18 days, milk 2.5 days. *Sheep*: slaughter 18 days, should not be used in sheep producing milk for human consumption. *Pigs*: slaughter 18 days
Dose. *Horses, cattle, sheep, pigs*: *by intramuscular injection*, 0.04 mL/kg

MFS **Linco-Spectin Premix** (Pharmacia & Upjohn) *UK*
Premix, lincomycin (as hydrochloride) 22 g, spectinomycin (as sulphate) 22 g/kg, for *pigs*; 2 kg, 20 kg
Withdrawal Periods. *Pigs*: slaughter 1 day
Dose. *Pigs*: enteritis, treatment, 2 kg of premix/tonne feed daily for 3 weeks; prophylaxis, 1–2 kg of premix/tonne feed during period of risk
Mycoplasmal pneumonia, prophylaxis, 1–2 kg of premix/tonne feed during period of risk
Mastitis, metritis, agalactia syndrome (MMA), treatment, 1–2 kg of premix/tonne feed daily for 5–10 days before and 2–3 weeks after farrowing

POM **Linco-Spectin 100 Soluble Powder** (Pharmacia & Upjohn) *UK*
Oral powder, for addition to drinking water, lincomycin (as hydrochloride) 33.3 g, spectinomycin (as sulphate) 66.7 g/150 g, for *poultry*; 150 g
Withdrawal Periods. *Poultry*: slaughter 2 days, should not be used in poultry producing eggs for human consumption
Dose. *Poultry*: 75 g of powder/100 litres drinking water

POM **Microfac HP** (Vericore LP) *UK*
Oral powder, for addition to feed, chlortetracycline 82 g, procaine benzylpenicillin 41 g, sulfadimidine 82 g/kg, for *pigs*; 2 kg, 20 kg
Withdrawal Periods. *Pigs*: slaughter 15 days
Dose. *Pigs*: 2 kg of powder/tonne feed

POM **Neopen** (Intervet) *UK*
Injection, neomycin (as sulphate) 100 mg, procaine benzylpenicillin 200 mg/mL, for *horses, sheep, pigs, dogs, cats*; 100 mL
Withdrawal Periods. Should not be used in *horses* intended for human consumption. *Sheep*: slaughter 70 days, should not be used in sheep producing milk for human consumption. *Pigs*: slaughter 60 days
Dose. *Horses, cattle, sheep, pigs*: *by intramuscular injection*, 0.05 mL/kg
Dogs, cats: *by intramuscular injection*, 0.1 mL/kg

POM **Orojet Lamb** (Fort Dodge) *UK*
Oral liquid, neomycin sulphate 70 mg, streptomycin sulphate 70 mg/unit dose, for *lambs*; 210-mL metered-dose applicator (1 unit dose = 1 mL)
Withdrawal Periods. *Lambs*: slaughter 28 days
Dose. *Lambs*: 1 unit dose/5 kg body-weight twice daily

POM **Pen & Strep** (Norbrook) *UK*
Injection, dihydrostreptomycin sulphate 250 mg, procaine benzylpenicillin 200 mg/mL, for *horses, cattle, sheep, pigs*; 50 mL, 100 mL
Withdrawal Periods. Should not be used in *horses* intended for human consumption. *Cattle*: slaughter 18 days, milk 2.5 days. *Sheep*: slaughter 18 days, should not be used in sheep producing milk for human consumption. *Pigs*: slaughter 18 days
Dose. *Horses, cattle, sheep, pigs*: by intramuscular injection, 0.04 mL/kg

POM **Penicillin/Streptomycin Injection** (Vericore VP) *UK*
Injection, dihydrostreptomycin sulphate 250 mg, procaine benzylpenicillin 200 mg/mL, for *horses, cattle, sheep, pigs*; 100 mL
Withdrawal Periods. Should not be used in *horses* intended for human consumption. *Cattle*: slaughter 18 days, milk 2.5 days. *Sheep*: slaughter 18 days, should not be used in sheep producing milk for human consumption. *Pigs*: slaughter 18 days
Dose. *Cattle, sheep, pigs*: by intramuscular injection, 0.04 mL/kg

POM **Stomorgyl 2** (Merial) *UK*
Tablets, coated, metronidazole 25 mg, spiramycin 46.7 mg, for *dogs, cats*
Dose. *Dogs, cats*: 1 tablet/2 kg body-weight once daily
Note. Tablets should not be broken or crushed

POM **Stomorgyl 10** (Merial) *UK*
Tablets, coated, metronidazole 125 mg, spiramycin 234.4 mg, for *dogs, cats*
Dose. *Dogs, cats*: 1 tablet/10 kg body-weight once daily
Note. Tablets should not be broken or crushed

POM **Stomorgyl 20** (Merial) *UK*
Tablets, coated, metronidazole 250 mg, spiramycin 469 mg, for *dogs, cats*; 100
Dose. *Dogs, cats*: 1 tablet/20 kg body-weight once daily
Note. Tablets should not be broken or crushed

POM **Streptacare** (Animalcare) *UK*
Injection, dihydrostreptomycin sulphate 250 mg, procaine benzylpenicillin 200 mg/mL, for *horses, cattle, sheep, pigs*; 100 mL
Withdrawal Periods. Should not be used in *horses* intended for human consumption. *Cattle*: slaughter 18 days, milk 60 hours. *Sheep*: slaughter 18 days, should not be used in sheep producing milk for human consumption. *Pigs*: slaughter 18 days
Dose. *Horses, cattle, sheep, pigs*: by intramuscular injection, 0.04 mL/kg

POM **Streptopen** (Schering-Plough) *UK*
Injection, dihydrostreptomycin (as sulphate) 250 mg, procaine benzylpenicillin 250 mg/mL, for *horses, cattle, sheep, pigs*; 30 mL, 100 mL
Withdrawal Periods. Should not be used in *horses* intended for human consumption. *Cattle*: slaughter 28 days, milk 2.5 days. *Sheep*: slaughter 28 days, should not be used in sheep producing milk for human consumption. *Pigs*: slaughter 28 days
Dose. *Horses, cattle, sheep, pigs*: by intramuscular injection, 0.04 mL/kg

POM **Strypen** (Merial) *UK*
Injection, dihydrostreptomycin sulphate 250 mg, procaine benzylpenicillin 200 mg/mL, for *cattle, sheep, pigs*; 100 mL
Withdrawal Periods. *Cattle*: slaughter 18 days, milk 2.5 days. *Sheep*: slaughter 18 days, should not be used in sheep producing milk for human consumption. *Pigs*: slaughter 18 days
Dose. *Cattle, sheep, pigs*: by intramuscular injection, 0.04 mL/kg

POM **Tylasul G50** (Elanco) *UK*
Premix, sulfadimidine 50 g, tylosin (as phosphate) 50 g/kg, for *pigs*; 2 kg
Withdrawal Periods. *Pigs*: slaughter 9 days
Dose. *Pigs*: 2 kg of premix/tonne feed

Australia

Indications. **Dose**. See manufacturer's information

Aquacaine S Injectable Suspension (Boehringer Ingelheim) *Austral.*
Injection, procaine benzylpenicillin 200 mg/mL and dihydrostreptomycin sulphate 250 mg/mL, for *cattle, horses, sheep, pigs, dogs, cats*
Withdrawal Periods. *Horses, sheep, pigs*: slaughter 30 days. *Cattle*: slaughter 30 days, milk 36 hours (single dose) or 72 hours (multiple dose)

Biodexamine (Intervet) *Austral.*
Injection, procaine benzylpenicillin 200 mg/mL, dihydrostreptomycin sulphate 250 mg, dexamethasone 1 mg, tripelennamine hydrochloride 10 mg, for *cattle, horses, sheep, pigs, dogs, cats*
Withdrawal Periods. *Horses, sheep, pigs*: slaughter 30 days. *Cattle*: slaughter 30 days, milk 36 hours (single dose) or 72 hours (multiple dose)

Delta Albaplex (Pharmacia & Upjohn) *Austral.*
Tablets, tetracycline hydrochloride 60 mg, novobiocin sodium 60 mg, prednisolone 1.5 mg, for *dogs, cats*

Delta Albaplex 3X (Pharmacia & Upjohn) *Austral.*
Tablets, tetracycline hydrochloride 180 mg, novobiocin sodium 180 mg, prednisolone 4.5 mg, for *dogs*

Depomycin (Intervet) *Austral.*
Injection, procaine benzylpenicillin 200 mg/mL, dihydrostreptomycin (as sulphate) 250 mg/mL, for *horses, cattle, sheep, pigs, dogs, cats*
Withdrawal Periods. *Horses, sheep, pigs*: slaughter 30 days. *Cattle*: slaughter 30 days, milk 36 hous (single dose) or 72 hours (multiple dose)

Hydropen (Pharmtech) *Austral.*
Injection, procaine benzylpenicillin 200 mg/mL, dihydrostreptomycin sulphate 250 mg/mL, for *horses, cattle, sheep, pigs, goats, dogs, cats*
Withdrawal Periods. *Horses, sheep, goats, pigs*: slaughter 30 days. *Cattle*: slaughter 30 days, milk 72 hours

Lincomix S Antibiotic Premix (Pharmacia & Upjohn) *Austral.*
Premix, lincomycin (as hydrochloride monohydrate) 44 g/kg and sulfadimidine 110 g/kg, for *pigs*
Withdrawal Periods. Slaughter 14 days

Linco-Spectin Antibiotic Premix (Pharmacia & Upjohn) *Austral.*
Premix, lincomycin (as hydrochloride monohydrate) 22 g/kg and spectinomycin (as sulphate tetrahydrate) 22 g/kg premix, for *pigs*
Withdrawal Periods. Slaughter 1 day

Linco-Spectin Antibiotic Soluble Powder (Pharmacia & Upjohn) *Austral.*
Powder, for addition to drinking water, lincomycin (as hydrochloride monohydrate) 222 g/kg and spectinomycin (as sulphate tetrahydrate) 445 g/kg powder, for *pigs, poultry*
Withdrawal Periods. *Pigs*: slaughter 8 days. *Poultry*: slaughter 10 days

Linco-Spectin Solution (Pharmacia & Upjohn) *Austral.*
Injection, lincomycin (as hydrochloride monohydrate) 50 mg/mL, spectinomycin (as sulphate tetrahydrate) 100 mg/mL, for *pigs, chickens, turkeys, dogs, cats*
Withdrawal Periods. *Pigs*: slaughter 21 days. *Poultry*: slaughter 10 days

Neomycin-Penicillin 100/200 (Intervet) *Austral.*
Injection, neomycin (as sulphate) 100 mg/mL, procaine benzylpenicillin 200 mg/ml, polyvinylpyrrolidone, for *horses, cattle, sheep, pigs, dogs, cats*
Withdrawal Periods. *Horses, pigs*: slaughter 100 days. *Cattle*: slaughter 35 days, milk 36 hours (single dose) or 72 hours (multiple dose). *Sheep*: slaughter 35 days

Neo-Terramycin 50/50 Soluble Powder (Pfizer) *Austral.*
Powder, for addition to drinking water, oxytetracycline hydrochloride 50 g/kg and neomycin sulphate 50 g/kg powder, for *poultry, pigs, sheep, cattle*
Withdrawal Periods. *Calves*: slaughter 5 days. *Cattle*: should not be used in cattle producing milk for human consumption. *Pigs*: slaughter 4 days. *Poultry*: slaughter 7 days, should not be used in poultry producing eggs for human consumption

Pen and Strep Injection (Novartis) *Austral.*
Injection, procaine benzylpenicillin 200 mg/mL, dihydrostreptomycin sulphate 250 mg/mL, for *horses, cattle, sheep, pigs, dogs, cats*

Withdrawal Periods. *Horses, sheep, pigs*: slaughter 30 days. *Cattle*: slaughter 30 days, milk 72 hours

Penstrep (Ilium) *Austral.*
Injection, procaine benzylpenicillin 200 mg/mL, dihydrostreptomycin sulphate 250 mg/mL, procaine hydrochloride 20 mg/mL, for *horses, cattle, sheep, pigs, dogs, cats*
Withdrawal Periods. *Horses, sheep, pigs*: slaughter 30 days. *Cattle*: slaughter 30 days, milk 36 hours (single dose) or 72 hours (multiple dose)

Stomorgyl (Merial) *Austral.*
Tablets, spiramycin/ metronidazole 150,000units/25 mg and 750,000 units/ 125 mg, for *dogs, cats*

Sulcin (Jurox) *Austral.*
Oral granules, sulfadimidine 375 mg, sulfadiazine 375 mg, streptomycin (as sulphate) 40 mg (with thiamine and riboflavine)/g granules, for *cattle, pigs*
Withdrawal Periods. Slaughter 14 days

Tylan 100 + Sulfa G (Elanco) *Austral.*
Premix, tylosin phosphate 100 g/kg, sulfadimidine 100 g/kg, for *pigs*
Withdrawal Periods. Slaughter 14 days

Eire
Indications. Dose. See manufacturer's information

Aurofac 20 (Whelehan) *Eire*
Oral powder, chlortetracycline hydrochloride 1.4 g, neomycin sulphate 0.7 g per 100 g of powder, for *calves*
Withdrawal Periods. Slaughter 75 days

Bactidiaryl Powder (Vetoquinol) *Eire*
Oral powder, neomycin (as sulphate) 500,000 units, tetracycline hydrochloride 250 mg, for *horses, cattle, sheep, goats, pigs*
Withdrawal Periods. Slaughter 8 days

Chanacin Plus (Chanelle) *Eire*
Tablets, phthalylsulfathiazole 2 g, streptomycin sulphate 0.5 g, for *calves*
Withdrawal Periods. Slaughter 28 days

Colamox Injectable Suspension (Virbac) *Eire*
Injection, amoxicillin (as trihydrate) 100 mg/mL, colistin (as sulfate) 250,000 units/mL, for *calves*
Withdrawal Periods. Slaughter 4 weeks

Cyfax HS Granular (Whelehan) *Eire*
Premix, chlortetracycline hydrochloride 73.2 g/kg, procaine penicillin 36.6 g/kg, sulfadimidine 73.2 g/kg, for *pigs*
Withdrawal Periods. Slaughter 15 days

Depomycin (Intervet) *Eire*
Injection, procaine benzylpenicillin 200 mg/mL, dihydrostreptomycin (as sulphate) 200 mg/mL, for *horses, cattle, sheep, pigs, dogs, cats*
Withdrawal Periods. Should not be used in *horses* intended for human consumption. *Cattle*: slaughter 21 days, milk 72 hours. *Sheep*: slaughter 35 days, should not be used in sheep producing milk for human consumption. *Pigs*: slaughter 21 days

Diet-Scour Soluble Powder (Virbac) *Eire*
Oral powder, per 70-g sachet: ampicillin (as trihydrate), colistin sulfate 1,000,000 units, for *calves*
Withdrawal Periods. Slaughter 3 days

Duphapen + Strep (Interchem) *Eire*
Injection, procaine benzylpenicillin 200 mg/mL, dihydrostreptomycin (as sulphate) 200 mg/mL, for *cattle, sheep, pigs*
Withdrawal Periods. *Cattle*: slaughter 18 days, milk 48 hours. *Sheep*: slaughter 18 days, should not be used in sheep producing milk for human consumption. *Pigs*: slaughter 18 days

KCN Injectable Solution (Virbac) *Eire*
Injection, kanamycin sulphate 50 mg/mL, colistin 100,000 units/mL, neomycin sulphate 50 mg/mL, for *horses, cattle, sheep, pigs, small animals*
Withdrawal Periods. *Horses, cattle, sheep, pigs*: slaughter 10 days. *Cattle, sheep*: milk 2 milkings

Linco-Spectin Premix (Pharmacia & Upjohn) *Eire*
Premix, lincomycin (as hydrochloride) 22 g/kg, spectinomycin (as sulphate) 22 g/kg, for *pigs*
Withdrawal Periods. Slaughter 24 hours

Linco-Spectin 100 Soluble Powder (Pharmacia & Upjohn) *Eire*
Oral powder, for addition to drinking water, lincomycin (as hydrochloride) 33.3 g, spectinomycin (as sulphate) 66.7 g/ pack, for *poultry*
Withdrawal Periods. Slaughter 48 hours

Linco-Spectin Sterile Solution (Pharmacia & Upjohn) *Eire*
Injection, lincomycin (as hydrochloride) 50 mg/mL, spectinomycin (as sulphate) 100 mg/mL, for *calves, pigs, dogs, cats*
Withdrawal Periods. *Calves*: slaughter 21 days. *Pigs*: slaughter 14 days

Neomycin Penicillin (Intervet) *Eire*
Injection, neomycin (as sulphate) 100 mg/mL, procaine penicillin 200 mg/ mL, for *cattle, pigs*
Withdrawal Periods. *Cattle*: slaughter 29 days, milk 3 days. *Pigs*: slaughter 39 days

Orojet Lamb (Fort Dodge) *Eire*
Oral liquid, neomycin sulphate 70 mg/mL, streptomycin sulphate 70 mg/mL, for *lambs*
Withdrawal Periods. Slaughter 28 days

Pen & Strep (Norbrook) *Eire*
Injection, dihydrostreptomycin (as sulphate) 200 mg/mL, procaine benzylpenicillin 200 mg/mL, for *cattle, sheep, pigs*
Withdrawal Periods. *Cattle*: slaughter 18 days, milk 48 hours. *Sheep*: slaughter 18 days, should not be used in sheep producing milk for human consumption. *Pigs*: slaughter 18 days

Penijectyl Injectable Suspension (Virbac) *Eire*
Injection, dihydrostreptomycin sulfate 200 mg/mL, procaine benzylpenicillin 200 mg/mL, for *cattle*
Withdrawal Periods. Slaughter 60 days, milk 84 hours

Pen/Strep Injection (Interpharm) *Eire*
Injection, procaine benzylpenicillin 200,000 iu/mL, dihydrostreptomycin sulphate 250 mg/mL, for *horses, cattle, sheep, goats, pigs, dogs, cats*
Withdrawal Periods. *Horses, cattle, sheep, goats, pigs*: slaughter 18 days. *Cattle*: milk 48 hours

Pentomycin (Univet) *Eire*
Injection, dihydrostreptomycin 200 mg/mL, procaine benzylpenicillin 200 mg/mL, for *cattle, sheep, pigs*
Withdrawal Periods. *Cattle*: slaughter 21 days, milk 72 hours. *Sheep*: slaughter 21 days, should not be used in sheep producing milk for human consumption. *Pigs*: slaughter 21 days

Strisul Vettabs (Rice Steele) *Eire*
Tablets, phthalylsulphathiazole 2.0 g, streptomycin sulphate 0.5 g, for *calves*
Withdrawal Periods. Slaughter 28 days

Tylasul G50 (Elanco) *Eire*
Premix, tylosin (as phosphate) 50 g/kg, sulphadimidine 50 g/kg, for *pigs*
Withdrawal Periods. Slaughter 9 days

Tylasul G10 (Elanco) *Eire*
Premix, tylosin (as phosphate) 100 g/kg, sulphadimidine 100 g/kg, for *pigs*
Withdrawal Periods. Slaughter 9 days

Tylasul G50 (Elanco) *Eire*
Premix, tylosin (as phosphate) 50 g/kg, sulphadimidine 50 g/kg, for *pigs*
Withdrawal Periods. Slaughter 9 days

Tylasul G100 (Elanco) *Eire*
Premix, tylosin (as phosphate) 100 g/kg, sulphadimidine 100 g/kg, for *pigs*
Withdrawal Periods. Slaughter 9 days

New Zealand
Indications. Dose. See manufacturer's information

Biodexamine (Chemavet) *NZ*
Injection, dexamethasone 1 mg/mL, dihydrostreptomycin (as sulphate) 250 mg/mL, procaine penicillin 200 000 units/mL, tripelennamine (as hydrochloride) 10 mg/mL, for *horses, cattle, sheep, pigs, dogs, cats*
Withdrawal Periods. *Horses, pigs*: slaughter 30 days. *Cattle, sheep*: slaughter 30 days, milk 3 days

Delta Albaplex (Pharmacia & Upjohn) *NZ*
Tablets, novobiocin (as sodium salt) 60 mg, prednisolone 1.5 mg, tetracycline (as hydrochloride) 60 mg, for *dogs, cats*

Depomycin (Chemavet) *NZ*
Injection, dihydrostreptomycin 200 mg/mL, procaine benzylpenicillin 200 000 units/mL, for *horses, cattle, sheep, pigs, dogs, cats*
Withdrawal Periods. *Horses, pigs*: slaughter 30 days. *Cattle, sheep*: slaughter 30 days, milk 48 hours (1 dose), 60 hours (2 doses), 72 hours (3 or more doses)

Dynamutilin-S (PCL) *NZ*
Premix, sulfadimidine 100 g/kg, tiamulin fumarate 25 g/kg, for *pigs*
Withdrawal Periods. Slaughter 15 days

Hydropen (Bomac) *NZ*
Injection, dihydrostreptomycin 250 mg/mL, procaine benzylpenicillin 200 mg/mL, for *horses, cattle, sheep, pigs, dogs, cats*
Withdrawal Periods. *Horses, pigs*: slaughter 30 days. *Cattle, sheep*: slaughter 30 days, milk 48 hours (1 dose), 60 hours (2 doses), 72 hours (3 or more doses)

Lincomix S Premix (Pharmacia & Upjohn) *NZ*
Premix, lincomycin (as hydrochloride) 44 g/kg, sulfadimidine 110 g/kg, for *pigs*
Withdrawal Periods. Slaughter 10 days

Linco-Spectin Premix (Pharmacia & Upjohn) *NZ*
Premix, lincomycin 22 g/kg, spectinomycin 22 g/kg, for *pigs*
Withdrawal Periods. Slaughter 1 day

Linco-Spectin Soluble Powder (Pharmacia & Upjohn) *NZ*
Oral powder, lincomycin 33.3 g/150 g, spectinomycin 66.7 g/150 g, for *pigs, poultry*
Withdrawal Periods. *Pigs*: slaughter 8 days. *Poultry*: slaughter 48 hours, should not be used in laying birds

Linco-Spectin Sterile Solution (Pharmacia & Upjohn) *NZ*
Injection, lincomycin (as hydrochloride) 50 mg/mL, spectinomycin (as sulphate) 100 mg/mL, for *pigs, dogs, cats, poultry*
Withdrawal Periods. *Pigs*: slaughter 21 days. *Poultry*: slaughter 21 days, should not be used in laying birds

Neomycin-Penicillin 100/200 (Chemavet) *NZ*
Injection, neomycin (as sulphate) 100 mg/mL, procaine benzylpenicillin 200 000 units/mL, for *horses, cattle, sheep, pigs, dogs, cats*
Withdrawal Periods. *Horses, pigs*: slaughter 30 days. *Cattle, sheep*: slaughter 30 days, milk 72 hours

Penodure S (Boehringer Ingelheim) *NZ*
Depot injection, dihydrostreptomycin (as sulphate) 250 mg/mL, benzathine benzylpenicillin 150 000 units/mL, procaine benzylpenicillin 150 000 units/mL, for *horses, cattle, sheep, pigs, dogs, cats*
Withdrawal Periods. *Horses, pigs*: slaughter 30 days. *Cattle, sheep*: slaughter 30 days, milk 108 hours

Penomycin 250/250 (Boehringer Ingelheim) *NZ*
Injection, dihydrostreptomycin (as sulphate) 250 mg/mL, procaine benzylpenicillin 250 000 units/mL, for *horses, cattle, sheep, pigs, dogs, cats*
Withdrawal Periods. *Horses, pigs*: slaughter 30 days. *Cattle, sheep*: slaughter 30 days, milk 48 hours (1 dose), 60 hours (2 doses), 72 hours (3 or more doses)

Penstrep LA (Bomac) *NZ*
Depot injection, benzathine benzylpenicillin 100 000 units/mL, dihydrostreptomycin 250 mg/mL, procaine benzylpenicillin 100 000 units/mL, for *horses, cattle, dogs, cats*
Withdrawal Periods. *Horses*: slaughter 30 days. *Cattle*: slaughter 30 days, milk 108 hours

Phoenix Pink Scour Tablets (Phoenix) *NZ*
Tablets, sulfadiazine 1.58 g, sulfamerazine 1.58 g, sulfapyridine 1.59 g, streptomycin sulphate 0.313 g, for *calves, sheep, goats*
Withdrawal Periods. *Calves*: slaughter 21 days. *Sheep, goats*: slaughter 21 days, should not be used in sheep or goats producing milk for human consumption

Propen S (Schering-Plough) *NZ*
Injection, benethamine benzylpenicillin 141.5 mg/mL, dihydrostreptomycin (as sulphate) 250 mg/mL, procaine benzylpenicillin 150 mg/mL, for *horses, cattle, sheep, pigs, dogs, cats*
Withdrawal Periods. *Horses, pigs*: slaughter 30 days. *Cattle, sheep*: slaughter 30 days, milk 132 hours

Stomorgyl 2 (Merial) *NZ*
Tablets, metronidazole 25 mg, spiramycin 150 000 units, for *dogs, cats*

Stomorgyl 10 (Merial) *NZ*
Tablets, metronidazole 125 mg, spiramycin 750 000 units, for *dogs, cats*

Stomorgyl 20 (Merial) *NZ*
Tablets, metronidazole 250 mg, spiramycin 1 500 000 units, for *dogs*

Strepcin (Stockguard) *NZ*
Injection, dihydrostreptomycin (as sulphate) 250 mg/mL, procaine benzylpenicillin 250 000 units/mL, for *horses, cattle, sheep, pigs, dogs, cats*
Withdrawal Periods. *Horses, pigs*: slaughter 30 days. *Cattle, sheep*: slaughter 30 days, milk 48 hours (1 dose), 60 hours (2 doses), 72 hours (3 or more doses)

Strepcin L.A. (Stockguard) *NZ*
Depot injection, benzathine benzylpenicillin 100 000 units/mL, dihydrostreptomycin (as sulphate) 250 mg/mL, procaine benzylpenicillin 100 000 units/mL, for *horses, cattle, sheep, pigs, dogs, cats*
Withdrawal Periods. *Horses, pigs*: slaughter 30 days. *Cattle, sheep*: slaughter 30 days, milk 108 hours

Streptopen 250/250 (Schering-Plough) *NZ*
Injection, dihydrostreptomycin (as sulphate) 250 mg/mL, procaine benzylpenicillin 250 000 units/mL, for *horses, cattle, sheep, pigs, dogs, cats*
Withdrawal Periods. *Horses, pigs*: slaughter 30 days. *Cattle, sheep*: slaughter 30 days, milk 72 hours

Streptopenicillin (Ethical) *NZ*
Injection, dihydrostreptomycin 250 mg/mL, procaine benzylpenicillin 200 000 units/mL, for *horses, cattle, sheep, goats, pigs, dogs, cats, poultry*
Withdrawal Periods. *Horses, pigs, poultry*: slaughter 30 days. *Cattle, sheep, goats*: slaughter 30 days, milk 96 hours

Strepvet 250 (Phoenix) *NZ*
Injection, dihydrostreptomycin (as sulphate) 250 mg/mL, procaine benzylpenicillin 250 000 units/mL, for *horses, cattle, sheep, pigs, dogs, cats*
Withdrawal Periods. *Horses, pigs*: slaughter 30 days. *Cattle, sheep*: slaughter 30 days, milk 48 hours (1 dose), 60 hours (2 doses), 72 hours (3 or more doses)

Strepvet L.A. (Phoenix) *NZ*
Depot injection, benzathine benzylpenicillin 100 000 units/mL, dihydrostreptomycin (as sulphate) 250 mg/mL, procaine benzylpenicillin 100 000 units/mL, for *horses, cattle, sheep, pigs, dogs, cats*
Withdrawal Periods. *Horses, pigs*: slaughter 30 days. *Cattle, sheep*: slaughter 30 days, milk 108 hours

Strinacin (Merial) *NZ*
Tablets, streptomycin sulphate 0.25 g, sulfadiazine 1.58 g, sulfamerazine 1.58 g, sulfapyridine 1.58 g, for *horses, cattle, sheep, goats, deer, pigs*
Withdrawal Periods. *Horses*: slaughter 180 days. *Cattle*: slaughter 14 days, should not be used in cattle producing milk for human consumption. *Sheep, goats, deer, pigs*: slaughter 14 days

Tetramutin (Reamor) *NZ*
Premix, chlortetracycline 100 g/kg, tiamulin fumarate 33.3 g/kg, for *pigs*
Withdrawal Periods. Slaughter 10 days

Tylasul-G Concentrate (Elanco) *NZ*
Premix, sulfadimidine 100 g/kg, tylosin (as phosphate) 100 g/kg, for *pigs*
Withdrawal Periods. Slaughter 15 days

USA

Albaplex (Pharmacia & Upjohn) *USA*
Tablets, tetracycline hydrochloride 60 mg, novobiocin sodium 60 mg, for *dogs*

Aureo 500 Granular (Roche Vitamins) *USA*
Premix, Chlortetracycline hydrochloride (as calcium complex) 8.8%, sulfadimidine 8.8%, penicillin (as procaine penicillin) 4.4%, for *pigs*
Withdrawal Periods. Slaughter 15 days

Aureo S 700 (Roche Vitamins) *USA*
Premix, chlortetracycline hydrochloride (as calcium complex) 7.7%, sulfamethazine 7.7%, for *cattle*
Withdrawal Periods. Slaughter 7 days

Aureo SP 250 (RocheVitamins) *USA*
Premix, chlortetracycline hydrochloride (as calcium complex) 2.2%, sulfadimidine 2.2%, penicillin (as procaine penicillin 1.1%, for *pigs*
Withdrawal Periods. Slaughter 15 days

Aureomycin Sulmet Soluble Powder (Fort Dodge) *USA*
Oral powder, for addition to drinking water, chlortetracycline hydrochloride (as bisulphate) 225.3 mg/kg, sulfadimidine 225.3 mg/kg, for *pigs*
Withdrawal Periods. Slaughter 5 days

Aureozol Granular (Roche Vitamins) *USA*
Premix, chlortetracycline hydrochloride (as calcium complex) 2.2%, sulfathiazole 2.2%, penicillin (as procaine penicillin) 1.1%; also preparation with 8.8%, 8.8% and 4.4% respectively, for *pigs*
Withdrawal Periods. Slaughter 7 days

CSP 250 Fermablend (Boehringer Ingelheim NOBL) *USA*
Premix, chlortetracycline 22 g/kg, sulfathiazole 22 g/kg, penicillin 11 g/kg feed, for *pigs*
Withdrawal Periods. Slaughter 7 days

Delta Albaplex (Pharmacia & Upjohn) *USA*
Tablets, tetracycline hydrochloride 60 mg, novobiocin (as sodium salt) 60 mg, prednisolone 1.5 mg, for *dogs*

L-S 50 (Pharmacia & Upjohn) *USA*
Oral powder, to add to drinking water, lincomycin 16.7 g and spectinomycin (as sulphate tetrahydrate) 33.3 g/ 75 g powder (packet), for *chickens*

Maxi Care NT (Land O'Lakes) *USA*
Premix, oxytetracycline 125 g/ton, neomycin (as sulphate) 250 mg/ton, for *cattle*
Withdrawal Periods. *Calves*: slaughter 30 days, should not be used in calves intended for veal production

Neo-Terramycin 100/50 (Pfizer) *USA*
Premix, oxytetracycline hydrochloride 110 g/kg premix, neomycin sulphate 220 g/kg premix, for *chickens, turkeys, pigs, cattle*
Withdrawal Periods. *Calves*: slaughter 0 or 7 days (depending on oxytet dose). *Pigs*: slaughter 5 days. *Chickens*: slaughter 5 days (broilers), slaughter 14 days (laying hens)

Neo-Terramycin 100/50D (Pfizer) *USA*
Premix, oxytetracycline hydrochloride 110 g/kg, neomycin 22 g/kg, for *cattle, pigs*
Withdrawal Periods. *Calves*: slaughter 30 days. *Pigs*: slaughter 5 or 10 days (depending on neomycin dose)

Neo-Terramycin 50/50 (Pfizer) *USA*
Premix, oxytetracycline hydrochloride 110 g/kg, neomycin sulphate 110 g/kg, for *chickens, turkeys, pigs, cattle*
Withdrawal Periods. *Calves*: slaughter 0 or 7 days (depending on oxytet dose). *Pigs*: slaughter 5 days. *Chickens*: slaughter 5 days (broilers), slaughter 14 days (laying hens).*Turkeys*: slaughter 14 days.

Neo-Terramycin 50/50D (Pfizer) *USA*
Premix, oxytetracycline hydrochloride 110 g/kg premix, neomycin (as sulphate) 110 g/kg premix, for *cattle, pigs*
Withdrawal Periods. *Calves*: slaughter 30 days. *Pigs*: slaughter 5 or 10 days (depending on neomycin dose)

Nursing Formula NT (Land O'Lakes) *USA*
Premix, oxytetracycline 125 g/ton; neomycin (as sulphate) 250 mg/ton, for *cattle*
Withdrawal Periods. *Calves*: should not be used in calves intended for veal production

Sav-A-Caf Scours Control 2 (IntAgra) *USA*
Oral powder, for reconstitution, neomycin (as neomycin sulphate) 200 mg/ 113.3 g powder, oxytetracycline hydrochloride 100mg/ 1133 g powder, for *cattle*
Withdrawal Periods. *Calves*: slaughter 30 days

Sav-A-Caf Scours Control Medicated Concentrate (IntAgra) *USA*
Oral powder, for reconstitution, neomycin 13.46 g/kg powder, oxytetracycline 6.73 g/kg powder, for *cattle*
Withdrawal Periods. *Calves*: slaughter 30 days

Tylan 40 Sulfa-G (Elanco) *USA*
Pellets (Premix), tylosin (as phosphate) 88 g/kg and sulfadimidine 88 g/kg, for *pigs*
Withdrawal Periods. Slaughter 15 days

1.1.13 Compound preparations for bacterial enteritis

Antibacterial drugs are unnecessary in most cases of bacterial gastro-enteritis and may be contra-indicated. Antidiarrhoeal drugs may give symptomatic relief but should not distract from the importance of giving oral or parenteral fluids (see section 16.1). Compound preparations may contain an antibacterial such as neomycin or colistin, an adsorbant such as kaolin or bismuth, and a gastro-intestinal motility modifier such as hyoscine.

Note. Compound antibacterial preparations are listed under 1.1.12

UK

POM **Kaobiotic Tablets** (Pharmacia & Upjohn) *UK*
Tablets, scored, neomycin (as sulphate) 5.68 mg, kaolin 729 mg, for *dogs, cats*; 500
Dose. *Dogs, cats*: *by mouth,* 1 tablet/4 kg daily in divided doses

Australia

Ensal (Jurox) *Austral.*
Oral suspension, phthalylsulfathiazole 250 mg, kaolin 500 mg, hyoscine methobromide 1 mg /5 mL (also contains monosodium glutamate and calcium and potassium gluconates, for *dogs, cats*

Gastrozine (Apex) *Austral.*
Oral liquid, trimethoprim 200 mg, sulfadiazine 1 g, hyoscine methobromide 10 mg, kaolin 11.3 g, pectin 1.38 g, bismuth carbonate 770 mg (+ vitamins, minerals and amino acids) / 100 mL, for *cattle, horses, sheep, goats, dogs*
Withdrawal Periods. *Horses, cattle, sheep, goats*: slaughter 14 days. *Cattle, sheep, goats*: milk 96 hours

Neobiotic P Pump Antibiotic (Pharmacia & Upjohn) *Austral.*
Oral suspension, neomycin sulphate 50 mg/ ml, hyoscine methobromide 0.25 mg/mL, for *pigs*
Withdrawal Periods. Slaughter 20 days

Neo-Sulcin Suspension (Jurox) *Austral.*
Oral suspension, sulfadiazine 1278 mg, sulfadimidine 852 mg, neomycin sulphate 54 mg, hyoscine methobromide 1.2 mg, kaolin 3.1 g, pectin 213 mg (+ thiamine and riboflavine) /30 mL, for *cattle, horses, sheep, goats, dogs, cats*

Withdrawal Periods. *Horses, cattle, sheep, goats*: slaughter 14 days. *Cattle, sheep, goats*: milk 36 hours (single dose), 72 hours (multiple dose)

Neo-Sulcin Tablets (Jurox) *Austral.*
Tablets, sulfadiazine 750 mg, sulfadimidine 750 mg, neomycin sulphate 250 mg, hyoscine methobromide 2 mg (+ thiamine and riboflavine), for *cattle, horses, pigs*
Withdrawal Periods. *Cattle*: slaughter 14 days, milk 36 hours (single dose) 72 hours (multiple dose). *Horses, pigs*: slaughter 14 days.

Scourban (Pharmtech) *Austral.*
Oral suspension, sulfadimidine 1065 mg, sulfadiazine 1065 mg, streptomycin sulphate 228 mg, neomycin sulphate 54 mg, hyoscine hydrobromide 1.2 mg, kaolin 3.1 g, pectin 159.6 mg (with electrolytes and glycine)/30 mL, for *horses, cattle, sheep, goats, dogs, cats*
Withdrawal Periods. *Horses, cattle, sheep, goats*: slaughter 14 days. *Cattle, sheep, goats*: milk 36 hours (single dose), 72 hours (multiple dose)

Scour-X (Jurox) *Austral.*
Oral suspension, sulfadiazine 1278 mg, sulfadimidine 852 mg, neomycin sulphate 54 mg, hyoscine methobromide 1.2 mg, kaolin 3.1 g, pectin 213 mg (with thiamine and riboflavine) /30 mL, for *cattle, sheep, horses, goats, dogs, cats*
Withdrawal Periods. *Horses, cattle, sheep, goats*: slaughter 14 days. *Cattle, sheep, goats*: milk 36 hours (single dose), 72 hours (multiple dose)

Strepto Sulcin Forte (Jurox) *Austral.*
Tablets, sulfadimidine 2400 mg, sulfadiazine 2400 mg, dihydrostreptomycin sulphate 350 mg, hyoscine methobromide 2 mg (with thiamine), for *cattle*
Withdrawal Periods. Slaughter 14 days, milk 72 hours

New Zealand

Ensal (Jurox) *NZ*
Oral suspension, hyoscine methylbromide 0.2 mg/mL, kaolin 100 mg/mL, phthalylsulfathiazole 50 mg/mL, electrolytes, for *dogs, cats*

Scourban Plus (Bomac) *NZ*
Oral solution, hyoscine hydrobromide 0.02 mg/mL, kaolin 103.3 mg/mL, neomycin sulphate 1.8 mg/mL, streptomycin sulphate 7.6 mg/mL, sulfadiazine 28.4 mg/mL, sulfadimidine 21.3 mg/mL, sulfaguanidine 21.3 mg/mL, electrolytes, glycine, pectin, for *horses, cattle, sheep, goats, pigs, dogs, cats*

Trisulfin (Bomac) *NZ*
Oral suspension, sulfadiazine 25 mg/mL, trimethoprim 5 mg/mL, kaolin 125 mg/mL, pectin, electrolytes, for *horses, cattle, sheep, goats, pigs, dogs, cats*
Withdrawal Periods. *Horses*: slaughter 28 days. *Cattle, pigs*: 14 days

Virbac Scour Mixture (Virbac) *NZ*
Oral suspension, hyoscine 0.044 mg/mL, kaolin 105 mg/mL, neomycin 10 mg/mL, sulfadiazine 21.3 mg/mL, sulfadimidine 21.3 mg/mL, sulfaguanidine 21.3 mg/mL, pectin, glycine, electrolytes, for *cattle, sheep, goats*
Withdrawal Periods. Slaughter 14 days, milk 72 hours

USA

Amforol (Fort Dodge) *USA*
Oral suspension, kanamycin (as sulphate) 100 mg/5 mL, bismuth subcarbonate 250 mg/5 mL, aluminium magnesium silicate 500 mg/5 mL, for *dogs*

Amforol (Fort Dodge) *USA*
Tablets, kanamycin (as sulphate) 100 mg, bismuth subcarbonate 250 mg, aluminium magnesium silicate 500 mg, for *dogs*

Entromycin Powder (Veterinary Specialities) *USA*
Oral powder, bacitracin methylene disalicylate 200 units, streptomycin (as sulphate) 20 mg, for *dogs*)

1.2 Antifungal drugs

Treatment of fungal infections may include either systemic or topical medication. Topical antifungal drugs are used for the treatment of fungal infections of the skin (see section 14.4.2), ear (see section 14.8), and eye (see section 12.2.2).

Systemic antifungal drugs are discussed below. Discussion of dermatophytosis (ringworm) and topical treatment is included in section 14.4.2. Griseofulvin is the main systemic medication used although ketoconazole or itraconazole are recommended for refractory cases.

Aspergillosis is caused by *Aspergillus fumigatus* infection and characterised by severe mucopurulent nasal discharge and epistaxis. Long-term systemic treatment such as ketoconazole has been used. Topical enilconazole (see section 14.4.2) by intrasinus administration is preferred. The frontal sinuses are trephined and irrigation tubes inserted. Enilconazole 10 mg/kg daily in 2 divided doses is diluted in sodium chloride 0.9% solution (to make up to 5 to 10 mL) and administered for 10 days.

Yeast infections include candidiasis (moniliasis) caused by *Candida albicans* and cryptococcosis caused by *Cryptococcus neoformans*. These are treated using systemic medication such as ketoconazole, amphotericin B, or amphotericin B in combination with flucytosine.

Griseofulvin is deposited in keratin precursor cells and concentrated in the stratum corneum of skin, hair, and nails thus preventing fungal invasion of newly formed cells. Griseofulvin is metabolised in the liver. In the dog and cat, absorption of griseofulvin is enhanced by administration with a fatty meal. Manufacturers may recommend treatment for 7 days but usually treatment for 3 to 4 weeks is required and extended periods of up to 12 weeks are often necessary. In dogs and cats, the usual dose may not be effective and a dose of 40–50 mg/kg daily♦ may be required. Griseofulvin may be teratogenic and therefore should not be administered to pregnant animals.

Ketoconazole, an imidazole compound, is active against fungi and yeasts and also against some Gram-positive bacteria. Ketoconazole is well absorbed by mouth and is the treatment of choice for systemic candidiasis. It is also used for refractory dermatophyte infections. Ketoconazole may interfere with the biosynthesis of steroid hormones and indeed may be used in the treatment of hyperadrenocorticism. Administration of ketoconazole with food may reduce the nausea associated with the drug. Prolonged administration of ketoconazole may cause liver damage and the drug may be teratogenic.

The related **itraconazole** may also be used in systemic candidiasis and is the drug of choice for refractory dermatophyte infections. Itraconazole appears to be much less hepatotoxic and associated with fewer side-effects than ketoconazole. It has minimal effect on steroid hormone concentrations.

Nystatin is not absorbed from the gastro-intestinal tract and may be given orally for the treatment of gastro-intestinal candidiasis.

Amphotericin is active against yeasts and fungi. Amphotericin B may cause renal damage and renal function should be monitored regularly during treatment.

Flucytosine is effective against systemic yeast infections but not against fungal infections. Resistance develops rapidly and therefore the use of flucytosine is restricted to combination therapy with amphotericin B. Flucytosine and amphotericin B are synergistic and may be given concurrently to delay the onset of resistance to flucytosine and for the treatment of systemic cryptococcosis. The dose of amphotericin B should be halved when used in combination with flucytosine. Flucytosine is distributed throughout the body and diffuses into the cerebrospinal fluid and thus is indicated for intracranial yeast infections.

Sodium iodide is used for fungal infections although the precise mechanism of action is unknown. It aids in resolution of granulomatous lesions in actinobacillosis, actinomycosis, and other fungal infections.

Insufficient information is available at present to provide guidance on the use of **terbinafine**.

AMPHOTERICIN
(Amphotericin B)

UK

Indications. Systemic yeast and fungal infections; leishmaniosis (see section 1.4.7)
Contra-indications. Renal impairment, see notes above
Side-effects. Nephrotoxicity
Warnings. Drug Interactions – see Appendix 1
Dose. *Dogs, cats*: fungal infections, *by intravenous infusion*, 0.15–1.0 mg/kg, given as amphotericin B 200 micrograms/mL solution, 3 times weekly
Note. Dose should be halved when used in combination with flucytosine

POM Ⓗ **Fungizone** (Squibb) *UK*
Intravenous infusion, powder for reconstitution, amphotericin (as sodium deoxycholate complex) 50 mg

FLUCYTOSINE

UK

Indications. Systemic yeast infections
Contra-indications. Renal and hepatic impairment, pregnant animals
Dose. *Dogs, cats*: *by mouth*, 100–200 mg/kg daily in 3–4 divided doses in combination with amphotericin B

POM Ⓗ **Flucytosine** (Non-proprietary) *UK*
Preparations of oral flucytosine are not generally available. A written order, stating case details, should be sent to Bell and Croydon to obtain a supply of the preparation

GRISEOFULVIN

UK

Indications. Dermatophyte infections
Contra-indications. Hepatic impairment, pregnant animals
Side-effects. High doses may cause hepatotoxicity, particularly in cats
Warnings. Preparations should be handled with caution by women of child-bearing age, operators should wear impervious gloves; Drug Interactions – see Appendix 1
Dose. *By mouth*.
Horses, donkeys: 10 mg/kg daily for 7 days
Dogs, cats: 15–20 mg/kg daily (**but see notes above**)

POM **Dufulvin Equine Paste** (Fort Dodge) *UK*
Oral paste, griseofulvin 1.5 mg/unit dose, for *horses*; 70-g metered-dose applicator (1 unit dose = 4.5 g paste)
Withdrawal Periods. Should not be used in *horses* intended for human consumption

POM **Dufulvin Granules** (Fort Dodge) *UK*
Oral granules, for addition to feed, griseofulvin 75 mg/g, for *horses*
Withdrawal Periods. Should not be used in *horses* intended for human consumption

POM **Equifulvin** (Boehringer Ingelheim) *UK*
Oral granules, for addition to feed, griseofulvin 75 mg/g, for *horses*
Withdrawal Periods. Should not be used in *horses* intended for human consumption

POM Ⓗ **Fulcin** (Zeneca) *UK*
Tablets, griseofulvin 125 mg, 500 mg
Oral suspension, griseofulvin 25 mg/mL

POM **Grisol-V** (Vétoquinol) *UK*
Oral granules, for addition to feed, griseofulvin 75 mg/g, for *horses*
Withdrawal Periods. Should not be used in *horses* intended for human consumption
Oral powder, for addition to feed, griseofulvin 75 mg/g, for *horses*
Withdrawal Periods. Should not be used in *horses* intended for human consumption

POM Ⓗ **Grisovin** (GlaxoWellcome) *UK*
Tablets, griseofulvin 125 mg, 500 mg

POM **Norofulvin Equine Paste** (Norbrook) *UK*
Oral paste, griseofulvin 1.5 g/unit dose, for *horses*; 70-g metered-dose applicator (1 unit dose = 4.5 g paste)
Withdrawal Periods. Should not be used in *horses* intended for human consumption

POM **Norofulvin Granules** (Norbrook) *UK*
Oral granules, for addition to feed, griseofulvin 75 mg/g, for *horses*
Withdrawal Periods. Should not be used in *horses* intended for human consumption

Eire

Indications. Ringworm
Dose. *By mouth*.
Horses: 10 mg/kg daily
Cattle: 7.5 mg/kg daily

Chanovin Medicated Pre-Mix (Chanelle) *Eire*
Oral powder, for addition to feed, griseofulvin 75 mg/g, for *horses, cattle*
Withdrawal Periods. *Horses*: slaughter 14 days. *Cattle*: slaughter 10 days, milk 6 days

Fungacide 7.5% w/w Premix (Univet) *Eire*
Premix, griseofulvin 75 mg/g, for *cattle*
Withdrawal Periods. Slaughter 5 days, should not be used in cattle producing milk for human consumption

Norofulvin Equine Paste (Norbrook) *Eire*
Oral paste, griseofulvin 33 1/3%, for *horses*
Withdrawal Periods. Should not be used in *horses* intended for human consumption

Norofulvin Granules (Norbrook) *Eire*
Oral granules, to mix with feed, griseofulvin 75 mg/g, for *horses, cattle*
Withdrawal Periods. Should not be used in *horses* intended for human consumption. *Cattle*: slaughter 5 days, milk 48 hours

Pharmafulvin Granules (Interpharm) *Eire*
Oral granules, for addition to feed, griseofulvin 75 mg/g, for *horses, cattle*
Withdrawal Periods. Should not be used in *horses* intended for human consumption. *Cattle*: slaughter 5 days, milk 48 hours

New Zealand

Indications. Ringworm; superficial dermatophyte infections

Contra-indications. Hepatic impairment, pregnant animals

Side-effects. High doses may cause hepatotoxicity, particularly in cats

Warnings. Preparations should be handled with caution by women of child-bearing age, operators should wear impervious gloves. Horses should not be raced until 48 hours after last treatment. Drug Interactions – see Appendix 1

Dose. *By mouth.*

Dogs, cats: 15–30 mg/kg

Griseovet (Virbac) *NZ*
Tablets, griseofulvin 120 mg, 480 mg, for *dogs, cats*

Grisovin (Schering-Plough) *NZ*
Tablets, griseofulvin 125 mg, for *dogs*

USA

Indications. Ringworm; superficial dermatophyte infections

Contra-indications. Hepatic impairment, pregnant animals

Side-effects. High doses may cause hepatotoxicity, particularly in cats

Warnings. Preparations should be handled with caution by women of child-bearing age, operators should wear impervious gloves. Horses should not be raced until 48 hours after last treatment. Drug Interactions – see Appendix 1

Dose. *By mouth.* See manufacturer's information

Fulvicin U/F (Schering-Plough) *USA*
Tablets, griseofulvin (microsize) 250 mg, 500 mg, for *dogs, cats*

Fulvicin-U/F (Schering-Plough) *USA*
Oral powder, griseofulvin (microsize) 2.5 g/15 g packet, for *horses*
Withdrawal Periods. Should not be used in *horses* intended for human consumption

---

ITRACONAZOLE

UK

Indications. Dermatophyte infections

Dose. *Dogs, cats*: *by mouth,* 10 mg/kg daily

POM Ⓗ **Sporanox** (Janssen-Cilag) *UK*
Capsules, itraconazole 100 mg; 4, 15
Oral liquid, itraconazole 10mg/mL

KETOCONAZOLE

UK

Indications. Systemic candidiasis, dermatophyte infections; hyperadrenocorticism (see section 7.6)

Contra-indications. Hepatic impairment, pregnant animals

Side-effects. Hepatotoxicity, anorexia, particularly in cats

Dose. *Dogs, cats*: skin conditions, *by mouth,* 10 mg/kg daily

POM Ⓗ **Nizoral** (Janssen-Cilag) *UK*
Tablets, scored, ketoconazole 200 mg; 30

NYSTATIN

UK

Indications. Alimentary candidiasis

Dose. *Dogs, cats*: *by mouth,* 100 000 units 4 times daily

POM Ⓗ **Nystatin** (Non-proprietary) *UK*
Oral suspension, nystatin 100 000 units/mL; 30 mL

POM Ⓗ **Nystan** (Squibb) *UK*
Tablets, s/c, nystatin 500 000 units; 56
Oral suspension, nystatin 100 000 units/mL; 30 mL

SODIUM IODIDE

Australia

Indications. Actinobacillosis, actinomycosis, fungal infections

Dose. *Cattle*: *by subcutaneous injection or slow intravenus infusion,* 66 mg/kg

Sodide (Parnell) *Austral.*
Injection, sodium iodide 500 mg/mL, for *cattle*
Withdrawal Periods. Slaughter 28 days, milk 10 days

USA

Indications. Actinobacillosis, actinomycosis,

Dose. *Cattle*: *by or slow intravenus infusion,* 66 mg/kg

Iodoject (Vetus) *USA*
Injection, sodium iodide 20 g/100 mL, for *cattle*
Withdrawal Periods. Should not be used in cattle producing milk for human consumption

Sodium Iodide (Pro Labs, VetTek) *USA*
Injection, sodium iodide 200 mg/mL, for *cattle*
Withdrawal Periods. Should not be used in cattle producing milk for human consumption

Sodium Iodide 20% (Western Veterinary Supplies) *USA*
Injection, sodium iodide 200 mg/mL, for *cattle*
Withdrawal Periods. Should not be used in cattle producing milk for human consumption

Sodium Iodide 20% Injection (Aspen, Butler, Phoenix, Vedco) *USA*
Injection, sodium iodide 200 mg/mL, for *cattle*
Withdrawal Periods. Should not be used in cattle producing milk for human consumption

---

1.3 Antiviral drugs

Although antiviral compounds are sometimes used for systemic infections such as feline immunodeficiency virus (FIV) infection, their main application in veterinary medicine is in ophthalmology, particularly for herpesvirus infections in cats and horses. Only limited data are available on the efficacy of antiviral compounds against veterinary viruses. Antiviral compounds are highly toxic, have a relatively narrow therapeutic index and should be used with great care.

Aciclovir has been used to treat both ocular and respiratory disease caused by feline herpesvirus 1 in cats. However published information on efficacy is equivocal and aciclovir has no activity against felid herpesvirus 1 in cell culture. Aciclovir appears to be more effective for conjunctivitis and keratitis caused by equine herpesvirus in horses; clinical improvement is usually seen within a few days. Aciclovir has also been used experimentally in equid herpesvirus 1 abortion outbreaks, but further studies are required before this regimen can be recommended.

Zidovudine has been used to treat cats with FIV infection. The drug produces at least temporary alleviation of clinical signs in a proportion of cats, and may increase both survival time and quality of life. However, zidovudine has no obvious effect on viraemia. Clinical improvement is generally observed 10 to 14 days after commencement of treatment. Zidovudine is less effective against feline leukaemia virus and has no clinical value at non-toxic doses. The drug can cause severe anaemia in cats, and possibly hepatotoxicity at high doses. The side-effects of long-term treatment with lower doses have not been ascertained.

In addition to specific antiviral compounds, drugs which may enhance the immune response are sometimes used either alone or in conjunction with antivirals to treat virus infections. These include interferons, levamisole (see section 2.1.1.3), and various other immune-stimulatory preparations. Immunoglobulins directed against specific viral infections are available for use in animals exposed to infection (see sections 18.1.8 and 18.4.9). Vaccines are rarely effective at controlling disease once infection has occurred (and certainly once clinical signs have developed) in an individual animal, although they will provide group protection.

Treatment of viral infections in animals usually consists of nursing, control of secondary bacterial infections, possibly analgesics, NSAIDs, and other symptomatic therapies.

ACICLOVIR

UK
Indications. **Dose**. See Prescribing for reptiles

POM Ⓗ **Aciclovir** (Non-proprietary) *UK*
Tablets, aciclovir 200 mg, 400 mg, 800 mg

AMANTADINE HYDROCHLORIDE
UK
Indications. **Dose**. See Prescribing for ferrets

POM Ⓗ **Symmetrel** (Alliance) *UK*
Capsules, amantadine hydrochloride 100 mg
Syrup, amantadine hydrochloride 10 mg/mL

ZIDOVUDINE
(Azidothymidine, AZT)

UK
Indications. Feline immunodeficiency virus infection in cats, particularly when clinical signs of immunodeficiency related disease are evident

Contra-indications. Renal impairment, hepatic impairment

Side-effects. Hepatotoxicity and anaemia in cats

Dose. *Cats*: *by mouth or by subcutaneous injection*, 5–10 mg/kg daily in 2–4 divided doses

POM Ⓗ **Retrovir** (GlaxoWellcome) *UK*
Syrup, zidovudine 10 mg/mL; 200 mL
Injection, zidovudine 10 mg/mL; 20 mL. For dilution and use as an intravenous infusion

1.4 Antiprotozoal drugs

1.4.1 Anticoccidials
1.4.2 Drugs for histomoniosis
1.4.3 Drugs for trichomoniosis
1.4.4 Drugs for babesiosis
1.4.5 Drugs for giardiosis
1.4.6 Drugs for hexamitiosis
1.4.7 Drugs for leishmaniosis
1.4.8 Drugs for theileriosis
1.4.9 Drugs for trypanosomosis

Protozoal infections affect many species; causative protozoa and effective drug treatments are listed in Table 1.3. Medicated feedingstuffs, that were previously authorised as PML in the UK, are now zootechnical feed additives authorised under and used in accordance with the relevant Annex entry of Directive 70/524/EEC (*The Feedingstuffs (Zootechnical Products) Regulations 1999*), as amended.

1.4.1 Anticoccidials

Coccidiosis is of major economic importance in the poultry industry, but other animals including calves, lambs, goats, pigs, dogs, cats, game birds, and rabbits may also be affected by the disease. The principal enteric coccidia affecting animals are *Eimeria* or *Isospora* spp. The protozoa invade the gut where their development damages the intestinal mucosa causing diarrhoea. Intestinal damage may occur before diagnosis of coccidiosis is possible. Disease prevention involves good husbandry and the use of anticoccidials. Anticoccidials may suppress development of asexual stages, sexual stages, or both. Drugs may act at different stages of the protozoal life-cycle.

In the poultry industry, it is usual to employ anticoccidials to control the disease in broiler birds and replacement stock. In broilers, anticoccidials are administered continuously until just before slaughter. In replacement stock, pullets that are reared on litter but are housed in cages for the laying cycle are medicated continuously until commencement of egg laying. Anticoccidials may interfere with egg quality and production, and with fertility. Prophylactic medication is therefore discontinued from the commencement of egg laying and some anticoccidials may only be indicated for use in broilers. In pullet rearing, where the birds are to be raised on litter, the use of subtherapeutic doses of anticoccidials allows a degree of parasite development enabling the birds to acquire immunity to reinfection.

Table 1.3 Drugs effective against protozoal infections[1]

	Protozoa	Antiprotozoals[2]
CATTLE		
Coccidiosis	*Eimeria* spp.	decoquinate, sulfadimidine
Babesiosis	*Babesia divergens*	imidocarb
Cryptosporidiosis	*Cryptosporidium*	halofuginone
SHEEP		
Coccidiosis	*Eimeria* spp.	decoquinate, diclazuril, sulfadimidine, sulfamethoxypyridazine
Toxoplasmosis	*Toxoplasma gondii*	decoquinate
PIGS		
Coccidiosis	*Isospora suis*	toltrazuril ◆
DOGS		
Giardiosis	*Giardia duodenalis*	fenbendazole (Panacur), metronidazole
Leishmaniosis	*Leishmania infantum*	allopurinol Ⓗ, amphotericin B Ⓗ, meglumine antimoniate Ⓗ, pentamidine Ⓗ, sodium stibogluconate Ⓗ
CATS		
Toxoplasmosis	*Toxoplasma gondii*	clindamycin ◆
Giardiosis	*Giardia duodenalis*	metronidazole
CHICKENS		
Intestinal and caecal coccidiosis	*Eimeria* spp.	clopidol, decoquinate, diclazuril, halofuginone, lasalocid, maduramicin, monensin, narasin, nicarbazin, robenidine, salinomycin, toltrazuril, amprolium + ethopabate (Amprolmix-UK), clopidol + methylbenzoquate (Lerbek), narasin + nicarbazin (Maxiban G160)
TURKEYS		
Intestinal and caecal coccidiosis	*Eimeria* spp.	diclazuril, halofuginone, lasalocid, maduramicin, monensin, robenidine, amprolium + ethopabate (Amprolmix-UK), clopidol + methylbenzoquate (Lerbek)
Histomoniosis	*Histomonas meleagridis*	dimetridazole, nifursol

Table 1.3 Drugs effective against protozoal infections[1]

	Protozoa	Antiprotozoals[2]
PIGEONS		
Coccidiosis	*Eimeria* spp	amprolium, clazuril, sulfadimethoxine
Trichomoniosis	*Trichomonas gallinae*	carnidazole, dimetridazole, metronidazole
GUINEA FOWL		
Coccidiosis	*Eimeria numida*	clopidol
Histomoniosis	*Histomonas meleagridis*	dimetridazole
PARTRIDGES, PHEASANTS		
Coccidiosis	*Eimeria* spp.	clopidol, lasalocid
Histomoniosis	*Histomonas meleagridis*	dimetridazole
Trichomoniosis	*Trichomonas* spp.	dimetridazole
Hexamitosis	*Spironucleus* spp.	dimetridazole
RABBITS		
Coccidiosis	*Eimeria* spp.	clopidol, robenidine

[1] infections and treatment used in the UK

[2] activity of anticoccidials against individual species of protozoa may vary

Continuous use of anticoccidials may lead to ineffective treatment due to drug-resistance in the parasite populations. Various strategies are employed in the poultry industry to avoid this problem, such as shuttle programmes using different drugs in the starter and grower rations, and rotation of drugs after several crops of broilers. Immunological control in pullets can also be achieved through use of an attenuated vaccine (see section 18.6.1).

In lambs, calves, and rabbits, continuous anticoccidial medication is used during periods of increased risk and stress. Drugs may also be administered to the ewe at the time of lambing to aid control of coccidiosis in the young.

The sulphonamides were among the first anticoccidials and are active against first and second stage schizonts, being coccidiostatic at low doses and coccidiocidal at higher doses.

Currently the most widely used compounds are the ionophore antibiotics, **monensin**, **narasin**, **salinomycin**, **maduramicin**, **semduramicin** and **lasalocid**, which prevent the development of first generation schizonts. These compounds are extremely toxic to horses. Ionophores such as monensin, narasin, and salinomycin may cause severe growth retardation when administered with tiamulin. Ionophores allow birds to develop immunity to coccidial protozoa and are used in replacement stock to be housed on litter.

Clopidol (meticlorpindol), **decoquinate**, and **methylbenzoquate** are 4-hydroxyquinolones that act on first generation schizonts. Clopidol is used either on its own or in combination with methylbenzoquate.

Dinitolmide and **nicarbazin** are dinitro compounds used to prevent coccidiosis. Dinitolmide affects first generation schizonts and nicarbazin affects second generation schizonts. **Robenidine** affects the late first generation and second stage schizonts. **Halofuginone** affects first and second generation schizonts. **Diclazuril** is active against various stages of the life cycle according to the particular species of coccidia.

Amprolium is used either on its own or in combination with **ethopabate** to achieve a broader spectrum of activity, effective for the prophylaxis and treatment of clinical outbreaks of coccidiosis. Both drugs act on first generation schizonts thereby preventing differentiation of merozoites.

Toltrazuril is a symmetrical triazone compound and is active against all intracellular stages of coccidia.

Treatment of coccidiosis in all species involves restoring body fluids, when practicable, and combating the causal organism with a suitable anticoccidial drug.

Infections with *Isospora* spp. may occasionally be responsible for disease in young dogs and cats. Clinical signs include diarrhoea, weight loss, reduced appetite, and dehydration. Treatment in dogs and cats with sulfadiazine with trimethoprim (co-trimazine) at a dose of 15 to 30 mg/kg twice daily for 6 days (once daily in animals weighing less than 4 kg) has been reported. Toltrazuril has been used for the treatment of *Isospora suis* in piglets♦.

Neosporosis is caused by *Neospora caninum*. The main clinical signs of infection consist of abortion in cattle and progressive paralysis in dogs. Treatment in dogs has included clindamycin♦ and sulfadiazine with trimethoprim (co-trimazine)♦.

Toxoplasmosis is an infection caused by *Toxoplasma gondii* with a wide host range including all domestic animals, birds, and man. The cat is the definitive host in which oocyst production occurs. Clinical signs of toxoplasmosis are rarely seen in cats. Treatment of toxoplasmosis in cats may be effected with clindamycin♦ (see section 1.1.4) at a dose of 25 mg/kg daily in divided doses for a minimum period of 2 weeks.

Clinical signs can be severe in intermediate hosts such as sheep and man, that usually become affected through infection derived from cat faeces. In humans, infection is relatively common but clinical signs usually develop only in the presence of immunodeficiency, in pregnancy, or in children. Routine hygiene measures prevent *Toxoplasma gondii* infection in humans. Further information is provided by:
•*The facts about toxoplasmosis.* Pet Health Council
•*Toxoplasmosis and your pet cat.* The Toxoplasmosis Trust.
In sheep, toxoplasmosis can cause heavy losses through early embryonic death, abortion, or the birth of weak, infected lambs. Control in sheep is through routine measures such as disposal of dead lambs, infected placentas, and disinfection of contaminated pens. Decoquinate is used in ewes during mid-pregnancy to prevent abortions and perinatal losses due to toxoplasmosis. Vaccination is available for use in non-pregnant ewes (see section 18.2.11.2).

Cryptosporidiosis is caused by parasites of the coccidial genus *Cryptosporidium* and occurs in a number of hosts including calves, lambs, and humans. Infection with *Cryptosporidium* also occurs in poultry, turkeys, and game birds, although the significance is not known. Disease is usually seen in neonates or immunocompromised individuals. Halofuginone is used for treatment i of cryptosporidiosis in calves. Cryptosporidiosis is a zoonotic disease.

AMPROLIUM HYDROCHLORIDE

UK
Indications. Treatment of coccidiosis

GSL **Coxoid** (Harkers) *UK*
Oral solution, for addition to drinking water, amprolium hydrochloride 38.4 mg/mL, for *pigeons*; 112 mL, 500 mL
Withdrawal Periods. Should not be used in *pigeons* intended for human consumption
Dose. *Pigeons*: *by addition to drinking water*, 112 mL for treatment of 30 birds

Australia
Indications. Coccidiosis
Dose. *Poultry, pigeons*: *by addition to drinking water*, 240 mg/L

Amprolium 200 (Controlled Medications) *Austral.*
Powder, for addition to drinking water, amprolium (as hydrochloride) 200 g/kg, for *chickens, turkeys, ducks, pigeons*
Withdrawal Periods. Slaughter withdrawal period nil

New Zealand
Indications. Coccidiosis
Dose. *Poultry*: *by addition to drinking water*, 60–240 mg/L

Coxiprol (PCL) *NZ*
Oral solution, amprolium 120 mg/mL, for *poultry*
Withdrawal Periods. Slaughter 5 days, eggs 10 days

CLAZURIL

UK
Indications. Treatment and prophylaxis of coccidiosis
Contra-indications. Concurrent administration of drugs that may cause emesis
Dose. *Pigeons*: *by mouth*, 2.5 mg

GSL **Appertex** (Harkers) *UK*
Tablets, clazuril 2.5 mg, for *pigeons*; 30
Withdrawal Periods. Should not be used in *pigeons* intended for human consumption

CLOPIDOL
(Meticlorpindol)

UK
Indications. Prophylaxis of coccidiosis
Contra-indications. Layer replacement stock from commencement of egg laying. Replacement stock to be housed on litter
Side-effects. Overdosage may cause inappetence
Warnings. Should not be mixed with other anticoccidials
Dose. *Poultry, game birds*: 125 g/tonne feed
Rabbits: 200 g/tonne feed

ZFA **Coyden 25 Anticoccidial Premix** (Merial) *UK*
Premix, clopidol 250 g/kg, for *broiler chickens, guinea fowl, rabbits*; 25 kg
Withdrawal Periods. *Chickens, guinea fowl, rabbits*: slaughter 5 days

MFS **Coyden 25 for Game Birds** (Merial) *UK*
Premix, clopidol 250 g/kg, for *pheasants, partridges*; 25 kg
Withdrawal Periods. *Pheasants, partridges*: slaughter 7 days, should not be used from laying age onwards

ZFA**Coyden Pure** (Merial) *UK*
Premix, clopidol, for *broiler chickens, guinea fowl, rabbits*; 25 kg
Withdrawal Periods. *Chickens, guinea fowl, rabbits*: slaughter 5 days, should not be used from laying age onwards

Eire

Indications. Coccidiosis
Contra-indications. Layer replacement stock from commencement of egg laying
Side-effects. Overdosage may cause inappetence
Warnings. Should not be mixed with other anticoccidials
Dose. *Poultry, game birds*: 125 g/tonne feed
Rabbits: 200 g/tonne feed

Coyden 25 Anticoccidial Premix (Merial) *Eire*
Premix, clopidol 25%, for *rabbits, chickens, guinea fowl*
Withdrawal Periods. Slaughter 5 days

DECOQUINATE

UK

Indications. Treatment and prophylaxis of coccidiosis in calves and lambs; prophylaxis of coccidiosis in chickens; prophylaxis of abortion due to toxoplasmosis in sheep
Warnings. See under Clopidol
Dose.
Calves: treatment of coccidiosis, 100 g/tonne feed *or* 1 mg/kg body-weight for 28 days
prophylaxis of coccidiosis, 50 g/tonne feed *or* 500 micrograms/kg body-weight for 28 days
Sheep. Ewes: prophylaxis of coccidiosis in lambs (given with concurrent medication in lambs), 50 g/tonne feed *or* 500 micrograms/kg body-weight for 28 days
prophylaxis of toxoplasmosis, 2 mg/kg body-weight daily for 14 weeks before lambing
Lambs: treatment and prophylaxis of coccidiosis, 100 g/tonne feed *or* 1 mg/kg body-weight for 28 days
Broiler chickens: 20–40 g/tonne feed

MFS **Deccox** (Forum) *UK*
Premix, decoquinate 60 g/kg, for *calves, sheep*
Withdrawal Periods. *Calves, sheep*: slaughter 1 day, should not be used in animals producing milk for human consumption

ZFA **Deccox Broilers** (Forum) *UK*
Premix, decoquinate 60 g/kg, for *broiler chickens*
Withdrawal Periods. Slaughter 3 days

Eire

Indications. Treatment and prophylaxis of coccidiosis
Warnings. Should not be mixed with other anticoccidials
Dose.
Calves: treatment of coccidiosis, 100 g/tonne feed
prophylaxis of coccidiosis, 50 g/tonne feed
Sheep. Ewes: prophylaxis of coccidiosis in lambs, 50 g/tonne feed
Lambs: treatment and prophylaxis of coccidiosis, 100 g/tonne feed

Deccox 2.5% (Merial) *Eire*
Oral powder, to mix with feed, decoquinate 25 g/kg, for *cattle, sheep*
Withdrawal Periods. Slaughter 1 day, should not be used in cattle or sheep producing milk for human consumption

Deccox (Merial) *Eire*
Oral powder, to mix with feed, decoquinate 60 g/kg, for *cattle, sheep*
Withdrawal Periods. Slaughter 1 day, should not be used in cattle or sheep producing milk for human consumption

New Zealand

Indications. Coccidiosis
Dose.
Cattle, sheep, goats: treatment and prophylaxis of coccidiosis, 100 g/tonne feed

Deccox (APS) *NZ*
Premix, decoquinate 100 g/kg, for *cattle, sheep, goats*
Withdrawal Periods. Slaughter withdrawal period nil, should not be used in cattle, sheep or goats producing milk for human consumption

USA

Indications. Coccidiosis
Warnings. Should not be mixed with other anticoccidials
Dose. *Cattle*: 500 micrograms/kg body-weight

Deccox (Alpharma) *USA*
Premix, decoquinate 59.84 g/kg premix, for *cattle, sheep, goats, chickens*
Withdrawal Periods. *Cattle*: should not be used in cattle producing milk for human consumption. *Chickens*: should not be used in chickens producing eggs for human consumption

Deccox (Alpharma) *USA*
Premix, decoquinate 59.84 g/kg premix, for *cattle, sheep, goats, chickens*
Withdrawal Periods. *Cattle*: should not be used in cattle producing milk for human consumption. *Chickens*: should not be used in chickens producing eggs for human consumption

DICLAZURIL

UK

Indications. Treatment and prophylaxis of coccidiosis in lambs, prophylaxis of coccidiosis in poultry
Side-effects. Rarely severe scouring
Warnings. See under Clopidol
Dose. *Lambs*: 1 mg/kg
Poultry: 1 g/tonne feed

ZFA **Clinacox** (Intervet) *UK*
Premix, diclazuril 5 g/kg, for *broiler chickens, turkeys up to 12 weeks of age*; 20 kg
Withdrawal Periods. *Chickens, turkeys*: slaughter 5 days

POM **Vecoxan** (Janssen) *UK*
Oral suspension, diclazuril 2.5 mg/mL, for *lambs*
Withdrawal Periods. Slaughter withdrawal period nil
Warnings. Product should be protected from frost

DINITOLMIDE
(Zoalene)

Australia

Indications. Coccidiosis
Contra-indications. Concurrent nitrofurans
Dose. *Boilers, replacement pullets*: 125 g/tonne feed
Turkeys: 190 g/tonne feed

D.O.T. (Dinitolmide) Feed Additive (CCD) *Austral.*
Powder, for addition to feed, dinitolmide 1000 g/kg powder, for *poultry*
Withdrawal Periods. Slaughter withdrawal period nil, should not be used in poultry producing eggs for human consumption

D.O.T. 250 Premix (CCD) *Austral.*
Premix, dinitolmide 250 g/kg premix, for *poultry*
Withdrawal Periods. Slaughter withdrawal period nil, should not be used in poultry producing eggs for human consumption

USA
Indications. Coccidiosis
Contra-indications. Concurrent nitrofurans
Dose. *Chickens*: 125 g/tonne feed
Turkeys: 187 g/tonne feed

Zoamix (Alpharma) *USA*
Premix, zoalene 25% premix, for *chickens, turkeys*
Withdrawal Periods. Should not be used in chickens and turkeys producing eggs for human consumption

HALOFUGINONE HYDROBROMIDE

UK
Indications. Prophylaxis of coccidiosis; treatment and prophylaxis of cryptosporidiosis in calves
Contra-indications. Side-effects. Warnings. See under Clopidol. Should not be used in poultry over 12 weeks of age; should not be given to calves with an empty stomach or with diarrhoea of more than 24 hours duration
Dose. *Calves*: *by mouth*, (<35 kg body-weight) 1 g/10 kg once daily; (35–45 kg body-weight) 4 g once daily; (45–60 kg body-weight) 6 g once daily; (>60 kg body-weight) 1 g/ 10 kg once daily. Give after feeding
Poultry: 3 g/tonne feed

POM **Halocur** (Intervet)
Oral solution, halofuginone 500 micrograms/mL, for *calves*
Withdrawal Periods. Slaughter 13 days

ZFA **Stenorol** (Intervet) *UK*
Premix, halofuginone hydrobromide 6 g/kg, for *broiler chickens, turkeys less than 12 weeks of age*; 25 kg
Withdrawal Periods. *Chickens, turkeys*: slaughter 5 days
Note. Not for use in laying hens, guinea fowl, or game birds

Eire
Indications. Coccidiosis
Contra-indications. Side-effects. Warnings. Concurrent other anticoccidials; should not be used in poultry over 12 weeks of age
Dose. *Poultry*: 3 g/tonne feed

Stenerol (Hoechst Roussel Vet) *Eire*
Premix, halofuginone hydrochloride 6 g/kg, for *broiler chickens, turkeys*
Withdrawal Periods. *Chickens*: slaughter 5 days. *Turkeys*: slaughter 7 days
Note. Not for use in laying hens, guinea fowl, or game birds

LASALOCID SODIUM

UK
Indications. Prophylaxis of coccidiosis
Contra-indications. Side-effects. Warnings. See under Clopidol
Dose. *Chickens*: 75–125 g/tonne feed (usual dose 90 g/ tonne for broiler chickens)
Turkeys: 90–125 g/tonne feed
Game birds: 90–120 g/tonne feed

MFS **Avatec 15% CC (Game Birds)** (Alpharma) *UK*
Premix, lasalocid sodium 150 g/kg, for *partridges, pheasants*
Withdrawal Periods. *Chickens, turkeys*: slaughter 5 days

ZFA **Avatec 15% CC Premix** (Alpharma) *UK*
Premix, lasalocid sodium 150 g/kg, for *broiler chickens, layer replacement chickens up to 16 weeks of age, turkeys up to 12 weeks of age*; 20 kg
Withdrawal Periods. *Game birds*: slaughter 7 days

Australia
Indications. Coccidiosis
Contra-indications. Horses
Dose. *Cattle*: 1 mg/kg daily
Chickens: 75–100 g/tonne feed
Turkeys: 90–125 g/tonne feed

Avatec 150 (Roche) *Austral.*
Premix, lasalocoid sodium 150 g/kg premix, for *poultry*
Withdrawal Periods. *Turkeys*: slaughter 3 days. *Broilers*: slaughter withdrawal period nil, should not be used in hens producing fertile eggs

Bovatec 150 (Roche) *Austral.*
Premix, lasalocoid sodium 150 g/kg, for *cattle*
Withdrawal Periods. Slaughter withdrawal period nil

Bovatec 200 Liquid (Roche) *Austral.*
Liquid, lasalocoid sodium 150 g/kg liquid, for *cattle*
Withdrawal Periods. Slaughter withdrawal period nil

New Zealand
Indications. Coccidiosis
Contra-indications. Laying or breeding hens
Dose. *Goats*: 1 mg/kg daily
Poultry: 75–100 g/tonne feed

Avatec (Roche) *NZ*
Premix, lasalocid sodium 150 g/kg, for *poultry*
Withdrawal Periods. Slaughter withdrawal period nil, should not be used within 14 days of commencment of laying

Bovatec (Roche) *NZ*
Premix, lasalocid sodium 150 g/kg, for *goats*
Withdrawal Periods. Should not be used in lactating animals

USA
Indications. Coccidiosis
Contra-indications. Horses
Dose. *Cattle*: 1mg/kg
Poultry: 75–100 g/tonne feed

Avatec (Roche Vitamins) *USA*
Premix, lasalocoid sodium 200 g/kg, for *chickens, turkeys*

Bovatec (Roche Vitamins) *USA*
Premix, lasalocoid sodium 15%, for *cattle*
Withdrawal Periods. *Cattle*: should not be used in calves intended for veal production

MADURAMICIN AMMONIUM

UK
Indications. Prophylaxis of coccidiosis
Contra-indications. Side-effects. Warnings. See under Clopidol; toxic to horses
Dose. *Poultry*: 500 g/tonne feed

ZFA **Cygro** (Alpharma)
Premix, maduramicin ammonium 10 g/kg, for *broiler chickens, turkeys*
Withdrawal Periods. *Poultry*: slaughter 5 days

Australia
Indications. Coccidiosis

Dose. *Poultry*: 500 g/tonne feed

Cygro 10 Anticoccidial Premix (Roche) *Austral.*
Premix, maduramicin 10 g/kg, for *chickens*
Withdrawal Periods. Slaughter withdrawal period nil, egg withdrawal period nil

MONENSIN

UK

Indications. Prophylaxis of coccidiosis in poultry; to improve growth-rate and feed conversion efficiency in cattle (see section 17.1)
Contra-indications. Side-effects. Warnings. See under Clopidol. Should not be given within 7 days of administration of tiamulin (see Drug Interactions – Appendix 1). Toxic to horses, should not be used in guinea fowl or other game birds
Dose. *Chickens*: coccidiosis, 100–120 g/tonne feed
Turkeys: coccidiosis, 90–100 g/tonne feed

PML Ecox 200 (ECO) UK
Premix, monensin (as monensin sodium) 100 g/kg, for *beef cattle* (see section 17.1), *poultry*
Withdrawal Periods. *Cattle*: slaughter withdrawal period nil. *Poultry*: slaughter 3 days

ZFA Elancoban G200 (Elanco) *UK*
Premix, monensin 200 g/kg, for *broiler chickens, layer replacement chickens up to 16 weeks of age, turkeys up to 16 weeks of age*; 25 kg
Withdrawal Periods. *Chickens, turkeys*: slaughter 3 days, should not be used in birds producing eggs for human consumption

Australia

Indications. Coccidiosis
Dose. *Cattle*: *by addition to feed,* 11–33 mg/kg
Poultry: coccidiosis, 100–120 g/tonne feed

Elancoban G (Elanco) *Austral.*
Premix, monensin sodium 100 g/kg premix, for *poultry*
Withdrawal Periods. Slaughter withdrawal period nil, should not be used in chickens producing eggs for human consumption

Rumensin 100 Premix (Elanco) *Austral.*
Premix, monensin sodium 100 g/kg premix, for *cattle, goats*
Withdrawal Periods. Slaughter withdrawal period nil, milk withdrawal period nil, milk should not be used for human consumption within 72 hours of calving

Rumensin 200 Premix (Elanco) *Austral.*
Premix, monensin sodium 200 g/kg premix, for *cattle, goats*
Withdrawal Periods. Slaughter withdrawal period nil, milk withdrawal period nil, milk should not be used for human consumption within 72 hours of calving

Eire

Indications. Prophylaxis of coccidiosis in poultry; to improve growth-rate and feed conversion efficiency in cattle (see section 17.1)
Contra-indications. Side-effects. Warnings. See under Clopidol. Should not be given within 7 days of administration of tiamulin (see Drug Interactions – Appendix 1). Toxic to horses, should not be used in guinea fowl or other game birds
Dose. *Chickens*: coccidiosis, 100–120 g/tonne feed
Turkeys: coccidiosis, 90–100 g/tonne feed

Elancoban G200 (Elanco) *Eire*
Premix, monensin 200 g/kg, for *poultry*
Withdrawal Periods. Slaughter 3 days

New Zealand

Indications. Coccidiosis

Elancoban 200 (Elanco) *NZ*
Premix, monensin sodium 200 g/kg, for *poultry*
Withdrawal Periods. Slaughter withdrawal period nil

Rumensin Premix (Elanco) *NZ*
Premix, monensin sodium 100 g/kg, for *cattle, sheep, goats*
Withdrawal Periods. Slaughter withdrawal period nil, milk withdrawal period nil

USA

Indications. Coccidiosis
Dose. *Cattle*: by addition to feed, 100–360 mg

Coban 60 (Elanco) *USA*
Premix, monesin (as sodium) 132g/kg premix, for *chickens, turkeys, quail*
Withdrawal Periods. Chickens: should not be used in chickens producing eggs for human consumption

Rumensin 80 (Elanco) *USA*
Premix, monesin (as sodium salt) 176 g/kg premix, for *cattle, goats*
Withdrawal Periods. Should not be used in cattle or goats producing milk for human consumption

NARASIN

UK

Indications. Prophylaxis of coccidiosis
Contra-indications. Side-effects. Warnings. See under Clopidol. Should not be given within 7 days of administration of tiamulin (see Drug Interactions – Appendix 1). Toxic to horses, should not be used in turkeys, guinea fowl or other game birds
Dose. *Poultry*: 70 g/tonne feed

ZFA Monteban G100 (Elanco) *UK*
Premix, narasin 100 g/kg, for *broiler chickens*; 25 kg
Withdrawal Periods. *Chickens*: slaughter 5 days, should not be used in birds producing eggs

Australia

Indications. Coccidiosis
Contra-indications. Concurrent administration of tiamulin; horses, turkeys, or game birds
Dose. *Poultry*: 60–80 g/tonne feed

Monteban 100 (Elanco) *Austral.*
Premix, narasin 100 g/kg, for *chickens*
Withdrawal Periods. Slaughter withdrawal period nil, should not be used in chickens producing eggs for human consumption

Eire

Indications. Coccidiosis
Contra-indications. Side-effects. Warnings. Concurrent Administration within 7 days of tiamulin; horses, turkeys, or guinea fowl
Dose. *Poultry*: 70 g/tonne feed

Monteban G100 (Elanco) *Eire*
Premix, narasin 100 g/kg, for *chickens*
Withdrawal Periods. Slaughter 5 days, should not be used in birds producing eggs for human consumption

New Zealand

Indications. Coccidiosis
Contra-indications. Concurrent administration of tiamulin or oleandomycin; horses or game birds
Dose. *Poultry*: 60–80 g/tonne feed

Monteban (Elanco) *NZ*
Premix, narasin 100 g/kg, for **chickens**
Withdrawal Periods. Slaughter withdrawal period nil, should not be used in laying chickens

USA

Indications. Coccidiosis
Contra-indications. Horses or turkeys

Monteban 45 (Elanco) *USA*
Premix, narasin 99 g/kg premix, for **chickens**

NICARBAZIN

UK

Indications. Prophylaxis of coccidiosis
Contra-indications. Side-effects. Warnings. See under Clopidol
Dose. *Poultry*: 100–125 g/tonne feed

ZFA **Carbigran** (Elanco) *UK*
Premix, nicarbazin 250 g/kg, for **broiler chickens up to 4 weeks of age**; 25 kg
Withdrawal Periods. **Chickens**: slaughter 9 days, should not be used in laying birds

ZFA **Nicarmix 25** (Eurotec) *UK*
Premix, nicarbazin 250 g/kg, for **broiler chickens**; 25 kg
Withdrawal Periods. **Chickens**: slaughter 9 days, should not be used in laying birds

Australia

Indications. Coccidiosis
Warnings. Caution in administration to broilers more than 28 days of age
Dose. *Poultry*: 125 g/tonne feed

Carbigran 250 (Elanco) *Austral.*
Premix, nicarbazin 250 g/kg premix, for **chickens**
Withdrawal Periods. Slaughter 4 days, should not be used in chickens producing eggs for human consumption

Cycarb 250 Anticoccidial Premix (Roche) *Austral.*
Premix, nicarbazin 250 g/kg premix, for **chickens**
Withdrawal Periods. Slaughter 4 days, should not be used in chickens producing eggs for human consumption

Keycarbazin (International Animal Health Products) *Austral.*
Premix, nicarbazin 1000 g/kg, for **poultry**
Withdrawal Periods. Slaughter 4 days, should not be used in poultry producing eggs for human consumption

Eire

Indications. Coccidiosis
Contra-indications. Concurrent administration of other anticoccidials
Dose. *Poultry*: 100–125 g/tonne feed

Carbigran Premix (Elanco) *Eire*
Premix, nicarbazin 250 g/kg, for **chickens**
Withdrawal Periods. Slaughter 9 days, should not be used in laying hens

New Zealand

Indications. Coccidiosis
Dose. *Poultry*: 125 g/tonne feed

Carbigran (Elanco) *NZ*
Premix, nicarbazin 250 g/kg, for **chickens**
Withdrawal Periods. Slaughter 5 days

ORMETOPRIM WITH SULFADIMETHOXINE

USA

Indications. Coccidiosis; ormetoprim/sulfadimethoxine-sensitive infections
Dose. Consult manufacturer's information

Rofenaid 40 (Roche Vitamins) *USA*
Premix, ormetoprim 150 mg/g, sulfadimethoxine 250 mg/g, for **chickens, turkeys, ducks**
Withdrawal Periods. Slaughter 5 days, should not be used in chickens, turkeys, ducks producing eggs for human consumption

ROBENIDINE HYDROCHLORIDE

UK

Indications. Prophylaxis of coccidiosis
Contra-indications. Side-effects. Warnings. See under Clopidol
Dose. *Poultry*: 33 g/tonne feed
Rabbits: 50–66 g/tonne feed

ZFA **Cycostat 66G** (Roche) *UK*
Premix, robenidine hydrochloride 66 g/kg, for **broiler chickens, turkeys, rabbits**; 20 kg
Withdrawal Periods. **Chickens, turkeys**: slaughter 5 days, should not be used in laying birds. **Rabbits**: slaughter 5 days

Australia

Indications. Coccidiosis
Dose. *Poultry*: 50 g/tonne feed

Cycostat 66 (Roche) *Austral.*
Premix, robenidine hydrochloride 66 g/kg, for **chickens**
Withdrawal Periods. Slaughter 5 days, should not be used in chickens producing eggs for human consumption

USA

Indications. Coccidiosis
Contra-indications. Use in feeds containing bentonite

Robenz (Roche Vitamins) *USA*
Medicated feed, robenidine hydrochloride 66 g/kg, for **chickens**
Withdrawal Periods. Slaughter 5 days, should not be used in layers

SALINOMYCIN SODIUM

UK

Indications. Prophylaxis of coccidiosis in poultry; to improve growth rate and feed conversion in pigs (see section 17.1)
Contra-indications. Side-effects. Warnings. See under Clopidol. Not to be given within 7 days of administration of tiamulin (see Drug Interactions – Appendix 1). Toxic to horses. Should not be used in turkeys, breeding birds
Dose. *Broiler chickens*: coccidiosis, 60 g/tonne feed
Replacement layer chickens: coccidiosis, 40 g/tonne feed

ZFA **Bio-Cox 120G** (Alpharma) *UK*
Premix, salinomycin sodium 120 g/kg, for **broiler chickens, replacement layer chickens, pigs** (see section 17.1)
Withdrawal Periods. *Chickens*: slaughter 5 days

ZFA **Sacox 120** (Intervet) *UK*
Premix, salinomycin sodium 120 g/kg, for **broiler chickens, replacement layer chickens up to 12 weeks of age**; 25 kg
Withdrawal Periods. *Chickens*: slaughter 5 days

PML **Sal-Eco 120** (ECO)
Premix, salinomycin sodium 120 g/kg, for **chickens**, pigs (see section 17.1)
Withdrawal Periods. *Pigs*: slaughter withdrawal period nil. *Poultry*: slaughter 5 days

ZFA **Salinomix 12 MG** (Eurotec)
Premix, salinomycin sodium 120 g/kg, for **broiler chickens**; 25 kg
Withdrawal Periods. *Chickens*: slaughter 5 days

Australia
Indications. Coccidiosis
Dose. *Cattle*: 15 g/tonne feed
Pigs: 25 g/tonne feed
Poultry: 60 g/tonne feed

Coxistat (Pfizer) *Austral.*
Premix, salinomycin 60 g/kg premix, for **chickens**
Withdrawal Periods. Slaughter withdrawal period nil, should not be used in chickens producing eggs for human consumption, should not be used in pullets within 7 days of start of egg production

Coxistac 120 (Pfizer) *Austral.*
Premix, salinomycin sodium 120 g/kg, for **poultry, pigs, cattle**
Withdrawal Periods. *Cattle*: slaughter withdrawal period nil, should not be used in cattle producing milk for human consumption. *Pigs*: slaughter withdrawal period nil. *Poultry*: slaughter withdrawal period nil, should not be used in chickens producing eggs for human consumption, should not be used in pullets within 7 days of onset of egg production

Posistac 60 (Pfizer) *Austral.*
Premix, salinomycin sodium 60 g/kg, for **chickens**
Withdrawal Periods. Slaughter withdrawal period nil, should not be used in chickens producing eggs for human consumption.

Sacox 120 (Hoechst Roussel Vet) *Austral.*
Premix, salinomycin sodium 120 g/kg, for **chickens**
Withdrawal Periods. Slaughter withdrawal period nil, should not be used in chickens producing eggs or within 7 days of producing eggs for human consumption.

Eire
Indications. Coccidiosis
Dose. *Poultry*: 40–60 g/tonne feed

Sacox 120 Premix (Hoechst Roussel Vet) *Eire*
Premix, salinomycin sodium 120 g/kg, for **chickens**
Withdrawal Periods. Slaughter 5 days

New Zealand
Indications. Coccidiosis
Dose. *Cattle*: 15 g/tonne feed
Pigs: 25 g/tonne feed
Poultry: 60 g/tonne feed

Coxistac 120 Anticoccidial Premix (Pfizer) *NZ*
Premix, salinomycin sodium 120 g/kg, for **cattle, pigs, poultry**
Withdrawal Periods. Slaughter withdrawal period nil, should not be used in birds within 7 days of commencement of laying

USA
Indications. Coccidiosis
Dose. Consult manufacturer's information
Poultry: 60 g/tonne feed

Bio-Cox 60 (Roche Vitamins) *USA*
Premix, salinomycin sodium (as salinomycin) 132 g/kg premix, for **chickens, quail**
Withdrawal Periods. Chickens: should not be used in chickens producing eggs for human consumption

SEMDURAMICIN

New Zealand
Indications. Coccidiosis
Dose. *Poultry*: 25 g/tonne feed

Aviax (Pfizer) *NZ*
Premix, semduramicin (as sodium salt) 50 g/kg, for **chickens**
Withdrawal Periods. Slaughter withdrawal period nil, should not be used in birds producing eggs for human consumption

USA
Indications. Coccidiosis
Dose. *Poultry*: 25 g/tonne feed

Aviax (Pfizer) *USA*
Premix, semduramicin 5%, for **chickens**
Withdrawal Periods. Should not be used in chickens producing eggs for human consumption

SULFADIMETHOXINE

UK
Indications. Treatment and prophylaxis of coccidiosis in pigeons
Contra-indications. Renal impairment; use during the breeding season
Warnings. Birds should not participate in races during treatment
Dose. *Pigeons*: see preparation details

POM **Coxi Plus** (Vetrepharm) *UK*
Oral powder, for addition to drinking water, sulfadimethoxine sodium anhydrous 1 g/sachet, for **racing pigeons**; 4-g sachet
Withdrawal Periods. Should not be used in *pigeons* intended for human consumption
Dose. *Pigeons*: (40 birds) *by addition to drinking water*, 1 sachet/2 litres water

USA
Indications. Coccidiosis in poultry; sulfadimethoxine-sensitive infections

Albon (Pfizer) *USA*
Solution, for addition to drinking water, sulfadimethoxine 125 mg/mL, for **cattle, chickens, turkeys**
Withdrawal Periods. *Cattle*: slaughter 7 days. *Chickens, turkeys*: slaughter 5 days.

Sulfadimethoxine Oral Solution (Aspen, Butler, DurVet, Vedco) *USA*
Oral solution, sulfadimethoxine 125 mg/mL, for **cattle, chickens, turkeys**
Withdrawal Periods. *Cattle*: slaughter 7 days, should not be used in calves intended for veal production. *Chickens, turkeys*: slaughter 5 days

Sulfadimethoxine Soluble Powder (DurVet, RXV, Vedco) *USA*
Oral powder, for addition to drinking water, sulfadimethoxine (as sodium salt) 94.6 g/107 g packet, for **cattle, chickens, turkeys**
Withdrawal Periods. *Cattle*: slaughter 7 days. *Chickens, turkeys*: slaughter 5 days

SULFADIMIDINE

UK

Indications. Treatment of coccidiosis in cattle and sheep; sulfadimidine-sensitive infections (see section 1.1.6.1)
Warnings. See under Clopidol
Dose. *Calves, lambs*: *by mouth or by subcutaneous or intravenous (preferred) injection*, initial dose 200 mg/kg then 100 mg/kg daily

See section 1.1.6.1 for preparation details and additional doses

SULFAMETHOXYPYRIDAZINE

UK

Indications. Treatment of coccidiosis in sheep; sulfamethoxypyridazine-sensitive infections (see section 1.1.6.1)
Warnings. See under Clopidol
Dose. *Sheep*: coccidiosis, *by subcutaneous or intramuscular injection*, 20 mg/kg daily

See section 1.1.6.1 for preparation details and additional doses

Eire

Indications. Sulfamethoxypyridazine-sensitive infections; coccidiosis in sheep

Midicel Parenteral (Pharmacia & Upjohn) *Eire*
Injection, sulfamethoxypyridazine 250 mg/mL, for *sheep, cattle*
Withdrawal Periods. *Cattle*: slaughter 7 days, milk 48 hours. *Sheep*: slaughter 7 days, should not be used in sheep producing milk for human consumption

SULFAQUINOXALINE

Australia

Indications. Coccidiosis
Dose. Consult manufacturer's information

Sulfa Quin (Inca) *Austral.*
Liquid, for addition to drinking water, sulfaquinoxaline 70 g/L, for *poultry*
Withdrawal Periods. Slaughter 14 days, should not be used in poultry producing eggs for human consumption

Sulfaquinoxaline Feed Additive Premix (CCD) *Austral.*
Premix, sulfaquinoxaline 1000 g/kg premix, for *chickens, turkeys*
Withdrawal Periods. *Chickens, turkeys*: slaughter 14 days, should not be used in poultry producing eggs for human consumption

USA

Indications. Coccidiosis
Dose. Consult manufacturer's information

Purina Liquid Sulfa-Nox (Purina Mills) *USA*
Solution, for addition to drinking water, sulfaquinoxaline 34.4 mg/g, for *cattle, sheep, poultry, rabbits*
Withdrawal Periods. *Cattle*: slaughter 10 days, should not be used in cattle producing milk for human consumption. *Sheep, rabbits, chickens, turkeys, pheasant, quail*: slaughter 10 days

Sulfa-Q 20% Concentrate (RXV) *USA*
Oral solution, for addition to drinking water, sulfaquinoxaline 20 g/100 mL, for *cattle, chickens, turkeys*
Withdrawal Periods. *Cattle*: slaughter 10 days, should not be used in cattle producing milk for human consumption. *Chickens, turkeys*: slaughter 10

days, should not be used in chickens or turkeys producing eggs for human consumption

Sul-Q-Nox (Russell) *USA*
Oral solution, for addition to drinking water, sulfaquinoxaline (as sodium and potassium salts) 319.2 mg/mL, for *cattle, chickens, turkeys*
Withdrawal Periods. *Cattle*: slaughter 10 days, should not be used in cattle producing milk for human consumption, should not be used in calves intended for val production. *Chickens, turkeys*: slaughter 10 days, should not be used in chickens or turkeys producing eggs for human consumption

SULFAQUINOXALINE with TRIMETHOPRIM

Indications. Treatment of coccidiosis in chickens; sulfadimidine/trimethoprim-sensitive infections (section 1.1.6.2)
Warnings. See under Clopidol
Dose. Expressed as sulfaquinoxaline + trimethoprim
Chickens: coccidiosis, *by addition to drinking water*, 30 mg/kg body-weight

See section 1.1.6.2 for preparation details

TOLTRAZURIL

UK

Indications. Treatment of coccidiosis in poultry; treatment of *Isospora suis* in piglets◆
Warnings. Alkaline solution, operators should wear adequate protective clothing
Dose. *Piglets*◆: *by mouth*, 25 mg/kg at 4 days of age
Poultry: *by addition to drinking water*, 7 mg/kg daily for 2 days

POM **Baycox 2.5%** (Bayer) *UK*
Solution, for addition to drinking water, toltrazuril 25 mg/mL, for *broiler breeder, layer replacement chickens*; 1 litre, 5 litres
Withdrawal Periods. *Chickens*: slaughter 21 days, should not be used in birds within 14 days of commencement of laying or in birds producing eggs for human consumption

Australia

Indications. Coccidiosis
Contra-indications. Use in galvinised or rusty iron water tanks
Dose. *Piglets*: *by mouth*, 50 mg
Poultry: *by addition to drinking water*, 6 mg/kg

Baycox Coccidiocide for Piglets (Bayer) *Austral.*
Oral solution, toltrazuril 50 mg/mL, for *pigs*
Withdrawal Periods. Slaughter 70 days

Baycox Coccidiocide Solution (Bayer) *Austral.*
Liquid, for addition to drinking water, toltrazuril 25 g/L, for *chickens*
Withdrawal Periods. Slaughter 14 days, should not be used in chickens producing eggs for human consumption

Eire

Indications. Treatment of coccidiosis in poultry; treatment of *Isospora suis* in piglets◆
Warnings. Alkaline solution, operators should wear adequate protective clothing
Dose. *Poultry*: *by addition to drinking water*, 25 g/1000 litres

Baycox 2.5% Solution (Bayer) *Eire*
Solution, for addition to drinking water, toltrazuril 25 mg/mL, for *chickens*
Withdrawal Periods. Slaughter withdrawal period 8 days, should not be used in birds producing eggs for human consumption

New Zealand

Indications. Coccidiosis
Dose. *Poultry: by addition to drinking water,* 25 g/1000 litres

Baycox (Bayer) *NZ*
Oral solution, toltrazuril 25 mg/mL, for *poultry*
Withdrawal Periods. Slaughter 14 days, should not be used in birds producing eggs for human consumption

---

COMPOUND ANTICOCCIDIAL PREPARATIONS

UK
Indications. Prophylaxis of coccidiosis

ZFA Amprol Plus (Merial) *UK*
Premix, amprolium hydrochloride 250 g/kg, ethopabate 16 g/kg, for *chickens, turkeys, guinea fowl;* 25 kg
Withdrawal Periods. *Chickens, turkeys, guinea fowl:* slaughter 3 days, should not be used from commencement of laying
Contra-indications. See under Clopidol
Dose. *Poultry, game birds:* 250–500 g premix/tonne feed

ZFA Lerbek (Merial) *UK*
Premix, clopidol 200 g, methylbenzoquate 16.7 g/kg, for *broiler and replacement chickens less than 16 weeks of age, turkeys less than 12 weeks of age;* 25 kg
Withdrawal Periods. *Chickens, turkeys:* slaughter 5 days
Dose. *Poultry:* 500 g premix/tonne feed

ZFA Maxiban G160 (Elanco) *UK*
Premix, narasin 80 g, nicarbazin 80 g/kg, for *broiler chickens;* 25 kg
Withdrawal Periods. *Chickens:* slaughter 5 days, should not be used in chickens producing eggs
Dose. *Poultry:* 500–625 g premix/tonne feed

Australia
Amprolmix-Plus Preparations (Merial) *Austral.*
Powder, amprolium 250 g/kg, ethopabate 16 g/kg, for coccidiosis in *chickens, turkeys*
Withdrawal Periods. Slaughter nil, should not be used in chickens and turkeys producing eggs for human consumption

Amprosol (Agrotech) *Austral.*
Powder, for addition to drinking water, amprolium 432 g/kg, ethopabate 28 g/kg, for coccidiosis in *poultry, pigeons, cage birds*
Withdrawal Periods. *Poultry, pigeons:* slaughter nil, should not be used in poultry producing eggs for human consumption

Coccivet (Vetafarm) *Austral.*
Liquid, for addition to drinking water, amprolium 80 g/L, ethopabate 5.1 g/L, for coccidiosis in *cage birds, pigeons*

Coxitrol (Controlled Medications) *Austral.*
Powder, for addition to drinking water, sulfaquinoxaline 145 g/kg, diaveridine 36.3 g/kg, menadione 3.6 g/kg, for coccidiosis in *poultry*
Withdrawal Periods. Slaughter 7 days, should not be used in poultry producing eggs for human consumption

DSM Coccidiostat Water Soluble Powder (CCD) *Austral.*
Powder, for addition to drinking water, diaveridine 36.6 mg/g, sulfaquinoxaline 145 mg/g, (vitamin K 3.6 mg/g), for coccidiosis in *poultry*
Withdrawal Periods. Slaughter 7 days, should not be used in chickens producing eggs for human consumption
Keystat Coccidiostat Solution (International Animal Health Products) *Austral.*
Liquid, for addition to drinking water, amprolium 216 g/L, ethopabate 14 g/L, for coccidiosis in *poultry*
Withdrawal Periods. Slaughter withdrawal period nil, should not be used in poultry producing eggs for human consumption

Keystat Powder (International Animal Health Products) *Austral.*
Premix, amprolium 250 g/kg, ethopabate 16 g/kg, for coccidiosis in *poultry*
Withdrawal Periods. Slaughter withdrawal period nil

Lerbek Premix (Merial) *Austral.*
Premix, clopidol 200 g/kg, methyl benzoquate 16.7 g/kg, for coccidiosis in *chickens*
Withdrawal Periods. Slaughter withdrawal period nil, should not be used in chickens producing eggs for human consumption

Maxiban (Elanco) *Austral.*
Premix, narasin 80 g/kg, nicarbazin 80 g.kg, for coccidiosis in *chickens*
Withdrawal Periods. Slaughter withdrawal period nil, should not be used in chickens producing eggs for human consumption

Solquin (International Animal Health Products) *Austral.*
Powder, for addition to drinking water, sulfaquinoxaline 145 g/kg, diaveridine 36.3 g/kg, menadione 3.6 g/kg, for coccidiosis in *poultry*
Withdrawal Periods. Should not be used in poultry producing eggs for human consumption

Toltro (Agrotech) *Austral.*
Powder, for addition to drinking water, diaveridine 36.3 g/kg, sulfaquinoxaline 147 g/kg, vitamin K 3.6 g/kg, for coccidiosis in *poultry*
Withdrawal Periods. Slaughter 7 days, should not be used in poultry producing eggs for human consumption

Eire
Lerbek Anticoccidial Premix (Merial) *Eire*
Premix, clopidol 20%, methyl benzoquate 1.67%, for coccidiosis in *chickens, turkeys*
Withdrawal Periods. Slaughter 5 days

Maxiban G160 (Elanco) *Eire*
Premix, narasin 80 g/kg, nicarbazin 80 g/kg, for coccidiosis in *chickens*
Withdrawal Periods. Slaughter 7 days

New Zealand
Maxiban (Elanco) *NZ*
Premix, narasin 80 g/kg, nicarbazin 80 g/kg, for coccidiosis in *chickens*
Withdrawal Periods. Slaughter 5 days

USA
Maxiban 72 (Elanco) *USA*
Premix, narasin 79.2 g/kg premix, nicarbazin 79.2 g/kg premix, for coccidiosis in *chickens*
Withdrawal Periods. Slaughter 5 days)

1.4.2 Drugs for histomoniosis

Dimetridazole and nifursol are used to prevent and treat infections caused by *Histomonas meleagridis* (blackhead) in turkeys, pheasants, partridges, and guinea fowl. Histomoniosis (histomoniasis) was most commonly seen in turkeys but is now more likely to be seen in game birds after they have been released.

Dimetridazole appears to interfere with RNA synthesis. Dimetridazole is included in Annex IV of Regulation 2377/90/EEC which effectively prohibits its use in food-producing species. However it is available in the UK as an authorised veterinary medicine (see also sections 1.4.3 and 1.4.6) for use in pheasants and partridges for health and welfare reasons; it may not be prescribed for any other food-producing species under the 'cascade'. Dimetridazole may be used as a zootechnical feed additive but only in accordance with Annex I of Directive 70/524/EEC; it is used for the prevention of blackhead in turkeys and guinea fowl.

Nifursol acts by causing damage to lipids and DNA within the cells.

DIMETRIDAZOLE

UK

Indications. Prophylaxis of histomoniosis in turkeys and guinea fowl; treatment and prophylaxis of histomoniosis in pheasants, and partridges; trichomoniosis (see section 1.4.3); hexamitosis (see section 1.4.6)

Contra-indications. Layer replacement stock from commencement of egg laying

Side-effects. Hyperexcitability, incoordination, and convulsions have been reported in turkeys with overdosage

Warnings. Should not be administered concurrently with other drugs for histomoniosis

Dose.

Turkeys: prophylaxis of histomoniosis, 100–200 g/tonne feed

Guinea fowl: prophylaxis of histomoniosis, 125–150 g/tonne feed

Pheasants, partridges: treatment of histomoniosis, 27 g/100 litres drinking water for 12 days *or* 54 g/100 litres drinking water for 3–5 days then 27 g/100 litres drinking water for treatment up to 12 days

prophylaxis of histomoniosis, 125–200 g/tonne feed; 12 g/100 litres drinking water for up to 15 days

MFS **Emtryl Premix for Game Birds** (Merial) *UK*
Premix, dimetridazole 225 g/kg, for *pheasants, partridges*; 10 kg
Withdrawal Periods. *Pheasants, partridges*: slaughter 28 days, should not be used from commencement of laying

MFS **Emtryl Pure for Game Birds** (Merial) *UK*
Oral powder, for addition to feed, dimetridazole 225 g/kg, for *pheasants, partridges*; 10 kg
Withdrawal Periods. *Pheasants, partridges*: slaughter 28 days, should not be used from commencement of laying

POM **Emtryl Soluble for Gamebirds** (Merial) *UK*
Oral powder, for addition to drinking water, dimetridazole 400 mg/g, for *pheasants, partridges*; 500 g
Withdrawal Periods. *Pheasants, partridges*: slaughter 28 days, should not be used from commencement of laying

ZFA **Sintodim 200** (Merial) *UK*
Premix, dimetridazole 200 g/kg, for *turkeys, guinea fowl*
Withdrawal Periods. Slaughter 5 days, should not be used from laying age onwards

Australia

Indications. Histomoniosis in turkeys and game birds; trichomoniosis in caged birds and pigeons; bacterial infections in pigs

Dose. Consult manufacturer's information

Dimetrasol (PCL) *NZ*
Oral powder, dimetridazole 400 mg/g, for *pigs, poultry, game birds, pigeons*
Withdrawal Periods. Slaughter 5 days. Should not be used in birds producing eggs for human consumption

Dimetridazole 225 Premix (CCD) *Austral.*
Premix, dimetridazole 225 g/kg premix, for *turkeys, chickens, pigs*
Withdrawal Periods. *Pigs*: slaughter 5 days. *Turkeys, chickens*: slaughter 5 days, should not be used in poultry producing eggs for human consumption

Dimetridazole Water Soluble Powder (CCD) *Austral.*
Powder, for addition to drinking water, dimetridazole 980 mg/g powder, for *pigs, turkeys, cage birds*
Withdrawal Periods. *Pigs*: slaughter 5 days. *Turkeys*: slaughter 5 day, should not be used in turkeys producing eggs for human consumption

Emtryl Premix (Rhône-Poulenc) *Austral.*
Premix, dimetridazole 200 g/kg premix, for *poultry, pigs*
Withdrawal Periods. *Pigs*: slaughter 5 days. *Turkeys, chickens*: slaughter 5 days, should not be used in poultry producing eggs for human consumption

Emtryl Soluble (Rhône-Poulenc) *Austral.*
Powder, for addition to drinking water, dimetridazole 400 g/kg powder, for *poultry, pigs, pigeons*
Withdrawal Periods. *Pigs*: slaughter 5 days. *Turkeys, chickens, pigeons*: slaughter 5 days, should not be used in poultry producing eggs for human consumption

Eire

Indications. Histomoniosis in turkeys and game birds; trichomoniosis in caged birds and pigeons; bacterial infections in pigs

Dose.

Turkeys: 100–200 g/tonne feed

Guinea fowl: 125–150 g/tonne feed

Emtryl Pure (Merial) *Eire*
Oral powder, to mix with feed, dimetridazole, for *turkeys, guinea fowl*
Withdrawal Periods. Slaughter 6 days

Emtryl Premix (Merial) *Eire*
Premix, dimetridazole 22.5%, for *turkeys, guinea fowl*
Withdrawal Periods. Slaughter 6 days

New Zealand

Indications. Trichomoniosis in pigeons; histomoniosis in game birds; bacterial infections in pigs

Dose. Consult manufacturer's information

Dimetrasol (PCL) *NZ*
Oral powder, dimetridazole 400 mg/g, for *pigs, poultry, game birds, pigeons*
Withdrawal Periods. Slaughter 5 days. Should not be used in birds producing eggs for human consumption

NIFURSOL

UK

Indications. Prophylaxis of histomoniosis
Dose. *Turkeys*: 50 g/tonne feed

ZFA **Salfuride 50** (Fort Dodge) *UK*
Premix, nifursol 500 g/kg, for *turkeys*; 25 kg
Withdrawal Periods. *Turkeys*: slaughter 5 days

1.4.3 Drugs for trichomoniosis

Trichomonads cause infection in a number of species of animals. Bovine trichomoniosis (trichomoniasis) is a venereal disease caused by *Tritrichomonas foetus*, and has been controlled in many countries by artificial insemination. Avian trichomoniosis occurs in two forms. Infection with *Trichomonas gallinae* (*T. columbae*) causes lesions in the mouth and upper respiratory tract (canker in pigeons, frounce in birds of prey). *Tetratrichomonas gallinarum* (*Trichomonas gallinarum*) has been incriminated as causing diarrhoea in pheasants, partridges, and other game birds.

5-Nitroimidazole drugs are used to treat a number of protozoal infections. **Metronidazole**, **ronidazole**, and **carnidazole** are thought to interact with DNA destroying its ability to act as a template for DNA and RNA synthesis; **dimetridazole** appears to act by interfering with RNA synthesis. Dimetridazole is included in Annex IV of Regulation 2377/90/EEC which effectively prohibits its use in food-producing species. However it is available in the UK as an authorised veterinary medicine (see also sections 1.4.2 and 1.4.6) for use pheasants and partridges for health and welfare reasons; it may not be prescribed for any other food-producing species under the 'cascade'. Dimetridazole may be used as a zootechnical feed additive but only in accordance with Annex I of Directive 70/524/EEC; it is used for the prevention of blackhead in turkeys and guinea fowl.

CARNIDAZOLE

UK

Indications. Treatment and prophylaxis of trichomoniosis
Dose. *Pigeons*: *by mouth,* (adult birds) 10 mg; (young birds) 5 mg

GSL **Spartrix** (Harkers) *UK*
Tablets, scored, carnidazole 10 mg, for *pigeons*; 50
Withdrawal Periods. Should not be used in *pigeons* intended for human consumption

Australia

Indications. Treatment and prophylaxis of trichomoniosis
Dose. *Pigeons*: *by mouth,* (adult birds) 10 mg; (young birds) 5 mg

Spartrix (Boehringer Ingelheim) *Austral.*
Tablets, carnidazole 10 mg, for *pigeons*
Withdrawal Periods. Should not be used in pigeons intended for human consumption.

USA

Indications. Treatment and prophylaxis of trichomoniosis
Dose. *Pigeons*: *by mouth,* (adult birds) 10 mg; (young birds) 5 mg

Carnidazole (Wildlife Pharm) *USA*
Tablets, carnidazole 10 mg, for *pigeons*

DIMETRIDAZOLE

UK

Indications. Treatment and prophylaxis of trichomoniosis in pheasants, and partridges; histomoniosis (see section 1.4.2); hexamitiosis (see section 1.4.6)
Dose. *Pheasants, partridges*: treatment of trichomoniosis, 27 g/100 litres drinking water for 12 days *or* 54 g/100 litres drinking water for 3–5 days then 27 g/100 litres drinking water for treatment up to 12 days
prophylaxis of trichomoniosis, 125–200 g/tonne feed; 12 g/100 litres drinking water for up to 15 days

MFS **Emtryl Premix for Game Birds** (Merial) *UK*
See section 1.4.2 for preparation details

MFS **Emtryl Pure for Game Birds** (Merial) *UK*
See section 1.4.2 for preparation details

POM **Emtryl Soluble for Gamebirds** (Merial) *UK*
See section 1.4.2 for preparation details

Australia

Indications. Trichomoniosis in caged birds; histomoniosis in turkeys; bacterial infections in pigs
Dose. Consult manufacturer's information

Dimetridazole Water Soluble Powder (CCD) *Austral.*
Powder, for addition to drinking water, dimetridazole 980 mg/g, for *pigs, turkeys, cage birds*
Withdrawal Periods. *Turkeys*: slaughter 5 day, should not be used in turkeys producing eggs for human consumption. *Pigs*: slaughter 5 days.

New Zealand

Indications. Trichomoniosis in pigeons; histomoniosis in turkeys and game birds; bacterial infections in pigs
Dose. Consult manufacturer's information

Dimetrasol (PCL) *NZ*
Oral powder, dimetridazole 400 mg/g, for *pigs, poultry, game birds, pigeons*
Withdrawal Periods. Slaughter 5 days. Should not be used in birds producing eggs for human consumption

METRONIDAZOLE

UK

Indications. Treatment of trichomoniosis; metronidazole-sensitive infections (see section 1.1.8); giardiosis (see section 1.4.5); hepatic encephalopathy ♦ (see section 3.10)
Dose. *Dogs, cats, birds*: trichomoniosis, *by mouth or by subcutaneous injection,* 20 mg/kg daily

POM **Torgyl Solution** (Merial) *UK*
See section 1.1.8 for preparation details

RONIDAZOLE

Australia

Indications. Trichomoniosis

Ronivet-s (Vetafarm) *Austral.*
Powder, for addition to drinking water, ronidazole 60 mg/g, for *cage birds, pigeons*
Withdrawal Periods. Should not be used in birds intended for human consumption.

1.4.4 Drugs for babesiosis

Infection caused by *Babesia* spp. occur in a number of species. Bovine babesiosis (redwater fever) is characterised by fever and intravascular haemolysis. Organisms involved include *Bab. bigemina*, *Bab. bovis*, and *Bab. divergens*. Transmission of the protozoa is by ticks and ectoparasitic control (see section 2.2) may assist in prevention of the disease in cattle.

Ovine babesiosis has been reported throughout Europe. *Bab. motasi* and *Bab. ovis* are both capable of causing either acute or chronic disease with symptoms similar to those seen in cattle.

Equine babesiosis (*Bab. equi* and *Bab. caballi*) is an occasional cause of severe clinical disease and mortality and is of importance to the international horse trade requiring strict control. Canine babesiosis (*Bab. canis*) is becoming increasingly widespread in the USA and Europe.

Imidocarb is effective against *Bab. divergens* infection. The drug appears to act directly on the parasite leading to an alteration in morphology. Imidocarb is excreted unchanged mainly in the urine. It is effective in preventing and treating bovine babesiosis without interfering with the development of immunity. **Diminazine** is an aromatic diamidine derivative related to pentamidine.

DIMINAZINE

Indications. Babesiosis; trypanosomosis
Dose. *Cattle:* trypanosomosis, *by intramuscular injection,* 3.5 mg/kg

Dogs: babesiosis, *by intramuscular injection,* 3.5–7.0 mg/kg as a single dose or 3 mg/kg twice daily for 6 days

IMIDOCARB DIPROPIONATE

Australia
Indications. Babesiosis; anaplasmosis
Dose. *Cattle*: babesiosis, treatment, *by subcutaneous injection*, 1.2 mg/kg
babesiosis prophylaxis, anaplasmosis, *by subcutaneous injection*, 3 mg/kg

Imizol (Coopers) *Austral.*
Injection, imidocarb dipropionate 120 mg/mL, for *cattle*
Withdrawal Periods. Slaughter 28 days, should not be used in cattle producing milk for human consumption

Eire
Indications. Babesiosis
Dose. *Cattle*: babesiosis, treatment, *by subcutaneous injection*, 1.2 mg/kg
babesiosis prophylaxis, *by subcutaneous injection*, 3 mg/kg

Imizol Injection (Schering-Plough) *Eire*
Injection, imidocarb dipropionate 12%, for *cattle*
Withdrawal Periods. Slaughter 90 days, milk 5 days

USA
Indications. Babesiosis
Dose. *Dogs*: *by subcutaneous or intramuscular injection*, 6 mg/kg

Imizol (Schering-Plough) *USA*
Injection, imidocarb dipropionate 120 mg/mL, for *dogs*

1.4.5 Drugs for giardiosis

Giardia spp. are flagellate protozoa commonly associated with human enteric infections, yet frequently overlooked as parasites of domestic animals. Infections in many animals are asymptomatic; where disease does occur, the signs include chronic diarrhoea, weight loss, lethargy, and failure to thrive. Giardiosis is a zoonotic disease.

Metronidazole is used for the treatment of giardiosis (giardiasis) in dogs and cats. **Fenbendazole** is also available for the treatment of giardiosis in adult dogs and puppies.

FENBENDAZOLE

UK
Indications. Treatment of giardiosis in dogs; endoparasites (see section 2.1.1.2)
Dose. *Dogs*: giardiosis, *by mouth*, 50 mg/kg daily for 3 days

PML **Panacur 2.5% Liquid** (Intervet)
See section 2.1.1.2 for preparation details

PML **Panacur 10% Liquid** (Intervet)
See section 2.1.1.2 for preparation details

PML **Panacur Paste** (Intervet)
See section 2.1.1.2 for preparation details

PML **Panacur Wormer** (Intervet)
See section 2.1.1.2 for preparation details

METRONIDAZOLE

UK
Indications. Treatment of giardiosis; metronidazole-sensitive infections (see section 1.1.8); trichomoniosis (see section 1.4.3); hepatic encephalopathy♦ (see section 3.10)
Dose. *Dogs, cats*: giardiosis, *by mouth or by subcutaneous injection*, 20 mg/kg daily

POM **Torgyl Solution** (Merial) *UK*
See section 1.1.8 for preparation details

1.4.6 Drugs for hexamitiosis

Spironucleus meleagridis (Hexamita meleagridis) is a flagellate protozoan causing an infectious catarrhal enteritis in birds. Infections in adult birds are usually asymptomatic but in young birds heavy losses can occur. **Dimetridazole** appears to interfere with RNA synthesis.

Dimetridazole is included in Annex IV of Regulation 2377/90/EEC which effectively prohibits its use in food-producing species. However it is available in the UK as an authorised veterinary medicine (see also sections 1.4.2 and 1.4.3) for use pheasants and partridges for health and welfare reasons; it may not be prescribed for any other food-producing species under the 'cascade'. Dimetridazole may be used as a zootechnical feed additive but only in accordance with Annex I of Directive 70/524/EEC; it is used for the prevention of blackhead in turkeys and guinea fowl.

DIMETRIDAZOLE

UK
Indications. Treatment and prophylaxis of hexamitiosis pheasants, and partridges; histomoniosis (see section 1.4.2); trichomoniosis (see section 1.4.3)

Dose. *Pheasants, partridges*: treatment of hexamitiosis, 27 g/100 litres drinking water for 12 days *or* 54 g/100 litres drinking water for 3–5 days then 27 g/100 litres drinking water for treatment up to 12 days
prophylaxis of hexamitiosis, 125–200 g/tonne feed; 12 g/100 litres drinking water for up to 15 days

MFS **Emtryl Premix for Game Birds** (Merial) *UK*
See section 1.4.2 for preparation details

MFS **Emtryl Pure for Game Birds** (Merial) *UK*
See section 1.4.2 for preparation details

POM **Emtryl Soluble for Gamebirds** (Merial) *UK*
See section 1.4.2 for preparation details

1.4.7 Drugs for leishmaniosis

Leishmania spp. are vector-borne protozoan parasites primarily affecting dogs. The protozoa are transmitted by various species of sandflies belonging to the genus *Phlebotomus*. In Mediterranean Europe, canine visceral leishmaniosis is caused by *L. infantum*. The disease is zoonotic with dogs acting as a reservoir host. Infection in dogs causes a chronic insidious systemic disease characterised by inappetance, hair loss, and enlarged lymph nodes, liver, and spleen. The disease often proves fatal. Cutaneous leishmaniosis in Europe is usually caused by *L. tropica* which manifests itself in dogs as ulcers and sores that heal to a scar after several months.

Pentavalent antimony compounds such as **meglumine antimonate** and **sodium stibogluconate** are active against amastigote stages but the mechanism of action is unknown. **Pentamidine**, an aromatic diamidine derivative, has been used against some species of *Leishmania* but can be extremely nephrotoxic and hepatotoxic. It acts by interfering with DNA and folate transformation and by inhibiting RNA and protein synthesis.

Treated animals often show clinical relapse. For unresponsive cases or relapses, **amphotericin B** may be of benefit for visceral leishmaniosis but can be nephrotoxic. Other reported treatments include **allopurinol**, which is usually administered in combination with pentavalent antimony compounds for the first month of treatment. The mechanism of action of allopurinol for leishmaniosis is thought to be due to its incorporation into the protozoal purine salvage pathway.This leads to the formation of a toxic analogue of adenosine triphosphate, which is incorporated into ribonucleic acid.

ALLOPURINOL

UK
Indications. Leishmaniosis; urate calculi (see section 9.4)
Side-effects. Erythema, hypersensitivity; predisposition to xanthine calculi
Warnings. Reduce dosage for patients with renal impairment
Dose. *Dogs*: leishmaniosis, *by mouth*, 20 mg/kg daily

See section 9.4 for preparation details

AMPHOTERICIN
(Amphotericin B)

UK
Indications. Leishmaniosis; systemic yeast and fungal infections (see section 1.2)
Contra-indications. Renal impairment, see notes above
Side-effects. Nephrotoxicity
Warnings. Drug Interactions – see Appendix 1
Dose. Leishmaniosis, *by intravenous infusion*, 0.5–1.0 mg/kg. Dose should be gradually increased from 5–10 mg daily

See section 1.2 for preparation details

MEGLUMINE ANTIMONATE
(Meglumine antimoniate)

Indications. Acute and chronic leishmaniosis
Dose. *Dogs*: *by subcutaneous or intramuscular injection*, 80–100 mg/kg daily

Glucantime (Merial) *Fr.*

Ⓗ preparations available in *Fr., Ital., Spain*

PENTAMIDINE ISETIONATE
(Pentamidine isethionate)

UK
Indications. Cutaneous and visceral leishmaniosis
Side-effects. Metabolic disturbances, hepatic impairment, haematological disorders
Warnings. Use with caution in animals with renal or hepatic impairment
Dose. *Dogs*: *by intramuscular injection*, 3–4 mg/kg on alternate days. Maximum course is 10 treatments

POM Ⓗ **Pentacarinat** (JHC) *UK*
Injection, powder for reconstitution, pentamidine isetionate 300 mg

SODIUM STIBOGLUCONATE

UK
Indications. Cutaneous and visceral leishmaniosis
Side-effects. Occasional anaphylactoid reaction, bradycardia, cardiac arrhythmias
Warnings. Renal impairment, hepatic impairment, risk of local thrombosis (see *Note* below)
Dose. See preparation details

POM Ⓗ **Pentostam** (GlaxoWellcome) *UK*
Injection, sodium stibogluconate equivalent to pentavalent antimony 100 mg/mL
Dose. *Dogs*: *by intravenous injection*, 0.1–0.2 mg/kg for maximum 20 days
Note. Injection should be administered slowly over 5 minutes

1.4.8 Drugs for theileriosis

A number of *Theileria* spp. have been reported in cattle and sheep, of which some are significant causes of disease in many tropical countries. The protozoa occur within lymphocytic and erythrocytic cells and are transmitted by the bites of various species of ticks. In cattle, *Theileria parva*

parva, the cause of East Coast fever, and *T. annulata*, the cause of Mediterranean Coast fever, are the main pathogenic species. In sheep, *T. lestoquardi* (*T.hirci*) is highly pathogenic. A more benign species of *Theleria* found throughout Europe is *T. ovis*.

Buparvaquone is a hydroxynapthoquinone used for the treatment of theileriosis in cattle. Napthoquinones are though to interfere with electron transport within mitochondria at the uboquinone level.

The tetracyclines (see section 1.1.2), **chlortetracycline** and **oxytetracycline**, are used for prophylaxis against *T. parva parva* and may reduce parasitaemia by arresting schizogony. Chlortetracycline is used at a dose of 1.5mg/kg orally for 28 days and oxytetracycline is given at a dose of 20 mg/kg intramuscularly once or twice, or 5 to 15 mg/kg intravenously.

BUPARVAQUONE

Indications. Theileriosis in cattle
Dose. *Cattle*: *by intramuscular injection*, 2.5–5.0 mg/kg

1.4.9 Drug for trypanosomosis

Trypanosomosis is an important disease of humans and domestic animals in parts of the tropics. A large number of species have been identified and can be broadly divided into two groups depending on the site of development in the insect vector. The salivarian trypanosomes, transmitted in the saliva of biting flies, are responsible for diseases such as African sleeping sickness in humans, and 'surra' and 'nagana' in domestic ruminants. The stercorarian trypanosomes, which are transmitted by contamination with infected insect faeces, cause diseases including Chagas' disease in humans in Central and South America and is transmitted by reduviid bugs.

Diminazine (see section 1.4.4) is an aromatic diamidine derivative related to pentamidine. **Isometamidium chloride** is used therapeutically and for prophylaxis. A dose of 0.5 to 2.0 mg/kg by intramuscular injection is used in cattle. These drugs appear to bind to parasite DNA and block DNA and RNA synthesis.

2   Drugs used in the treatment and control of
PARASITIC INFECTIONS

Contributors:
Professor D E Jacobs BVMS, PhD, FRCVS, FRCPath
Professor M A Taylor BVMS, PhD, CBiol, MIBiol, MRCVS

Parasitic infections are caused by helminths, arthropods, and protozoa. The latter group is considered in section 1.4. Control of parasites of animals, birds, fish (see Prescribing for fish), and bees (see Prescribing for invertebrates) is essential for both their welfare and to maximise production. The control of some infections is particularly important for public health reasons; for example, they may have zoonotic potential or cause condemnation of offal or the carcass at the slaughterhouse. In this chapter, drug treatment is discussed under the following headings:

2.1 Endoparasiticides
2.2 Ectoparasiticides

Notes on endectocides, such as avermectins and milbemycins, are included in each section because they have activity against a range of parasites in both categories.

2.1 Endoparasiticides

2.1.1 Drugs for roundworms (nematodes)
2.1.2 Drugs for tapeworms (cestodes)
2.1.3 Drugs for flukes (trematodes)
2.1.4 Compound endoparasiticides

Anthelmintics are used prophylactically and also to treat acute and chronic infections. Control measures reduce worm burdens, enhance productivity, and substantially reduce the build-up of infective worm larvae on the pasture or eggs in the environment.

Some endoparasiticide preparations contain cobalt and selenium. These ingredients should be regarded as nutritional adjuncts, rather than substitutes for other measures to correct mineral deficiencies.

The three major groups of helminths are the roundworms (nematodes), tapeworms (cestodes), and flukes (trematodes). The biological characteristics of these groups are often sufficiently disparate to necessitate anthelmintics with different modes of action. Even within a group there is sufficient diversity to limit the spectrum of activity of many drugs, the choice being further complicated by the fact that the various developmental stages of the parasites may not be equally susceptible. The nature and composition of the target population must therefore be known in order to select the most appropriate preparation.

Table 2.1 outlines drugs that are effective against common endoparasitic infections in the UK in horses, ruminants, pigs, dogs, cats, poultry, game birds, and pigeons. Different formulations of a preparation may be indicated for different parasites.

2.1.1 Drugs for roundworms (nematodes)

2.1.1.1 Avermectins and milbemycins
2.1.1.2 Benzimidazoles
2.1.1.3 Imidazothiazoles
2.1.1.4 Organophosphorus compounds
2.1.1.5 Tetrahydropyrimidines
2.1.1.6 Other drugs for roundworms

The roundworms form a large and complex group and infections may be caused by a single or multiple species. Infections should be controlled by suitable hygiene and strategic prophylactic treatment based on a knowledge of the epidemiology of the infection. Both specific and broad-spectrum treatments are used. The latter are also used in cases where it is difficult to make a definitive diagnosis without undue delay or to maximise the production benefits of prophylactic treatment.

In order to minimise the possibility of development of resistance, the chemical class of drugs used should be changed from year to year. To assist in the planning of anthelmintic rotation programmes, labels on worming products for farm animals display one of the following symbols to denote the chemical group of the active ingredient:

*   **1-BZ** benzimidazoles, probenzimidazoles
*   **2-LM** imidazothiazoles, tetrahydropyrimidines
*   **3-AV** avermectins, milbemycins.

Compounds within each of the above categories have similar modes of action. If resistance develops to one drug, then other drugs in the same category will normally show side- or cross-resistance.

Information on control of anthelmintic resistance may be found in *Anthelmintic resistance of worms in sheep and goats, practical help on avoidance* CVL/NOAH, 1993. See also under Benzimidazoles (section 2.1.1.2)

Equidae

Equidae harbour a wider variety of nematodes than any other domesticated animal. Strongylid and ascarid infections commonly cause ill-thrift, diarrhoea, and sometimes colic in horses and donkeys. Migrating *Strongylus vulgaris* larvae damage the cranial mesenteric artery causing equine verminous arteritis. *Dictyocaulus* infection may cause lung lesions and although it generally causes few ill effects in donkeys unless they carry a heavy worm burden, it may affect ponies and horses if they graze alongside; control of this parasite necessitates treatment of donkeys with an appropriate anthelminthic and inclusion in a regular dosing regimen for all equines.

In general, gastro-intestinal nematodes may be controlled by regular dosing of all horses, for example every 6 to 13 weeks throughout spring, summer, and autumn, and every 3 months during winter. More or less frequent administration may be required depending on risk factors such as the graz-

Table 2.1 Drugs effective against common endoparasitic infections[1]

	Parasite	Endoparasiticides
EQUIDAE (consult individual monographs because some preparations are not suitable for all species)		
Gastro-intestinal roundworms	*Parascaris, Strongylus,* Cyathostomes, *Oxyuris*	febantel, fenbendazole, ivermectin, mebendazole, moxidectin, oxibendazole, pyrantel
	Strongyloides	fenbendazole, ivermectin, moxidectin, oxibendazole
	Migrating strongyles	fenbendazole, ivermectin, moxidectin
Horse bots	*Gasterophilus*	haloxon, ivermectin, moxidectin
Lungworms	*Dictyocaulus*	ivermectin, mebendazole
Tapeworms	*Anoplocephala perfoliata*	pyrantel, praziquantel ♦
	Anoplocephaloides mammillana	praziquantel ♦
Liver flukes	*Fasciola*	triclabendazole ♦
RUMINANTS (consult individual monographs because some preparations are not suitable for all species)		
Gastro-intestinal roundworms	*Bunostomum, Chabertia, Cooperia, Haemonchus, Nematodirus, Oesophagostomum, Ostertagia (Teladorsagia), Strongyloides, Trichostrongylus*	abamectin, albendazole, closantel (*Haemonchus* only), doramectin, eprinomectin, febantel, fenbendazole, ivermectin, levamisole, mebendazole, morantel, moxidectin, netobimin, nitroxinil (*Bunostomum, Haemonchus, Oesophagostomum* only), oxfendazole, thiophanate
	Type II ostertagiosis	abamectin, albendazole, doramectin, eprinomectin, fenbendazole, ivermectin, moxidectin, netobimin, oxfendazole, thiophanate
Lungworms	*Dictyocaulus*	abamectin, albendazole, doramectin, eprinomectin, febantel, fenbendazole, ivermectin, levamisole, mebendazole, moxidectin, netobimin, oxfendazole
	Protostrongylus	ivermectin (by injection)
Sheep nasal bots	*Oestrus ovis*	closantel, doramectin, ivermectin
Tapeworms	*Moniezia*	albendazole, febantel, fenbendazole, mebendazole, netobimin, oxfendazole
Liver flukes	*Fasciola*	
	1–12 weeks	closantel, nitroxinil, triclabendazole

Table 2.1 Drugs effective against common endoparasitic infections[1]

	Parasite	Endoparasiticides
Liver flukes	Fasciola	
	adult	albendazole, clorsulon, closantel, netobimin, nitroxinil, triclabendazole
	Dicrocoelium	netobimin

PIGS

	Parasite	Endoparasiticides
Gastro-intestinal roundworms	Oesophagostomum, Ascaris, Hyostrongylus	doramectin, febantel, fenbendazole, flubendazole, ivermectin, thiophanate
	Trichuris	doramectin (adult worms), fenbendazole, flubendazole, thiophanate
	Strongyloides	doramectin, ivermectin
Lungworms	Metastrongylus	doramectin, fenbendazole, flubendazole, ivermectin

DOGS and CATS (consult individual monographs because some preparations are not suitable for both species)

	Parasite	Endoparasiticides
Gastro-intestinal roundworms	Ancylostoma, Toxocara, Toxascaris, Uncinaria	fenbendazole, mebendazole, nitroscanate, piperazine, pyrantel, selamectin
	Trichuris	fenbendazole, mebendazole
	Transplacental roundworm transmission in dogs	fenbendazole
Lungworms	Oslerus	fenbendazole
	Angiostrongylus	fenbendazole ♦, levamisole ♦
	Aelurostrongylus	fenbendazole
Tapeworms	Echinococcus	mebendazole, praziquantel
	Dipylidium	dichlorophen, nitroscanate, praziquantel
	Taenia	dichlorophen, fenbendazole, mebendazole, nitroscanate, praziquantel

Table 2.1 Drugs effective against common endoparasitic infections[1]

	Parasite	Endoparasiticides
Heartworms	Dirofilaria	
	prophylaxis in dogs for export	ivermectin[2], milbemycin oxime[2], moxidectin[2], selamectin
	treatment in imported dogs (**seek specialist advice before treatment**)	
	adults	levamisole ◆, melarsomine[2], thiacetarsamide[2]
	microfilariae	dithiazanine[2], levamisole ◆

POULTRY

	Parasite	Endoparasiticides
Gastro-intestinal roundworms	Amidostomum, Ascaridia, Capillaria, Heterakis, Trichostrongylus	flubendazole
Gapeworms	Syngamus	flubendazole
Tapeworms	Raillietina	flubendazole

GAME BIRDS (consult individual monographs because some preparations are not suitable for all species)

	Parasite	Endoparasiticides
Gastro-intestinal roundworms	Amidostomum, Ascaridia, Capillaria, Heterakis	flubendazole
	Trichostrongylus	fenbendazole, flubendazole
Gapeworms	Syngamus	flubendazole
Tapeworms	Raillietina	flubendazole

PIGEONS

	Parasite	Endoparasiticides
Gastro-intestinal roundworms	Ascaridia	febantel, fenbendazole, levamisole, piperazine
	Capillaria	febantel, fenbendazole, levamisole

[1] infections and treatment used in the UK
[2] specific veterinary-authorised preparations not available in the UK

ing history and the stocking rate. Newly acquired animals are usually treated with a broad-spectrum anthelmintic, although presence of encysted cyathostomes may reduce efficacy of therapy. Avermectins and milbemycins, particularly moxidectin, may give a longer period of protection than other chemical groups. A 5-day course of treatment with fenbendazole in early winter is claimed to reduce the risk of larval cyathostomosis, which is associated with the resumed development of hypobiotic larvae.

Reliance on anthelmintics can be reduced by regular removal of faeces from paddocks. Faecal egg-counts should be used to monitor the adequacy of worming programmes.

Ruminants

In ruminants, parasitic gastro-enteritis and parasitic bronchitis (husk) are the main clinical disorders caused by adult nematodes.

Ostertagia larvae may undergo an arrested development within the host when environmental conditions are adverse to the survival of free-living stages. Type II ostertagiosis is caused by these larvae emerging from a prolonged hypobiotic state. They have a reduced metabolic rate and are relatively resistant to anthelmintic attack.

Most forms of parasitic gastro-enteritis in ruminants tend to occur in the second half of the summer, although Type II ostertagiosis occurs in late winter and spring, and nematodirosis in lambs occurs in late spring. Routine control entails repeated use of anthelmintics during spring and summer and at housing, but to prevent or delay resistance problems, unnecessary treatments should be avoided. The dosing interval is determined by the stocking density, pasture contamination, and the particular anthelmintic. Certain avermectin and milbemycin preparations prevent infective larvae from establishing for some time after treatment. This provides a period of protection from re-infection, the duration of which varies with the drug, formulation, host and worm species (see section 2.1.1.1).

This property of avermectins and milbemycins has been used for the design of strategic control programmes for *cattle*. When set-stocked calves are given 2 or 3 carefully timed anthelmintic doses at or after turnout, there is a substantial reduction in the build up of infective gastro-intestinal and lungworm larvae on the pasture throughout the grazing season. A similar effect can be obtained by the use of modified-release (continuous or pulse-release) intra-ruminal devices that provide medication over a period of 90 to 135 days, although not all are effective against lungworm. These systems will break down if untreated stock are grazed on the clean pasture or if treated animals are subsequently put onto contaminated pasture. There is concern that some prophylactic measures for calves are so effective that there may not always be sufficient antigenic stimulation to ensure full development of immunity. Animals may be at risk if put onto heavily contaminated pasture towards the end of a long grazing season, or in their second year. An alternative prophylactic approach is to give a mid-July dose and move the stock to aftermath grazing or other clean pasture. If there is no option but to graze calves on heavily con-

taminated pasture, repeated avermectin or milbemycin treatment or an intra-ruminal device can be given later in the season.

Medicated feed blocks are sometimes used for general worm control but the accuracy of individual dosing by this method is uncertain.

Preventive measures in *sheep* are more complicated and often less satisfactory. The ewe acts as an additional source of infection to the lamb and a pre-lambing treatment is therefore necessary to eliminate the peri-parturient rise in faecal egg-counts. Routine dosing programmes for lambs should comply with CVL/NOAH guidelines for preventing and avoiding resistance. Reliance on anthelmintics can be reduced by alternating grazing between cattle and sheep, as few parasites can survive in the wrong host, although problems have arisen in some areas because *Nematodirus battus* can be transmitted through calves to cause disease in lambs the following year. Additional treatment of lambs in spring may be necessary to prevent nematodirosis, especially if a high-risk season is anticipated due to climatic conditions.

The control of nematode infections in *goats* is further complicated by the fact that they do not develop an effective immunity and therefore remain susceptible throughout their lives. They also tend to metabolise some anthelmintics more quickly than sheep and so doses and treatment intervals cannot be extrapolated from one species to the other. For example, the recommended dose of albendazole for sheep is 5 mg/kg and for goats is 10 mg/kg. This higher dose entails withdrawal periods of at least 7 days for milk and 28 days for meat, but lower doses may be ineffective and may encourage the onset of resistance. Similarly, levamisole♦ has to be given at an elevated dosage of up to 12 mg/kg. Levamisole may be toxic in goats and should be used with caution in this species; treatment by injection is contra-indicated. Ivermectin may be given as an oral formulation at a dose of 200 micrograms/kg. The frequency of occurrence of resistance and the range of anthelmintics involved are greater in goats than sheep. It is important therefore that an integrated approach to worm control is adopted with minimal reliance on anthelmintics.

Pigs

In pigs, *Hyostrongylus*, *Trichuris*, and lungworms are almost exclusively found in animals kept outdoors, as is the swine kidney worm, *Stephanurus dentatus*, but this does not occur in the UK being largely confined to tropical and subtropical regions. *Ascaris* and *Oesophagostomum* are common even in intensively kept pigs, the former mainly in younger animals, and the latter particularly in breeding stock. They can both cause production losses.

The choice of drug for roundworms affecting extensively farmed animals is restricted, but a wider variety is available for housed stock. For convenience and economy, pig anthelmintics are usually administered as a single dose in the form of a feed dressing or in medicated feed over a period of days. Ivermectin and doramectin can be given by injection. Weaners may be treated before moving to fattening pens and again 8 weeks later. Sows are dosed shortly before farrowing. Boars are dosed regularly at intervals of about 6 months. Alternatively, all pigs in a building may be treated simultaneously at intervals determined by monitoring faecal egg-counts.

Dogs and cats

Roundworm infections are common in dogs and cats. Most puppies carry prenatally acquired *Toxocara* infection. This roundworm is of zoonotic importance and is harmful to the puppy. When infective eggs of *Toxocara canis* are swallowed by humans, the larvae migrate to various sites and may rarely result in unilateral impairment of vision. Therefore routine worming of puppies from an early age is essential together with removal of faeces. For guidance, puppies should ideally be wormed fortnightly from 2 weeks of age until 12 weeks of age. A similar result may be achieved with fenbendazole given during the third and sixth weeks of life. A reduced dosage regimen is required because benzimadazoles are more effective against larval ascarids than piperazine and prevent faecal egg-output for a longer period. Ease of application is an important criterion for the choice of product in very young pups.

Older dogs may harbour somatic *Toxocara* larvae in various tissues. These are not killed by routine worming and become active in late pregnancy to migrate across the placenta and into the milk. Pre- and post-natal transmission can be controlled with a special regimen of fenbendazole treatments given to the bitch in late pregnancy (see section 2.1.1.2). This prophylactic programme will also prevent the transfer of *Ancylostoma* larvae via the milk. This hookworm is rare in the UK but is a frequent cause of anaemia, particularly in puppies, in warmer climates.

As kittens are infected by *Toxocara cati* via the milk but not prenatally, routine worming commences at 4 to 6 weeks of age followed by further doses every 3 weeks up to the age of 4 months.

Toxascaris, Uncinaria (hookworm), and *Trichuris* (whipworm) are acquired later in life and are associated mainly with large kennel establishments and contaminated exercise areas. *Trichuris*, which causes intermittent diarrhoea, is particularly difficult to treat and repeated dosing may be necessary.

For routine control of common gastro-intestinal roundworms, adults should normally be treated every few months. Lactating bitches, however, commonly harbour patent *Toxocara* infections and should be treated at 3-week intervals until the puppies are weaned.

There are few authorised treatments for lungworm infections in dogs and cats. *Angiostrongylus* infections usually respond to levamisole♦ but fenbendazole♦ may be safer although its efficacy is less well documented. *Oslerus* (*Filaroides*) and *Aelurostrongylus* can be serious pathogens of dogs and cats respectively. Each can be controlled with fenbendazole given over several days (see section 2.1.1.2). The course of treatment may have to be repeated in some cases.

Fortunately, canine heartworm disease (dirofilariosis) is not endemic in the UK but cases do occur among imported dogs. It is a major cause of morbidity and premature death in dogs in endemic areas such as parts of Italy, North America, and many tropical and subtropical countries. Cats are sometimes infected. Affected animals initially show exercise intolerance due to progressive heart failure and organ dysfunction, but acute cases occasionally occur. Melarsomine may be used for treatment. This drug does not have a veterinary marketing authorisation in the UK and therefore may only be supplied under a Special Treatment Authorisation from the VMD. **Specialist advice should be sought before treating *Dirofilaria* infections.** Dogs travelling to affected countries can be protected on arrival with monthly treatments of ivermectin♦, moxidectin♦, milbemycin oxime, or selamectin♦. Diethylcarbamazine, which has to be given daily during and subsequent to the mosquito season, is still used in some countries.

Birds

Poultry and **game birds** are treated for gastro-intestinal roundworm, gapeworm, and tapeworm infections. Helminth infection is less of a problem in poultry reared indoors because of their lack of contact with intermediate hosts. Breeding birds are treated before laying. Rearing birds are dosed 3 weeks after placing on infected ground, maintenance doses being given every 6 to 8 weeks. **Pigeons** are treated routinely for gastro-intestinal roundworm infections each year 2 weeks before their first race and before pairing. **Ostriches** are routinely wormed at 6, 12, and 24 months of age and as adults.

2.1.1.1 Avermectins and milbemycins

Preparations for farm animals that contain avermectins, including **abamectin**, **doramectin**, **eprinomectin**, and **ivermectin**, and milbemycins such as **milbemycin** and **moxidectin** are labelled with the symbol 3-AV. These are natural or semi-natural macrocyclic lactone fermentation products of strains of, respectively *Streptomyces avermitilis* and *Streptomyces cyanogriseus*. They interfere with parasite nerve transmission by opening chloride channels in the post-synaptic membrane. They are effective against a wide range of nematode species and developmental stages, but have no activity against trematodes or cestodes. They are termed endectocides because they are also active against many ectoparasites (see section 2.2.1.1). As yet, resistance to this group in the UK is confined to some goat farms.

In addition to killing an existing parasite population, the avermectins and milbemycins prevent re-infection for a period after treatment. The duration of activity is affected by the lipophilicity of the molecule, the formulation, the route of administration, the host and worm species. In cattle, for example, different preparations provide a duration of activity against *Ostertagia* for 14 to 35 days. Corresponding figures for *Cooperia* are 0 to 28 days and for *Dictyocaulus* 28 to 42 days. In sheep, abomasal worms may be controlled for 5 weeks with moxidectin. This phenomenon is utilised in strategic programmes for the prevention of parasitic gastro-enteritis and bronchitis in calves (see section 2.1.1

Ruminants). For example, ivermectin is given at 3, 8, and 13 weeks after turnout, or doramectin is given at turnout and again 8 weeks later. Because of their persistence, however, avermectins and milbemycins are not recommended for use in lactating animals or for a prescribed period before calving. An exception is eprinomectin which has an unusually low milk:plasma coefficient, allowing a zero milk withholding period in dairy cows.

Ivermectin given to sows before farrowing effectively controls transmission of *Strongyloides ransomi* via the milk. Horses carrying heavy infections of *Onchocerca* may develop transient oedema and pruritus following treatment. This may be due to the sudden death of large numbers of microfilariae in the skin.

A new avermectin, **selamectin**, has recently been introduced for heartworm propylaxis and ectoparasite control in dogs and cats. It also has activity against *Toxocara* in dogs and cats and hookworm in cats.

Ivermectin is sometimes used for control of lungworms and ectoparasites in dogs♦ and cats♦ **but should be used with extreme caution**. Toxicity is predominantly seen in rough-haired Collies but has also occurred in other breeds. The clinical signs of toxicity are ataxia, depression, tremors, recumbency, and mydriasis; fatalities may occur. Similar clinical signs have been reported in cases of moxidectin overdosage in dogs due to ingestion of preparations authorised for horses.

ABAMECTIN

UK

Indications. Endoparasites. Gastro-intestinal roundworms and lungworms in cattle; Type II ostertagiosis in cattle Ectoparasites. See section 2.2.1.1

Contra-indications. Administration to calves less than 16 weeks of age

Side-effects. Transient discomfort and swelling at injection site

Dose. *Cattle*: *by subcutaneous injection*, 200 micrograms/kg

PML **Enzec Injection for Cattle** (Merial) *UK*
Injection, abamectin 10 mg/mL, for *cattle*
Withdrawal Periods. Cattle: slaughter 42 days, should not be used in cattle producing milk for human consumption

Australia

Indications. Endoparasites. Gastro-intestinal roundworms and lungworms in horses, cattle, sheep
Ectoparasites. See section 2.2.1.1

Contra-indications. Administration to calves less than 16 weeks of age, foals less than 6 weeks of age

Side-effects. Transient discomfort and swelling at injection site

Dose. *Horses*: *by mouth,* 200 micrograms/kg
Cattle: *by subcutaneous injection*, 200 micrograms/kg
by 'pour-on' application, 500 micrograms/kg
Sheep: *by mouth*, 200 micrograms/kg

Avomec Antiparasitic Injection for Cattle (Merial) *Austral*
Injection, abamectin 10 g/L, for *cattle*
Withdrawal Periods. *Cattle*: slaughter 30 days, should not be used in cattle producing milk for human consumption.

Duotin Antiparasitic Injection for Cattle (Nufarm) *Austral*
Injection, abamectin 10 g/L, for *cattle*
Withdrawal Periods. *Cattle*: slaughter 30 days, milk 30 days

Equiminth (Virbac) *Austral*
Oral paste, abamectin 3.7 mg/g, for *horses*

Paramectin Broad Spectrum Oral Antiparasitic Solution for Sheep (Dover) *Austral*
Oral solution, abamectin 0.9 mg/mL, for *sheep*
Withdrawal Periods. *Sheep*: slaughter 28 days, should not be used in sheep producing milk for human consumption

Paramectin Injection for Cattle (Dover) *Austral*
Injection, abamectin10 mg/mL, for *cattle*
Withdrawal Periods. *Cattle*: slaughter 30 days, milk 30 days

Rycomectin Antiparasitic Cattle Injection (Novartis) *Austral*
Injection, abamectin 10 mg/mL, for *cattle*
Withdrawal Periods. *Cattle*: slaughter 30 days, should not be used in cattle producing milk for human consumption, should not be used within 30 days of calving in dairy cattle

Rycomectin Oral Endectocide for Sheep and Lambs (Novartis) *Austral*
Oral solution, abamectin, for *sheep*
Withdrawal Periods. *Sheep*: slaughter 14 days, should not be used in sheep producing milk for human consumption

Virbamec Antiparasitic Injection for Cattle (Virbac) *Austral*
Injection, abamectin 10 mg/mL, for *cattle*
Withdrawal Periods. Cattle: slaughter 30 days, should not be used in cattle producing milk for human consumption, should not be used within 30 days of calving in dairy cattle

Virbamec for Sheep (Virbac) *Austral*
Oral solution, abamectin 0.8 g/L, for *sheep*
Withdrawal Periods. Sheep: slaughter 14 days, should not be used in sheep producing milk for human consumption

Virbamec Pour on for Cattle (Virbac) *Austral*
Solution, pour-on, abamectin 5 mg/mL, for *cattle >50 kg body-weight*
Withdrawal Periods. *Cattle*: slaughter 35 days, should not be used in cattle producing milk for human consumption

Eire

Indications. Endoparasites. Gastro-intestinal roundworms and lungworms in cattle; Type II ostertagiosis in cattle Ectoparasites. See section 2.2.1.1

Contra-indications. Administration to calves less than 16 weeks of age

Side-effects. Transient discomfort and swelling at injection site

Dose. *Cattle*: *by subcutaneous injection*, 200 micrograms/kg

Enzec Injection for Cattle (Janssen) *Eire*
Injection, abamectin 10 mg/mL, for *cattle*
Withdrawal Periods. Cattle: slaughter 45 days, should not be used in cattle producing milk for human consumption or within 28 days prior to calving

New Zealand

Indications. Endoparasites. Gastro-intestinal roundworms and lungworms in horses, cattle, sheep
Ectoparasites. See section 2.2.1.1

Contra-indications. Administration to calves less than 16 weeks of age, foals less than 6 weeks of age, lambs less than 6 weeks of age

Side-effects. Transient discomfort and swelling at injection site

Dose. *Horses*: *by mouth,* 200 micrograms/kg

Cattle: *by subcutaneous injection,* 200 micrograms/kg

by 'pour-on' application, 500 micrograms/kg

Sheep: *by mouth,* 200 micrograms/kg

by subcutaneous injection, 200 micrograms/kg

Duotin (Merial) *NZ*
Injection, abamectin 10 mg/mL, for *cattle*
Withdrawal Periods. Slaughter 49 days, should not be used in cattle producing milk for human consumption

Equell (Virbac) *NZ*
Oral paste, abamectin 4 mg/mL, for *horses*
Withdrawal Periods. Slaughter 28 days

Genesis Hi Mineral for Sheep (Ancare) *NZ*
Oral solution, abamectin 1 mg/mL in a mineral formulation, for *sheep*
Withdrawal Periods. Slaughter 14 days, should not be used in sheep producing milk for human consumption

Genesis Injection (Ancare) *NZ*
Injection, abamectin 10 mg/mL, for *cattle, sheep*
Withdrawal Periods. Slaughter 49 days, should not be used in cattle or sheep producing milk for human consumption

Genesis Pour-on for Cattle & Deer (Ancare) *NZ*
Solution, pour-on, abamectin 10 mg/mL, for *cattle, deer*
Withdrawal Periods. *Cattle*: slaughter 35 days, milk withdrawal period nil. *Deer*: slaughter 28 days

Rycomectin (Novartis) *NZ*
Oral solution, abamectin 0.8 mg/mL, for *sheep*
Withdrawal Periods. Slaughter 21 days, should not be used in sheep producing milk for human consumption

Rycomectin Mineralised Plus Selenium (Novartis) *NZ*
Oral solution, abamectin 0.8 mg/mL, selenium 0.4 mg/mL in a mineral formulation, for *sheep*
Withdrawal Periods. Slaughter 21 days, should not be used in sheep producing milk for human consumption

DORAMECTIN

UK

Indications. Endoparasites. Gastro-intestinal roundworms and lungworms in ruminants and pigs; Type II ostertagiosis in cattle; nasal bots in sheep

Ectoparasites. See section 2.2.1.1

Dose. *Cattle*: *by 'pour-on' application,* 500 micrograms/kg

by subcutaneous injection, 200 micrograms/kg

Sheep: roundworms, nasal bots, *by intramuscular injection,* 200 micrograms/kg

Nematodirosis, *by intramuscular injection,* 300 micrograms/kg

Pigs: *by intramuscular injection,* 300 micrograms/kg

PML Dectomax Injectable Solution for Cattle and Sheep(Pfizer) *UK*
Injection, doramectin 10 mg/mL, for *cattle, sheep*; 50 mL, 200 mL, 500 mL
Withdrawal Periods. *Cattle*: slaughter 42 days, should not be used in cattle producing milk for human consumption, or dairy cows within 60 days before calving. *Sheep*: slaughter 56 days, should not be used in sheep producing milk for human consumption

PML Dectomax Injection for Pigs (Pfizer) *UK*
Injection, doramectin 10 mg/mL, for *pigs*; 200 mL, 500 mL
Withdrawal Periods. *Pigs*: slaughter 49 days

PML Dectomax Pour-On (Pfizer) *UK*
Solution, 'pour-on', doramectin 5 mg/mL, for *cattle*
Withdrawal Periods. *Cattle*: slaughter 35 days, should not be used in cattle producing milk for human consumption or on dairy cows within 60 days before calving

Australia

Indications. Endoparasites. Gastro-intestinal roundworms and lungworms in cattle

Ectoparasites. See section 2.2.1.1

Dose. *Cattle*: *by 'pour-on' application,* 500 micrograms/kg

by subcutaneous injection, 200 micrograms/kg

Dectomax Injectable (Pfizer) *Austral*
Injection, doramectin 10 mg/mL in oil base, for *cattle*
Withdrawal Periods. *Cattle*: slaughter 49 days, should not be used in cattle producing milk for human consumption

Dectomax Pour-On (Pfizer) *Austral*
Solution, pour-on, doramectin 5 g/L, for *cattle*
Withdrawal Periods. *Cattle*: slaughter 42 days, should not be used in cattle producing milk for human consumption

Eire

Indications. Endoparasites. Gastro-intestinal roundworms and lungworms in ruminants; Type II ostertagiosis in cattle; nasal bots in sheep

Ectoparasites. See section 2.2.1.1

Side-effects. Rarely, necrotic lesions at site of administration of 'pour-on' solution

Warnings. Caution with timing for treatment for *Hypoderma*

Dose. *Cattle*: *by 'pour-on' application,* 500 micrograms/kg

by subcutaneous injection, 200 micrograms/kg

Sheep: roundworms, nasal bots, *by intramuscular injection,* 200 micrograms/kg

Dectomax Injectable Solution (Pfizer) *Eire*
Injection, doramectin 10 mg/mL, for *cattle, sheep*
Withdrawal Periods. *Cattle*:slaughter 42 days, should not be used in cattle producing milk for human consumption or within 60 days prior to calving. *Sheep*: slaughter 35 days, should not be used in sheep producing milk for human consumption or 70 days prior to lambing

Dectomax Pour-on (Pfizer) *Eire*
Solution, pour-on, doramectin 5 mg/mL, for *cattle*
Withdrawal Periods. Slaughter 35 days, should not be used in cattle producing milk for human consumption or within 60 days prior to calving

New Zealand

Indications. Endoparasites. Gastro-intestinal roundworms and lungworms in cattle; Type II ostertagiosis in cattle

Ectoparasites. See section 2.2.1.1 - lice, mites on cattle

Contra-indications. Treatment with a 'pour-on' formulation when hide or hair is wet

Dose. *Cattle*: *by 'pour-on' application,* 500 micrograms/kg

by subcutaneous injection, 200 micrograms/kg

Dectomax (Pfizer) *NZ*
Injection, doramectin 10 mg/mL, for *cattle*
Withdrawal Periods. Slaughter 49 days, should not be used in cattle producing milk for human consumption

Dectomax Pour-on (Pfizer) *NZ*
Solution, pour-on, doramectin 5 mg/mL, for *cattle*
Withdrawal Periods. Slaughter 49 days, should not be used in cattle producing milk for human consumption

USA

Indications. Endoparasites. Gastro-intestinal roundworms and lungworms in cattle and pigs; Type II ostertagiosis in cattle;
Ectoparasites. See section 2.2.1.1
Contra-indications. Treatment with a 'pour-on' formulation when hide or hair is wet or rain is expected
Warnings. Caution with timing for treatment for *Hypoderma*
Dose. *Cattle*: *by 'pour-on' application*, 500 micrograms/kg
by subcutaneous or intramuscular injection, 200 micrograms/kg
Pigs: *by intramuscular injection*, 300 micrograms/kg

Dectomax (Pfizer) *USA*
Injection, doramectin 10 mg/mL, for *cattle, pigs*
Withdrawal Periods. *Cattle*: slaughter 35 days, should not be used in cattle producing milk for human consumption, should not be used in calves intended for veal production. *Pigs*: slaughter 24 days

Dectomax Pour-On (Pfizer) *USA*
Solution, pour-on, doramectin 5 mg/mL, for *cattle*
Withdrawal Periods. *Cattle*: slaughter 45 days, should not be used on cattle producing milk for human consumption, should not be used on calves intended for veal production

EPRINOMECTIN

UK

Indications. Endoparasites. Gastro-intestinal roundworms and lungworms in cattle; Type II ostertagiosis in cattle
Ectoparasites. See section 2.2.1.1
Contra-indications. Administration to areas of backline covered with mud or faeces
Dose. *Cattle*: *by 'pour-on' application*, 500 micrograms/kg

POM **Eprinex** (Merial) *UK*
Solution, 'pour-on', eprinomectin 5 mg/mL, for *beef cattle, dairy cattle*; 250 mL, 1 litre, other sizes available
Withdrawal Periods. *Cattle*: slaughter 15 days, milk withdrawal period nil

Australia

Indications. Endoparasites. Gastro-intestinal roundworms and lungworms in cattle; Type II ostertagiosis in cattle
Ectoparasites. See section 2.2.1.1
Dose. *Cattle*: *by 'pour-on' application*, 500 micrograms/kg

Ivomec Eprinex Pour-On (Merial) *Austral*
Solution, pour-on, eprinomectin 5 g/L, for *cattle, deer*
Withdrawal Periods. *Cattle*: slaughter withdrawal period nil, milk withdrawal period nil. *Red deer*: slaughter withdrawal period nil

Eire

Indications. Endoparasites. Gastro-intestinal roundworms and lungworms in cattle; Type II ostertagiosis in cattle

Ectoparasites. See section 2.2.1.1
Contra-indications. Administration to areas of backline covered with mud or faeces
Dose. *Cattle*: *by 'pour-on' application*, 500 micrograms/kg

Eprinex Pour-on for Beef and Dairy Cattle (Merial) *Eire*
Solution, pour-on, eprinomectin 0.5%, for *cattle*
Withdrawal Periods. Slaughter 17 days, milk withdrawal period nil

New Zealand

Indications. Endoparasites. Gastro-intestinal roundworms and lungworms in cattle; Type II ostertagiosis in cattle
Ectoparasites. See section 2.2.1.1
Contra-indications. Administration to areas of backline covered with mud or faeces
Side-effects. Occasionally skin scurf
Dose. *Cattle*: *by 'pour-on' application*, 500 micrograms/kg

Ivomec Eprinex Pour-on for Cattle & Deer (Merial) *NZ*
Solution, pour-on, eprinomectin 0.5%, for *cattle, deer*
Withdrawal Periods. *Cattle*: slaughter 14 days, milk withdrawal period nil.
Deer: slaughter 14 days

USA

Indications. Endoparasites. Gastro-intestinal roundworms and lungworms in cattle; Type II ostertagiosis in cattle
Ectoparasites. See section 2.2.1.1
Contra-indications. Administration to areas of backline covered with mud or faeces
Dose. *Cattle*: *by 'pour-on' application*, 500 micrograms/kg

Ivomec Eprinex Pour-On For Beef And Dairy Cattle (Merial) *USA*
Solution, pour-on, eprinomectin 5 mg/mL, for *cattle*
Withdrawal Periods. *Cattle*: slaughter withdrawal period nil, milk withdrawal period nil

IVERMECTIN

UK

Indications. Endoparasites. Gastro-intestinal roundworms and lungworms in horses, ruminants, and pigs; Type II ostertagiosis in ruminants; horse bots; nasal bots in sheep
Ectoparasites. See section 2.2.1.1
Contra-indications. Administration of ruminal boluses to non-ruminating cattle, administration to calves less than 12 weeks of age
Side-effects. Occasional coughing in sheep and goats after oral treatment; occasional transient oedema and pruritus in horses; transient pain after injection in sheep
Warnings. If cattle are vaccinated against lungworm, the ruminal bolus should not be administered until 14 days after the second dose of vaccine
Dose.
Horses: *by mouth*, 200 micrograms/kg
Cattle: *by 'pour-on' application*, 500 micrograms/kg
by subcutaneous injection, 200 micrograms/kg
see also modified-release oral preparations below
Sheep: *by mouth or by subcutaneous injection*, 200 micrograms/kg
Goats: *by mouth*, 200 micrograms/kg
Pigs: *by addition to feed*, 100 micrograms/kg daily for 7 days

by subcutaneous injection, 300 micrograms/kg

PML Eqvalan (Merial) *UK*
Oral paste, ivermectin 20 mg/division, for *horses, donkeys*; 6.42-g metered-dose applicator
Withdrawal Periods. *Horses, donkeys:* slaughter 21 days
Dose. *Horses: by mouth,* 1 division of paste/100 kg body-weight

PML Furexel (Janssen) *UK*
Oral paste, ivermectin 20 mg/division, for *horses*; 6.42-g metered-dose applicator
Withdrawal Periods. *Horses:* slaughter 21 days
Dose. *Horses: by mouth,* 1 division of paste/100 kg body-weight

PML Ivomec Classic Pour-On for Cattle (Merial) *UK*
Solution, 'pour-on', ivermectin 5 mg/mL, for *beef cattle, non-lactating dairy cattle*; 250 mL, 1 litre, 2.5 litres
Withdrawal Periods. *Cattle:* slaughter 28 days, should not be used on cattle producing milk for human consumption or on dairy cows, including pregnant heifers, within 60 days before calving

PML Ivomec Injection for Cattle and Sheep (Merial) *UK*
Injection, ivermectin 10 mg/mL, for *beef cattle, non-lactating dairy cattle, sheep*; 50 mL, 200 mL, 500 mL
Withdrawal Periods. *Cattle:* slaughter 35 days, should not be used in cattle producing milk for human consumption or in dairy cows, including pregnant heifers, within 60 days before calving. *Sheep:* slaughter 42 days, should not be used in sheep producing milk for human consumption

PML Ivomec Injection for Pigs (Merial) *UK*
Injection, ivermectin 10 mg/mL, for *pigs*; 100 mL, 200 mL, 500 mL
Withdrawal Periods. *Pigs:* slaughter 28 days

PML Ivomec Premix for Pigs (Merial) *UK*
Premix, ivermectin, 6 g/kg, for *growing and adult pigs*; 5 kg
Withdrawal Periods. *Pigs:* slaughter 7 days

PML Ivomec SR Bolus (Merial) *UK*
Ruminal bolus, m/r, ivermectin 1.72 g delivered over 135 days, for *cattle 3 months of age and over, and 100-400 kg body-weight*; 12
Withdrawal Periods. *Cattle:* slaughter 180 days, should not be used in cattle producing milk for human consumption
Note. Should not be administered to dairy heifers within 180 days of calving. If calving occurs within 180 days of treatment, milk withdrawal period is 180 days
Dose. *Cattle:* (100–400 kg body-weight) one 1.72-g bolus

PML Oramec (Merial) *UK*
Oral solution, ivermectin 800 micrograms/mL, for *sheep, goats*
Withdrawal Periods. *Sheep, goats:* slaughter 14 days, milk 14 days. Should not be used in animals within 28 days of commencement of lactation if milk is to be used for human consumption

PML Panomec Injection for Cattle, Sheep and Pigs (Merial) *UK*
Oral paste, ivermectin 10 mg/mL, for *cattle, sheep, pigs*
Withdrawal Periods. *Cattle:* slaughter 35 days, should not be used in cattle producing milk for human consumption or in dairy cows, including pregnant heifers, within 60 days before calving. *Sheep:* slaughter 42 days, should not be used in sheep producing milk for human consumption. *Pigs:* slaughter 28 days

PML Panomec Paste for Horses (Merial) *UK*
Oral paste, ivermectin 20 mg/division, for *horses*; 6.42-g metered dose applicator
Withdrawal Periods. *Horses:* slaughter 21 days

PML Rycomec Drench (Young's) *UK*
Oral solution, ivermectin 800 micrograms/mL, for *sheep, goats*
Withdrawal Periods. *Sheep, goats:* slaughter 14 days, milk 14 days. Should not be used in animals within 28 days before lambing if milk is to be used for human consumption

PML Rycomec Injection (Young's) *UK*
Injection, ivermectin 10 mg/mL, for *sheep*
Withdrawal Periods. *Sheep:* slaughter 42 days, should not be used in sheep producing milk for human consumption

PML Noromectin (Norbrook) *UK*
Injection, ivermectin 10 mg/mL, for *beef cattle, non-lactating dairy cattle*
Withdrawal Periods. *Cattle:* slaughter 35 days, should not be used in cattle producing milk for human consumption or in dairy cows, including pregnant heifers, within 60 days before calving

PML Noromectin Pour-On (Norbrook) *UK*
Solution, 'pour-on', ivermectin 5 mg/mL, for *beef cattle, non-lactating dairy cattle*
Withdrawal Periods. *Cattle:* slaughter 28 days, should not be used on cattle producing milk for human consumption or on dairy cows, including pregnant heifers, within 60 days before calving

PML Panomec (Merial) *UK*
Injection, ivermectin 10 mg/mL, for *beef cattle, non-lactating dairy cattle, sheep, pigs*; 50 mL, 200 mL, 500 mL
Withdrawal Periods. *Cattle:* slaughter 35 days, should not be used in cattle producing milk for human consumption or in dairy cows, including pregnant heifers, within 60 days before calving. *Sheep:* slaughter 42 days, should not be used in sheep producing milk for human consumption. *Pigs:* slaughter 28 days

PML Virbamec Injectable Solution (Virbac) *UK*
Injection, ivermectin 10 mg/mL, for *beef cattle, non-lactating dairy cattle*
Withdrawal Periods. *Cattle:* slaughter 35 days, should not be used in cattle producing milk for human consumption or in dairy cows, including pregnant heifers, within 60 days before calving

Australia

Indications. Endoparasites. Gastro-intestinal roundworms and lungworms in horses, ruminants, and pigs; hookworm in cats; Type II ostertagiosis in ruminants; horse bots; nasal bots in sheep; heartworm (prophylaxis) in dogs and cats Ectoparasites. See section 2.2.1.1

Contra-indications. Administration of damaged ruminal boluses to sheep; in general, treatment with a 'pour-on' formulation when hide or hair is wet or rain fall less than 2 hours after treatment

Warnings. Occasionally transient oedema and pruritus in horses. Care with administration of ruminal boluses to sheep; cats should be examined for existing heartworm infection before starting treatment

Dose. *Horses: by mouth,* 200 micrograms/kg
Cattle: by 'pour-on' application, 500 micrograms/kg
by subcutaneous injection, 200 micrograms/kg
Sheep: by mouth , 200 micrograms/kg
Pigs: by addition to feed, 100 micrograms/kg
by subcutaneous injection, 300 micrograms/kg
Dogs: by mouth, 6 micrograms/kg
Cats: by mouth, 24 micrograms/kg

Baymec Pour On for Cattle (Bayer) *Austral*
Solution, pour-on, ivermectin 5 mg/mL, for *cattle*
Withdrawal Periods. *Cattle:* slaughter 42 days, should not be used in cattle producing milk for human consumption

Equimec (Merial) *Austral*
Oral paste, ivermectin 18.7 g/kg paste, for *horses*
Withdrawal Periods. *Horses:* slaughter 21 days

Equimec Tubing Liquid (Merial) *Austral*
Oral solution, ivermectin 10 g/L, for *horses*
Withdrawal Periods. *Horses:* slaughter 21 days

Heartgard 30 (Merial) *Austral*
Tablets, ivermectin 68 micrograms, 136 micrograms, 272 micrograms, for *dogs*

Heartgard 30 FX (Merial) *Austral*
Chewable beef portions, ivermectin 55 micrograms, 165 micrograms, for *cats*

Ivomec Antiparasitic Injection for Cattle (Merial) *Austral*
Injection, ivermectin 10 g/L, for *cattle*
Withdrawal Periods. *Cattle*: slaughter 42 days, should not be used in cattle producing milk for human consumption, or in dairy cattle within 28 days of calving

Ivomec Antiparasitic Injection for Pigs (Merial) *Austral*
Injection, ivermectin 10 g/L, for *pigs*
Withdrawal Periods. *Pigs*: slaughter 28 days

Ivomec Liquid for Sheep (Merial) *Austral*
Oral solution, ivermectin 0.8 g/L, for *sheep*
Withdrawal Periods. *Sheep*: slaughter 21 days, should not be used within 28 days of lambing or during lactation if milk is to be used for human consumption

Ivomec Maximizer (Merial) *Austral*
Capsules(ruminal boluses), ivermectin 80 mg (weaner) and 160 mg (adult), for *sheep*
Withdrawal Periods. *Sheep*: slaughter 126 days, should not be used in sheep producing milk for human consumption

Ivomec Pour-On for Cattle (Merial) *Austral*
Solution, pour-on, ivermectin 5 mg/mL, for *cattle*
Withdrawal Periods. *Cattle*: slaughter 42 days, should not be used within 28 days of calving or during lactation if milk is to be used for human consumption

Ivomec Premix for Pigs (Merial) *Austral*
Premix, ivermectin 6 g/kg premix, for *pigs*
Withdrawal Periods. *Pigs*: slaughter 7 days

Ivomec-RV for Sheep (Merial) *Austral*
Oral solution, ivermectin 2 g/L, for *sheep*
Withdrawal Periods. *Sheep*: slaughter 21 days, should not be used within 28 days of lambing or during lactation if milk is to be used for human consumption

Numectin 100 (Nufarm) *Austral*
Capsules(ruminal boluses), ivermectin 80 mg (weaner) and 160 mg (adult), for *sheep*
Withdrawal Periods. *Sheep*: slaughter 126 days, should not be used in sheep producing milk for human consumption

Numectin Liquid for Sheep (Nufarm) *Austral*
Oral solution, ivermectin 0.8 g/L, for *sheep*
Withdrawal Periods. *Sheep*: slaughter 21 days, milk 28 days

Totectin Paste (Vetsearch) *Austral*
Oral paste, ivermectin 120 mg/6.42 g paste, for *horses*

Eire

Indications. Endoparasites. Gastro-intestinal roundworms and lungworms in horses, ruminants, and pigs; Type II ostertagiosis in ruminants; horse bots; nasal bots in sheep Ectoparasites. See section 2.2.1.1
Contra-indications. Administration of ruminal boluses to non-ruminating cattle, administration to calves less than 12 weeks of age; in general, treatment with a 'pour-on' formulation when hide or hair is wet or rain is expected (although established infections of *Ostertagia* or *Dictycaulus* are not affected)
Warnings. Occasionally transient oedema and pruritus in horses. If cattle are vaccinated against lungworm, the ruminal bolus should not be administered until 14 days after the second dose of vaccine
Dose.
Horses: by mouth, 200 micrograms/kg

Cattle: by 'pour-on' application, 500 micrograms/kg
by mouth or subcutaneous injection, 200 micrograms/kg
Sheep: by mouth or by subcutaneous injection, 200 micrograms/kg
Pigs: by addition to feed, 100 micrograms/kg
by subcutaneous injection, 300 micrograms/kg

Furexel (Janssen) *Eire*
Oral paste, ivermectin 1.87%, for *horses*
Withdrawal Periods. Slaughter 21 days

Eqvalan Paste for Horses (Merial) *Eire*
Oral paste, ivermectin 1.87%, for *horses*
Withdrawal Periods. Slaughter 21 days

Ivomec Drench for Cattle (Merial) *Eire*
Oral drench, ivermectin 0.4%, for *cattle*
Withdrawal Periods. Slaughter 10 days, should not be used in cattle producing milk for human consumption, or in dairy cows within 28 days prior to calving

Ivomec Classic Injection for Cattle and Sheep (Merial) *Eire*
Injection, ivermectin 1%, for *cattle, sheep*
Withdrawal Periods. *Cattle*: slaughter 21 days, should not be used in cattle producing milk for human consumption or in dairy cows within 28 days prior to calving. *Sheep*: slaughter 21 days, should not be used in sheep within 21 days before lambing if milk is to be used for human consumption

Ivomec Injection for Pigs (Merial) *Eire*
Injection, ivermectin 1%, for *pigs*
Withdrawal Periods. Slaughter 28 days

Ivomec Classic Pour-on for Cattle (Merial) *Eire*
Solution, pour-on, ivermectin 0.5%, for *cattle*
Withdrawal Periods. Slaughter 28 days, should not be used in cattle within 28 days before calving if milk is to be used for human consumption

Ivomec Premix for Pigs (Merial) *Eire*
Premix, ivermectin 0.6%, for *pigs*
Withdrawal Periods. Slaughter 5 days

Ivomec SR Bolus for Cattle (Merial) *Eire*
Ruminal boluses, ivermectin 1.72 g, for *cattle*
Withdrawal Periods. Slaughter 180 days, should not be used in cattle producing milk for human consumption
Dose. *Cattle*: one bolus

Oramec Drench for Sheep (Merial) *Eire*
Oral drench, ivermectin 0.08%, for *sheep*
Withdrawal Periods. Slaughter 14 days, milk 28 days

Panomec Injection for Cattle, Sheep and Pigs (Merial) *Eire*
Injection, ivermectin 1%, for *cattle, sheep, pigs*
Withdrawal Periods. *Cattle*: slaughter 21 days, should not be used in cattle producing milk for human consumption or in dairy cows within 28 days prior to calving. *Sheep*: slaughter 21 days, should not be used in sheep within 21 days before lambing if milk is to be used for human consumption. *Pigs*: slaughter 28 days

New Zealand

Indications. Endoparasites. Gastro-intestinal roundworms and lungworms in horses, ruminants, and pigs; Type II ostertagiosis in ruminants; horse bots; nasal bots in sheep Ectoparasites. See section 2.2.1.1
Contra-indications. Administration of ruminal boluses to non-ruminating cattle, administration to calves less than 12 weeks of age; in general, treatment with a 'pour-on' formulation when hide or hair is wet or rain fall less than 2 hours after treatment
Side-effects. Occasional transient discomfort and swelling at injection site in cattle and pigs

Warnings. Care with administration of ruminal boluses to sheep

Dose. *Horses*: *by mouth*, 200 micrograms/kg

Cattle: *by 'pour-on' application*, 500 micrograms/kg

by mouth or by subcutaneous injection, 200 micrograms/kg

Sheep, goats: *by mouth* , 200 micrograms/kg

Pigs: *by subcutaneous injection*, 300 micrograms/kg

Eqvalan (Merial) *NZ*
Oral paste, ivermectin 18.7 mg/g, for *horses*
Withdrawal Periods. Slaughter 14 days

Ivomec Injection for Cattle & Pigs (Merial) *NZ*
Injection, ivermectin 10 mg/mL, for *cattle, pigs*
Withdrawal Periods. *Cattle*: slaughter 49 days, should not be used in cattle producing milk for human consumption. *Pigs*: slaughter 28 days

Ivomec Liquid for Sheep & Goats (Merial) *NZ*
Oral solution, ivermectin 0.8 mg/mL, for *sheep, goats*
Withdrawal Periods. *Sheep*: slaughter 10 days, should not be used in sheep producing milk for human consumption. *Goats*: slaughter 14 days, should not be used in goats producing milk for human consumption

Ivomec Liquid with Selenium for Sheep & Goats (Merial) *NZ*
Oral solution, ivermectin 0.8 mg/mL, selenium 4 mg/mL, for *sheep, goats*
Withdrawal Periods. *Sheep*: slaughter 10 days, should not be used in sheep producing milk for human consumption. *Goats*: slaughter 14 days, should not be used in goats producing milk for human consumption

Ivomec Maximiser CR for Lambs (Merial) *NZ*
Capsules, ivermectin 80 mg, for *lambs more than 20 kg body-weight*
Withdrawal Periods. Slaughter 126 days
Dose. *Lambs*: *by mouth*, (20–40 kg body-weight) 1 capsule

Ivomec Maximiser CR for Sheep (Merial) *NZ*
Capsules, ivermectin 160 mg, for *sheep more than 40 kg body-weight*
Withdrawal Periods. Slaughter 126 days, should not be used in sheep producing milk for human consumption
Dose. *Sheep*: *by mouth*, (40–80 kg body-weight)1 capsule; (>80 kg body-weight) 2 capsules

Ivomec Oral Solution for Cattle (Merial) *NZ*
Oral solution, ivermectin 4 mg/mL, for *cattle*
Withdrawal Periods. Slaughter 21 days, should not be used in cattle producing milk for human consumption

Ivomec Pour-on for Cattle & Deer (Merial) *NZ*
Solution, pour-on, ivermectin 0.5%, for *cattle, deer*
Withdrawal Periods. *Cattle*: slaughter 35 days, should not be used in cattle producing milk for human consumption. *Deer*: slaughter 28 days

Ivomec SR Bolus for Cattle (Merial) *NZ*
Ruminal boluses, ivermectin 1.72 g, for *cattle 100–400 kg body-weight*
Withdrawal Periods. Slaughter 180 days, should not be administered to cattle producing milk for human consumption
Dose. *Cattle*: *by mouth*, 1 bolus

Stockman (Nufarm) *NZ*
Capsules, ivermectin 160 mg, for *sheep more than 40 kg body-weight*
Withdrawal Periods. Slaughter 126 days, should not be used in sheep producing milk for human consumption
Dose. *Sheep*: *by mouth*, (40–80 kg body-weight) 1 capsule; (>80 kg body-weight) 2 capsules

Stockman Jnr (Nufarm) *NZ*
Capsules, ivermectin 80 mg, for *sheep more than 20 kg body-weight*
Withdrawal Periods. Slaughter 126 days, should not be used in sheep producing milk for human consumption
Dose. *Sheep*: *by mouth*, (20–40 kg body-weight) 1 capsule

USA

Indications. Endoparasites. Gastro-intestinal roundworms and lungworms in horses, ruminants, and pigs; Type II ostertagiosis in ruminants; horse bots; nasal bots in sheep; heartworm prophylaxis in dogs and cats; hookworms in cats Ectoparasites. See section 2.2.1.1

Contra-indications. Administration of ruminal boluses to non-ruminating cattle, administration to calves less than 12 weeks of age; in general, treatment with a 'pour-on' formulation when hide or hair is wet or rain is expected to wet cattle within 6 hours after treatment

Warnings. Occasionally transient oedema and pruritus in horses; dogs and cats should be examined for existing heartworm infection before starting treatment

Dose.

Horses: *by mouth*, 200 micrograms/kg

Cattle: *by 'pour-on' application*, 500 micrograms/kg

by subcutaneous injection, 200 micrograms/kg

Sheep: *by mouth* , 200 micrograms/kg

Pigs: *by addition to feed*, 100 micrograms/kg

by subcutaneous injection, 300 micrograms/kg

Dogs: *by mouth*, 6 micrograms/kg

Cats: *by mouth*, 24 micrograms/kg

Double Impact (AgriLabs) *USA*
Injection, ivermectin 1%, for *cattle, pigs, reindeer*
Withdrawal Periods. *Cattle*: slaughter 35 days, should not be used in cattle producing milk for human consumption. *Pigs*: slaughter 18 days. *Reindeer*: slaughter 8 weeks

Eqvalan Liquid for Horses (Merial) *USA*
Oral solution, ivermectin 10 mg/mL, for *horses*
Withdrawal Periods. Should not be used in *horses* intended for human consumption

Eqvalan Paste 1.87% (Merial) *USA*
Oral paste, ivermectin 1.87% , for *horses*
Withdrawal Periods. Should not be used in *horses* intended for human consumption

Heartgard Chewables (Merial) *USA*
Tablets, ivermectin 68, 136, 272 micrograms, for *dogs more than 6 weeks of age*

Heartgard Tablets (Merial) *USA*
Tablets, ivermectin 68, 136, 272 micrograms, for *dogs more than 6 weeks of age*

Heartgard for Cats (Merial) *USA*
Tablets, ivermectin 55, 165 micrograms, for *cats more than 6 weeks of age*

Ivomec Injection For Cattle And Swine (Merial) *USA*
Injection, ivermectin 1%, for *cattle, pigs, reindeer, bison*
Withdrawal Periods. *Cattle*: slaughter 35 days, should not be used in cattle producing milk for human consumption. *Pigs*: slaughter 18 days. *Reindeer, bison*: slaughter 8 weeks

Ivomec Injection For Grower And Feeded Pigs (Merial) *USA*
Injection, ivermectin 0.27%, for *pigs*
Withdrawal Periods. Slaughter 18 days

Ivomec Injection For Swine (Merial) *USA*
Injection, ivermectin 1%, for *pigs*
Withdrawal Periods. Slaughter 18 days

Ivomec Pour-On For Cattle (Merial) *USA*
Solution, pour-on, ivermectin 5 mg/mL, for *cattle*
Withdrawal Periods. Slaughter 48 days, should not be used in cattle producing milk for human consumption.

Ivomec Premix For Swine (Merial) *USA*
Premix, ivermectin 0.6%, for *pigs*
Withdrawal Periods. Slaughter 5 days

Ivomec Sheep Drench (Merial) *USA*
Oral solution, ivermectin 0.08%, for *sheep*
Withdrawal Periods. Slaughter 11 days

Ivomec SR Bolus For Cattle (Merial) *USA*
Ruminal boluses, ivermectin 1.72 g, for *cattle*
Withdrawal Periods. Slaughter 180 days, shouldnot be used in cattle producing milk for human consumption
Dose. *Cattle*: *by mouth*, (125–300 kg body-weight) 1 bolus

Top Line (AgriLabs) *USA*
Solution, pour-on, ivermectin 5 mg/mL, for *cattle*
Withdrawal Periods. Slaughter 48 days, dhould not be used in cattle producing milk for human consumption

MILBEMYCIN

Australia
Indications. Endoparasites. Gastro-intestinal roundworms and heartworm prophylaxis in dogs
Contra-indications. Administration to puppies less than 2 weeks of age
Warnings. It is recommended that dogs are examined and treated for existing heartworm infection before starting treatment
Dose. *Dogs*: *by mouth*, 500 micrograms/kg

Interceptor Flavour Tabs for Dogs (Novartis) *Austral*
Tablets, milbemycin oxime 2.3 mg, 5.75 mg, 11.5 mg, 23 mg, for *dogs*

USA
Indications. Endoparasites. Gastro-intestinal roundworms and heartworm prophylaxis in dogs
Contra-indications. Administration to puppies less than 4 weeks of age and 1 kg body-weight
Warnings. It is recommended that dogs are examined and treated for existing heartworm infection before starting treatment
Dose. *Dogs*: *by mouth*, 500 micrograms/kg

Interceptor Flavor Tabs (Novartis) *USA*
Tablets, milbemycin oxime 2.3 mg, 5.75 mg, 11.5 mg and 23 mg, for *dogs*

MOXIDECTIN

UK
Indications. Endoparasites. Gastro-intestinal roundworms in horses and ruminants; lungworms in ruminants; Type II ostertagiosis in cattle; horse bots; nasal bots in sheep
Ectoparasites. See section 2.2.1.1
Contra-indications. Administration to calves less than 8 weeks of age; administration to foals less than 4 months of age; injection in sheep previously vaccinated against footrot
Dose.
Horses, ponies: *by mouth*, 400 micrograms/kg
Cattle: *by 'pour-on' application*, 500 micrograms/kg
by subcutaneous injection, 200 micrograms/kg
Sheep: *by mouth or by subcutaneous injection*, 200 micrograms/kg

PML **Cydectin 0.1% Oral Drench for Sheep** (Fort Dodge) *UK*
Oral solution, moxidectin 1 mg/mL, for *sheep*; 1 litre, 2.5 litres, 5 litres
Withdrawal Periods. *Sheep*: slaughter 14 days, should not be used in sheep producing milk for human consumption or industrial purposes during lactation or the dry period

PML **Cydectin 0.5% Pour-On for Cattle** (Fort Dodge) *UK*
Solution, 'pour-on', moxidectin 5 mg/mL, for *cattle*
Withdrawal Periods. *Cattle*: slaughter 14 days, should not be used in cattle producing milk for human consumption or industrial purposes or on dairy cows within 60 days before calving

PML **Cydectin 1% Injectable Solution for Sheep** (Fort Dodge) *UK*
Injection, moxidectin 10 mg/mL, for *sheep*
Withdrawal Periods. *Sheep*: slaughter 70 days, should not be used in sheep producing milk for human consumption or industrial purposes

PML **Cydectin 1% Injection for Cattle** (Fort Dodge) *UK*
Injection, moxidectin 10 mg/mL, for *cattle more than 8 weeks of age*
Withdrawal Periods. *Cattle*: slaughter 45 days, should not be used in cattle producing milk for human consumption or industrial purposes or within 60 days before calving

PML **Equest** (Fort Dodge) *UK*
Oral gel, moxidectin 18.92 mg/g, for *horses, ponies*
Withdrawal Periods. *Horses*: slaughter 32 days

Australia
Indications. Endoparasites. Gastro-intestinal roundworms and lungworms in ruminants; Type II ostertagiosis in cattle; gastro-intestinal roundworms in horses; horse bots; heartworm prophylaxis in dogs
Ectoparasites. See section 2.2.1.1
Contra-indications. Administration to puppies less than 4 weeks of age; administration to goats
Warnings. It is recommended that dogs are examined for existing heartworm infection before starting treatment
Dose.
Horses: *by mouth*, 400 micrograms/kg
Cattle: *by 'pour-on' application*, 500 micrograms/kg
Sheep: *by mouth*, 200 micrograms/kg
Dogs: *by mouth*, 3 micrograms/kg

Cydectin LV Drench for Sheep (Fort Dodge) *Austral*
Oral solution, moxidectin 2 g/L, for *sheep*
Withdrawal Periods. *Sheep*: slaughter 7 days, should not be used in sheep producing milk for human consumption

Cydectin Oral Drench for Sheep (Fort Dodge) *Austral*
Oral solution, moxidectin 1 g/L, for *sheep*
Withdrawal Periods. *Sheep*: slaughter 7 days, should not be used in sheep producing milk for human consumption

Cydectin Pour-On for Cattle and Red Deer (Fort Dodge) *Austral*
Solution, pour-on, moxidectin 5 g/L, for *cattle, red deer*
Withdrawal Periods. *Cattle*: slaughter withdrawal period nil, milk withdrawal period nil. *Red deer*: slaughter withdrawal period nil.

Cydectin Se Oral Drench for Sheep (Fort Dodge) *Austral*
Oral solution, moxidectin 1 mg/mL, selenium (as sodium selenate) 0.5 mg/mL, for *sheep*
Withdrawal Periods. *Sheep*: slaughter 7 days, should not be used in sheep producing milk for human consumption

Equest Gel (Fort Dodge) *Austral*
Oral gel, moxidectin 20 g/L, for *horses*
Withdrawal Periods. *Horses*: slaughter 28 days

Proheart (Fort Dodge) *Austral*
Tablets, moxidectin 30 micrograms, 68 micrograms, 136 micrograms, 204 micrograms, for *dogs*

Eire
Indications. Endoparasites. Gastro-intestinal roundworms and lungworms in ruminants; Type II ostertagiosis in cattle; nasal bots in sheep; horse bots

Ectoparasites. See section 2.2.1.1

Contra-indications. Administration of injectable solution to calves less than 8 weeks of age; administration to foals less than 4 months of age

Dose.

Horses: *by mouth*, 400 micrograms/kg

Cattle: *by 'pour-on' application*, 500 micrograms/kg *by subcutaneous injection*, 200 micrograms/kg

Sheep: *by mouth or by subcutaneous injection*, 200 micrograms/kg

Cydectin 1% Injectable Solution for Sheep (Whelehan) *Eire*
Injection, moxidectin 10 g/L, for *sheep*
Withdrawal Periods. Slaughter 40 days, should not be used in sheep producing milk for human consumption or in dairy sheep within 60 days of lambing

Cydectin 0.1% Oral Drench for Sheep (Whelehan) *Eire*
Oral solution, moxidectin 1 g/L, for *sheep*
Withdrawal Periods. Slaughter 14 days, should not be used in sheep producing milk for human consumption

Cydectin 0.5% Pour-On for Cattle (Whelehan) *Eire*
Solution, pour-on, moxidectin 5 g/L, for *cattle*
Withdrawal Periods. Slaughter 14 days, should not be used in cattle producing milk for human consumption or in cattle within 60 days before calving

Cydectin 1% Injectable Solution for Cattle (Whelehan) *Eire*
Injection, moxidectin 10 g/L, for *cattle*
Withdrawal Periods. Slaughter 45 days, should not be used in cattle producing milk for human consumption

Equest Oral Gel (Whelehan) *Eire*
Oral gel, moxidectin 18.92 mg/g, for *horses, ponies*
Withdrawal Periods. *Horses*: slaughter 32 days

New Zealand

Indications. Endoparasites. Gastro-intestinal roundworms and lungworms in ruminants; Type II ostertagiosis in cattle; gastro-intestinal roundworms in horses; horse bots; nasal bots in sheep
Ectoparasites. See section 2.2.1.1

Contra-indications. Administration to sheep that have been vaccinated against footrot

Dose.

Horses: *by mouth*, 400 micrograms/kg

Cattle: *by 'pour-on' application*, 500 micrograms/kg *by subcutaneous injection*, 200 micrograms/kg

Sheep: *by mouth or by subcutaneous injection*, 200 micrograms/kg

Cydectin Injection (Fort Dodge) *NZ*
Injection, moxidectin 10 mg/mL, for *cattle, sheep*
Withdrawal Periods. *Cattle*: slaughter 35 days, milk 28 days. *Sheep*: slaughter 28 days, milk 28 days

Cydectin Oral Drench (Fort Dodge) *NZ*
Oral solution, moxidectin 1 mg/mL, for *sheep*
Withdrawal Periods. Slaughter 10 days, should not be used in sheep producing milk for human consumption

Cydectin Pour On (Fort Dodge) *NZ*
Solution, pour-on, moxidectin 5 g/L, for *cattle, deer*
Withdrawal Periods. *Cattle*: slaughter 28 days, milk withdrawal period nil. *Deer*: slaughter 21 days

Cydectin S (Fort Dodge) *NZ*
Oral solution, moxidectin 1 mg/mL, selenium 0.5 mg/mL, for *sheep*
Withdrawal Periods. Slaughter 10 days, should not be used in sheep producing milk for human consumption

Equest (Fort Dodge) *NZ*
Gel, moxidectin 230 mg/syringe, for *horses*
Withdrawal Periods. Slaughter 60 days

Vetdectin Injection (Fort Dodge) *NZ*
Injection, moxidectin 10 mg/mL, for *cattle, sheep*
Withdrawal Periods. *Cattle*: slaughter 35 days, milk 28 days. *Sheep*: slaughter 28 days, milk 28 days

Vetdectin Oral Drench (Fort Dodge) *NZ*
Oral solution, moxidectin 1 mg/mL, for *sheep*
Withdrawal Periods. Slaughter 10 days, should not be used in sheep producing milk for human consumption

Vetdectin Pour On (Fort Dodge) *NZ*
Solution, pour-on, moxidectin 5 g/L, for *cattle, deer*
Withdrawal Periods. *Cattle*: slaughter 28 days, milk withdrawal period nil. *Deer*: slaughter 21 days

Vetdectin S (Fort Dodge) *NZ*
Oral solution, moxidectin 1 mg/mL, selenium 0.5 mg/mL, for *sheep*
Withdrawal Periods. Slaughter 10 days, should not be used in sheep producing milk for human consumption

USA

Indications. Endoparasites. Gastro-intestinal roundworms and lungworms in cattle; Type II ostertagiosis in cattle; gastro-intestinal roundworms in horses; horse bots; heartworm prophylaxis in dogs
Ectoparasites. See section 2.2.1.1

Contra-indications. Administration to puppies less than 8 weeks of age; administration to horses less than 4 months of age

Warnings. Dogs should be examined for existing heartworm infection before starting treatment

Dose.

Horses: *by mouth*, 400 micrograms/kg

Cattle: *by 'pour-on' application*, 500 micrograms/kg

Dogs: *by mouth*, 3 micrograms/kg

Cydectin Pour-On (Fort Dodge) *USA*
Solution, pour-on, moxidectin 5 mg/mL, for *cattle*
Withdrawal Periods. *Cattle*: slaughter withdrawal period nil, should not be used on cattle producing milk for human consumption, should not be used on calves intended for veal production

Proheart (Fort Dodge) *USA*
Tablets, moxidectin 30, 68, and 136 micrograms, for *dogs*

Quest 2% Equine Oral Gel (Fort Dodge) *USA*
Oral gel, moxidectin 20 mg/mL, for *horses*
Withdrawal Periods. *Horses*: should not be used in horses intended for human consumption

SELAMECTIN

UK

Indications. Endoparasites. Gastro-intestinal roundworms and heartworm prophylaxis in dogs and cats
Ectoparasites. See section 2.2.1.1

Contra-indications. Administration to puppies and kittens less than 6 weeks of age; application when hair coat is wet

Warnings. Do not allow treated animals to bathe in water courses until at least 2 hours after treatment, Keep children away from treated animals for at least 30 minutes after application or until hair coat is dry

Dose. *Dogs, cats*: *by 'spot-on' application*, 6 mg/kg

POM **Stronghold** (Pfizer) *UK*
Solution, 'spot-on', selamectin 15 mg, 30 mg, 45mg, 60 mg, 120 mg, 240 mg/dose applicator, for *dogs, cats*

USA

Indications. Endoparasites. Gastro-intestinal roundworms and heartworm prophylaxis in dogs and cats
Ectoparasites. See section 2.2.1.1
Contra-indications. Administration to puppies and kittens less than 6 weeks of age; application when hair coat is wet
Side-effects. Transient localised alopecia at application site; rarely vomiting, diarrhoea, anorexia, lethargy, salivation, tachypnoea, muscle tremors
Warnings. Do not allow treated animals to bathe in water courses until at least 2 hours after treatment; dogs should be tested for existing heartworm infection before treatment
Dose. *Dogs, cats*: *by 'spot-on' application*, 6 mg/kg

POM **Revolution** (Pfizer) *USA*
Solution, 'spot-on', selamectin 15 mg, 30 mg, 45mg, 60 mg, 120 mg, 240 mg/dose applicator, for *dogs and cats more than 6 weeks of age*

2.1.1.2 Benzimidazoles

Benzimidazoles such as **albendazole, fenbendazole, flubendazole, mebendazole, oxfendazole, oxibendazole** and **tiabendazole** have a similar mode of action. They disrupt parasite energy metabolism by binding to tubulin, a protein required for the uptake of nutrients and other functions. **Febantel**, **netobimin**, and **thiophanate** are probenzimidazoles, which are converted to fenbendazole, albendazole, and lobendazole, respectively, in the body. Products containing benzimidazoles or probenzimidazoles are labelled with the symbol 1-BZ.
The anthelmintic activity of the benzimidazoles is related to the duration of therapeutic blood concentrations. Doses may need to be repeated in pigs, dogs, and cats, while single doses are sufficient in ruminants and horses because the rumen or large intestine acts as a drug reservoir.
Most benzimidazoles are effective against larval and adult roundworms, and albendazole, febantel, fenbendazole, oxfendazole, and oxibendazole are also ovicidal. Fenbendazole is used in pregnant and lactating bitches to reduce roundworm infection in puppies. Fenbendazole is used for lungworm infection in dogs and cats. Albendazole, febantel, fenbendazole, mebendazole, netobimin, and oxfendazole are also effective against tapeworms (see section 2.1.2), and some are also active against adult liver flukes at a higher dosage (see section 2.1.3). **Triclabendazole** is effective against both immature and adult flukes (see section 2.1.3) but has no activity against nematodes.
Some benzimidazoles such as albendazole have been found to be teratogenic in the early stages of pregnancy. These should be used with caution or avoided at mating or during early pregnancy.
Strains of *Haemonchus* and *Ostertagia* (*Teladorsagia*) in goats and sheep, and of cyathostomes in horses have been found with varying degrees of resistance to the benzimidazoles, particularly in the south of England. Resistance to one benzimidazole confers side-resistance to other drugs in the same chemical group. The onset of resistance can be delayed or prevented if precautions are taken to administer the correct dose based on the accurately determined weight of the animal, to use the minimum number of treatments necessary, to rotate the class of anthelmintic used annually, and to ensure purchased animals are not infected with resistant strains. Any newly-acquired animals should be treated, and then kept off pasture until faecal egg counts have fallen to zero. Sheep and goats should not be kept on the same land because resistant strains develop more readily in goats, and may then infect sheep. Regular monitoring for resistance and control strategies based on sound epidemiological principles are important.

ALBENDAZOLE

UK

Indications. Gastro-intestinal roundworms, lungworms, tapeworms (see section 2.1.2), and adult *Fasciola* (see section 2.1.3) in cattle, sheep; Type II ostertagiosis; gastro-intestinal roundworms and lungworms in goats♦ and deer♦
Contra-indications. Concurrent administration of other ruminal boluses, treatment of ewes at a dosage of 7.5 mg/kg during the mating period and until 1 month after rams are removed
Warnings. Care not to exceed 'fluke and worm dose' in cows during first month of pregnancy; coughing for some weeks after treatment in cattle suffering from severe lung damage at time of treatment
Dose. *By mouth.*
Cattle: roundworms and tapeworms, 7.5 mg/kg
Adult flukes, roundworms, and tapeworms, 10 mg/kg
Sheep: roundworms and tapeworms, 5 mg/kg
Adult flukes, roundworms, and tapeworms, 7.5 mg/kg
Goats♦, deer♦: roundworms, 10 mg/kg

Note. For therapeutic purposes albendazole and albendazole oxide may be considered equivalent in effect

PML **Albenil Low Dose** (Virbac) *UK*
Oral suspension, albendazole 100 mg/mL, cobalt (as sulphate) 2.5 mg/mL, selenium (as sodium selenite) 1.08 mg/mL, for *cattle, sheep*
Withdrawal Periods. *Cattle*: slaughter 14 days, milk 2.5 days. *Sheep*: slaughter 4 days, should not be used in sheep producing milk for human consumption

PML **Albenil SC** (Virbac) *UK*
Oral suspension, albendazole 25 mg/mL, cobalt (as sulphate) 620 micrograms/mL, selenium (as sodium selenite) 270 micrograms/mL, for *cattle, sheep*
Withdrawal Periods. *Cattle*: slaughter 14 days, milk 2.5 days. *Sheep*: slaughter 4 days, should not be used in sheep producing milk for human consumption

PML **Albex 2.5%** (Chanelle) *UK*
Oral suspension, albendazole 25 mg/mL, for *cattle, sheep*
Withdrawal Periods. *Cattle*: slaughter 14 days, milk 2.5 days. *Sheep*: slaughter 4 days, should not be used in sheep producing milk for human consumption

PML **Albex 10%** (Chanelle) *UK*
Oral suspension, albendazole 100 mg/mL, for *cattle, sheep*; 1 litre, 2.5 litres, 5 litres
Withdrawal Periods. *Cattle*: slaughter 14 days, milk 2.5 days. *Sheep*: slaughter 4 days, should not be used in sheep producing milk for human consumption

PML **Allverm 4%** (Crown) *UK*
Oral suspension, albendazole oxide 40 mg, hydrated cobalt sulphate 28.8 mg, hydrated sodium selenate 3 mg/mL, for *sheep*; 1 litre, 2.5 litres
Withdrawal Periods. *Sheep*: slaughter 3 days, should not be used in sheep producing milk for human consumption

PML **Allverm 15%** (Crown) *UK*
Oral suspension, albendazole oxide 150 mg/mL, for *cattle*; 1 litre, 2.5 litres
Withdrawal Periods. *Cattle*: slaughter 14 days, milk 3 days

PML **Endospec 2.5% SC** (Bimeda) *UK*
Oral suspension, albendazole 25 mg, cobalt (as sulphate) 2.5 mg, selenium (as sodium selenite) 1.08 mg/mL, for *cattle, sheep*
Withdrawal Periods. *Cattle*: slaughter 14 days, milk 2.5 days. *Sheep*: slaughter 4 days, should not be used in sheep producing milk for human consumption

PML **Endospec 10% SC** (Bimeda) *UK*
Oral suspension, albendazole 100 mg, cobalt (as sulphate) 620 micrograms, selenium (as sodium selenite) 270 micrograms/mL, for *cattle, sheep*
Withdrawal Periods. *Cattle*: slaughter 14 days, milk 2.5 days. *Sheep*: slaughter 4 days, should not be used in sheep producing milk for human consumption

PML **Rycoben Cattle** (Young's) *UK*
Oral suspension, albendazole oxide 75 mg, hydrated cobalt sulphate 54 mg, hydrated sodium selenate 5.7 mg/mL, for *cattle*
Withdrawal Periods. *Cattle*: slaughter 14 days, milk 3 days

PML **Rycoben SC for Sheep** (Young's) *UK*
Oral suspension, albendazole oxide 25 mg, hydrated cobalt sulphate 18 mg, hydrated sodium selenate 1.9 mg/mL, for *sheep*
Withdrawal Periods. *Sheep*: slaughter 10 days, should not be used in sheep producing milk for human consumption

PML **Tramazole 2.5%** (Tulivin) *UK*
Oral suspension, albendazole 25 mg/mL, for *cattle, sheep*; 2.5 litres, 5 litres
Withdrawal Periods. *Cattle*: slaughter 14 days, milk 2.5 days. *Sheep*: slaughter 4 days, should not be used in sheep producing milk for human consumption

PML **Valbazen 2.5% SC Total Spectrum Wormer** (Pfizer) *UK*
Oral suspension, albendazole 25 mg, cobalt 630 micrograms, selenium 270 micrograms/mL, for *sheep*; 2.5 litres, 5 litres, 10 litres
Withdrawal Periods. *Sheep*: slaughter 8 days, should not be used in sheep producing milk for human consumption

PML **Valbazen 10% Total Spectrum Wormer** (Pfizer) *UK*
Oral suspension, albendazole 100 mg/mL, for *cattle, sheep*; 1 litre, 2.5 litres, 5 litres
Withdrawal Periods. *Cattle*: slaughter 14 days, milk 3 days. *Sheep*: slaughter 8 days, should not be used in sheep producing milk for human consumption

PML **Wormaway Albendazole 2.5% SC** (DiverseyLever) *UK*
Oral suspension, albendazole 25 mg, cobalt (as sulphate) 620 micrograms, selenium (as sodium selenite) 270 micrograms/mL, for *cattle, sheep*; 1 litre, 2.5 litres, 5 litres, 10 litres
Withdrawal Periods. Cattle: slaughter 14 days, milk 2.5 days. *Sheep*: slaughter 4 days, should not be used in sheep producing milk for human consumption

Australia
Indications. Gastro-intestinal roundworms, lungworms, tapeworms, and adult *Fasciola* in ruminants; Type II ostertagiosis
Dose. *By mouth*.
Cattle: roundworms and tapeworms, 7.5 mg/kg
Adult flukes, 10 mg/kg

Sheep, goats: roundworms and tapeworms, 3.8–4.0 mg/kg
Adult flukes, 4.75–5.0 mg/kg

Alben (Virbac) *Austral*
Liquid, albendazole 19 g/L, for *sheep, goats*
Withdrawal Periods. Slaughter 10 days, should not be used in goats or sheep producing milk for human consumption

Captec Extender 100 Controlled Release Worm Control Capsule for Adult Sheep (Nufarm) *Austral*
Ruminal bolus (= *capsule*), albendazole 3.85 g, for *sheep 35–65 kg body-weight*
Withdrawal Periods. Slaughter withdrawal period nil
Dose. *Sheep*: *by mouth*, 1 capsule/ 35–65 kg body-weight

Captec Extender Junior Controlled Release AnthelminticCapsule for Young Sheep (Nufarm) *Austral*
Ruminal bolus (= *capsule*), albendazole 2.1 g, for *sheep 20–40 kg boy-weight*
Withdrawal Periods. Slaughter withdrawal period nil
Dose. *Sheep*: *by mouth*, 1 capsule/ 20–40 kg body-weight

Nemadet Broad Spectrum Cattle Drench (Nufarm) *Austral*
Oral suspension, albendazole 112.5 g/L, for *cattle*
Withdrawal Periods. Slaughter 10 days, should not be used in animals producing milk for human consumption.

Nemadet Oral Anthelmintic Drench for Lambs, Sheep and Goats (Nufarm) *Austral*
Oral suspension, albendazole 19 g/L, for *sheep, goats*
Withdrawal Periods. Slaughter 10 days, should not be used in goats or sheep producing milk for human consumption

Rycoben (Novartis) *Austral*
Oral solution, albendazole oxide 40 g/L, for *sheep*
Withdrawal Periods. Slaughter10 days

Strategik Broad Spectrum Lamb, Weaner and Sheep Drench (Dover) *Austral*
Oral solution, albendazole 19 g/L, for *sheep*
Withdrawal Periods. Slaughter 10 days

Strategik Mini-dose Worming Drench for Cattle (Dover) *Austral*
Oral solution, albendazole 112.5 g/L, for *cattle*
Withdrawal Periods. Slaughter 10 days, should not be used in animals producing milk for human consumption

Valbazen Broad Spectrum Mini-Dose Cattle Drench (Pfizer) *Austral*
Oral solution, albendazole 112.5 g/L, for *cattle*
Withdrawal Periods. Slaughter 10 days, should not be used in animals producing milk for human consumption

Valbazen Broad Spectrum Sheep, Lamb and Goat Drench (Pfizer) *Austral*
Oral Solution, albendazole 19 mg/mL, for *sheep, goats*
Withdrawal Periods. *Sheep:* slaughter 10 days. *Goats*: slaughter 10 days, should not be used in goats producing milk for human consumption

Eire
Indications. Gastro-intestinal roundworms, lungworms, tapeworms, and adult *Fasciola* in ruminants; Type II ostertagiosis
Contra-indications. Treatment of ewes at a dosage of 7.5 mg/kg during the mating period and until 1 month after rams are removed
Dose. *By mouth*.
Cattle: roundworms and tapeworms, 7.5 mg/kg
Adult flukes, 10 mg/kg
Sheep: roundworms and tapeworms, 5 mg/kg
Adult flukes, 7.5 mg/kg

Albex 2.5% (Chanelle) *Eire*
Oral suspension, albendazole 25 mg/mL, for *cattle, sheep*
Withdrawal Periods. *Cattle*: slaughter 14 days, milk 60 hours. *Sheep*: slaughter 4 days, should not be used in sheep producing milk for human consumption

Albex 10% (Chanelle) *Eire*
Oral suspension, albendazole 100 mg/mL, for *cattle, sheep*
Withdrawal Periods. *Cattle*: slaughter 14 days, milk 60 hours. *Sheep*: slaughter 4 days, should not be used in sheep producing milk for human consumption

Young's Rycoben Drench for Cattle (Cypharm) *Eire*
Oral suspension, albendazole oxide 75 mg/mL, cobalt sulphate 54 mg/mL, sodium selenate 5.7 mg/mL, for *cattle*
Withdrawal Periods. Slaughter 14 days, milk 72 hours

Young's Rycoben Drench for Sheep (Cypharm) *Eire*
Oral suspension, albendazole oxide 25 mg/mL, cobalt sulphate 18 mg/mL, sodium selenate 1.9 mg/mL, for *sheep*
Withdrawal Periods. Slaughter 10 days, should not be used in sheep producing milk for human consumption

Valbazen 2.5% Total Spectrum Wormer (Pfizer) *Eire*
Oral suspension, albendazole 25 mg/mL, for *cattle, sheep*
Withdrawal Periods. *Cattle*: slaughter 14 days, milk 72 hours. *Sheep*: slaughter 10 days, milk 72 hours

Valbazen 10% Total Spectrum Wormer (Pfizer) *Eire*
Oral suspension, albendazole 100 mg/mL, for *cattle*
Withdrawal Periods. Slaughter 14 days, milk 72 hours

Valbazen Cattle Wormer Pellets (Pfizer) *Eire*
Oral pellets, albendazole 30 mg/g, for *cattle*
Withdrawal Periods. Slaughter 14 days, milk 72 hours

New Zealand

Indications. Gastro-intestinal roundworms, lungworms, tapeworms, and adult *Fasciola* in ruminants; Type II ostertagiosis
Dose. *By mouth*.
Cattle, goats: roundworms and tapeworms, 7.5 mg/kg
Adult flukes, 10 mg/kg
Sheep: roundworms and tapeworms, 3.8 mg/kg
Adult flukes, 4.75 mg/kg

Albendazole C (Ancare) *NZ*
Oral suspension, albendazole 150 mg/mL, selenium 1.47 mg/mL, for *cattle, deer*
Withdrawal Periods. *Cattle*: slaughter 14 days, should not be used in cattle producing milk for human consumption. *Deer*: slaughter 14 days

Albendazole Sheep (Ancare) *NZ*
Oral suspension, albendazole 23.8 mg/mL, for *sheep*
Withdrawal Periods. Slaughter 7 days, should not be used in sheep producing milk for human consumption

Albendazole Sheep Hi-mineral (Ancare) *NZ*
Oral suspension, albendazole 23.8 mg/mL in a mineral formulation, for *sheep*
Withdrawal Periods. Slaughter 7 days, should not be used in sheep producing milk for human consumption

Extender 100 (Nufarm) *NZ*
Ruminal boluses (= capsules), albendazole 3.85 g, for *sheep more than 35 kg body-weight*
Withdrawal Periods. Slaughter withdrawal period nil, milk withdrawal period nil
Dose. *Sheep*: by mouth, 1 capsule/ 35–65 kg body-weight

Extender Jnr (Nufarm) *NZ*
Capsules, albendazole 2.1 g, for *sheep more than 20 kg body-weight*
Withdrawal Periods. Slaughter withdrawal period nil, milk withdrawal period nil
Dose. *Sheep*: by mouth, 1 capsule/ 20–40 kg body-weight

Nemadet Extra (Nufarm) *NZ*
Oral suspension, albendazole 19 mg/mL in a mineral formulation, for *sheep*
Withdrawal Periods. Slaughter 7 days

Rycoben Cattle & Deer (Novartis) *NZ*
Oral suspension, ricobendazole 150 mg/mL, for *cattle, deer*
Withdrawal Periods. *Cattle*: slaughter 4 days, milk 36 hours. *Deer*: slaughter 14 days

Rycoben Cattle and Deer Mineralised Plus Selenium (Novartis) *NZ*
Oral suspension, ricobendazole 150 mg/mL, selenium (as sodium salt) 1.5 mg/mL, for *cattle, deer*
Withdrawal Periods. *Cattle*: slaughter 4 days, milk 36 hours. *Deer*: slaughter 14 days

Rycoben Sheep & Lamb (Novartis) *NZ*
Oral suspension, ricobendazole 20 mg/mL, for *sheep*
Withdrawal Periods. Slaughter 5 days, should not be used in sheep producing milk for human consumption

Rycoben Sheep & Lamb Mineralised Plus Selenium (Novartis) *NZ*
Oral suspension, ricobendazole 20 mg/mL, selenium (as sodium salt) 0.4 mg/mL, for *sheep*
Withdrawal Periods. Slaughter 5 days, should not be used in sheep producing milk for human consumption

Valbazen Mineralised Cattle (Pfizer) *NZ*
Oral suspension, albendazole 150 mg/mL, selenium 1.5 mg/mL in a mineral formulation, for *cattle, deer*
Withdrawal Periods. *Cattle*: slaughter 7 days, milk 48 hours. *Deer*: slaughter 7 days

Valbazen Mineralised Sheep (Pfizer) *NZ*
Oral suspension, albendazole 25 mg/mL, selenium 0.5 mg/mL in a mineral formulation, for *sheep*
Withdrawal Periods. Slaughter 7 days, should not be used in sheep producing milk for human consumption

Valbazen Sheep (Pfizer) *NZ*
Oral suspension, albendazole 25 mg/mL, for *cattle, sheep, goats, deer*
Withdrawal Periods. *Cattle*: slaughter 7 days, milk 48 hours. *Sheep*: slaughter 7 days, should not be used in sheep producing milk for human consumption. *Goats*: slaughter 7 days, milk 72 hours. *Deer*: slaughter 7 days

USA

Indications. Gastro-intestinal roundworms, lungworms, tapeworms, and adult *Fasciola* in cattle; Type II ostertagiosis
Contra-indications. Treatment of cows during first 45 days of pregnancy and for 45 days after removal of bulls
Dose. *Cattle*: *by mouth*, roundworms, tapeworms, adult flukes, 10 mg/kg

Valbazen (Pfizer) *USA*
Oral paste, albendazole 300 mg/mL, for *cattle*
Withdrawal Periods. Slaughter 27 days, should not be used in cattle producing milk for human consumption

Valbazen (Pfizer) *USA*
Oral suspension, albendazole 113.6 mg/mL, for *cattle*
Withdrawal Periods. Slaughter 27 days, should not be used in cattle producing milk for human consumption

FEBANTEL

UK

Indications. Gastro-intestinal roundworms in horses, ruminants, pigs, and pigeons; lungworms in ruminants; tapeworms in sheep (see section 2.1.2)

Dose. *By mouth.*
Horses: 6 mg/kg
Cattle: 7.5 mg/kg
Sheep, pigs: 5 mg/kg

PML **Bayverm 2.5% Suspension** (Bayer) *UK*
Oral suspension, febantel 25 mg/mL, for *cattle, sheep*; 5 litres
Withdrawal Periods. *Cattle*: slaughter 35 days, milk 4 days. *Sheep*: slaughter
14 days, should not be used in sheep producing milk for human consumption
Note. Available as twin-pack with Pardevit

PML **Bayverm Armadose** (Bayer) *UK*
Oral suspension, febantel 100 mg/mL, for *sheep*; 500 mL
Withdrawal Periods. *Sheep*: slaughter 14 days, should not be used in sheep
producing milk for human consumption

PML **Bayverm Pellets 1.9%** (Bayer) *UK*
Pellets, for use alone or by addition to feed on a herd basis, febantel 19 mg/g,
for *horses, cattle, sheep, pigs*; 2 kg
Note. For medication of individual animals, body-weight should be more
than 50 kg
Withdrawal Periods. Should not be used in *horses* intended for human consumption. *Cattle*: slaughter 35 days, milk 4 days. *Sheep*: slaughter 14 days,
should not be used in sheep producing milk for human consumption. *Pigs*:
slaughter 35 days

FENBENDAZOLE

UK
Indications. Gastro-intestinal roundworms in horses, ruminants, pigs, dogs, cats, and pigeons; Type II ostertagiosis;
transplacental roundworm transmission in dogs; lungworms
in ruminants, pigs, dogs, and cats; *Trichostrongylus tenuis*
in grouse; tapeworms (see section 2.1.2) in ruminants; *Taenia* in dogs and cats; *Giardia* in dogs (Panacur, see section
1.4)
Contra-indications. Administration within 14 days of
treatment for liver fluke, administration of ruminal boluses
to non-ruminating cattle or cattle less than 100 kg body-
weight and 3 months of age, concurrent administration of
other ruminal boluses, treatment of grouse after March
Warnings. If cattle are vaccinated against lungworm, the
ruminal bolus should not be administered until 14 days after
the second dose of vaccine; treatment of pigeons when rearing young and during the main moult not recommended
Dose. *By mouth.*
Horses: roundworms, 7.5 mg/kg as a single dose
Larval *Trichonema* (cyathostomes), 30 mg/kg as a single
dose *or* 7.5 mg/kg daily for 5 days
Migrating strongyles, 60 mg/kg as a single dose *or* 7.5 mg/
kg daily for 5 days
Strongyloides westeri in foals, 50 mg/kg as a single dose
Cattle: 7.5 mg/kg as a single dose *or* in divided doses over 5
or 10 days (may not be effective against *Trichuris, Strongy-
loides*)

see also modified-release oral preparations below
Sheep: 5 mg/kg as a single dose
Pigs: roundworms, 5 mg/kg as a single dose
Trichuris, Metastrongylus apri, 5 mg/kg in divided doses
over 7 days
Dogs: roundworms, tapeworms, *Giardia*,
treatment, (adults) 50 mg/kg daily for 3 days
prophylaxis, (<6 months of age) 50 mg/kg daily for 3 days;
(adults) 100 mg/kg as a single dose
Transplacental transmission, 25 mg/kg daily from day 40 of
pregnancy until 2 days post partum
Lungworms, 50 mg/kg daily for 7 days
Cats: roundworms, tapeworms,
treatment, (adults) 50 mg/kg daily for 3 days
prophylaxis, (<6 months of age) 50 mg/kg daily for 3 days;
(adults) 100 mg/kg as a single dose
Pregnant queens, 100 mg/kg as a single dose
Lungworms, 50 mg/kg daily for 3 days
Grouse: *Trichostrongylus, by addition to feed*, 7–10 mg/kg
body-weight given in divided doses over 14 days; 1 kg/
tonne feed
Pigeons: 20 mg/kg
Exotic species ♦: contact manufacturer for further details

PML **Curazole 5% Oral Drench** (Tulivin) *UK*
Oral suspension, fenbendazole 50 mg/mL, for *cattle*
Withdrawal Periods. *Cattle*: slaughter 28 days, milk 3 days

MFSX **Curazole 5% Powder** (Tulivin) *UK*
Oral powder, for addition to feed, 50 mg/g, for *pigs*
Withdrawal Periods. *Pigs*: slaughter 10 days

PML **Curazole 10% Oral Drench** (Tulivin) *UK*
Oral suspension, fenbendazole 100 mg/mL, for *cattle*
Withdrawal Periods. *Cattle*: slaughter 28 days, milk 3 days

GSL **Easy to Use Wormer** (Bob Martin) *UK*
Oral granules, fenbendazole 220 mg/g, for dogs, cats; 1 g, 4 g

PML **Fenzol 5.0%** (Norbrook) *UK*
Oral suspension, fenbendazole 50 mg/mL, for *cattle, sheep*
Withdrawal Periods. *Cattle*: slaughter 12 days, milk 5 days. *Sheep*: slaughter
14 days, should not be used in sheep producing milk for human consumption

PML **Flexadin** (Vétoquinol) *UK*
Oral suspension, fenbendazole 100 mg/mL, for *cattle*; 1 litre, 5 litres
Withdrawal Periods. *Cattle*: slaughter 28 days, milk 3 days

MFSX **Flexadin 5% Premix** (Vétoquinol) *UK*
Premix, fenbendazole 50 g/kg, for *pigs*
Withdrawal Periods. *Pigs*: slaughter 10 days

PML **Granofen Wormer for Dogs and Cats** (Virbac) *UK*
Oral granules, fenbendazole 220 mg/g, for *dogs, cats*; 1 g, 2 g, 4 g

PML **Multiwurma-F Granules** (Day Son & Hewitt)
Oral granules, fenbendazole 220 mg/g, for *horses, other equines*
Withdrawal Periods. Should not be used in *horses* intended for human con-
sumption

PML **Panacur 1.5%** (Intervet) *UK*
Pellets, fenbendazole 15 mg/g, for *cattle, pigs*; 2.5 kg, 5 kg
Withdrawal Periods. *Cattle*: slaughter 19 days, milk 7 days. *Pigs*: slaughter 3
days

PML **Panacur 2.5% Liquid** (Intervet) *UK*
Oral suspension, fenbendazole 25 mg/mL, for *dogs, cats*; 100 mL

PML **Panacur 2.5% Suspension** (Intervet) *UK*
Oral suspension, fenbendazole 25 mg/mL, for *cattle, sheep*
Withdrawal Periods. *Cattle*: slaughter 12 days, milk 5 days. *Sheep*: slaughter 19 days, milk 7 days

MFSX **Panacur 4% Powder** (Intervet)
Oral powder, for addition to feed, fenbendazole 40 mg/g, for *cattle, pigs, grouse*; 2.5 kg, 25 kg
Withdrawal Periods. *Cattle*: slaughter 14 days, milk 7 days. *Pigs*: slaughter 3 days

PML **Panacur 10% Liquid** (Intervet) *UK*
Oral suspension, fenbendazole 100 mg/mL, for *dogs, cats*; 100 mL

PML **Panacur 10% Suspension** (Intervet) *UK*
Oral suspension, fenbendazole 100 mg/mL, for *horses, cattle, sheep*
Withdrawal Periods. Should not be used in *horses* intended for human consumption. *Cattle*: slaughter 12 days, milk 5 days. *Sheep*: slaughter 19 days, milk 7 days

PML **Panacur Bolus** (Intervet) *UK*
Ruminal bolus, m/r, fenbendazole 12 g delivered for up to 140 days, for *cattle 100–300 kg body-weight*; 10
Withdrawal Periods. *Cattle*: slaughter 200 days, should not be used in cattle producing milk for human consumption or dairy heifers within 200 days before calving
Dose. *Cattle*: one 12-g bolus

GSL **Panacur Capsules** (Intervet) *UK*
Capsules, fenbendazole 8 mg, for *pigeons more than 2 months of age*; 25
Withdrawal Periods. Should not be used in *pigeons* intended for human consumption
Dose. *Pigeons*: *by mouth,* 1 capsule/bird

PML **Panacur Equine Granules** (Intervet) *UK*
Oral granules, for addition to feed, fenbendazole 220 mg/g, for *horses, other equines*; 10.2 g, 1 kg
Withdrawal Periods. Should not be used in *horses* intended for human consumption

PML **Panacur Equine Guard** (Intervet) *UK*
Oral suspension, for addition to feed, fenbendazole 100 mg/mL, for *horses, other equines*; 225 mL
Withdrawal Periods. Should not be used in *horses* intended for human consumption

PML **Panacur Equine Paste** (Intervet) *UK*
Oral paste, fenbendazole 187 mg/g, for *horses, other equines*; 24-g dose applicator
Withdrawal Periods. Should not be used in *horses* intended for human consumption

PML **Panacur Granules** (Intervet) *UK*
Oral granules, for addition to feed, fenbendazole 220 mg/g, for *dogs, cats*

PML **Panacur Paste** (Intervet) *UK*
Oral paste, fenbendazole 187 mg/g, for *dogs, cats*; 5-g dose applicator

PML **Panacur SC 2.5%** (Intervet)
Oral suspension, fenbendazole 25 mg, cobalt 940 micrograms, selenium 400 micrograms/mL, for *sheep*
Withdrawal Periods. *Sheep*: slaughter 19 days, milk 7 days

PML **Panacur SC 5%** (Intervet) *UK*
Oral suspension, fenbendazole 50 mg, cobalt 10 mg, selenium 1.6 mg/mL, for *cattle, sheep*; 1 litre, 2.5 litres
Withdrawal Periods. *Cattle*: slaughter 12 days, milk 5 days. *Sheep*: slaughter 19 days, milk 7 days

PML **Panacur SC 10%** (Intervet) *UK*
Oral suspension, fenbendazole 100 mg, cobalt 20 mg, selenium 3.2 mg/mL, for *cattle, sheep*
Withdrawal Periods. *Cattle*: slaughter 12 days, milk 5 days. *Sheep*: slaughter 19 days, milk 7 days

PML **Wormaway Feben** (DiverseyLever)
Oral suspension, fenbendazole 25 mg/mL, for *cattle, sheep*; 2.5 litres, 5 litres, 10 litres

Withdrawal Periods. *Cattle, sheep*: slaughter 28 days, should not be used in cattle, sheep producing milk for human consumption

PML **Wormaway Feben 10** (DiverseyLever) *UK*
Oral suspension, fenbendazole 100 mg/mL, for *cattle*; 2.5 litres
Withdrawal Periods. *Cattle*: slaughter 28 days, should not be used in cattle producing milk for human consumption

PML **Wormaway Feben SC** (DiverseyLever) *UK*
Oral suspension, fenbendazole 25 mg, cobalt (as sulphate) 7.2 mg, selenium (as sodium sesquestrate) 400 micrograms/mL, for *sheep*
Withdrawal Periods. *Sheep*: slaughter 21 days, should not be used in sheep producing milk for human consumption

GSL **Worming Granules for Cats** (Sherley's)
Oral granules, fenbendazole 220 mg/g, for *cats more than 6 months of age*

GSL **Worming Granules for Dogs** (Sherley's)
Oral granules, fenbendazole 220 mg/g, for *dogs more than 6 months of age*

PML **Zerofen 2.5%** (Chanelle) *UK*
Oral suspension, fenbendazole 25 mg/mL, for *cattle, sheep*
Withdrawal Periods. *Cattle*: slaughter 14 days, milk 4 days. *Sheep*: slaughter 21 days, should not be used in sheep producing milk for human consumption

MFSX **Zerofen 4%** (Chanelle) *UK*
Oral powder, for addition to feed, fenbendazole 40 mg/g, for *pigs*
Withdrawal Periods. *Pigs*: slaughter 21 days

PML **Zerofen 10%** (Chanelle) *UK*
Oral solution, fenbendazole 100 mg/mL, for *cattle, sheep*
Withdrawal Periods. *Cattle*: slaughter 14 days, milk 4 days. *Sheep*: slaughter 21 days, should not be used in sheep producing milk for human consumption

PML **Zerofen 22%** (Chanelle) *UK*
Oral granules, for addition to feed, fenbendazole 220 mg/g, for *dogs, cats*

PML **Zerofen 22% Granules (Horse Wormer)** (Chanelle) *UK*
Oral granules, fenbendazole 220 mg/g, for *horses*
Withdrawal Periods. Slaughter 35 days

Australia
Indications. Gastro-intestinal roundworms in horses and ruminants; lungworms and tapeworms in ruminants
Contra-indications. Administration within 7 days of bromsalans
Dose. *By mouth.*
Horses: 10 mg/kg
Strongyloides westeri, 50 mg/kg
Cattle: 7.5 mg/kg
Sheep, goats: 5 mg/kg

Fenbendazole (Western Stock Distributors) *Austral*
Oral solution, fenbendazole 25 g/L, for *cattle, sheep, goats*
Withdrawal Periods. *Cattle, sheep*: slaughter 14 days. *Goats*: milk 24 hours

Fenbendazole 100 (Western Stock Distributors) *Austral*
Oral solution, fenbendazole 100 g/L, for *horses, cattle*
Withdrawal Periods. *Horses*: slaughter 28 days. *Cattle*: slaughter 14 days

Fencare 25 (Virbac) *Austral*
Liquid, fenbendazole 25 g/L, for *sheep, cattle*
Withdrawal Periods. *Cattle*: slaughter 21 days, milk withdrawal period nil. *Sheep*: slaughter 21 days

Fencare 100 (Virbac) *Austral*
Liquid, fenbendazole 100 g/L, for *horses, cattle*
Withdrawal Periods. *Horses*: slaughter 28 days. *Cattle*: slaughter 21 days

Mineralised Fencare (Virbac) *Austral*
Oral solution, fenbendazole 25 g/L (with minerals), for *cattle, sheep*
Withdrawal Periods. *Cattle*: slaughter 21 days, milk withdrawal period nil. *Sheep*: slaughter 21 days.

Panacur 25 (Hoechst Roussel) *Austral*
Oral solution, fenbendazole 25 g/L, for *sheep, goats, cattle*
Withdrawal Periods. *Cattle*: slaughter 14 days, milk withdrawal period nil.
Sheep: slaughter 14 days. *Goats*: slaughter 14 days, milk 24 hours

Panacur 100 (Hoechst Roussel) *Austral*
Oral solution, fenbendazole 100 g/L, for *horses, cattle*
Withdrawal Periods. *Horses*: slaughter 28 days. *Cattle*: slaughter 14 days, milk withdrawal period nil

Eire

Indications. Gastro-intestinal roundworms in horses, ruminants, pigs, dogs, cats, and pigeons; Type II ostertagiosis; transplacental roundworm transmission in dogs; lungworms in horses, ruminants, pigs, dogs, and cats; tapeworms in ruminants, dogs, and cats; *Giardia* in dogs (Panacur, see section 1.4)

Contra-indications. Concurrent administration of bromsalans; Administration within 14 days of treatment for liver fluke, administration of ruminal boluses to non-ruminating cattle or cattle less than 3 months of age, concurrent administration of other ruminal boluses, treatment of grouse after March, treatment of pigeons when rearing young and during the main moult

Warnings. If cattle are vaccinated against lungworm, the ruminal bolus should not be administered until 14 days after the second dose of vaccine

Dose. *By mouth.*
Horses: roundworms, 7.5 mg/kg
Larval *Trichonema* (cyathostomes), 30 mg/kg
Migrating strongyles, 60 mg/kg as a single dose *or* 7.5 mg/kg daily for 5 days
Cattle: 7.5 mg/kg
Sheep, pigs: 5 mg/kg
Dogs: roundworms, tapeworms, *Giardia*,
prophylaxis, (<6 months of age) 50 mg/kg daily for 3 days; (adults) 100 mg/kg as a single dose
Transplacental transmission, 25 mg/kg daily from day 40 of pregnancy until 2 days post partum
Cats: roundworms, tapeworms,
prophylaxis, (<6 months of age) 50 mg/kg daily for 3 days; (adults) 100 mg/kg as a single dose
Pigeons: 20 mg/kg

Curazole 2.5% Oral Drench (Univet) *Eire*
Oral solution, fenbendazole 25 mg/mL, for *sheep*
Withdrawal Periods. Slaughter 14 days, should not be used in sheep producing milk for human consumption

Curazole 5% Oral Drench (Univet) *Eire*
Oral solution, fenbendazole 50 mg/mL, for *cattle, sheep*
Withdrawal Periods. *Cattle*: slaughter 14 days, milk 72 hours. *Sheep*: slaughter 14 days, should not be used in sheep producing milk for human consumption

Curazole 5% W/W Powder (Univet) *Eire*
Powder, for addition to feed, fenbendazole 50 g/kg, for *pigs*
Withdrawal Periods. *Pigs*: slaughter 10 days

Curazole 10% Oral Drench (Univet) *Eire*
Oral solution, fenbendazole 100 mg/mL, for *cattle*
Withdrawal Periods. Slaughter 28 days, milk 5 days

Forazole (Foran) *Eire*
Oral suspension, fenbendazole 100 mg/mL, for *horses*
Withdrawal Periods. Slaughter 45 days

Orazole (Foran) *Eire*
Oral suspension, fenbendazole 100 mg/mL, for *cattle*
Withdrawal Periods. Slaughter 28 days, milk 5 days

Parazole (Foran) *Eire*
Oral suspension, fenbendazole 100 mg/mL, for *dogs, cats*

Panacur 1.5% Pellets (Hoechst Roussel Vet) *Eire*
Pellets, fenbendazole 15 mg/g, for *pigs*
Withdrawal Periods. Slaughter 14 days

Panacur 4% Powder (Hoechst Roussel Vet) *Eire*
Oral powder, to mix with feed, fenbendazole 0.04 g/g, for *pigs*
Withdrawal Periods. Slaughter 14 days

Panacur 10% Suspension (Hoechst Roussel Vet) *Eire*
Oral suspension, fenbendazole 100 mg/mL, for *horses, cattle*
Withdrawal Periods. Should not be used in *horses* intended for human consumption. *Cattle*: slaughter 14 days, milk 72 hours

Panacur 22% Horse Granules (Hoechst Roussel Vet) *Eire*
Oral granules, fenbendazole 0.22 g/g, for *horses, donkeys*
Withdrawal Periods. Slaughter 14 days

Panacur Equine Guard (Hoechst Roussel Vet) *Eire*
Oral suspension, fenbendazole 100 mg/mL, for *horses*
Withdrawal Periods. Slaughter 14 days

Panacur Capsules for Pigeons (Hoechst Roussel Vet) *Eire*
Capsules, fendbendazole 8 mg, for *pigeons*
Withdrawal Periods. Should not be used in pigeons intended for human consumption

Panacur Paste (Hoechst Roussel Vet) *Eire*
Oral paste, fenbendazole 0.187 g/g in oral syringes containing 24 g, for *horses*
Withdrawal Periods. Slaughter 14 days

Panacur SC 2.5% Sheep Suspension (Hoechst Roussel Vet) *Eire*
Oral suspension, fenbendazole 25 mg/mL, for *sheep*
Withdrawal Periods. Slaughter 14 days

Panacur SC 10% Suspension (Hoechst Roussel Vet) *Eire*
Oral suspension, fenbendazole 100 mg/mL, for *cattle*
Withdrawal Periods. Slaughter 14 days, milk 72 hours

Panacur SR Bolus (Hoechst Roussel Vet) *Eire*
Ruminal bolus, fenbendazole 12 g/bolus, for *cattle*
Withdrawal Periods. Slaughter 199 days, should not be used in cattle producing milk for human consumption
Dose. *Cattle*: one bolus

Panacur Wormer (for Cats and Dogs) (Hoechst Roussel Vet) *Eire*
Oral granules, fenbendazole 0.22 g/g, for *dogs, cats*

Zerofen 2.5% (Chanelle) *Eire*
Oral suspension, fenbendazole 25 mg/mL, for *cattle, sheep*
Withdrawal Periods. Slaughter 14 days, milk 72 hours

Zerofen 10% (Chanelle) *Eire*
Oral suspension, fenbendazole 100 mg/mL, for *cattle*
Withdrawal Periods. Slaughter 14 days, milk 72 hours

Zerofen 4% Powder (Chanelle) *Eire*
Oral powder, to mix with feed, fenbendazole 4%, for *pigs*
Withdrawal Periods. Slaughter 14 days

Zerofen 22% Granules - Small Animal (Chanelle) *Eire*
Oral granules, to mix with feed, fenbendazole 0.22 g/g, for *dogs, cats*

New Zealand

Indications. Gastro-intestinal roundworms in horses and ruminants; lungworms and tapeworms in ruminants
Contra-indications. Administration within 7 days of bromsalans

Dose. *By mouth.*
Horses, cattle: 7.5 mg/kg
Sheep, goats: 5 mg/kg

Axilur 10 (Animal Health) *NZ*
Oral suspension, fenbendazole 100 mg/mL, for *horses, cattle, sheep, goats, deer*
Withdrawal Periods. *Horses, deer*: slaughter 10 days. *Cattle, sheep, goats*: slaughter 10 days, milk 96 hours

Fenben (Ancare) *NZ*
Oral suspension, fenbendazole 25 mg/mL, for *cattle, sheep*
Withdrawal Periods. Slaughter 10 days, should not be used in cattle or sheep producing milk for human consumption

Fenben Hi-Mineral (Ancare) *NZ*
Oral suspension, fenbendazole 25 mg/mL in a mineral formulation, for *cattle, sheep*
Withdrawal Periods. Slaughter 10 days, should not be used in cattle or sheep producing milk for human consumption

Panacur (Novartis) *NZ*
Oral suspension, fenbendazole 25 mg/mL, for *sheep*
Withdrawal Periods. Slaughter 10 days, milk 96 hours

Panacur 100 (Novartis) *NZ*
Oral suspension, fenbendazole 100 mg/mL, for *horses, cattle, sheep, deer*
Withdrawal Periods. *Horses*: slaughter 28 days. *Cattle, sheep*: slaughter 10 days, milk 96 hours. *Deer*: slaughter 10 days

Panacur 100 Mineralised Plus Selenium (Novartis) *NZ*
Oral suspension, fenbendazole 100 mg/mL, selenium 1 mg/mL in a mineral formulation, for *horses, cattle, sheep, deer*
Withdrawal Periods. *Horses*: slaughter 28 days. *Cattle, sheep*: slaughter 10 days, milk 96 hours. *Deer*: slaughter 10 days

Panacur Mineralised (Novartis) *NZ*
Oral suspension, fenbendazole 25 mg/mL in a mineral formulation, for *sheep*
Withdrawal Periods. Slaughter 10 days, milk 96 hours

Panacur Mineralised Plus Selenium (Novartis) *NZ*
Oral suspension, fenbendazole 25 mg/mL, selenium 0.5 mg/mL in a mineral formulation, for *sheep*
Withdrawal Periods. Slaughter 10 days, milk 96 hours

USA

Indications. Gastro-intestinal roundworms in horses, ruminants, pigs, and dogs; lungworms in ruminants, pigs, and dogs; tapeworms in ruminants and dogs
Contra-indications. Administration within 14 days of the hunting season
Dose. *By mouth.*
Horses, cattle: 5–10 mg/kg
Pigs: *by addition to feed*, 9 mg/kg
Dogs: prophylaxis, 50 mg/kg daily for 3 days

Panacur (Hoechst-Roussel) *USA*
Granules, fenbendazole 222 mg/g granules, for *horses*
Withdrawal Periods. Should not be used in horses intended for human consumption

Panacur (Hoechst-Roussel) *USA*
Suspension, fenbendazole 100 mg/mL, for *horses*
Withdrawal Periods. Should not be used in horses intended for human consumption

Panacur (Hoechst-Roussel) *USA*
Oral paste, fenbendazole 100 mg/g, for *horses*
Withdrawal Periods. Should not be used in horses intended for human consumption

Panacur (Hoechst-Roussel) *USA*
Granules, fenbendazole 222 mg/g granules, for *dogs, carniverous/omniverous Felidae and Ursidae*

Panacur (Hoechst-Roussel) *USA*
Oral paste, fenbendazole 100 mg/g, for *cattle*
Withdrawal Periods. Slaughter 8 days, should not be used in cattle producing milk for human consumption

Panacur (Hoechst-Roussel) *USA*
Suspension, fenbendazole 100 mg/mL, for *cattle*
Withdrawal Periods. Slaughter 8 days, should not be used in cattle producing milk for human consumption

Safe-Guard (Hoechst-Roussel) *USA*
Supplement block, fenbendazole 1.65 g/kg block, for *cattle*
Withdrawal Periods. Slaughter 11 days

Safe-Guard EZ Scoop Swine Dewormer (Hoechst-Roussel) *USA*
Premix, fenbendazole 1.8%, for *pigs*

Safe-Guard (Hoechst-Roussel) *USA*
Medicated feed, fenbendazole 4.18 g/kg feed, for *cattle*
Withdrawal Periods. Slaughter 13 days, should not be used in cattle producing milk for human consumption

Safe-Guard Premix (Hoechst-Roussel) *USA*
Medicated feed, fenbendazole, for *zoo and wildlife ruminants sheep (big horn), feral pigs*

Safe-Guard Sweetlix Blocks (Hoechst-Roussel) *USA*
Supplement block, fenbendazole 20%, for *beef cattle*
Withdrawal Periods. *Cattle*: slaughter 16 days

Safe-Guard Top Dress Pellets (Hoechst-Roussel) *USA*
Pellets, fenbendazole 5 g/kg pellets, for *cattle*
Withdrawal Periods. Slaughter 13 days, should not be used in cattle producing milk for human consumption

FLUBENDAZOLE

UK

Indications. Gastro-intestinal roundworms and lungworms in pigs; gastro-intestinal roundworms, gapeworms, and tapeworms in poultry and game birds
Dose. *By addition to feed.*
Pigs: 5 mg/kg body-weight as a single dose
30 g/tonne feed for 5 or 10 days
Chickens: roundworms, 30 g/tonne feed for 7 days
Tapeworms, 60 g/tonne feed for 7 days
Turkeys: 20 g/tonne feed for 7 days
Geese: roundworms, 30 g/tonne feed for 7 days
Tapeworms, 60 g/tonne feed for 7 days
Game birds: 60 g/tonne feed for 7 days

MFSX **Flubenol Individual Treatment Pack** (Janssen) *UK*
Oral powder, for addition to feed, flubendazole 50 mg/g, for *pigs*; 600 g
Withdrawal Periods. *Pigs*: slaughter 7 days

MFSX **Flubenol Premix Pack** (Janssen) *UK*
Premix, flubendazole 50 mg/g, for *pigs*; 25 kg
Withdrawal Periods. *Pigs*: slaughter 7 days

MFSX **Flubenvet Intermediate** (Janssen) *UK*
Oral powder, for addition to feed, flubendazole 25 mg/g, for *chickens, turkeys, geese, partridges, pheasants*; 2.4 kg
Withdrawal Periods. *Poultry*, slaughter 7 days, egg withdrawal period nil.
Game birds: slaughter 7 days, eggs 7 days

Australia

Indications. Gastro-intestinal roundworms and tapeworms (*Taenia*) in dogs and cats
Side-effects. Transient salivation in cats
Dose. *Dogs, cats*: *by mouth*, 22 mg/kg

Flubenol (Boehringer Ingelheim) *Austral*
Oral paste, flubendazole 44 mg/mL, for *dogs, cats*

Eire

Indications. Gastro-intestinal roundworms and lungworms in pigs
Dose. *By addition to feed.*
Pigs: 5 mg/kg body-weight as a single dose
30 g/tonne feed for 5 or 10 days

Flubenol Premix Pack (Janssen) *Eire*
Oral powder, to mix with feed, flubendazole 50 g/kg, for *pigs*
Withdrawal Periods. *Pigs*: slaughter 7 days

Flubenol Individual Treatment Pack (Janssen) *Eire*
Oral powder, to mix with feed, flubendazole 5% (50 mg/g), for *pigs*
Withdrawal Periods. *Pigs*:slaughter 7 days

New Zealand

Indications. Gastro-intestinal roundworms and lungworms in pigs; gastro-intestinal roundworms, gapeworms, and tapeworms in poultry
Dose. *By addition to feed.*
Pigs: 30 g/tonne feed for 5 or 10 days
Poultry: 30 g/tonne feed for 7 days

Flubenol 5% (Nutritech) *NZ*
Oral powder, flubendazole 50 g/kg, for *pigs, poultry*
Withdrawal Periods. *Pigs*: slaughter 7 days. *Poultry*: slaughter withdrawal period nil

---

MEBENDAZOLE

UK

Indications. Gastro-intestinal roundworms in horses, donkeys, sheep, dogs, and cats; lungworms in donkeys and sheep; tapeworms (see section 2.1.2) in sheep; *Echinococcus* and *Taenia* in dogs and cats
Contra-indications. Administration during first 4 months of pregnancy in donkeys for treatment for *Dictyocaulus*. Manufacturer does not recommend administration to pigeons or parrots
Side-effects. Occasional mild diarrhoea
Dose. *By mouth.*
Horses: roundworms, 5–10 mg/kg
Donkeys: *Dictyocaulus arnfieldi*, 15–20 mg/kg daily for 5 days
Sheep: 15 mg/kg
Dogs, cats: roundworms, (puppies, kittens) 50 mg twice daily for 2 days; (>2 kg body-weight) 100 mg twice daily for 2 days
roundworms and tapeworms, (<2 kg body-weight) 50 mg twice daily for 5 days; (>2 kg body-weight) 100 mg twice daily for 5 days; (dogs >30 kg body-weight) 200 mg twice daily for 5 days

PML **Chanazole SC** (Chanelle) *UK*
Oral suspension, mebendazole 50 mg, cobalt (as sulphate) 4 mg, selenium (as sodium selenite) 400 micrograms/mL, for *sheep*; 1 litre, 5 litres
Withdrawal Periods. *Sheep*: slaughter 14 days, should not be used in sheep producing milk for human consumption

PML **Ovitelmin S & C** (Janssen) *UK*
Oral suspension, mebendazole 50 mg, cobalt (as sulphate) 430 micrograms, sodium (as selenite) 340 micrograms/mL, for *sheep*; 1 litre, 5 litres
Withdrawal Periods. *Sheep*: slaughter 7 days, milk 1 day

PML **Telmin** (Janssen) *UK*
Oral granules, for addition to feed, mebendazole 100 mg/g, for *horses, donkeys*; 20 g
Withdrawal Periods. Should not be used in *horses, donkeys* intended for human consumption

PML **Telmin KH** (Janssen) *UK*
Tablets, to prepare an oral solution, mebendazole 100 mg, for *dogs, cats*; 10

PML **Telmin Paste** (Janssen) *UK*
Oral paste, mebendazole 200 mg/g, for *horses, donkeys*; 20-g dose applicator
Withdrawal Periods. Should not be used for *horses, donkeys* intended for human consumption
Dose. *Horses*: (100–200 kg body-weight) ¼ dose applicator; (200–400 kg body-weight) ½ dose applicator; (400–800 kg body-weight) 1 dose applicator

Australia

Indications. Gastro-intestinal roundworms in horses and sheep; lungworms in sheep
Dose. *By mouth.*
Horses: 9 mg/kg
Sheep: 12.5 mg/kg

Benzicare (Virbac) *Austral*
Liquid, mebendazole 50 g/L, for *sheep*
Withdrawal Periods. Slaughter 7 days

Telmin Horse Wormer Granules (Boehringer Ingelheim) *Austral*
Oral granules, mebendazole 100 mg/g granules, for *horses*
Withdrawal Periods. Slaughter 28 days

Telmin Horse Wormer Paste (Boehringer Ingelheim) *Austral*
Oral paste, mebendazole 200 mg/g paste, for *horses*
Withdrawal Periods. Slaughter 28 days

Eire

Indications. Gastro-intestinal roundworms in horses, donkeys, and sheep; lungworms in donkeys and sheep; tapeworms in sheep;
Contra-indications. Administration during first 4 months of pregnancy in donkeys treated for *Dictyocaulus*
Dose. *By mouth.*
Horses, donkeys: roundworms, 5–10 mg/kg
Dictyocaulus arnfieldi in donkeys, 15–20 mg/kg daily for 5 days
Sheep: 15 mg/kg

Chanazole (Chanelle) *Eire*
Oral suspension, mebendazole 50 mg/mL, for *sheep*
Withdrawal Periods. Slaughter 14 days, should not be used in sheep producing milk for human consumption

Chanazole SC (Chanelle) *Eire*
Oral suspension, mebendazole 50 mg/mL, selenium 0.4 mg/mL, cobalt 4 mg/mL, for *sheep*
Withdrawal Periods. Slaughter 14 days, should not be used in sheep producing milk for human consumption

Ovitelmin S&C (Janssen) *Eire*
Oral suspension, mebendazole 50 mg/mL (also contains cobalt and selenium), for *sheep*
Withdrawal Periods. Slaughter 7 days, milk 24 hours

Pharmamin SC (Interpharm) *Eire*
Oral suspension, mebendazole 50 mg/mL, for *sheep*
Withdrawal Periods. Slaughter 14 days

Telmin Paste (Janssen) *Eire*
Oral paste, mebendazole 4 g/syringe, for *horses, donkeys*
Withdrawal Periods. Slaughter 28 days

NETOBIMIN

UK

Indications. Gastro-intestinal roundworms, lungworms, tapeworms (see section 2.1.2), and adult flukes (see section 2.1.3) in ruminants; Type II ostertagiosis
Contra-indications. Administration during first 7 weeks of pregnancy in cattle, first 5 weeks of pregnancy in sheep
Dose. *By mouth.*
Cattle: roundworms, tapeworms, 7.5 mg/kg
Type II ostertagiosis, adult flukes, 20 mg/kg
Sheep: roundworms, tapeworms, Type II ostertagiosis, 7.5 mg/kg
Adult flukes, 20 mg/kg

PML **Hapadex Cattle Wormer** (Schering-Plough) *UK*
Oral suspension, netobimin 150 mg/mL, for *cattle*; 1 litre
Withdrawal Periods. *Cattle*: slaughter 10 days, milk 2 days

PML **Hapadex Sheep Wormer** (Schering-Plough) *UK*
Oral suspension, netobimin 50 mg/mL, for *sheep*; 1 litre, 5 litres
Withdrawal Periods. *Sheep*: slaughter 5 days, milk 3 days

Australia

Indications. Gastro-intestinal roundworms and tapeworms in caged birds and pigeons
Contra-indications. Administration during first 7 weeks of pregnancy in cattle, first 5 weeks of pregnancy in sheep
Dose. *By addition to drinking water.*
Pigeons: 140 mg (4g of powder)/800 mL; one 56-g tablet/100 mL
Other birds: 140 mg (4g of powder)/400 mL; one 56-g tablet/100 mL

Hapavet (Vetafarm) *Austral*
Powder, for addition to drinking water, netobimin 35 mg/g, for *caged birds, pigeons*
Withdrawal Periods. Should not be used in birds intended for human consumption
Tablets, for addition to drinking water, netobimin 56 mg, for *caged birds, pigeons*
Withdrawal Periods. Should not be used in birds intended for human consumption

Eire

Indications. Gastro-intestinal roundworms, lungworms, tapeworms (see section 2.1.2), and adult flukes (see section 2.1.3) in ruminants; Type II ostertagiosis
Contra-indications. Administration during first 7 weeks of pregnancy in cattle, first 5 weeks of pregnancy in sheep
Dose. *By mouth.*
Cattle: roundworms, tapeworms, 7.5 mg/kg

Type II ostertagiosis, adult flukes, 20 mg/kg
Sheep: roundworms, tapeworms, Type II ostertagiosis, 7.5 mg/kg
Adult flukes, 20 mg/kg

Hapadex Cattle Wormer (Schering-Plough) *Eire*
Oral suspension, netobimin 150 mg/mL, for *cattle*
Withdrawal Periods. Slaughter 10 days, milk 48 hours

Hapadex Sheep Wormer (Schering-Plough) *Eire*
Oral suspension, netobimin 50 mg/mL, for *sheep*
Withdrawal Periods. Slaughter 5 days, milk 72 hours

OXFENDAZOLE

UK

Indications. Gastro-intestinal roundworms, lungworms, and tapeworms (see section 2.1.2) in ruminants; Type II ostertagiosis
Contra-indications. Administration of ruminal boluses to non-ruminating cattle or calves less than 12 weeks of age, concurrent administration of other ruminal boluses (except as specified by manufacturer)
Warnings. If cattle are vaccinated against lungworm, the ruminal bolus should not be administered until 10 to 14 days after the second dose of vaccine
Dose. *By mouth.*
Cattle: 4.5 mg/kg as a single dose
modified-release preparations, (100–400 kg body-weight) 1 ruminal bolus
Sheep: 5 mg/kg as a single dose

PML **Autoworm Finisher** (Schering-Plough) *UK*
Ruminal bolus, m/r, comprising 5 tablets each containing oxfendazole 1.25 g (= total oxfendazole 6.25 g) released at 3-week intervals starting 21 days after administration, for *grazing cattle 100–400 kg body-weight*; 12
Withdrawal Periods. *Cattle*: slaughter 6 months, should not be used in cattle producing milk for human consumption nor in cattle 6 months before calving which precedes the production of milk for human consumption
Dose. *Cattle*: (100–400 kg body-weight) one ruminal bolus

PML **Autoworm First Grazer** (Schering-Plough) *UK*
Ruminal bolus, m/r, comprising 7 tablets each containing oxfendazole 1.25 g (= total oxfendazole 8.75 g) released at 3-week intervals starting 21 days after administration, for *cattle in their first grazing season 100–400 kg body-weight*; 12
Withdrawal Periods. *Cattle*: slaughter 6 months, should not be used in cattle producing milk for human consumption nor in cattle 6 months before calving which precedes the production of milk for human consumption
Dose. *Cattle*: (100–400 kg body-weight) one ruminal bolus

PML **Autoworm Ready Pulse** (Schering-Plough) *UK*
Ruminal bolus, m/r, comprising 7 tablets each containing oxfendazole 1.25 g (= total oxfendazole 8.75 g) released on day of treatment and then at 3-week intervals, for *grazing cattle 100–400 kg body-weight*; 12
Withdrawal Periods. *Cattle*: slaughter 6 months, should not be used in cattle producing milk for human consumption nor in cattle 6 months before calving which precedes the production of milk for human consumption
Dose. *Cattle*: (100–400 kg body-weight) one ruminal bolus

PML **Bovex 2.265%** (Chanelle) *UK*
Oral suspension, oxfendazole 22.65 mg/mL, for *cattle, sheep*
Withdrawal Periods. *Cattle*: slaughter 14 days, milk 3.5 days. *Sheep*: slaughter 21 days, should not be used in sheep producing milk for human consumption

PML **Parafend 5.0% SC** (Norbrook) *UK*
Oral suspension, oxfendazole 50 mg, cobalt (as sulphate) 3.69 mg, selenium (as sodium selenate) 1.1 mg/mL, for *sheep*; 500 mL, 1 litre, other sizes available
Withdrawal Periods. *Sheep:* slaughter 21 days, should not be used in sheep producing milk for human consumption

PML **Parafend** (Norbrook) *UK*
Oral suspension, oxfendazole 22.65 mg/mL, for *sheep*
Withdrawal Periods. *Sheep:* slaughter 21 days, should not be used in sheep producing milk for human consumption

PML **Parafend LV (New Formula)** (Norbrook) *UK*
Oral suspension, oxfendazole 90.6 mg/mL, for *cattle, sheep*
Withdrawal Periods. *Cattle, sheep:* slaughter 21 days, should not be used in cattle, sheep producing milk for human consumption

PML **Performex 5.0% SC** (Novartis) *UK*
Oral suspension, oxfendazole 50 mg, cobalt (as sulphate) 3.69 mg, selenium (as sodium selenate) 1.1 mg/mL, for *sheep*
Withdrawal Periods. Slaughter 21 days, should not be used in sheep producing milk for human consumption

PML **Systamex 2.265** (Schering-Plough) *UK*
Oral suspension, oxfendazole 22.65 mg/mL, for *cattle, sheep*
Withdrawal Periods. *Cattle:* slaughter 28 days, milk 5 days. *Sheep:* slaughter 10 days, should not be used in sheep producing milk for human consumption

PML **Systamex 906** (Schering-Plough) *UK*
Oral suspension, oxfendazole 90.6 mg/mL, for *cattle, sheep*
Withdrawal Periods. *Cattle:* slaughter 28 days, milk 5 days. *Sheep:* slaughter 21 days, should not be used in sheep producing milk for human consumption

PML **Systamex SC** (Schering-Plough) *UK*
Oral suspension, oxfendazole 22.65 mg, cobalt (as sulphate) 1.67 mg, selenium (as sodium selenate) 500 micrograms/mL, for *cattle, sheep*
Withdrawal Periods. *Cattle:* slaughter 28 days, milk 5 days. *Sheep:* slaughter 10 days, should not be used in sheep producing milk for human consumption

Australia
Indications. Gastro-intestinal roundworms in horses and ruminants; lungworms and tapeworms in ruminants
Contra-indications. Administration within 7 days of bromsalans; concurrent treatment with copper sulphate or copper bisulfide; concurrent treatment with rafoxanide in sheep on grain concentrate feed; intraruminal injection in calves less than 12 weeks of age
Dose.
Horses: *by mouth,* 10 mg/kg
Cattle: *by mouth or intraruminal injection,* 4.5–5.0 mg/kg
Sheep, goats: *by mouth,* 4.5 mg/kg

Benzelmin Anthelmintic Paste for Horses (Jurox) *Austral*
Oral paste, oxfendazole 185 g/kg paste, for *horses*
Withdrawal Periods. Slaughter 28 days

Benzelmin Anthelmintic Suspension (Jurox) *Austral*
Oral suspension, oxfendazole 200 g/L, for *horses*
Withdrawal Periods. Slaughter 28 days

Farnam Worma Drench (International Animal Health Products) *Austral*
Oral solution, oxfendazole 100 g/L, for *horses, cattle*
Withdrawal Periods. *Horses:* slaughter 28 days. *Cattle:* slaughter 8 days

Oxazole Concentrated Worming Drench for Cattle and Horses (Dover) *Austral*
Oral solution, oxfendazole 90.6 g/L, for *cattle, horses*
Withdrawal Periods. *Horses:* slaughter 28 days. *Cattle:* slaughter 8 days, milk withdrawal period nil

Oxazole Worming Drench for Sheep, Lambs and Goats (Dover) *Austral*
Oral solution, oxfendazole 22.65 g/L, for *sheep, goats*
Withdrawal Periods. Slaughter 10 days, should not be used in goats or sheep producing milk for human consumption

Oxfen (Virbac) *Austral*
Oral suspension, oxfendazole 22.6 g/L, for *sheep, goats*
Withdrawal Periods. *Sheep:* slaughter 10 days. *Goats:* slaughter 10 days, should not be used in goats producing milk for human consumption

Oxfen C (Virbac) *Austral*
Oral suspension, oxfendazole 90.6 g/L, for *cattle*
Withdrawal Periods. Slaughter 8 days, milk withdrawal period nil

Oxfen L V (Virbac) *Austral*
Oral suspension, oxfendazole 45.3 g/L, for *cattle, goats*
Withdrawal Periods. *Cattle:* slaughter 10 days, milk withdrawal period nil. *Goats:* slaughter 10 days, should not be used in goats producing milk for human consumption.

Systamex Concentrated Drench (Coopers) *Austral*
Oral solution, oxfendazole 90.6 g/L, for *horses, cattle*
Withdrawal Periods. *Horses:* slaughter 28 days. *Cattle:* slaughter 8 days

Systamex Oral (Coopers) *Austral*
Oral solution, oxfendazole 45.3 g/L, for *cattle*
Withdrawal Periods. Slaughter 8 days, milk withdrawal period nil

Systamex Rumen Injection Cattle Wormer (Coopers) *Austral*
Rumen injection, oxfendazole 225 g/L, for *cattle >12 weeks of age*
Withdrawal Periods. Slaughter 8 days

Eire
Indications. Gastro-intestinal roundworms, lungworms, and tapeworms in ruminants
Contra-indications. Administration of ruminal boluses to non-ruminating cattle or calves less than 12 weeks of age, concurrent administration of other ruminal boluses (except as specified by manufacturer)
Warnings. If cattle are vaccinated against lungworm, the ruminal bolus should not be administered until 10–14 days after the second dose of vaccine
Dose. *By mouth.*
Cattle: 4.5 mg/kg; see also preparations details
Sheep: 5 mg/kg

Bovex 2.265% (Chanelle) *Eire*
Oral suspension, oxfendazole 22.65 mg/mL, for *cattle, sheep*
Withdrawal Periods. *Cattle:* slaughter 14 days, milk 84 hours. *Sheep:* slaughter 21 days, milk 84 hours

Parafend 2.265% (Norbrook) *Eire*
Oral suspension, oxfendazole 2.265%, for *cattle, sheep*
Withdrawal Periods. *Cattle:* slaughter 14 days, milk 48 hours. *Sheep:* slaughter 14 days, should not be used in sheep producing milk for human consumption

Parafend 9.06% (Norbrook) *Eire*
Oral suspension, oxfendazole 9.06%, for *cattle, sheep*
Withdrawal Periods. *Cattle:* slaughter 14 days, milk 48 hours. *Sheep:* slaughter 14 days, should not be used in sheep producing milk for human consumption

Repidose Mid Season Pulse Release Bolus with Systamex Cattle Wormer (Schering-Plough) *Eire*
Tablets, oxfendazole 1.25 g, for *cattle 200–400 kg body-weight*
Withdrawal Periods. Slaughter 6 months, should not be used in cattle producing milk for human consumption, or within 6 months of expected calving
Dose. One bolus

Repidose Pulse Release Bolus with Systamex Cattle Wormer (Schering-Plough) *Eire*
Tablets, oxfendazole 750 mg, for *cattle 100–250 kg body-weight*

Withdrawal Periods. Slaughter 6 months, should not be used in cattle producing milk for human consumption
Dose. One bolus

Systamex 2.265 (Schering-Plough) *Eire*
Oral suspension, oxfendazole 22.65 mg/mL, for *cattle, sheep*
Withdrawal Periods. *Cattle*: slaughter 28 days, milk 5 days. *Sheep*: slaughter 21 days, should not be used in sheep producing milk for human consumption

Systamex 906 (Schering-Plough) *Eire*
Oral suspension, oxfendazole 90.6 mg/mL, for *cattle, sheep*
Withdrawal Periods. *Cattle*: slaughter 28 days, milk 5 days. *Sheep*: slaughter 21 days, should not be used in sheep producing milk for human consumption

Vetazole 2.265% (Vetoquinol) *Eire*
Oral suspension, oxfendazole 2.265%, for *cattle, sheep*
Withdrawal Periods. *Cattle*: slaughter 14 days, milk 48 hours. *Sheep*: slaughter 14 days, should not be used in sheep producing milk for human consumption.

New Zealand
Indications. Gastro-intestinal roundworms in horses and ruminants; lungworms and tapeworms in ruminants; flukes in sheep
Contra-indications. Concurrent treatment with bromsalans or copper sulphate
Side-effects. Rarely slight scurfiness thickening of skin with pour-on formulation
Dose. *Horses*: *by mouth*, 10 mg/kg
Cattle: *by mouth*, 4.5 mg/kg
by 'pour-on' application, 15 mg/kg
Sheep, goats: *by mouth*, 4.5 mg/kg

Bomatak-C (Bomac) *NZ*
Oral suspension, oxfendazole 90.6 mg/mL, for *cattle, sheep, goats, deer*
Withdrawal Periods. *Cattle, sheep, goats*: slaughter 10 days, milk 72 hours. *Deer*: slaughter 10 days

Bomatak-C Mineralised (Bomac) *NZ*
Oral suspension, oxfendazole 90.6 mg/mL in a mineral formulation, for *cattle, sheep, goats, deer*
Withdrawal Periods. *Cattle, sheep, goats*: slaughter 10 days, milk 72 hours. *Deer*: slaughter 10 days

Bomatak-S (Bomac) *NZ*
Oral suspension, oxfendazole 22.7 mg/mL, for *cattle, sheep, goats, deer*
Withdrawal Periods. *Cattle, sheep, goats*: slaughter 10 days, milk 72 hours. *Deer*: slaughter 10 days

Bomatak-S Mineralised (Bomac) *NZ*
Oral suspension, oxfendazole 22.7 mg/mL in a mineral formulation, for *cattle, sheep, goats, deer*
Withdrawal Periods. *Cattle, sheep, goats*: slaughter 10 days, milk 72 hours. *Deer*: slaughter 10 days

Bomatak White-Stripe (Bomac) *NZ*
Suspension, pour-on, oxfendazole 75 mg/mL, for *cattle*
Withdrawal Periods. Slaughter 21 days, milk 7 days

Double Strength Oxfen Hi-Mineral (Ancare) *NZ*
Oral suspension, oxfendazole 45.3 mg/mL in a mineral formulation, for *cattle, sheep, goats, deer*
Withdrawal Periods. *Cattle, sheep, goats*: slaughter 10 days, milk 5 days. *Deer*: slaughter 10 days

Eradox (Novartis) *NZ*
Oral suspension, oxfendazole 22.65 mg/mL, for *cattle, sheep*
Withdrawal Periods. *Cattle*: slaughter 10 days, milk 3 days. *Sheep*: slaughter 10 days, milk 6 days

Eradox Low Volume (Novartis) *NZ*
Oral suspension, oxfendazole 90.6 mg/mL, for *cattle, sheep*
Withdrawal Periods. Slaughter 10 days, milk 3 days

Eradox Low Volume Mineralised Plus Selenium (Novartis) *NZ*
Oral suspension, oxfendazole 90.6 mg/mL, selenium 2 mg/mL in a mineral formulation, for *cattle, sheep*
Withdrawal Periods. Slaughter 10 days, milk 3 days

Eradox Mineralised Plus Selenium (Novartis) *NZ*
Oral suspension, oxfendazole 22.65 mg/mL, selenium 0.5 mg/mL in a mineral formulation, for *cattle, sheep*
Withdrawal Periods. *Cattle*: slaughter 10 days, milk 3 days. *Sheep*: slaughter 10 days, milk 6 days

Oxfen (Ancare) *NZ*
Oral solution, oxfendazole 22.65 mg/mL, for *cattle, sheep, goats, deer*
Withdrawal Periods. *Cattle, sheep, goats*: slaughter 10 days, milk 5 days. *Deer*: slaughter 10 days

Oxfen C (Ancare) *NZ*
Oral suspension, oxfendazole 90.6 mg/mL, for *cattle, deer*
Withdrawal Periods. *Cattle*: slaughter 10 days, milk 5 days. *Deer*: slaughter 10 days

Oxfen C Hi-Mineral (Ancare) *NZ*
Oral suspension, oxfendazole 90.6 mg/mL in a mineral formulation, for *cattle, deer*
Withdrawal Periods. *Cattle*: slaughter 10 days, milk 5 days. *Deer*: slaughter 10 days

Oxfen Hi-Mineral (Ancare) *NZ*
Oral suspension, oxfendazole 22.65 mg/mL in a mineral formulation, for *cattle, sheep, goats, deer*
Withdrawal Periods. *Cattle, sheep, goats*: slaughter 10 days, milk 5 days. *Deer*: slaughter 10 days

Spectre (Schering-Plough) *NZ*
Oral suspension, oxfendazole 45.3 mg/mL, for *cattle, sheep, deer*
Withdrawal Periods. *Cattle*: slaughter 10 days, milk 72 hours. *Sheep*: slaughter 10 days, milk 144 hours. *Deer*: slaughter 10 days

Spectre Selenised (Schering-Plough) *NZ*
Oral suspension, oxfendazole 45.3 mg/mL, sodium selenate 1 mg/mL in a mineral formulation, for *cattle, sheep, deer*
Withdrawal Periods. *Cattle*: slaughter 10 days, milk 72 hours. *Sheep*: slaughter 10 days, milk 144 hours. *Deer*: slaughter 10 days

Systamex Low Dose (Schering-Plough) *NZ*
Oral suspension, oxfendazole 90.6 mg/mL, for *horses, cattle, deer*
Withdrawal Periods. *Horses*: slaughter 20 days. *Cattle*: slaughter 10 days, milk 72 hours. *Deer*: slaughter 10 days

Systamex Low Dose Selenised (Schering-Plough) *NZ*
Oral suspension, oxfendazole 90.6 mg/mL in a mineral formulation, for *cattle, deer*
Withdrawal Periods. *Cattle*: slaughter 10 days, milk 72 hours. *Deer*: slaughter 10 days

Systamex Mineralised (Schering-Plough) *NZ*
Oral suspension, oxfendazole 22.65 mg/mL in a mineral formulation, for *cattle, sheep, deer*

Systamex Oral Drench (Schering-Plough) *NZ*
Oral suspension, oxfendazole 22.65 mg/mL, for *cattle, sheep, deer*
Withdrawal Periods. *Cattle*: slaughter 10 days, milk 72 hours. *Sheep*: slaughter 10 days, milk 144 hours. *Deer*: slaughter 10 days

Systamex Selenised (Schering-Plough) *NZ*
Oral suspension, oxfendazole 22.65 mg/mL in a mineral formulation, for *cattle, sheep, deer*
Withdrawal Periods. *Cattle*: slaughter 10 days, milk 72 hours. Sheep: slaughter 10 days, milk 144 hours. Deer: slaughter 10 days

USA
Indications. Gastro-intestinal roundworms in horses and cattle; lungworms and tapeworms in cattle
Dose. *By mouth*.
Horses: 10 mg/kg
Cattle: 4.5 mg/kg

Benzelmin Paste (Fort Dodge) *USA*
Oral paste, oxfendazole 4.5 g/12 g, 27 g/72 g, for **horses**
Withdrawal Periods. Should not be used in **horses** intended for human consumption

Benzelmin Suspension (Fort Dodge) *USA*
Oral suspension, oxfendazole 90.6 mg/mL, for **horses**
Withdrawal Periods. Should not be used in **horses** intended for human consumption

Synanthic Bovine Dewormer Paste 18.5% (Fort Dodge) *USA*
Oral paste, oxfendazole 185 mg/g paste, for **cattle**
Withdrawal Periods. Slaughter 11 days, should not be used in cattle producing milk for human consumption.

Synanthic Bovine Dewormer Suspension, (9.06%) (Fort Dodge) *USA*
Oral suspension, oxfendazole 90.06 mg/mL, for **cattle**
Withdrawal Periods. Slaughter 7 days, should not be used in cattle producing milk for human consumption

Synanthic Bovine Dewormer Suspension, (22.5%) (Fort Dodge) *USA*
Oral suspension, oxfendazole 225 mg/mL, for **cattle**
Withdrawal Periods. Slaughter 7 days, should not be used in cattle producing milk for human consumption

OXIBENDAZOLE

UK
Indications. Gastro-intestinal roundworms in horses
Dose. *Horses*: roundworms, *by mouth,* 10 mg/kg
Strongyloides westeri, by mouth, 15 mg/kg

PML **Lincoln Horse and Pony Wormer** (Battle Hayward & Bower) *UK*
Oral paste, oxibendazole 1 g/division, for **horses**; 17-g metered-dose applicator
Withdrawal Periods. Should not be used in **horses** intended for human consumption

Australia
Indications. Gastro-intestinal roundworms in horses
Dose. *By mouth.*
Horses: 10 mg/kg
Foals up to 6 months of age: *Strongyloides westeri*, 15 mg/kg

Anthelcide EQ (Ranvet) *Austral*
Oral suspension, oxibendazole 100 g/L, for **horses**
Withdrawal Periods. *Horses*: slaughter 28 days

Oximinth Horse Worming Paste (Virbac) *Austral*
Oral paste, oxibendazole 1 g/5 mL, for **horses**
Withdrawal Periods. *Horses*: slaughter 28 days

Eire
Indications. Gastro-intestinal roundworms in pigs
Dose. *Pigs*: *alone or by addition to feed (pellets)*, 15 mg/kg body-weight

Loditac 3% (Pfizer) *Eire*
Oral pellets, oxibendazole 30 mg/g, for **pigs**
Withdrawal Periods. Slaughter 14 days

USA
Indications. Gastro-intestinal roundworms in horses
Dose. *By mouth.*
Horses: 10 mg/kg
Foals up to 6 months of age: *Strongyloides westeri*, 15 mg/kg

Anthelcide EQ (Pfizer) *USA*
Oral paste, oxibendazole 22.7%, for **horses**
Withdrawal Periods. Should not be used in **horses** intended for human consumption

Anthelcide EQ (Pfizer) *USA*
Oral suspension, oxibendazole 10%, for **horses**
Withdrawal Periods. Should not be used in **horses** intended for human consumption

THIOPHANATE

UK
Indications. Gastro-intestinal roundworms in ruminants and pigs; Type II ostertagiosis
Dose. See preparation details

PML **Nemafax 14** (Merial) *UK*
Oral powder, for addition to feed, thiophanate 225 g/kg, for **cattle, sheep, goats, pigs**; 10 kg
Withdrawal Periods. *Cattle, sheep, goats*: slaughter 7 days, milk 3 days. *Pigs*: slaughter 7 days
Dose. *Cattle, sheep, goats*: 9 kg of thiophanate/tonne feed as a single dose *or* 2.8 kg of thiophanate/tonne feed daily for 5 days *or* 675 g of thiophanate/tonne feed daily for 20 days
Pigs: 2.25–4.5 kg of thiophanate/tonne feed as a single dose *or* 150–450 g of thiophanate/tonne feed daily for 14 days

Australia
Indications. Gastro-intestinal roundworms in pigs
Dose. *Pigs*: 450 g of thiophanate/tonne feed

Nemafax 14 (Rhône-Poulenc) *Austral*
Oral powder, thiophanate 225 g/kg powder, for **pigs**
Withdrawal Periods. Slaughter 14 days

New Zealand
Indications. Gastro-intestinal roundworms in pigs
Dose. *Pigs*: 225–450 g of thiophanate/tonne feed

Nemafax Pig Wormer (PCL) *NZ*
Premix, thiophanate 225 g/kg, for **pigs**
Withdrawal Periods. Slaughter 7 days

TIABENDAZOLE
(Thiabendazole)

UK
Indications. Dose. See Prescribing for amphibians

POM Ⓗ **Mintezol** (MSD) *UK*
Tablets, tiabendazole 500 mg

2.1.1.3 Imidazothiazoles

Levamisole and **tetramisole** are imidazothiazoles that act by interfering with parasite nerve transmission causing muscular paralysis and rapid expulsion. Products containing imidazothiazoles are labelled with the symbol 2-LM. Levamisole is the active isomer of tetramisole and is therefore more potent and has a wider safety margin.

Levamisole is effective against adult and larval gastro-intestinal roundworm and lungworm infections. The margin of safety of levamisole is relatively low in animals, especially in horses♦ and dogs♦. The clinical signs of toxicity include salivation and muscle tremors. Resistance to levamisole is emerging as a problem on some sheep farms in the UK.

Levamisole also modulates cell-mediated immune responses by restoring depressed T-cell function. The term 'immunostimulant' has often been used; it is appropriate only so far as restoration of depressed response is concerned; stimulation above normal does not seem to occur.

LEVAMISOLE

UK
Indications. Gastro-intestinal roundworms in ruminants and pigeons; lungworms in ruminants and dogs♦; heartworm treatment in dogs♦ (seek specialist advice); immune stimulation♦

Contra-indications. Administration within 14 days of treatment with organophosphorus compounds or diethylcarbamazine. (However, may be treated with phosmet or dichlorvos for warble fly concurrently.) Application of 'pour-on' formulations to wet animals and prevent exposure to rain for 1 hour after treatment

Side-effects. Transient coughing; overdosage may cause transient muscle tremors, salivation, nervous symptoms, and colic; occasional skin irritation and epidermal flaking at pour-on application site; vomiting in pigeons; slight reaction at injection site

Warnings. Operators should wear protective clothing. Levamisole may cause idiosyncratic reactions and serious blood disorders in a small number of people. Seek medical advice immediately if dizziness, nausea, vomiting, abdominal discomfort, sore mouth or throat, or fever occur during or shortly after product application.

Dose. *Horses*♦: immune stimulation, *by mouth*, 6.5 mg/kg daily for 14 days
by intramuscular injection, 5.5 mg/kg
Cattle: roundworms, *by mouth or by subcutaneous injection*, 7.5 mg/kg
by 'pour-on' application, 10 mg/kg
Sheep: roundworms, *by mouth or by subcutaneous injection*, 7.5 mg/kg
Goats♦: roundworms, *by mouth,* 12 mg/kg but should be used with caution
Dogs♦: *Angiostrongylus, by mouth,* 7.5 mg/kg daily for 2 days, then 10 mg/kg daily for 2 days
Immune stimulation, *by mouth,* 0.5–2.0 mg/kg every 2–3 days
Pigeons: roundworms, *by mouth,* 20 mg

PML **Anthelpor 20** (Young's) *UK*
Solution, 'pour-on', levamisole 200 mg/mL, for *cattle*; 500 mL, 2.5 litres
Withdrawal Periods. *Cattle*: slaughter 22 days, should not be used on cattle producing milk for human consumption
Note. Use Endecto dosing gun for administration

PML **Armadose Breakwormer** (Bayer) *UK*
Oral solution, levamisole hydrochloride 75 mg/mL, for *cattle, sheep*; 500 mL
Withdrawal Periods. *Cattle, sheep*: slaughter 18 days, should not be used in cattle, sheep producing milk for human consumption

PML **Chanaverm 1.5%** (Chanelle) *UK*
Oral solution, levamisole hydrochloride 15 mg/mL, for *cattle, sheep*
Withdrawal Periods. *Cattle, sheep*: slaughter 18 days, should not be used in cattle or sheep producing milk for human consumption

PML **Chanaverm 7.5%** (Chanelle) *UK*
Oral solution, levamisole hydrochloride 75 mg/mL, for *cattle, sheep*
Withdrawal Periods. *Cattle, sheep*: slaughter 18 days, should not be used in cattle or sheep producing milk for human consumption

PML **Decazole Forte** (Bimeda) *UK*
Oral solution, levamisole hydrochloride 75 mg/mL, for *cattle, sheep*
Withdrawal Periods. *Cattle, sheep*: slaughter 28 days, should not be used in cattle, sheep producing milk for human consumption

PML **Levacide 3% Drench** (Norbrook) *UK*
Oral solution, levamisole hydrochloride 30 mg/mL, for *cattle, sheep*
Withdrawal Periods. *Cattle*: slaughter 14 days, should not be used in cattle producing milk for human consumption. *Sheep*: slaughter 21 days, should not be used in sheep producing milk for human consumption

PML **Levacide Low Volume** (Norbrook) *UK*
Oral solution, levamisole hydrochloride 75 mg/mL, for *cattle, sheep*
Withdrawal Periods. *Cattle*: slaughter 14 days, should not be used in cattle producing milk for human consumption. *Sheep*: slaughter 21 days, should not be used in sheep producing milk for human consumption

PML **Levacide Worm Drench** (Norbrook) *UK*
Oral solution, levamisole hydrochloride 15 mg/mL, for *cattle, sheep*
Withdrawal Periods. *Cattle*: slaughter 14 days, should not be used in cattle producing milk for human consumption. *Sheep*: slaughter 21 days, should not be used in sheep producing milk for human consumption

PML **Levacide** (Norbrook) *UK*
Injection, levamisole hydrochloride 75 mg/mL, for *cattle, sheep*
Withdrawal Periods. *Cattle*: slaughter 14 days, should not be used in cattle producing milk for human consumption. *Sheep*: slaughter 28 days, should not be used in sheep producing milk for human consumption

PML **Levacide Pour-on** (Norbrook) *UK*
Solution, 'pour-on', levamisole 200 mg/mL, for *cattle*; 500 mL, 2.5 litres
Withdrawal Periods. *Cattle*: slaughter 21 days, should not be used on cattle producing milk for human consumption

PML **Levacur SC** (Intervet) *UK*
Oral solution, levamisole hydrochloride 30 mg, cobalt (as sulphate heptahydrate) 1.6 mg, selenium (as sodium selenate) 320 micrograms/mL, for *cattle, sheep*; 2.5 litres, 5 litres
Withdrawal Periods. *Cattle*: slaughter 7 days, should not be used in cattle producing milk for human consumption. *Sheep*: slaughter 10 days, should not be used in sheep producing milk for human consumption

PML **Levadin 15 Drench** (Vétoquinol) *UK*
Oral solution, levamisole 15 mg/mL, for *cattle, sheep*; 5 litres
Withdrawal Periods. *Cattle*: slaughter 14 days, should not be used in cattle producing milk for human consumption. *Sheep*: slaughter 21 days, should not be used in sheep producing milk for human consumption

PML **Levadin 75** (Vétoquinol) *UK*
Injection, levamisole hydrochloride 75 mg/mL, for *cattle, sheep*; 100 mL, 250 mL, 500 mL
Withdrawal Periods. *Cattle*: slaughter 14 days, should not be used in cattle producing milk for human consumption. *Sheep*: slaughter 21 days, should not be used in sheep producing milk for human consumption

PML **Nilverm Gold** (Schering-Plough) *UK*
Oral solution, levamisole hydrochloride 30 mg/mL, for *cattle, sheep*
Withdrawal Periods. *Cattle*: slaughter 7 days, should not be used in cattle producing milk for human consumption. *Sheep*: slaughter 10 days, should not be used in sheep producing milk for human consumption

PML **Nilverm Super Drench** (Schering-Plough) *UK*
Oral solution, levamisole hydrochloride 30 mg, cobalt sulphate heptahydrate 7.64 mg, sodium selenate 766 micrograms/mL, for *cattle, sheep*
Withdrawal Periods. *Cattle*: slaughter 7 days, should not be used in cattle producing milk for human consumption. *Sheep*: slaughter 10 days, should not be used in sheep producing milk for human consumption

PML **Niratil Pour-On** (Virbac) *UK*
Solution, 'pour-on', levamisole 200 mg/mL, for *cattle*; 500 mL, 2.5 litres
Withdrawal Periods. *Cattle*: slaughter 35 days, should not be used on cattle producing milk for human consumption

PML **Ripercol 3.2%** (Janssen) *UK*
Oral solution, levamisole hydrochloride 32 mg/mL, for *sheep*; 1 litre, 5 litres
Withdrawal Periods. *Sheep*: slaughter 10 days, should not be used in sheep producing milk for human consumption

PML **Ripercol Pour-on** (Janssen) *UK*
Solution, 'pour-on', levamisole 200 mg/mL, for *cattle*
Withdrawal Periods. *Cattle*: slaughter 22 days, should not be used on cattle producing milk for human consumption

GSL **Spartakon** (Harkers) *UK*
Tablets, scored, levamisole (as hydrochloride) 20 mg, for *pigeons*; 50
Withdrawal Periods. Should not be used in *birds* intended for human consumption
Dose. *Pigeons*: *by mouth*, 1 tablet/bird

PML **Sure LD** (Young's) *UK*
Oral solution, levamisole hydrochloride 75 mg/mL, for *cattle, sheep*
Withdrawal Periods. *Cattle*: slaughter 18 days, should not be used in cattle producing milk for human consumption. *Sheep*: slaughter 21 days, should not be used in sheep producing milk for human consumption

PML **Vermisole** (Bimeda) *UK*
Injection, levamisole hydrochloride 75 mg/mL, for *cattle, sheep*; 250 mL
Withdrawal Periods. *Cattle, sheep*: slaughter 28 days, should not be used in cattle, sheep producing milk for human consumption

PML **Wormaway Levam** (DiverseyLever) *UK*
Oral solution, levamisole hydrochloride 75 mg/mL, for *cattle, sheep*
Withdrawal Periods. *Cattle, sheep*: slaughter 28 days, should not be used in cattle, sheep producing milk for human consumption

PML **Wormaway Levamisole Injection** (Diversey Lever) *UK*
Injection, levamisole hydrochloride 75 mg/mL, for *cattle, sheep*; 500 mL
Withdrawal Periods. *Cattle, sheep*: slaughter 28 days, should not be used in cattle, sheep producing milk for human consumption

Australia

Indications. Gastro-intestinal roundworms in ruminants, pigs, birds; lungworms in ruminants; gapeworms in birds
Contra-indications. Carbon tetrachloride within 72 hours of treatment; dogs or horses; treatment of birds in hot dry weather, stressed birds, during the breeding or racing season, birds with young
Side-effects. Transient excitement, tremors, and salivation in cattle with overdosage; vomiting in birds
Warnings. Care in weak or pregnant animals; care in parrots
Dose.
Cattle: *by mouth*, 8 mg/kg
by subcutaneous injection, 6 mg/kg
by 'pour-on' application, 10 mg/kg
Sheep: *by mouth*, 8 mg/kg
by subcutaneous injection, 6 mg/kg
Pigs: *by mouth*, 8 mg/kg
Poultry, birds: dosages vary, consult manufacturer's information

Avitrol Bird Wormer Syrup Concentrate (Mavlab) *Austral*
Syrup, levamisole hydrochloride 10 mg/mL, for *cage birds*
Withdrawal Periods. Slaughter 7 days

Avitrol Bird Wormer Tablets (Mavlab) *Austral*
Tablets, levamisole hydrochloride 20 mg, for *cage birds*
Withdrawal Periods. Slaughter 7 days

Citarin Pour On (Bayer) *Austral*
Solution, pour-on, levamisole 200 mg/L, for *cattle*
Withdrawal Periods. Slaughter 3 days, milk 24 hours

Injectable Levamisole (Novartis) *Austral*
Injection, levamisole (as phosphate) 60 g/L, for *cattle, sheep*
Withdrawal Periods. Slaughter 3 days

Levamisole (Nufarm) *Austral*
Oral solution, levamisole hydrochloride 32 g/L, for *cattle, sheep*
Withdrawal Periods. *Cattle*: slaughter 3 days, milk withdrawal period nil. *Sheep*: slaughter 3 days

Levamisole (Western Stock Distributors) *Austral*
Oral solution, levamisole hydrochloride 32 g/L, for *cattle, sheep*
Withdrawal Periods. Slaughter 3 days

Levamisole 80 (Nufarm) *Austral*
Oral solution, levamisole hydrochloride 80 g/L, for *cattle, sheep*

Levamisole Concentrate (Controlled Medications) *Austral*
Powder, for addition to drinking water, levamisole hydrochloride 995 g/kg, for *poultry*
Withdrawal Periods. Slaughter 7 days, egg withdrawal period nil

Levamisole Gold (Virbac) *Austral*
Oral solution, levamisole hydrochloride 32 g/L, for *cattle, sheep*
Withdrawal Periods. *Cattle*: slaughter 3 days, should not be used in cattle producing milk for human consumption. *Sheep*: slaughter 3 days

Levamisole Gold Low Volume (Virbac) *Austral*
Oral solution, levamisole hydrochloride 75 g/L, for *cattle, sheep*
Withdrawal Periods. *Cattle*: slaughter 3 days, should not be used in cattle producing milk for human consumption. *Sheep*: slaughter 3 days

Levamisole Oral Anthelmintic for Sheep and Cattle (Novartis) *Austral*
Oral solution, levamisole hydrochloride 32 g/L, for *cattle, sheep*
Withdrawal Periods. Slaughter 3 days

Levamisole Poultry Wormer (CCD) *Austral*
Powder, for addition to drinking water, levamisole hydrochloride 850 mg/kg, for *poultry, pigeons, cage birds*
Withdrawal Periods. Slaughter 7 days

Levamisole Pour-On (Virbac) *Austral*
Solution, pour-on, levamisole 200 g/L, for *cattle*
Withdrawal Periods. Slaughter 3 days, milk 24 hours

Levipor (Novartis) *Austral*
Solution, pour-on, levamisole 20%, for *cattle*
Withdrawal Periods. Slaughter 3 days, milk withdrawal period nil

Low Volume Levamisole Oral Anthelmintic (Novartis) *Austral*
Oral solution, levamisole hydrochloride 80 g/L, for *cattle, sheep*
Withdrawal Periods. Slaughter 3 days

Low Volume Levamisole with Selenium (Novartis) *Austral*
Oral solution, levamisole 80 g/L, selenium (as sodium selenate) 1 g/L, for *cattle, sheep*
Withdrawal Periods. Slaughter 3 days

LV Levamisole (Western Stock Distributors) *Austral*
Oral solution, levamisole hydrochloride 80 g/L, for *cattle, sheep*
Withdrawal Periods. Slaughter 3 days

Mineralised Levamisole (Virbac) *Austral*
Oral solution, levamisole hydrochloride 80 mg/mL (with minerals), for *cattle, sheep*
Withdrawal Periods. *Cattle*: slaughter withdrawal period nil, should not be used in cattle producing milk for human consumption

Nilverm Injection (Coopers) *Austral*
Injection, levamisole (as phosphate) 60 g/L, for *cattle, sheep*
Withdrawal Periods. *Cattle*: slaughter 3 days, milk withdrawal period nil. *Sheep*: slaughter 3 days

Nilverm LV (Coopers) *Austral*
Oral solution, levamisole hydrochloride 80 g/L, for *cattle, sheep*
Withdrawal Periods. *Cattle*: slaughter 3 days, milk withdrawal period nil. *Sheep*: slaughter 3 days

Nilverm Oral (Coopers) *Austral*
Oral solution, levamisole hydrochloride 32 g/L, for *cattle, sheep*
Withdrawal Periods. *Cattle*: slaughter 3 days, milk withdrawal period nil. *Sheep*: slaughter 3 days

Nilverm Pig and Poultry Wormer (Coopers) *Austral*
Oral solution, levamisole hydrochloride 16 g/L, for *pigs, poultry*
Withdrawal Periods. *Pigs*: slaughter 3 days. *Poultry*: Slaughter 7 days, egg withdrawal period nil

Nilverm Pour On Cattle Wormer (Coopers) *Austral*
Solution, pour-on, levamisole 125 g/L, for *cattle*
Withdrawal Periods. Slaughter 3 days, milk withdrawal period nil

Ripercol Soluble Powder (Pfizer) *Austral*
Oral powder, for drench, levamisole hydrochloride 999 g/kg powder, for *sheep*
Withdrawal Periods. Slaughter 3 days, should not be used in sheep producing milk for human consumption

Eire

Indications. Gastro-intestinal roundworms in ruminants and pigs; lungworms in ruminants
Contra-indications. Administration within 14 days of treatment with organophosphorus compounds or diethylcarbamazine; hypersensitivity to levamisole; application of 'pour-on' formulations to wet animals
Side-effects. Overdosage may cause transient muscle tremors, salivation, nervous symptoms; transientreaction at injection site; occasional vomiting in pigs
Warnings. Care in heavily pregnant animals
Dose.
Cattle: *by mouth or by subcutaneous injection*, 7.5 mg/kg *by 'pour-on' application*, 10 mg/kg
Sheep, goats: *by mouth or by subcutaneous injection*, 7.5 mg/kg
Pigs: *by subcutaneous injection*, 7.5 mg/kg

Ascara Worm Drench (Univet) *Eire*
Oral solution, levamisole hydrochloride 15 mg/mL, for *cattle*
Withdrawal Periods. Slaughter 28 days, should not be used in cattle producing milk for human consumption

Ascaraject (Univet) *Eire*
Injection, levamisole hydrochloride 75 mg/mL, for *cattle*
Withdrawal Periods. Slaughter 28 days, should not be used in cattle producing milk for human consumption

Boverm (Foran) *Eire*
Oral solution, levamisole hydrochloride 15 mg/mL, for *cattle, sheep*
Withdrawal Periods. Slaughter 35 days, should not be used in cattle or sheep producing milk for human consumption

Cahlverm Worm Drench (Co-operative Animal Health) *Eire*
Oral solution, levamisole hydrochloride 15 mg/mL, for *cattle, sheep*
Withdrawal Periods. Slaughter 28 days

Chanaverm 7.5% (Chanelle) *Eire*
Oral solution, levamisole hydrochloride 75 mg/mL, for *cattle, sheep*
Withdrawal Periods. Slaughter 18 days, should not be used in cattle or sheep producing milk for human consumption

Chanaverm Plus (Chanelle) *Eire*
Oral solution, levamisole hydrochloride 15 mg/mL, cobalt sulphate 3.8 mg/mL, for *cattle, sheep*
Withdrawal Periods. Slaughter 18 days, should not be used in cattle or sheep producing milk for human consumption

Duphalevasole Injection (Interchem) *Eire*
Injection, levamisole hydrochloride 75mg/mL, for *cattle, sheep*
Withdrawal Periods. *Cattle*: slaughter 14 days, milk 84 hours. *Sheep*: slaughter 14 days, should not be used in sheep producing milk for human consumption

Levacide 1.5% SC Worm Drench (Norbrook) *Eire*
Oral solution, levamisole hydrochloride 1.5% (also contains selenium and cobalt), for *cattle, sheep*
Withdrawal Periods. Slaughter 14 days, should not be used in cattle or sheep producing milk for human consumption

Levacide Injection (Norbrook) *Eire*
Injection, levamisole hydrochloride 7.5%, for *cattle, sheep*
Withdrawal Periods. Slaughter 14 days, should not be used in cattle or sheep producing milk for human consumption

Levacide Low Volume (Norbrook) *Eire*
Oral solution, levamisole hydrochloride 7.5%, for *cattle, sheep*
Withdrawal Periods. Slaughter 14 days, should not be used in cattle or sheep producing milk for human consumption

Levacide Pour-On (Norbrook) *Eire*
Solution, pour-on, levamisole 200 mg/mL, for *cattle*
Withdrawal Periods. Slaughter 21 days, should not be used in cattle producing milk for human consumption

Levapharm Injection (Interpharm) *Eire*
Injection, levamisole hydrochloride 75 mg/mL, for *cattle, sheep, pigs*
Withdrawal Periods. *Cattle, sheep*: slaughter 14 days, should not be used in cattle or sheep producing milk for human consumption. *Pigs*: slaughter 5 days

Levapharm Plus Worm Drench (Interpharm) *Eire*
Oral drench, levamisole hydrochloride 15 mg/mL, for *cattle, sheep, goats*
Withdrawal Periods. *Cattle, sheep*: slaughter 14 days, should not be used in cattle or sheep producing milk for human consumption. *Goats*: slaughter 14 days

Nilverm Plus (Schering-Plough) *Eire*
Oral suspension, levamisole hydrochloride 15 mg/mL (also contains cobalt), for *cattle, sheep*
Withdrawal Periods. *Cattle*: slaughter 7 days, should not be used in cattle producing milk for human consumption. *Sheep*: slaughter 10 days, should not be used in sheep producing milk for human consumption

Ripercol Pour On (Janssen) *Eire*
Solution, pour-on, levamisole 200 mg/mL, for *cattle*
Withdrawal Periods. Slaughter 21 days, should not be used in cattle producing milk for human consumption

New Zealand

Indications. Gastro-intestinal roundworms and lungworms in ruminants
Contra-indications. Hepatic impairment; concurrent organophosphorus compounds, within 72 hours of carbon tetrachloride; pour-n formulation on animals that are wet
Warnings. Care in pregnant animals
Dose.
Cattle: *by mouth*, 8 mg/kg
by 'pour-on' application, 10 mg/kg
Sheep: *by mouth*, 8 mg/kg

All-Min Levamisole (Nufarm) *NZ*
Oral solution, levamisole hydrochloride 40 mg/mL in a mineral formulation, for *cattle, sheep*
Withdrawal Periods. Slaughter 10 days, milk 24 hours

Anthelpor (Novartis) *NZ*
Solution, pour-on, levamisole 200 g/litre, for *cattle*
Withdrawal Periods. Slaughter 10 days, milk 24 hours

Centor (Schering-Plough) *NZ*
Oral solution, levamisole hydrochloride 80 mg/mL, for *cattle, sheep*
Withdrawal Periods. Slaughter 10 days, milk 24 hours

Centor Selenised (Schering-Plough) *NZ*
Oral solution, levamisole hydrochloride 80 mg/mL in a mineral formulation, for *cattle, sheep*
Withdrawal Periods. Slaughter 10 days, milk 24 hours

Citarin-L (Bayer) *NZ*
Oral solution, levamisole 40 mg/mL, for *cattle, sheep*
Withdrawal Periods. Slaughter 10 days, milk 24 hours

Endozole (Novartis) *NZ*
Oral suspension, levamisole hydrochloride 40 mg/mL, for *cattle, sheep*
Withdrawal Periods. Slaughter 10 days, milk 96 hours

Endozole Mineralised Plus Selenium (Novartis) *NZ*
Oral suspension, levamisole hydrochloride 40 mg/mL, selenium 0.5 mg/mL in a mineral formulation, for *cattle, sheep*
Withdrawal Periods. Slaughter 10 days, milk 96 hours

Levicare (Ancare) *NZ*
Oral solution, levamisole 40 mg/mL, for *cattle, sheep*
Withdrawal Periods. Slaughter 10 days, milk 24 hours

Levicare Hi-Mineral (Ancare) *NZ*
Oral solution, levamisole 40 mg/mL in a mineral formulation, for *cattle, sheep*
Withdrawal Periods. Slaughter 10 days, milk 24 hours

Nilverm (Schering-Plough) *NZ*
Oral solution, levamisole hydrochloride 40 mg/mL, for *cattle, sheep*
Withdrawal Periods. *Cattle*: slaughter 10 days, milk 24 hours. *Sheep*: slaughter 10 days, should not be used in sheep producing milk for human consumption

Nilverm Mineralised (Schering-Plough) *NZ*
Oral solution, levamisole hydrochloride 40 mg/mL in a mineral formulation, for *cattle, sheep*
Withdrawal Periods. *Cattle*: slaughter 10 days, milk 2 days. *Sheep*: slaughter 10 days, should not be used in sheep producing milk for human consumption

Nilverm Selenised (Schering-Plough) *NZ*
Oral solution, levamisole hydrochloride 40 mg/mL, sodium selenate 0.5 mg/mL, in a mineral formulation, for *cattle, sheep*
Withdrawal Periods. *Cattle*: slaughter 10 days, milk 24 hours. *Sheep*: slaughter 10 days, should not be used in sheep producing milk for human consumption

Rycozole (Novartis) *NZ*
Oral solution, levamisole hydrochloride 40 mg/mL, for *cattle, sheep*
Withdrawal Periods. Slaughter 10 days, milk 24 hours

Rycozole Mineralised Plus Selenium (Novartis) *NZ*
Oral solution, levamisole hydrochloride 40 mg/mL, selenium (as sodium salt) 0.5 mg/mL in a mineral formulation, for *cattle, sheep*
Withdrawal Periods. Slaughter 10 days, milk 24 hours

Vermatak (Bomac) *NZ*
Oral solution, levamisole hydrochloride 40 mg/mL, for *cattle, sheep*
Withdrawal Periods. Slaughter 10 days, milk 24 hours

Vermatak Mineralised (Bomac) *NZ*
Oral solution, levamisole hydrochloride 40 mg/mL in a mineral formulation, for *cattle, sheep*
Withdrawal Periods. Slaughter 10 days, should not be used in cattle or sheep producing milk for human consumption

USA

Indications. Gastro-intestinal roundworms and lungworms in ruminants and pigs

Contra-indications. Pour-on formulation on animals that are wet
Side-effects. Transient salivation or foaming at the muzzle; coughing and vomiting in pigs; skin flaking at pour-on application site
Dose.
Cattle: *by mouth*, 8 mg/kg
by subcutaneous injection, 6 mg/kg
by 'pour-on' application, 10 mg/kg
Sheep: *by mouth*, 8 mg/kg
Pigs: *by mouth*, 8 mg/kg

Aspen Brand of Levamisole Phosphate (Aspen) *USA*
Injection, levamisole hydrochloride (as phosphate) 136.5 mg/mL, for *cattle*
Withdrawal Periods. Slaughter 7 days, should not be used in cattle producing milk for human consumption

Levamisole (AgriLabs) *USA*
Powder, for reconstitution and addition to drinking water, levamisole hydrochloride 18.15 g, for *pigs*
Withdrawal Periods. Slaughter 3 days

Levamisole Phosphate (AgriLabs) *USA*
Injection, levamisole hydrochloride (as equivalent phosphate) 136.5 mg/mL, for *cattle*
Withdrawal Periods. Slaughter 7 days, should not be used in cattle producing milk for human consumption

Levasole Cattle Wormer Boluses (Schering-Plough) *USA*
Tablets, levamisole hydrochloride 2.19 g, for *cattle*
Withdrawal Periods. Slaughter 2 days, should not be used in cattle producing milk for human consumption
Dose: 0.5–1.5 tablets (depending on body-weight)

Levasole Injectable Solution 13.65% (Schering-Plough) *USA*
Injection, levamisole hydrochloride (as equivalent phosphate) 136.5 mg/mL, for *cattle*
Withdrawal Periods. Slaughter 7 days, should not be used in cattle producing milk for human consumption

Levasole Sheep Wormer Boluses (Schering-Plough) *USA*
Tablets, levamisole hydrochloride 184 mg, for *sheep*
Withdrawal Periods. Slaughter 3 days

Levasole Soluble Drench Powder (Schering-Plough) *USA*
Powder, for solution, levamisole hydrochloride 544.5 g, for *cattle, sheep*
Withdrawal Periods. *Cattle*: slaughter 2 days, should not be used in cattle producing milk for human consumption. *Sheep*: slaughter 3 days

Levasole Soluble Drench Powder (Schering-Plough) *USA*
Powder, for solution, levamisole hydrochloride 11.7 g, for *sheep*
Withdrawal Periods. Slaughter 3 days

Levasole Soluble Pig Wormer (Schering-Plough) *USA*
Powder, for solution, levamisole hydrochloride 18.15 g, for *pigs*
Withdrawal Periods. Slaughter 3 days

Prohibit (AgriLabs) *USA*
Powder, for oral solution, levamisole 544.5 g/bottle (for 3 L solution), for *cattle, sheep*
Withdrawal Periods. *Cattle*: slaughter 2 days, should not be used in cattle producing milk for human consumption. *Sheep*: slaughter 3 days

Totalon (Schering-Plough) *USA*
Solution, pour-on, levamisole 200 mg/mL, for *cattle*
Withdrawal Periods. Slaughter 9 days; should not beused in cattle producing milk for human consumption

Tramisol Cattle Wormer Oblets (Schering-Plough) *USA*
Tablets, levamisole 2.19 g/oblet (tablet), for *cattle*
Withdrawal Periods. Slaughter 2 days, should not be used in cattle producing milk for human consumption.
Dose: 0.5–1.5 tablets (depending on body-weight)

Tramisol Hog Wormer Mix (Schering-Plough) *USA*
Premix, levamisole hydrochloride (as resinate) 5.806 g/58.01g, for *pigs*
Withdrawal Periods. Slaughter 3 days

Tramisol Injectable Solution 13.65% (Schering-Plough) *USA*
Injection, levamisole hydrochloride (as phosphate) 136.5 mg/mL, for *cattle*
Withdrawal Periods. Slaughter 7 days, should not be used in cattle producing milk for human consumption

Tramisol Sheep Wormer Oblets (Schering-Plough) *USA*
Tablets, levamisole 0.184 g, for *sheep*
Withdrawal Periods. Slaughter 3 days

Tramisol Soluble Drench Powder (Schering-Plough) *USA*
Powder, for drench solution, levamisole hydrochloride 46.8 g/52 g packet, for *cattle, sheep*
Withdrawal Periods. *Cattle*: slaughter 2 days. *Sheep*: slaughter 3 days

Tramisol Soluble Drench Powder (Schering-Plough) *USA*
Powder, for drench solution, levamisole hydrochloride 11.7 g/13 g packet, for *sheep*
Withdrawal Periods. Slaughter 3 days

Tramisol Soluble Pig Wormer (Schering-Plough) *USA*
Powder, for addition to drinking water, levamisole hydrochloride 18.15 g/20.17 g, for *pigs*
Withdrawal Periods. Slaughter 3 days

Tramisol Type A Medicated Article (Schering-Plough) *USA*
Premix, levamisole hydrochloride (as resinate) 227 g/ 454 g premix (50%), for *pigs, cattle*
Withdrawal Periods. *Cattle*: slaughter 2 days, should not be used in cattle producing milk for human consumption. *Pigs*: slaughter 3 days.

2.1.1.4 Organophosphorus compounds

Haloxon, dichlorvos, naftalofos, and **metrifonate** are organophosphorus compounds. They act by inhibiting cholinesterase thereby interfering with neuromuscular transmission in the parasite. They are effective against adult gastro-intestinal roundworms and bots, but ineffective against migrating larvae, tapeworms, or flukes. Clinical signs of toxicity such as salivation and diarrhoea may occasionally occur, particularly in foals. If used as a feed dressing, birds and other animals must not have access to uneaten residues. These compounds should not be given if other anticholinesterases are in use, for example for ectoparasite or environmental insect control.

DICHLORVOS

USA
Indications. Gastro-intestinal roundworms in pigs and dogs
Contra-indications. Do not allow poultry access to feed or faeces from treated pigs; concurrent use with other anthelmintics, muscle relaxants, or tranquilisers; dogs with severe constipation, hepatic impairment, infectious disease, or infected with heartworm
Warnings. Dogs more than 1 year of age from endemic heartworm areas hould be examined for heartworm infection before treatment
Dose. *Pigs*: (>32 kg body-weight) 1.46 g
Dogs: by mouth, 26.4–33.0 mg/kg

Atgard C Swine Wormer (Boehringer Ingelheim NOBL) *USA*
Premix, dichlorvos 9.6%, for *pigs*
Withdrawal Periods. Slaughter withdrawal period nil

Task (Boehringer Ingelheim Vetmedica) *USA*
Pellets, dichlorvos 136 mg, 204 mg, 544 mg, for *dogs*
Capsules, dichlorvos 68 mg, 136 mg, 204 mg, for *dogs*

METRIFONATE
(Metriphonate, Trichlorfon)

Australia
Indications. Gastro-intestinal roundworms in cattle; horse bots
Contra-indications. Administration to mares during last 6 weeks of pregnancy
Dose. *Horses*: 2 g/65 kg body-weight
Cattle: Reconstitute 10 g in 100 mL water. Administer 7.5 mL reconstituted solution/10 kg body-weight

Neguvon Soluble Powder Anthelmintic, Boticide (Bayer) *Austral*
Oral powder, metrifonate 800 g/kg powder, for *horses, cattle*
Withdrawal Periods. *Horses*: slaughter 28 days. *Cattle*: slaughter 5 days, should not be used in cattle producing milk for human consumption

New Zealand
Indications. Endoparasites. Gastro-intestinal roundworms in horses, sheep, and pigs; nasal bots in sheep; horse bots Ectoparasites. See section 2.2.1.5
Contra-indications. Administration to mares during last 6 weeks of pregnancy
Dose. For horses and sheep, reconstitute 15 g powder in 150 mL water.
Horses: 15 mL reconstituted solution/45 kg body-weight
Sheep: 10–45 mL reconstituted solution (depending on body-weight)
Pigs: by addition to feed, 2.5 g of powder/45 kg body-weight

Neguvon 98% (Bayer) *NZ*
Powder for oral solution or spray, metrifonate 980 g/kg, for *horses, sheep, pigs, poultry*
Withdrawal Periods. Slaughter 24 hours

NAFTALOFOS
(Naphthalophos)

Australia
Indications. Gastro-intestinal roundworms in sheep
Contra-indications. Administration to lambs <6kg body-weight or animals affectedby lupinosis

Rametin Sheep Drench (Bayer) *Austral*
Oral powder, for drench, naftalofos 800 g/kg powder, for *sheep*
Withdrawal Periods. *Sheep*: slaughter 7 days

2.1.1.5 Tetrahydropyrimidines

Tetrahydropyrimidines, such as **morantel, oxantel,** and **pyrantel**, interfere with parasitic nerve transmission as cholinergic stimulants, leading to neuromuscular paralysis. Products containing tetrahydropyrimidines are labelled with the symbol 2-LM. These drugs are effective against adult and larval gastro-intestinal roundworms. Pyrantel is also effective at an increased dose against tapeworms in horses.

Morantel is available as a modified-release ruminal bolus. A negligible amount of drug is absorbed systemically by this route.

MORANTEL

UK

Indications. Gastro-intestinal roundworms in ruminants
Contra-indications. Concurrent administration of other ruminal boluses, administration of ruminal boluses to non-ruminating cattle, administration to calves less than 100 kg body-weight and less than 4 months of age, administration less than 14 days after lungworm vaccine
Dose. See preparation details

PML **Exhelm** (Pfizer) *UK*
Oral suspension, morantel (as citrate monohydrate) 29.7 mg/mL, for *sheep*; 1 litre, 2.5 litres, 5 litres
Withdrawal Periods. *Sheep*: slaughter 3 days, should not be used in sheep producing milk for human consumption
Dose. *Sheep*: by mouth, 5.94 mg (0.2 mL)/kg

PML **Paratect Flex Sustained Release Bolus** (Pfizer) *UK*
Ruminal bolus, m/r, morantel (as tartrate) 11.8 g delivered for at least 90 days, for *cattle more than 100 kg body-weight*; 20
Withdrawal Periods. *Cattle*: slaughter withdrawal period nil, milk withdrawal period nil
Dose. *Cattle*: (>100 kg body-weight) one 11.8-g ruminal bolus

Australia

Indications. Gastro-intestinal roundworms in horses, sheep, goats, and pigs; tapeworm in horses
Contra-indications. Administration to foals less than 1 week of age
Dose. *Horses*: by mouth, 10 mg/kg
Sheep, goats: by mouth, 10 mg/kg
Pigs: by addition to feed, 30 g/tonne feed

Equiban Granules (Pfizer) *Austral*
Oral granules, morantel tartrate 115 mg/g, for *horses*
Withdrawal Periods. *Horses*: slaughter 28 days

Equiban Paste (Pfizer) *Austral*
Oral paste, morantel tartrate 150 mg/mL, for *horses*
Withdrawal Periods. *Horses*: slaughter 28 days

Goat and Sheep Wormer (Vetsearch) *Austral*
Oral paste, morantel citrate 30 mg/mL, for *sheep, goats*
Withdrawal Periods. *Goats, sheep*: slaughter 7 days, should not be used in goats and sheep producing milk for human consumption

Wormtec 30 Pig Wormer (Pfizer) *Austral*
Premix, morantel citrate 30 g/kg premix, for *pigs*
Withdrawal Periods. Slaughter withdrawal period nil

Eire

Indications. Gastro-intestinal roundworms and lungworms in cattle
Contra-indications. Administration of ruminal boluses to non-ruminating cattle, administration to calves less than 4 months of age and 100 kg body-weight, administration less than 14 days after lungworm vaccine
Dose. *Cattle*: (>100 kg body-weight) one 11.8-g bolus

Paratect Flex Sustained Release Bolus (Pfizer) *Eire*
Ruminal bolus, morantel (as tartrate) 11.8 g, for *cattle*
Withdrawal Periods. Slaughter withdrawal period nil, milk withdrawal period nil

New Zealand

Indications. Gastro-intestinal roundworms in horses, ruminants, and pigs; tapeworms in horses
Dose. *Horses:* by mouth, 10 mg/kg
Cattle, sheep: by mouth, 10 mg/kg
Pigs: by addition to feed, 30 g/tonne feed

Exhelm-E (Pfizer) *NZ*
Oral suspension, morantel citrate 40 mg/mL, for *cattle, sheep*
Withdrawal Periods. Slaughter 7 days, milk 24 hours

Paraminth Paste (Pfizer) *NZ*
Oral paste, morantel tartrate 150 mg/g, for *horses*

Wormtec 30 (Pfizer) *NZ*
Premix, morantel citrate 30 g/kg, for *pigs*
Withdrawal Periods. Slaughter 14 days

USA

Indications. Gastro-intestinal roundworms in ruminants
Contra-indications. Administration in feeds containing bentonite
Dose. *Cattle, goats*: by addition to feed, 9.68 mg/kg

Rumatel (Pfizer) *USA*
Premix, morantel tartrate 194 mg/g, for *cattle, goats*
Withdrawal Periods. *Cattle*: slaughter 14 days, milk withdrawal period nil.
Goats: slaughter 30 days, milk withdrawal period nil

PYRANTEL EMBONATE
(Pyrantel pamoate)

Note. Pyrantel embonate 2.9 g = pyrantel base 1 g

UK

Indications. Gastro-intestinal roundworms in horses and dogs; tapeworms (see section 2.1.2) in horses
Contra-indications. Foals less than 4 weeks of age; concurrent administration of levamisole, piperazine
Dose. By mouth.
Horses: roundworms, 19 mg/kg
Anoplocephala perfoliata, 38 mg/kg
Dogs: 14.4 mg/kg (= 5 mg pyrantel base/kg)

PML **Pyratape P** (Intervet) *UK*
Oral paste, pyrantel embonate 400 mg/g, for *horses, donkeys, ponies*; 28.5 g dose applicator
Withdrawal Periods. Should not be used in *horses* intended for human consumption

PML **Strongid Caramel** (Pfizer) *UK*
Oral paste, pyrantel embonate 439 mg/g, for *horses and ponies more than 4 weeks of age*; 26-g dose applicator
Withdrawal Periods. Should not be used in *horses* intended for human consumption

PML **Strongid Paste for Dogs** (Pfizer) *UK*
Oral paste, pyrantel base 10 mg/division, for *dogs*; 16-g metered dose applicator

PML **Strongid-P Granules** (Pfizer) *UK*
Oral granules, for addition to feed, to prepare an oral solution, or for administration by gavage, pyrantel embonate 767 mg/g, for *horses and ponies more than 4 weeks of age*; 7.43 g, 1.5 kg
Withdrawal Periods. Should not be used in *horses* intended for human consumption

Australia

Indications. Gastro-intestinal roundworms in dogs
Dose. *Dogs*: *by mouth*, 14.4 mg/kg

Canex (Pfizer) *Austral*
Tablets, pyrantel embonate 143 mg, for *dogs*

Canex Puppy Suspension (Pfizer) *Austral*
Oral suspension, pyrantel embonate 14.4 mg/mL, for *dogs*

Exelpet Palatable Puppy Worming Suspension (Excelpet) *Austral*
Oral suspension, pyrantel embonate 14.4 mg/mL, for *dogs*

Worm Ban (Troy) *Austral*
Oral suspension, pyrantel embonate 14.4.mg/mL, for *dogs*

Eire

Indications. Gastro-intestinal roundworms in horses and dogs; tapeworms in horses
Contra-indications. Foals less than 4 weeks of age
Dose. *By mouth*.
Horses: roundworms, 19 mg/kg
Anoplocephala perfoliata, 38 mg/kg
Dogs: 14.4 mg/kg (= 5 mg pyrantel base/kg)

Pyratape P (Hoechst Roussel) *Eire*
Oral paste, pyrantel embonate 11.4 g/28.5 g oral syringe, for *horses*
Withdrawal Periods. Slaughter 7 days

Strongid Paste for Dogs (Pfizer) *Eire*
Oral paste, pyrantel 7.5 mg/g, for *dogs*

Strongid-P Granules (Pfizer) *Eire*
Oral granules, to mix with feed, pyrantel embonate 346 mg/g, for *horses*
Withdrawal Periods. Should not be used in *horses* intended for human consumption

Strongid-P Paste (Pfizer) *Eire*
Oral paste, pyrantel embonate 11.41 g/26.00 g paste, for *horses*
Withdrawal Periods. Should not be used in *horses* intended for human consumption

New Zealand

Indications. Gastro-intestinal roundworms in dogs and cats
Dose. *By mouth*.
Dogs: 14.4 mg/kg (= 5 mg pyrantel base/kg)
Cats: 50 mg/kg (=20 mg pyrantel base/kg)

Cancare (Ancare) *NZ*
Tablets, pyrantel embonate 100 mg, for *dogs, cats*

Canex Puppy (Pfizer) *NZ*
Oral suspension, pyrantel embonate 14.4 mg/mL, for *dogs*

Wormicide (Virbac) *NZ*
Tablets, pyrantel (as embonate) 50 mg or 100 mg, for *dogs, cats*

USA

Indications. Gastro-intestinal roundworms in horses, pigs, and dogs
Contra-indications. Administration to pigs in feed containing bentonite
Side-effects. Increased respiration rate, profuse sweating, or incoordination in horses
Dose. *By mouth or addition to feed*.
Horses: 6.6 mg pyrantel base/kg *or* 12.5 mg pyrantel tartrate/kg
Dogs: 5 mg pyrantel base/kg

Banminth (Pfizer) *USA*
Premix, pyrantel tartrate 106 g/kg, for *pigs*
Withdrawal Periods. Slaughter 1 day

Equi-Phar Horse & Colt Wormer (Vedco) *USA*
Premix, pyrantel tartrate 12.5 g/kg, for *horses*
Withdrawal Periods. Should not be used in *horses* intended for human consumption

Horsecare Horse & Colt Wormer (DurVet) *USA*
Premix, pyrantel tartrate 1.25%, for *horses*
Withdrawal Periods. Should not be used in *horses* intended for human consumption

Nemex-2 (Pfizer) *USA*
Oral suspension, pyrantel (as embonate) 4.54 mg/mL, for *dogs*

Nemex Tabs (Pfizer) *USA*
Tablets, pyrantel (as embonate) 113.5 mg, for *dogs*

Purina Colt and Horse Wormer (Purina Mills) *USA*
Medicated feed, pyrantel tartrate 12.5 g/kg, for *horses*
Withdrawal Periods. Should not be used in *horses* intended for human consumption

Pyrantel 4.54 (Eudaemonic) *USA*
Oral suspension, pyrantel (as embonate) 4.54 mg/mL, for *dogs*

Pyratabs (Fort Dodge) *USA*
Tablets, pyrantel (as embonate) 22.7 mg, 113.5 mg, for *dogs*

Strongid C (Pfizer) *USA*
Pellets, pyrantel tartrate 10.56 g/kg, for *horses*
Withdrawal Periods. Should not be used in *horses* intended for human consumption

Strongid C 2X (Pfizer) *USA*
Pellets, pyrantel tartrate 21.12 g/kg, for *horses*
Withdrawal Periods. Should not be used in *horses* intended for human consumption

Strongid Paste (Pfizer) *USA*
Oral paste, pyrantel (as embonate) 180 mg/mL, for *horses*
Withdrawal Periods. Should not be used in *horses* intended for human consumption

Strongid T (Pfizer) *USA*
Oral suspension, pyrantel (as embonate) 50 mg/mL, for *horses*
Withdrawal Periods. Should not be used in *horses* intended for human consumption

Sure Shot Liquid Wormer (Performer) *USA*
Oral liquid, pyrantel (as embonate) 2.27 mg/mL, for *dogs*

2.1.1.6 Other drugs for roundworms

Piperazine and **diethylcarbamazine** modify neurotransmission in parasites causing relaxation and subsequent expulsion of helminths. Piperazine is used for treatment of some gastro-intestinal roundworms such as *Toxocara, Toxascaris*, and *Uncinaria* in dogs and cats. Piperazine has little activity against larval *Toxocara* in puppies and is ineffective against lungworms or tapeworms. Large doses of the drug are required for hookworm infection. In the treatment of kittens and small puppies, particular care should be taken to assess body-weight accurately to minimise the risk of ataxia due to overdosing. Benzimidazoles (see section 2.1.1.2) are more effective against larval ascarids than piperazine and therefore prevent faecal egg-output for a longer period. **Diethylcarbamazine** is active against adult ascarids but is more frequently used as a heartworm prophylactic. It must not be given to dogs with microfilaraemia because a hypersensitivity reaction sometimes occurs.

Nitroscanate is used for the control of roundworms and tapeworms (see section 2.1.2) in dogs. **Nitroxinil** is used for the treatment of some roundworm and adult and immature fluke infections (see section 2.1.3). **Closantel**, in addition to its use for treatment of fluke infections, can be used for the treatment of benzimidazole-resistant *Haemonchus* infections in sheep (see section 2.1.3).

Arsenamide, melarsomine and **thiacetarsamide** are arsenical derivatives used for the treatment of canine dirofilariosis. Thiacetarsamide was the standard treatment for adult heartworm infection in dogs for many years. It is hepatotoxic and nephrotoxic and should be used with caution. Liver and kidney function tests should be performed before initiating treatment. Debilitated dogs should first be treated symptomatically to improve their physical condition. The drug is administered intravenously; oedematous swelling and skin sloughing may occur if the drug is deposited subcutaneously. The recently introduced melarsomine is given by deep intramuscular injection. It is more effective and safer than thiacetarsamide but needs to be used with care. **Specialist advice should be sought before treating** *Dirofilaria* **infections.**

Disophenol is a narrow-spectrum compound active against adult hookworms in dogs. It has a narrow safety margin. It is also effective against the gapeworm *Syngamus trachea* in poultry.

Hygromycin B is a fermentation product used as a feed additive which, over a period of weeks, gives moderately effective control of gastro-intestinal roundworms in pigs and poultry. Continuous feeding may lead to deafness in pigs.

DIETHYLCARBAMAZINE

Australia

Indications. Heartworm prophylaxis in dogs
Contra-indications. Administration to dogs infected with circulating microfilariae; administration to dogs less than 4 weeks of age
Warnings. Dogs more than 6 months of age should be tested for circulating microfilariae before treatment
Dose. *Dogs: by mouth*, 5.5–6.0 mg/kg

Dimmitrol (Mavlab) *Austral*
Tablets, diethylcarbamazine citrate 50 mg, 200 mg, 400 mg, for *dogs*
Syrup, diethylcarbamazine citrate 60 mg/mL, for *dogs*

Dirozine (Jurox) *Austral*
Tablets, diethylcarbamazine citrate 200 mg, for *dogs*
Syrup, diethylcarbamazine citrate 60 mg/mL, for *dogs*

Exelpet Ezy-Dose Palatable Heartworm Prevention Capsules (Excelpet) *Austral*
Capsules, diethylcarbamazine citrate 50 mg, 200 mg, for *dogs*

Exelpet Heartworm Prevention Tablets (Excelpet) *Austral*
Tablets, diethylcarbamazine citrate 200 mg, for *dogs*

Exelpet Palatable Heartworm Prevention Syrup for Dogs (Excelpet) *Austral*
Syrup, diethylcarbamazine citrate 60 mg/mL, for *dogs*

Fido's Dec-Tab (Mavlab) *Austral*
Tablets, diethylcarbamazine 50 mg, 200 mg, 400 mg, for *dogs*

Fido's Dec-Lik (Mavlab) *Austral*
Syrup, diethylcarbamazine 60 mg/mL, for *dogs*

Filar Heartworm Tablets (David) *Austral*
Tablets, diethylcarbamazine citrate 200 mg, 400 mg, for *dogs*

Filaribits (Dover) *Austral*
Tablets, diethylcarbamazine citrate 60 mg, 180 mg, for *dogs*

Heartworm Palatable Tablets (Ilium, Troy) *Austral*
Tablets, diethylcarbamazine cirate 200 mg, for *dogs*

Heartworm Syrup (Troy) *Austral*
Syrup, diethylcarbamazine 60 mg/mL, for *dogs*

USA

Indications. Heartworm prophylaxis in dogs; gastro-intestinal roundworms in dogs and cats
Contra-indications. Administration to dogs infected with adult heartworms
Warnings. Dogs on prophylactic treatment should be tested for circulating microfilariae every 6 months; dogs with established heartworm infections should receive prior treatment with adulticidal and microfilaricidal drugs
Dose. *By mouth.*
Dogs: heartworm prophylaxis, 5.5–6.6 mg/kg daily
Roundworms, 110 mg/kg given in 2 divided doses at an interval of 8–12 hours *or* 55–110 mg/kg as a single dose
Cats: roundworms, 55–110 mg/kg as a single dose

Carbam (Osborn) *USA*
Tablets, diethylcarbamazine citrate 50 mg, 100 mg, 200 mg, 300 mg, 400 mg, for *dogs, cats*

Diethylcarbamazine Citrate Tablets (Global) *USA*
Tablets, diethylcarbamazine citrate 200 mg and 400 mg, for *dogs, cats*

Filaribits (Pfizer) *USA*
Tablets, diethylcarbamazine citrate 60 mg, 120 mg and 180 mg, for *dogs*

Nemacide Oral Syrup (Boehringer Ingelheim Vetmedica) *USA*
Syrup, diethylcarbamazine citrate 60 mg/mL, for *dogs*

Nemacide Tablets (Boehringer Ingelheim Vetmedica) *USA*
Tablets, diethylcarbamazine citrate 50 mg, 100 mg, 200 mg, 300 mg, 400 mg, for *dogs*

HYGROMYCIN B

Australia

Indications. Gastro-intestinal roundworms in pigs and poultry
Dose. *Pigs, poultry*: *by addition to feed*, 13.2 g/tonne feed

Hygromix 13 (Elanco) *Austral*
Premix, hygromycin B 13.2 g/kg, for *pigs*
Withdrawal Periods. Slaughter 2 days

Hygromix 13 (Elanco) *Austral*
Premix, hygromycin B 13.2 g/kg, for *poultry*
Withdrawal Periods. Slaughter 2 days

New Zealand

Indications. Gastro-intestinal roundworms in pigs and poultry

Side-effects. Possible reduced response to sound after prolonged treatment
Dose. *Pigs, chickens*: *by addition to feed*, 13.2 g/tonne feed

Hygromix-13 (Elanco) *NZ*
Premix, hygromycin B 13.2 g/kg, for *pigs, chickens*
Withdrawal Periods. *Pigs*: slaughter 15 days. *Chickens*: slaughter 3 days

USA

Indications. Gastro-intestinal roundworms in pigs and poultry
Dose. *Pigs, chickens*: *by addition to feed*, 8–12 g/tonne feed

Hygromix 8 (Elanco) *USA*
Premix, hygromycin B 17.6 g/kg, for *pigs, chickens*
Withdrawal Periods. *Pigs*: slaughter 15 days. *Chickens*: slaughter 3 days

MELARSOMINE

Australia

Indications. Heartworm treatment in dogs
Contra-indications. Pregnant animals
Side-effects. Transient pain at injection site, transient anorexia, agitation, tremor, salivation after injection. Pyrexia, anorexia, and depression after first week of treatment. Fatigue, depression, anorexia, polypnoea, and dyspnoea 7–20 days after treatment
Warnings. Severe heartworm infection (caval syndrome) should be treated surgically and medical treatment initiated 1–2 months later

Immiticide Canine Heartworm Treatment (Merial) *Austral*
Injection, powder for reconstitution, melarsomine dihydrochloride 25 mg/mL, for *dogs*

USA

Indications. Heartworm treatment in dogs
Contra-indications. Severe heartworm infection (caval syndrome)
Side-effects. Transient pain at injection site, transient anorexia, coughing, panting, vomiting, salivation, pyrexia, depression, and lung congestion
Warnings. Safety in breeding, lactating, or pregnant animals has not been established
Dose. *Dogs*: *by intramuscular injection*, 2.5 mg/kg, repeat after 24 hours. Repeat course after 4 months *or* 2.5 mg/kg asa single dose, repeat twice after 4 months at an interval of 24 hours

Immiticide (Merial) *USA*
Injection, powder for reconstitution, melarsomine dihydrochloride 25 mg/mL, for *dogs*

NITROSCANATE

UK

Indications. Gastro-intestinal roundworms, tapeworms (see section 2.1.2) in dogs
Side-effects. Occasional vomiting with high dosage

Warnings. Nitroscanate is irritant and tablets should not be crushed, broken, or divided
Dose. *Dogs*: *by mouth*, 50 mg/kg, given with a little food but on an empty stomach

GSL **All in One Wormer** (Bob Martin) *UK*
Tablets, nitroscanate 100 mg, 500 mg, for *dogs*; 100-mg tablets 4; 500-mg tablets 3

GSL **Lopatol 100** (Novartis) *UK*
Tablets, f/c, nitroscanate 100 mg, for *dogs up to 6 kg body-weight*; 100

GSL **Lopatol 500** (Novartis) *UK*
Tablets, f/c, nitroscanate 500 mg, for *dogs*; 100

GSL **Nitroscanate 100** (Millpledge) *UK*
Tablets, f/c, nitroscanate 100 mg, for *dogs*

GSL **Nitroscanate 500** (Millpledge) *UK*
Tablets, f/c, nitroscanate 500 mg, for *dogs*

GSL **One Dose Wormer** (Sherley's) *UK*
Tablets, f/c, nitroscanate 100 mg, 500 mg, for *dogs*; 100-mg tablets 3, 6; 500-mg tablets 2, 4

GSL **Troscan 100** (Chanelle) *UK*
Tablets, f/c, nitroscanate 100 mg, for *dogs*; 4, 6, 100

GSL **Troscan 500** (Chanelle) *UK*
Tablets, f/c, nitroscanate 500 mg, for *dogs*; 4, 60

Eire

Indications. Gastro-intestinal roundworms and tapeworms in dogs
Side-effects. Occasional vomiting
Warnings. Nitroscanate is irritant and tablets should not be crushed, broken, or divided
Dose. *Dogs*: *by mouth*, 50 mg/kg, given with a little food but on an empty stomach

Lopatol 100 & 500 (Novartis) *Eire*
Tablets, nitroscanate 100 mg, 500 mg, for *dogs*

Troscan 100 & 500 (Chanelle) *Eire*
Tablets, nitroscanate 100 mg, 500 mg, for *dogs*

PIPERAZINE

UK

Indications. Gastro-intestinal roundworms in dogs, cats, and pigeons
Contra-indications. Renal impairment
Warnings. Overdosage may cause vomiting, diarrhoea, and ataxia in dogs and cats; care in animals with history of epilepsy or severe renal impairment; pregnant animals
Dose. Expressed as piperazine hydrate. *By mouth*.
Dogs, cats: *Toxocara, Toxascaris*, 80–100 mg/kg
Ancylostoma, Uncinaria, 120–240 mg/kg
Pigeons: *Ascaridia*, see preparation details

Note. 100 mg piperazine hydrate = 120 mg piperazine adipate = 125 mg piperazine citrate = 104 mg piperazine phosphate

GSL **Biozine** (Harkers) *UK*
Oral powder, for addition to drinking water, piperazine (as dihydrochloride) 510 mg/g, for *ornamental pigeons*; 3.7-g sachet
Withdrawal Periods. Should not be used in *pigeons* intended for human consumption
Dose. *Pigeons*: (30 birds) one 3.7-g sachet/litre drinking water

GSL **Canovel Palatable Wormer** (Pfizer) *UK*
Tablets, piperazine phosphate 416 mg, for *dogs*; 4, 12, 100

GSL **Catovel Palatable Wormer** (Pfizer) *UK*
Tablets, piperazine phosphate 416 mg, for *cats*; 4

GSL **Easy Round Wormer for Kittens** (Johnson's) *UK*
Tablets, piperazine phosphate 104 mg, for *cats*; 12
Contra-indications. Kittens less than 6 weeks of age

GSL **Easy Round Wormer for Puppies** (Johnson's) *UK*
Tablets, piperazine phosphate 416 mg, for *dogs*; 8
Contra-indications. Puppies less than 2 weeks of age

GSL **Endorid** (Pfizer) *UK*
Tablets, scored, piperazine phosphate 416 mg, for *dogs, cats*; 12, 500

GSL **Kitten Easy-Worm Syrup** (Johnson's) *UK*
Oral syrup, piperazine hydrate 58 mg/mL, for *cats*; 50 mL
Contra-indications. Kittens less than 6 weeks of age

GSL **Palatable Roundworm Tablets** (Johnson's) *UK*
Tablets, piperazine phosphate 416 mg, for *dogs, cats*; 8

GSL **Palatable Worming Tablets** (Sherley's) *UK*
Tablets, piperazine citrate 220 mg, for *dogs, cats*; 12

GSL **Piperazine Citrate BP(Vet)** (Distributed by Millpledge) *UK*
Tablets, piperazine citrate 500 mg, for *dogs, cats*; 500

GSL **Piperazine Citrate Tablets** (Arnolds) *UK*
Tablets, piperazine citrate 500 mg, for *dogs and cats more than 2.5 kg body-weight*; 500

GSL **Piperazine Citrate Tablets BP** (Battle Hayward & Bower) *UK*
Tablets, scored, piperazine citrate 500 mg, for *dogs and cats more than 1.25 kg body-weight*; 6, 24

GSL **Piperazine Citrate Worm Tablets** (Loveridge) *UK*
Tablets, scored, piperazine citrate 500 mg, for *dogs and cats more than 1.25 kg body-weight*; 500

GSL **Puppy Easy-Worm Syrup** (Johnson's) *UK*
Oral syrup, piperazine hydrate 58 mg/mL, for *dogs*; 50 mL
Contra-indications. Puppies less than 4 weeks of age

GSL **Roundworm Tablets** (Bob Martin) *UK*
Tablets, scored, piperazine (as citrate) 105 mg, for *dogs more than 2 weeks of age and 1.2 kg body-weight*; 8

GSL **Roundworm Tablets for Cats** (Bob Martin) *UK*
Tablets, scored, piperazine (as citrate) 105 mg, for *cats more than 2 weeks of age and 1.2 kg body-weight*; 4

GSL **Ruby Oral Wormer Syrup** (Spencer) *UK*
Syrup, piperazine 100 mg/mL, for *puppies*; 50 mL

GSL **Worming Cream** (Sherley's) *UK*
Oral paste, piperazine citrate 250 mg/g, for *dogs, cats*; 18-g dose applicator
Contra-indications. Puppies and kittens less than 2 weeks of age

GSL **Worming Syrup** (Sherley's) *UK*
Oral syrup, piperazine citrate 80 mg/mL, for *dogs, cats*; 45-mL dose applicator
Contra-indications. Puppies and kittens less than 2 weeks of age

Australia
Indications. Gastro-intestinal roundworms in horses, pigs, dogs, cats, and birds
Dose. *By mouth*. Dosages vary, consult manufacturer's information

Pip A Tabs (Apex) *Austral*
Tablets, piperazine adipate 500 mg, for *dogs, cats*

PC Powder (Pharmachem) *Austral*
Oral powder, piperazine citrate, for *horses, pigs, dogs, cats, poultry*

Pip-Cit Syrup (Apex) *Austral*
Syrup, piperazine citrate 140 mg/mL, for *dogs, cats, birds*

Piperazine Solution (Pharmachem) *Austral*
Liquid, for dilution, piperazine citrate 450 g/L, for *pigs, poultry, pigeons, cage birds*

Piperazine Solution for Pigeons (Inca) *Austral*
Solution, piperazine citrate 217 g/L, for *pigeons*

Piperazine Solution for Poultry and Pigs (Inca) *Austral*
Liquid, piperazine 172.5 g/L, for *pigs, poultry*

Piperazine Tablets for Pigeons (Inca) *Austral*
Tablets, piperazine citrate 213.5 mg, for *pigeons*

Piperazine Water Soluble Powder (CCD) *Austral*
Powder, for addition to drinking water, piperazine 530 mg/g, for *poultry*

Piperazine Worm Powder (Virbac) *Austral*
Oral powder, piperazine citrate 1 g/kg, for *horses, pigs*

Puppy and Kitten Worm Syrup (Troy) *Austral*
Syrup, piperazine citrate 1 g/10 mL, for *dogs, cats*

USA
Indications. Gastro-intestinal roundworms in horses, cattle, sheep, pigs, dogs, cats, poultry
Contra-indications. Renal impairment
Warnings. Overdosage may cause vomiting, diarrhoea, and ataxia in dogs and cats
Dose. *By mouth*. Dosages vary, consult manufacturer's information

Kennel Wormer (Happy Jack) *USA*
Powder, for addition to feed, piperazine adipate 100% equivalent to piperazine base 37%, for *dogs*

Pig Swig (LeGear) *USA*
Solution, for addition to drinking water, piperazine (as monohydrochloride) 17 g/100 mL, for *pigs, chickens*

Pipa-Tabs (Vet-A-Mix) *USA*
Tablets, piperazine (as dihydrochloride) 50 mg, 250 mg, for *dogs, cats*

Piperazine-17 (AgriLabs, AgriPharm) *USA*
Solution, for addition to drinking water, piperazine (as sulphate) 17 g/100 mL, for *horses, pigs, dogs, cats, chicken, turkeys*

Piperazine-17% Medicated (DurVet) *USA*
Solution, for addition to drinking water, piperazine (as sulphate) 17 g/100 mL, for *horses, pigs, dogs, cats, chickens, turkeys*

**Piperazine-17% ** (RXV) *USA*
Solution, for addition to drinking water, piperazine (as sulphate) 17 g/100 mL, for *horses, pigs, dogs, cats, chickens, turkeys*

Piperazine-34 (AgriLabs) *USA*
Solution, for addition to drinking water, piperazine (as sulphate) 34 g/100 mL, for *horses, pigs, dogs, cats, chickens, turkeys*

Piperazine-34% Medicated (DurVet) *USA*
Solution, for addition to drinking water, piperazine (as sulphate) 34 g/100 mL, for *horses, pigs, dogs, cats, chickens, turkeys*

**Piperazine-34% ** (RXV) *USA*
Solution, for addition to drinking water, piperazine (as sulphate) 34 g/100 mL, for *horses, pigs, dogs, cats, chickens, turkeys*

Piperazine 34% Solution (Vedco) *USA*
Solution, for addition to drinking water, piperazine (as sulphate) 34 g/100 mL, for *horses, pigs, dogs, cats, chickens, turkeys*

Pip-Pop 320 (Vet-A-Mix) *USA*
Powder, for addition to drinking water, piperazine (as dihydrochloride) 320 g, for *horses, cattle, sheep, pigs, dogs, cats, chickens, turkeys*

Puppy Paste (Happy Jack) *USA*
Oral paste, piperazine (as adipate) 37%, for *dogs*

Purina Liquid Wormer (Purina Mills) *USA*
Solution, for addition to drinking water , piperazine (as monohydrochloride) 16%, for *pigs, poultry*

2.1.2 Drugs for tapeworms (cestodes)

Although adult tapeworms do not usually cause discernible disease, treatment is often necessary for public health purposes, to prevent disease due to larval stages in farm livestock, to minimise meat inspection losses, and for aesthetic reasons in dogs and cats.

Diagnosis of infected animals is difficult and often relies on the chance observation of a passed segment, the morphology of which is used for generic identification. Care is needed in assessing the success of treatment. A mass of tapeworm strobilae may be passed after use of a relatively ineffective product, but this is of no benefit if the scolices are left to re-grow. Conversely, a lack of evidence of expulsion of segments may be due to dissolution of the dead tapeworm within the alimentary tract.

All tapeworms have an indirect life-cycle and preventive measures often include control of arthropods. Information on effective drugs for treatment is given in Table 2.1 at the beginning of the chapter.

Heavy infections of *Anoplocephala* in horses may be a predisposing factor in some colics. Pasture-living mites are the intermediate hosts and therefore infection is unlikely in permanently stabled horses. Horses are usually treated in midsummer and again in early autumn.

Moniezia infection is mostly seen in lambs and calves during their first summer on pasture but rarely causes ill-effect, except perhaps for a marginal influence on growth. Infections are often lost spontaneously in the summer and are not common in older animals. Free-living mites on the pasture are the intermediate hosts and prevention of re-infection is thus impossible. Control of *Moniezia,* if required, includes treatment in late spring or early summer and again in autumn.

Dipylidium, Echinococcus, and *Taenia* affect dogs. *Dipylidium* and *Taenia* affect cats. The choice of anthelmintic and advice on preventing re-infection are dependent on accurate identification of the tapeworm involved. The long-term control of *Dipylidium* tapeworm includes elimination of fleas and lice (see sections 2.2), the intermediate hosts. Dogs are infected with *Taenia* by ingesting the larval forms (metacestodes) in undercooked meat or viscera from sheep or rabbits. Cats are infected by hunting small mammals. Treatments are usually given every 6 months for the routine control of *Taenia* and *Dipylidium.* If animals are persistently re-infected, the treatment interval has to be reduced and advice given, as appropriate, on feeding or flea control. The metacestodes of the two British strains of *Echinococcus* are found in the viscera of sheep and horses, respectively. The sheep strain is a potential zoonosis and dogs in

endemic areas should be treated with praziquantel every 6 weeks to ensure that no infective eggs are passed. Another species, *Echinococcus multilocularis* is also zoonotic but fortunately does not occur in the UK. The cyst form of this species infiltrates tissues by budding externally and thus infection in humans is very serious.

Praziquantel is effective against all tapeworms in dogs and cats and is preferred in most *Echinococcus* control programmes because it kills all intestinal forms of the parasite. It acts by inducing calcium ion influx across the parasite tegument causing immediate muscular spasm. The tegument is disrupted making it more easily attacked by proteolytic enzymes. Therefore, whole tapeworms are very rarely passed in the faeces; only disintegrated and partially digested fragments are seen. Under the *Pet Travel Scheme,* implemented in the UK, 24 to 48 hours before embarkation for the UK, animals must be treated against *Echinococcus multilocularis* with praziquantel. Other requirement for bringing pet dogs and cats without being placed under quarantine are given under section 18.4.6. Praziquantel is also active against *Moniezia* in sheep♦ and against *Anoplocephala* and *Anoplocephaloides* in horses♦.

Epsiprantel is an anthelmintic closely related to praziquantel but has marginally lower efficacy against immature *Echinococcus.*

Dichlorophen and **nitroscanate** (see section 2.1.1.6) are effective against *Taenia* and *Dipylidium* but have limited efficacy against *Echinococcus.*

Pyrantel (see section 2.1.1.5) is effective against *Anoplocephala perfoliata* in horses at twice the dose required for roundworms; it is not effective against *Anoplocephaloides mammillana.*

Various **benzimidazoles** (see section 2.1.1.2), including albendazole, febantel, fenbendazole, mebendazole, netobimin, and oxfendazole are effective for tapeworm control in ruminants. Fenbendazole and mebendazole also control some tapeworms in dogs and cats.

Niclosamide acts by uncoupling oxidative phosphorylation, thereby interfering with adenosine triphosphate production. It has little efficacy against *Echinococcus* and variable activity against *Dipylidium.*

DICHLOROPHEN

UK

Indications. *Dipylidium* and *Taenia* in dogs and cats
Side-effects. Rarely salivation, vomiting, anorexia, hyperaesthesia, and loss of co-ordination including limb weakness and unsteadiness
Dose. *Dogs, cats*: *by mouth,* 200 mg/kg

GSL **Canovel Tapewormer** (Pfizer) *UK*
Tablets, dichlorophen 750 mg, for *dogs*; 4

GSL **Catovel Tapewormer** (Pfizer) *UK*
Tablets, dichlorophen 750 mg, for *cats*; 4

GSL **Dichlorophen Tablets BP** (Battle Hayward & Bower) *UK*
Tablets, scored, dichlorophen 500 mg, for *dogs and cats more than 1.25 kg body-weight and more than 6 months of age*; 6, 24

GSL **Easy Tape Wormer for Cats** (Johnson's) *UK*
Tablets, dichlorophen 250 mg, for *cats*; 6
Contra-indications. Cats less than 6 months of age, pregnant or nursing queens

GSL **Easy Tape Wormer for Dogs** (Johnson's) *UK*
Tablets, dichlorophen 500 mg, for *dogs*; 8
Contra-indications. Dogs less than 6 months of age, pregnant or nursing bitches

GSL **Flavoured Tapeworm Tablets** (Johnson's) *UK*
Tablets, dichlorophen 500 mg, for *dogs, cats*; 12
Contra-indications. Dogs or cats less than 6 months of age, pregnant or nursing bitches or queens

GSL **Kitzyme Veterinary Tapewormer** (Seven Seas)
Tablets, scored, dichlorophen 750 mg, for *cats more than 900 g body-weight*; 4
Note. Consult a veterinarian before treating cats less than 6 months of age or pregnant animals

GSL **Tapeworm Tablets** (Bob Martin) *UK*
Tablets, dichlorophen 500 mg, for *dogs*; 12
Contra-indications. Dogs less than 6 months of age

GSL **Tapeworm Tablets for Cats** (Bob Martin) *UK*
Tablets, dichlorophen 250 mg, for *cats*; 8
Contra-indications. Cats less than 6 months of age

GSL **Vetzyme Veterinary Tapewormer** (Seven Seas) *UK*
Tablets, scored, dichlorophen 750 mg, for *dogs more than 1.75 kg body-weight*; 4, 12
Note. Consult a veterinarian before treating dogs less than 6 months of age or pregnant animals

USA

Indications. *Dipylidium* and *Taenia* in dogs
Side-effects. Vomiting, diarrhoea
Dose. *Dogs*: *by mouth*, 1g/4.54 kg. Withhold solid food and milk for 12 hours before and 4 hours after treatment

Happy Jack Tapeworm Tablets (Happy Jack) *USA*
Tablets, dichlorophen 1 g, for *dogs*

EPSIPRANTEL

USA

Indications. *Dipylidium* and *Taenia* in dogs and cats
Warnings. Safety in pregnant or breeding animals has not been established
Dose. *Dogs*: *by mouth*, 5.5 mg/kg
Cats: *by mouth*, 2.75 mg/kg

Cestex (Pfizer) *USA*
Tablets, epsiprantel 12.5 mg, 25 mg, 50 mg and 100 mg, for *dogs, cats*
Withdrawal Periods. n/a

NICLOSAMIDE

UK

Indications. **Dose**. See Prescribing for amphibians

POM Ⓗ **Yomesan** (Bayer) *UK*
Tablets, niclosamide 500 mg

New Zealand

Indications. Tapeworms in lambs
Warnings. Safety in pregnant or breeding animals has not been established

Mansonil-M (Bayer) *NZ*
Oral powder, to prepare an oral solution, niclosamide 790 g/kg, for **lambs**
Withdrawal Periods. Slaughter 4 days
Dose. *Lambs*: *by mouth*, reconstitute 500 g powder in 3.75 litres water. Give 6–15mL reconstituted solution/animal (depending on body-weight)

PRAZIQUANTEL

UK

Indications. Tapeworms in horses♦, sheep♦, dogs and cats
Contra-indications. Unweaned puppies or kittens; injection in hounds
Side-effects. Occasional pain on subcutaneous injection
Dose. *Horses*♦: *by mouth*, 1 mg/kg
Sheep♦: *by mouth*, 3.75 mg/kg
Dogs, cats: *by mouth*, 5 mg/kg
by subcutaneous or intramuscular injection, 5.68 mg/kg (0.1 mL/kg)

Droncit (Bayer) *UK*
GSL *Tablets*, scored, praziquantel 50 mg, for *dogs, cats*; 20
POM *Injection*, praziquantel 56.8 mg/mL, for *dogs, cats*; 10 mL

Australia

Indications. Tapeworms in dogs and cats
Contra-indications. Feeding offal of any species to dogs
Dose. *By mouth*. Dosages vary, for guidance:
Dogs: tapeworm prophylaxis, 2.5–5.0 mg/kg
Echinococcus treatment, 5 mg/kg
Spirometra erinacei, 20 mg/kg
Cats: tapeworms, 2.5–5.0 mg/kg

Bay-O-Pet Droncit Tapeworm & Hydatid Control for Dogs (Bayer) *Austral*
Tablets, praziquantel 50 mg, for *dogs*

Droncit Tapeworm & Hydatid Control for Dogs (Bayer) *Austral*
Tablets, praziquantel 50 mg, for *dogs*

Paratak (Pharmtech) *Austral*
Tablets, praziquantel 50 mg, for *dogs, cats*

Popantel Tapeworm Tablets for Dogs and Cats (Jurox) *Austral*
Tablets, praziquantel 50 mg, for *dogs, cats*

Tapewormer for Dogs and Cats (Virbac) *Austral*
Tablets, praziquantel 50 mg, for *dogs, cats*

Eire

Indications. Tapeworms in dogs and cats
Contra-indications. Unweaned puppies or kittens
Dose. *Dogs, cats*: *by mouth*, 5 mg/kg

Droncit Tablets (Bayer) *Eire*
Tablets, praziquantel 50 mg, for *dogs, cats*

New Zealand

Indications. Tapeworms in horses, sheep, dogs and cats
Dose.
Horses: *by mouth*, 0.5 mg/kg
Sheep: *by mouth*, 3.75–7.5 mg/kg
Dogs: tapeworm prophylaxis, *by mouth*, 2.5 mg/kg
by subcutaneous or intramuscular injection, 2.84 mg/kg (0.05 mL/kg)
Echinococcus treatment, *by mouth*, 5 mg/kg

by intramuscular injection, 5.68 mg/kg (0.1 mL/kg)
Cats: tapeworms, 2.5–5.0 mg/kg

Adtape (Ancare) *NZ*
Oral solution, praziquantel 37.5 mg/mL, for *horses, sheep*
Withdrawal Periods. *Horses*: slaughter 7 days. *Sheep*: slaughter 7 days, milk 28 days

Droncit Solution (Bayer) *NZ*
Injection, praziquantel 56.8 mg/mL, for *dogs, cats*

Droncit Tablets (Bayer) *NZ*
Tablets, praziquantel 50 mg, for *dogs, cats*

Paratak (Bomac) *NZ*
Tablets, praziquantel 50 mg, for *dogs, cats*

Vetcare Tapewormer (Ancare) *NZ*
Tablets, praziquantel 50 mg, for *dogs, cats*

Wormicide Tape (Virbac) *NZ*
Tablets, praziquantel 50 mg, 100 mg, for *dogs, cats*

USA

Indications. Tapeworms in dogs and cats
Contra-indications. Puppies less than 4 weeks of age; kittens less than 6 weeks of age
Dose. *Dogs*: *by mouth or by subcutaneous or intramuscular injection*, 17–170 mg (depending on body-weight), 17–170
Cats: *by mouth or by subcutaneous or intramuscular injection*, 11.5–34.5 mg (depending on body-weight)

Droncit (Bayer) *USA*
Tablets, praziquantel 34 mg, for *dogs*

Droncit (Bayer) *USA*
Tablets, praziquantel 23 mg, for *cats*

Droncit (Bayer) *USA*
Injection, praziquantel 56.8 mg/mL, for *dogs, cats*

2.1.3 Drugs for flukes (trematodes)

The liver fluke *Fasciola hepatica* is endemic in many wet regions and mainly affects ruminants kept in or originating from such areas. The intermediate host is a small mud snail, *Lymnaea truncatula*. The acute disease, which occurs in autumn and early winter, is caused by immature *F. hepatica* destroying the liver parenchyma, while the chronic form in the early months of the year results from the feeding activities of adult flukes in the bile ducts. Both acute and chronic forms of fasciolosis occur in sheep, but only the latter in cattle. Horses are more resistant to fasciolosis but occasionally show clinical signs of ill thrift. Patent liver fluke infection occurs in donkeys and treatment with triclabendazole♦ has proved effective.
Treatment may be therapeutic or prophylactic. For acute disease in young animals the drug dose should be repeated after 5 to 6 weeks. To prevent infection, all animals exposed to fluke-infested pastures during the fluke season should be treated regularly at intervals dependent on the area, climatic conditions, and the particular product and there should be restricted access to contaminated areas during the high risk periods of autumn and winter. Control of the mud snail includes drainage, fencing off of wetter areas, and using molluscicide sprays. The risk of disease varies from year to year and a monitoring system assists the choice of an appropriate level of control.
Care is required in the choice of fasciolicide because few are active against all stages of parasitic development. See Table 2.1 in the introduction to section 2.1, and drug monographs for information on drug treatment.
The lancet fluke, *Dicrocoelium dendriticum*, passes through various land snails and ants. This fluke affects cattle and sheep although infection in the UK is largely restricted to the Hebrides.
Benzimidazoles (see section 2.1.1.2) active against *Fasciola* include albendazole and netobimin, which are effective against adult stages. Netobimin is also effective against adult *Dicrocoelium dendriticum*. **Triclabendazole** is highly effective against all liver stages of *Fasciola*. Liver fluke resistant to triclabendazole have recently been found on a small number of farms in the UK.
Nitroxinil is effective against adult flukes and at a higher dosage, immature flukes and also *Haemonchus* in cattle and sheep, and *Oesophagostomum* and *Bunostomum* in cattle but should not be regarded or used as a broad spectrum anthelmintic. **Closantel** is effective against adult and immature flukes, *Oestrus ovis,* and *Haemonchus contortus*. This drug acts by uncoupling oxidative phosphorylation. It binds strongly to plasma proteins and therefore its activity against nematodes is restricted to those that suck blood. **Clorsulon** is a sulphonamide and competitive inhibitor of enzymes important for energy metabolism in flukes. It is used in cattle for control of liver fluke.
Oxyclozanide is mainly active against adult flukes. The drug is distributed to the liver, kidney, and intestines and is excreted in the bile.
Bithionol is a chlorinated bis-phenol with bactericidal and anthelmintic properties and **bromofenofos** is a bis-phenol derivative; both are active against flukes. **Rafoxanide** is a salicylanilide active against adult and immature flukes aged 6 to 8 weeks and older.

CLOSANTEL

UK

Indications. Immature and adult *Fasciola*, nasal bots, and *Haemonchus* in sheep
Dose. *Sheep*: *by mouth,* 10 mg/kg

PML **Flukiver** (Janssen) *UK*
Oral suspension, closantel 50 mg/mL, for *sheep*; 1 litre, 2.5 litres, 5 litres
Withdrawal Periods. *Sheep*: slaughter 42 days, should not be used in sheep producing milk or milk products for human consumption

PML **Flukol** (Young's) *UK*
Oral suspension, closantel 50 mg/mL, for *sheep*; 1 litre, 2.5 litres, 5 litres
Withdrawal Periods. *Sheep*: slaughter 42 days, should not be used in sheep producing milk or milk products for human consumption

Australia

Indications. Immature and adult *Fasciola*, nasal bots, and *Haemonchus* in sheep
Dose. *Sheep*: *by mouth,* 7.5 mg/kg

Closantel (Western Stock Distributors) *Austral*
Oral solution, closantel 37.5 g/L, for *sheep*
Withdrawal Periods. Slaughter 28 days

Closicare (Virbac) *Austral*
Oral solution, closantel 37.5 g/L, for *sheep*
Withdrawal Periods. Slaughter 28 days

Razar Plus (Coopers) *Austral*
Oral solution, closantel 37.5 g/L, sodium selenate 1.2 g/L, for *sheep*
Withdrawal Periods. Slaughter 28 days

Seponver (Pfizer) *Austral*
Oral solution, closantel 37.5 g/L, for *sheep*
Withdrawal Periods. Slaughter 28 days

Sustain (Dover) *Austral*
Oral solution, closantel 37.5 g/L, for *sheep*
Withdrawal Periods. Slaughter 28 days

Eire

Indications. Immature and adult *Fasciola* and some gastro-intestinal roundworms in ruminants, nasal bots in sheep, warbles in cattle
Dose. *Cattle*: *by subcutaneous injection*, roundworms, flukes, 2.5 mg/kg, warbles, 5 mg/kg
Sheep: *by mouth,* 10 mg/kg
by subcutaneous injection, Strongyloides, flukes, 5 mg/kg
Haemonchus, Oesophagostomum, nasal bots, 2.5 mg/kg

Flukiver (Janssen) *Eire*
Oral suspension, closantel (as closantel sodium) 50 mg/mL, for *sheep*
Withdrawal Periods. Slaughter 42 days, should not be used in sheep producing milk for human consumption

Flukiver 5 Injection (Janssen) *Eire*
Injection, closantel (as closantel sodium) 50 mg/mL, for *cattle, sheep*
Withdrawal Periods. Slaughter 56 days, milk 56 days

NITROXINIL
(Nitroxynil)

UK
Indications. Immature and adult *Fasciola* and some gastro-intestinal roundworms in ruminants
Side-effects. Solution may stain wool if accidental spillage occurs; transient swelling at injection site in cattle
Dose.
Cattle: *by subcutaneous injection*, 10 mg/kg
Sheep: *by subcutaneous injection*, 10 mg/kg
Acute fascioliosis, *by subcutaneous injection*, up to 15 mg/kg

PML **Trodax 34%** (Merial) *UK*
Injection, nitroxinil 340 mg/mL, for *cattle, sheep*; 100 mL, 250 mL, 1 litre
Withdrawal Periods. *Cattle*: slaughter 60 days, should not be used in cattle producing milk for human consumption. *Sheep*: slaughter 60 days
Note. Dairy cattle should be treated at least 15 days before calving

Australia
Indications. Immature and adult *Fasciola* and some gastro-intestinal roundworms in ruminants;
Dose. *By subcutaneous injection.*
Cattle: 10 mg/kg
Sheep: 10 mg/kg

Trodax (Merial) *Austral*
Injection, nitroxinil (as eglumine) 340 g/L, for *sheep, cattle*
Withdrawal Periods. *Cattle*: slaughter 28 days, should not be used in cattle producing milk for human consumption. *Sheep*: slaughter 28 days

Eire
Indications. Immature and adult *Fasciola* and some gastro-intestinal roundworms in ruminants
Side-effects. Solution may stain wool if accidental spillage occurs; transient swelling at injection site in cattle
Dose. *By subcutaneous injection.*
Cattle: 10 mg/kg
Sheep: 10 mg/kg
Acute fascioliosis, up to 15 mg/kg

Deldrax 34% (Intervet) *Eire*
Injection, nitroxynil 34%, for *cattle, sheep*
Withdrawal Periods. *Cattle*: slaughter 30 days, should not be used in cattle producing milk for human consumption. *Sheep*: slaughter 30 days

Trodax 34% (Merial) *Eire*
Injection, nitroxynil (as eglumine salt) 340 mg/mL, for *cattle, sheep*
Withdrawal Periods. *Cattle*: slaughter 60 days, should not be used in cattle producing milk for human consumption. *Sheep*: slaughter 60 days

OXYCLOZANIDE

Eire
Indications. Adult *Fasciola* in ruminants
Side-effects. Occasional increased defecation and inappetance in cattle; occasional reduction in milk yield in cattle
Dose. *By mouth.*
Cattle: 10 mg/kg
Sheep: 15 mg/kg

Zanil Fluke Drench (Schering-Plough) *Eire*
Oral suspension, oxyclozanide 34 mg/mL, for *cattle, sheep*
Withdrawal Periods. *Cattle*: slaughter 28 days, milk 3 days. *Sheep*: slaughter 28 days, should not be used in sheep producing milk for human consumption

RAFOXANIDE

Eire
Indications. *Fasciola* in ruminants; nasal bots in sheep
Side-effects. Occasional increased defecation and inappetance in cattle; occasional reduction in milk yield in cattle
Dose. *By mouth*. Dosages vary.
Cattle: 11.25 mg/kg
Sheep: 7.5 mg/kg *or* 11.25 mg/kg (depending on preparation)

Flukex 3% w/v Oral Drench (Univet) *Eire*
Oral solution, rafoxanide 30 mg/mL, for *cattle, sheep*
Withdrawal Periods. Slaughter 60 days, should not be used in cattle or sheep producing milk for human consumption

Ridafluke (Chanelle) *Eire*
Oral suspension, rafoxanide 3%, for *cattle, sheep*
Withdrawal Periods. Slaughter 60 days, should not be used in cattle or sheep producing milk for human consumption

TRICLABENDAZOLE

UK

Indications. Immature and adult *Fasciola* in horses♦ and ruminants
Dose. *By mouth.*
Horses♦, cattle: 12 mg/kg
Sheep: 10 mg/kg

PML **Fasinex 5%** (Novartis) *UK*
Oral suspension, triclabendazole 50 mg/mL, for *sheep*
Withdrawal Periods. *Sheep*: slaughter 56 days, should not be used in sheep producing milk for human consumption

PML **Fasinex 10%** (Novartis) *UK*
Oral suspension, triclabendazole 100 mg/mL, for *cattle*
Withdrawal Periods. *Cattle*: slaughter 28 days, should not be used in cattle producing milk for human consumption or in dairy cows within 7 days of calving

Australia

Indications. Immature and adult *Fasciola* in ruminants
Warnings. It is recommended to vaccinate against black disease in affected areas
Dose. *By mouth.*
Cattle: 12 mg/kg
Sheep, goats: 10 mg/kg

Fasinex 50 (Novartis) *Austral*
Liquid, triclabendazole 50 g/L, for *cattle, sheep, goats*
Withdrawal Periods. Slaughter 28 days, should not be used in cattle, sheep or goats producing milk for human consumption

Fasinex 120 (Novartis) *Austral*
Liquid, triclabendazole 120 g/L, for *cattle, sheep*
Withdrawal Periods. Slaughter 28 days, should not be used in cattle or sheep producing milk for human consumption

Eire

Indications. Immature and adult *Fasciola* in ruminants
Warnings. It is recommended to vaccinate against black disease in affected areas
Dose. *By mouth.*
Cattle: 12 mg/kg
Sheep: 10 mg/kg

Fasinex 5% (Novartis) *Eire*
Oral solution, triclabendazole 5%, for *sheep*
Withdrawal Periods. Slaughter 42 days, milk 7 days

Fasinex 10% (Novartis) *Eire*
Oral solution, triclabendazole 10%, for *cattle*
Withdrawal Periods. Slaughter 42 days, should not be used in cattle producing milk for human consumption or within 14 days of calving

New Zealand

Indications. Immature and adult *Fasciola* in ruminants
Warnings. It is recommended to vaccinate against black disease in affected areas
Dose. *By mouth.*
Cattle, sheep, goats: 10 mg/kg

Fasinex 10 (Novartis) *NZ*
Oral suspension, triclabendazole 100 mg/mL, for *cattle, sheep, goats*
Withdrawal Periods. Slaughter 28 days, should not be used in cattle, sheep or goats producing milk for human consumption

2.1.4 Compound endoparasiticides

Multiple parasitic infections are the rule rather than the exception in domesticated animals. Most preparations in this category are combinations of drugs with complementary properties to attain an extended range of activity. For example, most combination endoparasiticide preparations for ruminants include a fasciolicide and a drug effective against roundworms. Similarly, combination preparations for dogs and cats generally give broad spectrum roundworm and tapeworm control. See sections 2.1.1 to 2.1.3 for specific drug information.

Many parasitic infections are seasonal and the prescriber should consider if it is pharmacologically sound to use a compound preparation at a time of year when one ingredient is redundant. An appropriate time for treatment of ewes is at prelambing to control both chronic fluke disease and inhibited or recently ingested nematodes. Otherwise, the use of a compound preparation is usually on an *ad hoc* basis when animals present evidence of infection with both types of parasite.

UK

PML **Combinex Cattle** (Novartis) *UK*
Oral suspension, levamisole hydrochloride 75 mg, triclabendazole 120 mg/mL, for roundworms and flukes in *cattle*; 2.2 litres
Withdrawal Periods. *Cattle*: slaughter 28 days, should not be used in cattle producing milk for human consumption or in dairy cows within 7 days of calving
Dose. *Cattle*: *by mouth,* 0.1 mL/kg

PML **Combinex Sheep** (Novartis) *UK*
Oral suspension, levamisole hydrochloride 37.5 mg, triclabendazole 50 mg/mL, for roundworms and flukes in *sheep*; 800 mL, 2.2 litres, 5 litres
Withdrawal Periods. *Sheep*: slaughter 28 days, should not be used in sheep producing milk for human consumption
Dose. *Sheep*: *by mouth,* 0.2 mL/kg

PML **Drontal Cat Tablets** (Bayer) *UK*
Tablets, scored, coated, praziquantel 20 mg, pyrantel embonate 230 mg, for roundworms and tapeworms in *cats*; 2, 20, 100
Contra-indications. Kittens less than 6 weeks of age, pregnant queens; concurrent administration of piperazine
Dose. *Cats*: *by mouth,* 1 tablet/4 kg

PML **Drontal Plus** (Bayer) *UK*
Tablets, febantel 150 mg, praziquantel 50 mg, pyrantel embonate 144 mg, for roundworms and tapeworms in *dogs*; 2, 20, 100
Contra-indications. Concurrent administration of piperazine; care in pregnant animals
Dose. *Dogs*: *by mouth,* 1 tablet/10 kg

PML **Drontal Puppy Suspension** (Bayer) *UK*
Oral suspension, febantel 15 mg/mL, pyrantel embonate 14.4 mg/mL, for roundworms in *puppies and dogs up to 1 year of age*
Contra-indications. Concurrent administration of piperazine
Dose. *Dogs*: *by mouth,* 1 ml/kg

GSL **Dual Wormer** (Bob Martin) *UK*
Tablets, (white) dichlorophen 250 mg, (yellow) piperazine citrate 297 mg, for *cats more than 1.2 kg body-weight*; 4 (yellow) + 4 (white)
Contra-indications. Cats less than 6 months of age
Dose. *Cats*: *by mouth,* see manufacturer's information

PML **Ivomec Super** (Merial) *UK*
Injection, clorsulon 100 mg, ivermectin 10 mg/mL, for roundworms, adult flukes, lice, mites, and warble fly larvae in *beef cattle, non-lactating dairy cattle*; 50 mL, 200 mL, other sizes available

Withdrawal Periods. *Cattle*: slaughter 28 days, should not be used in cattle producing milk for human consumption or in dairy cows within 28 days before calving
Dose. *Cattle*: *by subcutaneous injection*, 0.02 mL/kg (1 mL/50 kg bodyweight)

GSL **Kitzyme Veterinary Combined Wormer** (Seven Seas) *UK*
Tablets, scored, (white) dichlorophen 750 mg, (blue) piperazine citrate 375 mg, for *cats more than 900 g body-weight and 6 months of age*; 2 (white) + 4 (blue)
Dose. *Cats*: *by mouth*, (depending on body weight) see manufacturer's information
Note. Consult a veterinarian before treating pregnant animals or animals with a history of epilepsy or renal impairment

PML **Levafas Fluke and Worm Drench** (Norbrook) *UK*
Oral suspension, levamisole hydrochloride 15 mg, oxyclozanide 30 mg/mL, for roundworms and flukes in *cattle, sheep*
Withdrawal Periods. *Cattle, sheep*: slaughter 28 days, should not be used in cattle, sheep producing milk for human consumption
Dose. *Cattle, sheep*: *by mouth*, 0.5 mL/kg

PML **Levafas Diamond** (Norbrook) *UK*
Oral suspension, levamisole hydrochloride 30 mg, oxyclozanide 60 mg/mL, for roundworms and flukes in *cattle, sheep*; 1 litre, 2.5 litres, 5 litres
Withdrawal Periods. *Cattle, sheep*: slaughter 28 days, should not be used in cattle, sheep producing milk for human consumption
Dose. *Cattle, sheep*: *by mouth*, 0.25 mL/kg

PML **Mebadown Super** (Janssen) *UK*
Oral solution, closantel 50 mg, mebendazole 75 mg/mL, for roundworms, tapeworms, flukes, and nasal bots in *sheep*; 1 litre, 2.5 litres, 5 litres
Withdrawal Periods. *Sheep*: slaughter 42 days, should not be used in sheep producing milk for human consumption
Dose. *Sheep*: *by mouth*, 0.2 mL/kg

GSL **Multiwormer for Cats** (Sherley's) *UK*
Tablets, (fawn) dichlorophen 250 mg, (pink) piperazine citrate 125 mg, for *cats*; 4 (fawn) +8 (pink)
Contra-indications. Kittens less than 6 months of age
Dose. *Cats*: *by mouth*, (depending on body weight) see manufacturer's information

GSL **Multiwormer for Dogs** (Sherley's) *UK*
Tablets, (fawn) dichlorophen 750 mg, (pink) piperazine citrate 375 mg, for *dogs*; 4 (fawn) +8 (pink), 12 (fawn) + 24 (pink)
Contra-indications. Puppies less than 6 months of age
Dose. *Dogs*: *by mouth*, (depending on body weight) see manufacturer's information

PML **Nilzan Drench Super** (Schering-Plough) *UK*
Oral suspension, levamisole hydrochloride 30 mg, oxyclozanide 60 mg, cobalt sulphate heptahydrate 7.64 mg, sodium selenate 766 micrograms/mL, for roundworms and flukes in *cattle, sheep*; 1 litre, 2.5 litres, 5 litres
Withdrawal Periods. *Cattle, sheep*: slaughter 28 days, should not be used in cattle, sheep producing milk for human consumption
Dose. *Cattle, sheep*: *by mouth*, 0.25 mL/kg

PML **Nilzan Gold** (Schering-Plough) *UK*
Oral suspension, levamisole hydrochloride 30 mg, oxyclozanide 60 mg/mL, for roundworms and flukes in *cattle, sheep*; 1 litre, 2.5 litres, 5 litres
Withdrawal Periods. *Cattle, sheep*: slaughter 28 days, should not be used in cattle, sheep producing milk for human consumption
Dose. *Cattle, sheep*: *by mouth*, 0.25 mL/kg

GSL **Pet Care Dual Action Worming Tablets for Dogs** (Armitage) *UK*
Tablets, dichlorophen 500 mg, piperazine citrate 500 mg, for *dogs*; 8 + 4
Dose. *Dogs*: *by mouth*, (depending on body weight) see manufacturer's information

GSL **Pet Care Dual Action Worming Tablets for Cats** (Armitage) *UK*
Tablets, dichlorophen 500 mg, piperazine citrate 500 mg, for *cats*; 4 + 2
Dose. *Cats*: *by mouth*, (depending on body weight) see manufacturer's information

PML **Supaverm** (Janssen) *UK*
Oral suspension, closantel 50 mg, mebendazole 75 mg/mL, for roundworms, tapeworms, flukes, and nasal bots in *sheep*; 1 litre, 2.5 litres, 5 litres
Withdrawal Periods. *Sheep*: slaughter 42 days, should not be used in sheep producing milk for human consumption
Dose. *Sheep*: *by mouth*, 0.2 mL/kg

PML **Systamex Plus Fluke SC** (Schering-Plough) *UK*
Oral suspension, oxfendazole 22.65 mg, oxyclozanide 62.5 mg, cobalt (as sulphate) 1.67 mg, selenium (as sodium selenate) 500 micrograms/mL, for roundworms, tapeworms, and flukes in *cattle, sheep*; 2.5 litres, 10 litres
Withdrawal Periods. *Cattle*: slaughter 28 days, milk 5 days. *Sheep*: slaughter 28 days, should not be used in sheep producing milk for human consumption
Dose. *Cattle, sheep*: *by mouth*, 0.2 mL/kg

GSL **Twin Wormer for Cats** (Johnson's) *UK*
Tablets, (yellow) dichlorophen 250 mg, (white) piperazine phosphate 104 mg, for *cats*; 18
Contra-indications. Cats less than 6 months of age, pregnant or nursing queens
Dose. *Cats*: *by mouth*, (depending on body weight) see manufacturer's information

GSL **Twin Wormer for Dogs** (Johnson's) *UK*
Tablets, (yellow) dichlorophen 500 mg, (white) piperazine phosphate 416 mg, for *dogs*; 12, 24
Contra-indications. Dogs less than 6 months of age, pregnant or nursing bitches
Dose. *Dogs*: *by mouth*, (depending on body weight) see manufacturer's information

GSL **Vetzyme Veterinary Combined Wormer** (Seven Seas) *UK*
Tablets, scored, (white) dichlorophen 750 mg, (blue) piperazine citrate 375 mg, for *dogs more than 1.8 kg body-weight and 6 months of age*; 4 (white) + 8 (blue), 12 (white) + 24 (blue)
Dose. *Dogs*: *by mouth*, (depending on body weight) see manufacturer's information
Note. Consult a veterinarian before treating pregnant animals or animals with a history of epilepsy or renal impairment

Australia

Ambex Two (Pharmtech) *Austral*
Tablets, levamisole hydrochloride 10 mg, niclosamide 200 mg, for roundworms and tapeworms in *dogs, cats*
Dose. *Dogs, cats*: *by mouth*, 1 tablet/2 kg body-weight

Ambex Five (Pharmtech) *Austral*
Tablets, levamisole hydrochloride 25 mg, niclosamide 500 mg, for roundworms and tapeworms in *dogs, cats*
Dose. *Dogs, cats*: *by mouth*, 1 tablet/5 kg body-weight

Ambex Ten (Pharmtech) *Austral*
Tablets, levamisole hydrochloride 50 mg, niclosamide 1 g, for roundworms and tapeworms in *dogs*
Dose. *Dogs*: *by mouth*, 1 tablet/10 kg body-weight

Ascarid Worming Tablets for Dogs and Cats (Pharmachem) *Austral*
Tablets, niclosamide 1 g, levamisole (as hydrochloride) 42.4 mg, for roundworms and tapeworms in *dogs, cats*
Dose. *Dogs, cats*: *by mouth*, 1 tablet/10 kg body-weight

Avitrol Plus Syrup (Mavlab) *Austral*
Syrup, levamisole 10 mg/mL, praziquantel 2 mg/mL, for roundworms, tapeworms, and gapeworms in *cage birds*
Withdrawal Periods. Slaughter 7 days

Avitrol Plus Tablets (Mavlab) *Austral*
Tablets, levamisole hydrochloride 20 mg, praziquantel 4 mg, for roundworms, tapeworms, and gapeworms in *cage birds*
Withdrawal Periods. Should not be used in *birds* intended for human consumption

Bay-O-Pet Drontal Allwormer Cat Pills (Bayer) *Austral*
Tablets, praziquantel 5 mg, febantel 25 mg, pyrantel embonate 57.5 mg, for roundworms and tapeworms in *cats*
Dose. *Cats*: *by mouth*, 1 tablet/kg body-weight

Bay-O-Pet Drontal Allwormer for Dogs (Bayer) *Austral*
Tablets, praziquantel 15 mg, febantel 75 mg, pyrantel embonate 43.2 mg (for small dogs); praziquantel 50 mg, febantel 250 mg, pyrantel embonate 144 mg (for dogs); praziquantel 175 mg, febantel 875 mg, pyrantel embonate 504 mg (large dogs), for roundworms and tapeworms in *dogs*
Dose. *Dogs*: *by mouth*, (depending on body-weight) see manufacturer information

Canatak (Pfizer) *Austral*
Tablets, pyrantel embonate 143 mg, oxantel embonate 543 mg, for roundworms *dogs*
Dose. *Dogs*: *by mouth*, 1 tablet/10 kg body-weight

Canex Cube (Pfizer) *Austral*
Cubes, pyrantel embonate 143 mg, oxantel embonate 543 mg, praziquantel 50 mg, for roundworms and tapeworms in *dogs*
Dose. *Dogs*: *by mouth*, 1 cube/10 kg body-weight

Canex Multi Spectrum All Wormer (Pfizer) *Austral*
Tablets, pyrantel embonate 143 mg, oxantel embonate 543 mg, praziquantel 50 mg (for dogs); pyrantel embonate 286 mg, oxantel embonate 1086 mg, praziquantel 100 mg (for large dogs), for *dogs*
Dose. *Dogs*: *by mouth*, 1 tablet/10 kg body-weight (dogs); 1 tablet/20 kg body-weight (large dogs)

Closal (Pfizer) *Austral*
Oral solution, albendazole 19 g/L, closantel 37.5 g/L, for roundworms, nasal bots, and flukes in *sheep*
Withdrawal Periods. Slaughter 28 days
Dose. *Sheep*: *by mouth*, 1 mL/5 kg body-weight

Combi Broad Spectrum Sheep & Lamb Drench with Selenium (Novartis) *Austral*
Oral solution, albendazole oxide 36 g/L, levamisole (as hydrochloride) 70 g/L, selenium (as sodium salt) 1 g/L, for roundworms and tapeworms in *sheep*
Withdrawal Periods. Slaughter 10 days, should not be used in sheep producing milk for human consumption
Dose. *Sheep*: *by mouth*, 1 mL/10 kg body-weight

Combination (Western Stock Distributors) *Austral*
Oral solution, fenbendazole 25 g/L, levamisole (as hydrochloride) 40 g/L, for roundworms and tapeworms in*sheep*
Withdrawal Periods. Slaughter 14 days, milk 3 days
Dose. *Sheep*: *by mouth*, 1 mL/5 kg body-weight

Decaflea (Dermcare-Vet) *Austral*
Tablets, cyromazine 300mg, diethylcarbamazine citrate 200 mg, for heartworm prophylaxis and fleas in *dogs*
Dose. *Dogs*: *by mouth*, (<7.5 kg bdy-weight) 0.25 tablet, (7.5–15 kg body-weight) 0.5 tablet, (15–30 kg body-weight) 1 tablet

Delquantel Worming Paste for cats (Delvet) *Austral*
Oral paste, pyrantel embonate 115 mg/mL, praziquantel 10 mg/mL, for roundworms and tapeworms in *cats*
Dose. *Cats*: *by mouth*, 0.5 mL/kg body-weight

Drontal Allwormer for Dogs (Bayer) *Austral*
Tablets, praziquantel 15 mg, febantel 75 mg, pyrantel embonate 43.2 mg (for small dogs); praziquantel 50 mg, febantel 250 mg, pyrantel embonate 144 mg (for dogs); praziquantel 175 mg, febantel 875 mg, pyrantel embonate 504 mg (large dogs), for roundworms and tapeworms in *dogs*
Dose. *Dogs*: *by mouth*, (depending on body-weight) see manufactuer information

Drontal Cat Allwormer (Bayer) *Austral*
Tablets, praziquantel 20 mg, pyrantel embonate 230 mg, for roundworms and tapeworms in *cats*
Dose. *Cats*: *by mouth*, (<2 kg body-weight) 0.5 tablet, (2.1–4 kg body-weight) 1 tablet, (>4 kg body-weight) 1 tablet/4 kg

Drontal Worming Suspension for Puppies and Small Dogs (Bayer) *Austral*
Oral suspension, febantel 15 mg/mL, pyrantel embonate 14.4 mg/mL, for roundworms in *dogs*
Dose. *Dogs*: *by mouth*, 1 mL/kg

D-Worm (Pharmachem) *Austral*
Tablets, niclosamide 1 g, levamisole (as hydrochloride) 42.4 mg, for roundworms and tapeworms in *dogs, cats*
Dose. *Dogs, cats*: *by mouth*, 1tablet/10 kg

Equimax (Virbac) *Austral*
Oral paste, abamectin 3.7 mg/g, praziquantel 46.2 mg/g, for roundworms, tapeworms, horse bots, and skin lesions due to ectoparasitic infestations in *horses*
Dose. *Horses*: *by mouth*, 1 mL/20 kg body-weight

Duocare (Virbac) *Austral*
Oral solution, levamisole (as hydrochloride) 40 g/L, fenbendazole 25 g/L, for roundworms and tapeworms in*sheep*
Withdrawal Periods. Slaughter 14 days, milk 3 days
Dose. *Sheep*: *by mouth*, 1 mL/5 kg body-weight

Equimax Liquid Allwormer (Virbac) *Austral*
Oral liquid, abamectin 0.8 g/L, praziquantel 10 g/L, for roundworms, tapeworms, horse bots, and skin lesions due to ectoparasitic infestations in *horses*
Withdrawal Periods. Slaughter 28 days
Dose. *Horses*: *by mouth*, 1 mL/4 kg body-weight

Exelpet All 4in 1 Intestinal Wormer for Dogs (Excelpet) *Austral*
Tablets, praziquantel 50 mg, pyrantel embonate 143 mg, oxantel embonate 543 mg, for roundworms and tapeworms in *dogs*
Dose. *Dogs*: *by mouth*, 1 tablet/10 kg body-weight

Exelpet All 4 in 1 Intestinal Wormer for Small Dogs (Excelpet) *Austral*
Tablets, praziquantel 25 mg, pyrantel embonate 71 mg, oxantel embonate 271 mg, for roundworms and tapeworms in *dogs*
Dose. *Dogs*: *by mouth*, 1 tablet/5 kg body-weight

Exelpet All Wormer Paste for Cats (Excelpet) *Austral*
Oral paste, pyrantel embonate 90 mg/g, niclosamide monohydrate 264 mg/g paste, for roundworms and tapeworms in *cats*
Dose. *Cats*: *by mouth*, 1 mg/kg

Exelpet All Wormer for Dogs/Large Dogs (Excelpet) *Austral*
Tablets, febantel 250 mg, pyrantel embonate 144 mg, praziquantel 50 mg (dogs), praziquantel 175 mg, pyrantel embonate 174.4 mg, febantel 875 mg (large dogs), for roundworms and tapeworms in *dogs*
Dose. *Dogs*: *by mouth*, (dogs) 1 tablet/10 kg body-weight, (large dogs) 1–3 tablets depending on body-weight

Exelpet Ezy-Dose Intestinal All Wormer for Dogs (Excelpet) *Austral*
Cubes, praziquantel 50 mg, pyrantel embonate 143 mg, oxantel embonate 543 mg, for roundworms and tapeworms in *dogs*
Dose. *Dogs*: *by mouth*, 1 cube/10 kg body-weight

Exelpet Palatable Worming Granules for Dogs (Excelpet) *Austral*
Oral granules, pyrantel embonate 150 mg/3 g, oxantel embonate 585 mg/3 g, niclosamide monohydrate 1107 mg/3 g granules, for *dogs*
Dose. *Dogs*: *by mouth*, 3 g/10 kg body-weight

Farnam Worma and Bot Paste (International Animal Health Products) *Austral*
Oral paste, oxfendazole 28.4 mg/g, metrifonate 454.4 mg/g, for roundworms and horses bots in *horses*
Withdrawal Periods. Slaughter 28 days
Dose. *Horses*: *by mouth*, 40 g/450 kg

Farnam Worma Paste (International Animal Health Products) *Austral*
Oral paste, oxfendazole 107.2 mg/g, piperazine (as dihydrochloride) 214.4 mg/g, for roundworms in *horses*
Withdrawal Periods. Slaughter 28 days
Dose. *Horses*: *by mouth*, 42 g/450 kg

Felex Plus All Wormer Paste (Pfizer) *Austral*
Oral paste, pyrantel embonate 90 mg/g, niclosamide monohydrate 264 mg/g, for roundworms and tapeworms in *cats*
Dose. *Cats*: *by mouth*, 2.56 g/4 kg body-weight

Fido's Closasole (Mavlab) *Austral*
Tablets, levamisole (as hydrochloride) 42.2 mg, niclosamide 1 g, for roundworms and tapeworms in *dogs, cats*
Dose. *Dogs, cats*: *by mouth*, 1 tablet/10 kg body-weight

Heartgard 30 Plus (Merial) *Austral*
Cubes, ivermectin 68 micrograms, pyrantel embonate 57 mg; ivermectin 136 micrograms, pyrantel 114 mg; ivermectin 272 micrograms, pyrantel 227 mg, for roundworms and heartworm prophylaxis in *dogs*
Dose. *Dogs*: *by mouth*, ivermectin 6 micrograms/kg, pyrantel 5 mg/kg

Ivomec Plus Antiparasitic Injection for Cattle (Merial) *Austral*
Injection, ivermectin 10 mg/mL, clorsulon 100 mg/mL, for roundworms, lungworms, lice, mites, and ticks in *cattle*
Withdrawal Periods. Slaughter 42 days, should not be used within 28 days of calving or during lactation if milk is to be used for human consumption
Dose. *Cattle*: *by subcutaneous injection*, 1 mL/50 kg

Nilzan LV (Coopers) *Austral*
Oral solution, levamisole hydrochloride 75 g/L, oxyclozanide 150 g/L, for roundworms, tapeworms, and flukes in *cattle, sheep*
Withdrawal Periods. *Cattle*: slaughter 14 days, milk withdrawal period nil. *Sheep*: slaughter 14 days.
Dose. *Cattle*: *by mouth*, 1mL/45 kg
Sheep: *by mouth*, 1 mL/10 kg

Oximinth Plus Horse Worming Paste (Virbac) *Austral*
Oral paste, oxibendazole 1 g/5 mL, dichlorvos 1 g/5 mL, for roundworms in *horses*
Withdrawal Periods. Slaughter 28 days
Dose. *Horses*: *by mouth*, 5 mL/100 kg

Paratak Plus (Pharmatech) *Austral*
Tablets, praziquantel 50 mg, pyrantel embonate 140 mg, oxantel embonate 545 mg, for roundworms and tapeworms in *dogs*
Dose. *Dogs*: *by mouth*, 1 tablet/10 kg body-weight

Parid V (Apex) *Austral*
Tablets, niclosamide 500 mg, levamisole hydrochloride 25 mg, for roundworms and tapeworms in *dogs, cats*
Dose. *Dogs*: *by mouth*, 1 tablet/5 kg body-weight
Cats: *by mouth*, 1 tablet/10 kg body-weight

Parid X (Apex) *Austral*
Tablets, niclosamide 1000 mg, levamisole hydrochloride 50 mg, for roundworms and tapeworms in *dogs*
Dose. *Dogs*: *by mouth*, 1 tablet/10 kg body-weight

Popantel Allwormer Tablets for Dogs/Large Dogs (Dover) *Austral*
Tablets, praziquantel 50 mg, oxantel embonate 542 mg, pyrantel embonate 143 mg (dogs), praziquantel 200 mg, oxantel embonate 2168 mg, pyrantel embonate 572 mg (large dogs), for roundworms and tapeworms in *dogs*
Dose. *Dogs*: *by mouth*, (dogs) 1 tablet/10 kg body-weight, (large dogs) 1tablet/40 kg body-weight

Salvo (Hoechst Roussel) *Austral*
Oral solution, fenbendazole 25 g/L, levamisole (as hydrochloride) 40 g/L, for roundworms and tapeworms in *sheep*
Withdrawal Periods. Slaughter 14 days, milk 3 days
Dose. *Sheep*: *by mouth*, 1 mL/5 kg body-weight

Scanda (Coopers) *Austral*
Oral solution, levamisole hydrochloride 80 g/L, oxfendazole 45.3 g/L, for roundworms and tapeworms in *sheep*
Withdrawal Periods. Slaughter 10 days.
Dose. *Sheep*: *by mouth*, 1 mL/10 kg body-weight

Sentinel (Novartis) *Austral*
Tablets, milbemycin oxime 2.3 mg, lufenuron 46 mg (very small dogs); milbemycin oxime 5.75 mg, lufenuron 115 mg (small dogs); milbemycin oxime 11.5 mg, lufenuron 230 mg (medium dogs); milbemycin oxime 23

mg, lufenuron 460 mg (large dogs), for roundworms, heartworm prophylaxis,and fleas in *dogs*
Dose. *Dogs*: *by mouth*, 1 tablet depending on body-weight

Strategy-T Paste (Vetsearch) *Austral*
Oral paste, oxfendazole 6 g/30 mL, pyrantel pamoate 7.8 g/30 mL, for roundworms and tapeworms in *horses*
Withdrawal Periods. Slaughter 28 days
Dose. *Horses*: *by mouth*, 5 mL/100 kg body-weight

Telmin Plus Horse Wormer with Boticide Granules (Boehringer Ingelheim) *Austral*
Oral granules, mebendazole 2 g/20 g, metrifonate 6 g/20 g granules, for roundworms and horse bots in *horses*
Withdrawal Periods. Slaughter 28 days
Dose. *Horses*: *by mouth*, (100–225 kg body-weight) 20 g, (>225 kg body-weight) 40 g; reduce dose for horses <100 kg body-weight

Telmin Plus Horse Wormer with Boticide Paste (Boehringer Ingelheim) *Austral*
Oral paste, mebendazole 5 g/40 g, metrifonate 15 g/40 g paste, for roundworms and horse bots in *horses*
Withdrawal Periods. Slaughter 28 days
Dose. *Horses*: *by mouth*, 40 g/565 kg body-weight

Two-Up (Nufarm) *Austral*
Oral solution, fenbendazole 25 g/L, levamisole (as hydrochloride) 40 g/L, for roundworms and tapeworms in *sheep*
Withdrawal Periods. Slaughter 14 days, milk 3 days
Dose. *Sheep*: *by mouth*, 1 mL/5 kg body-weight

Virbac First Drench (Virbac) *Austral*
Oral solution, levamisole hydrochloride 37.5 g/L, praziquantel 18.8 g/L, for roundworms and tapeworms in *sheep*
Withdrawal Periods. Slaughter 3 days
Dose. *Sheep*: *by mouth*, 1 mL/5 kg body-weight

Vita Verm Plus (Virbac) *Austral*
Tablets, niclosamide 500 mg, levamisole hydrochloride 25 mg, for roundworms and tapeworms in *dogs*
Dose. *Dogs*: *by mouth*, 1 tablet/5 kg body-weight

Eire

Bovermplus (Foran) *Eire*
Oral suspension, levamisole hydrochloride 15 mg/mL, bithionol sulphoxide 80 mg/mL, for roundworms in *cattle, sheep*
Withdrawal Periods. Slaughter 60 days, should not be used in cattle or sheep producing milk for human consumption
Dose. *Cattle, sheep*: *by mouth*, 1 mL/2 kg body-weight

Chan Broad Spec (Chanelle) *Eire*
Oral suspension, rafoxanide 225 mg/mL, levamisole hydrochloride 15 mg/mL, for roundworms and fluke in *cattle, sheep*
Withdrawal Periods. Slaughter 60 days, should not be used in cattle or sheep producing milk for human consumption
Dose. *Cattle, sheep*: *by mouth*, 1 mL/2 kg body-weight

Curafluke Oral Drench (Univet) *Eire*
Oral solution, fenbendazole 50 mg/mL, rafoxanide 50 mg/mL, for roundworms and fluke *cattle, sheep*
Withdrawal Periods. Slaughter 60 days, should not be used in cattle or sheep producing milk for human consumption
Dose. *Cattle*: *by mouth*, 2.25 mL/10 kg body-weight
Sheep: *by mouth*, 1.5 mL/10 kg body-weight

Drontal Cat Tablets (Bayer) *Eire*
Tablets, pyrantel embonate 230 mg, praziquantel 20 mg, for roundworms and tapeworms in *cats*
Dose. *Cats*: *by mouth*, 1 tablet/4 kg body-weight

Drontal Plus Tablets (Bayer) *Eire*
Tablets, praziquantel 50 mg, pyrantel embonate 144 mg, febantel 150 mg, for roundworms and tapeworms in *dogs*
Dose. *Dogs*: *by mouth*, 1 tablet/10 kg body-weight

Duphabendazole (Interchem) *Eire*
Oral solution, oxibendazole 2.5 g/25 mL, dichlorvos 5 g/25 mL, for **horses**
Dose. *Horses*: *by mouth*, 5 mL/100 kg body-weight

Endex (Cattle) (Novartis) *Eire*
Oral solution, levamisole hydrochloride 75 mg/mL, triclabendazole 120 mg/mL, for roundworms and fluke in **cattle**
Withdrawal Periods. Slaughter 42 days, should not be used in cattle producing milk for human consumption
Dose. *Cattle*: *by mouth*, 1 mL/10 kg body-weight

Endex (Sheep) (Novartis) *Eire*
Oral solution, levamisole hydrochloride 37.5 mg/mL, triclabendazole 50 mg/mL, for roundworms and flukes in **sheep**
Withdrawal Periods. Slaughter 42 days, should not be used in sheep producing milk for human consumption
Dose. *Sheep*: *by mouth*, 1 mL/5 kg body-weight

Equiminthe Plus Horse Wormer (Virbac) *Eire*
Oral paste, per 25-ml syringe: oxibendazole 5 g, dichlorvos 5 g, for **horses**
Withdrawal Periods. Slaughter 28 days
Dose. *Horses*: *by mouth*, 5 mL/100 kg body-weight

Ivomec Super Injection for Cattle (Merial) *Eire*
Injection, ivermectin 10 mg/mL, clorsulon 100mg/mL, for roundworms, warbles, mites, and lice in **cattle**
Withdrawal Periods. Slaughter 28 days, should not be used in cattle porducing milk for human consumption, should not be used in cattle within 28 days before calving if milk is to be used for human consumption
Dose. *Cattle*: *by subcutaneous injection*, 1 mL/50 kg body-weight

Levafas C Fluke and Worm Drench (Norbrook) *Eire*
Oral solution, levamisole hydrochloride 15 mg/mL, oxyclozanide 30 mg/mL, (also contains selenium and cobalt), for roundworms in **cattle, sheep**
Withdrawal Periods. Slaughter 28 days, should not be used in cattle or sheep producing milk for human consumption
Dose. *Cattle, sheep*: *by mouth*, 1 mL/2 kg body-weight

Levafas Diamond Fluke and Worm Drench (Norbrook) *Eire*
Oral solution, levamisole hydrochloride 30 mg/mL, oxyclozanide 60mg/mL, for roundworms in **cattle, sheep**
Withdrawal Periods. Slaughter 28 days, should not be used in cattle or sheep producing milk for human consumption
Dose. *Cattle, sheep*: *by mouth*, 25 mL/100 kg body-weight

Nilzan Drench Plus (Schering-Plough) *Eire*
Oral suspension, levamisole hydrochloride 15 mg/mL, oxyclozanide 30 mg/mL (also contains cobalt), for roundworms in **cattle, sheep**
Withdrawal Periods. Slaughter 28 days, should not be used in cattle or sheep producing milk for human consumption
Dose. *Cattle, sheep*: *by mouth*, 1 mL/2 kg body-weight

Panafluke (Hoechst Roussel Vet) *Eire*
Oral suspension, rafoxanide 45 mg/mL, fenbendazole 30 mg/mL, for roundworms and fluke in **cattle, sheep**
Withdrawal Periods. Slaughter 60 days, should not be used in cattle or sheep producing milk for human consumption
Dose. *Cattle, sheep*: *by mouth*, 2.5 mL/10 kg body-weight

Rafazole (Chanelle) *Eire*
Oral suspension, rafoxanide 30 mg/mL, levamisole hydrochloride 30 mg/mL, for roundworms and flukes in **cattle, sheep**
Withdrawal Periods. Slaughter 60 days, should not be used in cattle or sheep producing milk for human consumption
Dose. *Cattle, sheep*: *by mouth*, 12.5 mL/50 kg body-weight

Stromiten Dogs Divisible Tablets (Vetoquinol) *Eire*
Tablets, levamisole (as hydrochloride) 16 mg, niclosamide 720 mg, for roundworms and tapewormsin **dogs**
Dose. *Dogs*: *by mouth*, 1 tablet/4 kg body-weight

Supaverm (Janssen) *Eire*
Oral suspension, closantel 50 mg/mL, mebendazole 75 mg/mL, for roundworms, fluke, and nasal bots in **sheep**
Withdrawal Periods. Slaughter 42 days, should not be used in sheep producing milk for human consumption
Dose. *Sheep*: *by mouth*, 1 mL/5 kg body-weight

Univet Multidose Fluke and Worm Drench (Univet) *Eire*
Oral solution, levamisole 15 mg/mL, rafoxanide 22.5 mg/mL, for roundworms and fluke in **cattle, sheep**
Withdrawal Periods. Slaughter 60 days, should not be used in cattle or sheep producing milk for human consumption
Dose. *Cattle, sheep*: *by mouth*, 1 mL/2 kg body-weight

New Zealand

Ambex Two (Bomac) *NZ*
Tablets, levamisole hydrochloride 10 mg, niclosamide 200 mg, for roundworms and tapeworms in **dogs, cats**
Dose. *Dogs, cats*: *by mouth*, 1 tablet/2 kg body-weight

Ambex Five (Bomac) *NZ*
Tablets, levamisole hydrochloride 25 mg, niclosamide 500 mg, for roundworms and tapeworms in **dogs, cats**
Dose. *Dogs, cats*: *by mouth*, 1 tablet/5 kg body-weight

Arrest (Ancare) *NZ*
Oral solution, albendazole 23.8 g/litre, levamisole hydrochloride 37.5 g/litre, for roundworms, tapeworms, and flukes in **sheep**
Withdrawal Periods. Slaughter 10 days, should not be used in sheep producing milk for human consumption
Dose. *Sheep*: *by mouth*, 1 mL/5 kg body-weight

Arrest C (Ancare) *NZ*
Oral solution, albendazole 100 g/litre, levamisole hydrochloride 75 g/litre, for roundworms, tapeworms, and flukes in **cattle**
Withdrawal Periods. Slaughter 14 days, should not be used in cattle producing milk for human consumption
Dose. *Cattle*: *by mouth*, 1 mL/10 kg body-weight

Arrest Hi-mineral (Ancare) *NZ*
Oral solution, albendazole 23.8 g/litre, levamisole hydrochloride 37.5 g/litre in a mineralised formulation, for roundworms, tapeworms, and flukes in **sheep**
Withdrawal Periods. Slaughter 10 days, should not be used in sheep producing milk for human consumption
Dose. *Sheep*: *by mouth*, 1 mL/5 kg body-weight

Cancare Plus (Ancare) *NZ*
Tablets, oxantel pamoate 760 mg, pyrantel pamoate 200 mg, for roundworms in **dogs**
Dose. *Dogs*: *by mouth*, 1 tablet/14 kg body-weight

Canex Cube Palatable All Wormer for Dogs (Pfizer) *NZ*
Tablets, oxantel embonate 542 mg, praziquantel 50 mg, pyrantel embonate 143 mg, for roundworms and tapeworms in **dogs**
Dose. *Dogs*: *by mouth*, 1 tablet/10 kg body-weight

Canex Multispectrum All Wormer for Medium/Large Dogs (Pfizer) *NZ*
Tablets, oxantel embonate 343 mg, praziquantel 50 mg, pyrantel embonate 143 mg (dogs), oxantel embonate 1086 mg, praziquantel 100 mg, pyrantel embonate 286 mg (large dogs), for roundworms and tapeworms in **dogs**
Dose. *Dogs*: *by mouth*, 1 tablet/20 kg body-weight (large dogs); 1 tablet/10 kg body-weight (medium dogs)

Canikat (Virbac) *NZ*
Oral paste, niclosamide 240 mg/mL, oxibendazole 45 mg/mL, for roundworms and tapeworms in **dogs, cats**
Dose. *Dogs, cats*: *by mouth*, 1mL/2 kg body-weigh

Closal (Pfizer) *NZ*
Oral solution, albendazole 19 mg/mL, closantel 37.5 mg/mL, for roundworms, nasal bots, and flukes in **sheep**
Withdrawal Periods. Slaughter 28 days, should not be used in sheep producing milk for human consumption
Dose. *Sheep*: *by mouth*, 1 mL/5 kg body-weight

Combitape (Novartis) *NZ*
Oral suspension, levamisole hydrochloride 37.5 mg/mL, praziquantel 18.8 mg/mL, albendazole 20 mg/mL, for roundworms, tapeworms, and flukes in **sheep**
Withdrawal Periods. Slaughter 10 days, should not be used in sheep producing milk for human consumption

Dose. *Sheep*: *by mouth*, roundworms, tapeworms, 1 mL/5 kg body-weight; flukes, 1 mL/4 kg body-weight

Combitape Mineralised Plus Selenium (Novartis) *NZ*
Oral suspension, levamisole hydrochloride 37.5 mg/mL, praziquantel 18.8 mg/mL, albendazole 20 mg/mL in a mineral formulation, for roundworms, tapeworms, and flukes in *sheep*
Withdrawal Periods. Slaughter 10 days, should not be used in sheep producing milk for human consumption
Dose. *Sheep*: *by mouth*, roundworms, tapeworms, 1 mL/5 kg body-weight; flukes, 1 mL/4 kg body-weight

Drontal Allwormer for Cats (Bayer) *NZ*
Tablets, praziquantel 20 mg, pyrantel embonate 230 mg, for roundworms and tapeworms in *cats*
Dose. *Cats*: *by mouth*, 1 tablet/4 kg body-weight

Drontal Allwormer for Large Dogs (Bayer) *NZ*
Tablets, febantel 875 mg, praziquantel 175 mg, pyrantel embonate 504 mg, for roundworms and tapeworms in *dogs*
Dose. *Dogs*: *by mouth*, 1 tablet/35 kg body-weight

Drontal Plus (Bayer) *NZ*
Tablets, febantel 150 mg, praziquantel 50 mg, pyrantel pamoate 145 mg, for roundworms and tapeworms in *dogs*
Dose. *Dogs*: *by mouth*, 0.5–4 tablet depending on body-weight

Endex Sheep (Novartis) *NZ*
Oral suspension, levamisole hydrochloride 37.5 mg/mL, triclabendazole 50 mg/mL, for roundworms and flukes in *sheep*
Withdrawal Periods. Slaughter 28 days, should not be used in sheep producing milk for human consumption
Dose. *Sheep*: *by mouth*, 1 mL/5 kg body-weight

Equiminth Plus (Virbac) *NZ*
Oral paste, dichlorvos 200 mg/mL, oxibendazole 200 mg/mL, for roundworms and horsebots in *horses*
Withdrawal Periods. Slaughter 28 days
Dose. *Horses*: *by mouth*, 5 mL/100 kg body-weight

Felex Plus All Wormer (Pfizer) *NZ*
Oral paste, niclosamide 267 mg/g, pyrantel pamoate 90 mg/g, for roundworms and tapeworms in *cats*
Dose. *Cats*: *by mouth*, 2.56 g/4 kg body-weight

First Drench (Ancare) *NZ*
Oral solution, albendazole 25 mg/mL, levamisole 37.5 mg/mL, praziquantel 18.8 mg/mL, for roundworms, tapeworms, and flukes in *sheep*
Withdrawal Periods. Slaughter 10 days, should not be used in sheep producing milk for human consumption
Dose. *Sheep*: *by mouth*, 1 mL/5 kg body-weight

First Drench Hi-mineral (Ancare) *NZ*
Oral solution, albendazole 25 mg/mL, levamisole 37.5 mg/mL, praziquantel 18.8 mg/mL in a mineral formulation, for roundworms, tapeworms, and flukes in *sheep*
Withdrawal Periods. Slaughter 10 days, should not be used in sheep producing milk for human consumption
Dose. *Sheep*: *by mouth*, 1 mL/5 kg body-weight

Genesis Horse Wormer (Ancare) *NZ*
Oral paste, abamectin 4 mg/mL, praziquantel 50 mg/mL, for roundworms, tapeworms, and horse bots in *horses*
Withdrawal Periods. Slaughter 28 days
Dose. *Horses*: *by mouth*, 1 mL/20 kg body-weight

Genesis Tape Hi Mineral for Lambs (Ancare) *NZ*
Oral solution, abamectin 1 mg/mL, praziquantel 18.8 mg/mL in a mineral formulation, for roundworms and tapeworms in *sheep*
Withdrawal Periods. Slaughter 14 days, should not be used in sheep producing milk for human consumption
Dose. *Sheep*: *by mouth*, 1 mL/5 kg body-weight

Ivomec Plus (Merial) *NZ*
Injection, ivermectin 10 mg/mL, clorsulon 100 mg/mL, for roundworms, flukes, and lice in *cattle*

Withdrawal Periods. Slaughter 49 days, should not be used in cattle producing milk for human consumption
Dose. *Cattle*: *by subcutaneous injection*, 1 mL/50 kg body-weight

Leviben (Novartis) *NZ*
Oral suspension, levamisole hydrochloride 37.5 mg/mL, albendazole 20 mg/mL, for roundworms, tapeworms, and flukes in *sheep*
Withdrawal Periods. Slaughter 21 days, should not be used in sheep producing milk for human consumption
Dose. *Sheep*: *by mouth*, roundworms, tapeworms, 1 mL/5 kg body-weight; flukes, 1 mL/4 kg body-weight

Leviben Mineralised Plus Selenium (Novartis) *NZ*
Oral suspension, levamisole hydrochloride 37.5 mg/mL, albendazole 20 mg/mL, selenium 0.4 mg/mL in a mineral formulation, for roundworms, tapeworms, and flukes in *sheep*
Withdrawal Periods. Slaughter 21 days, should not be used in sheep producing milk for human consumption
Dose. *Sheep*: *by mouth*, roundworms, tapeworms, 1 mL/5 kg body-weight; flukes, 1 mL/4 kg body-weight

Levitape (Ancare) *NZ*
Oral suspension, levamisole 37.5 mg/mL, praziquantel 18.8 mg/mL, for roundworms and tapeworms in *lambs*
Withdrawal Periods. Slaughter 10 days
Dose. *Sheep*: *by mouth*, 1 mL/5 kg body-weight

Levitape Hi-Mineral (Ancare) *NZ*
Oral suspension, levamisole 37.5 mg/mL, praziquantel 18.8 mg/mL in a mineral formulation, for roundworms and tapeworms in *lambs*
Withdrawal Periods. Slaughter 10 days
Dose. *Sheep*: *by mouth*, 1 mL/5 kg body-weight

Nilzan (Schering-Plough) *NZ*
Oral suspension, levamisole hydrochloride 40 mg/mL, oxyclozanide 75 mg/mL, for roundworms, tapeworms, flukes in *cattle, sheep*
Withdrawal Periods. *Cattle*: slaughter 21 days, milk 24 hours. *Sheep*: slaughter 21 days, should not be used in sheep producing milk for human consumption
Dose. *Cattle*: *by mouth*, 1 mL/5 kg body-weight
Sheep: *by mouth*, 1 mL/6 kg body-weight

Paratak Plus (Bomac) *NZ*
Tablets, oxantel pamoate 545 mg, praziquantel 50 mg, pyrantel pamoate 140 mg, for roundworms and tapeworms in *dogs*
Dose. *Dogs*: *by mouth*, 1 tablet/10 kg body-weigh

Paratak Plus 35 (Bomac) *NZ*
Tablets, oxantel pamoate 1907 mg, praziquantel 175 mg, pyrantel pamoate 490 mg, for roundworms and tapeworms in *dogs*
Dose. *Dogs*: *by mouth*, 1 tablet/35 kg body-weigh

Rintal + Neguvon Paste (Bayer) *NZ*
Oral paste, febantel 71.2 g/kg, metrifonate 355.7 g/kg, for roundworms and horse bots in *horses*
Withdrawal Periods. Slaughter 28 days
Dose. *Horses*: *by mouth*, 38 g/450 kg body-weight

Rycomectin Abatape (Novartis) *NZ*
Oral solution, abamectin 0.8 mg/mL, praziquantel 15.04 mg/mL, for roundworms and tapeworms in *sheep*
Withdrawal Periods. Slaughter 21 days, should not be used in sheep producing milk for human consumption
Dose. *Sheep*: *by mouth*, 1 mL/4 kg body-weight

Rycotape (Novartis) *NZ*
Oral suspension, levamisole hydrochloride 37.5 mg/mL, praziquantel 18.8 mg/mL, for roundworms and tapeworms in *sheep*
Withdrawal Periods. Slaughter 10 days, should not be used in sheep producing milk for human consumption
Dose. *Sheep*: *by mouth*, 1 mL/5 kg body-weight

Rycotape Mineralised Plus Selenium (Novartis) *NZ*
Oral suspension, levamisole hydrochloride 37.5 mg/mL, praziquantel 18.8 mg/mL, selenium (as sodium salt) 0.5 mg/mL in a mineral formulation, for roundworms and tapeworms in *sheep*

Withdrawal Periods. Slaughter 10 days, milk 24 hours
Dose. *Sheep: by mouth*, 1 mL/5 kg body-weight

Scanda (Schering-Plough) *NZ*
Oral solution, levamisole hydrochloride 80 mg/mL, oxfendazole 45.3 mg/mL, for roundworms in *cattle*, for roundworms, tapeworms, and flukes in *sheep*
Withdrawal Periods. *Cattle*: slaughter 10 days, milk 144 hours. *Sheep*: slaughter 10 days, should not be used in sheep producing milk for human consumption
Dose. *Cattle, sheep: by mouth*, 1 mL/10 kg body-weight

Scanda Selenised (Schering-Plough) *NZ*
Oral solution, levamisole hydrochloride 80 mg/mL, oxfendazole 45.3 mg/mL, sodium selenate 1 mg/mL in a mineral formulation, for roundworms in *cattle*, for roundworms, tapeworms, and flukes in *sheep*
Withdrawal Periods. *Cattle*: slaughter 10 days, milk 144 hours. *Sheep*: slaughter 10 days, should not be used in sheep producing milk for human consumption
Dose. *Cattle, sheep: by mouth*, 1 mL/10 kg body-weight

Tandem (Novartis) *NZ*
Oral suspension, fenbendazole 25 mg/mL, levamisole 47.2 mg/mL, for roundworms and tapeworms in *sheep*
Withdrawal Periods. Slaughter 10 days, milk 96 hours
Dose. *Sheep: by mouth*, 1 mL/5 kg body-weight

Tandem Mineralised (Novartis) *NZ*
Oral suspension, fenbendazole 25 mg/mL, levamisole 47.2 mg/mL in a mineral formulation, for roundworms and tapeworms in *sheep*
Withdrawal Periods. Slaughter 10 days, milk 96 hours
Dose. *Sheep: by mouth*, 1 mL/5 kg body-weight

Tandem Mineralised Plus Selenium (Novartis) *NZ*
Oral suspension, fenbendazole 25 mg/mL, levamisole 47.2 mg/mL, selenium 0.5 mg/mL in a mineral formulation, for roundworms and tapeworms in *sheep*
Withdrawal Periods. Slaughter 10 days, milk 96 hours
Dose. *Sheep: by mouth*, 1 mL/5 kg body-weight

Valbazen Combo (Pfizer) *NZ*
Oral solution, albendazole 23.8 mg/mL, levamisole hydrochloride 37.5 mg/mL in a mineral formulation, for roundworms and flukes in *sheep*
Withdrawal Periods. Slaughter 10 days, should not be used in sheep producing milk for human consumption
Dose. *Sheep: by mouth*, 1 mL/5 kg body-weight

USA

Drontal (Bayer) *USA*
Tablets, praziquantel 18.2 mg, pyrantel (as embonate) 72.6 mg, for roundworms and tapeworms in *cats*
Dose. *Cats: by mouth*, 0.25–2.0 tablets depending on body-weigh

Drontal Plus (Bayer) *USA*
Tablets, praziquantel 22.7 mg, pyrantel (as embonate) 22.7 mg, febantel 113.4 (small dogs); praziquantel 68 mg, pyrantel (as embonate) 68 mg, febantel 340.2 mg (medium to large dogs), for roundworms and tapeworms in *dogs*
Dose. *Dogs: by mouth*, 0.5–2.5 tablets depending on body-weigh (small dogs); 1–4 tablets depending on body-weight (medium to large dogs)

Ivomec Plus Injection (Merial) *USA*
Injection, clorsulon 100 mg/mL, ivermectin 10 mg/mL, for roundworms, flukes, mites, and lice in *cattle*
Withdrawal Periods. Slaughter 49 days, should not be used in cattle producing milk for human consumption
Dose. *Cattle: by subcutaneous injection*, 1 mL/50 kg body-weight

RM Paraciticide-10 (Merial) *USA*
Oral paste, febantel 34 mg/mL, praziquantel 3.4 mg/mL, for roundworms and tapeworms in *dogs, cats*
Dose. *Dogs, cats: by mouth*, 0.3 mL/kg body-weight

Sentinel (Novartis) *USA*
Tablets, milbemycin oxime 2.3 mg, lufenuron 46 mg; milbemycin oxime 5.75 mg, lufenuron 115 mg; milbemycin oxime 11.5mg, lufenuron 230 mg;

milbemycin oxime 23 mg, lufenuron 460 mg, for roundworms, heartworm prophylaxis,and fleas in *dogs*
Dose. *Dogs: by mouth*, 1 tablet/4.6 kg body-weight

Filaribits Plus (Pfizer) *USA*
Tablets, diethylcarbamazine citrate 60 mg, oxibendazole 45mg; diethylcarbamazine citrate 120mg, oxibendazole 91 mg; diethylcarbamazine citrate 180 mg, oxibendazole 136 mg, for roundwormsand heartworm prophylaxis in *dogs*

Heartgard Plus Chewables (Merial) *USA*
Tablets, ivermectin 68 micrograms, pyrantel (as embonate) 57 mg; ivermectin 136 micrograms, pyrantel 114 mg; ivermectin 272 micrograms, pyrantel 227 mg, for *dogs*

Tri-Wormer (Performer) *USA*
Capsules, toluene 4.8 g and dichlorophen 4 g, for roundworms and tapeworms in *dogs*
Dose. *Dogs: by mouth*, 1capsule/18.2 kg body-weight

2.2 Ectoparasiticides

2.2.1 Ectoparasiticides
2.2.2 Insect growth regulators
2.2.3 Compound preparations for ectoparasites
2.2.4 Sheep dips
2.2.5 Fly repellents
2.2.6 Environmental control of ectoparasites

Ectoparasites can cause severe irritation and be responsible for loss of condition, disease, and in farm animals, production deficits due to weight loss, reduced milk yield, or damage to the hide or fleece.

The use of ectoparasiticides often depends on the conditions under which the animals are kept as well as the species of ectoparasite causing the infestation. In many cases, the expected ectoparasitic challenge may be predicted. For example, there will be a rise in tick populations in the spring and autumn, increased numbers of blowfly in late spring and early summer, warble fly oviposition from May to July, and the possible increase of lice on winter-housed stock and hill sheep. These can be countered by strategic therapeutic and prophylactic use of ectoparasiticides. In contrast, parasitism of intensively housed stock or companion animals, where transmission is by contact, is not 'seasonal' and requires diagnosis as infestations may go unnoticed for some time. In these situations, control measures should be included in routine hygiene programmes to treat the animals and, where necessary, the housing.

It is advisable that if no parasite control programme has been used before, or has been allowed to lapse, the whole herd or flock should be treated. All new additions to the herd or flock should be isolated and treated before mixing with the established stock. Empty premises should be thoroughly cleaned and then disinfested.

Equidae

Horses are susceptible to various flies, lice, and mites. The blood-sucking fly that seriously affects horses is *Stomoxys*, the 'stable fly'. In addition to the severe irritation caused by its bite, the fly is also an intermediate host of the nematode *Habronema*, which infects horses. Infected flies modify their feeding habits, larvae pass from the mouth parts and are swallowed, or flies are swallowed whole. Flies that cause worry to horses are mainly the non-biting flies *Hydrotaea* and *Musca*.

Horse bots are larvae of the flies of several species of the genus *Gasterophilus*. The noise of the flies causes worry to horses. *G. intestinalis* lays its eggs on the horse's front legs. The eggs hatch as a result of the increase in temperature caused by the licking or grooming action of the animal. The other species lay their eggs in or near the mouth. Hatched larvae either enter the mouth or are transferred via the tongue to penetrate it or the buccal mucosa. Some aspects of the life cycle of *Gasterophilus* are not fully known but the larvae of all species ultimately reach the stomach where they remain for several months. The infection cannot be diagnosed, by parasitological means, once the larvae are located in the stomach or intestines but areas around the mouth may be examined for parasite eggs, the pharynx for larvae, and the stomach by gastroscopy. Infection is controlled by frequent grooming to remove eggs before they hatch. Alternatively, warm water containing insecticide may be applied to the forelimbs and mouth area; this encourages the eggs to hatch and the drug then kills the larvae. Treatment of larvae in the stomach is traditionally given twice yearly; initially after adult fly activity has ceased and again during late winter (see section 2.1 for preparation details).

Culicoides spp. are midges that give rise to 'sweetitch' ('Queensland itch'), a dermatitis resulting from hypersensitivity to the saliva of this insect. Preventative measures to reduce exposure to midges during the summer months include the application of fly repellents, spraying with insecticides, or stabling before the afternoon and overnight. Treatment in severe cases involves the administration of oral or parenteral corticosteroids (see section 7.2.1) supported by the application of topical corticosteroid and anti-bacterial creams (see section 14.2.1) or antipruritic preparations (see section 14.5.1).

Lice can be identified in the mane and at the base of the tail during early infestation. Later they become more generalised. *Bovicola* (*Damalinia*) spp., the biting louse, causes hair loss and irritation with consequent rubbing. Animals infested with the sucking louse *Haematopinus* spp. will lose condition and anaemia can result.

Sarcoptes spp., a mite that burrows into the skin, is first observed on the head, neck, and shoulders, while the non-burrowing mite *Psoroptes* spp. is found on either the body or the ears. *Chorioptes* spp. can be found on the lower legs and hocks. All will cause irritation, rubbing, scratching, restlessness, and hair loss. Treatment for mite infestation is usually in autumn or winter.

Cattle

Cattle are susceptible to attacks by various flies. The blood-sucking flies of the genera *Stomoxys* and *Haematobia* are common parasites of cattle. The biting fly *Haematobia irritans*, the 'horn fly', causes intense irritation. *Hydrotaea irritans* is not a biting fly but the female can abrade skin and the fly does cause worry to cattle, sheep, and goats by feeding on ocular and nasal secretions. Skin lesions and weight loss may result. In addition, *Hydrotaea irritans* appears to be a major factor in the transmission of bacteria that cause summer mastitis. Some species of muscids, for example *Musca autumnalis*, have been implicated in the transmission of *Moraxella bovis* (infectious bovine keratoconjunctivitis, 'pinkeye', New Forest Disease). Others, including *Morellia*, occur on vegetation but may be attracted to sweat and mucus on cattle and horses, and cause fly-worry in late summer. *Musca domestica* also affects cattle similarly. Fly control is usually from late spring until autumn. Insecticide impregnated ear tags (see section 2.2.4), applied at the start of the grazing season, can give full season protection. Alternatively, insecticides or fly repellents may be applied at regular intervals or at anticipated periods of peak fly activity.

Biting midges, *Simulium* spp., breed in running water. They may cause eye lesions in cattle. Only the adult female sucks blood, whereas both male and female biting 'stable flies' *Stomoxys calcitrans* feed on blood, which can be very painful for cattle and other species, such as horses (see also above). Treatment should be anticipated for peak activity in summer.

Warble flies ('cattle grubs'), *Hypoderma*, affecting cattle and also deer, are active particularly during the warm summer months. The adult fly makes a characteristic noise, which causes excessive worry to animals as the flies approach to lay their eggs. The larvae penetrate rapidly into the animal and migrate towards the diaphragm spending the winter months in the spinal canal or the oesophageal area. In the following year the mature larvae locate in the back forming a perforated warble, which ultimately downgrades the hide. *Hypoderma* is a notifiable disease in the UK. It is now almost eradicated from the UK. Traditionally, treatment for *Hypoderma* is in the autumn when lice may also be controlled. Systemic organophosphorus parasiticides should be used at the appropriate time and use is contra-indicated when serious adverse effects may result due to the location of the parasite within the animal's body. Dead larvae in the proximity of the spinal column or oesophagus may result in either paraplegia, or bloat, respectively.

Sucking lice found on cattle include *Haematopinus*, *Linognathus*, and the more uncommon *Solenopotes*. Lice will be found on different areas of the body depending upon the species: Linognathidae prefer the head, neck, and dewlap. The chewing louse, *Bovicola bovis* (*Damalinia bovis*) may be present on most of the upper parts of the animal's body.

Chorioptic mange is due to the mite *Chorioptes bovis*, which is prevalent in winter. *Chorioptes bovis* and *Psoroptes ovis* var *bovis* can spread over the body from the base of the tail. *Sarcoptes scabiei* var *bovis* causes sarcoptic mange but infestations are uncommon. It is usually present on the head and neck but may occur elsewhere on the body.

Ticks are blood feeders and species affecting cattle and sheep include *Ixodes*, *Dermacentor*, and *Haemaphysalis*. In tropical climates a number of tick species belonging to the genera *Amblyomma*, *Boophilus*, *Hyalomma*, and *Rhipicephalus* are important as vectors of a number of major diseases worldwide. In Britain, *Ixodes ricinus* transmits babesiosis (redwater), louping ill, and tick-borne fever. *Dermacentor reticulatus* is occasionally found in southern England and Wales, and transmits equine and canine babesiosis. *Haemaphysalis punctata*, found in the same general areas as *Dermacentor* transmits *Babesia major* in Britain. Treatment just before the tick population rise is advocated, particularly in sheep (see below), with additional treatments, especially in cattle, according to the duration of challenge. Although challenge can be anticipated, the persistence of many ectoparasiticides on hair is less than on wool therefore repeat treatments may be necessary on cattle.

Sheep and goats

One of the main ectoparasites infesting sheep is calliphorine larval myiosis. Species of flies responsible are *Lucilia*, *Phormia*, and some *Calliphora*. Calliphorine myiosis may be complex and an initial strike may lead to further strikes and result in large wounds. Affected sheep have identifiable characteristics and odour. Feed intake is reduced and their condition deteriorates leading to reduced meat, milk, and fleece production and finally death. The use of insecticides immediately before fly challenge and certainly during the peak challenge in late spring and early summer is advised. Clipping wool from the area around the tail and breech can help reduce fly strike in this area.

Hydrotaea irritans, the 'head fly', causes considerable worry to sheep. Frequently, a large number of flies will attack an individual animal, concentrating around the head and taking advantage of any abrasion or secretion on the skin, particularly around the horns and eyes.

Infestation with sheep nasal bots *Oestrus ovis*, results in the condition 'false gid'. The viviparous females deposit larvae around the animal's nostrils. During this process, large numbers of flies may attack, causing the sheep to panic. The fly may also affect goats. The larvae crawl up the nose into the sinuses and irritate the mucosae. This results in the discharge of mucus exudate on which the larvae feed. Dead larvae may give rise to secondary bacterial infection with occasional mortality. When development is complete, the larvae crawl out from the nostrils and pupate on the ground. See section 2.1 for details of treatment of nasal bots with anthelmintics.

Melophagus ovinus, the sheep ked, lives in the wool and feeds by sucking blood; heavy infestations may cause anaemia. Generally, production loss is associated with irritation leading to wool damage and staining. Chewing and sucking lice lead to wool and skin damage, and sucking lice to body fluid loss. Louse infestations are characterised by constant itching, rubbing, tagging, and biting of the fleece. Sucking lice found on sheep include the face louse *Linognathus ovillus* and the foot louse *Linognathus pedalus*. The prevalence of chewing lice *Bovicola (Damalinia) ovis* has increased throughout Britain in recent years. Lice and keds are controlled by the ectoparasiticides used for fly, tick, and scab control and generally do not need specific treatment unless identified as a major problem. Frequent treatments have led to a serious resistance problem in some countries. It is important not to dip unnecessarily nor at an ineffective drug concentration. Goats may be treated in winter; care should be taken.

The sheep scab mite, *Psoroptes ovis*, is an economically important ectoparasite that occurs in sheep. In Britain, this disease is the subject of *The Sheep Scab Order 1997* (SI 1997/968), which is based on the treatment of infected sheep or those that may have been exposed to the mite, rather than the compulsory dipping of the national flock, as previously required by MAFF. Guidelines have been published on the treatment and flock management: MAFF. *Sheep Scab.* 1994 PB1927 and MAFF. *Sheep Scab: Protect your flock.* 1995 PB2354. Farmers should not send infected sheep to market or slaughter, and should follow the manufacturer's instructions on treatment to avoid temporary suppression of the disease.

The mites are able to survive in the environment for about 2 weeks and may be present on fences, in buildings, vehicles, and trailers. The mites are spread by physical contact with infested sheep. Treated stock should be kept off grazed pastures for about 3 weeks. *Psoroptes* mites suck lymph by piercing the epidermis, causing a serious allergic response followed by crust formation. There is marked variation in the response of sheep to the allergen. Animals become restless, and wool is pulled out by scratching or biting, or simply falls out. This is a continuous process as scab mites migrate away from the initial infective foci. Death can result from scab mite infestations.

Psoroptes infestations are most prevalent in autumn and winter. Treatment is by dipping in an ectoparasiticide (see section 2.2.4). Dimpylate (diazinon), flumethrin, and propetamphos-containing dips treat and prevent scab infestations. Cypermethrin-containing dips are effective for treatment only. The emergence of populations of mites resistant to either propetamphos or flumethrin may limit the choice of sheep dip. As an alternative, infestations may be treated with injectable ivermectin administered as 2 doses given at an interval of 7 days, or injectable moxidectin as 2 doses given at an interval of 10 days, or injectable doramectin given as a single dose. Ivermectin and doramectin are effective for treatment of existing infestations.

Mange due to *Sarcoptes* spp. is usually limited to the head in sheep; the area of infestation is more generalised in the goat. Chorioptic mange in sheep is now believed to be the result of infection with *Chorioptes bovis*, and lesions occur on the pasterns and interdigital spaces.

Ixodes ricinus transmits louping ill and tick-borne fever in sheep. Lambs should initially be treated twice with an interval of 3 weeks between treatments. Adult sheep should have at least 3 weeks wool growth when treated to ensure residual protection. Treatment should anticipate the tick rise and, if the level of challenge is high, a further treatment approximately 6 weeks later may be needed. The life cycle of the sheep tick may extend over 3 years and the location of flocks in the UK is important when considering challenge and treatment. It is generally considered that ticks feed from March until June in north-east England and north-east Scotland but in Wales, Ireland, Cumbria, western Scotland, and southern and western England there appears to be a tendency to feed also between August and November.

Pigs

There are two main ectoparasites of intensively and extensively housed pigs, the burrowing mange mite *Sarcoptes scabiei* var *suis* and the sucking louse *Haematopinus suis*. Both parasites cause restlessness, rubbing, and scratching with consequent skin abrasion, encrustation, and hair loss. The skin may become thickened and consequent open lesions may lead to secondary infections and loss of body fluids. Mange can adversely affect production efficiency in growing stock and cause erratic suckling patterns in nursing sows. Infection may lead to carcass downgrading due to skin rash. Ideally the ectoparasiticides used should control both mange and lice. Prophylactic use includes treatment of sows as they enter the farrowing house, young pigs at weaning, and boars every 2 to 3 months.

Dogs and cats

Control of ectoparasites on dogs and cats is greatly dependent upon the diligence of the owner. Ticks, lice, and fleas may be noticed by the owner. Microscopic parasitic mites or allergic conditions due to ectoparasites are initially only apparent from the dermatological conditions they cause.

Ctenocephalides felis more commonly infests dogs and cats than *C. canis*. The adult flea feeds and breeds on the animal. Flea eggs are shed from the animal's coat and develop in the environment. The flea emerges as an adult when favourable conditions are present and usually when a suitable host is nearby. Flea control includes elimination of adult fleas on the animal and reduction of developmental stages and emerging adult fleas in the environment by prevention of adult fleas producing viable eggs, using an insecticide (see section 2.2.2.7) on the animal's bedding, and vacuuming regularly. In animals that have developed an allergy to fleas, it is particularly important that control is aimed at reducing the number of fleas biting the animal. Many preparations are unsuitable for dogs and cats less than 12 weeks of age. Fipronil spray may be used on puppies and kittens more than 2 days of age or fleas may be manually removed with a fine-toothed comb in very young animals.

Lice infestation on dogs is due to *Trichodectes*, a biting louse, and is considered more prevalent than lice on cats.

Localised or generalised demodectic mange, *Demodex*, transmitted by contact, can be severely traumatic to the dog. Demodectic mange is commonly associated with immunosuppression in dogs and maintenance treatment may need to be continued for a long period in such animals. Sarcoptic mange, *Sarcoptes*, also occurs in the dog. Other mites infesting companion animals include *Notoedres*, notoedric mange, now rarely seen in the UK, which principally affects cats' ears and face but may be more generalised, and otodectic mange, *Otodectes*, which affects aural and facial areas of both dogs and cats (see also section 14.8). It is important to choose an ectoparasiticide that is indicated for

use in cats as some drugs, such as benzyl benzoate, are contra-indicated in this species.

Neotrombicula autumnalis (harvest mite) is a free-living mite found in wooded and grassed areas. Animals may become infested with the larvae, particularly on the feet and head, resulting in mild to severe pruritic lesions. Treatment is aimed at killing the larvae and should be repeated if re-infestation occurs.

Ticks, *Ixodes* spp., may be found on dogs and cats that are exercised in infested woodland or open areas. Dogs and cats are affected mainly on the head, face, ears, and legs. Individual ticks may be removed manually but large numbers may have to be treated with an acaricide. In some parts of the world, ticks are responsible for the transmission of canine babesiosis (*Bab. canis*, *Bab. gibsoni*), tropical canine pancytopaenia (*Ehrlichia canis*), and various bacterial and rickettsial diseases. In the UK, under the *Pet Travel Scheme*, 24 to 48 hours before embarkation for the UK, animals must be treated against ticks. However, to prevent an animal becoming infected with tick-borne diseases, it is recommended that animals are also treated for ticks before and during the period outside the UK. Other requirements for bringing pet dogs and cats without being placed under quarantine are given under section 18.4.6.

Birds

Common ectoparasites infesting **poultry** in the UK include poultry red mite *Dermanyssus gallinae*, northern fowl mite *Ornithonyssus*, lice, and the soft tick *Argas persicus*. Most production involving poultry for meat or eggs is intensive, therefore broiler houses or laying houses should be disinfested when they are cleared at the end of each batch of birds. Lice and mites affect **pigeons**, and lofts should be routinely disinfested.

Ectoparasiticide formulation and application. Table 2.2 outlines drugs that are available in the UK and effective against common ectoparasitic infections in the UK in horses, ruminants, pigs, dogs, cats, poultry, and pigeons. Ectoparasiticides are available for systemic administration and for topical application by various methods including by dip, spray, 'pour-on', 'spot-on', dusting powder, collar, and tag. Different formulations of a drug preparation may be indicated for different parasites.

Typically, formulations used in ectoparasite control for livestock are liquid concentrates requiring dilution with water to produce an emulsion for application. Traditionally, to ensure wetting to the skin, sheep are dipped, while other livestock are sprayed. However, more convenient ready-for-use 'pour-on' and 'spot-on' application methods provide the farmer with a broad choice of systems depending upon individual circumstances, for example, availability of spraying, dipping, and animal handling facilities, in addition to staff numbers required for such operations.

The volume of solution of 'pour-on' formulations used may depend on the size of the animal and the type of infestation. Solutions may be applied along the dorsal midline for fly infestation, to the top of the head and around the base of the horns for headfly infestation, or to the site of the lesion for blowfly strike. In general, 'pour-on' solutions should not be applied to the base of the tail in lambs as this may interfere with ewe-lamb recognition. 'Spot-on' formulations are applied to a single site on the dorsal midline behind the shoulders or to the base of the poll of the head.

Tapes and tags are used for fly control in extensive husbandry systems on animals that are not gathered on a regular basis. These should be removed when no longer efficacious (as described by the manufacturer) in order to prevent exposure of ectoparasites to sub-lethal drug dosage, resulting in resistant strains. Tags are attached to one or both ears of cattle. It is preferable to apply tags to the whole herd. The period of fly challenge in the UK is generally from June until September and for optimum protection the tags should be attached to the animal shortly before required. The insecticide is released onto the animal and spreads over its surface. Most tags act for up to 4 to 5 months and are used on dairy and beef cattle and calves. Tags should be removed at the end of the fly season or before slaughter. Bands are used on horses. They are attached to the browband or head collar and left in place for approximately 4 months.

Emulsifiable concentrates for dilution with water are also applied to dogs, particularly for demodectic and sarcoptic mange control, to ensure penetration to the skin of the active ingredient. Shampooing and washing of cats is rarely undertaken due to poor patient compliance. 'Spot-on' formulations are available for use on dogs and cats. The medication should be applied to an area where the animal is unable to lick it off, such as the back of the neck. The coat is parted to allow visibility of the skin because the solution should be applied to the skin rather than the fur. Excessive wetting of the fur should be avoided.

Spray formulations are used on dogs and cats although cats, in particular, may not tolerate the noise of aerosol spraying; powders, foams, or pump sprays may be preferred. To apply a spray, the animal's coat should be combed or brushed the wrong way and the spray applied to the roots of the fur and the skin from a distance of 15 to 20 cm. Care should be taken to avoid spraying the eyes, nose, and mouth. In general, the animal should be kept away from fires and other sources of heat for at least 30 minutes following spraying and until the coat is totally dry. Similarly, before application of a powder, the animal's fur should be raised and the powder applied close to the skin. Powders should only be applied when the coat is dry. Some ectoparasiticides are available as tablets, oral solution, or injection for dogs and cats.

Insecticidal collars for dogs and cats work on the same principle of insecticide dispersion as tags and should be worn at all times. The collar should be applied to fit loosely around the animal's neck; elasticated collars are available for cats. Some authorities do not recommend that cats wear collars because it has been found that elasticated collars may allow the animal to put its jaw or leg through the collar and then sustain injury. Children should not be allowed to handle or play with the collar, and animals should not be allowed to chew it. Occasionally animals show an allergic reaction to collars and the collar should be removed immediately if this is evident. Owners should be directed to read the *Owner Information Leaflet* insert which provides information on the drugs contained in the collar and human and animal safety precautions. Some flea collars contain agents such as organophosphorus compounds and the legal category of flea collars is to be reviewed.

2.2.1 Ectoparasiticides

2.2.1.1 Amidines
2.2.1.2 Avermectins and milbemycins
2.2.1.3 Carbamates
2.2.1.4 Nitroguanidines
2.2.1.5 Organophosphorus compounds
2.2.1.6 Phenylpyrazoles
2.2.1.7 Pyrethrins and synthetic pyrethroids
2.2.1.8 Other ectoparasiticides

Ectoparasiticides are available that act systemically and may be given parenterally or applied topically, either by the 'pour-on' technique where a solution of the drug is poured along the animal's dorsal midline, or by the 'spot-on' method in which all the specified amount of solution is applied to a small area on the head or back, as directed by the manufacturer. Some of the applied drug is absorbed percutaneously and taken up into the circulatory system.

Other ectoparasiticides are applied and act topically (information on sheep dips is given in section 2.2.3). There are many formulations of topical ectoparasiticides available and the preparation of choice will depend on the animal, owner compliance, and environment. In general, different preparations should not be used concurrently or within 7 days of treatment.

2.2.2.1 Amidines

Amitraz acts at octopamine receptor sites in ectoparasites giving rise to increased nervous activity. There is no requirement for removal of mange scabs before treatment.

Idiosyncratic reactions have been reported in Chihuahuas, and preparations containing amitraz should not be used on this breed nor on dogs with heat stress. In horses, amitraz may cause a reduction in gastro-intestinal motility resulting in impaction of the large intestine; amitraz should not be used on this species. Amitraz should not be used on cats.

AMITRAZ

UK

Indications. Lice, mites, and ticks on cattle; keds, lice, and ticks on sheep; lice and mites on pigs; *Demodex* and *Sarcoptes* on dogs

Contra-indications. Horses, Chihuahuas, cats, or dogs in heat stress; puppies less than 12 weeks of age, pregnant or

Table 2.2 Drugs effective against common ectoparasitic infections[1]

	Parasite	Ectoparasiticides
HORSES		
Flies	Haematobia, Hydrotaea, Musca, Stomoxys	cypermethrin, permethrin
Biting midges	Culicoides	benzyl benzoate, permethrin, pyrethrins
Lice	Bovicola, Haematopinus	cypermethrin, permethrin, pyrethrins
Mites	Psoroptes, Sarcoptes	ivermectin♦
	Chorioptes	selenium sulphide♦ (see section 14.5.1)
Horse bot	Gasterophilus	(haloxon, ivermectin) see section 2.1
RUMINANTS (some preparations are not suitable for all ruminant species, please consult individual monographs)		
Flies	Hydrotaea, Morellia, Musca, Simulium, Stomoxys	cypermethrin, deltamethrin, fenvalerate, permethrin
	Haematobia	doramectin 'pour-on', ivermectin 'pour-on', moxidectin 'pour-on'
Blowfly larvae	Calliphora, Lucilia	cypermethrin, cyromazine, deltamethrin, dimpylate (diazinon)
Warble flies	Hypoderma	abamectin, doramectin, eprinomectin, ivermectin, moxidectin, phosmet
Sheep keds	Melophagus ovinus	amitraz, deltamethrin, dimpylate (diazinon), flumethrin,
Lice	Bovicola, Haematopinus, Linognathus, Solenopotes	abamectin, amitraz, cypermethrin, deltamethrin, dimpylate (diazinon), doramectin, eprinomectin, fenthion, fenvalerate, flumethrin, ivermectin, moxidectin, permethrin, phosmet, propetamphos
Mites	Chorioptes, Sarcoptes	abamectin, amitraz, doramectin, eprinomectin, ivermectin, moxidectin, permethrin, phosmet
	Psoroptes	abamectin , cypermethrin, dimpylate (diazinon), doramectin , flumethrin, ivermectin , moxidectin
Ticks	Ixodes, Dermacentor, Haemaphysalis	amitraz, cypermethrin, deltamethrin, dimpylate (diazinon), flumethrin
Sheep nasal bot	Oestrus ovis	(closantel, doramectin, ivermectin, moxidectin) see section 2.1

Table 2.2 Drugs effective against common ectoparasitic infections[1]

	Parasite	Ectoparasiticides
PIGS		
Lice	Haematopinus	amitraz, doramectin, ivermectin, phosmet
Mites	Sarcoptes	amitraz, doramectin, ivermectin, phosmet
DOGS and CATS (some preparations are not suitable for both species, please consult individual monographs)		
Fleas	Ctenocephalides	carbaril, dimpylate (diazinon), dichlorvos + fenitrothion, fenthion, fenvalerate, fipronil, flumethrin + propoxur, imidacloprid, lufenuron, permethrin, propoxur, pyrethrins, selamectin
Lice	Felicola, Trichodectes	fipronil♦, permethrin♦, pyrethrins♦
Mites	Cheyletiella	fipronil♦
	Demodex (dogs)	amitraz, ivermectin♦
	Sarcoptes (dogs)	amitraz, fipronil♦, selamectin
	Notoedres (cats)	ivermectin♦
	Otodectes	selamectin, see also section 14.7
	Neotrombicula, Pneumonyssoides	dichlorvos + fenitrothion♦, fipronil♦, propoxur♦
Ticks	Ixodes, Rhipicephalus	dimpylate (diazinon), fenvalerate, fipronil, flumethrin + propoxur, permethrin, selamectin♦
POULTRY		
Mites	Dermanyssus	cypermethrin
Lice	Lipeurus, Goniocotes, Gonoides, Menopon, Menacanthus	fipronil♦
PIGEONS		
Lice	Columbicola	permethrin, pyrethrins
	Goniocotes	permethrin
Mites	Cnemidocoptes, Dermanyssus	pyrethrins
	Megninia, Pterolichus	permethrin

[1] infections and treatment used in the UK

lactating bitches; concurrent treatment with other insecticides

Side-effects. Occasional transient sedation, lethargy, CNS depression, bradycardia, slow shallow breathing in dogs

Warnings. Maintenance therapy may be required for a long period in immunosuppressed dogs; to avoid sunburn, pigs kept outdoors should not be exposed to intense sunlight on day of treatment

Dose.

Cattle: *by spray*, 0.025% solution

Sheep: *by dip*, 0.05% solution

Pigs: *by spray*, 0.05% solution

by 'pour-on' application, (100–180 kg body-weight) 40 mL on dorsal midline and 5 mL into each ear of 2% solution, (180–240 kg body-weight) 60 mL on dorsal midline and 5 mL into each ear of 2% solution

Dogs: *by wash*,

demodectic mange, 0.05% solution

sarcoptic mange, 0.025% solution

Rabbits ♦, *rodents* ♦: contact manufacturer for information on dosage

POM **Aludex** (Intervet) *UK*
Liquid concentrate, amitraz 5%, for *dogs*; 50 mL. To be diluted before use
Dilute 1 volume in 100 volumes water (= amitraz 0.05%)
Dilute 1 volume in 200 volumes water (= amitraz 0.025%)

PML **Taktic** (Intervet) *UK*
Liquid or dip concentrate, amitraz 12.5%, for *cattle, sheep , pigs*; 1 litre, 5 litres. To be diluted before use
Withdrawal Periods. *Cattle*: slaughter 1 day, milk 2 days. *Sheep*: slaughter 21 days, should not be used on sheep producing milk for human consumption. *Pigs*: slaughter 8 days
Dilute 1 volume in 250 volumes water (= amitraz 0.05%)
Dilute 1 volume in 500 volumes water (= amitraz 0.025%)
Dipwash. Dilute 1 volume in 250 volumes water (= amitraz 0.05%)
Replenisher. Dilute 1 volume in 167 volumes water and add to dipwash after each fall in volume of 20%

PML **Topline** (Intervet) *UK*
Solution, 'pour-on', amitraz 2%, for *pigs*; 3 litres
Withdrawal Periods. *Pigs*: slaughter 7 days

Australia

Indications. Ticks on ruminants and dogs; mites on pigs and dogs

Contra-indications. Manufacturer does not recommend use on horses, Chihuahuas, cats, or dogs in heat stress; puppies less than 3 months of age

Dose. See manufacturer's information

Amitik EC (Coopers) *Austral*
Topical spray, amitraz 125 g/L, for *cattle, sheep, goats, deer, circus animals, pigs*
Withdrawal Periods. Slaughter withdrawal period nil

Amitik EC Cattle and Pig Spray (Coopers) *Austral*
Topical spray, amitraz 125 g/L, for *cattle, pigs*
Withdrawal Periods. *Cattle*: slaughter withdrawal period nil, milk withdrawal period nil. *Pigs*: slaughter withdrawal period nil

Amitik WP (Coopers) *Austral*
Spray or dip, amitraz 500 g/kg, for *cattle, sheep, goats, deer, circus animals*
Withdrawal Periods. Slaughter withdrawal period nil

Deltaderm Demadex-Acaricidal Dog Wash (Delvet) *Austral*
Liquid concentrate, amitraz 50 g/L, for *dogs*

Ectodex EC (Hoechst Roussel) *Austral*
Liquid concentrate, amitraz 50 g/L, for *dogs*

Nu-Tic EC (Nufarm) *Austral*
Liquid concentrate, amitraz 125 g/L, for *cattle, sheep, goats, deer, circus animals, pigs*
Withdrawal Periods. Slaughter withdrawal period nil

Preventic 2 Month Tick Collar for Dogs (Virbac) *Austral*
Collar, amitraz 90 g/kg, for *dogs*

Taktic EC (Hoechst Roussel) *Austral*
Liquid concentrate, amitraz 125 g/L, for *cattle, sheep, goats, deer, circus animals, pigs*
Withdrawal Periods. Slaughter withdrawal period nil

Taktic Topline (Hoechst Roussel) *Austral*
Solution, pour-on, amitraz 20 g/L, for *pigs*
Withdrawal Periods. Slaughter 7 days

Taktic WP (Hoechst Roussel) *Austral*
Liquid concentrate, amitraz 500 g/kg, for *cattle, sheep, goats, deer, circus animals*
Withdrawal Periods. Slaughter withdrawal period nil

Eire

Indications. Lice, mites, and ticks on cattle; keds, lice, and ticks on sheep; lice and mites on pigs; mites on dogs

Contra-indications. Manufacturer does not recommend use on horses, Chihuahuas, cats, or dogs in heat stress; puppies less than 12 weeks of age, pregnant or lactating bitches; concurrent treatment with other insecticides

Side-effects. Occasional transient sedation, lethargy, CNS depression, bradycardia, slow shallow breathing in dogs

Warnings. To avoid sunburn, pigs kept outdoors should not be exposed to intense sunlight on day of treatment

Dose. See manufacturer's information

Aludex (Hoechst Roussel Vet) *Eire*
Liqud concentrate, amitraz 5%, for *dogs*

Taktic (Hoechst Roussel Vet) *Eire*
Spray or dip, amitraz 125 g/L, for *cattle, sheep, goats, pigs*
Withdrawal Periods. *Cattle*: slaughter 24 hours, milk 48 hours. *Sheep*: slaughter 21 days, should not be used in sheep producing milk for human consumption. *Goats*: slaughter 28 days, should not be used in goats producing milk for human consumption. *Pigs*: slaughter 7 days

Topline (Hoechst Roussel Vet) *Eire*
Solution, pour-on, amitraz 2%, for *pigs*
Withdrawal Periods. Slaughter 7 days

New Zealand

Indications. Ticks on cattle and dogs; mites on pigs and dogs; lice on pigs

Contra-indications. Chihuahuas or dogs in heat stress; handling of animals before coat is air dry; horses

Dose. See manufacturer's information

Ectodex EC (Animal Health) *NZ*
Liquid concentrate, amitraz 5%, for *dogs*

Taktic (Animal Health) *NZ*
Liquid concentrate, amitraz (formamidine) 125 g/litre, for *cattle, pigs*
Withdrawal Periods. *Cattle*: slaughter 24 hours, milk 24 hours. *Pigs*: slaughter 24 hours

Preventic Tick Collar for Dogs (Virbac) *NZ*
Collar, amitraz 9%, for *dogs*

USA

Indications. Ticks on cattle and dogs; mites on pigs and dogs; lice on pigs

Contra-indications. Manufacturer does not recommend use on horses; puppies less than 4 months of age; breeding or pregnant dogs

Dose. See manufacturer's information

Mitaban (Pharmacia & Upjohn) *USA*
Liquid concentrate, amitraz 19.9 %, for *dogs*

Point-Guard (Hoechst-Roussel) *USA*
Solution, pour-on, amitraz 2%, for *pigs*

Preventic Tick Collar For Dogs (Allerderm/Virbac) *USA*
Collar, amitraz 2%, for *dogs*

Taktic (Hoechst-Roussel) *USA*
Solution, for dilution, amitraz 12.5%, for *cattle, pigs*
Withdrawal Periods. Pigs: slaughter 3 days

2.2.1.2 Avermectins and milbemycins

Avermectins such as **abamectin**, **doramectin**, **eprinomectin**, and **ivermectin**, and the structurally related milbemycins such as **moxidectin** are active against a wide range of immature and mature nematodes and arthropods. The avermectin, **selamectin**, has been formulated for use in dogs and cats with activity against ectoparasites and endoparasites. These drugs are carried to all parts of the body in the circulation and therefore sucking lice and some mange mites are eliminated in addition to endoparasites.

They may be used for the control of sucking lice in cattle although complete elimination of biting species, for example *Bovicola* does not occur. For the control of lice infestation in pigs, re-treatment after 3 weeks may be necessary.

They are also effective in cattle against the mange mites *Psoroptes bovis* and *Sarcoptes scabiei* var *bovis* and may assist in control of *Chorioptes* although complete elimination does not occur. For the treatment of *Psoroptes ovis* (sheep scab) 2 injections of ivermectin should be administered at an interval of 7 days, or 2 injections of moxidectin at an interval of 10 days, or a single injection of doramectin in order to treat the clinical signs of scab and to eliminate living mites. No protection is afforded after treatment. Following treatment, sheep must be moved to fresh pasture which has not carried sheep during the previous 14 to 16 days. *Psoroptes* and *Sarcoptes* in horses♦ may be controlled with ivermectin.

Otodectes in cats may be treated with selamectin and *Notoedres* and *Demodex* in dogs♦ may be controlled with ivermectin but should be used with great caution because toxicity and fatalities may occur. Ivermection should not be administered to Collies.

Avermectins and milbemycins are also effective against warbles in cattle. Ivermectin and moxidectin administered by 'pour-on' on cattle aids in protection against *Haematobia irritans* for up to 35 days after treatment; doramectin for up to 42 days.

ABAMECTIN

UK

Indications. Ectoparasites. Warble-fly larvae, mites, and lice on cattle
Endoparasites. See section 2.1.1.1

See section 2.1.1.1 for preparation details

Australia

Indications. Ectoparasites. *Culicoides* on horses; horse bots; lice and ticks on cattle; mites on sheep; nasal bots
Endoparasites. See section 2.1.1.1

See section 2.1.1.1 for preparation details

Eire

Indications. Ectoparasites. Warble-fly larvae, mites, and lice on cattle
Endoparasites. See section 2.1.1.1

See section 2.1.1.1 for preparation details

New Zealand

Indications. Ectoparasites. Horse bots; lice on cattle
Endoparasites. See section 2.1.1.1

See section 2.1.1.1 for preparation details

DORAMECTIN

UK

Indications. Ectoparasites. Warble-fly larvae, mites, lice, horn flies ('pour-on') on cattle; mites and lice on pigs; ; *Psoroptes ovis* on sheep
Endoparasites. See section 2.1.1.1
Warnings. Treated infected and untreated uninfected sheep should not be incontact for 14 days
Dose. *Cattle*: see section 2.1.1.1
Sheep: *Psoroptes ovis, by intramuscular injection*, 300 mg/kg
Pigs: see section 2.1.1.1

See section 2.1.1.1 for preparation details

Australia

Indications. Ectoparasites. Mites, ticks, flies, and lice on cattle
Endoparasites. See section 2.1.1.1

See section 2.1.1.1 for preparation details

Eire

Indications. Ectoparasites. Warble fly larvae, mites, flies and lice on cattle; nasal bots and *Psoroptes ovis* on sheep
Endoparasites. See section 2.1.1.1

See section 2.1.1.1 for preparation details

New Zealand

Indications. Ectoparasites. Mites and lice on cattle
Endoparasites. See section 2.1.1.1

See section 2.1.1.1 for preparation details

USA

Indications. Ectoparasites. Warble-fly larvae, mites, and lice on cattle; mites and lice pigs
Endoparasites. See section 2.1.1.1

See section 2.1.1.1 for preparation details

EPRINOMECTIN

UK

Indications. Ectoparasites. Warble-fly larvae, mites, and lice on cattle
Endoparasites. See section 2.1.1.1
Dose. *See* section 2.1.1.1

See section 2.1.1.1 for preparation details

Australia

Indications. Ectoparasites. Mites, ticks, flies, and lice on cattle
Endoparasites. See section 2.1.1.1

See section 2.1.1.1 for preparation details

Eire

Indications. Ectoparasites. Warble-fly larvae, mites, and lice on cattle
Endoparasites. See section 2.1.1.1

See section 2.1.1.1 for preparation details

New Zealand

Indications. Ectoparasites. Mites and lice on cattle
Endoparasites. See section 2.1.1.1

See section 2.1.1.1 for preparation details

USA

Indications. Ectoparasites. Mites, flies, and lice on cattle
Endoparasites. See section 2.1.1.1

See section 2.1.1.1 for preparation details

IVERMECTIN

UK

Indications. Ectoparasites. Mites and lice on pigs; warble-fly larvae, mites, lice, and horn flies ('pour-on') on cattle; *Psoroptes* on sheep; mites on horses ♦, dogs ♦, and cats ♦
Endoparasites. See section 2.1.1.1
Contra-indications. Administration of ruminal boluses to non-ruminating cattle; administration to calves less than 12 weeks of age; in general, treatment with a 'pour-on' formulation when hide or hair is wet or rain is expected; direct application of 'pour-on' formulation to mange scabs or areas contaminated with mud or dung
Warnings. If cattle are vaccinated against lungworm, the ruminal bolus should not be given until 14 days after the second dose of vaccine. Serious side-effects and fatalities may be seen in some dogs ♦ treated with ivermectin for

Demodex; treated infected and untreated uninfected sheep should not be incontact for 7 days
Dose.
Horses ♦, cattle, pigs: see section 2.1.1.1
Sheep: *Psoroptes, by subcutaneous injection*, 200 micrograms/kg, repeat after 7 days
Dogs ♦: *by mouth*, 200–600 micrograms/kg daily
Cats ♦: *Notoedres, by subcutaneous injection*, 400 micrograms/kg

See sections 2.1.1.1 and 2.1.4 for preparation details

Australia

Indications. Ectoparasites. Mites, flies, ticks, and lice on cattle; mites and lice on pigs; mites on sheep
Endoparasites. See section 2.1.1.1

See sections 2.1.1.1 for preparation details

Eire

Indications. Ectoparasites. Mites and lice on ruminants and pigs; warble-fly larvae on cattle
Endoparasites. See section 2.1.1.1

See section 2.1.1.1 for preparation details

USA

Indications. Ectoparasites. Mites, ticks, and flies on cattle and pigs
Endoparasites. See section 2.1.1.1

See section 2.1.1.1 for preparation details

MOXIDECTIN

UK

Indications. Ectoparasites. Mites, lice, warble-fly larvae and horn flies on cattle; *Psoroptes ovis* on sheep
Endoparasites. See section 2.1.1.1
Contra-indications. Administration to calves less than 8 weeks of age
Warnings. Treated infected and untreated uninfected sheep should not be incontact for 12 days
Dose. *Cattle*: see section 2.1.1.1
Sheep: *Psoroptes ovis, by subcutaneous injection*, 200 micrograms/kg, repeat after 10 days for treatment

See section 2.1.1.1 for preparation details

Australia

Indications. Ectoparasites. Horse bots; mites and ticks on cattle; mites on sheep
Endoparasites. See section 2.1.1.1

See section 2.1.1.1 for preparation details

Eire

Indications. Ectoparasites. Mites, lice, warble-fly larvae, and horn flies on cattle; *Psoroptes ovis* on sheep
Endoparasites. See section 2.1.1.1

See section 2.1.1.1 for preparation details

New Zealand

Indications. Ectoparasites. Mites and lice on cattle and pigs; mites and keds on sheep
Endoparasites. See section 2.1.1.1

See section 2.1.1.1 for preparation details

USA

Indications. Ectoparasites. Mites, lice, warble-fly larvae, and horn flies on cattle
Endoparasites. See section 2.1.1.1

See section 2.1.1.1 for preparation details

SELAMECTIN

UK

Indications. Ectoparasites. Fleas and sarcoptic mange mites on dogs; fleas and *Otodectes* on cats
Endoparasites. See section 2.1.1.1

See section 2.1.1.1 for preparation details

USA

Indications. Ectoparasites. Fleas, ticks, and sarcoptic mange mites on dogs; fleas and *Otodectes* on cats
Endoparasites. See section 2.1.1.1

See section 2.1.1.1 for preparation details

2.2.2.2 Carbamates

Bendiocarb, **carbaril**, and **propoxur** are carbamates. These drugs cause inhibition of cholinesterase at the parasite nerve synapses but unlike organophosphorus compounds are spontaneously reversible. Carbaril may be carcinogenic and care should be taken by operators when handling carbaril-containing products.

BENDIOCARB

Australia

Indications. Lice and flies on cattle
Contra-indications. Concurrent use of carbamates or organophosphorus compounds

Bovicare Pour On Louse Treatment (Virbac) *Austral*
Solution, pour-on, bendiocarb 20 g/L, for *cattle*
Withdrawal Periods. Slaughter withdrawal period nil, milk withdrawal period nil

Ficam Gold Cattle Dust (Bayer) *Austral*
Dusting powder, bendiocarb 10 g/kg powder, for *cattle*

CARBARIL
(Carbaryl)

UK

Indications. Fleas on dogs and cats
Contra-indications. Use of other ectoparasiticides concurrently or within 7 days of removal of collar; puppies or kittens less than 6 months of age, nursing bitches or queens

Side-effects. Occasional skin irritation and alopecia
Warnings. Children should not be allowed to play with collar

GSL **Cat Flea Collar** (Johnson's) *UK*
Carbaril 5%

GSL **Dog Flea Collar** (Johnson's) *UK*
Carbaril 5%

GSL **Secto Cat Flea Collar** (Sinclair) *UK*
Carbaril 5%

GSL **Secto Dog Flea Collar** (Sinclair) *UK*
Carbaril 5%

Australia

Indications. Lice, ticks, mites, *Culicoides* on horses; fleas, ticks, lice, and mites on dogs and cats

7-Dust (Troy) *Austral*
Dusting powder, carbaril 50 g/kg, for *dogs, cats*

G-Wizz Insecticidal Block (Joseph Lyddy) *Austral*
Block shampoo, carbaril 37.2 g/kg, for *horses*

Fido's Fre-Itch Flea Powder (Mavlab) *Austral*
Dusting powder, carbaril 50 g/kg, for *dogs, cats*

Fido's Fre-Itch Flea Shampoo (Mavlab) *Austral*
Shampoo, carbaril 10 g/L, for *dogs, cats*

Skatta-7 Tick Flea Louse Powder (David) *Austral*
Dusting powder, carbaril 50 g/kg, for *dogs, cats*

Y-Itch medicated Lotion (Joseph Lyddy) *Austral*
Lotion, zinc oxide 55.6 g/kg, sulphur 22 g/kg, lanolin 0.6 g/kg, menthol 5.9 g/kg, carbaril 2.2 g/kg, camphor 0.6 g/kg, for *horses*

USA

Indications. Fleas, ticks, and lice on dogs and cats

2.5X Flea & Tick Powder (Vedco) *USA*
Dusting powder, carbaril 12.5%, for *dogs*

Adams Carbaryl Flea & Tick Shampoo (Pfizer) *USA*
Shampoo, carbaril 0.5%, for *cats, dogs*

Flea & Tick Powder (Performer) *USA*
Dusting powder, carbaril 12.5%, methoxychlor 0.25%, for *dogs, cats*

Flea-Tick Powder II (Happy Jack) *USA*
Dusting powder, carbaril 5%, for *dogs, cats*

Mycodex Pet Shampoo with Carbaryl (Pfizer) *USA*
Shampoo, carbaril 0.5%, for *cats, dogs*

Ritter's Tick and Flea Powder (Ritter) *USA*
Dusting powder, carbaril 12.5%, methoxychlor 0.25%, for *dogs, cats*

PROPOXUR

UK

Indications. Fleas on dogs and cats
Contra-indications. Concurrent or use within 7 days of other ectoparasiticides; puppies or kittens less than 12 weeks of age, nursing bitches or queens
Side-effects. Occasional skin irritation and alopecia with collar
Warnings. Children should not be allowed to play with collar; animals should not be allowed to chew the collar

GSL **Big Red Flea Spray** (Sherley's) *UK*
Aerosol spray, propoxur 0.25%, for *dogs, cats*; 153 g

PML **Negasunt** (Bayer) *UK*
See section 14.2.1 under Sulphanilamide for preparation details

GSL **Vet-Kem Breakaway Flea Collar for Cats** (Ceva) *UK*
Propoxur 10%

GSL **Vet-Kem Flea Collar for Dogs** (Ceva) *UK*
Propoxur 10%

Australia
Indications. Fleas and ticks on dogs and cats
Contra-indications. Concurrent use of other ectoparasiticides; collar on kittens less than 8 weeks of age
Warnings. Children should not be allowed to play with collar; animals should not be allowed to chew collar

Bay-O-Pet Flea Powder for Dogs & Cats (Bayer) *Austral*
Dusting powder, propoxur 10 g/kg, for *dogs, cats*

Bay-O-Pet Flea & Tick Spray for Dogs & Cats (Bayer) *Austral*
Spray (aerosol), propoxur 2.5 g/kg, for *dogs, cats*

Bay-O-Pet Flea Collar for Cats (Bayer) *Austral*
Collar, propxur 94 g/kg, for *cats*

Eire
Indications. Fleas on dogs and cats
Contra-indications. Concurrent or use within 7 days of other ectoparasiticides; puppies or kittens less than 12 weeks of age, nursing bitches or queens
Warnings. Children should not be allowed to play with collar; animals should not be allowed to chew collar

Bolfo Flea Collars for Large Dogs (Bayer) *Eire*
Collar, propoxur 9.4%, for *dogs*

Vet-Kem Breakaway Flea Collar for Cats (Interpharm) *Eire*
Collar, propoxur 10%, for *cats*

Vet-Kem Flea Collar for Dogs (Interpharm) *Eire*
Collar, propoxur 10%, for *dogs*

New Zealand
Indications. Fleas and ticks on dogs and cats
Contra-indications. Concurrent use of other ectoparasiticides; collar on puppies or kittens less than 12 weeks of age
Warnings. Children should not be allowed to play with collar; animals should not be allowed to chew collar

Bayer Flea Powder (Bayer) *NZ*
Dusting powder, propoxur 10 g/kg, for *dogs, cats*

Bayer 5 Month Flea and Tick Collar for Cats (Bayer) *NZ*
Collar, propoxur 9.4%, for *cats*

Bayer 5 Month Flea and Tick Collar for Dogs (Bayer) *NZ*
Collar, propoxur 9.4%, for *dogs*

2.2.1.4 Nitroguanidines

Imidacloprid is a chloronicotinyl nitroguanide that acts by binding to nicotinic acetycholine receptors in the insect CNS leading to inhibition of cholinergic transmission resulting in paralysis and death. Imidacloprid provides protection against re-infestation of fleas for up to one month in dogs and cats. It is not necessary to treat puppies or kittens of less than 8 weeks of age because treatment of nursing bitches and queens controls flea infestation on both dam and litter. Imidacloprid-containing 'spot-on' products rapidly kill fleas and therefore the incidence of flea allergy dermatitis is reduced.

IMIDACLOPRID

UK
Indications. Fleas on dogs and cats; reduced incidence of flea allergy dermatitis
Contra-indications. Recently treated animals should not groom each other; puppies or kittens less than 8 weeks of age
Side-effects. Transient salivation if the animal licks the application site immediately after treatment
Warnings. Efficacy reduced if animal becomes markedly wet
Dose. By 'spot-on' application.
Dogs: (up to 4 kg body-weight) 0.4 mL, (4–10 kg body-weight) 1.0 mL, (10–25 kg body-weight) 2.5 mL, (25–40 kg body-weight) 4.0 mL, (>40 kg body-weight) two 4.0 mL
Cats: (up to 4 kg body-weight) 0.4 mL, (>4 kg body-weight) 0.8 mL

POM **Advantage 40, 80 for Cats** (Bayer) *UK*
Solution, 'spot-on', imidacloprid 10%, for *cats*; 0.4 mL, 0.8 mL

POM **Advantage 40, 100, 250, 400 for Dogs** (Bayer) *UK*
Solution, 'spot-on', imidacloprid 10%, for *dogs*; 0.4 mL, 1 mL, 2.5 mL, 4.0 mL

Australia
Indications. Fleas on dogs and cats
Dose. By 'spot-on' application.
Dogs: (up to 4 kg body-weight) 0.4 mL, (4–10 kg body-weight) 1.0 mL, (10–25 kg body-weight) 2.5 mL, (>25 kg body-weight) 4.0 mL
Cats: (up to 4 kg body-weight) 0.4 mL, (>4 kg body-weight) 0.8 mL

Advantage for Dogs and Cats (Bayer) *Austral*
Solution, spot-on, imidacloprid 100 g/L, for *dogs, cats*

Eire
Indications. Fleas on dogs and cats; reduced incidence of flea allergy dermatitis
Contra-indications. Recently treated animals should not groom each other
Side-effects. Transient salivation if the animal licks the application site immediately after treatment
Warnings. Efficacy reduced if animal becomes markedly wet
Dose. By 'spot-on' application.
Dogs: (up to 4 kg body-weight) 0.4 mL, (4–10 kg body-weight) 1.0 mL, (10–25 kg body-weight) 2.5 mL, (25–40 kg body-weight) 4.0 mL, (>40 kg body-weight) two 4.0 mL
Cats: (up to 4 kg body-weight) 0.5 mL, (>4 kg body-weight) 0.8 mL

Advantage 40, 100, 250, 400 for Dogs (Bayer) *Eire*
Solution, spot-on, imdacloprid 10%, for *dogs*

Advantage 40, 80 for Cats (Bayer) *Eire*
Solution, spot-on, imdacloprid 10%, for *cats*

New Zealand

Indications. Fleas on dogs and cats
Side-effects. Transient salivation if the animal licks the application site immediately after treatment
Dose. *By 'spot-on' application.*
Dogs: (up to 4 kg body-weight) 0.4 mL, (4–10 kg body-weight) 1.0 mL, (10–25 kg body-weight) 2.5 mL, (>25 kg body-weight) 4.0 mL
Cats: (up to 4 kg body-weight) 0.4 mL, (>4 kg body-weight) 0.8 mL

Advantage Flea Adulticide for Cats (Bayer) *NZ*
Solution, spot-on, imidacloprid 10%L, for *cats*

Advantage Flea Adulticide for Dogs (Bayer) *NZ*
Solution, spot-on, imidacloprid 10%, for *dogs*

USA

Indications. Fleas on dogs and cats; reduced incidence of flea allergy dermatitis
Contra-indications. Puppies less than 7 weeks of age; kittens less than 8 weeks of age
Dose. *By 'spot-on' application.*
Dogs: (up to 4 kg body-weight) 0.4 mL, (4–10 kg body-weight) 1.0 mL, (10–25 kg body-weight) 2.5 mL, (>25 kg body-weight) 4.0 mL
Cats: (up to 4 kg body-weight) 0.5 mL, (>4 kg body-weight) 0.8 mL

Advantage Topical Solution for Cats and Kittens (Bayer) *USA*
Solution, spot-on, imidacloprid 9.1%, for *cats*

Advantage Topical Solution for Dogs and Puppies (Bayer) *USA*
Solution, spot-on, imidacloprid 9.1%, for *dogs*

2.2.1.5 Organophosphorus compounds

Organophosphorus compounds inhibit cholinesterase, thereby interfering with neuromuscular transmission in the ectoparasite. Topical acting organophosphorus compounds include **azamethiphos, chlorpyrifos, clofenvinfos, coumafos, dichlorvos, dimpylate** (diazinon), **ethion, fenitrothion, heptenophos, malathion, metrifonate, phoxim, propetamphos, temefos,** and **tetrachlorvinphos.**
Dimpylate (diazinon) and propetamphos are approved for use in the control of sheep scab in the UK. Both are also effective against blowfly larvae, keds, lice, and ticks. Dimpylate (diazinon) and propetamphos provide residual action; dimpylate (diazinon) gives longer residual protection than propetamphos. These compounds are strongly lipophilic and replenishment according to the manufactuer's recommendations must be adhered to in order to prevent inadequate concentration in the dip bath.
Collars containing dimpylate and esters of fatty acids as a conditioner are available. The effect of the drug on fleas can be seen within a few hours and that on ticks within 5 days. Collars are effective for about 4 months.

Cythioate is an orally administered organophosphorus compound. Cythioate is absorbed from the gastro-intestinal tract within 2 to 3 hours of administration. Ectoparasites are killed when they ingest body fluids containing cythioate.
Fenthion, famphur, and **phosmet** are systemically acting organophosphorus compounds. Such compounds applied by either the 'pour-on' or 'spot-on' method. Fenthion, for example, is absorbed percutaneously over an 8 hour period. A proportion is absorbed into the circulation and is widely distributed in the body so in warble-fly treatments all larval stages within the body are destroyed. Therefore treatment in cattle should not be carried out between December and March because larvae are in the spinal cord and oesophageal area during this period and destruction of the parasites may cause side-effects. Dead larvae may give rise to severe local oedematous lesions. Systemic insecticidal action persists for some time, for example for about 4 weeks in dogs and cats and fleas approaching the animal to feed will be killed. Additional measures to control adult fleas and developmental stages in the environment should be undertaken (see section 2.2.5).

Parasiticides may be toxic to animals and the operator. Care should be taken with dosage and handling of the product. The recommendations for storage, use, and disposal of unused materials and containers should be followed. For guidance and information, see:
- MAFF/HSE. *Code of practice for the safe use of pesticides on farms and holdings.* London: HMSO, 1998. PB3528
- *Animal medicines: A user's guide.* NOAH, 1995
- Control of Substances Hazardous to Health (COSHH) Regulations 1994.

Acute overdosage or overexposure to organophosphorus compounds in animals and humans is characterised by abdominal pain, diarrhoea, salivation, muscular tremors, and pupil constriction. Death may occur from respiratory failure. Acetylcholine accumulates at muscarinic and nicotinic receptors, which are subsequently overstimulated. Treatment is aimed at inhibiting the muscarinic effects of acetylcholine with a competitive antagonist such as atropine (see Treatment of poisoning). Manufacturer's literature should be consulted. Chronic exposure may lead to damage to the nervous system and clinical signs including headaches, anxiety, and irritability in operators.
Although most organophosphorus compounds are not persistent in the environment, they may be toxic to humans, livestock, and wildlife, and adequate precautions should be taken to avoid environmental contamination.

AZAMETHIPHOS

UK
See Prescribing for fish

Australia

Indications. Lice and mites on poultry
Contra-indications. Birds less than 1 week of age; concurrent use of other insecticides

Alfacron 500 (Novartis) *Austral*
Powder, for spray, azamethiphos 500 g/kg powder, for *poultry, premises*
Withdrawal Periods. Slaughter 1 day, egg withdrawal period nil

> Operators should take care when handling or using preparations containing organophosphorus compounds. Personal protective equipment should be worn. Care should be taken to avoid inhalation of powder or spray and any skin contamination should be washed off immediately. Cases of ill health among sheep handlers claimed to arise from exposure to organophosphorus-containing dips have been reported. Operators should wear protective clothing when applying treating and handling freshly treated animals.

CHLORPYRIFOS

Australia

Indications. Fleas and ticks on dogs; fleas on cats
Contra-indications. Concurrent use of other ectoparasiticides; collar on puppies or kittens less than 12 weeks of age
Warnings. Children should not be allowed to play with collar; animals should not be allowed to chew collar

Exelpet No Fleas Continuous Spray (Exelpet) *Austral*
Spray, chlorpyrifos 2.1 g/L, for *dogs*
Contra-indications. Concurrent or use within 14 days of other organophosphorus compounds; puppies less than 16 weeks of age; cats; pregnant or nursing bitches

Exelpet Red 5 Month Flea Collar for Dogs (Exelpet) *Austral*
Collar, chlorpyrifos 80 g/kg, for *dogs*

Exelpet Red 8 Month Collar for Cats (Exelpet) *Austral*
Collar, chlorpyrifos 40 g/kg, for *cats*

Vet-Kem LONG LIFE Flea Cat Collar (Novartis) *Austral*
Collar, chlorpyrifos 40 g/kg, for *cats*

Vet-Kem LONG LIFE Flea Dog Collar (Novartis) *Austral*
Collar, chlorpyrifos 80 g/kg, for *dogs*

Zodiac LONG LIFE Flea Cat Collar (Novartis) *Austral*
Collar, chlorpyrifos 40 g/kg, for *cats*

Zodiac LONG LIFE Flea and Tick Dog Collar (Novartis) *Austral*
Collar, chlorpyrifos 80 g/kg, for *dogs*

New Zealand

Indications. Fleas and ticks on dogs; fleas on cats; lice, keds, and flystrike on sheep
Contra-indications. Concurrent use of other ectoparasiticides
Warnings. Children should not be allowed to play with collar; animals should not be allowed to chew collar; remove collar if signs of irritation occur; in sheep, allow 2 months between dipping treatment and shearing

Vet-Kem Long Life Flea and Tick Collar for Cats (Bayer) *NZ*
Collar, chlorpyrifos 4.3%, for *cats*

Vet-Kem Long Life Flea and Tick Collar for Dogs (Bayer) *NZ*
Collar, chlorpyrifos 8.4%, for *dogs*

Xterminate 10 (Ancare) *NZ*
Dip concentrate, chlorpyrifos 100 g/litre, for *sheep*
Withdrawal Periods. Slaughter 21 days, should not be used in sheep producing milk for human consumption

USA

Indications. Fleas, ticks, and mites on dogs and cats
Contra-indications. Concurrent use of other ectoparasiticides; puppies or kittens less than 12 weeks of age; dip on cats or nursing bitches
Warnings. Children should not be allowed to play with collar; animals should not be allowed to chew collar

3-X Flea, Tick & Mange Collar for Cats (Happy Jack) *USA*
Collar, chlorpyrifos 3%, for *cats*

3-x Flea, Tick & Mange Collar for Dogs (Happy Jack) *USA*
Collar, chlorpyrifos 9%, for *dogs*

Ban-Guard Dip For Dogs (Allerderm/Virbac) *USA*
Solution, spot-on, chlorpyrifos 3.84%, for *dogs*

Dursban Dip For Dogs (Davis, Vedco) *USA*
Dip concentrate, chlorpyrifos 4.85%, for *dogs*

Enduracide Dip for Dogs (Happy Jack) *USA*
Dip concentrate, chlorpyrifos 4.85%, for *dogs*

Flea & Tick Dip For Dogs (Performer) *USA*
Dip concentrate, chlorpyrifos 4.85%, for *dogs*

Paracide II Shampoo (Happy Jack) *USA*
Shampoo, chlorpyrifos 0.125%, for *dogs*

Pet Care 11-Month Flea Collar For Dogs (DurVet) *USA*
Collar, chlorpyrifos 8%, for *dogs*

Pet Care Dip For Dogs (DurVet) *USA*
Dip concentrate, chlorpyrifos 3.84%, for *dogs*

Sardex (Happy Jack) *USA*
Topical spray, chlorpyrifos 0.2%, for *dogs*

Streaker (Happy Jack) *USA*
Solution, spot-on, chlorpyrifos 0.5%, for *dogs*

CLOFENVINFOS
(Chlorfenvinphos)

Australia

Indications. Blowfly strike on sheep; flies on horses, cattle
Contra-indications. Use within 10 days of dipping with other organophosphorus compounds on cattle

Aerosol Sheep Dressing (Western Stock Distributors) *Austral*
Aerosol spray, dibutyl phthalate 20 g/kh, chlorfenvinphos, for *sheep*
Withdrawal Periods. Slaughter 7 days

Chlorfenvinphos 100 (Western Stock Distributors) *Austral*
Liquid concentrate, chlorfenvinphos, for *sheep*
Withdrawal Periods. Slaughter 3 days

Defiance 'S' (Fort Dodge) *Austral*
Topical spray, chlorfenvinphos 2.5 g/L, for *horses, cattle, sheep*
Withdrawal Periods. *Horses*: slaughter 3 days. *Cattle*: slaughter 3 days, do not apply to udders of cattle producing milk for human consumption. *Sheep*: slaughter 3 days, should not be used on sheep producing milk for human consumption.

Supona Buffalo Fly Insecticide (Fort Dodge) *Austral*
Solution, chlorfenvinphos 200g/L, for *cattle*
Withdrawal Periods. Slaughter withdrawal period nil, should not be used on cattle producing milk for human consumption.

Suprex 100 (Coopers) *Austral*
Liquid concentrate, chorfenvinphos 1000 g/L, for *sheep*
Withdrawal Periods. Slaughter 3 days

New Zealand
Indications. Lice, keds, blowfly strike on sheep
Contra-indications. Concurrent use of other organophosphorus compounds

Fly Strike Dressing (FIL) *NZ*
Solution, pour-on or spray, chlorfenvinphos 10 g/litre, for *sheep*

Supreme (Schering-Plough) *NZ*
Dip or spray concentrate, chlorfenvinphos 1000 g/litre, for *sheep*
Withdrawal Periods. Slaughter 21 days, should not be used in sheep producing milk for human consumption

COUMAFOS
(Coumaphos)

Australia
Indications. Fleas and ticks on dogs; lice and *Culicoides* on horses
Contra-indications. Concurrent use of organophosphorus-compounds or carbamates; cats; puppies less than 3 months of age, nursing bitches

Bay-O-Pet Asuntol Dog and Horse Rinse (Bayer) *Austral*
Liquid concentrate, coumafos 50 g/L, for *horses, dogs*

Bay-O-Pet Asuntol Flea & Tick Dog Rinse (Bayer) *Austral*
Liquid concentrate, coumafos 50 g/L, for *dogs*

Bay-O-Pet Asuntol Flea Soap for Dogs (Bayer) *Austral*
Soap, coumafos 10 g/kg, for *dogs*

Exelpet Dog Wash (Exelpet) *Austral*
Liquid concentrate, coumafos 50 g/L, for *dogs*

New Zealand
Indications. Fleas, ticks on dogs; lice on horses, cattle, sheep, pigs, and dogs; ticks, keds, and blowfly strike on sheep; mites on pigs
Contra-indications. Cats; puppies less than 3 months of age
Side-effects. Colic, diarrhoea, sweating, muscle tremors, ataxia, salivation

Asuntol Dog and Horse Wash (Bayer) *NZ*
Liquid concentrate, coumafos 50 g/litre, for *horses, dogs*

Asuntol Lice and Flystrike Powder (Bayer) *NZ*
Dusting powder, coumafos 10 g/kg, for *horses, sheep*
Withdrawal Periods. *Horses*: slaughter 180 days. *Sheep*: slaughter 14 days

Asuntol Liquid (Bayer) *NZ*
Liquid concentrate, coumafos 160 g/litre, for *horses, cattle, sheep, pigs, dogs*
Withdrawal Periods. *Horses, pigs*: slaughter 7 days. *Cattle, sheep*: slaughter 7 days, milk 3 days

Asuntol Medicated Dog Soap (Bayer) *NZ*
Medicated soap, coumafos 10 g/kg, for *dogs*

Asuntol Powder (Bayer) *NZ*
Powder for dip, coumafos 500 g/kg, for *sheep*
Withdrawal Periods. Slaughter 7 days, milk 3 days

USA
Indications. Lice on cattle and pigs; flies on cattle and horses

Co-Ral (Bayer) *USA*
Topical solution, coumafos 11.6%, for *horses, cattle, pigs*
Withdrawal Periods. Should not be used on *horses* intended for human consumption. *Cattle*: slaughter withdrawal period nil, milk withdrawal period nil

Co-Ral 1% Dust (AgriLabs) *USA*
Dusting powder, coumafos 1%, for *cattle, pigs*
Withdrawal Periods. Slaughter withdrawal period nil, milk withdrawal period nil

Co-Ral Fly and Tick Spray (Bayer) *USA*
Topical spray, coumafos 5.8%, for *horses, cattle, pigs*
Withdrawal Periods. Should not be used on *horses* intended for human consumption. Cattle: slaughter withdrawal period nil, milk withdrawal period nil

Prozap Zipcide (Loveland) *USA*
Dusting powder, coumafos 1%, for *cattle, pigs, bedding*

CYTHIOATE

Australia
Indications. Fleas, ticks, and mange mites on dogs; fleas on cats
Contra-indications. Concurrent use of other organophosphorus compounds; pregnant or lactating dogs or cats
Dose. *By mouth.*
Dogs: 3 mg/kg
Cats: 1.5 mg/kg

Exelpet Fleaban Liquid for Cats and Small Dogs (Exelpet) *Austral*
Liquid concentrate, cythioate 15 mg/mL, for *dogs, cats*

Exelpet Fleaban Tablets (Exelpet) *Austral*
Tablets, cythioate 30 mg, for *dogs, cats*

Proban (Boehringer Ingelheim) *Austral*
Tablets, cythioate 30 mg, for *dogs, cats*

Proban (Boehringer Ingelheim) *Austral*
Oral solution, cythioate 15 mg/mL, for *dogs, cats*

New Zealand
Indications. Fleas on cats
Contra-indications. Concurrent use of other organophosphorus compounds; pregnant cats
Dose. *Cats: by mouth*, 1.5 mg/kg

Cyflee Liquid for Cats (Bomac) *NZ*
Oral solution, cythioate 15 mg/mL, for *cats*

DICHLORVOS

USA
Indications. Flies on horses and cattle

Prozap Beef & Dairy Cattle Spray RTU (Loveland) *USA*
Topical spray, dichlorvos 0.92%, related cpds 0.08%, for *cattle, premises*

1% Vapona Insecticide (DurVet) *USA*
Topical spray, dichlorvos 0.93%, related cpds 0.07%, for *horses, cattle, premises*

Vapona Concentrate Insecticide (Boehringer Ingelheim Vetmedica) *USA*
Liquid for dilution, dichlorvos 40.2%, related cpds 3%, for *cattle, premises*
Withdrawal Periods. Slaughter 1 day, milk withdrawal period nil

DIMPYLATE
(Diazinon)

UK

Indications. Blowfly strike, keds, lice, *Psoroptes*, and ticks on sheep; fleas and ticks on dogs; fleas on cats
Contra-indications. Administration of an organophosphorus compound within 14 days of dipping; puppies less than 12 weeks of age; cats less than 6 months of age, aged cats, nursing bitches or queens. Concurrent use of other ectoparasiticides or within 7 days of removal of collar
Side-effects. Occasional skin irritation and alopecia with collar
Warnings. Some dimpylate (diazinon)-containing dip concentrates contain epichlorhydrin 1%; adequate ventilation should be provided for operators working continuously with these preparations. Doctors should be aware of possible clinical signs associated with exposure to organophosporus compounds
Warnings. Children should not be allowed to play with the collar; animals should not be allowed to chew the collar

PML All Seasons Fly and Scab Dip (Schering-Plough) *UK*
Dip concentrate, dimpylate (diazinon) 16%, for *sheep*. To be diluted before use
Withdrawal Periods. *Sheep*: slaughter 35 days, should not be used on sheep producing milk for human consumption
Dipwash. Dilute dip concentrate 1 volume in 400 volumes water
Replenisher. Dilute dip concentrate 1.5 volumes in 400 volumes water and replenish water to original volume after each 20 sheep dipped

GSL Bounders Dog Flea Collar (Sinclair) *UK*
Dimpylate (diazinon) 15%

GSL Canovel Doublecare Insecticidal Collar (Pfizer) *UK*
Dimpylate (diazinon) 15%, essential fatty acid esters 5%, for *dogs*

GSL Cat Flea Collar (Plastic) (Sherley's) *UK*
Dimpylate (diazinon) 15%

GSL Catovel Doublecare Elasticated Insecticidal Collar (Pfizer) *UK*
Dimpylate (diazinon) 15%, essential fatty acid esters 5%, for *cats*

GSL Catovel Prettycare Insecticidal Collar (Pfizer) *UK*
Dimpylate (diazinon) 15%, for *cats*

GSL Derasect Insecticidal Collar (Pfizer) *UK*
Dimpylate (diazinon) 15%, essential fatty acid esters 5%, for *dogs*

GSL Derasect Elasticated Flea Collar (Pfizer) *UK*
Dimpylate (diazinon) 15%, essential fatty acid esters 5%, for *cats*

PML Diazadip All Seasons (Bayer) *UK*
Dip concentrate, dimpylate (diazinon) 60%, for *sheep*; 2.5 litres, 5 litres. To be diluted before use
Withdrawal Periods. *Sheep*: slaughter 35 days, should not be used on sheep producing milk for human consumption
Dipwash. Dilute dip concentrate 300 mL in 450 litres water
Replenisher. Add 200 mL (for bath <2250 mL) or 300 mL (for bath >2250) after every 40 sheep dipped and replenish water to original volume

PML Deosan Diazinon Dip (DiverseyLever) *UK*
Dip concentrate, dimpylate (diazinon) 60%, for *sheep*. To be diluted before use
Withdrawal Periods. *Sheep*: slaughter 35 days, should not be used on sheep producing milk for human consumption

Dipwash. Dilute dip concentrate 600 mL in 900 litres water
Replenisher. Add 200 mL (for bath <2250 litres) after every 40 sheep dipped and replenish water to original volume. Add 500 mL (for bath >2250 litres) after every 100 sheep dipped and replenish water to original volume

GSL Dog Flea Collar (Plastic) (Sherley's) *UK*
Dimpylate (diazinon) 15%

GSL Flea Collar for Cats (Bob Martin) *UK*
Dimpylate (diazinon) 15%

GSL Flea Collar for Dogs (Bob Martin) *UK*
Dimpylate (diazinon) 15%

GSL Flea Guard for Cats (Johnson's) *UK*
Collar, dimpylate (diazinon) 15%

GSL Flea Guard for Dogs (Johnson's) *UK*
Collar, dimpylate (diazinon) 15%

PML Osmonds Gold Fleece Sheep Dip (Bimeda, Virbac) *UK*
Dip concentrate, dimpylate (diazinon) 60%, for *sheep*; 1 litre, 5 litres. To be diluted before use
Withdrawal Periods. *Sheep*: slaughter 35 days, should not be used on sheep producing milk for human consumption
Dipwash. Dilute dip concentrate 600 mL in 900 litres water
Replenisher. *Replenisher*. Add 200 mL (for bath <2250 litres) after every 40 sheep dipped and replenish water to original volume. Add 500 mL (for bath >2250 litres) after every 100 sheep dipped and replenish water to original volume

PML Paracide Plus (Battle Hayward & Bower) *UK*
Dip concentrate, dimpylate (diazinon) 16%, for *sheep*; 2 litres, 5 litres, 10 litres. To be diluted before use
Withdrawal Periods. *Sheep*: slaughter 14 days
Dipwash. Dilute 1 volume in 400 volumes water
Replenisher. Dilute 1.5 volumes in 400 volumes water and add to dipwash after every 20 sheep dipped

GSL Pet Care Plastic Flea Band for Dogs (Armitage) *UK*
Collar, dimpylate (diazinon) 15%, for *dogs*

GSL Pet Care Plastic Flea Band for Cats (Armitage) *UK*
Collar, dimpylate (diazinon) 15%, for *cats*

GSL Prevender Insecticidal Collar for Dogs/Large Dogs (Virbac) *UK*
Dimpylate (diazinon) 15%, for *dogs*

GSL Preventef Elasticated Flea Collar (Virbac) *UK*
Dimpylate (diazinon) 15%, essential fatty acid esters 5%, for *cats*

GSL Preventef Insecticidal Collar for Dogs/Large Dogs (Virbac) *UK*
Dimpylate (diazinon) 15%, essential fatty acid esters 5%, for *dogs*

Australia

Indications. Blowfly strike, keds, lice on sheep; lice and flies on cattle; lice and mange mites on pigs; fleas on cats; fleas, ticks, lice, sarcoptic mange mites on dogs
Contra-indications. Use of concentrate to pregnant or nursing bitches or puppies less than 3 months of age; collar on puppies or kittens less than 6 months of age; treatment for lice less than 6 weeks before lambing or on ewes with lambs at foot; sheep that have not been cleanly shorn or with wounds or heavy grass seed infestation
Warnings. Children should not be allowed to play with collar; animals should not be allowed to chew collar

5 Month Flea Collar for Cats (Virbac) *Austral*
Collar, dimpylate 150 g/kg, for *cats*

5 Month Flea Collar for Dogs (Virbac) *Austral*
Collar, dimpylate 150 g/kg, for *dogs*

Diatrol (Ilium) *Austral*
Liquid concentrate, dimpylate150 g/L, for *dogs*

Diazinon (Western Stock Distributors) *Austral*
Liquid concentrate, dimpylate 200 g/L, for *cattle, sheep, goats, pigs*
Withdrawal Periods. *Cattle*: slaughter 3 days. *Goats*: slaughter 14 days, milk 48 hours. *Sheep, pigs*: slaughter 14 days

Di-Jet (Coopers) *Austral*
Liquid concentrate, dimpylate 200 g/L, for *cattle, sheep, goats, pigs*
Withdrawal Periods. *Cattle*: slaughter 3 days. *Goats*: slaughter 14 days, milk 48 hours. *Sheep, pigs*: slaughter 14 days

Eureka Gold OP Spray-On (Novartis) *Austral*
Spray concentrate, dimpylate 93.3 g/L, for *sheep*
Withdrawal Periods. Slaughter 21 days, should not be used on sheep producing milk for human consumption

Exelpet Water Resistant 5 Month Flea Collar (Exelpet) *Austral*
Collar, dimpylate 150 g/kg, for *dogs, cats*

Exelpet Yard and Kennel Flea Control Concentrate (Exelpet) *Austral*
Liquid concentrate, dimpylate 200 g/L, for *dogs, premises*

Jetdip (Virbac) *Austral*
Liquid concentrate, dimpylate 200 g/L, for *sheep*
Withdrawal Periods. Slaughter 14 days

KFM Blowfly Dressing (Nufarm) *Austral*
Liquid concentrate, dimpylate 3 g/l, for *sheep*
Withdrawal Periods. Slaughter 14 days

Kleen-Dok with Diazinon (Virbac) *Austral*
Solution, dimpylate 1 g/L, for *cattle, sheep*
Withdrawal Periods. Slaughter 14 days

Mulesing and Fly Strike Powder (Virbac) *Austral*
Dusting powder, dimpylate 20 g/kg, for *cattle, sheep*
Withdrawal Periods. Cattle: slaughter 3 days. Sheep: slaughter 14 days

Nucidol 200 Dog Wash (Novartis) *Austral*
Liquid concentrate, dimpylate 200 g/L, for *dogs, premises*

Nucidol 200 EC (Novartis) *Austral*
Liquid concentrate, dimpylate 200 g/L, for *horses, cattle, pigs, dogs, goats, premises*
Withdrawal Periods. *Cattle, horses*: slaughter 3 days. *Pigs, goats*: slaughter 14 days

Petcare Preventef 5 Month Flea Collar for Dogs (Virbac) *Austral*
Collar, dimpylate 150 g/kg, for *dogs*

Petcare Preventef 5 Month Flea Collar for Cats (Virbac) *Austral*
Collar, dimpylate 150 g/kg, for *cats*

Spike Insecticidal Cattle Ear Tags (Novartis) *Austral*
Ear tags, dimpylate 200 g/kg, for *cattle*
Withdrawal Periods. Slaughter withdrawal period nil, milk withdrawal period nil, remove ear tags before slaughter

Topclip Blue Shield (Novartis) *Austral*
Liquid concentrate, dimpylate 200 g/L, for *sheep*
Withdrawal Periods. Sheep: slaughter 14 days, wool 2 months, should not be used on sheep producing milk for human consumption

Virbac Working Dog 7 Month Waterproof Flea Collar for Dogs (Virbac) *Austral*
Collar, dimpylate 150 g/kg, for *dogs*

Eire
Indications. Blowfly strike, keds, lice, and *Psoroptes* on sheep; lice, mange mites, and ticks on cattle; fleas and ticks on dogs
Contra-indications. Collar on puppies less than 6 months of age

Warnings. Children should not be allowed to play with the collar; animals should not be allowed to chew the collar

All Seasons Fly and Scab Dip, Coopers (Schering-Plough) *Eire*
Dip concentrate, dimpylate 16%, for *sheep*
Withdrawal Periods. Slaughter 35 days, should not be used on sheep producing milk for human consumption

Gullivers Flea and Tick Collar for Dogs (Chanelle) *Eire*
Collar, diazinon 15%, for *dogs*

Nucidol 600EC Winter Dip (Novartis) *Eire*
Dip concentrate, diazinon 600 g/L, for *sheep*

Tixol Coopers (Schering-Plough) *Eire*
Liquid concentrate, dimpylate 4%, for *cattle*
Withdrawal Periods. Slaughter 14 days, milk 7 days

Topclip Gold Shield (Novartis) *Eire*
Dip concentrate, diazinon 60%, for *sheep*
Withdrawal Periods. Slaughter 14 days

Winter Dip 200, Coopers (Schering-Plough) *Eire*
Dip concentrate, dimpylate, for *sheep*
Withdrawal Periods. Slaughter 28 days, should not be used in sheep producing milk for human consumption

New Zealand
Indications. Flystrike on horses; blowfly strike, keds, lice on sheep; fleas, ticks, and flystrike on dogs; fleas on cats;

Diazinon 40 (Novartis) *NZ*
Dip concentrate, dimpylate 400 g/litre, for *sheep*
Withdrawal Periods. Slaughter 21 days

Diazinon 40 Sheep Dip (Nufarm) *NZ*
Dip concentrate, dimpylate 400 g/litre, for *sheep*
Withdrawal Periods. Slaughter 21 days

Eureka Gold (Novartis) *NZ*
Liquid concentrate, dimpylate 93.3 g/litre, for *sheep*
Withdrawal Periods. Slaughter 21 days, should not be used in sheep producing milk for human consumption

Fleatrol 5 Month Insecticidal Collar for Cats (Virbac) *NZ*
Collar, dimpylate 15%, for *cats*

Fleatrol 5 Month Insecticidal Collar for Dogs (Virbac) *NZ*
Collar, dimpylate 15%, for *dogs*

Jetting Fluid (FIL) *NZ*
Dip concentrate, dimpylate 400 g/litre, for *sheep*
Withdrawal Periods. Slaughter 21 days, should not be used in sheep producing milk for human consumption

Preventef 5 Month Insecticidal Collar for Cats (Virbac) *NZ*
Collar, dimpylate 15%, for *cats*

Preventef 5 Month Insecticidal Collar for Dogs (Virbac) *NZ*
Collar, dimpylate 15%, for *dogs*

Strike Powder (FIL) *NZ*
Dusting powder, dimpylate 20 g/kg, for *horses, sheep, dogs*
Withdrawal Periods. *Horses, sheep*: slaughter 28 days

Topclip 40 (Novartis) *NZ*
Dip concentrate, dimpylate 40%, for *sheep*
Withdrawal Periods. Slaughter 21 days, should not be used in sheep producing milk for human consumption

USA
Indications. Flies, lice, and ticks on cattle; keds and lice on sheep; fleas and ticks on dogs and cats

Bovagard Insecticide Cattle Ear Tag (Y-Tex) *USA*
Tags (ear), dimpylate 21.4&, for *cattle*
Withdrawal Periods. Cattle: should not be used on cattle producing milk for human consumption

Cutter 1 Insecticide Cattle Ear Tag (Bayer) *USA*
Tags (ear), dimpylate 40%, for *cattle*
Withdrawal Periods. Remove tag before slaughter

Dryzon WP (Y-Tex) *USA*
Powder, for solution, dimpylate 50%, for *sheep*
Withdrawal Periods. Slaughter 14 days

Escort 300 (Schering-Plough) *USA*
Collar, dimpylate 15%, for *dogs*

Escort 300 (Schering-Plough) *USA*
Collar, dimpylate 15%, for *cats*

Escort Plus (Schering-Plough) *USA*
Collar, dimpylate, for *dogs, cats*

Escort Signal (Schering-Plough) *USA*
Collar, dimpylate 15%, for *dogs, cats*

New Z Diazinon Insecticide Cattle Ear Tags (Farnam) *USA*
Tags (ear), dimpylate 18%, piperonyl butoxide 2%, for *cattle*
Withdrawal Periods. Remove tags before slaughter

Optimizer Insecticide Calf Ear Tags (Y-Tex) *USA*
Tags (ear), dimpylate 21.4%, for *cattle*
Withdrawal Periods. Remove tags before slaughter

Optimizer Insecticide Cattle Ear Tags (Y-Tex) *USA*
Tags (ear), dimpylate 21.4%, for *cattle*
Withdrawal Periods. Remove tags before slaughter

Patriot Insecticide Cattle Ear Tag (Boehringer Ingelheim Vetmedica) *USA*
Tags (ear), dimpylate 40%, for *cattle*
Withdrawal Periods. Catle: should not be used in cattle producing milk for human consumption, remove tags before slaughter

Pet Care 5-Month Flea Collar For Cats (DurVet) *USA*
Collar, dimpylate 15%, for *cats*

Preventef Flea and Tick Collar For Cats With EFA (Allerderm/Virbac) *USA*
Collar, dimpylate 11%, for *cats*

Preventef Flea and Tick Collar For Dogs With EFA (Allerderm/Virbac) *USA*
Collar, dimpylate 11%, for *dogs*

ETHION

USA
Indications. Flies and ticks on cattle

Commando Insecticide Cattle Ear Tag (Boehringer Ingelheim Vetmedica) *USA*
Tags (ear), ethion 36%, for *cattle*
Withdrawal Periods. Remove tag prior to slaughter

FAMPHUR

Australia
Indications. Lice on cattle
Contra-indications. Use within 3 days of other organic phosphorus agent

Warbex (Coopers) *Austral*
Solution, pour-on, famphur 125 g/L, for *cattle*
Withdrawal Periods. Slaughter 14 days, should not be used on cattle producing milk for human consumption

New Zealand
Indications. Lice on cattle
Side-effects. Alopecia at site of application

Warbex (Schering-Plough) *NZ*
Solution, pour-on, famphur 125 g/litre, for *cattle*
Withdrawal Periods. Slaughter 35 days, should not be used in cattle producing milk for human consumption

USA
Indications. Lice and warble-fly larvae on cattle
Contra-indications. Calves less than 3 months of age; Brahman bulls
Warnings. Treat for warble-fly larvae at appropriate time

Warbex (Schering-Plough) *USA*
Solution, pour-on, famphur 13.2%, for *cattle*
Withdrawal Periods. Cattle: slaughter 35 days, should not be used in cattle producing milk for human consumption.

FENTHION

UK
Indications. Fleas on dogs and cats
Contra-indications. Dogs less than 6 months of age, cats less than 1 year of age; dogs less than 3 kg body-weight, cats less than 2 kg body-weight; pregnant dogs or cats less than 1 week before expected date of parturition. Treatment within 10–14 days before or after other organophosphorus compounds or other anticholinesterase compounds (see Drug Interactions – Appendix 1), levamisole, phenothiazine derivatives, muscle relaxants, or diethylcarbamazine citrate.
Side-effects. Occasionally cats show clinical signs of excitment after treatment
Warnings. Dogs and cats should not be handled for 8 hours after application of the preparation and recently treated animals should not be allowed to sleep in the same location as their owners, especially children; use with caution in renal or hepatic impairment. Multi-use operators should wear protective rubber gloves
Dose. *Dogs*: *by 'spot-on' application*, (3–10 kg body-weight) 80 mg, (11–25 kg body-weight) 200 mg, (26–50 kg body-weight) 400 mg, (>50 kg body-weight) 600 mg
Cats: *by 'spot-on' application*, 30 mg

POM **Tiguvon 10** (Bayer) *UK*
Solution, 'spot-on', fenthion 100 mg/mL, for *cats*; 0.3 mL

POM **Tiguvon 20** (Bayer) *UK*
Solution, 'spot-on', fenthion 200 mg/mL, for *dogs*; 0.4 mL, (Tiguvon 20L) 1 mL

Australia
Indications. Lice on cattle; fleas on dogs
Contra-indications. Cats; use within 14 days of other insecticidal tratment on dogs; bathing of dogs within 2 days of treatment; puppies less than 4 months of age; dogs less than 2.5 kg body-weight; chihuahuas; pregnant or nursing bitches

Bay-O-Pet Spotton Flea Control (Bayer) *Austral*
Solution, spot-on, fenthion 100 g/L, 200 g/L, for *dogs*

Exelpet Flea Liquidator (Exelpet) *Austral*
Solution, spot-on, fenthion 100 g/L, 200 g/L, for *dogs*

Tiguvon Pour-On Cattle Lice Insecticide (Bayer) *Austral*
Solution, pour-on, fenthion 20 g/L, for *cattle*
Withdrawal Periods. Slaughter 10 days, should not be used on cattle producing milk for human consumption

Tiguvon Spot-On Cattle Lice Insecticide (Bayer) *Austral*
Solution, spot-on, fenthion 200 g/L, for *cattle*
Withdrawal Periods. Slaughter 10 days, should not be used on cattle producing milk for human consumption

Eire
Indications. Lice, warble-fly larvae on cattle; fleas on dogs and cats
Contra-indications. Cats less than 1 year of age; cats less than 2 kg body-weight; puppies less than 6 months of age; pregnant bitches or queens within 1 week of expected parturition; concurrent or treatment within 10 days with other flea control agents, organophosphus compounds, phenothiazine derivatives, muscle relaxants
Warnings. Dogs and cats should not be handled for 8 hours after application of the preparation and recently treated animals should not be allowed to sleep in the same location as their owners, especially children; use with caution in renal or hepatic impairment.

Tiguvon 10 (Bayer) *Eire*
Solution, spot-on, fenthion 10%, for *cats*

Tiguvon 20, 20L (Bayer) *Eire*
Solution, spot-on, fenthion 20%, for *dogs*

Tiguvon Spot-on 20% (Bayer) *Eire*
Solution, spot-on, fenthion 20 g/100 mL, for *cattle*
Withdrawal Periods. Slaughter 21 days, milk 5 days

New Zealand
Indications. Lice on cattle; fleas on dogs and cats
Contra-indications. Puppies less than 4 months of age; cats less than 1 year of age; cats less than 2 kg body-weight; cats within one week of expected parturition; calves less than 6 weeks of age; use within 14 days with other flea control agents in dogs; use within 28 days with other flea control agents in cats; use within 10 days of tranquiliser treatment in dogs and cats

Spotton for Cats (Bayer) *NZ*
Solution, spot-on, fenthion 100 mg/mL, for *cats*

Spotton for Dogs (Bayer) *NZ*
Solution, spot-on, fenthion 200 mg/mL, for *dogs*

Tiguvon Pour-on (Bayer) *NZ*
Solution, pour-on, fenthion 2%, for *cattle*
Withdrawal Periods. Slaughter 21 days, milk 24 hours

Tiguvon Spot-on (Bayer) *NZ*
Solution, spot-on, fenthion 20%, for *cattle*
Withdrawal Periods. Slaughter 21 days, milk 24 hours

USA
Indications. Lice, warble-fly larvae, and flies on cattle; lice on pigs
Contra-indications. Pour-on or spot-on on calves less than 3 months of age

Warnings. Treatment for warble-fly larvae should be during appropriate period

Cutter Blue (Bayer) *USA*
Tags (ear), fenthion 20 %, piperonyl butoxide 15%, for *cattle*
Withdrawal Periods. Remove tag prior to slaughter

Lysoff Pour-On (Bayer) *USA*
Solution,pour-on, fenthion 7.6%, for *cattle*
Withdrawal Periods. Slaughter 21 days (or 35 days if second or third application is used), should not be used on cattle producing milk for human consumption

Spotton (Bayer) *USA*
Solution, spot-on , fenthion 20%, for *cattle*
Withdrawal Periods. Slaughter 45 days, do not use on cattle producing milk for human consumption, should not be used on calves intended for veal production

Tiguvon (Bayer) *USA*
Solution, pour-on, fenthion 3%, for *cattle*
Withdrawal Periods. Slaughter 35 days (or 45 days after 2nd treatment for louse control), should not be used on cattle producing milk for human consumption

Tiguvon (Bayer) *USA*
Solution, pour-on, fenthion 3%, for *pigs*
Withdrawal Periods. Slaughter 14 days

MALATHION
(Maldison)

Australia
Indications. Fleas, lice, ticks, and sarcoptic mange mites on dogs and cats; red mites on birds; lice on horses, cattle, and pigs
Contra-indications. Puppies or kittens less than 3 months of age; pregnant or lactating animals

Di-Flea Flea and Tick Rinse and Yard Spray (Jurox) *Austral*
Spray, maldison 200 g/L, for *dogs, cats*

Malaban Wash Concentrate (Inca) *Austral*
Liquid concentrate, malathion 200 g/L, for *dogs, cats, aviaries*

Malatroy (Troy) *Austral*
Liquid concentrate, malathion 200 g/L, for *dogs, cats, birds*

Maldison 50 (Pharmachem) *Austral*
Liquid concentrate, maldison 500 g/L, for *horses, cattle, pigs, dogs, cats, poultry, premises*

New Zealand
Indications. Fleas, lice, ticks, and mites on dogs and cats; red mites and lice on birds; lice on cattle

Parasite Spray (Ethical) *NZ*
Spray concentrate, malathion 500 g/litre, for *cattle, dogs, cats, poultry*
Withdrawal Periods. Poultry: slaughter 24 hours, eggs 24 hours

USA
Indications. Fleas, lice, ticks, and mites on dogs and cats; red mites and lice on birds; lice on cattle

Prozap Malathion 57EC (Loveland) *USA*
Topical spray, malathion 57%, for *horses, cattle, sheep, goats, pigs, dogs, cats, poultry*

METRIFONATE
(Metriphonate, Trichlorfon)

New Zealand
Indications. Lice and mange mites on pigs and chickens

See section 2.1.1.4 for preparation details

NALED

Indications. Fleas and ticks on dogs

Performer (Performer) *USA*
Collar, naled 15 % , for *dogs*

PHOXIM

Eire
Indications. *Psoroptes*, lice, keds, and ticks on sheep
Contra-indications. Treatment within 14 days of other organophosphorus compounds

Sebacil 50% Emulsifiable Concentrate (Bayer) *Eire*
Plunge dip solution, phoxim 50%, for *sheep*
Withdrawal Periods. Slaughter 5 weeks, should not be used in sheep producing milk for human consumption

PHOSMET

UK
Indications. Warble-fly larvae, lice, and mites on cattle; mites and lice on pigs
Contra-indications. Calves less than 3 months of age; treatment between December 1 and March 14 in cattle, see notes above; application of 'pour-on' when animals are wet. See also under Fenthion
Dose. *Cattle*: by 'pour-on' application.
Lice, 10 mg/kg, repeat after 10–14 days
Mites and warble-fly larvae, 20 mg/kg as a single dose
Pigs: by 'pour-on' application, 20 mg/kg as a single dose

PML Dermol Plus (Crown) *UK*
Solution, 'pour-on', phosmet 200 mg/mL, for *cattle*; 1 litre
Withdrawal Periods. *Cattle*: slaughter 14 days, milk 2 days

PML Porect (Crown) *UK*
Solution, 'pour-on', phosmet 200 mg/mL, for *pigs*
Withdrawal Periods. *Pigs*: slaughter 35 days

PML Poron 20 (Young's) *UK*
Solution, 'pour-on', phosmet 200 mg/mL, for *cattle*; 500 mL, 1 litre
Withdrawal Periods. *Cattle*: slaughter 14 days
Note. Animals producing milk for human consumption should be treated immediately after milking, which should be at least 6 hours before the next milking

Australia
Indications. Lice on cattle; lice and mange mites on pigs
Contra-indications. Use of other organophosphorus compounds or levamisole within 14 days of treatment in pigs; concurrent use of organophosphorus compounds in cattle

Porect (Pfizer) *Austral*
Solution, pour-on, phosmet 188 g/L, for *pigs*
Withdrawal Periods. Slaughter 28 days

Poron (Novartis) *Austral*
Solution, pour-on, phosmet 10 %, for *cattle*
Withdrawal Periods. Slaughter withdrawal period nil

Eire
Indications. Lice, mange mites, and warble fly larvae on cattle
Contra-indications. Use of other organophosphorus compounds, levamisole, or diethylcarbamazine within 14 days of treatment

Young's Poron 20 (Cypharm) *Eire*
Solution, pour-on, phosmet 20%, for *cattle*
Withdrawal Periods. Slaughter 14 days, milk 6 hours

New Zealand
Indications. Lice and mange mites on pigs
Contra-indications. Use of other organophosphorus compounds or levamisole within 14 days of treatment

Porect (Pfizer) *NZ*
Solution, pour-on, phosmet 20%, for *pigs*
Withdrawal Periods. Slaughter 28 days

USA
Indications. Lice, ticks, flies,and sarcoptic mange mites on cattle; lice and mange mites on pigs; fleas, ticks, and sarcoptic mange on dogs
Contra-indications. Concurrent use of cholinesterase inhibiting agents

Del-Phos Emulsifiable Liquid Insecticide (Schering-Plough) *USA*
Topical spray, phosmet 11.6%, for *cattle, pigs*
Withdrawal Periods. *Cattle*: slaughter 3 days (depends of spray conc), should not be used on cattle producing milk for human consumption. *Pigs*: slaughter one day

Paramite Sponge-On or Dip for Dogs (Hoechst-Roussel) *USA*
Dip concentrate, phosmet 11.6%, for *dogs*

ProTICall Derma-Dip (Schering-Plough) *USA*
Dip concentrate, phosmet 11.6%, for *dogs*

PROPETAMPHOS

Australia
Indications. Blowfly strike, keds and lice on sheep
Contra-indications. Dipping more than 6 weeks after shearing or within 2 weeks after shearing; dipping heavily grass seed infested sheep or heavily pregnant ewes

Deadmag (Novartis) *Austral*
Liquid concentrate, propetamphos 14.4 g/L, for *sheep*
Withdrawal Periods. Slaughter 14 days

Ectomort Plus Lanolin (Novartis) *Austral*
Dip or spray concentrate, propetamphos 360 g/L, for *sheep*
Withdrawal Periods. Slaughter 14 days

Magget (Novartis) *Austral*
Solution, pour-on, propetamphos 0.72 g/L, for *sheep*
Withdrawal Periods. Slaughter 14 days

Mules 'N Mark II Blowfly Dressing (Nufarm) *Austral*
Topical solution, propetamphos 0.5 g/L, for *sheep*
Withdrawal Periods. Slaughter 14 days

Seraphos 360 (Nufarm) *Austral*
Dip concentrate, propetamphos 360 g/L, for *sheep*
Withdrawal Periods. Slaughter 14 days

Eire
Indications. Blowfly larvae (blowfly strike), keds, lice, *Psoroptes*, and ticks on sheep

Young's Ectomort Sheep Dip (Cypharm) *Eire*
Dip concentrate, propetamphos 8%, for *sheep*
Withdrawal Periods. Slaughter 14 days, should not be used on sheep producing milk for human consumption

New Zealand
Indications. Lice on cattle; blowfly strike, keds, ticks, and lice on sheep
Contra-indications. Calves less than 50 kg body-weight; concurrent use of other organophosphorus compounds in cattle; goats

Destruct (Novartis) *NZ*
Solution, pour-on, propetamphos 100 g/litre, for *cattle*
Withdrawal Periods. Slaughter 3 days, milk 5 days

Maggo (Novartis) *NZ*
Liquid concentrate, propetamphos 16 g/litre, for *sheep*
Withdrawal Periods. Slaughter 14 days

Seraphos 500 (Novartis) *NZ*
Dip concentrate, propetamphos 160 g/litre, for *sheep*
Withdrawal Periods. Slaughter 14 days, should not be used in sheep producing milk for human consumption

Seraphos 1250 (Novartis) *NZ*
Dip concentrate, propetamphos 400 g/litre, for *sheep*
Withdrawal Periods. Slaughter 14 days, should not be used in sheep producing milk for human consumption

TEMEFOS
(Temephos)

Australia
Indications. Lice on sheep; fleas on dogs and cats
Contra-indications. Use of liquid concentrate on pregnant or lactating cats and dogs or concurrent use of other organophosphorus compounds

Assassin Sheep Dip (Coopers) *Austral*
Sheep dip, temefos 350 g/L, for *sheep*
Withdrawal Periods. Slaughter 14 days

Exelpet Flea Kill Powder for Cats, Dogs, Kittens & Puppies (Exelpet) *Austral*
Dusting powder, temefos 20 mg/g, for *dogs, cats*

Exelpet Flea Kill Rinse Concentrate for Dogs & Cats (Exelpet) *Austral*
Liquid concentrate, temefos 100 mg/mL, for *dogs, cats*

New Zealand
Indications. Lice on sheep and cattle
Contra-indications. Pour-on within 3 days of other organophosphorus compounds

Assassin Sheep Dip (Schering-Plough) *NZ*
Dip concentrate, temefos 350 g/litre, for *sheep*
Withdrawal Periods. Slaughter 35 days, should not be used in sheep producing milk for human consumption

Lypor (Fort Dodge) *NZ*
Solution, pour-on, temefos 20%, for *cattle*
Withdrawal Periods. Slaughter 10 days, milk 14 days

Tempor (Ancare) *NZ*
Solution, pour-on, temefos 20%, for *cattle*
Withdrawal Periods. Slaughter 10 days, should not be used in cattle producing milk for human consumption

Vengeance (Fort Dodge) *NZ*
Solution, pour-on, temefos 20%, for *cattle*
Withdrawal Periods. Slaughter 10 days, milk 14 days

TETRACHLORVINPHOS

USA
Indications. Lice and flies on cattle; lice on pigs; lice and mites on chickens

Prozap Dust'R (Loveland) *USA*
Dusting powder, tetrachlorvinphos 3%, for *cattle, pigs, chickens*

Rabon 3% Dust (AgriLabs) *USA*
Dusting powder, tetrachlorvinphos 3%, for *cattle, pigs*
Withdrawal Periods. Slaughter withdrawal period nil

Rabon 3% Livestock Dust (DurVet) *USA*
Dusting powder, tetrachlorvinphos 3%, for *cattle, pigs*
Withdrawal Periods. Slaughter withdrawal period nil

Rabon 50 WP Insecticide (Boehringer Ingelheim Vetmedica) *USA*
Topical spray, tetrachlorvinphos 50%, for *cattle, poultry, premises*

2.2.1.6 Phenylpyrazoles

Fipronil is a phenylpyrazole that acts by blocking the action of the neurotransmitter gamma-amino-butyric acid resulting in rapid death of the invertebrate. Adult fleas are killed before egg laying is possible and therefore environmental challenge is reduced. Depending on the environmental population, fipronil spray provides protection against re-infestation of fleas for up to 3 months in dogs and up to 2 months in cats. Fipronil 'spot-on' provides protection against re-infestation of fleas for up to 2 months in dogs and up to 5 weeks in cats. Tick control in dogs lasts for up to 4 weeks. Fipronil spray (100 mL, delivering 0.5 mL/actuation) is safe to use in puppies and kittens more than 2 days of age.

FIPRONIL
Indications. Fleas and ticks on dogs and cats; spray may aid in control of lice♦, *Sarcoptes*♦, *Cheyletiella*♦, and *Neotrombicula*♦ on dogs and cats
Contra-indications. Puppies and kittens less than 2 days of age (spray); bathing animals within 2 days of treatment; rabbits
Side-effects. Transient hypersalivation if cat licks 'spot-on' application area
Warnings. Safety of spot-on in puppies less than 10 weeks of age and kittens less than 12 weeks of age not established; recently treated animals should not be handled until dry and should not be allowed to sleep with humans, especially children

Dose. *Dogs*: *by 'spot-on' application,* (up to 10 kg body-weight) 0.67 mL (10–20 kg body-weight) 1.34 mL, (20–40 kg body-weight) 2.68 mL, (>40 kg body-weight) 4.02 mL *by spray application,* see manufacturer's information
Cats: *by 'spot-on' application,* 0.5 mL
by spray application, see manufacturer's information

POM **Frontline Spray** (Merial) *UK*
Spray, fipronil 0.25%, for *dogs, cats*; 100 mL, 250 mL

POM **Frontline Spot On Cat** (Merial) *UK*
Solution, 'spot-on', fipronil 10%, for *cats*; 0.5 mL

POM **Frontline Spot On Dog** (Merial) *UK*
Solution, 'spot-on', fipronil 10%, for *dogs*; 0.67 mL, 1.34 mL, 2.68 mL, 4.02 mL

Australia
Indications. Fleas and ticks on dogs and cats
Contra-indications. Spot-on on puppies and kittens less than 12 weeks of age

Frontline Spray (Troy) *Austral*
Spray (pump), fipronil 2.5 g/L, for *dogs, cats*

Frontline Top Spot Cat (Troy) *Austral*
Solution, spot-on, fipronil 100 g/L, for *cats*

Frontline Top Spot Dog (Troy) *Austral*
Solution, spot-on, fipronil 100 g/L, for *dogs*

Eire
Indications. Fleas on dogs and cats; ticks on dogs
Contra-indications. Puppies and kittens less than 2 days of age (spray); bathing animals within 2 days of treatment
Warnings. Safety of spot-on in puppies less than 10 weeks of age and kittens less than 12 weeks of age not established; treated animals should not be handled until dry

Frontline Spray (Merial) *Eire*
Spray, fipronil 0.25%, for *dogs, cats*

Frontline Spot On Cat (Merial) *Eire*
Solution, spot-on, fipronil 10%, for *cats*

Frontline Spot On Dog (Merial) *Eire*
Solution, spot-on, fipronil 10%, for *dogs*

New Zealand
Indications. Fleas and ticks on dogs and cats
Contra-indications. Puppies and kittens less than 2 days of age (spray)
Warnings. Safety of spot-on in puppies less than 10 weeks of age and kittens less than 12 weeks of age not established

Frontline Spray (Merial) *NZ*
Spray, fipronil 0.25%, for *dogs, cats*

Frontline Top Spot (Merial) *NZ*
Solution, spot-on, fipronil 10%, for *dogs, cats*

USA
Indications. Fleas and ticks on dogs and cats
Contra-indications. Puppies less than 8 weeks (spray) or 10 weeks (spot-on) of age; kittens less than 8 weeks (spray) or 12 weeks (spot-on)

Frontline Spray Treatment (Merial) *USA*
Topical spray, fipronil 0.29%, for *dogs, cats*

Frontline Top Spot for Cats (Merial) *USA*
Solution, spot-on, fipronil 9.7%, for *cats*

Frontline Top Spot for Dogs (Merial) *USA*
Solution, spot-on, fipronil 9.7%, for *dogs*

2.2.1.7 Pyrethrins and synthetic pyrethroids

Natural **pyrethrins** extracted from pyrethrum flowers and the synthetic pyrethroids **bioallethrin, cyhalothrin, cypermethrin, deltamethrin, fenvalerate, flumethrin, lambda-cyhalothrin, phenothrin,** and **permethrin** exert their action on the sodium channels of parasite nerve axons, causing initial excitement then paralysis.

Pyrethrum extract, prepared from pyrethrum flower, contains about 25% of pyrethrins. Some preparations contain pyrethrins together with piperonyl butoxide with which they are synergistic. Piperonyl butoxide inhibits the microsomal system of some arthropods and has been shown to be effective against some mites.

The content of some synthetic pyrethroid preparations is expressed in terms of the drug isomers. For example, cypermethrin preparations may contain varying proportions of their *cis:trans* isomers, for example 60:40 or 80:20. Cypermethrin (*cis:trans* 60:40) 2.5% is equivalent to cypermethrin (*cis:trans* 80:20) 1.25%.

Some pyrethrins such as permethrin appear to repel flea feeding and may be able to prevent the flea biting and therefore assist in the control of allergic dermatitis.

Cypermethrin-containing 'pour-on' preparations for sheep may be used for the prevention and treatment of blowfly strike. Protection against blowfly is only provided at the site of application for 6 to 8 weeks. Cyermethrin- and flumethrin-containing sheep dips are authorised for use against sheep scab in the UK. Cypermethrin is effective against many ectoparasites. Animals should be dipped twice at an interval of 14 days for *Psoroptes*. After treatment sheep should be moved to pasture that has not carried sheep for 16 days. Flumethrin has residual action and is effective against keds, lice, ticks, and *Psorptes* but not blowfly strike.

Cypermethrin ear tags are attached to the back of the ear in cattle and provide protection for up to 5 months. Permethrin-containing ear tags are available that are effective for up to 5 months. One tag will provide general fly control; 2 tags are required when fly infestation is likely to be severe. Tags containing second and third generation synthetic pyrethroids are used to control biting and nuisance flies on cattle. High fly populations are associated with summer mastitis and infectious bovine keratoconjunctivitis (New Forest Disease). Other measures such as dry cow therapy (see section 11.1.2) and treatment of udder and teat lesions (see section 11.2) should also be used to prevent summer mastitis.

BIOALLETHRIN

USA

Indications. Fleas and ticks on dogs and cats

Duocide Shampoo (Allerderm/Virbac) *USA*
Shampoo, bioallethrin 0.08%, related cpds 0.006%, phenothrin 0.025%, n-octyl bicycloheptene dicarboximide 0.4%, for *dogs, cats*

Mycodex Sensicare Flea & Tick Shampoo (Pfizer) *USA*
Shampoo, bioallethrin 0.12%, piperonyl butoxide 0.5%, for *dogs, cats*

CYFLUTHRIN

USA

Indications. Flies, lice, and ticks on cattle

Cutter Gold (Bayer) *USA*
Tags (ear), cyfluthrin 10%, for *cattle*
Withdrawal Periods. Remove tag prior to slaughter

Cylence (Bayer) *USA*
Solution, pour-on, cyfluthrin 1%, for *cattle*

CYHALOTHRIN

Eire

Indications. Lice on cattle
Side-effects. Transient, mild discomfort

Spot On CY, Coopers (Schering-Plough) *Eire*
Solution, spot-on, cyhalothrin 2%, for *cattle*
Withdrawal Periods. Slaughter 7 days, milk withdrawal period nil

New Zealand

Indications. Lice and keds on sheep

Grenade (Schering-Plough) *NZ*
Dip concentrate, cyhalothrin 5%, for *sheep*
Withdrawal Periods. Slaughter withdrawal period nil, should not be used in sheep producing milk for human consumption

CYPERMETHRIN

UK

Indications. Flies on horses and cattle; lice on horses, cattle and goats; blowfly strike, biting lice, ticks, headflies, and *Psoroptes* (dip) on sheep; red mites on poultry
Contra-indications. Treatment of lambs less than one week of age or treatment of animals during hot weather
Side-effects. 'Pour-on' preparations should not be applied to the tail region of lambs because this could interfere with ewe-lamb recognition
Warnings. Wash udders of sprayed animals before milking and apply only to unbroken lesions

PML Auriplak Fly and Scab Dip (Virbac) *UK*
Dip concentrate, cypermethrin (*cis:trans* 80:20) 10%, for *sheep*; 1 litre, 2.5 litres, 5 litres. To be diluted before use
Withdrawal Periods. *Sheep*: slaughter 12 days, should not be used on sheep producing milk for human consumption
Dipwash. Blowfly, keds, lice, ticks, *Psoroptes*. Dilute 1 volume in 500 volumes water. Repeat after 14 days for *Psoroptes*
Replenisher. Dilute 1 volume in 500 volumes water and add to dipwash after each 50 sheep dipped

PML Barricade 5% EC (Sorex) *UK*
Liquid concentrate, cypermethrin 5%, for *horses, ponies, poultry*; 1 litre. To be diluted before use
Withdrawal Periods. Should not be used on *horses* intended for human consumption. *Poultry*: slaughter 21 days, egg withdrawal period nil
Dilute 1 volume with 50 volumes water (= cypermethrin 0.1%)
Dilute 1 volume with 100 volumes water (= cypermethrin 0.05%)
Dose. *Horses*: by spray, 125–500 mL of 0.1% solution
Poultry: by spray, 20 mL of 0.05% solution

PML Crovect (Crown) *UK*
Solution, 'pour-on', cypermethrin (*cis:trans* 80:20) 1.25%, for *sheep*; 500 mL, 2.5 litres, 5 litres
Withdrawal Periods. *Sheep*: slaughter 3 days, should not be used on sheep producing milk for human consumption
Dose. *Sheep*: by 'pour-on' application (unless otherwise indicated).
Blowfly larvae, treatment, 5–10 mL on affected area; prophylaxis, by spray, (>12.5 kg body-weight and < 25 kg body-weight) 20 mL, (25–40 kg body-weight) 30 mL, (>40 kg body-weight) 40 mL
Headflies, 5 mL
Lice, 0.25 mL/kg (maximum 20 mL)
Ticks, (<10 kg body-weight) 5 mL then, after 3 weeks, 10 mL, (>10 kg body-weight) 0.5 mL/kg (maximum 40 mL)

PML Crovect Dip (Crown) *UK*
Dip concentrate, cypermethrin 10%, for *sheep*; 1 litre, 2.5 litres, 5 litres. To be diluted before use
Withdrawal Periods. *Sheep*: slaughter withdrawal period nil, should not be used on sheep producing milk for human consumption
Dipwash. Blowfly, *Psoroptes*. Dilute 1 volume in 400 volumes water. Repeat after 14 days for *Psoroptes*
Replenisher. Dilute 1 volume in 300 volumes water and add to dipwash after each fall in volume of 10%
Dipwash. Lice, ticks. Dilute 1 volume in 1000 volumes water
Replenisher. Dilute 1 volume in 660 volumes water and add to dipwash after each fall in volume of 10%

PML Deosan Deosect (Fort Dodge) *UK*
Liquid concentrate, cypermethrin (*cis:trans* 50:50) 5%, for *horses, poultry*; 250 mL, 1 litre. To be diluted before use
Withdrawal Periods. Should not be used on *horses, ponies* intended for human consumption. *Poultry*: slaughter 21 days, egg withdrawal period nil
Dilute 1 volume with 50 volumes water (= cypermethrin 0.1%)
Dilute 1 volume with 100 volumes water (= cypermethrin 0.05%)
Dose. *Horses*: by spray, 500 mL of 0.1% solution
Ponies: by spray, 125 mL of 0.1% solution
Poultry: by spray, 20 mL/bird of 0.05% solution

PML Deosan Dysect 'Pour-on' (Fort Dodge) *UK*
Solution, 'pour-on', alphacypermethrin 1.5%, for *cattle*; 250 mL, 1 litre
Withdrawal Periods. *Cattle*: slaughter 28 days, milk withdrawal period nil
Dose. *Cattle*: by 'pour-on' application, 10 mL

PML Deosan Flectron Fly Tags (Fort Dodge) *UK*
Ear tags, cypermethrin (*cis:trans* 50:50) 93.5%, for *cattle*; 10
Withdrawal Periods. *Cattle*: slaughter withdrawal period nil, milk withdrawal period nil
Note. Tags should be removed before slaughter

PML Ecofleece Sheep Dip (Bimeda) *UK*
Dip concentrate, cypermethrin (high *cis*) 10%, for *sheep*. To be diluted before use
Withdrawal Periods. *Sheep*: slaughter 12 days, should not be used on sheep producing milk for human consumption
Dipwash and Replenisher. Blowfly, keds, lice, ticks, *Psoroptes*. Dilute 1 volume in 500 volumes water

PML Provinec (Vericore VP) *UK*
Solution, 'pour-on', cypermethrin (*cis:trans* 80:20) 1.25%, for *sheep more than 1 week of age*; 2.5 litres, 5 litres
Withdrawal Periods. *Sheep*: slaughter 3 days, should not be used on sheep producing milk for human consumption
Dose. *Sheep*: by 'pour-on' application (unless otherwise indicated).
Blowfly larvae, treatment, 5–10 mL on affected area; prophylaxis, by spray, (>12.5 kg body-weight and <25 kg body-weight) 20 mL, (25–40 kg body-weight) 30 mL, (>40 kg bodyweight) 40 mL

Headflies, 5 mL
Lice, 0.25 mL/kg (maximum 20 mL)
Ticks, (<10 kg body-weight) 5 mL then, after 3 weeks, 10 mL, (>10 kg body-weight) 0.5 mL/kg (maximum 40 mL)

PML Renegade (Sorex) *UK*
Solution, 'pour-on', alphacypermethrin 1.5%, for *cattle*; 500 mL, 1 litre
Withdrawal Periods. *Cattle*: slaughter 28 days, milk withdrawal period nil
Dose. *Cattle*: by 'pour-on' application, 10 mL

PML Robust (Young's) *UK*
Dip concentrate, cypermethrin (high *cis*) 10%, for *sheep*. To be diluted before use
Withdrawal Periods. *Sheep*: slaughter withdrawal period nil, should not be used on sheep producing milk for human consumption
Dipwash. Blowfly, *Psoroptes*. Dilute 1 volume in 400 volumes water. Repeat after 14 days for *Psoroptes*
Replenisher. Dilute 1 volume in 300 volumes water and add to dipwash after each fall in volume of 10%
Dipwash. Lice, ticks. Dilute 1 volume in 1000 volumes water
Replenisher. Dilute 1 volume in 660 volumes water and add to dipwash after each fall in volume of 10%

PML Vector (Young's) *UK*
Solution, 'pour-on', cypermethrin (*cis:trans* 80:20) 1.25%, for *sheep*
Withdrawal Periods. *Sheep*: slaughter 3 days, should not be used on sheep producing milk for human consumption
Dose. *Sheep*: by 'pour-on' application (unless otherwise indicated).
Blowfly larvae, treatment, 5–10 mL on affected area; prophylaxis, *by spray*, (>12.5 kg body-weight and < 25 kg body-weight) 20 mL, (25–40 kg body-weight) 30 mL, (>40 kg body-weight) 40 mL
Headflies, 5 mL
Lice, 0.25 mL/kg
Ticks, (<10 kg body-weight) 5 mL then, after 3 weeks, 10 mL; (>10 kg body-weight) 0.5 mL/kg (maximum 40 mL)

Australia

Indications. Lice, keds, and blowfly strike on sheep; *Haematobia* on cattle; fleas and ticks on dogs; fleas on cats
Contra-indications. In general, application of pour-on solution more than 24 hours after shearing; application on sheep that cannot be closely shorn; ewes within 6 weeks before lambing or with lambs at foot; application to cattle within 3 weeks of treatment with a synthetic pyrethroid; application of dip to grass seed infected sheep or sheep with wounds

Cypafly (Novartis) *Austral*
Liquid concentrate, cypermethrin 237 mg/mL, for *cattle*
Withdrawal Periods. Slaughter 3 days, should not be used on cattle producing milk for human consumption.

Cypercare Off-Shears Pour-On Bodylice Treatment (Virbac) *Austral*
Solution, pour-on, cypermethrin 25 g/L, for *sheep*
Withdrawal Periods. Slaughter 3 days

Cypon (Novartis) *Austral*
Solution, pour-on, cypermethrin 25 g/L, for *sheep*
Withdrawal Periods. Slaughter 3 days

Di-Flea Dog and Cat Insecticidal Shampoo (Jurox) *Austral*
Shampoo, cypermethrin 1 g/L, piperonyl butoxide 10 g/L, for *dogs, cats*

Di-Flea Insecticidal Rinse for Dogs (Jurox) *Austral*
Liquid concentrate, cypermethrin 20 g/L, piperonyl butoxide 20 g/L, for *dogs*
Contra-indications. Cats; puppies less than 3 months of age

Duracide (Pfizer) *Austral*
Suspension, pour-on, cypermethrin 20 g/L, for *sheep*
Withdrawal Periods. Slaughter withdrawal period nil

Kleenklip (Virbac) *Austral*
Solution, pour-on, cypermethrin 25 g/L, piperonyl butoxide 100 g/l, for *sheep*
Withdrawal Periods. Slaughter withdrawal period nil

Outflank Off-Shears Pour-On Sheep Lice Treatment (Fort Dodge) *Austral*
Solution, pour-on, cypermethrin 25 g/L, for *sheep*
Withdrawal Periods. Slaughter withdrawal period nil, should not be used on animals producing milk for human consumption or processing

Robust (Novartis) *Austral*
Dip concentrate, cypermethrin 47 mg/mL, for *sheep*
Withdrawal Periods. Slaughter 7 days

Spurt (Western Stock Distributors) *Austral*
Solution, pour-on, cypermethrin 25 g/L, for *sheep*
Withdrawal Periods. Slaughter withdrawal period nil

Vanquish Long Wool (Pfizer) *Austral*
Solution, pour-on, cypermethrin 50 g/L, for *sheep*
Withdrawal Periods. Slaughter withdrawal period nil

Eire

Indications. Flies and lice on cattle; flies, lice, ticks, and blowfly strike on sheep
Contra-indications. Lambs less than 1 week of age

Flectron Fly Tags (Whelehan) *Eire*
Ear tag, cypermethrin 8.5%, for *cattle*
Withdrawal Periods. Remove tag before slaughter, milk withdrawal period nil

Renegade Pour-on (Whelehan) *Eire*
Solution, pour-on, alphacypermethrin 1.5%, for *cattle*
Withdrawal Periods. Slaughter 14 days, milk withdrawal period nil

Vector (Cypharm) *Eire*
Solution, pour-on, cypermethrin (cis:trans 80:20) 1.25%, for *sheep*
Withdrawal Periods. Slaughter 3 days, should not be used on sheep producing milk for human consumption

New Zealand

Indications. Lice, keds, and blowfly strike on sheep; lice on goats
Contra-indications. In general, application of pour-on solution more than 24 hours after shearing; application on sheep that cannot be closely shorn; ewes within 6 weeks before lambing or with lambs at foot; application of dip to grass seed infected sheep or sheep with wounds

Avalanche (Novartis) *NZ*
Spray, cypermethrin 50 g/litre, for *sheep*
Withdrawal Periods. Slaughter 10 days, should not be used in sheep producing milk for human consumption

Cypafly (Novartis) *NZ*
Solution, pour-on, cypermethrin 25 g/litre, for *sheep, goats*
Withdrawal Periods. Slaughter 7 days, milk withdrawal period nil

Cypercare (Ancare) *NZ*
Solution, pour-on, cypermethrin 25 g/litre, for *sheep, goats*
Withdrawal Periods. Slaughter 14 days, should not be used in sheep or goats producing milk for human consumption

Cypor (Novartis) *NZ*
Solution, pour-on, cypermethrin 12.5 g/litre, for *sheep, goats*
Withdrawal Periods. Slaughter 7 days, milk withdrawal period nil

Duracide (Pfizer) *NZ*
Solution, pour-on, alphacypermethrin 20 g/litre, for *sheep*
Withdrawal Periods. Slaughter 21 days

Ectomin 100 EC (Novartis) *NZ*
Dip concentrate, cypermethrin 100 g/litre, for *sheep*
Withdrawal Periods. Slaughter withdrawal period nil, should not be used in sheep producing milk for human consumption

Vanquish Long Wool (Pfizer) *NZ*
Solution, pour-on, alphacypermethrin 50 g/litre, for *sheep*

USA

Indications. Flies, ticks, and lice on cattle

Zetagard (Y-Tex) *USA*
Tags (ear), cypermethrin 10%, piperonyl butoxide 20%, for *cattle*
Withdrawal Periods. Remove tags before slaughter

DELTAMETHRIN

UK

Indications. Lice and flies on cattle; headflies, blowfly strike, keds, lice, and ticks on sheep
Side-effects. Minor signs of discomfort with some cattle up to 48 hours after treatment
Warnings. Some operators may experience transient tingling sensation on skin contact. Operators should wear protective clothing and avoid handling recently treated animals
Dose. *Cattle*: by 'spot-on' application, 10 mL of 1% solution
Sheep: by 'spot-on' application, 5 mL of 1% solution; *lambs*: 2.5 mL

PML **Spot On Insecticide, Coopers** (Schering-Plough) *UK*
Solution, 'spot-on', deltamethrin 1%, for *cattle*, *sheep*
Withdrawal Periods. *Cattle*: slaughter 3 days, milk withdrawal period nil. *Sheep*: slaughter 7 days, should not be used on sheep producing milk for human consumption

Australia

Indications. Lice, ticks, and flies on cattle; lice and keds on sheep and goats
Contra-indications. Ewes less than 6 weeks before lambing; sheep that cannot be cleanly shorn

Arrest (Coopers) *Austral*
Soultion, pour-on, deltamethrin 7.5 g/L, for *cattle*
Withdrawal Periods. Slaughter withdrawal period nil

Arrest Easy-Dose (Coopers) *Austral*
Soultion, pour-on, deltamethrin 15 g/L, for *cattle*
Withdrawal Periods. Slaughter withdrawal period nil

Clout (Coopers) *Austral*
Solution, pour-on, deltamethrin 10 g/L, for *sheep*
Withdrawal Periods. Slaughter 3 days

Clout-S (Coopers) *Austral*
Suspension, pour-on, deltamethrin 10 g/L , for *sheep, goats*
Withdrawal Periods. *Sheep*: slaughter 3 days. *Goats*: slaughter 3 days, should not be used on goats producing milk for human consumption

Coopafly (Coopers) *Austral*
Solution, pour-on, deltamethrin 25 g/L, hydrocarbon liquid 485 g/L as solvent, for *cattle*
Withdrawal Periods. Slaughter withdrawal period nil

Tixafly (Coopers) *Austral*
Liquid concentrate, deltamethrin 25 g/L, ethion 125 g/L, for *cattle*
Withdrawal Periods. Slaughter withdrawal period nil, should not be used on cattle producing milk for human consumption

Eire

Indications. Lice and flies on cattle; lice, ticks, blowfly strike, and keds on sheep; lice on pigs
Side-effects. Lacrimation and minor signs of discomfort 48 hours after treatment in cattle

Butox Pour-On (Hoechst Roussel Vet) *Eire*
Solution, pour-on, deltamethrin 0.75%, for *cattle, sheep*
Withdrawal Periods. *Cattle*: slaughter 3 days, milk withdrawal period nil. *Sheep*: slaughter 7 days, milk withdrawal period nil

Spot On Insecticide, Coopers (Schering-Plough) *Eire*
Solution, spot-on, deltamethrin 1%, for *cattle, sheep, pigs*
Withdrawal Periods. *Cattle*: slaughter 1 day, milk withdrawal period nil. *Sheep*: slaughter 3 days, should not be used on sheep producing milk for human consumption. *Pigs*: slaughter 14 days

New Zealand

Indications. Lice and flies on cattle; lice and keds on sheep; lice on goats
Side-effects. Rarely irritation 48–72 hours after treatment; do not repeat treatment on these animals

Stampede Easy Dose (Schering-Plough) *NZ*
Solution, pour-on, deltamethrin 15 g/litre, for *cattle*
Withdrawal Periods. Slaughter 28 days, milk withdrawal period nil

Wipe-out (Schering-Plough) *NZ*
Solution, pour-on, deltamethrin 1%, for *sheep, goats*
Withdrawal Periods. Slaughter 3 days, should not be used in sheep or goats producing milk for human consumption

FENVALERATE

UK

Indications. Flies and lice on cattle; fleas and ticks on dogs and cats
Contra-indications. Puppies less than 12 weeks of age, nursing bitches; cats less than 6 months of age, pregnant and nursing queens
Warnings. Avoid direct contamination of milk and milking machine
Dose. See preparation details

PML **Deosan Flyaway** (Fort Dodge) *UK*
Liquid concentrate, fenvalerate 10%, for *cattle*; 500 mL. To be diluted before use
Withdrawal Periods. *Cattle*: slaughter 1 day, milk withdrawal period nil
Dilute 1 volume with 100 volumes water (= fenvalerate 1%)
Dose. *Cattle*: by spray, (adults) 500 mL of 1% solution; *calves*: 250 mL of 1% solution

Australia

Indications. *Culicoides* on horses, flies on cattle
Contra-indications. Use within 3 weeks after other synthetic pyrethroid treatment

Sumifly Buffalo Fly Insecticide (Fort Dodge) *Austral*
Liquid concentrate, fenvalerate 200 g/L, for *horses, cattle*
Withdrawal Periods. *Horses*: slaughter withdrawal period nil. *Cattle*: slaughter withdrawal period nil, milk withdrawal period nil.

USA

Indications. *F*lies, ticks, and lice on cattle

Ectrin Insecticide (Boehringer Ingelheim Vetmedica) *USA*
Solution, concentrate, fenvalerate 10%, for **horses, sheep, goats, pigs**

Ectrin Insecticidal Cattle Ear Tag (Boehringer Ingelheim Vetmedica) *USA*
Tags (ear), fenvalerate 8%, related cpds 0.6%, for **cattle**
Withdrawal Periods. Remove tags before slaughter

FLUMETHRIN

UK

Indications. *Psoroptes*, ticks, lice,keds on sheep

PML **Bayticol Scab and Tick Dip** (Bayer) *UK*
Dip concentrate, flumethrin 6%, for **sheep**; 1 litre. To be diluted before use
Withdrawal Periods. **Sheep**: slaughter withdrawal period nil, milk withdrawal period nil
Note. Lactating dairy sheep should be treated after milking is completed
Dipwash. Treatment and prophylaxis of *Psoroptes*, keds, lice, and ticks. Dilute 1 volume in 900 volumes water. Repeat after 14 days
Replenisher. Dilute 1 volume in 900 volumes water and add to dipwash as necessary
Dipwash. Prophylaxis of *Psoroptes*. Dilute 1 volume in 1360 volumes water
Replenisher. Dilute 1 volume in 1360 volumes water and add to dipwash as necessary
Bacteriostat
Solution, powder for reconstitution, copper sulphate; 50 g
Reconstitute 50 g of powder in each 228 litres dipwash

GSL **Bayvarol** (Bayer)
See Prescribing for invertebrates

Australia

Indications. *F*lies and ticks on cattle; ticks on horses

Bayticol Cattle Dip and Spray (Bayer) *Austral*
Liquid concentrate, flumethrin 75 g/L, for **horses, cattle**
Withdrawal Periods. Slaughter withdrawal period nil

Bayticol Pour-On Cattle Tickicide (Bayer) *Austral*
Solution, pour-on, flumethrin 10 g/L, for **cattle**
Withdrawal Periods. Slaughter withdrawal period nil

Eire

Indications. Lice, ticks, *Psoroptes* on cattle

Bayticol 1% Pour-on (Bayer) *Eire*
Solution, pour-on, flumethrin 1%, for **cattle**
Withdrawal Periods. Slaughter withdrawal period nil, milk withdrawal period nil

New Zealand

Indications. Ticks on cattle

Bayticol Pour-on Tickicide (Bayer) *NZ*
Solution, pour-on, flumethrin 1%, for **cattle, deer**
Withdrawal Periods. **Cattle**: slaughter withdrawal period nil, milk withdrawal period nil. **Deer**: slaughter withdrawal period nil

LAMBDACYHALOTHRIN

USA

Indications. Flies and lice on cattle

Saber Extra (Schering-Plough) *USA*
Tags (ear), lambdacyhalothrin 10%, piperonyl butoxide 13%, for **cattle**
Withdrawal Periods. Remove tags before slaughter

Saber Pour-On Insecticide (Schering-Plough) *USA*
Solution, pour-on, lambdacyhalothrin 1%, for **cattle**
Withdrawal Periods.Should not be used on cattle producing milk for human consumption, should not be used on calves intended for veal production

PERMETHRIN

UK

Indications. *Culicoides* and flies on horses; lice on donkeys; flies, mites, and lice on cattle; fleas and ticks on dogs and cats; lice and mites on pigeons; lice♦ on dogs and cats
Contra-indications. Treatment of calves under one week of age; unless otherwise indicated puppies or kittens less than 12 weeks of age, nursing bitches or queens, pigeons less than 1 month of age
Side-effects. Occasional skin irritation and alopecia in animals wearing insecticidal collars and 'spot-on' formulations
Warnings. For 'spot-on' and 'pour-on' applications for dogs: dogs should be treated in the evening, treated area should not be handled for 3–6 hours and dogs should not be allowed to go swimming for 12 hours after application. Treated dogs should not be allowed to sleep with people, especially children. Care should be taken to ensure that other animals do not lick the preparation off treated dogs Children should not be allowed to play with collar. Cats may show signs of hyperaesthesia with excitability, twitching, and collapse if overdosage occurs; remove collar if signs of irritation occur
Dose. See preparation details

PML **Auriplak** (Virbac) *UK*
Ear tags, permethrin (*cis:trans* 40:60) 1.2 g, for **cattle**; 20
Withdrawal Periods. **Cattle**: slaughter withdrawal period nil, milk withdrawal period nil
Note. Tags should be removed before slaughter

GSL **Canovel Flea Drops** (Pfizer) *UK*
Solution, 'spot-on', permethrin (*cis:trans* 80:20) 4%, for **dogs**; 1 mL, 5 mL

GSL **Canovel Insecticidal Powder** (Pfizer) *UK*
Dusting powder, permethrin (*cis:trans* 40:60) 1%, for **dogs**; 150 g

GSL **Canovel Insecticidal Shampoo** (Pfizer) *UK*
Shampoo, permethrin (*cis:trans* 40:60) 1%, for **dogs**; 200 mL

GSL **Cat Flea Collar (Felt)** (Sherley's) *UK*
Permethrin (cis:trans 40:60) 456 mg

GSL **Cat Flea Collar (Felt-Reflective)** (Sherley's) *UK*
Permethrin (cis:trans 40:60) 456 mg

GSL **Catovel Insecticidal Powder** (Pfizer) *UK*
Dusting powder, permethrin (*cis:trans* 40:60) 1%, for **cats**; 150 g

GSL **Companion Flea Powder** (Battle Hayward & Bower) *UK*
Dusting powder, permethrin (*cis:trans* 25:75) 1.05%, for **dogs, cats**; 85 g
GSL **Companion Insecticidal Shampoo** (Battle Hayward & Bower) *UK*
Liquid concentrate, permethrin 1.05%, for **dogs, cats**; 240 mL. To be diluted before use

GSL **Defencare Shampoo** (Virbac) *UK*
Shampoo, permethrin (*cis:trans* 40:60) 1%, for **dogs**; 200 mL

GSL **Defencat Insecticidal Foam for Cats** (Virbac) *UK*
Aerosol foam, permethrin (*cis:trans* 40:60) 0.72%, for **cats**; 150 mL
Contra-indications. Kittens less than 4 months of age, nursing queens
Dose. **Cats**: apply a ball of foam of approximately 8 cm in diameter/kg body-weight. Operators should wear household or rubber gloves

GSL Exspot (Schering-Plough) *UK*
Solution, 'spot-on', permethrin (*cis:trans* 40:60) 65%, for *dogs*; 1 mL
Contra-indications. Puppies less than 2 weeks of age; cats
Dose. *Dogs: by 'spot-on' application*, (up to 15 kg body-weight) 1 mL; (>15 kg body-weight) 2 mL. Do not re-apply until at least 7 days

GSL Flea & Tick Spot On (Bob Martin) *UK*
Solution, 'spot-on', permethrin (*cis:trans* 25:75) 65%, for *dogs*; 1 mL
Contra-indications. Puppies less than 2 weeks of age; cats
Dose. *Dogs: by 'spot-on' application*, (up to 15 kg body-weight) 1 mL; (>15 kg body-weight) 2 mL. Do not re-apply until at least 7 days

GSL Fly Repellent Plus for Horses, Coopers (Schering-Plough) *UK*
See section 2.2.5 for preparation details

PML Flypor (Crown) *UK*
Solution, 'pour-on', permethrin (*cis:trans* 80:20) 4%, for *cattle*
Withdrawal Periods. *Cattle*: slaughter 3 days, milk withdrawal period nil (see note)
Note. Animals producing milk for human consumption should be treated immediately after milking, which should be at least 6 hours before next milking
Dose. *Cattle: by 'pour-on' application*, 0.1 mL/kg

GSL Fussy Puss Cat Flea Collar (Sinclair) *UK*
Permethrin 8%

GSL Head-To-Tail Flea Powder, Coopers (Schering-Plough) *UK*
Dusting powder, permethrin (*cis:trans* 25:75) 1.05%, for *dogs, cats*; 85 g
Contra-indications. Kittens less than 2 weeks of age

GSL Insecticidal Shampoo (Sherley's) *UK*
Shampoo, permethrin (*cis:trans* 40:60) 0.2%, for *dogs*; 100 mL, 250 mL

GSL Lincoln Lice Control Plus (Battle Hayward & Bower) *UK*
Liquid, citronellol 2%, permethrin (*cis:trans* 25:75) 1.05%, for *horses*; 250 mL, 600 mL. Use undiluted
Withdrawal Periods. Should not be used on *horses* intended for human consumption

GSL Lincoln Sweet Itch Control (Battle Hayward & Bower) *UK*
Liquid, citronellol 2%, permethrin (*cis:trans* 25:75) 1.05%, for *horses*; 250 mL, 600 mL. Use undiluted
Withdrawal Periods. Should not be used on *horses* intended for human consumption

GSL Louse Powder (Arnolds) *UK*
Dusting powder, permethrin (*cis:trans* 25:75) 1%, for *horses*; 150 g
Withdrawal Periods. Should not be used on *horses* intended for human consumption

GSL Natura Elasticated Insecticidal Collar for Cats (Virbac) *UK*
Permethrin (*cis:trans* 40:60) 8%, essential fatty acid esters, for *cats*

GSL Natura Insecticidal Collar for Dogs (Virbac) *UK*
Permethrin (*cis:trans* 40:60) 8%, essential fatty acid esters, for *dogs*

GSL Permethrin Flea Powder (Johnson's) *UK*
Dusting powder, permethrin (*cis:trans* 25:75) 1.05%, for *dogs, cats*; 75 g

GSL Permethrin Flea Powder (Sherley's) *UK*
Dusting powder, permethrin (*cis:trans* 25:75) 1%, for *dogs, cats*; 80 g

GSL Permethrin Flea Shampoo (Johnson's) *UK*
Shampoo, permethrin (*cis:trans* 25:75) 1.05%, for *dogs*; 125 mL
GSL Pet Care Felt Flea Collar for Cats (Armitage) *UK*
Permethrin 456 mg

PML Ridect Pour-On (Pfizer) *UK*
Solution, 'pour-on', permethrin (*cis:trans* 80:20) 4%, for *cattle more than 1 week of age*; 1 litre
Withdrawal Periods. *Cattle*: slaughter 3 days, milk withdrawal period nil (see note)
Note. Animals producing milk for human consumption should be treated immediately after milking, which should be at least 6 hours before next milking
Dose. *Cattle: by 'pour-on' application*, 0.1 mL/kg

GSL Secto Flea Powder (Sinclair) *UK*
Dusting powder, permethrin (*cis:trans* 25:75) 1.05%, for *dogs, cats*; 80 g

PML Swift (Young's) *UK*
Solution, 'pour-on', permethrin (*cis:trans* 80:20) 4%, for *cattle*; 1 litre, 2.5 litres
Withdrawal Periods. *Cattle*: slaughter 3 days, milk withdrawal period nil (see note)
Note. Animals producing milk for human consumption should be treated immediately after milking, which should be at least 6 hours before next milking
Dose. *Cattle: by 'pour-on' application*, 0.1 mL/kg

GSL Switch (Day, Son & Hewitt) *UK*
Solution, 'pour-on', permethrin (*cis:trans* 80:20) 4%, for *horses, donkeys*
Withdrawal Periods. Should not be used on *horses, donkeys* intended for human consumption
Dose. *Horses, donkeys: by 'pour-on' application*, 0.1 mL/kg (maximum 40 mL)

GSL Vetzyme JDS Insecticidal Shampoo (Seven Seas) *UK*
Shampoo, permethrin 1%, for *dogs*; 125 mL, 250 mL, other sizes available

Australia

Indications. *Culicoides* and flies on horses; flies on cattle; fleas and ticks on dogs; fleas on cats

Care 4 Month Flea Collar for Kittens and Cats (Virbac) *Austral*
Collar, permethrin 80 g/kg (with eucalyptus oil, pennyroyal oil, essential fatty acids), for *cats*

Care 4 Month Flea & Tick Collar for Small Dogs & Puppies (Virbac) *Austral*
Collar, permethrin 80 g/kg (with eucalyptus oil, pennyroyal oil, essential fatty acids), for *dogs*

Care Flea Shampoo for Dogs (Virbac) *Austral*
Shampoo, permethrin 10 g/L, for *dogs*

Care Long Acting Spray (Virbac) *Austral*
Spray (pump), permethrin 20 g/L, for *dogs*

Care Permethrin Foam Mousse for Flea Control on Dogs (Virbac) *Austral*
Mousse (aerosol), permethrin 0.8% in a foam base, for *dogs*

Exelpet No Fleas Powder for Dogs & Puppies (Exelpet) *Austral*
Dusting powder, permethrin 10 g/kg, for *dogs*

Exelpet Red 4 Month Flea Collar for Cats & Kittens (Exelpet) *Austral*
Collar, permethrin 80 mg/g, for *cats*

Exelpet Red 4 Month Flea Collar for Dogs & Puppies (Exelpet) *Austral*
Collar, permethrin 80 g/kg, for *dogs*

Exetick (Schering-Plough) *Austral*
Solution, pour-on, permethrin 650 g/L, for *dogs*

Permoxin Insecticidal Spray & Rinse Concentrate for Dogs & Horses (Dermcare-Vet) *Austral*
Liquid concentrate, permethrin 40 g/L, for *horses, dogs*
Withdrawal Periods. Slaughter 28 days

Permoxin Insecticidal Spray & Rinse Livestock Concentrate fo Cattle, Horses & Dogs (Dermcare-Vet) *Austral*
Liquid concentrate, permethrin 40 g/L, for *horses, cattle, dogs*
Withdrawal Periods. *Horses*: slaughter 28 days.

Quick-Kill Rinse or Spray Concentrate for Fleas on Dogs and Flies on Horses (Pharmachem) *Austral*
Liquid concentrate, permethrin 40 g/L, for *horses, dogs*

Swift (Novartis) *Austral*
Solution, pour-on, permethrin 40 g/L, for *horses*
Withdrawal Periods. Slaughter 28 days

Eire

Indications. *Culicoides* on horses; flies, lice, and mange mites on cattle

Crown Louse Powder (Cypharm) *Eire*
Dusting powder, permethrin (cis:trans 80:20) 0.5%, for *cattle*
Withdrawal Periods. Slaughter withdrawal period nil, milk 12 hours

Ridect (Pfizer) *Eire*
Solution, pour-on, permethrin (cis:trans 80:20) 4%, for *cattle*
Withdrawal Periods. Slaughter 3 days, milk 6 hours

Swift (Cypharm) *Eire*
Solution, pour-on, permethrin (cis:trans 80:20) 4%, for *cattle*
Withdrawal Periods. Slaughter 3 days, milk 6 hours

Switch (Cypharm) *Eire*
Solution, pour-on, permethrin, for *horses*
Withdrawal Periods. Should not be used on *horses* intended for human consumption

New Zealand

Indications. Flies on horses and cattle; fleas and ticks on dogs; fleas on cats

Ecto-soothe (Virbac) *NZ*
Shampoo, permethrin 10 g/litre, for *dogs*

Fleatrol 30 (Virbac) *NZ*
Liquid concentrate, permethrin 50 g/litre, for *dogs*

Exelpet Flea and Tick Kill Concentrate (Exelpet) *Austral*
Liquid concentrate, permethrin 40 g/L, for *dogs*

Fleatrol L.A. Spray (Virbac) *NZ*
Spray, permethrin 20 g/litre, for *dogs*

Fleatrol Mousse (Virbac) *NZ*
Mousse, permethrin 0.8%, for *cats*

Fleatrol Powder (Virbac) *NZ*
Dusting powder, permethrin 1%, for *dogs, cats*

Permoxin Concentrate (Phoenix) *NZ*
Liquid concentrate, permethrin 40 g/litre, for *horses, cattle, dogs*

Permoxin Dry Spray (Phoenix) *NZ*
Spray, permethrin 1 g/litre, for *horses, cattle, dogs*

USA

Indications. Lice and flies on horses and cattle; lice and keds on sheep; lice on pigs; fleas, lice, and ticks on dogs; fleas and ticks on cats; mites on poultry

Atroban 11% EC (Schering-Plough) *USA*
Topical spray, permethrin 11%, for *horses, cattle, goats, sheep, pigs, chickens*
Withdrawal Periods. Should not be used on *horses* intended for human consumption. *Cattle*: use only after milking is complete

Atroban 42.5% EC (Schering-Plough) *USA*
Topical spray, permethrin 42.5%, for *horses, cattle, sheep, goats, pigs, chickens*

Atroban Delice Pour-on (Schering-Plough) *USA*
Solution, pour-on, permethrin %, for *cattle, sheep*
Withdrawal Periods. Should not be used on *cattle* producing milk for human consumption

Atroban Extra (Schering-Plough) *USA*
Tags (ear), permethrin 10%, piperonyl butoxide 13%, for *cattle*

Back Side (AgriLabs) *USA*
Solution, pour-on, permethrin 1% , for *cattle, sheep*

Back Side Plus (AgriLabs) *USA*
Solution, pour-on, permethrin 1%, piperonyl butoxide 1%, for *cattle, sheep*

Boss Pour-On Insecticide (Schering-Plough) *USA*
Solution, pour-on, permethrin 5%, for *cattle, sheep*
Withdrawal Periods. Should not be used on *cattle* producing milk for human consumption

Brute Pour-On For Cattle (Y-Tex) *USA*
Solution, pour-on, permethrin 10%, for *cattle*
Withdrawal Periods. Slaughter withdrawal period nil, milk withdrawal period nil

Buzz-Off II (Bio-Ceutic) *USA*
Topical spray, permethrin 0.5%, for *horses*

Catron IV (Boehringer Ingelheim Vetmedica) *USA*
Topical spray, permethrin 0.5%, for *horses, cattle, sheep, goats, pigs*
Withdrawal Periods. *Pigs*: slaughter 5 days

Defend Flea & Tick Cream Rinse (Schering-Plough) *USA*
Topical solution, permethrin 0.5%, for *dogs, cats*

Defend Exspot Insecticide For Dogs (Schering-Plough) *USA*
Solution, spot-on, permethrin 65%, for *dogs*

Durasect (Pfizer) *USA*
Solution, pour-on, permethrin 1%, for *cattle, sheep, goats*

Ectiban D (DurVet) *USA*
Dusting powder, permethrin 0.25%, for *cattle, pigs, chickens*

Ectiban Delice (DurVet) *USA*
Solution, pour-on, permethrin 1%, for *cattle, sheep*

Ectiban EC (DurVet) *USA*
Spray concentrate, permethrin 5.7%, for *horses, cattle, sheep, chickens*
Withdrawal Periods. Should not be used on *horses* intended for human consumption. *Cattle*: only use in lactating dairy cows after milking is complete. *Pigs*: slaughter 5 days.

Equi-Phar Horse Fly Spray & Rub (Vedco) *USA*
Topical spray, permethrin 0.5%, for *horses*

Equine Spray (Anchor) *USA*
Topical spray, permethrin 0.5%, for *horses*

Escort P (Schering-Plough) *USA*
Collar, permethrin 8%, for *dogs, cats*

Exit Insecticide (RXV) *USA*
Solution, pour-on, permethrin 1%, for *cattle, sheep*

Exit II Synergised Formula Insecticide (RXV) *USA*
Solution, pour-on, permethrin 1%, piperonyl butoxide 1%, for *cattle, sheep*

Gardstar 40% EC (Y-Tex) *USA*
Solution, concentrate, permethrin 40%, for *horses, cattle, sheep, goats, pigs, dogs, chickens*

Gardstar Plus Insecticide Ear Tag (Y-Tex) *USA*
Tags (ear), permethrin 10%, for *cattle*
Withdrawal Periods. Slaughter withdrawal period nil, tags should be removed before slaughter

Horsecare Permeth 5 Fly Spray (DurVet) *USA*
Topical spray, permethrin 0.5%, for *horses*

New Z Permethrin Insecticide Cattle ear Tags (Farnam) *USA*
Tags (ear), permethrin 10%, for *cattle*
Withdrawal Periods. Remove tags before slaughter

Permectrin II (Aspen) *USA*
Topical spray, permethrin 10%, for *horses, cattle, sheep, pigs, chickens, dogs, premises*

Permectrin II Dairy Cattle and Barn Spray (Boehringer Ingelheim Vetmedica) *USA*
Topical spray, permethrin 10%, for *horses, cattle, sheep, pigs, chickens, dogs, premises*

Permectrin II Insecticide (Boehringer Ingelheim Vetmedica) *USA*
Topical spray, permethrin 10%, for *horses, cattle, sheep, pigs, chickens, dogs, premises*

Permectrin CDS Pour-On (Boehringer Ingelheim Vetmedica) *USA*
Solution, pour-on, permethrin 7.4%, piperonyl butoxide 7.4%, for *cattle, premises*
Withdrawal Periods. Should not be used on *cattle* producing milk for human consumption

Permectrin Dairy Cattle & Swine Dust (Boehringer Ingelheim Vetmedica) *USA*
Dusting powder, permethrin 0.25%, for *cattle, pigs, chickens*

Permectrin Livestock & Litter Dust (Boehringer Ingelheim Vetmedica) *USA*
Dusting powder, permethrin 0.25%, for *cattle, pigs, chickens*

Permectrin Pet, Yard and Kennel Spray (Anchor, Bio-Ceutic) *USA*
Topical spray, permethrin 10%, for *dogs, premises*

Permectrin Pour-On Insecticide (Boehringer Ingelheim Vetmedica) *USA*
Solution, pour-on, permethrin 1%, for *cattle, sheep*

Permethrin (AgriLabs) *USA*
Dusting powder, permethrin 25%, for *horses, cattle, pigs, cats, dogs*
Withdrawal Periods. *Pigs*: slaughter 5 days

Permethrin 10% (DurVet) *USA*
Topical spray, permethrin 10%, for *horses, cattle, sheep, goats, pigs, dogs, cats, chickens, premises*
Withdrawal Periods. *Pigs*: slaughter 5 days

Preventic LA Flea & Tick Spray For Dogs (Allerderm/Virbac) *USA*
Topical spray, permethrin 2%, for *dogs*

ProTICall Insecticeide Coat Conditioner (Schering-Plough) *USA*
Solution, permethrin 0.5%, for *dogs, cats*

ProTICall Insecticide For Dogs (Schering-Plough) *USA*
Solution, spot-on , permethrin 65%, for *dogs*

ProTICall Permethrin Dip (Schering-Plough) *USA*
Dip concentrate, permethrin 3.2%, for *dogs*

Prozap Drycide (Loveland) *USA*
Dusting powder, permethrin 0.25%, for *horses, cattle, pigs, dogs, cats, chickens*

Prozap Insectrin Dust (Loveland) *USA*
Dusting powder, permethrin 0.25%, for *horses, cattle, pigs, chickens, dogs, cats*

Prozap Insectrin X (Loveland) *USA*
Spray, permethrin 10%, for *horses, cattle, sheep, goats, dogs, premises*

Python (Y-Tex) *USA*
Tags (ear), permethrin 10%, piperonyl butoxide 20%, for *cattle*
Withdrawal Periods. Slaughter withdrawal period nil, remove tags before slaughter

Repel-A-Cide Dip (Happy Jack) *USA*
Dip concentrate, permethrin 3.2%, related cpds 0.28%, N-octyl bicycloheptene dicarboximide 15%, for *dogs, cats*

Synerkyl Creme Rinse (DVM) *USA*
Lotion, permethrin 0.5%, for *dogs, cats*

Synerkyl Shampoo (DVM) *USA*
Shampoo, permethrin 0.1%, related cpds 0.009%, pyrethrins 0.05%, N-octyl cycloheptene dicarboximide 0.5%, for *dogs, cats*

PYRETHRINS

UK
Indications. *Culicoides*, flies, and lice on horses; lice and mites on pigeons and caged birds; fleas and lice♦ on dogs and cats
Contra-indications. Unless otherwise stated, puppies or kittens less than 12 weeks of age, nursing bitches or queens

GSL **Anti-Mite & Insect Spray** (Johnson's) *UK*
Aerosol spray, piperonyl butoxide 1%, pyrethrins 0.2%, for *caged birds, pigeons*; 100 mL, 150 mL, 300 mL
Withdrawal Periods. Should not be used on *pigeons* intended for human consumption

GSL **Anti-Pest Insect Spray** (Johnson's) *UK*
Aerosol spray, piperonyl butoxide 1%, pyrethrins 0.2%, for *dogs, cats, pigeons*; 150 mL, 250 mL
Withdrawal Periods. Should not be used on *pigeons* intended for human consumption

GSL **Anti-Scratch Powder** (Johnson's) *UK*
Dusting powder, piperonyl butoxide 0.8%, pyrethrins 0.1%, for *dogs, cats*; 55 g

Canovel Insecticidal Spray (Pfizer) *UK*
Aerosol spray, piperonyl butoxide 1%, pyrethrins 0.1%, for *dogs*; 165 mL

GSL **Cat Flea Preparations** (Johnson's) *UK*
Dusting powder, piperonyl butoxide 0.8%, pyrethrins 0.1%, for *cats*; 55 g
Non-aerosol spray, piperonyl butoxide 1.25%, pyrethrins 0.25%, for *cats*; 100 mL

GSL **Dermoline Shampoo** (Day Son & Hewitt) *UK*
Liquid concentrate, piperonyl butoxide 0.08%, pyrethrum extract 0.04% (= pyrethrins 0.01%), for *horses*. To be diluted before use
Withdrawal Periods. *Horses*: slaughter 28 days
Dilute 1 volume with 10 volumes water for initial cleansing then use undiluted

GSL **Dog Flea Preparations** (Johnson's) *UK*
Dusting powder, piperonyl butoxide 0.8%, pyrethrins 0.1%, for *dogs*; 55 g, 110 g
Non-aerosol spray, piperonyl butoxide 1.25%, pyrethrins 0.25%, for *dogs*; 100 mL
Aerosol spray, piperonyl butoxide 1%, pyrethrins 0.2%, for *dogs*; 150 mL, 250 mL
Shampoo, piperonyl butoxide 0.49%, pyrethrins 0.05%, for *dogs*; 110 mL, 200 mL, other sizes available

GSL **Flea & Tick Spray Plus** (Bob Martin) *UK*
Spray, piperonyl butoxide (free and encapsulated) 1.3%, pyrethrins (free and encapsulated) 0.21%, for *dogs, cats*; 325 g

GSL **Flea Killing Mousse** (Bob Martin) *UK*
Foam, piperonyl butoxide (free and encapsulated) 1.3%, pyrethrins (free and encapsulated) 0.15%, for *cats*; 150 g

GSL **Flea Powder** (Bob Martin) *UK*
Dusting powder, piperonyl butoxide 0.8%, pyrethrins 0.1%, for *dogs, cats*; 100 g

GSL **Flea Shampoo** (Bob Martin) *UK*
Shampoo, piperonyl butoxide 0.49%, pyrethrins 0.04%, for *dogs*; 250 mL

GSL **Flea Spray** (Bob Martin) *UK*
Aerosol spray, piperonyl butoxide 1.57%, pyrethrins 0.32%, for *dogs*; 150 mL

GSL **Flea Spray** (Sherley's) *UK*
Spray, piperonyl butoxide 1.5%, pyrethrum extract 1.2% (= pyrethrins 0.3%), for *dogs, cats*; 150 mL
Contra-indications. Puppies or kittens less than 6 months of age

GSL **Pet Care Flea Powder for Cats** (Armitage) *UK*
Dusting powder, piperonyl butoxide 0.8%, pyrethrins 0.1%, for *cats*; 80 g

GSL **Pet Care Flea Powder for Dogs** (Armitage) *UK*
Dusting powder, piperonyl butoxide 0.8%, pyrethrins 0.1%, for *dogs*; 80 g

GSL **Pet Care Flea Spray for Cats** (Armitage) *UK*
Aerosol spray, piperonyl butoxide, pyrethrum extract 0.125%, for *cats*; 150 mL

GSL **Pet Care Flea Spray for Dogs** (Armitage) *UK*
Aerosol spray, piperonyl butoxide 0.6%, pyrethrum extract 0.125%, for *dogs*; 150 mL

GSL **Kil-Pest** (Johnson's) *UK*
Dusting powder, piperonyl butoxide 0.8%, pyrethrins 0.1%, for *dogs, cats, pigeons, caged birds*; 55 g, 110 g
Withdrawal Periods. Should not be used on *pigeons* intended for human consumption

GSL **Kitzyme Flearid Insecticidal Spray** (Seven Seas) *UK*
Aerosol spray, piperonyl butoxide 0.6%, pyrethrins 0.125%, for *cats*; 150 mL, 200 mL

GSL **Kitzyme Insecticidal Flea Powder** (Seven Seas) *UK*
Dusting powder, piperonyl butoxide 0.6%, pyrethrum extract 0.4% (= pyrethrins 0.1%), for *cats*; 50 g

GSL **Original Extra Tail** (Kalium) *UK*
Finger spray, diethyltoluamide 4.5%, piperonyl butoxide 0.6%, pyrethrins 0.075%, for *horses*; 250 mL
Liquid, diethyltoluamide 4.5%, piperonyl butoxide 0.6%, pyrethrins 0.075%, for *horses*; 250 mL, 500 mL, 1 litre

GSL **Otodex Insecticidal Shampoo** (Petlife) *UK*
Piperonyl butoxide 0.08%, pyrethrum extract 0.04% (= pyrethrins 0.01%), for *dogs*; 250 mL, 5 litres, 25 litres

GSL **Pigeon Insect Preparations** (Johnson's) *UK*
Dusting powder, piperonyl butoxide 0.8%, pyrethrins 0.1%, for *pigeons*
Withdrawal Periods. Should not be used on *pigeons* intended for human consumption
Aerosol spray, piperonyl butoxide 1%, pyrethrins 0.2%, for *pigeons*; 250 mL
Withdrawal Periods. Should not be used on *pigeons* intended for human consumption

GSL **Puppy Flea Powder** (Johnson's) *UK*
Dusting powder, piperonyl butoxide 0.8%, pyrethrins 0.1%, for *dogs*; 55 g

GSL **Radiol Insecticidal Shampoo** (Battle Hayward & Bower) *UK*
Shampoo, piperonyl butoxide 0.08%, pyrethrum extract 0.04%, for *horses*; 500 mL
Withdrawal Periods. Should not be used on *horses* intended for human consumption

GSL **Rid-Mite** (Johnson's) *UK*
Dusting powder, piperonyl butoxide 0.8%, pyrethrins 0.1%, for *caged birds, pigeons*; 55 g, 110 g
Withdrawal Periods. Should not be used on *pigeons* intended for human consumption

GSL **Ruby Paragard** (Spencer) *UK*
Spray, piperonyl butoxide 0.8%, pyrethrins 0.1%, for *dogs, cats, pigeons*; 150 mL
Withdrawal Periods. Should not be used on *pigeons* intended for human consumption

GSL **Scaly Lotion** (Johnson's) *UK*
Lotion, piperonyl butoxide 1%, pyrethrins 0.1%, for *caged birds*; 15 mL

GSL **Secto Cat Flea Spray** (Sinclair) *UK*
Spray, piperonyl butoxide 1.25%, pyrethrins 0.25%, for *cats*; 150 mL

GSL **Secto Dog and Cat Flea Powder** (Sinclair) *UK*
Dusting powder, piperonyl butoxide 0.8%, pyrethrins 0.1%, for *dogs, cats*; 80 g

GSL **Secto Flea Spray for Dogs** (Sinclair) *UK*
Spray, piperonyl butoxide 0.6%, pyrethrins 0.125%, for *dogs*; 150 mL

GSL **Secto Insecticidal Shampoo** (Sinclair) *UK*
Shampoo, piperonyl butoxide 0.49%, pyrethrins 0.19%, for *dogs*; 250 mL

GSL **Silent Flea Spray** (Bob Martin) *UK*
Spray, piperonyl butoxide 2.45%, pyrethrins 0.5%, for *dogs, cats*; 150 mL

GSL **Sweet Itch Lotion** (Day Son & Hewitt) *UK*
Piperonyl butoxide 0.5%, pyrethrum extract 0.4% (= pyrethrins 0.1%), for *horses*; 500 mL, 5 litres
Withdrawal Periods. Should not be used on *horses* intended for human consumption

GSL **Vetzyme Flearid Insecticidal Spray** (Seven Seas) *UK*
Aerosol spray, piperonyl butoxide 0.6%, pyrethrins 0.125%, for *dogs*; 150 mL, 200 mL, 300 mL

GSL **Vetzyme Insecticidal Flea Powder** (Seven Seas) *UK*
Dusting powder, piperonyl butoxide 0.6%, pyrethrum extract 0.4% (= pyrethrins 0.1%), for *dogs*; 50 g

GSL **Vivapet Flea Spray for Cats** (Seven Seas) *UK*
Aerosol spray, piperonyl butoxide 0.6%, pyrethrins 0.125%, for *cats*; 150 mL, 200 mL

GSL **Vivapet Flea Spray for Dogs** (Seven Seas) *UK*
Aerosol spray, piperonyl butoxide 0.6%, pyrethrins 0.125%, for *dogs*; 150 mL, 200 mL, 300 mL

Australia
Indications. *Fleas, lice, and ticks on dogs and cats*

Care Herbal Flea Rinse for Dogs and Cats (Virbac) *Austral*
Liquid concentrate, pyrethrins 5 g/L, piperonyl butoxide 20 g/L, linalool oil 100 g/L, for *dogs, cats*

Care Herbal Foam Mousse for Flea Control on Cats (Virbac) *Austral*
Mousse (aerosol), pyrethrins 1 g/kg, piperonyl butoxide 10 g/kg, linalool oil 5 g/kg, for *cats*

Coalfoam (Pharmachem) *Austral*
Solution, coal tar 2.5 mL, pyrethrins 250 mg, piperonyl butoxide 2.5 g, carbaril 2.5 g, all in 250 mL, for *dogs, cats*

Di-Flea Ovakill Insecticidal Spray for Cats and Dogs (Jurox) *Austral*
Spray (pump), pyrethrins 1.8 g/L, N-octyl bicycloheptene dicarboximide 6 g/L, pipeonyl butoxide 3.6 g/L, S-methoprene 2 g/L, for *dogs, cats*

Di-Flea Puppy and Kitten Insecticidal Shampoo (Jurox) *Austral*
Shampoo, pyrethrins 1g/L, piperonyl butoxide 10 g/L, for *dogs, cats*

Di-Flea Rapid Dry Insecticidal Spray for Dogs and Cats (Jurox) *Austral*
Spray (pump), pyrethrins 1 g/L, piperonyl butoxide 5 g/L, methylated spirits 750 mL/L as solvent, for *dogs, cats*

Exelpet Flea Control Powder for Cats (Exelpet) *Austral*
Dusting powder, pyrethrins 2.5 g/L, piperonyl butoxide 20 g/L, for *cats*

Exelpet Flea Control Powder for Dogs (Exelpet) *Austral*
Dusting powder, pyrethrins 2.5 g/L, piperonyl butoxide 20 g/L, for *dogs*

Exelpet Flea Control Shampoo (Exelpet) *Austral*
Shampoo, pyrethrins 1 g/L, piperonyl butoxide 1.6 g/L, N-octyl bicycloheptene dicarboximide 2.6 g/L, for *dogs*

Exelpet Flea Control Soap (Exelpet) *Austral*
Soap, pyrethrins 2 g/kg, piperonyl butoxide 18 g/kg, dichlorophen 9.7 g/kg, for *dogs*

Exelpet Pyrethrin Flea Knockdown Spray (Exelpet) *Austral*
Spray (pump), pyrethrins 1 g/L, piperonyl butoxide 10 g/L, for *dogs, cats*

Exelpet Pyrethrin Flea Fly Repellent Cream (Exelpet) *Austral*
Cream, pyrethrins 2 mg/g, piperonyl butoxide 10 mg/g, di-N-propyl isocinchomeronate 25 mg/g, for *dogs*

Fido's Fre-Itch Pyrethrin Shampoo (Mavlab) *Austral*
Shampoo, pyrethrins 1 g/L, piperonyl butoxide 10 g/L, for *dogs, cats*

Fido's Fre-Itch Quick-Dry Insecticidal Spray (Mavlab) *Austral*
Spray, pyrethrins 1.8 g/L, piperonyl butoxide 3.6 g/L, N-octyl bicicloheptene dicarboximide 6 g/l, for *dogs, cats*

Fido's Fre-Itch CPP Flea Powder (Mavlab) *Austral*
Dusting powder, piperonyl butoxide 10 g/kg, pyrethrins 1 g/kg, carbaril 50 g/kg, for *dogs, cats*

Fido's Fre-Itch Rinse Concentrate (Mavlab) *Austral*
Liquid concentrate, pyrethrins 10 g/L, piperonyl butoxide 18 g/L, N-octyl bicicloheptene dicarboximide 30 g/L, for *dogs, cats, cage birds*

Fleatrol Plus Quick Dry Insecticidal Spray (Mavlab) *Austral*
Spray, N-octyl bicicloheptene dicarboximide 6 g/L, piperonyl butoxide 3.6 g/L, methoprene 4 g/L, pyrethrins 1.8 g/L, for *dogs, cats*

Ovicide (Ilium) *Austral*
Spray, methoprene 4 g/L, pyrethrins, 1.8 g/L, N-octyl bicicloheptene dicarboximide 6 g/l, piperonyl butoxide 3.6 g/L, for *dogs, cats*

Pet Gloss Shampoo (Troy) *Austral*
Shampoo, pyrethrins 1 g/L, piperonyl butoxide 10 g/L, for *dogs, cats*

Quick-Kill Eclipse (Pharmachem) *Austral*
Spray, pyrethrins 1.8 g/L, piperonyl butoxide 3.6 g/L, N-octyl bicicloheptene dicarboximide 6 g/l, methoprene 4 g/L, for *cats, dogs*

Quick-Kill Flea Strike (Pharmachem) *Austral*
Spray, pyrethrins 1.8 g/L, piperonyl butoxide 3.6 g/L, N-octyl bicicloheptene dicarboximide 6 g/L, for *dogs, cats*

Quick-Kill Rinse Concentrate for Fleas, Ticks, Lice (Pharmachem) *Austral*
Liquid concentrate, pyrethrins 10 g/L, piperonyl butoxide 18 g/L, N-octyl bicicloheptene dicarboximide 30 g/L, for *dogs, cats, cage birds, premises*

Sectalin Insecticidal Shampoo for Dogs & Cats (Ilium) *Austral*
Shampoo, piperonyl botoxide 10 g/L, pyrethrins 1 g/L (with eucalyptus oil, lanolin, detergent base), for *dogs, cats*

Troy IGR (Troy) *Austral*
Spray, methoprene 4 g/L, pyrethrins, 1.8 g/L, N-octyl bicicloheptene dicarboximide 6 g/l, piperonyl butoxide 3.6 g/L, for *dogs, cats*

Vet-kem Insecticidal Antiseptic Shampoo (Novartis) *Austral*
Shampoo, pyrethrins 1 g/L, piperonyl butoxide 10 g/L, chloroxylenol 2.6 g/L, for *dogs, cats*

Vet-kem Ovitrol Insecticidal Spray for Cats and Dogs (Novartis) *Austral*
Spray, pyrethrins 1.8 g/L, piperonyl butoxide 3.6 g/L, N-octyl bicicloheptene dicarboximide 6 g/L, methoprene 2 g/L, for *cats, dogs*

Vet-kem Ovitrol Rinse (Novartis) *Austral*
Liquid concentrate, methoprene 34 g/L, pyrethrins 19 g/L, piperonyl butoxide 48 g/L, N-octyl bicicloheptene dicarboximide 58 g/L, for *dogs, cats*

Zodiac Flea Proof Rinse (Novartis) *Austral*
Liquid concentrate, methoprene 34 g/L, pyrethrins 19 g/L, piperonyl butoxide 48 g/L, N-octyl bicicloheptene dicarboximide 58 g/L, for *dogs, cats*

Zodiac Flea Proof Spray for Cats and Dogs (Novartis) *Austral*
Spray (pump), methoprene 2 g/L, pyrethrins 1.8 g/L, piperonyl butoxide 3.6 g/L, N-octyl bicicloheptene dicarboximide 6 g/L, for *dogs, cats*

Zodiac Insecticidal Antiseptic Shampoo (Novartis) *Austral*
Shampoo, pyrethrins 1 g/L, piperonyl butoxide 10 g/L, chloroxylenol 2.6 g/L, for *dogs, cats*

Eire
Indications. *F*leas on dogs

Gullivers Flea Shampoo (Chanelle) *Eire*
shampoo, pyrethrin 0.05%, piperonyl butoxide 0.5%, for *dogs*

New Zealand
Indications. *F*leas and lice on dogs and cats

Fleatrol Shampoo (Virbac) *NZ*
Shampoo, piperonyl butoxide 1.2%, pyrethrin 0.12%, for *dogs*

Vet-Kem Flea Kill (Bayer) *NZ*
Spray, n-octyl bicicloheptene dicarboxamide 0.6%, piperonyl butoxide 0.36%, pyrethrins 0.18%, for *dogs, cats*

Vet-Kem Insecticidal Antiseptic Shampoo (Bayer) *NZ*
Shampoo, n-octyl bicicloheptene dicarboxamide 0.26%, piperonyl butoxide 1.0%, pyrethrins 0.1%, for *dogs, cats*

USA
Indications. Flies on horses; flies, fleas, lice, ear mites, and ticks on dogs and cats

Adams Flea and Tick Dust II (Pfizer) *USA*
Dusting powder, pyrethrins 0.10%, piperonyl butoxide 1%, carbaril 12.5%, for *dog, cats*

Adams Flea and Tick Mist (Pfizer) *USA*
Topical spray, pyrethrins 0.15%, piperonyl butoxide 1.5%, N-octyl bicycloheptene dicarboxamide 0.5%, di n-propyl isocichomeronate 0.5%, for *horses, dogs, cats*

Adams Flea & Tick Mist With Sykillstop (Pfizer) *USA*
Topical spray, pyrethrins 0.15%, piperonyl butoxide 1.5%, pyriproxyfen 0.15%, N-octyl bicicloheptene dicarboxamide 0.5%, for *dogs, cats*

Adams Flea and Tick Shampoo (Pfizer) *USA*
Shampoo, pyrethrins 0.15%, piperonyl butoxide 1.5%, N-octyl bicicloheptene dicarboxamide 0.5%, for *dogs, cats*

Adams Fly Repellent Lotion (Pfizer) *USA*
Lotion, pyrethrins 0.15%, piperonyl butoxide 1.5%, N-octyl bicicloheptene dicarboxamide 0.5%, di n-propyl isocichomeronate 1%, for *horses*
Withdrawal Periods. Should not be used on horses intended for human consumption

Adams Gold Flea And Tick Shampoo (Pfizer) *USA*
Shampoo, pyrethrins 0.15%, piperonyl butoxide 1.5%, for *dogs, cats*

Adams Gold Flea & Tick Shampoo (Pfizer) *USA*
Shampoo, pyrethrins 0.15%, piperonyl butoxide 1.5%, for *cats*

Adams Pyrethrin Dip (Pfizer) *USA*
Topical solution, pyrethrins 0.7%, piperonyl butoxide 3.74%, N-octyl bicycloheptene dicarboxamide 5.7%, di-n-propyl isocinchomeronate 1.94%, for *dogs, cats*

Adams Water Based Flea & Tick Mist (Pfizer) *USA*
Topical spray, pyrethrins 0.2%, piperonyl butoxide 0.75%, N-octyl bicycloheptene dicarboxamide 2%, for *dogs, cats*

Brilliance Flea & Tick Shampoo (First Priority) *USA*
Shampoo, pyrethrins 0.1%, piperonyl butoxide 1%, for *dogs, cats*

Buzz Off (Bio-Ceutic) *USA*
Solution, spot-on, butoxypolypropylene glycol 10 %, methoxychlor 0.5%, piperonyl butoxide 0.5%, pyrethrins 0.5%, for *horses*
Withdrawal Periods. Should not be used on *horses* intended for human consumption

Davis Pyrethrins (Davis) *USA*
Liquid concentrate, pyrethrins 7.5%, piperonyl butoxide 75%, for *dogs, cats*

Defend Flea & Tick Emollient Oatmeal Shampoo (Schering-Plough) *USA*
Shampoo, pyrethrins 0.05%, piperonyl butoxide 0.5%, for *dogs, cats*

Defend Just-For-Cats Flea & Tick Foam (Schering-Plough) *USA*
Aerosol foam, pyrethrins 0.15%, piperonyl butoxide 0.7%, N-octyl bicycloheptene dicarboximide, 0.34%, for *dogs, cats*

Defend Just-For-Cats Spray (Schering-Plough) *USA*
Topical spray, pyrethrins 0.15%, piperonyl butoxide 1.5%, n-octyl bicyclohepene dicarboximide 1%, for *cats*

Ecto-Foam (Allerderm/Virbac) *USA*
Aerosol foam, pyrethrins 0.15%, piperonyl butoxide 0.7%, N-octyl bicyclohepene dicarboximide 0.34%, for *dogs, cats*

Ectokyl 3X Flea and Tick Shampoo (DVM) *USA*
Shampoo, pyrethrins 0.15%, piperonyl butoxide 1%, N-octyl bicycloheptene dicarboximide 0.5%, di-n-propyl isocinchomeronate 0.5%, for *dogs, cats*

Ectokyl 3X Spray-On Flea& Tick Shampoo (DVM) *USA*
Shampoo, pyrethrins 0.15%, piperonyl butoxide 1%, N-octyl bocycloheptene dicarboximide 0.5%, di-n-propyl isocinchomeronate 0.5%, for *dogs, cats*

Ecto-Soothe (Allerderm/Virbac) *USA*
Shampoo, pyrethrins 0.05%, piperonyl butoxide 0.5%, for *dogs, cats*

Ecto-Soothe 3X (Allerderm/Virbac) *USA*
Shampoo, pyrethrins 0.15%, piperonyl butoxide 1.5%, n-octyl bicycloheptene dicarboximide 0.5%, for *dogs, cats*

Flea & Tick Aqua-Mist (Davis) *USA*
Topical spray, pyrethrins 0.05%, piperonyl butoxide).5%, permethrin 0.05%, for *horses, dogs, cats*

Flea & Tick Mist (Davis) *USA*
Topical spray, pyrethrins 0.15%, piperonyl butoxide 1%, N-octyl bicycloheptene dicarboximide 0.5%, di-n-propyl isocinchomeronate 0.5%, for *horses, dogs, cats*

Flea and Tick Shampoo Plus (Hoechst-Roussel) *USA*
Shampoo, pyrethrins 0.15%, piperonyl butoxide 1%, N-octyl bicycloheptene dicarboximide 0.5%, di-n-propyl isocinchomeronate 0.5%, for *dogs, cats*

Flea And Tick Spray (Vedco) *USA*
Topical Spray, pyrethrins 0.15%, piperonyl butoxide 1.5%, N-octyl bicycloheptene dicarboximide 0.5%, for *horses, dogs, cats*

Horse Spray & Rub-on (Anchor) *USA*
Topical spray, butoxypolypropylene glycol 10%, methoxychlor 0.5%, piperonyl butoxide 0.5%, pyrethrins 0.05%, for *horses*
Withdrawal Periods. Should not be used on *horses* intended for human consumption

KC Fleapoo Dip (K.C.Pharmacal) *USA*
Dip concentrate, pyrethrins 0.3%, piperonyl butoxide 3%, for *dogs, cats*

KC Fleapoo Shampoo (K.C.Pharmacal) *USA*
Shampoo, pyrethrins 0.15%, piperonyl butoxide 1%, N-octyl bicycloheptene dicarboximide 0.5%, for *dogs, cats*

Mycodex All-In-One (Pfizer) *USA*
Topical spray, pyrethrins 0.15%, pyriproxyfen 0.15%, piperonyl butoxide 1.5%, N-octyl bicycloheptene dicarboximide 0.5%, for *dogs, cats*

Mycodex Fast Act Flea & Tick Dip (Pfizer) *USA*
Dip concentrate, pyrethrins 0.97%, piperonyl butoxide 3.74%, N-octyl bicycloheptene dicarboximide 5.7%, di-n-propyl isocinchomeronate 1.94%, for *dogs, cats*

Mycodex Pet Shampoo with pyrethrins (Pfizer) *USA*
Shampoo, pyrethrins 0.15%, piperonyl butoxide 1.5%, for *dogs, cats*

Mycodex Sensicare Flea 7 tick Spray (Pfizer) *USA*
Topical spray, pyrethrins 0.2%, piperonyl butoxide 2%, for *dogs, cats*

Nolvacide Insecticide Shampoo (Fort Dodge) *USA*
Shampoo, pyrethrins 0.045%, piperonyl butoxide 0.09%, N-octyl bicycloheptene dicarboximide 0.15%, for *dogs, cats*

Onex Wound dressing (Happy Jack) *USA*
Ointment, pyrethrins 0.2%, piperonyl butoxide 0.5%, di-n-propyl isocinchomeronate 1%, for *horses, dogs*

Paranol Flea-Tick Dip (Happy Jack) *USA*
Dip concentrate, pyrethrins 1.18%, piperonyl butoxide 11.84%, for *cats*

Pet Care Ear Mite Lotion And Repellent (DurVet) *USA*
Lotion, pyrethrins 0.15%, piperonyl butoxide 1%, for *horses, dogs, cats*
Withdrawal Periods. Should not be used on *horses* intended for human consumption

Pet Care Fast Kill Flea & Tick Spray for Dogs & Cats (DurVet) *USA*
Topical spray, pyrethrins 0.15%, piperonyl butoxide 1.5%, N-octyl bicycloheptene dicarboximide 0.5%, di-n-propyl isocinchomeronate 0.5%, for *horses, cats, dogs*
Withdrawal Periods. Should not be used on *horses* intended for human consumption

Pet Care Flea & Tick Shampoo For Dogs & Cats (DurVet) *USA*
Shampoo, pyrethrins 0.05%, piperonyl butoxide 0.5%, for *dogs, cats*

Pet Care Pyrethrin Dip (DurVet) *USA*
Dip concentrate, pyrethrins 0.3%, piperonyl butoxide 3%, for *dogs, cats*

Pet-Guard Insecticide Gel With Sunscreen (Allerderm/Virbac) *USA*
Gel, pyrethrins 0.1%, piperonyl butoxide 1%, N-octyl bicycloheptene dicarboximide 0.5% butoxypolypropylene glycol 10%, for *dogs, cats*

Pro Edge Horse Spray & Wipe (Aspen) *USA*
Topical spray, pyrethrins 0.06%, piperonyl butoxide 0.6%, for *horses, dogs, cats*

ProTICall Oatmeal 3X Insecticide Shampoo (Schering-Plough) *USA*
Shampoo, pyrethrins 0.15%, piperonyl butoxide 1.5%, N-octyl bicycloheptene dicarboximide 0.5%, for *dogs, cats*

Prozap (Loveland) *USA*
Topical spray, pyrethrins 0.1%, piperonyl butoxide 1% , for *horses, cattle, kennels*

Py-Kil Dip (Davis) *USA*
Dip concentrate, pyrethrins 0.33%, piperonyl butoxide 0.67%, N-octyl bicycloheptene dicarboximide 1.11%, for *dogs, cats*

Pyrethrin Dip (Allerderm/Virbac) *USA*
Dip concentrate, pyrethrins 1%, piperonyl butoxide 4%, N-octyl bicycloheptene dicarboximide 6%, di-n-propyl isocinchomeronate 4%, for *dogs, cats*

Pyrethrin Dip (Vedco) *USA*
Dip concentrate, pyrethrins 0.33%, piperonyl butoxide 0.67%, N-octyl bicycloheptene dicarboximide 1.11%, for *dogs, cats*

Pyrethrin Dip & Spray (Davis) *USA*
Dip concentrate, pyrethrins 3%, piperonyl butoxide 30%, for *dogs, cats, premises*

Pyrethrin Plus (DurVet) *USA*
Topical spray, pyrethrins 0.1%, piperonyl butoxide 1%, for *cattle*

Pyrethrin Plus Shampoo (Vedco) *USA*
Shampoo, pyrethrins 0.15%, piperonyl butoxide 1.5%, N-octyl bicycloheptene dicarboximide 0.5%, for *dogs, cats*

Quick Kill Flea and Tick Spray (Performer) *USA*
Topical spray, pyrethrins 0.15%, piperonyl butoxide 1%, N-octyl bicycloheptene dicarboximide 0.5%, di-n-propyl isocinchomeronate 0.5%, for *cats, dogs, bedding*

Ritter's Flea & Tick Spray (Ritter) *USA*
Topical spray, pyrethrins 0.15%, piperonyl butoxide 1.5%, N-octyl bicycloheptene dicarboximide 0.5%, di-n-propyl isocinchomeronate 0.5% petroleum distillate 1.35%, for *horses, cats, dogs*

Sungro Flea-Zy Pet Shampoo (Sungro) *USA*
Shampoo, pyrethrins 0.05%, piperonyl butoxide 0.5%, for *dogs, cats*

Synerkyl Pet Dip (DVM) *USA*
Dip concentrate, pyrethrins 18%, piperonyl butoxide 11.84%, for *dogs, cats*

Synerkyl Pet Mousse (DVM) *USA*
Mousse, pyrethrins 0.082%, piperonyl butoxide 0.825%, for *dogs, cats*

Triple Pyrethrins Flea & Tick Shampoo (Davis) *USA*
Shampoo, pyrethrins 0.15%, piperonyl butoxide 1%, N-octyl bicycloheptene dicarboximide 0.5%, di-n-propyl isocinchomeronate 0.5%, for *dogs, cats*

Ultrum Feline Flea & Tick Mousse (Hoechst-Roussel) *USA*
Mousse, pyrethrins 0.082%, piperonyl butoxide 0.825%, for *cats*

VIP Fly Repellent Ointment (VPL) *USA*
Ointment, butoxypolypropylene glycol 10%, piperonyl butoxide 1%, pyrethrins 0.15%, for *dogs, cats*

X-Pel (Happy Jack) *USA*
Topical spray, pyrethrins 0.36%, piperonyl butoxide 0.72%, N-octyl bicycloheptne dicarboximide 1.2%, butoxypolypropylene glycol 5%, for *horses, dogs*

2.2.1.8 Other ectoparasiticides

Benzyl benzoate is used for control of sweet itch caused by hypersensitivity to *Culicoides* midges.
Lindane (gamma benzene hexachloride) is an organochlorine compound which is banned from use in many countries including the UK.
Closantel is used for fluke infections. Ticks such as *Ixodes ricinus* which are feeding on sheep at the time of treatment with closantel are likely to produce less viable eggs.

BENZYL BENZOATE

UK

Indications. *Culicoides* on horses
Contra-indications. Should not be used on cats

GSL **Killitch** (Carr & Day & Martin) *UK*
Lotion, benzyl benzoate 25%, for *horses*; 500 mL, 1 litre
Withdrawal Periods. Should not be used on *horses* intended for human consumption

GSL **Sweet Itch Plus** (Pettifer) *UK*
Liquid, benzyl benzoate 25%, for *horses*; 500 mL, 1 litre

USA

Indications. Control of sarcoptic mange on dogs
Contra-indications. Cats or rabbits; puppiesless than 3 months of age, nursing bitches

Mange Treatment (LeGear) *USA*
Liquid, benzyl benzoate 36%, for *dogs*

LINDANE

USA

Indications. Control of fleas, ticks, and sarcoptic mange on dogs; ticks and screw worm on livestock
Contra-indications. Cats or toy dog breeds; puppies less than 4 months of age, nursing bitches; calves lessthan 3 months of age

Kennel Dip (Happy Jack) *USA*
Dip concentrate, lindane 12.89%, for *dogs*

Screw Worm Aerosol-L (AgriLabs) *USA*
Pressurised aerosol, lindane 3%, for *horses, cattle, sheep, goats, pigs, chickens, cats, dogs, premises*
Withdrawal Periods. Should not be used on cattle producing milk for human consumption

RESMETHRIN

Indications. Fleas on dogs and cats

Durakyl Shampoo (DVM) *USA*
Shampoo, resmethrin 0.25%, for *dogs, cats*

Ectokyl Puppy & Kitten Shampoo (DVM) *USA*
Shampoo, resmethrin 0.25%, for *dogs, cats*

ROTENONE

Australia

Indications. Lice and mites on sheep
Contra-indications. Lambs less than 10 weeks of age; sheep with wounds or heavy grass seed load**

Flockmaster (Western Stock Distributors) *Austral*
Dip powder, rotenone 15 g/kg, magnesium fluorosilicate 405 g/kg, sulphur 309 g/kg, for *sheep*
Withdrawal Periods. Slaughter 1 day

Rotomite (Novartis) *Austral*
Liquid concentrate, rotenone 56 g/L, for *sheep*
Withdrawal Periods. Slaughter 7 days

2.2.2 Insect growth regulators

2.2.2.1 Benzoylphenyl urea derivatives
2.2.2.2 Juvenile hormone analogues
2.2.2.3 Triazine and pyrimidine derivatives

Insect growth regulators (IGRs) are a group of chemical compounds that do not kill the target parasite directly but interfere with its growth and development. IGRs act mainly on immature stages of the parasite and as such are not usually suitable for the rapid control of established adult populations of parasites. With heavy infestation of adult bloodsucking parasites, IGRs may need to be combined with adulticides for the first few treatments. Where parasites show a clear seasonal pattern, IGRs can be applied at the start of the parasite season as a preventative. Based on their mode of action IGRs can be classified as chitin inhibitors, juvenile hormone analogues, and others.

2.2.2.1 Benzoylphenyl urea derivatives

Diflubenzuron, fluazuron, and **lufenuron** are a benzoylphenyl urea derivatives.
Lufenuron is used for the control of fleas of dogs and cats. Lufenuron accumulates in fat tissue allowing subsequent slow release. Fleas take up the drug through the blood and transfer it to their eggs. The formation of larval chitin structures is blocked by interference with the assembly of chitin chains and microfilrils thereby inhibiting the development of flea larvae and providing environmental control of the flea population. No viable eggs are produced 24 hours after administration. For oral administration, the drug must be administered in the food to allow sufficient time for absorption from the stomach. Injectable treatment is given at six-monthly intervals to cats and oral treatment is given to dogs or cats once monthly during summer, commencing 2 months before fleas become active. Insecticides that kill adult fleas may be required if there is an initial heavy infestation and in cases of severe hypersensitivity.

Diflubenzuron is available for blowfly control in sheep. It is also active against flies and lice. The drug is highly lipophilic with low solubility in water and is available as an emulsifiable concentrate for use as a dip or shower or for spraying after dilution. It provides 12 to 14 weeks protection against flystrike.

Fluazuron is a tick development inhibitor providing long-term protection against the one-host tick *Boophilus microplus*.

DIFLUBENZURON

Australia

Indications. Lice, blowfly strike prevention on sheep
Contra-indications. Dipping of sheep within 10 days after shearing; dipping of heavily pregnant sheep
Warnings. Operators should wear protective clothing

Fleececare (Hoechst Roussel) *Austral*
Dip concentrate, diflubenzuron 250 g/L, for *sheep*
Withdrawal Periods. Slaughter withdrawal period nil, wool 6 months, milk withdrawal period nil

Strike (Coopers) *Austral*
Dip concentrate, diflubenzuron 250 g/L, for *sheep*
Withdrawal Periods. Slaughter withdrawal period nil, wool 6 months.

New Zealand

Indications. Lice, blowfly strike prevention on sheep
Contra-indications. Treatment of existing flystrike
Warnings. Operators should wear protective clothing as for handling other ectoparasiticides

Blitz (Schering-Plough) *NZ*
Dip concentrate, diflubenzuron 250 g/litre, for *sheep*
Withdrawal Periods. Slaughter withdrawal period nil

Fleececare (Ancare) *NZ*
Dip concentrate, diflubenzuron 250 g/litre, for *sheep*
Withdrawal Periods. Slaughter withdrawal period nil, milk withdrawal period nil

Zenith (Novartis) *NZ*
Dip concentrate, diflubenzuron 250 g/litre, for *sheep*
Withdrawal Periods. Slaughter withdrawal period nil

FLUAZURON

Australia

Indications. Ticks on cattle
Contra-indications. Pregnant cattle within 6 weeks of calving
Warnings. Operators should wear protective clothing

Acatak Pour-On Tick Development Inhibitor (Novartis) *Austral*
Soultion, pour-on, fluazuron 25 g/L, for *cattle*
Withdrawal Periods. Slaughter 6 weeks, should not be used on cattle producing milk for human consumtpion

LUFENURON

UK

Indications. Prevention of flea infestation and treatment of flea allergy dermatitis in dogs and cats

Contra-indications. Injection in dogs; administration to unweaned puppies and kittens
Side-effects. Transient painless swelling at injection site for a few weeks; rarely transient lethargy after injection
Dose. *Dogs*: *by addition to feed*, 10 mg/kg
Cats: *by subcutaneous injection*, 10 mg/kg *or* (up to 4 kg body-weight) 0.4 mL; (>4 kg body-weight) 0.8 mL
by addition to feed, 30 mg/kg *or* (up to 4.5 kg body-weight) 133 mg; (> 4.5 kg body-weight) 266 mg

POM **Program 40/80 Injectable for Cats** (Novartis) *UK*
Injection, lufenuron 40 mg/0.4 mL, for *cats less than 4 kg body-weight*; 0.4 mL-syringe
Injection, lufenuron 80 mg/0.8 mL, for *cats equal to or more than 4 kg body-weight*; 0.8-mL syringe

POM **Program Suspension for Cats** (Novartis) *UK*
Oral suspension, lufenuron 133 mg/applicator, for *cats up to 4.5 kg body-weight*; 1.9-g dose applicator
Oral suspension, lufenuron 266 mg/applicator, for *cats more than 4.5 kg body-weight*; 3.8-g dose applicator

POM **Program Tablets for Dogs** (Novartis) *UK*
Tablets, lufenuron 23.1 mg, 67.8 mg, 204.9 mg, 409.8 mg, for *dogs*; 6

Australia

Indications. Fleas on dogs and cats
Dose. *Dogs*: *by addition to feed*, 10 mg/kg
Cats: *by subcutaneous injection*, 10 mg/kg
by addition to feed, 30 mg/kg

Program (Novartis) *Austral*
Tablets, lufenuron, 67.8 mg, 204.9 mg, 409.8 mg, for *dogs*

Program (Novartis) *Austral*
Oral suspension, lufenuron,133 mg, 266 mg, for *cats*

Program (Novartis) *Austral*
Injection, lufenuron, 40 mg and 80 mg/single use syringe, for *cats*

Eire

Indications. Fleas on dogs and cats
Dose. *Dogs*: *by addition to feed*, 10 mg/kg
Cats: *by addition to feed*, 30 mg/kg

Program Suspension for Cats (Novartis) *Eire*
Oral suspension, to mix with feed, lufenuron 7%, for *cats*

Program Suspension for Dogs (Novartis) *Eire*
Tablets, lufenuron 67.8 mg, 204.9 mg, 409.8 mg, for *dogs*

New Zealand

Indications. Fleas on dogs and cats
Dose. *Dogs*: *by addition to feed*, 10 mg/kg
Cats: *by subcutaneous injection*, 10 mg/kg
by addition to feed, 30 mg/kg

Program (Novartis) *NZ*
Tablets, lufenuron 67.8 mg, 204.9 mg, 409.8 mg, for *dogs*

Program 40, 80 (Novartis) *NZ*
Injection, lufenuron 100 mg/mL, for *cats*

Program Liquid (Novartis) *NZ*
Oral suspension, lufenuron 70 mg/g, for *cats*

USA

Indications. Fleas on dogs and cats

Dose. *Dogs*: *by addition to feed*, 10 mg/kg
Cats: *by subcutaneous injection*, 10 mg/kg
by addition to feed, 30 mg/kg

Program Cat Tablets (Novartis) *USA*
Tablets, lufenuron 90 mg, 204.9 mg, for *cats*

Program Suspension (Novartis) *USA*
Suspension, lufenuron 135 mg, 270 mg, for *cats*

Program Tablets (Novartis) *USA*
Tablets, lufenoron 45 mg, 90 mg, 204.9 mg, 409.8 mg, for *dogs*

Program 6 Month Injectable for Cats (Novartis) *USA*
Injection, lufenuron 100 mg/mL, for *cats*

TRIFLUMURON

Australia
Indications. Lice on sheep
Contra-indications. Existing flystrike infection; treatment of wet sheep

Zapp Pour-On Lousicide for Sheep (Bayer) *Austral*
Solution, pour-on, triflumuron 25 g/L, for *sheep*
Withdrawal Periods. Slaughter 14 days

New Zealand
Indications. Lice, flystrike on sheep
Contra-indications. Use on unshorn lambs more than 2 months of age; sheep with concurrent infections that cannot be shorn cleanly; mixing of treated sheep and uninfested sheep for at least 4 weeks after treatment, or infested sheep

Zapp (Bayer) *NZ*
Solution, pour-on, triflumuron 25 g/litre, for *sheep*
Withdrawal Periods. Slaughter 60 days

2.2.2.2 Juvenile hormone analogues

The juvenile hormone analogues, **methoprene** and **pyriproxyfen** mimic the activity of naturally occurring juvenile hormones and prevent metamorphosis to the adult stage.

METHOPRENE

UK
See section 2.2.5 for preparations

Australia
Indications. Fleas on dogs and cats
Warnings. Remove collar if signs of irritation occur

Vet-Kem Ovitrol Flea Egg Collar for Dogs and Puppies (Novartis) *Austral*
Collar, methoprene 10 g/kg, for *dogs*

Vet-Kem Ovitrol Flea Egg Collar for Cats and Kittens (Novartis) *Austral*
Collar, methoprene 20 g/kg, for *cats*

New Zealand
Indications. Fleas on dogs and cats
Warnings. Remove collar if signs of irritation occur

Vet-Kem Ovitrol Cat Collar (Bayer) *NZ*
Collar, methoprene 2%, for *cats*

Vet-Kem Ovitrol Dog Collar (Bayer) *NZ*
Collar, methoprene 10%, for *dogs*

PYRIPROXYFEN

Australia
Indications. Fleas on cats
Contra-indications. Kittens less than 3 months of age
Warnings. Remove collar if signs of irritation occur

Bodygard Band for Cats (Virbac) *Austral*
Collar, pyriproxyfen 0.5%, for *cats*

New Zealand
Indications. Fleas on cats

Bodyguard 12-month IGR Cat Flea Collar (Virbac) *NZ*
Collar, pyriproxyfen 5 mg/g, for *cats*

USA
Indications. Fleas on dogs and cats
Contra-indications. Puppies or kittens less than 3 months of age

Breakthru!-IGR Nylar Stripe-On (VPL) *USA*
Solution, spot-on, pyriproxyfen 5.3%, for *cats*

Virbac Knockout IGR Flea Collar for Cats & Kittens (Allerderm/Virbac) *USA*
Collar, pyriproxyfen 0.5%, for *cats*

Virbac Knockout IGR Flea Collar for Dogs & Puppies (Allerderm/Virbac) *USA*
Collar, pyriproxyfen 0.5%, for *dogs*

2.2.2.3 Triazine and pyrimidine derivatives

Cyromazine (a triazine derivative) and **dicyclanil** (a pyrimidine derivative) have a similar mode of action and appear to inhibit the deposition of chitin into the cuticle.

Cyromazine is effective for prevention of blowfly strike on sheep and lambs. The use of a 'pour-on' preparation of cyromazine has the advantage that efficacy is not dependent upon factors such as weather, fleece length, or whether the fleece is wet or dry. In addition, the persistence of the drug is such that control can be maintained for up to 10 weeks after a single application. The drug spreads to give full body protection. It is applied before an anticipated challenge. Other drugs, for example, sheep dips containing dimpylate (diazinon) or propetamphos, and selected formulations containing cypermethrin with blowfly larvae control recommendations, should be used to treat established myiosis.

CYROMAZINE

UK
Indications. Prevention of blowfly strike on sheep
Dose. *Sheep*: *by 'pour-on' application*, 15–50 mL of 6% solution depending on body-weight
Local application, 7.5–25 mL depending on body-weight

PML **Vetrazin** (Novartis) *UK*
Solution, 'pour-on', cyromazine 6%, for *sheep*; 2.2 litres, 5 litres
Withdrawal Periods. *Sheep*: slaughter 3 days, should not be used on sheep producing milk for human consumption

Australia
Indications. Blowfly strike on sheep
Contra-iIndications. Use on open wounds or sheep with less than 6 weeks wool; dipping of sheep heavily infested with grass seeds

Jetcon Australian Sheep Blowfly Treatment (Nufarm) *Austral*
Liquid concentrate, cyromazine 500 g/L, for *sheep*
Withdrawal Periods. Slaughter 7 days

Vetrazin (Novartis) *Austral*
Dip concentrate, cyromazine 500 g/L, for *sheep*
Withdrawal Periods. Slaughter 7 days, should not be used on sheep producing milk for human consumption

Vetrazin (Novartis) *Austral*
Spray, cyromazine 60 g/L, for *sheep*
Withdrawal Periods. Slaughter 7 days, should not be used on sheep producing milk for human consumption

Eire
Indications. Blowfly strike on sheep

Vetrazin Pour-on (Novartis) *Eire*
Solution, pour-on, cyromazine 6%, for *sheep*
Withdrawal Periods. Slaughter 3 days, should not be used on sheep producing milk for human consumption

New Zealand
Indications. Blowfly strike on sheep

Vetrazin Spray-on (Novartis) *NZ*
Spray, cyromazine 6%, for *sheep*
Withdrawal Periods. Slaughter 21 days, should not be used on sheep producing milk for human consumption

Vetrazin Liquid (Novartis) *NZ*
Dip concentrate, cyromazine 50%, for *sheep*
Withdrawal Periods. Slaughter 7 days, should not be used on sheep producing milk for human consumption

DICYCLANIL

New Zealand
Indications. Blowfly strike on sheep

Clik (Novartis) *NZ*
Spray, dicyclanil 50 g/litre, for *sheep*
Withdrawal Periods. Slaughter 35 days (wool length greater than 5 cm), 56 days (if treated after shearing), should not be used on sheep producing milk for human consumption

2.2.3 Compound preparations for ectoparasites

UK
PML **Negasunt** (Bayer) *UK*
See section 14.4.1 under Sulphanilamide for preparation details

PML **Nuvan Top** (Novartis) *UK*
Aerosol spray, dichlorvos 0.2%, fenitrothion 0.8%, for fleas on *dogs, cats*; 105 g

Contra-indications. Puppies less than 7 weeks of age, kittens less than 8 weeks of age, nursing bitches or queens

Australia
4-in-1 Liquid Sheep Dip (Coopers) *Austral*
Liquid concentrate, rotenone 15 g/L/ piperonyl butoxide 7.2 g/L, dimpylate 60 g/L, for lice, keds, mites, and blowfly strike on *sheep*
Withdrawal Periods. Slaughter 14 days

Amidaz 4 in 1 Liquid Dip (Coopers) *Austral*
Sheep dip, amitraz 125 g/L, dimpylate 200 g/L, for lice, keds, mites, and blowfly strike on *sheep*, lice and mites on *goats*
Withdrawal Periods. *Sheep*: slaughter 21 days. *Goats*: slaughter 21 days, should not be used on goats producing milk for human consumption

Avian Insect Liquidator (Vetafarm) *Austral*
Liquid concentrate, permethrin 25 g/L, piperonyl butoxide 125 g/L, methoprene 0.4 g/L, for lice on *cage birds*

Blaze (Coopers) *Austral*
Solution, pour-on, cypermethrin 144 g/L, dimpylate 96 g/L, for lice and blowfly on *sheep*
Withdrawal Periods. Slaughter 14 days, wool 3 months

Blockade-S (Coopers) *Austral*
Liquid concentrate, cypermethrin 25 g/L, chlorfenvinphos 138 g/L, for lice and ticks on *horses, cattle, goats, sheep, deer, working dogs*
Withdrawal Periods. *Cattle*: slaughter 8 days

Barricade 'S' Cattle Dip and Spray (Fort Dodge) *Austral*
Spray or dip, cypermethrin 25 g/L, chlorfenvinphos 138 g/L, for lice and ticks *horses, cattle, goats, sheep, deer, working dogs*
Withdrawal Periods. *Cattle*: slaughter 8 days

Bay-O-Pet Flea Control Spray for Dogs and Cats (Bayer) *Austral*
Spray, S-methoprene 2 g/L, pyrethrins 1.8 g/L, piperonyl butoxide 3.6 g/L, N-octylbicycloheptene dicarboximide 6 g/L, for fleas and ticks on *dogs, cats*

Bay-O-Pet Kiltix Tick & Flea Collar for Dogs (Bayer) *Austral*
Collar, flumethrin 22.5 g/kg, propoxur 100 g/kg, for fleas and ticks on *dogs*

Duogard Band for Cats (Virbac) *Austral*
Collar, pyriproxyfen 2.5 g/kg, dimpylate 150 g/kg, for fleas on *cats*

Duogard Band for Dogs (Virbac) *Austral*
Collar, pyriproxyfen 2.5 g/kg, dimpylate 150 g/kg, for fleas on *dogs*

Duogard Line-on (Virbac) *NZ*
Solution, spot-on, permethrin 400 mg/mL, pyriproxyfen 3 mg/mL, for fleas and ticks on *dogs*

Fly-Strike Powder (Coopers) *Austral*
Dusting powder, dimpylate 15 g/kg, piperonyl butoxide 0.8 g/kg, pyrethrins,1 g/kg, for flystrike on *cattle, sheep, pigs, goats*
Withdrawal Periods. *Sheep, pigs, goats*: slaughter 14 days. *Cattle*: slaughter 3 days

Flystrike Powder (Western Stock Distributors) *Austral*
Dusting powder, dimpylate 15 g/kg, piperonyl butoxide 0.8 g/kg, pyrethrins,1 g/kg, for *cattle, sheep, pigs, goats*
Withdrawal Periods. *Sheep, pigs, goats*: slaughter 14 days. *Cattle*: slaughter 3 days

Grenade Plus Rotenone Sheep Dip (Coopers) *Austral*
Liquid concentrate, cyhalothrin 16 g/L, rotenone 40 g/L, for lice, keds, and mites on *sheep*
Withdrawal Periods. Slaughter withdrawal period nil

Jetdip 4-in-1 (Virbac) *Austral*
Liquid concentrate, dimpylate 80 g/L, rotenone 15 g/L, piperonyl butoxide 9 g/L, for lice, keds, mites, and blowfly strike on *sheep*
Withdrawal Periods. Slaughter 14 days, wool 2 months

Keydust (International Animal Health) *Austral*
Dusting powder, carbaril 40 g/kg, maldison 10 g/kg, for fleas, lice, and ticks on *dogs, cats, birds, rabbits, guinea pigs, mice*
Withdrawal Periods. Chickens: slaughter withdrawal period nil

Mulesing Powder (Coopers) *Austral*
Dusting powder, dimpylate 15 g/kg, piperonyl butoxide 0.8 g/kg, pyrethrins,1 g/kg, for *cattle, sheep, pigs, goats,*
Withdrawal Periods. *Cattle*: slaughter 3 days. *Sheep, pigs, goats*: slaughter 14 days

Mulesing Powder (Western Stock Distributors) *Austral*
Dusting powder, dimpylate 15 g/kg, piperonyl butoxide 0.8 g/kg, pyrethrins,1 g/kg, for *cattle, sheep, pigs, goats*
Withdrawal Periods. *Cattle*: slaughter 3 days, should not be used on teats of animals producing milk for human consumption. *Sheep, goats, pigs*: slaughter 14 days, should not be used on the teats of sheep or goats producing milk for human consumption

Protect-A-Dog 'Double Impact' (Virbac) *Austral*
Spray (pump), permethrin 20 g/L, pyriproxifen 0.2 g/L, for *dogs*

Supreme Sheep Dip with Lanolin (Novartis) *Austral*
Liquid concentrate, cypermthrin 7.6 g/L, rotenone 28 g/L, for lice, mites, and keds on *sheep, goats*
Withdrawal Periods. Sheep, goats: slaughter withdrawal period nil

Vet-Kem Ovitrol (Bayer) *NZ*
Spray, methoprene 0.2%, n-octyl bicycloheptene dicarboximide 0.6%, piperonyl butoxide 0.36%, pyrethrins 0.18%, for fleas and ticks on *dogs, cats*

Vet-Kem Ovitrol Rinse (Bayer) *NZ*
Liquid concentrate, methoprene 34g/litre, n-octyl bicycloheptene dicarboximide 58 g/litre, piperonyl butoxide 48 g/litre, pyrethrins 19 g/litre, for fleas and ticks on *dogs, cats*

Eire

Kiltix Dog Collar (Bayer) *Eire*
Collar, propoxur 10% , flumethrin 2.5%, for fleas and ticks on *dogs*

Nuvan Top (Novartis) *Eire*
Spray, dichlorvos 0.2%, fenitrothion 0.8%, for fleas, lice, ticks, and mites on *dogs, cats*

New Zealand

Duogard 5-Month Flea Collars (Virbac) *NZ*
Collar, dimpylate (diazinon) 150 mg/g, pyriproxyfen 2.5 mg/g, for fleas on *dogs, cats*

Fleatrol I.G.R. Spray (Virbac) *NZ*
Spray, methoprene 4 g/litre, n-octylbicycloheptene dicarboxamide 6 g/litre, piperonyl butoxide 4 g/litre, pyrethrins 1.8 g/litre,, for fleas on *dogs, cats*

Flypel (Ancare) *NZ*
Spray, chlorpyrifos 10 g/litre, cypermethrin 100 g/litre, for lice, keds, and blowfly strike on *sheep*
Withdrawal Periods. Slaughter 14 days

Negasunt (Bayer) *NZ*
Powder, coumafos 3%, propoxur 2%, sulfanilamide 5%, for repelling flies

Nuvan Top (Bomac) *NZ*
Spray, dichlorvos 0.215%, fenitrothion 0.845%, for fleas, lice, and ticks on *dogs, cats*

Pouracide NF (Jurox) *NZ*
Solution, pour-on or spray, alphamethrin 0.7%, piperonyl butoxide 7.5%, tetrachlorvinphos 2%, for lice and flies on *cattle*
Withdrawal Periods. Slaughter 7 days, milk withdrawal period nil

USA

Adams Fly Repellent Concentrate (Pfizer) *USA*
Topical spray, permethrin 1%, pyrethrins 0.5%, piperonyl butoxide 1.85%, n-octyl bicycloheptene dicarboxamide 3.1%, di-n-propyl isocinchomeronate 1.25%, for *horses*
Withdrawal Periods. Should not be used on *horses* intended for human consumption

Adams Fly Spray And Repellent (Pfizer) *USA*
Topical spray, permethrin 0.2%, pyrethrins 0.2%, piperonyl butoxide 0.5%, n-octyl bicycloheptene dicarboxamide 2%, di-n-propyl isocinchomeronate 1%, butoxypolypropylene glycol 5%, for *horses*
Withdrawal Periods. Should not be used on *horses* intended for human consumption

Aqua 14 Flea & Tick Spray (Vedco) *USA*
Topical spray, pyrethrins 0.112%, permethrin 0.101%, related cpds 0.009%, for fleas and ticks on *dogs, cats*

Breakthru With Nylar Spot-On For Dogs (VPL) *USA*
Solution, spot-on, permethrin 45%, pyriproxyfen 5%, for fleas and ticks on *dogs*

DD-33 Flea & Tick Spray (Happy Jack) *USA*
Topical spray, pyrethrins 0.112%, permethrin 0.101%, related compounds 0.009%, for fleas and ticks on *dogs, cats*

Diaphos Insecticide Cattle Ear Tag (Y-Tex) *USA*
Tags (ear), dimpylate 30%, chlorpyriphos 10%, for flies, ticks and lice on *cattle*
Withdrawal Periods. Remove tags before slaughter

Duocide L.A. (Allerderm/Virbac) *USA*
Topical spray, pyrethrins 0.112%, permethrin 0.1%, related cpds 0.008%, N-octyl bicycloheptene dicarboximide 1%, for *dogs, cats*

Duogard Shampoo (Virbac) *NZ*
Shampoo, permethrin 10 g/litre, pyriproxyfen 0.5 g/litre, for fleas on *dogs*

Duradip (Davis) *USA*
Topical spray, rotenone 11%, pyrethrins 0.8%, for fleas, lice, ticks on *dogs*

KC 14-Day Flea & Tick Mist With Aloe (K.C.Pharmacal) *USA*
Topical spray, pyrethrins 0.056%, permethrin 0.05%, related cpds 0.004%, for fleas, lice, and ticks on *dogs, cats*

Max-Con Insecticide Ear Tag (Y-Tex) *USA*
Tags (ear), cypermethrin 7%, chlorpyrifos 5%, piperonyl butoxide and related cpds 3.5%, for flies, ticks and lice on *cattle*

No-Hop Flea-Tick Spray (Happy Jack) *USA*
Topical spray, pyrethrins 0.056%, permethrin 0.05%, related cpds 0.004%, for fleas and ticks on *dogs, cats*

Ovi-Spot Plus Topical Flea & Tick Control (Hoechst-Roussel) *USA*
Solution, spot-on , permethrin 45%, methoprene 2.9%, for fleas and ticks on *dogs*

Ovitrol Plus Compete Flea Collar for Cats and Kittens (Hoechst-Roussel) *USA*
Collar, tetrachlorvinphos 14.55%, methoprene 1.02%, for fleas and ticks on *cats*

Ovitrol Plus II Complete Flea & Tick Collar for Dogs and Puppies (Hoechst-Roussel) *USA*
Collar, methoprene 1%, chlorpyrifos 8.1%, for fleas and ticks on *dogs*

Performer-Eliminator (Performer) *USA*
Collar, naled 15%, propoxur 4.2%, for fleas and ticks on *dogs*

Pet Care Flea and Tick Spray (DurVet) *USA*
Topical spray, chlorpyrifos 0.225%, pyrethrins 0.05%, piperonyl butoxide 0.1%, N-octyl bicycloheptene dicarboximide 0.168%, for fleas on *dogs*
Withdrawal Periods. Slaughter withdrawal period nil, remove tags before slaughter

Ravap E.C. (Boehringer Ingelheim Vetmedica) *USA*
Topical spray, tetrachlorvinphos 23%, dichlorvos 5.3%, related cpds 0.4%, for ticks, fleas, flies, and lice on *cattle, chickens*
Withdrawal Periods. Cattle: apply at least 20 min before or after milking

Ritter's WB-14 Flea & Tick Spray (Ritter) *USA*
Topical spray, pyrethrins 0.112%, permethrin 0.101%, related cpds 0.009%, for *dogs, cats*

Surekill (IntAgra) *USA*
Liquid, pyrethrins 0.05%, piperonyl butoxide 0.1%, dichlorvos 0.465%, related cpds 0.035%, for flies on *cattle*
Withdrawal Periods. Cattle: apply 20 to 30 min before milking (do not spray on udders of lactating dairy cows)

Synerkyl AQ (DVM) *USA*
Topical spray, pyrethrins 0.112%, permethrin 0.101%, related cpds 0.009%, for fleas and ticks on *dogs, cats*

Synerkyl Pet Spray (DVM) *USA*
Topical spray, permethrin 0.1%, related cpds 0.009%, pyrethrins 0.05%, N-octyl cycloheptene dicarboximide 0.5%, for fleas and ticks on *dogs, cats*

Virbac long Acting Knockout Spray (Allerderm/Virbac) *USA*
Topical spray, pyriproxyfen 0.05%, permethrin 2%, for fleas and ticks on *dogs*

War Paint Roll-On Insecticidal Paste (Loveland) *USA*
Paste, roll-on, permethrin 7%, related cpds 0.6%, piperonyl butoxide 14%, N-Octyl bicycloheptene dicarboximide 21%, for *horses*
Withdrawal Periods. Should not be used on *horses* intended for human consumption

Warrior Insecticide Cattle Ear Tag (Y-Tex) *USA*
Tags (ear), dimpylate 30%, chlorpyrifos 10%, for ticks, lice and flies on *cattle*
Withdrawal Periods. Slaughter withdrawal period nil, remove tags before slaughter, should not be used on cattle producing milk for human consumption

2.2.4 Sheep dips

Dipping is the most common method of applying an ectoparasiticide to sheep. In the UK, the amidine, amitraz (see section 2.2.1.1), the synthetic pyrethroids cypermethrin and flumethrin (see section 2.2.1.7), and the organophosphorus compounds dimpylate and propetamphos (see section 2.2.1.5) are available as sheep dips; other organophosphorus compounds, cyhalothrin, cyromazine, and diflubenzuron are also available as sheep dips in other countries. See relevant sections for preparation details. Some products may be applied by shower for the treatment of some ectoparasitic infestations and are formulated for such use in some countries. Shower applications should not be used for the treatment of mite infestations of sheep.

In the UK, the sale and supply of sheep dips is regulated. Agricultural merchants must ensure that anyone purchasing sheep dips (organophosphorus compounds and non-organophosphorus compounds) is the holder of a Certificate of Competence in the Safe Use of Sheep Dips issued by the National Proficiency Tests Council. Alternatively, the purchaser may be an employer of, or acting on behalf of, someone who has such a certificate. To ensure good practice and continued availability of these dips, the RPSGB and RCVS have requested that pharmacists and veterinarians comply with the legislation when supplying clients and for their own use. Pharmacists are advised to record or keep a copy of the Certificate of Competence so that it may be seen by an inspector. Sheep dipping continues to be regulated by inspection by officials from the HSE and be subject to the requirements of the COSHH regulations.

Dip management. Certain principles need to be followed to ensure the correct use of sheep dips, the most fundamental being to know the capacity of the dip bath so that the amount of concentrate required for a particular dipping programme can be calculated accurately. This should not be more than is required for immediate use.

The dipwash should be prepared according to the manufacturer's directions. The dipwash should be stirred thoroughly before dipping and on each occasion when dipping is interrupted. Replenishment should be made using volume drop or head count, carefully following the manufacturer's recommendations on concentration required. The dipwash depletion per animal depends upon the fleece length. The volume of the dipwash should not fall below 75% of original volume.

Attention should be paid to the prevention of post-dipping lameness caused by *Erysipelothrix rhusiopathiae*. The dip should be prepared in a clean bath and any surface residues removed at regular intervals. Excessively fouled dipwashes should be discarded and manufacturers may recommend limitation of the number of sheep dipped to one for each 2 litres of dipwash, after which the bath should be emptied and refilled with fresh dipwash. Alternatively, dip formulations may be bacteriostatic or bactericidal, or manufacturers may advise addition of a disinfectant or bacteriostat to the dipwash at the end of a day's dipping. Thiram or copper sulphate are commonly used as disinfectants.

Dipping. To ensure a reasonable level of residual protection, sheep should have at least 3 weeks of wool growth before dipping. Extremes of weather should be avoided and dipping is inadvisable when it is raining or the sheep have wet fleeces. Also, sheep that are hot, tired, thirsty, or which have recently been fed should be allowed time to stabilise before dipping.

Where possible, lambs should be dipped separately from ewes with attention being paid to pairing-up ewes and lambs after dipping. It is recommended that rams and fat sheep are dipped separately. Care should be taken to reduce immersion shock. In addition, although it is necessary to immerse the sheep's head while dipping (as indicated below) the animal's head should not be restrained in that position because it may swallow or inhale the dipwash.

When dipping for blowfly larvae, keds, lice, mange mites, and ticks, the body of the sheep should be kept immersed until the fleece is completely saturated with the wash. Thirty seconds should be sufficient. For treatment of *Psoroptes ovis* (sheep scab) immersion for one minute is required to ensure full penetration of the 'scab' layer. The head should be immersed once or twice allowing the animal to breathe between immersions.

Sheep should be allowed to drain in an open space, preferably in the shade, but not in an enclosed building.

In Britain, *The Sheep Scab Order 1986* has been replaced by *The Sheep Scab Order 1997* (SI 1997/968), but existing legislation for Northern Ireland, *The Sheep Scab (Northern*

Ireland) Order 1970, as amended, is still in place. This deregulation of previous sheep scab control measures has led to an increase in the number of outbreaks of the disease. Owing to the importance of this highly contagious disease, manufacturer's directions should be carefully followed to prevent residual infestation leading to new outbreaks. When used in scab control, approved dips should not be used in conjunction with any other dip and the dipwash must be prepared and replenished correctly.

Dimpylate (diazinon), propetamphos, cypermethrin, flumethrin, and doramectin, ivermectin, or moxidectin (by injection) are authorised for use against sheep scab in the UK. Cypermethrin and flumethrin dips should be repeated after about 14 days. Cypermethrin affords no protection against reinfestation. Dimpylate (diazinon), propetamphos, and flumethrin provide a minimum of 3 weeks protection depending on the length of fleece when treated. Two injections of ivermectin at an interval of 7 days or two injections of moxidectin or a single injection of doramectin should be administered in order to treat the clinical signs of scab and to eliminate living mites.

Storage. All dip concentrates should be stored in their original containers, kept out of reach of children, and not mixed with other dip concentrates or washes unless otherwise directed by the manufacturer. Dips are for external treatment only.

Disposal. In the UK, the disposal of dips must be in accordance with an authorisation granted under *The Groundwater Regulations 1998 (SI 1998/2746)*. Soakaways are no longer acceptable for disposal of spent sheep dips. Degradation treatments are available. Sodium hydrochloride based treatment is used for cypermethrin-containing dips. Dips containing dimpylate (diazinon) or flumethrin can be hydrolysed with slaked lime (hydrated lime), and sodium hypochlorite 10% is used for propetamphos-containing dips. Manufacturers should be contacted for further information. Degraded dipwash can be disposed of by a reputable waste contractor or by spraying on suitable land as recommended by the manufacturer.

The Sheep Dip and Textiles Working Group of the Environmental Agency recommends that dips and pour-ons are not used on sheep within at least three months of shearing or slaughter. This is to minimise the amount of dip chemicals being discharged to rivers via sewerage treatment works after processing of fleeces and skins.

Protection of operators. Detail concerning Personal Protective Equipment (PPE) is the subject of the National Proficiency Tests Council (NPTC) certificate of competence and the advisory literature cited in this section. Readers should ensure that they consult current literature. The following can only be considered as a guide. A boiler suit or similar clothing made of strong cotton or similar material, wellington boots, strong gauntlet length nitrile or PVC gloves, waterproof leggings (worn outside the wellingtons), a bib apron (or waterproof coat), a face shield, and a hat, are necessary for those procedures involving measuring out the dip concentrate and mixing the bath for both the initial charge and top up, plunging sheep, emptying the dip, and disposal of wash. A boiler suit, wellingtons, waterproof trousers or leggings, and a bib apron, should provide sufficient protection for putting sheep into the dip bath. It should not be necessary to handle the sheep immediately after dipping because they should be simply shepherded out of draining pens onto pasture. All handling tasks should be done prior to dipping. All waterproof clothing should be resistant to penetration by chemicals, should be washed thoroughly after each day's dipping, and kept in good condition.

Overalls and wellingtons should be worn when handling sheep during the weeks after dipping, and it must be remembered to wash hands afterwards. Again this should only be taken as a guide for handling sheep after they have returned to pasture and the detail on PPE for such operations is the subject of material associated with the NPTC programme and supplementary literature. Precautions should be taken to minimise accidental splashing. For example, pen-gates should be remotely operated. Operator work stations should be provided with the means to treat people who may be injured or become unwell, particularly in isolated locations, and with washing facilities, that is, clean water and soap available close to the dipping area. (For further details, readers are advised to consult appropriate literature).

Parasiticides may be toxic to animals and the operator. Care should be taken with dosage and handling of the product. The recommendations for storage, use, and disposal of unused materials and containers should be followed. For guidance and information, see:

- MAFF/HSE. *Code of practice for the safe use of pesticides on farms and other holdings*. London: HMSO, 1998. PB3528
- NOAH. *Animal medicines: A user's guide.*1995
- Control of Substances Hazardous to Health (COSHH) Regulations 1994
- NOAH. *Guidelines for the disposal of used sheep dip and containers*. 1990
- VMD. *The safe handling and disposal of sheep dips: Advisory notes for farmers*. 1992
- HSE, VMD, EA, SEPA. *Sheep Dipping*. 1998: AS29 (rev2)
- NOAH, VMD. *Safe use of organophosphorus sheep dips: Important instructions for farmers and operators*. April, 1993
- VMD. *Handle sheep dips with care: Guidance sheet on disposal*. PB0645
- DANI. *Water: preventing pollution from sheep dip*. 1991.

2.2.5 Fly repellents

Citronella oil, **diethyltoluamide**, and **dimethyl phthalate** are the active ingredients of fly repellents. These preparations are used mainly on horses and cattle to reduce *Culicoides* attack and prevent worry by nuisance flies such as

Musca and *Hydrotaea*. Preparations containing permethrin are also effective against biting lice *Bovicola equi (Damalinia equi)*.

The preparations are generally applied on the basis of need rather than anticipating challenge. Time of challenge may vary from year to year, and with preceding and current weather.

UK

Battle's Head Fly Protection (Battle Hayward & Bower) *UK*
Liquid, diethyltoluamide 6.6%, dimethyl phthalate 16.6%, for *sheep*

Extra Tail (Kalium) *UK*
Liquid, diethyltoluamide 10%, dimethyl phthalate 10%, citronella 3%, for *horses*; 250 mL, 500 mL, 1 litre

GSL Fly Repellent Plus for Horses, Coopers (Schering-Plough) *UK*
Liquid, citronellol 2%, permethrin (*cis:trans* 25:75) 1.05%, for *horses*; 600 mL
Withdrawal Periods. Should not be used on *horses* intended for human consumption

GSL Lincoln Fly Repellent Plus (Battle Hayward & Bower) *UK*
Liquid, citronellol 2%, permethrin (*cis:trans* 25:75) 1.05%, for *horses*; 250 mL, 600 mL. Use undiluted
Withdrawal Periods. Should not be used on *horses* intended for human consumption

Summer Fly Cream (Battle Hayward & Bower) *UK*
Cream, diethyltoluamide 5%, for *sheep*; 400 g

2.2.6 Environmental control of ectoparasites

To control the population of ectoparasites in the environment several methods may be employed. Flea environmental challenge may be controlled by use of insect growth regulators (see section 2.2.2) or fipronil (see section 2.2.1.6) that inhibit reproduction. Alternatively, chemicals may be applied to the environment to kill adult stages or prevent larval development.

These insecticides are used to eradicate crawling and flying arthropods from an environment. They are employed in poultry houses, intensive livestock houses, and refuse depots to control flies, in pigeon lofts and poultry houses to control mites and beetles, and in the home mainly to control fleas. Arthropods breed in buildings and, in many cases, infest the animal or bird only when the arthropods concerned need to feed. Therefore it is an advantage to minimise the number of pests in the environment before the building is used to accommodate animals. Some insecticides can be used in buildings that would not be suitable for direct application to the animal. Therefore, in general **the following preparations are not for use on animals**. Regular vacuuming helps reduce the build-up of a flea population in a domestic environment.

UK

Many preparations are available. This is not a comprehensive list.

Acclaim Plus Flea Control (Ceva) *UK*
Aerosol spray, methoprene 0.18%, permethrin 0.567%; 340 g
Note. Not for use on animals

Alfacron 10WP (Novartis) *UK*
Solution, powder for reconstitution, azamethiphos 10%; 1 kg
Reconstitute 100 g azamethiphos (1 kg powder) in 7.5 litres water (spray) or in 500 mL water (paint-on)
Note. Not for use on animals

Alfadex (Novartis) *UK*
Solution, pyrethrins 0.075%; 5 litres
Note. Not for use on animals

Arrest (Arnolds) *UK*
Spray, bioallethrin 0.1%, methoprene 0.1%, permethrin 0.5%
Note. Not for use on animals

Ban Mite (Johnson's) *UK*
Liquid concentrate, malathion 60%; 100 mL. To be diluted before use
Dilute 15 mL in 1 litre water
Note. Not for use on animals

Canovel Pet Bedding & Household Spray (Pfizer) *UK*
Aerosol spray, methoprene 0.03%, piperonyl butoxide 1%, pyrethrins 0.1%; 200 g
Note. Not for use on animals

Carpet Flea Guard (Johnson's) *UK*
Powder, permethrin 0.5%; 200 g
Note. Not for use on animals

Defest II (Sherley's) *UK*
Aerosol spray, bioallethrin 0.1%, permethrin (*cis:trans* 25:75) 0.5%; 400 mL
Note. Not for use on animals

Duramitex (Harkers) *UK*
Liquid concentrate, malathion 60%; 140 mL. To be diluted before use
Dilute 140 mL in 9 litres water
Note. Not for use on animals

Flea Bomb (Bob Martin) *UK*
Permethrin smoke for home use
1 device per 3m x 4 m x 2m room
Note. Not for use on animals

Flea Buster (Sherley's) *UK*
Dusting powder, orthoboric acid 64%; 200 g
Note. Not for use on animals

Flea Fogger Plus (Bob Martin) *UK*
Total release aerosol, bioallethrin 0.1%, methoprene 0.15%, permethrin 0.5%
Note. Not for use on animals

Flea Kill Powder (Bob Martin) *UK*
Dusting powder, permethrin 0.53%; 250 g
Note. Not for use on animals

Fleegard (Bayer) *UK*
Aerosol spray, bioallethrin 0.1%, permethrin 0.5%; 500 mL
Note. Not for use on animals

Flego (Sherley's) *UK*
Aerosol spray, cyromazine 3.11%, permethrin 0.64%; 150 mL
Note. Not for use on animals

POM Frontline (Merial) *UK*
See section 2.2.1.6 for preparation details

Home Flea Kill Powder (Bob Martin) *UK*
Dusting powder, bendiocarb 0.5%
Note. Not for use on animals

Home Flea Spray Plus (Bob Martin) *UK*
Aerosol spray, permethrin 0.5%; 200 mL
Note. Not for use on animals

Household Flea Spray (Johnson's) *UK*
Aerosol spray, permethrin 0.25%, pyrethrins 0.1%; 150 mL, 250 mL
Note. Not for use on animals

Indorex (Virbac) *UK*
Aerosol spray, permethrin 0.93%, pyriproxyfen 0.02%
Note. Not for use on animals

Littac (Sorex) *UK*
Liquid concentrate, alphacypermethrin 1.47%; 1 litre. To be diluted before use
Dilute 100 mL in 2.5 litres water and apply with knapsack sprayer
Note. Not for use on animals

Microshield Household Flea Spray (Bob Martin) *UK*
Spray, bioallethrin 0.1%, RS-methoprene 0.1%, permethrin 0.5%; 450 mL
Note. Not for use on animals

Neporex 2SG (Novartis) *UK*
Granules, or to prepare a solution, cyramazine 2%; 1 kg
Apply 250 g powder per 10m^2
Note. Not for use on animals

Nuvan 500EC (Novartis) *UK*
Liquid concentrate, dichlorvos 50%; 1 litre. To be diluted before use
Dilute with water according to manufacturer's instructions and apply by spray
Note. Not for use on animals

Nuvan Staykil (Novartis) *UK*
Aerosol spray, dichlorvos 0.5%, iodofenphos 2%; 600 g
Note. Not for use on animals

POM **Program** (Novartis) *UK*
See section 2.2.2.1 for preparation details

Rug-de-Bug (Sherley's) *UK*
Powder, permethrin 0.5%; 200 g
Note. Not for use on animals

Secto Flea Free (Sinclair) *UK*
Dusting powder, permethrin 0.5%; 200 g, 500 g
Note. Not for use on animals

Secto Household Flea Spray (Sinclair) *UK*
Aerosol spray, permethrin 0.25%, pyrethrins 0.1%; 250 mL, 500 mL
Note. Not for use on animals

Super Fly Spray (Sorex) *UK*
Aerosol spray, phenothrin 0.25%, tetramethrin 0.1%; 450 mL
Note. Not for use on animals

Taktic Buildings Spray (Intervet) *UK*
Liquid concentrate, amitraz 12.5%. To be diluted before use
Dilute 80 mL in 10 litres water
Note. Not for use on animals

Turbair Kilsect Super (Pan Brittanica) *UK*
Solution, bromophos 5%, resmethrin 0.3%; 1 litre
Note. Not for use on animals

3 Drugs acting on the
GASTRO-INTESTINAL SYSTEM

Contributors:
D H Grove-White BVSc, DBR, FRCVS
P-J M Noble BVM&S, BSc, MRCVS
D J Taylor MA, VetMB, PhD, MRCVS
J P Walmsley MA, VetMB, CertEO, DipECVS, MRCVS

3.1 Antidiarrhoeal drugs

In diarrhoea there is a net failure of intestinal uptake of water and sodium, which is sufficient to overwhelm the compensatory capacity of the colon and results in the production of faeces with a higher than normal fluid content. This net failure in water and electrolyte uptake may be due to hypersecretion, reduced absorption, or both. Its deleterious effects on the animal are primarily metabolic in nature with dehydration and acidosis being of major importance and ultimately life threatening.

The causative agents of diarrhoea are numerous and include dietary imbalance or hypersensitivity, infections due to viruses, bacteria, yeasts, protozoa, or endoparasites, ingestion of toxins, small intestinal bacterial overgrowth, neoplasia, lymphangiectasia, villous atrophy, chronic inflammatory bowel disease, granulomatous enteritis and colitis-X in horses, exocrine pancreatic insufficiency, and stress. Diarrhoea may also result as a side-effect of drug treatment.

Treatment of diarrhoea should be directed at the cause but due to the multi-factorial aetiology of the condition, the causative agent(s) cannot always be ascertained; this is especially the case in acute diarrhoea in individual animals. Symptomatic treatment is therefore important and includes bowel rest and correction of fluid, electrolyte, and acid-base disturbances.

Fluid therapy, oral or parenteral, is of prime importance. In the majority of cases oral fluids will suffice but in severe cases, parenteral fluids will be required. Consideration should be given to the choice of oral fluid used especially with regard to the alkalinising potential and sodium concentration (on which depends the rehydrating ability of the fluid). Parenteral solutions should be isotonic with adequate bicarbonate yields, for example Hartmann's solution.

Food is usually withheld for 24 hours in dogs and cats and oral electrolyte replacement solutions (see section 16.1.1) are provided. This is followed by a low fat hypoallergenic diet with a highly digestible carbohydrate source and gradual re-introduction to normal feed. There is debate about withholding food or milk during oral fluid therapy in calves but it is suggested that witholding milk for more than 24 hours is contra-indicated in view of the villous atrophy that such starvation may produce. Hyperosmotic oral solutions that contain the amino acid glutamine (Glutalyte, Norbrook) are available. These limit the deleterious effects on gut structure and energy balance caused by withholding food or milk for a short period by minimising villous atrophy and assisting in repair in addition to improving fluid and electrolyte absorption. In view of the hypertonicity, these solutions should only be used in calves and not in other species in which they have not been evaluated.

Antibacterials are also often employed for the treatment of diarrhoea, but their use is controversial in some situations. Where diseases that result in diarrhoea (for example, salmonellosis in calves, watery mouth in lambs, post weaning enteritis and swine dysentery in pigs) are clearly identifiable clinically or following post mortem examination of members of an affected group, the group should be treated immediately with the appropriate antimicrobial and fluid therapy as necessary.

In some species, diseases causing diarrhoea are well defined and treatment protocols have been established, for example swine dysentery. In species where diarrhoeal disease is less well defined, antibacterials (see section 1.1) that are poorly absorbed from the gastro-intestinal tract may be given and may be included in compound preparations with adsorbents (see section 1.1.12). Antibacterials, that are absorbed systemically, are particularly indicated in acute haemorrhagic diarrhoea, and when there is evidence of sepsis because this suggests bacterial invasion of the intestinal mucosa. Antibacterials are also indicated if a known pathogen is cultured from the faeces, when biopsy shows enteroadherent bacteria, or in canine small intestinal bacterial overgrowth.

However, the routine use of antibacterials in the treatment of unidentified diarrhoea is not warranted because many of the infectious agents involved are viral or protozoal. Treatment should be considered if the condition is life threatening or occurring in a species in which individual nursing cannot be given. Animals with salmonellosis or *Campylobacter* infection may remain carriers following treatment and antimicrobial resistance may be selected in pathogens or normal flora and plasmid-mediated transferable multiple drug resistance encouraged where antimicrobials are given in inappropriate circumstances. Potential toxic effects such as reduced lactase activity have been seen with oral neomycin or tetracycline therapy. Prolonged antibacterial treatment for diarrhoea may result in alteration of the gastro-intestinal flora, secondary bacterial proliferation, and exacerbation of clinical signs.

Ruminal extract, probiotics, and yoghurt have been used to re-establish gastro-intestinal microbes after antibacterial therapy. Probiotics, for example Broilact (Orion; distributed by Forum) for poultry and Provita Protect, Provita Eurotech (see section 17.3) for calves, have proven to be particularly useful. It is not known whether probiotics may be helpful in dogs and cats with diarrhoea.

Vaccines (see Chapter 18) are available for the prevention of diarrhoea due to bacteria such as *E. coli, Salmonella* spp., and *Clostridium* spp. and viral infections including rotavirus, panleucopenia, and parvovirus.

3.1.1 Adsorbents

Adsorbents, given by mouth, adsorb toxins from the gastro-intestinal tract and thereby may prevent irritation and erosion of the mucosa. They may also adsorb other drugs such as lincomycin, and reduce their efficacy (see Drug Interactions – Appendix 1). Adsorbents also increase the bulk of the faeces. However, they have little or no effect on fluid or electrolyte losses and their value is doubtful.

Bismuth salts, **charcoal** (see also Treatment of poisoning), **zinc oxide**, and **kaolin** are available in single ingredient products, or compound preparations with antacids and electrolytes for the treatment of non-specific diarrhoea. Kaolin does not adsorb *E. coli* enterotoxins and therefore has limited use in neonatal diarrhoea and may even be contra-indicated. Bismuth salts and activated charcoal may adsorb these toxins. Some absorption of salicylate will occur from administration of bismuth salicylate; care should be taken with administration to cats (see Prescribing for dogs and cats).

Ispaghula husk and sterculia (see section 3.6.2) are used in the treatment of diarrhoea because of their ability to absorb water and increase faecal mass. Adequate fluid intake should be maintained.

UK

Indications. Non-specific diarrhoea
Contra-indications. Concurrent oral treatment
Dose. See preparation details

GSL **BCK** (Fort Dodge) *UK*
Oral granules, by addition to feed, bismuth subnitrate 39.2 mg/g, calcium phosphate 49 mg/g, charcoal 402 mg/g, light kaolin 420 mg/g, for *dogs, cats*
Dose. *Dogs, cats*: *by mouth*, 1–3 heaped 5-mL spoonfuls (6–18 g) 2–3 times daily

GSL **Diarrhoea Tablets** (Bob Martin) *UK*
Tablets, bismuth carbonate 32.5 mg, catechu powder 65 mg, prepared chalk 210 mg, rhubarb powder 16.5 mg, for *dogs*; 10
Dose. *Dogs*: *by mouth*, 1–3 tablets (depending on body-weight) 3–4 times daily

GSL **Diarrhoea Tablets** (Johnson's) *UK*
Tablets, bismuth carbonate 30 mg, calcium carbonate 240 mg, for *dogs, cats*; 12
Contra-indications. Puppies or kittens less than 12 weeks of age
Dose. *By mouth*.
Dogs: 1–4 tablets daily (depending on body-weight)
Cats: ½–1 tablet twice daily

GSL **Forgastrin** (Arnolds) *UK*
Oral powder, for addition to feed or to prepare an oral suspension, attapulgite 730 mg/g, bone charcoal 270 mg/g, for *cattle, pigs*; 250 g, 2.5 kg
Withdrawal Periods. Slaughter withdrawal period nil, milk withdrawal period nil
Dose. *By mouth*.
Horses ♦: 3–4 tablespoonfuls (45–60 g) 3 times daily
Cattle: 3–4 tablespoonfuls (45–60 g) 3 times daily
calves: 1–2 tablespoonfuls (15–30 g) 3 times daily
Pigs: 2–3 5-mL spoonfuls (6–10 g) 3 times daily; *piglets*: dissolve three 5-mL spoonfuls (10 g) in 60 mL water. Administer 5 mL daily

GSL **Kaogel V** (Pharmacia & Upjohn) *UK*
Oral suspension, light kaolin 200 mg/mL, pectin 4.3 mg/mL, for *calves, dogs*; 2.25 litres
Withdrawal Periods. *Calves*: slaughter withdrawal period nil
Dose. *By mouth*.
Horses ♦: 1 mL/kg daily
Calves, dogs: 1–2 mL/kg 2–3 times daily

P Ⓗ **Pepto-Bismol** (Proctor & Gamble) *UK*
Oral suspension, bismuth subsalicylate 17.52 mg/mL; 120 mL, 240 mL
Dose. *By mouth*.
Horses: 1 mL/kg 2–3 times daily
Dogs, cats: 1–3 mL/kg daily in divided doses

MFS **Pig Zinpremix** (Roche) *UK*
Oral powder, zinc oxide 100%, for *pigs*
Withdrawal Periods. *Pigs*: slaughter 28 days
Dose. *Pigs*: 3.1 kg/tonne feed daily for up to 14 days

GSL **Stat** (Intervet) *UK*
Oral suspension, calcium chloride (as hexahydrate) 11.97 mg/mL, dried aluminium hydroxide gel 19.3 mg/mL, light kaolin 108 mg/mL, magnesium chloride (as hexahydrate) 1 mg/mL, potassium acetate 3.3 mg/mL, sodium acetate (as trihydrate) 19.8 mg/mL, sodium chloride 18.1 mg/mL, for *cattle, sheep, pigs, dogs, cats*; 1 litre
Withdrawal Periods. Slaughter withdrawal period nil, milk withdrawal period nil
Dose. *By mouth*, repeat 2–3 times daily.
Cattle, sheep, pigs: (<100 kg body-weight) 20–100 mL, (100–250 kg body-weight) 100–200 mL, (250–400 kg body-weight) 200–300 mL, (>400 kg body-weight) 300–500 mL
Dogs: (large) 20 mL, (others) 5–10 mL
Cats: 5–10 mL

MFS **ZincoTec** (Nutec) *UK*
Oral powder, zinc oxide 100%, for *pigs*
Withdrawal Periods. *Pigs*: slaughter 28 days
Dose. *Pigs*: 3.1 kg/tonne feed daily for up to 14 days

Australia

Indications. Non-specific diarrhoea
Contra-indications. Concurrent oral treatment
Side-effects. Darkened faeces with bismuth-containing preparations

Antidiarrhoea Powder (Parnell) *Austral.*
Powder, reconstitute as oral solution with water, catechu 30 g/kg, kaolin, calcium carbonate, for *horses, cattle, pigs sheep, goats*
Withdrawal Periods. *Horses, cattle, pigs, sheep, goats*: slaughter withdrawal period nil
Dose. *horses, cattle*: 450 g of powder (1 sachet)/ 450 kg body-weight once daily; *calves*: 110–150 g of powder/50 kg body-weight once daily
Sheep, goats: 150 g of powder/50 kg body-weight once daily
Pigs: 225 g of powder/100 kg body-weight once daily

Direa Tablets (Mavlab) *Austral.*
Tablets, crospovidone, for *cats, dogs*
Dose. *Dogs, cats*: *by mouth*, 1 tablet/ 10 kg twice daily for 3–4 days

Peptosyl (RWR) *Austral.*
Oral suspension, bismuth salicylate 17.5 mg/mL, bentonite, for *dogs, horses*
Withdrawal Periods. *Horses*: slaughter 28 days
Dose. *Horses, dogs*: *by mouth*, 0.25-0.5 mL/kg
Warnings. Safety in pregnant animals has not been established

Gastro-Enteric Mixture (Apex) *Austral.*
Oral liquid, kaolin 3.75 g, pectin 375 mg, aluminium hydroxide 175 mg, bismuth subcarbonate 275 mg / 30 mL, for *cattle, horses, dogs, cats*
Withdrawal Periods. *Horses, calves*: slaughter withdrawal period nil
Dose. *Horses, calves*: 25 mL/10 kg body-weight in divided doses

Eire
Indications. Non-specific diarrhoea
Dose. See preparation details

Kaogel V (Pharmacia & Upjohn) *Eire*
Oral suspension, light kaolin 200 mg/mL, pectin 4.3 mg/mL, for *calves, dogs*
Withdrawal Periods. *Calves*: slaughter withdrawal period nil
Dose. *Calves, dogs*: *by mouth*, 1–2 mL/kg 2–3 times daily

New Zealand
Indications. Non-specific diarrhoea
Contra-indications. Gastro-intestinal obstruction, torsion, or penetration
Dose. See preparation details

Bismosal (Virbac) *NZ*
Oral suspension, bismuth salicylate 17.5 mg/mL, sodium bentonite 3.33 mg/mL, for *horses, dogs*
Withdrawal Periods. *Horses*: slaughter 28 days
Dose. *Horses*: *by mouth*, 0.5–1.0 mL/kg 4 times daily for 12–24 hours, then twice daily for 2–3 days
Dogs: *by mouth*, 0.25–0.5 mL/kg 4 times daily for 12–24 hours, then twice daily for 2–3 days
Contra-indications. Gastro-intestinal ulceration; severe renal impairment

Diarrhoea Powder (Parnell) *NZ*
Oral powder, powdered catechu 30 g/kg, kaolin 485 g/kg, for *horses, cattle, sheep, goats, pigs*
Dose. *Horses, cattle*: *by mouth*, 450 g daily for 2–3 days; *calves*, 110–150 g daily for 2–3 days
Sheep, goats: *by mouth*, 150 g daily for 2–3 days
Pigs: *by mouth*, 225 g daily for 2–3 days

Peptosyl (Vetpharm) *NZ*
Oral suspension, bismuth salicylate, sodium bentonite, for *horses, dogs*
Withdrawal Periods. *Horses*: slaughter 28 days
Dose. *Horses*: *by mouth*, 0.5–1.0 mL/kg 4 times daily for 12–24 hours, then twice daily for 2–3 days
Dogs: *by mouth*, 0.25–0.5 mL/kg 4 times daily for 12–24 hours, then twice daily for 2–3 days

Scour Powder (Bomac) *NZ*
Oral solution, powder for reconstitution, chalk, kaolin, catechu, ferrous sulphate, for *cattle*
Withdrawal Periods. Slaughter withdrawal period nil, milk withdrawal period nil
Dose. *Cattle*: as an oral solution, 240 g; *calves, as an oral solution*, 60 g

Phoenix Diarrhoea Powder (Phoenix) *NZ*
Oral powder, powdered catechu, kaolin, for *horses, cattle, sheep, goats, pigs*
Dose. *Horses, cattle*: *by mouth*, 450 g daily for 2–3 days; *calves*, 112.5–150 g daily for 2–3 days
Sheep, goats: *by mouth*, 150 g daily for 2–3 days
Pigs: *by mouth*, 225 g daily for 2–3 days

USA
Indications. Non-specific diarrhoea
Side-effects. Darkened faeces with bismuth-containing preparations
Dose. See preparation details

Ana-Sorb (Wendt) *USA*
Tablets, aluminium magnesium silicate, carob powder, pectin, magnesium trisilicate, colloidal aluminium silicate, for *horses, cattle*
Withdrawal Periods. *Cattle*: milk withdrawal nil
Dose. *Horses, cattle*: *by mouth*, 2–3 tablets every 4 hours

Anti-diarrheal Calf Bolus (AgriLabs) *USA*
Tablets, aluminium magnesium silicate, carob flour, pectin, magnesium trisilicate, for *horses, cattle*
Dose. *Foals, calves*: *by mouth*, 2 tablets every 4–6 hours

Bismukote Suspension (RXV) *USA*
Oral suspension, bismuth subsalicylate 1.75%, for *cattle, horses, dogs, cats*
Withdrawal Periods. Slaughter withdrawal period nil
Dose. *Horses, cattle*: *by mouth*, 180–300 mL every 2–3 hours; *foals, calves*: 90–120 mL every 2–3 hours
Dogs, cats: *by mouth*, 15–45 mL every 1–3 hours

Bismukote Paste (Vedco) *USA*
Oral paste, bismuth subsalicylate 5%, 10%, for *dogs*
Dose. *Dogs*: *by mouth*, 22 mg/kg 3–4 timesdaily

Bismupaste D5 (Vedco) *USA*
Oral paste, bismuth subsalicylate 5% (plus magnesium aluminium silicate), for *dogs*
Dose. *Dogs*: *by mouth*, 22 mg/kg 3–4 timesdaily

Bismupaste D10 (Vedco) *USA*
Oral paste, bismuth subsalicylate 10% (plus magnesium aluminium silicate), for *dogs*
Dose. *Dogs*: *by mouth*, 22 mg/kg 3–4 timesdaily

Bismupaste E20 (Vedco) *USA*
Oral paste, bismuth subsalicylate 20% (plus magnesium aluminium silicate), for *horses*
Dose. *Horses*: *by mouth*, 22 mg/kg 3–4 timesdaily

Bismusal Suspension (RXV) *USA*
Oral suspension, bismuth subsalicylate 1.75%, for *cattle, horses, dogs, cats*
Withdrawal Periods. Slaughter withdrawal period nil
Dose. *Horses, cattle*: *by mouth*, 180–300 mL every 2–3 hours; *foals, calves*: 90–120 mL every 2–3 hours
Dogs, cats: *by mouth*, 15–45 mL every 1–3 hours

Bismusol (First Priority) *USA*
Oral suspension, bismuth subsalicylate 1.75%, for *cattle, horses, dogs, cats*
Dose. *Horses, cattle*: *by mouth*, 180–300 mL every 2–3 hours; *foals, calves*: 90–120 mL every 2–3 hours
Dogs, cats: *by mouth*, 15–45 mL every 1–3 hours
Contra-indications. *Pregnant animals*

Boltan III (Butler) *USA*
Tablets, kaolin 9.6 g, for *horses, cattle*
Dose. *Horses, cattle*: *by mouth*, 2–3 tablets 2–3 times daily

Corrective Suspension (Phoenix) *USA*
Oral suspension, bismuth subsalicylate 1.75%, for *cattle, horses, dogs, cats*
Dose. *Horses, cattle*: *by mouth*, 180–300 mL every 2–3 hours; *foals, calves*: 90–120 mL every 2–3 hours
Dogs, cats: *by mouth*, 15–45 mL every 1–3 hours

Equi-Phar Bismukote Paste (Vedco) *USA*
Oral paste, bismuth subsalicylate 1 g/ 5 mL paste, for *horses*
Dose. *Horses*: *by mouth*, 22 mg/kg 3–4 timesdaily

Gastro-Cote (Butler) *USA*
Oral solution, bismuth subsalicylate 1.75%, for *horses, cattle, dogs, cats*
Dose. *Horses, cattle*: *by mouth*, 180–300 mL every 2–3 hours; *foals, calves*: 90–120 mL every 2–3 hours
Dogs, cats: *by mouth*, 15–45 mL every 1–3 hours

Gastro-Sorb Bolus (Butler) *USA*
Tablets, attapulgite, pectin, magnesium trisilicate, carob, for *horses, cattle, dogs, cats*
Dose. *Horses, cattle*: *by mouth*, 2 tablets every 4–6hours for up to 3 days; *foals, calves*: 1 tablet every 4–6hours for up to 3 days

Gastro-Sorb Calf Bolus (Butler) *USA*
Tablets, attapulgite, pectin, magnesium trisilicate, carob, for *horses, cattle*
Dose. *Foals, calves*: *by mouth*, 1 tablet every 4–6hours for up to 3 days

Intesti-Sorb Bolus (AgriPharm, RXV) *USA*
Tablets, attapulgite, pectin, magnesium trisilicate, carob, for *cattle, horses*,
Dose. *Horses*: *by mouth*, 0.5–1 tablet every 4 hours
Cattle: *by mouth*, 1–1.5 tablets every 4 hours

Intesti-Sorb Calf Bolus (AgriPharm, RXV) *USA*
Tablets, attapulgite, pectin, magnesium trisilicate, carob, for *cattle, horses*
Dose. *Foals, calves*: *by mouth*, 1 tablet every 4 hours for up to 3 days

K-P-Sol (Evsco) *USA*
Oral suspension, kaolin 0.23 g/mL, pectin 8.6 mg/mL, for *dogs, cats*
Dose. *Dogs, cats*: *by mouth*, 1.1–2.2 mL/kg every 6 hours or as needed for up to 5 days

Kao-Pec (AgriLabs) *USA*
Oral suspension, kaolin 200 mg/mL, pectin 4 mg/mL, for *horses, cattle, dogs, cats*
Dose. *Horses, cattle*: *by mouth*, 180–300 mL every 2–3 hours; *foals, calves*: 90–120 mL every 2–3 hours
Dogs, cats: *by mouth*, 15–45 mL every 1–3 hours

Kao-Pect (Phoenix) *USA*
Oral suspension, kaolin 200 mg/mL, pectin 4 mg/mL, for *horses, cattle, dogs, cats*
Dose. *Horses, cattle*: *by mouth*, 180–300 mL every 2–3 hours; *foals, calves*: 90–120 mL every 2–3 hours
Dogs, cats: *by mouth*, 15–45 mL every 1–3 hours

Kaolin-Pectin (DurVet, Wendt) *USA*
Oral suspension, kaolin 193 mg/mL, pectin 8.9 mg/mL, for *horses, cattle, dogs, cats*
Dose. *Horses, cattle*: *by mouth*, 180–300 mL every 2–3 hours; *foals, calves*: 90–120 mL every 2–3 hours
Dogs, cats: *by mouth*, 15–45 mL every 1–3 hours

Kaolin-Pectin Plus (AgriPharm, RXV) *USA*
Oral suspension, kaolin 193 mg/mL, pectin 4.3 mg/mL, for *horses, cattle*,
Dose. *Horses, cattle*: *by mouth*, 180–300 mL; *foals, calves*: 90–120 mL

Kaolin Pectin Suspension (Vedco) *USA*
Oral suspension, kaolin 193 mg/mL, pectin 4.3 mg/mL, for *dogs, cats*
Dose. *Dogs, cats*: *by mouth*, 15–45 mL

Kaopectolin (Aspen) *USA*
Oral suspension, kaolin 193 mg/mL, pectin 4.3 mg/mL, for *horses, cattle, dogs, cats*
Dose. *Horses, cattle*: *by mouth*, 180–300 mL; *foals, calves*: 90–120 mL
Dogs, cats: *by mouth*, 15–45 mL

Kaopectolin (Butler) *USA*
Oral suspension, kaolin 200 mg/mL, pectin 4 mg/mL, for *horses, cattle, dogs, cats*
Dose. *Horses, cattle*: *by mouth*, 180–300 mL every 2–3 hours; *foals, calves*: 90–120 mL every 2–3 hours
Dogs, cats: *by mouth*, 15–45 mL every 1–3 hours

Maxi Sorb Calf Bolus (DurVet) *USA*
Tablets, attapulgite, pectin, magnesium trisilicate, carob, for *cattle, horses*
Dose. *Foals, calves*: *by mouth*, 2 tablets every 4–6 hours for up to 3 days

MVT Powder (Butler) *USA*
Oral powder, for solution, magnesium hydroxide 65%, kaolin 35 %, for *cattle, sheep*
Withdrawal Periods. Milk 24 hours
Dose. *Cattle*: *by mouth or stomach tube*, 293 g magnesium hydroxide and 156 g kaolin/3.785 litres water
Sheep, goats: one-eighth to one-quarter of dose for cattle

PalaBIS (VRX) *USA*
Tablets, bismuth subsalicylate 262 mg, for *dogs*
Dose. *Dogs, cats*: *by mouth*, 17.5–52.5 mg/kg daily in 3–4 divided doses

Palapectate (VRX) *USA*
Tablets, attapulgite 750 mg, for *dogs*
Dose. *Dogs, cats*: *by mouth*, 25–50 mg/kg every 2–6 hours, or after every loose stool

Scour Out II (Wendt) *USA*
Tablets, attapulgite, carob powder, pectin, magnesium trisilicate, for *cattle*
Dose. *Cattle*: *by mouth*, 1–2 tablets 2–3 times daily

Veda-Sorb Bolus (Vedco) *USA*
Tablets, attapulgite, carob, pectin, magnesium trisilicate, for *cattle, horses*
Dose. *Cattle*: *by mouth*, 2–3 tablets every 4 hours

Veda-Sorb JR Bolus (Vedco) *USA*
Tablets, attapulgite, carob, pectin, magnesium trisilicate, for *cattle, horses*
Dose. *Foals, calves*: *by mouth*, 2 tablets every 4–6 hours

3.1.2 Antidiarrhoeal drugs that reduce motility

The use of drugs to stimulate or reduce intestinal motility in patients with diarrhoea is controversial. The diarrhoea may be accompanied by hypomotility rather than hypermotility. Also, in patients with diarrhoea due to entero-invasive bacteria, the diarrhoea may be considered as a protective response in eliminating pathogens and attempts to delay passage of gut contents may be contra-indicated because the toxins remain in the lumen for a prolonged period and the severity of the condition is increased.

Intestinal transit time is determined by the ratio between peristalsis and segmentation contractions. Antimuscarinics (anticholinergics) reduce both peristalsis and segmental contractions causing an open tube effect and may increase the severity of diarrhoea. Opioids are more effective for the treatment of diarrhoea because they reduce intestinal propulsive activity and increase segmental contractions and therefore prolong intestinal transit time.

Diphenoxylate, **codeine**, and **loperamide** are opioid derivatives that are used in the treatment of non-specific acute and chronic diarrhoea. Some authorities indicate that these drugs are contra-indicated for the treatment of diarrhoea due to infection with invasive bacteria. Diphenoxylate is well absorbed from the gastro-intestinal tract, whereas loperamide is only partially absorbed. Both drugs are metabolised in the liver. Loperamide may be of value in hypersecretory diarrhoea (because it has been shown in humans to inhibit cholera toxin induced hypersecretion). Diphenoxylate and loperamide should be used with care in cats because they may cause excitability on overdose in this species. In dogs, these drugs may be sedative; loperamide less so than diphenoxylate. Loperamide may be used in horses. Diphenoxylate is available in combination with a low dose of atropine (co-phenotrope). However, the atropine in this combination product has no pharmacological effect on the gut.

CODEINE PHOSPHATE

UK

Indications. Non-specific diarrhoea; non-productive cough (see section 5.4); analgesia (see section 6.3)
Contra-indications. Respiratory conditions with excess airway secretion, conditions causing CNS depression, hepatic impairment
Side-effects. Sedation, ataxia, respiratory depression
Dose. Non-specific diarrhoea, *by mouth.*
Horses: 1–3 mg/kg 3 times daily
Dogs: 200–500 micrograms/kg 3 times daily

See section 5.5 for preparation details

DIPHENOXYLATE with ATROPINE

(Co-phenotrope: preparations of diphenoxylate hydrochloride and atropine sulphate in the proportions, by weight, 100 parts to 1 part respectively)

UK

Indications. Non-specific diarrhoea
Side-effects. Constipation
Warnings. Care on administration to cats, see Prescribing for dogs and cats
Dose. Expressed as diphenoxylate, *by mouth.*
Dogs: 100–200 micrograms/kg 2–3 times daily
Cats: 50–100 micrograms/kg twice daily

POM Ⓗ **Lomotil** (Searle) *UK*
Tablets, diphenoxylate hydrochloride 2.5 mg, atropine sulphate 25 micrograms; 100, 500, 1000

LOPERAMIDE HYDROCHLORIDE

UK

Indications. Non-specific diarrhoea
Side-effects. **Warnings**. See under Diphenoxylate
Dose. *By mouth.*
Horses: 100–200 micrograms/kg 4 times daily
Dogs: 100–200 micrograms/kg 2–3 times daily
Cats: 80–160 micrograms/kg twice daily

POM Ⓗ **Loperamide** (Non-proprietary) *UK*
Capsules, loperamide hydrochloride 2 mg
Note. P if authorised and labelled for treatment of acute diarrhoea

P Ⓗ **Arret** (Johnson & Johnson MSD) *UK*
Capsules, loperamide hydrochloride 2 mg; 6, 12, 18

P Ⓗ **Diasorb** (Norton Consumer) *UK*
Capsules, loperamide hydrochloride 2 mg; 6, 12

P Ⓗ **Diocalm Ultra** (SSL International) *UK*
Capsules, loperamide hydrochloride 2 mg; 6, 12

POM Ⓗ **Imodium** (Janssen-Cilag) *UK*
Capsules, loperamide hydrochloride 2 mg; 30
Syrup, loperamide hydrochloride 200 micrograms/mL; 100 mL
Note. P if authorised and labelled for treatment of acute diarrhoea

3.1.3 Drugs used in the treatment of chronic diarrhoea

Chronic diarrhoea may be caused by dietary imbalance, small intestinal disease (for example, villous atrophy, inflammatory bowel disease, lymphangiectasia, and small intestinal bacterial overgrowth), parasitism, exocrine pancreatic insufficiency (see section 3.9), colitis, or occur as a result of other systemic disease.

Sulfasalazine is used in the management of chronic colitis. Intestinal bacteria split the compound into 5-aminosalicylate and sulfapyridine. The aminosalicylate becomes concentrated in the gastro-intestinal wall where it exerts its anti-inflammatory effect. The active component of **mesalazine** and **olsalazine** is 5-aminosalicylate. The most common side-effects of sulfasalazine are anorexia and vomiting. Keratoconjunctivitis sicca may occur with prolonged use and is often irreversible. This side-effect has been attributed primarily to the sulfapyridine moiety, but is occasionally seen with drugs containing 5-aminosalicylate only. Care should be taken with administration to cats (see Prescribing for dogs and cats).

Corticosteroids can be used in the control of inflammatory bowel disease including lymphocytic-plasmacytic or eosinophilic infiltrates of the small or large bowel in dogs and cats. They are also used in horses. **Prednisolone** (see section 7.2.1) is given at a dose of 1 to 2 mg/kg once or twice daily for up to 2 months, and reduced to the lowest effective dose administered on alternate days in dogs. In cats, an initial dose of 1 to 4 mg/kg once or twice daily is used. In horses, prednisolone may be used for chronic granulomatous enteritis at a dose of 0.5 to 1.0 mg/kg or **dexamethasone**, at a dose of 20–200 micrograms/kg once daily given by mouth, is also appropriate. NSAIDs (see section 10.1) such as **flunixin** may be of value in ameliorating gastro-intestinal inflammation and reducing hypersecretion in neonatal calf diarrhoea. NSAIDs should not be used in hypovolaemic patients due to the risk of inducing renal failure.

Antibacterials may be required to control small intestinal bacterial overgrowth in dogs. Oxytetracycline (10 to 20 mg/kg 3 times daily by mouth♦) is the drug of first choice. If response is inadequate, metronidazole (20 mg/kg twice daily by mouth♦) or tylosin (20 mg/kg twice daily by mouth♦) can be used. Treatment is given for at least 4 weeks and long-term antibacterial therapy may be required in some dogs. Metronidazole may also have an effect on cell-mediated immunity and has been used as adjunctive treatment in refractory inflammatory bowel disease in dogs and cats and in colitis.

Azathioprine (see section 13.2) is used in the management of severe inflammatory bowel disease. It is used as an adjunct to corticosteroids or to enable a reduction in the dosage of corticosteroids where side-effects are unacceptable. In dogs, an initial dose of 2 mg/kg once daily is given by mouth followed by a gradually tapered dose to 0.5 to 1.0 mg/kg on alternate days. In cats, the reported dosage is 300 to 500 micrograms/kg on alternate days; the occurrence of side-effects is higher in cats. Corticosteroids and azathioprine are given on alternate days. The white blood cell counts should be monitored when the drug is given daily. Dietetic pet foods (see section 16.8) may also assist in the management of colitis in dogs and cats. Patients with mild to moderate chronic idiopathic colitis may respond to dietary management alone, using a highly digestible diet containing a selected protein source that the animal has not been exposed to recently. Some animals may benefit from the use of diets containing either a fermentable or non-fermentable fibre source.

MESALAZINE

UK
Indications. Treatment of chronic colitis and maintenance of remission
Contra-indications. Renal impairment
Side-effects. Prolonged administration may cause keratoconjunctivitis sicca although less commonly than sulfasalazine
Warnings. Monitor Schirmer tear test at 1–3 month intervals
Dose. *Dogs*: *by mouth*, 10–20 mg/kg twice daily

POM Ⓗ **Asacol** (SmithKline Beecham) *UK*
Tablets, e/c, mesalazine 400 mg; 120

POM Ⓗ **Salofalk** (Cortecs) *UK*
Tablets, e/c, mesalazine 250 mg; 100

OLSALAZINE SODIUM

UK
Indications. Treatment of chronic colitis and maintenance of remission
Contra-indications. Renal impairment
Side-effects. Prolonged administration may cause keratoconjunctivitis sicca although less commonly than sulfasalazine
Warnings. Monitor Schirmer tear test at 1–3 month intervals
Dose. *Dogs*: *by mouth*, 10–20 mg/kg twice daily

POM Ⓗ **Dipentum** (Pharmacia & Upjohn) *UK*
Tablets, scored, olsalazine sodium 500 mg; 60
Capsules, olsalazine sodium 250 mg; 100

SULFASALAZINE
(Sulphasalazine)

UK
Indications. Treatment of chronic colitis and maintenance of remission
Side-effects. Prolonged administration may cause keratoconjunctivitis sicca
Warnings. Monitor Schirmer tear test at 1–3 month intervals
Dose. *By mouth*.
Dogs: 15–30 mg/kg 3 times daily until response then reduce to lowest effective maintenance dose. Dose may be increased up to 50 mg/kg 3 times daily if required
Cats: 10–20 mg/kg once daily

POM Ⓗ **Sulfasalazine** (Non-proprietary) *UK*
Tablets, sulfasalazine 500 mg

POM Ⓗ **Salazopyrin** (Pharmacia & Upjohn) *UK*
Tablets, scored, sulfasalazine 500 mg; 100, 300
Oral suspension, sulfasalazine 50 mg/mL; 500 mL

3.2 Drugs used in the treatment of bloat

Acute ruminal distension can result in compromise of respiratory and cardiovascular function, and requires urgent treatment. In dogs, gastric dilatation/torsion is a surgical emergency with adjunctive therapy given as necessary. In ruminants, medical treatment, with or without surgical intervention, may be effective depending on the type of bloat.

Ruminal tympany or bloat is the accumulation of gas in the rumen in a stable foam (frothy bloat) or as free gas. In the majority of cases, free gas bloat is secondary to other diseases such as oesophagitis, oesophageal foreign body or other oesophageal obstruction, vagal nerve lesions, ruminitis, tetanus, and ruminal acidosis. Frothy bloat is dietary in origin and occurs when leguminous plants or high grain diets, which contain foam-forming agents, are ingested. In frothy bloat a stable foam is produced which traps the gases of fermentation. Small gas bubbles are unable to coalesce thereby preventing their removal by eructation. The production of insufficient saliva, which is alkaline, may also exacerbate frothy bloat.

Treatment of free gas bloat includes ruminal intubation or trocharisation to allow the release of gas. Medical treatment of frothy bloat requires the administration of an antifoaming agent to break down the stable foam. **Oils** such as sunflower oil or arachis oil (peanut oil) are given via stomach tube at a dose of 250 mL for cattle and 50 mL for sheep. Traditionally, turpentine oil and linseed oil have been used to treat bloat and may still play a role in cases induced by grain overload. Turpentine oil may taint meat and milk and is readily absorbed from the gastro-intestinal tract and skin. Absorption may lead to clinical signs of renal and gastro-intestinal toxicity including colic, diarrhoea, incoordination, and excitement, followed by coma. Fish oils stabilise the foam and are contra-indicated in the treatment of frothy bloat. Paraffinic oil may be administered to the animal or applied to the pasture.

Poloxalene is a nonionic surfactant used for the treatment and prevention of frothy bloat. Silicones such as **dimeticone** reduce the surface tension of gas bubbles causing them to coalesce. It is used in the treatment of frothy bloat. **Sodium bicarbonate** may also be used for the treatment of frothy bloat at a dose of 150 to 200 g dissolved in one litre of water given via stomach tube to cause alkalinosis of ruminal contents. Caution should be exercised because further gas production may occur.

The prevention and control of bloat includes limited pasture access, avoiding finely milled feeds, and maintaining a high fibre content in the diet. Antifoaming substances may be included in the feed, drinking water, or sprayed on the crops.

DIMETICONE
(Dimethicone)

UK
Indications. Frothy bloat

GSL **Battles Bloat Remedy** (Battle Hayward & Bower)
Oral liquid, dimethicone 1%, for *cattle*
Withdrawal Periods. Slaughter withdrawal period nil, milk withdrawal period nil
Dose. *Cattle*: *by mouth*, 50 –100 mL

GSL **Birp** (Arnolds)
Oral liquid, dimeticone emulsion BVetC 65, for *cattle*; 100 mL
Dose. *Cattle*: *by mouth*, 100 mL

Eire
Indications. Frothy bloat

E.M.S. Bloat Treatment (Foran) *Eire*
Oral solution, activated dimeticone (simethicone) 3.6%, for *cattle, sheep*
Withdrawal Periods. Slaughter withdrawal period nil, milk withdrawal period nil
Dose. *Cattle*: *by mouth*, 100 mL mixed with 500 mL water
Sheep, *by mouth*, 25 mL mixed with 100 mL water

USA
Indications. Flatulence in dogs

Nutrived Flatulex Chewable Tablets (Vedco) *USA*
Tablets, activated dimeticone (simethicone) 80 mg, for *dogs*
Dose. *Dogs*: *by mouth*, 1–4 tablets (depending on body-weight) after each feeding and at bedtime

DOCUSATE

Australia
Indications. Bloat

Tympanyl (Intervet) *Austral.*
Liquid, docusate sodium 290 mg, carbomers 21 mg, soya bean oil 64.4 mL, triethanolamine 21 mg, polysorbate 80, 5.2 mL, sodium hydroxide 0.6 mg / 100 mL, for *cattle, horses* (see section 3.6.4), *sheep* (see section 3.6.4)
Dose. *Cattle*: *by mouth or stomach tube*, 350 mL

USA
Indications. Frothy bloat, faecal softener
Contra-indications. Concurrent administration of mineral oil or other drugs

Bloat Release (AgriLabs) *USA*
Oral emulsion, docusate sodium 8 mg/mL, for *cattle, sheep, goats*
Withdrawal Periods. *Cattle, sheep, goats*: slaughter 3 days, milk 96 hours
Dose. *Cattle*: *by mouth or stomach tube*, 2.88 g
Calves, sheep, goats: *by mouth or stomach tube*, 1.44 g

Bloat Treatment (Butler, DurVet) *USA*
Oral emulsion, docusate sodium 8 mg/mL, for *cattle, sheep, goats*
Dose. *Cattle*: *by mouth or stomach tube*, 2.88 g
Calves, sheep, goats: *by mouth or stomach tube*, 1.44 g

Bloat Treatment (AgriPharm, RXV) *USA*
Oral emulsion, docusate sodium 8 mg/mL, for *cattle, sheep, goats*
Withdrawal Periods. *Cattle, sheep, goats*: slaughter 3 days, milk 96 hours
Dose. *Cattle*: *by mouth or stomach tube*, 2.88 g
Calves, sheep, goats: *by mouth or stomach tube*, 1.44 g

LINSEED OIL

UK
Indications. Frothy bloat, in combination with turpentine oil
Dose. *Cattle*: 0.6–1.2 litres
Sheep: 100–250 mL

PARAFFINIC OIL

Australia
Indications. Frothy bloat
Dose. See preparation details

Anti-Bloat Oil (Australian Petroleum) *Austral.*
Liquid, highly refined paraffinic oil 822 g/L (970 mL/L), for *cattle*
Withdrawal Periods. *Cattle*: slaughter withdrawal period nil, milk withdrawal period nil
Dose. *Cattle*: *by mouth*, 110–140 mL oral solution *or* 70 mL applied to flank of cow at each milking
by addition to drinking water, 100 mL/cow
by addition to feed in stall, 100 mL/cow

Anti-Bloat Oil (Mobil Oil) *Austral.*
Liquid, highly refined paraffinic oil 820 g/L (970 mL/L), for *cattle*
Dose. *Cattle*: *by mouth*, 55–85 mL in 100 mL water
by addition to feed, 55–85 mL/cow

Pasture Spray Oil (Austral.ian Petroleum) *Austral.*
Liquid, highly refined emulsifiable paraffinic oil, for *cattle*
Withdrawal Periods. *Cattle*: slaughter withdrawal period nil, milk withdrawal period nil
Dose. *Cattle*: *by mouth*, 110–140 mL oral solution *or* 70 mL applied to flank of cow at each milking. May also be applied to pasture (see data sheet)

POLOXALENE

UK
Indications. Treatment and prevention of frothy bloat

PML **Bloat Guard Drench** (Agrimin) *UK*
Oral liquid, poloxalene 833 mg/mL, for *cattle*; 60 mL. To be diluted before use
Withdrawal Periods. *Cattle*: slaughter 3 days, milk 24 hours
Dose. *Cattle*: treatment, (up to 227 kg body-weight) 30 mL diluted in 500 mL water given as oral solution; (>227 kg body-weight) 60 mL diluted in 500 mL water given as oral solution
Treatment, severe cases , (up to 227 kg body-weight) 30 mL diluted in 4.5 litres water given by stomach tube; (>227 kg body-weight) 60 mL diluted in 4.5 litres water given by stomach tube

PML **Bloat Guard Premix** (Agrimin)
Premix, poloxalene 530 mg/g, for *cattle*; 25 kg
Withdrawal Periods. *Cattle*: slaughter 3 days, milk withdrawal period nil
Dose. *Cattle*: prevention, *by addition to feed*, 22 mg of poloxalene/kg body-weight daily given 2–3 days before and throughout period of risk. May be increased to 44 mg of poloxalene/kg if high risk

Australia
Indications. Bloat

Bloat Master (Nutrimol) *Austral.*
Liquid, aliphatic alcohol propoxylate ethoxylate polyether 969 g/L, for *cattle*
Withdrawal Periods. *Cattle*: slaughter withdrawal period nil, milk withdrawal period nil
Dose. *Cattle*: *by addition to feed*, 5–12 mL twice daily
by mouth, 25 mL in 200–300 mL water

Milkwell Trough-Add (Wells) *Austral.*
Liquid, polyalkalene glycol block co-polymer 960 g/L (with dye indicator), for *cattle*
Dose. *Cattle*: *by addition to drinking water*, 30 mL/90 litres water, then 30 mL/10 cows twice daily
by mouth, 15–30 mL in 30–60 mL water

USA

Indications. Bloat

Bloat Guard Liquid (Pfizer) *USA*
Oral liquid, poloxalene 99.5%, for *cattle*
Dose. *Cattle*: *by addition to liquid feed*, 1.65–2.2%w/w

Bloat Guard (Pfizer) *USA*
Top dressing, poloxalene 53%, for *cattle*
Dose. *Cattle*: *by addition to feed*, 22–44 mg/kg body-weight/day

Bloat Guard (Pfizer) *USA*
Premix, poloxalene 53%, for *cattle*
Dose. *Cattle*: *by addition to feed*, 22–44 mg/kg body-weight/day

Therabloat (Pfizer) *USA*
Oral solution, poloxalene 25 g/30 mL, for *cattle*
Dose. *Cattle*: *by mouth*, 25–50 g in 473.2 mL water
by stomach tube, 25–50 g in 3.785 litres water

TURPENTINE OIL

UK

Indications. Frothy bloat, in combination with linseed oil
Warnings. May taint meat and milk; see notes above
Dose. *Cattle*: 15–60 mL
Sheep: 3–15 mL

3.3 Drugs used in the treatment of equine colic

Colic describes the clinical sign of abdominal pain, particularly in horses. The most frequent causes of colic signs are intestinal problems. The aetiology of these is very diverse and in many cases poorly understood. Recognised factors are diet changes, overfeeding, sand ingestion, and parasites including strongyles, ascarids, and tapeworms. Stress, changes in stabling and levels of activity, dental problems, certain feeds, and climatic changes have also been implicated. Free access to pasture, a grain free diet, and good quality hay are factors known to decrease the incidence of colic. Differential diagnoses include exertional rhabdomyolysis, laminitis, and peritonitis.

A careful clinical evaluation is required to determine whether the horse has a simple, non-strangulating obstruction that will require medical therapy or a strangulating obstruction that is already causing, or has the potential to cause, intestinal infarction and will require surgery. Rectal examination will help to reach a definitive diagnosis in some cases. A thorough assessment of the cardiovascular

parameters is vital for detection of developing endotoxaemia.

Following initial treatment, the patient should be re-evaluated after two hours and sooner if the animal's condition deteriorates. Surgical cases should be referred promptly. If sedation is necessary for transport, xylazine (see section 6.1.3) is suitable. The NSAID, flunixin meglumine, decreases endotoxic shock and does not reduce gastro–intestinal motility but is effective for up to 8 hours. Therefore flunixin meglumine should not be used in the colic case unless surgery has definitely been decided upon (or decided against) because this drug may mask clinical signs until it is too late for successful surgery. Acepromazine is contra-indicated for patients with colic because of its hypotensive properties.

Analgesics are required for treatment. These should have minimal adverse effects on the cardiovascular system and, except in spasmodic colic, on gastro-intestinal motility. NSAIDs may be used and phenylbutazone combined with ramifenazone (Tomanol) is effective without having significant adverse effects. Opioid analgesics are employed (see section 6.3). Butorphanol provides more consistent results than methadone or pethidine and has minimal cardiovascular effects at lower dosages. Butorphanol has been shown to decrease propulsive bowel motility when given in repeated doses. Xylazine and detomidine are effective although quite short acting; detomidine being of greater duration of action. Both reduce intestinal motility and cause a transient fall in blood pressure. Care should be taken to avoid overmedication. Whenever gastric distension is suspected, decompression is essential.

Spasmodic colic is best treated with **antispasmodics** such as Buscopan Compositum, which contains hyoscine butylbromide and metamizole (see section 10.3).

Patients with pelvic flexure impactions should be given **laxatives** such as liquid paraffin (see section 3.6.1) 4 litres/450 kg body-weight. Concurrent analgesia is usually required because oils may take 24 hours or longer to be effective. Ispaghula or psyllium (see section 3.6.2) may be useful agents for the treatment of sand impaction in horses.

In all cases of colic, adequate **fluid therapy** (see section 16.1.2), given intravenously, should be administered as necessary. Horses with severe hypovolaemia may be treated with hypertonic saline (sodium chloride 7.2%) at the rate of 4 to 6 mL/kg given over 15 minutes. This must be followed with 15 to 20 litres of intravenous isotonic fluids within 2 hours until the horse is stabilised. Hypertonic saline is contra-indicated if there is impaired renal function or in horses suffering from exhaustion or water deprivation.

Since most risk factors for colic are unproven, it is difficult to offer accurate advice on prevention. Helminth management for both roundworm and tapeworm should be considered. It is important to ensure that the horse is receiving appropriate feeds in a regular routine and that the animal has no dental problems. A study of the general management and potential stress problems such as changes in stable or exercise routine may be helpful.

3.4 Anti-emetics

3.4.1 Drugs used in the treatment of non-specific vomiting

3.4.2 Drugs used in the prevention of motion sickness

Vomiting follows stimulation of the vomiting centre in the medulla and the closely associated chemoreceptor trigger zone which is sensitive to many drugs and to certain metabolic disturbances. Stimulation of the vomiting centre also occurs following activation of other areas such as the vestibular apparatus of the ear as in motion sickness. Vomiting may be due to systemic or metabolic disorders in addition to gastro-intestinal disease; the causative agent should be ascertained before treatment is commenced. If vomiting is prolonged, dehydration, hypokalaemia, and alkalosis may occur and replacement fluids and electrolytes may be necessary (see 16.1.2).

3.4.1 Drugs used in the treatment of non-specific vomiting

Nausea and vomiting in gastro-intestinal disease may be due to stimulation of a variety of receptors. Anti-emetic therapy in patients with gastro-intestinal disease is therefore best initiated with a broad-spectrum anti-emetic drug.

Alpha$_2$-adrenergic blocking drugs (alpha$_2$-adrenergic antagonists) such as **acepromazine**, **chlorpromazine** and **prochlorperazine** are often used initially in undiagnosed vomiting because they have a broad spectrum of anti-emetic activity, acting at both the chemoreceptor trigger zone and the vomiting centre. Hypotension and sedation are potential side-effects and use of phenothiazines should be avoided in hypovolaemic animals.

Metoclopramide is a dopamine D$_2$ and 5HT$_3$ receptor antagonist, which acts at both the chemoreceptor trigger zone and gastro-intestinal smooth muscle. It increases motility of the gastro-intestinal tract without affecting gastric acid secretion, and is especially useful to facilitate gastric emptying in dogs and cats. It should not be used if there is suspicion of gastric or intestinal foreign body.

Metoclopramide may cause restlessness and excitement in certain individuals at the usual dose; in these dogs and cats a lower dose such as 250–500 micrograms/kg 3–4 times daily by mouth or by intramuscular or intravenous injection is recommended.

Cisapride (see section 3.7) facilitates gastric emptying in dogs and cats and is used if gastric retention related vomiting does not respond to metoclopramide.

Erythromycin at sub-antimicrobial dosages also improves gastric emptying in dogs and cats and may be used where gastric retention is suspected.

Vomiting due to uraemia has both central and peripheral components. The central component is associated with activation of the chemoreceptor trigger zone and is best treated with metoclopramide. The peripheral component is associated with uraemic gastritis and is treated with H$_2$-receptor antagonists such as cimetidine (see section 3.8.2) at a dose of 2.5 to 5.0 mg/kg 2 to 3 times daily by mouth and gastroprotectants for example sucralfate (see section 3.8.2) 0.25 to 1.0 g 3 times daily in dogs or 250 mg 2 to 3 times daily in cats.

CHLORPROMAZINE HYDROCHLORIDE

UK

Indications. Gastritis; prevention of motion sickness

Contra-indications. Renal or hepatic impairment

Side-effects. May cause drowsiness, hypotension

Warnings. Owing to the risk of contact sensitisation, operators should avoid direct contact with chlorpromazine; tablets should not be crushed and solutions should be handled with care.

Dose. *Dogs, cats*.

Motion sickness, *by mouth*, 0.5–1.0 mg/kg

Gastritis, *by subcutaneous or intramuscular injection*, 200–400 micrograms/kg 3 times daily

by intravenous injection, 50 micrograms/kg 3–4 times daily

POM Ⓗ **Chlorpromazine** (Non-proprietary) *UK*
Tablets, coated, chlorpromazine hydrochloride 10 mg, 25 mg, 50 mg, 100 mg
Oral solution, chlorpromazine hydrochloride 5 mg/mL, 20 mg/mL; 100 mL
Injection, chlorpromazine hydrochloride 25 mg/mL; 1 mL, 2 mL

POM Ⓗ **Largactil** (Hawthorn) *UK*
Tablets, f/c, chlorpromazine hydrochloride 10 mg, 25 mg, 50 mg, 100 mg
Syrup, chlorpromazine hydrochloride 5 mg/mL, 20 mg/mL; 100 mL
Injection, chlorpromazine hydrochloride 25 mg/mL; 2 mL

METOCLOPRAMIDE HYDROCHLORIDE

UK

Indications. Vomiting due to gastritis, oesophageal reflux; ruminal atony, paralytic ileus; see notes above

Contra-indications. Gastric outlet obstruction

Side-effects. Occasional transient incoordination and excitement

Warnings. Manufacturer does not recommend administration to animals in early stages of pregnancy; caution with administration to epileptics; Drug Interactions – see Appendix 1

Dose.

Horses: *by intravenous infusion*, 40 micrograms/kg per hour

Cattle: initial dose *by intravenous injection*, 0.5–1.0 mg/kg then *by intramuscular injection*, 0.5–1.0 mg/kg twice daily (maximum 2 doses by intramuscular injection)

calves: *by intravenous injection*, 0.5–1.0 mg/kg

Dogs, cats: *by mouth or by subcutaneous, intramuscular, or intravenous injection*, 0.5–1.0 mg/kg daily. May be administered twice daily if required.

May cause excitement in certain individuals, see also notes and dose above

by intravenous infusion, 1–2 mg/kg daily

POM Ⓗ **Metoclopramide** (Non-proprietary) *UK*
Tablets, metoclopramide 10 mg
Oral solution, metoclopramide hydrochloride 1 mg/mL; 100 mL
Injection, metoclopramide 5 mg/mL

POM Ⓗ **Maxolon** (Monmouth) *UK*
Syrup, metoclopramide hydrochloride 1 mg/mL; 200 mL
Paediatric liquid, metoclopramide hydrochloride 1 mg/mL; 15 mL

POM Ⓗ **Maxolon High Dose** (Monmouth) *UK*
Intravenous infusion, metoclopramide hydrochloride 5 mg/mL; 20 mL. For dilution and use as an intravenous infusion

Australia
Indications. Gastro-intestinal disease, post-operative vomiting
Warnings. Caution when concurrent treatment is given
Dose. *Dogs, cats*: *by mouth or by intramuscular or intravenous injection*, 0.5–1.0 mg/kg 3–4 times daily. May be administered twice daily if required.

Metomide Anti-Emetic Injection (Delvet) *Austral.*
Injection, metoclopramide hydrochloride 5 mg/mL, for *dogs, cats*

Metomide Anti-Emetic Tablets (Delvet) *Austral.*
Tablets, metoclopramide hydrochloride 10 mg, for *dogs, cats*

PROCHLORPERAZINE

UK
Indications. Gastritis; prevention of motion sickness
Side-effects. May cause drowsiness, hypotension
Dose. *Dogs, cats*.
Motion sickness, *by mouth*, up to 500 micrograms/kg
Gastritis, *by intramuscular (preferred) injection*, 100–500 micrograms/kg 3–4 times daily
by intravenous injection, 50 micrograms/kg 3–4 times daily

POM Ⓗ **Prochlorperazine** (Non-proprietary) *UK*
Tablets, prochlorperazine maleate 5 mg

POM Ⓗ **Stemetil** (Castlemead) *UK*
Tablets, prochlorperazine maleate 5 mg
Syrup, prochlorperazine mesilate 1 mg/mL; 100 mL
Injection, prochlorperazine mesilate 12.5 mg/mL; 1 mL, 2 mL

3.4.2 Drugs used in the prevention of motion sickness

Motion sickness is believed to arise from stimulation of the labyrinthine structures in the inner ear.

In dogs, motion sickness may be treated with H_1-histaminergic antagonists such as **diphenhydramine**. **Cyclizine** is an antihistamine. It acts directly on the neural pathways arising in the vestibular apparatus. The action of cyclizine may last for 8 to 12 hours.

Acepromazine, chlorpromazine (see section 3.4.1), and **prochlorperazine** (see section 3.4.1) are phenothiazine derivatives which have alpha$_2$-adrenergic blocking activity. They are broad-spectrum anti-emetics which can also be used because their sedative properties may be of additional benefit in controlling motion sickness. In cats, chlorpromazine appears to be the more effective drug. Acepromazine (see section 6.1.1) 0.5 to 1.0 mg/kg by mouth, 15 to 30 minutes before a light meal is used for preventing motion sickness in dogs and cats. Acepromazine is effective for up to 24 hours.

CYCLIZINE HYDROCHLORIDE

UK
Indications. Prevention of motion sickness
Side-effects. May cause drowsiness
Dose. *Dogs*: *by mouth*, 25–100 mg daily in divided doses

P Ⓗ **Valoid** (GlaxoWellcome) *UK*
Tablets, scored, cyclizine hydrochloride 50 mg; 100

DIPHENHYDRAMINE

UK
Indications. Prevention of motion sickness
Dose. *Dogs*. *by mouth*, 2–4 mg/kg 3 times daily

See section 14.2.2 for preparation details

3.5 Emetics

Vomiting is a protective reflex that occurs effectively only in certain species. True emesis is not possible in horses, ruminants, rabbits, and rodents. Regurgitation may occur in these species but is indicative of severe illness.

In other species emesis may be induced, if the animal has ingested a poisonous or undesirable substance within the previous 1 to 2 hours, in order to empty the stomach and so minimise further absorption of toxin. See also Treatment of poisoning.

Ipecacuanha has an irritant action on the gastro-intestinal tract and may be used to induce emesis in dogs and cats. However, its effectiveness is unpredictable. In cases of poisoning, ipecacuanha syrup should not be used in conjunction with activated charcoal because the effectiveness of the charcoal is reduced. **Apomorphine** is also used to induce emesis in cases of poisoning.

Although **not** generally recommended, in an emergency information on emesis may be given to the owner. Crystalline **washing soda** (sodium carbonate), **salt** (sodium chloride), or **mustard** deposited over the back of the tongue and swallowed can cause vomiting.

Xylazine (see section 6.1.3) 200 micrograms/kg♦ by intravenous injection has been used in dogs and cats for inducing emesis; administration at this dose should not cause undue sedation.

IPECACUANHA

UK
Indications. Induction of emesis
Contra-indications. Poisoning with corrosive compounds or petroleum products (risk of aspiration); shock; see notes above
Side-effects. Cardiac effects if absorbed
Dose. *Dogs, cats*: 1–2 mL/kg. Maximum dose 15 mL for dogs

P Ⓗ **Paediatric Ipecacuanha Emetic Mixture** (Non-proprietary) *UK*
Ipecacuanha liquid extract 0.7 mL, hydrochloric acid 0.025 mL, glycerol 1 mL, syrup to 10 mL

3.6 Laxatives

3.6.1 Lubricant laxatives
3.6.2 Bulk-forming laxatives
3.6.3 Osmotic laxatives
3.6.4 Stimulant laxatives
3.6.5 Bowel cleansers

Laxatives loosen the bowel contents and induce defaecation. Drugs that have a stimulant effect on the intestines are known as purgatives or cathartics. The degree of intestinal stimulation is usually dose related.

3.6.1 Lubricant laxatives

Lubricant laxatives soften and lubricate the faecal mass, which allows expulsion. **Liquid paraffin** and **white soft paraffin** are commonly used and are thought generally safe, although prolonged use may cause problems. Lubricant laxatives line the mucosal surface and may inhibit the absorption of fat-soluble vitamins, other nutrients, or drugs. Absorption of small amounts of paraffin may lead to granulomatous lesions in the intestinal wall and the liver. Paraffins are not effective for chronic constipation or severe impactions.

Liquid paraffin may be used in the treatment of equine colic due to impaction. When liquid paraffin is administered to ruminants it should be mixed with ginger or mustard (except when given by stomach tube) in order to prevent inhalation. Oral dosing in horses is contra-indicated. Liquid paraffin may be mixed with food or sugar for administration to dogs and cats.

PARAFFINS

UK

Indications. Constipation; 'fur-balls'
Contra-indications. Prolonged use especially in young animals
Side-effects. Reduced absorption of nutrients; granulomatous lesions may develop with prolonged use
Warnings. Accidental administration into the trachea and bronchial tree may lead to lipid pneumonitis

Katalax (Vericore VP) *UK*
Oral paste, white soft paraffin 474 mg/g, for *cats*; 20 g
Dose. *Cats*: *by mouth*, ½–1 inch of paste 1–2 times daily

GSL Liquid Paraffin *UK*
Dose. By mouth.
Horses, cattle: 3–4 litres/450 kg body-weight; *foals*: 200–400 mL
Dogs: 2–60 mL
Cats: 2–10 mL

Australia

Indications. Constipation; 'fur-balls'
Contra-indications. Prolonged use especially in young animals
Side-effects. Reduced absorption of nutrients; granulomatous lesions may develop with prolonged use
Warnings. Prolonged use may lead to vitamin deficiency

Cat-Lax (Novartis) *Austral.*
Oral paste, white soft paraffin 33.331 g, malt syrup 33.331 g, lecithin 1.406 g, cod liver oil 1.134 g, caramel 0.422 g, vitamin E 0.0446 g and biotin 0.02 g in 70 g paste, for *cats*
Dose. *Cats*: *by mouth*, 2–3 cm of paste daily or 2–3 times weekly

Exelpet Tasty Furball Remover for Cats (Exelpet) *Austral..*
Oral paste, white soft paraffin 33.33 g/ 70 g paste (also contains malt syrup, lecethin, cod liver oil, caramel, biotin), for *cats*
Dose. *Cats*: *by mouth*, 2–3 cm of paste daily or 2–3 times weekly

Furlax (Pharmtech) *Austral.*
Oral paste, white soft paraffin 3.23 g, liquid paraffin 750 mg, codliver oil 250 mg, vitamin E 20 mg / 5 g paste, for *cats, small dogs*
Dose. *Dogs, cats*: *by mouth*, 5 g daily

Laxapet (Troy) *Austral.*
Oral paste, liquid paraffin 400 mg/g, for *cats, dogs*
Dose. *Dogs*: *by mouth*, 15–30 g (depending on size of dog) 2–3 times a week
Cats: *by mouth*, ingested fur, 5 g daily for 2–3 days, then 2.5 g 2–3 times weekly; laxative, 2.5 g 2–3 times weekly

New Zealand

Indications. Constipation; 'fur-balls'

Cat-lax (Pet Elite) *NZ*
Oral paste, white soft paraffin 474 mg/g, for *cats*
Dose. *Cats*: *by mouth*, 2–3 cm of paste daily or 2–3 times weekly

Furlax (Bomac) *NZ*
Oral paste, paraffin oils, cod liver oil , vitamin E , for *cats*
Dose. *Cats*: *by mouth*, 2 inch *(5 g)* of paste daily or 1–2 times weekly

USA

Indications. Constipation; 'fur-balls'
Contra-indications. Prolonged use especially in young animals
Side-effects. Reduced absorption of nutrients with prolonged use
Warnings. Accidental administration into the trachea and bronchial tree may lead to lipid pneumonitis

Cat Lax (Pharmaderm) *USA*
Oral paste, white soft paraffin 0.1%, for *cats*
Dose. *Cats*: *by mouth*, 1 inch of paste daily or 2–3 times weekly

Mineral Oil (AgriPharm, DurVet, First Priority, Vedco) *USA*
Oral liquid, liquid paraffin, for *horses, cattle, sheep, pigs, dogs*
Dose. *Horses, cattle*: *by mouth*, 946 mL
Sheep: *by mouth*, 150 mL
Pigs: *by mouth*, 473 mL
Dogs: *by mouth*, 30–60 mL

Mineral Oil (First Priority) *USA*
Oral liquid, liquid paraffin, for *horses, cattle, sheep, pigs, dogs*
Dose. *Horses, cattle*: *by mouth*, 473 mL
Sheep: *by mouth*, 150 mL
Pigs: *by mouth*, 473 mL
Dogs: *by mouth*, 30–60 mL

Mineral Oil 95 V (Butler) *USA*
Oral liquid, liquid paraffin, for *horses, cattle, sheep, pigs, dogs*
Dose. *Horses, cattle*: *by mouth*, 473 mL
Sheep: *by mouth*, 150 mL
Pigs: *by mouth*, 473 mL
Dogs: *by mouth*, 30–60 mL

Mineral Oil USP (Aspen) *USA*
Oral liquid, liquid paraffin, for *horses, cattle, sheep, pigs, dogs*
Dose. *Horses, cattle*: *by mouth*, 1.893–3.785 L
Sheep, goats, pigs: *by mouth*, 473–946 mL
Dogs: *by mouth*, 15–60 mL

Mineral Oil Light (AgriLabs) *USA*
Oral liquid, light liquid paraffin, for *cattle, horses, sheep, goats, pigs, dogs*
Dose. *Horses, cattle*: *by mouth*, 946 mL
Sheep: *by mouth*, 150 mL
Pigs: *by mouth*, 473 mL
Dogs: *by mouth*, 30–60 mL

Veterinary Mineral Oil (RXV) *USA*
Oral liquid, mineral oil, for *horses, cattle, sheep, pigs, dogs*
Dose. *Horses, cattle*: *by mouth*, 946 mL
Sheep: *by mouth*, 150 mL
Pigs: *by mouth*, 473 mL
Dogs: *by mouth*, 30–60 mL

3.6.2 Bulk-forming laxatives

Ispaghula and **sterculia** take up water in the gastro-intestinal tract, thereby increasing the volume of the faeces and promoting peristalsis. They are used in the management of chronic constipation and when excessive rectal straining is to be avoided, such as following surgery for perineal hernia repair or anal sac removal. Due to their ability to increase faecal mass they are also used in the control of diarrhoea. Ispaghula or sterculia (rather than bran) are used in patients that cannot tolerate gluten-containing diets. Ispaghula may be a useful agent for the treatment of sand impaction in horses.

Bran provides water-insoluble fibre and is obtained from the outer layer of cereal grains, usually wheat. It is also used to treat chronic constipation. Unprocessed wheat bran contains approximately 40% wheat fibre. As a guide, for dogs and cats, 1 to 2 tablespoonfuls of unprocessed bran are given per 450-g can of food consumed.

Adequate fluid intake should be provided when using bulk laxatives to avoid dehydration and consequent worsening of constipation leading to intestinal obstruction.

BRAN

UK

Indications. Constipation
Contra-indications. Abdominal pain, vomiting, intestinal obstruction
Side-effects. Flatulence, abdominal distension
Warnings. Water must be available at all times

Nutrifyba (Ceva) *UK*
Oral powder, wheat fibre 80%, for *dogs, cats*; 3.5 g, 250 g
Dose. *By addition to food*.
Dogs: 1.75–7.0 g of powder daily
Cats: 1.75 g of powder daily

ISPAGHULA HUSK

UK

Indications. Constipation
Contra-indications. **Side-effects**. **Warnings**. See under Bran

GSL Ⓗ **Isogel** (Pfizer Consumer Healthcare) *UK*
Oral granules, ispaghula husk 90%; 150 g, 300 g
Dose. *By addition to food*.
Horses: 75 g/450 kg body-weight 1–2 times daily for 2 weeks
Dogs: one to three 5-mL spoonfuls 1–2 times daily
Cats: one 5-mL spoonful 1–2 times daily

METHYLCELLULOSE

Australia

Indications. Constipation
Dose. *Dogs*: *by addition to feed*, 0.5–5.0 g daily
Cats: *by addition to feed*, 0.5–1.0 g daily

Methylcellulose (Apex) *Austral.*
Oral powder, methylcellulose, for *cats, dogs*

PSYLLIUM

Australia

Indications. Constipation

Nutra Vet Natural Fibre (Nutra Vet) *Austral.*
Oral powder, psyllium fibre 98%, for *cats, dogs*
Dose. *Dogs, cats*: *by addition to feed*, 1–6 teaspoonfuls/meal depending on body-weight

USA

Indications. Constipation; prevention of sand colic

Equi-Phar Sweet Psyllium (Vedco) *USA*
Premix, psyllium 100%, for *horses*
Withdrawal Periods. Should not be used in *horses* intended for human consumption
Dose. *Horses*: *by addition to feed*, psyllium 113 g daily for 3 days. Discontinue for 3 days, then use for 3 days. Repeat cycle for total of 30 days

Equine Enteric Colloid (Techmix) *USA*
Oral colloid, psyllium, for *horses*

Equine Psyllium (First Priority) *USA*
Oral colloid, psyllium hydrophilic mucilloid 100%, for *horses*
Dose. *Horses*: *by addition to feed*, psyllium 113 g daily for 3 days. Discontinue for 3 days, then use for 3 days. Repeat cycle for total of 30 days

Goldvet Laxative and Digestive Aid Granules (Landco) *USA*
Oral granules, psyllium husks 100 mg, bran 100 mg, both per 3 g scoop
Dose. One 3-g scoop/9 kg body-weight

STERCULIA

UK

Indications. Constipation; diarrhoea (see section 3.1.1)
Contra-indications. **Side-effects**. **Warnings**. See under Bran

GSL **Peridale Capsules** (Arnolds) *UK*
Capsules, sterculia 118 mg, for *cats*; 100
Dose. *Cats*: *by mouth*, 118 mg twice daily; *kittens*: 118 mg daily

GSL **Peridale Granules** (Arnolds) *UK*
Oral granules, sterculia 980 mg/g, for *dogs*; 175 g
Dose. *Dogs*: *by mouth or by addition to food*, (up to 5 kg body-weight) ½ 5-mL spoonful (1.5 g) daily, (5–15 kg body-weight) one 5-mL spoonful (3 g) 1–2 times daily, (>15 kg body-weight) one heaped 5-mL spoonful (6 g) 1–2 times daily

GSL **Peridale Paste** (Arnolds) *UK*
Oral paste, sterculia 120 mg/dose, for *cats*; metered-dose applicator
Dose. *Cats*: *by mouth*, 120 mg twice daily; *kittens*: 120 mg daily

New Zealand

Indications. Constipation; diarrhoea (see section 3.1.1)

Peridale Capsules (Bomac) *NZ*
Capsules, sterculia 118 mg, for *cats*
Dose. *Cats*: *by mouth*, 1–2 capsules daily

Peridale Granules (Bomac) *NZ*
Oral granules, sterculia 98 g/100 g, for *dogs*
Dose. *Dogs*: *by mouth or by addition to food,* (up to 5 kg body-weight) ½ 5-mL spoonful (1.5 g) daily, (5–15 kg body-weight) one 5-mL spoonful (3 g) 1–2 times daily, (>15 kg body-weight) one heaped 5-mL spoonful (6 g) 1–2 times daily

3.6.3 Osmotic laxatives

Osmotic laxatives are hypertonic solutions of poorly absorbed substances that retain water and promote its movement from the tissues into the intestinal lumen. The resulting bowel distension promotes peristalsis. Fluid should be available throughout treatment. These drugs are particularly contra-indicated as laxatives in dehydrated animals and should not be used in patients with renal failure.

Magnesium sulphate (Epsom salts) is effective within 3 to 12 hours in monogastric animals and after 12 to 18 hours in ruminants. **Sodium sulphate** (Glauber's salt) may be preferred because it has a less purgative and more predictable action.

Lactulose is not absorbed from the gastro-intestinal tract. It produces an osmotic diarrhoea of low faecal pH, discourages the proliferation of ammonia-producing organisms, and reduces absorption of ammonia. It is therefore also useful in the treatment of hepatic encephalopathy (see section 3.10).

Impacted rectal and colonic contents are best resolved by the use of an enema. Warm, soapy water solutions soften and break up the faecal mass. Intestinal distension will stimulate contractions of the gut wall.

Proprietary enema preparations containing **phosphates** or **sodium citrate** act as osmotic laxatives and are used to treat constipation, and evacuation of the bowel prior to surgery or radiographic examination. Phosphate-containing enemas cause electrolyte abnormalities, such as hyperphosphataemia or hypocalcaemia, in small dogs and cats and their use is contra-indicated in these animals.

LACTULOSE

UK

Indications. Constipation; hepatic encephalopathy (see section 3.10)
Contra-indications. Intestinal obstruction

P (H) **Lactulose** (Non-proprietary) *UK*
Oral solution, lactulose 0.62–0.74 g/mL, other ketoses; 200 mL
Dose. *By mouth*.
Horses: hepatic encephalopathy, 0.3 mL/kg 3–4 times daily
Dogs: constipation, 0.25–0.5 mL/kg 2–3 times daily (according to individual's response)
Hepatic encephalopathy, 0.5 mL/kg 3–4 times daily
Cats: constipation, 2.5–5.0 mL/animal 2–3 times daily
Hepatic encephalopathy, 0.25 mL/kg twice daily
Enema.
Dogs: hepatic encephalopathy, 5–15 mL with twice volume of water, administered 3 times daily

MAGNESIUM SALTS

UK

Indications. Constipation

GSL **Magnesium Hydroxide Mixture (Milk of Magnesia)** *UK*
Magnesium oxide (hydrated) about 80 mg/mL
Dose. *By mouth*.
Dogs: 5–10 mL
Cats: 2–6 mL

GSL **Magnesium Sulphate (Epsom salts)** *UK*
Dose. By mouth.
Horses: 1 g/kg body-weight given in 4 litres water
Cattle: 250–500 g
Pigs: 25–125 g
Dogs: 5–25 g
Cats: 2–5 g

USA

Indications. Mild constipation
Warnings. Avoid frequent or continual use

Carmilax Bolets (Pfizer) *USA*
Tablets, magesium hydroxide 27 g, for *cattle*
Withdrawal Periods. Should not be used in cattle intended for human consumption, milk 12 hours,
Dose. *Cattle*: *by mouth*, 1 g/kg (max. 162 g)

Carmilax Powder (Pfizer) *USA*
Oral solution, powder for reconstitution, magnesium hydroxide 794.2 g/kg of powder, for *cattle*
Withdrawal Periods. Should not be used in cattle intended for human consumption, milk 12 hours,
Dose. *Cattle*: *by mouth*, 1 g/kg given as solution containing 95 g/litre

Laxade Bolus (RXV) *USA*
Tablets, magnesium oxide 17.9 g, for *cattle*
Withdrawal Periods. Milk 1 day
Dose. *Cattle*: *by mouth*, 35.8–71.6 g

Laxade Powder (AgriPharm) *USA*
Oral powder, for solution, magnesium hydroxide 65%, for *cattle, sheep, goats*
Withdrawal Periods. Milk 12 hours
Dose. *Cattle*: *by mouth or stomach tube*, 293 g magnesium hydroxide/ 3.785 litres water
Sheep, goats: one-eighth to one-quarter of dose for cattle

Laxade Powder (RXV) *USA*
Oral powder, for solution, magnesium hydroxide 65%, for *cattle*
Dose. *Cattle*: *by mouth or stomach tube*, 293 g magnesium hydroxide/ 3.785 litres water

Magnalax Boluses (Aspen) *USA*
Tablets, magnesium oxide 17.9 g, for *cattle, sheep, goats*
Dose. *Cattle, sheep, goats*: *by mouth*, 35.8–71.6 g

Magnalax Bolus (Phoenix) *USA*
Tablets, magnesium oxide 17.9 g, for *cattle, sheep, goats*
Dose. *Cattle, sheep, goats*: *by mouth*, 2–4 tablets

Magnalax Bolus (Vedco) *USA*
Tablets, magnesium hydroxide 27 g, for *cattle*
Dose. *Cattle*: *by mouth*, 2–4 tablets

Magnalax Powder (Phoenix) *USA*
Oral solution, powder for reconsitution, magnesium hydroxide 65%, for *cattle, sheep, goats*
Withdrawal Periods. Milk 12 hours
Dose. *Cattle*: *by mouth or stomach tube*, 293 g magnesium hydroxide/ 3.785 litres water
Sheep, goats: one-eighth to one-quarter of dose for cattle

Magnalax Powder (Vedco) *USA*
Oral powder, for solution, magnesium hydroxide 65%, for *cattle, sheep, goats*
Dose. *Cattle*: *by mouth or stomach tube*, 293 g magnesium hydroxide/ 3.785 litres water
Sheep, goats: one-eighth to one-quarter of dose for cattle

Magne-Lax (Wendt) *USA*
Tablets, magnesium hydroxide 24 g, for *cattle*
Dose. *Cattle*: *by mouth*, 2–4 tablets

MVT Bolus (Butler) *USA*
Tablets, magnesium oxide 17.9 g, for *ruminants*
Dose. *Cattle*: *by mouth*, 2–4 tablets

MVT Powder (Butler) *USA*
Oral powder, for solution, magnesium hydroxide 65%, kaolin 35 %, for *cattle, sheep*
Withdrawal Periods. Milk 24 hours
Dose. *Cattle*: *by mouth or stomach tube*, 293 g magnesium hydroxide and 156 g kaolin/3.785 litres water
Sheep, goats: one-eighth to one-quarter of dose for cattle

Polymag bolus (Butler) *USA*
Tablets, magnesium hydroxide 90 g, for *cattle*
Dose. *Cattle*: *by mouth*, 2–4 tablets

Polyox II Bolus (Osborn, Vedco) *USA*
Tablets, magnesium hydroxide 5.4 g, for *cattle*
Dose. *Cattle*: *by mouth*, 2–4 tablets

Polyox Powder (Osborn) *USA*
Oral powder, for solution, magnesium hydroxide 106 g/pack, for *cattle*
Dose. *Cattle*: *by mouth*, 53–106 g magnesium hydroxide in water

Polyox Powder (Vedco) *USA*
Oral powder, for solution, magnesium hydroxide 96 g/pack, for *cattle*
Dose. *Cattle*: *by mouth*, 48–96 g magnesium hydroxide in water

Rumalax Bolus (AgriLabs) *USA*
Tablets, magnesium hydroxide 27 g, for *cattle*
Dose. *Cattle*: *by mouth*, 2–4 tablets

Rumen Boluses (DurVet) *USA*
Tablets, magnesium hydroxide 27 g, for *cattle*
Dose. *Cattle*: *by mouth*, 2–4 tablets

PHOSPHATES (RECTAL)

UK
Indications. Rectal impaction
Contra-indications. Cats, small dogs
Dose.
Dogs: (5–10 kg body-weight) ½ enema; (>10 kg body-weight) ½–1 enema as necessary

P Ⓗ **Fletchers' Phosphate Enema** (Pharmax) *UK*
Sodium acid phosphate 12.8 g, sodium phosphate 10.24 g/128 mL; 128-mL single dose bottle

SODIUM CITRATE (RECTAL)

UK
Indications. Rectal use in constipation
Dose. *Dogs, cats*: one enema as necessary

P Ⓗ **Micolette Micro-Enema** (Dexcel) *UK*
Sodium citrate 450 mg, sodium lauryl sulphoacetate 45 mg, glycerol 625 mg/5 mL with citric acid, potassium sorbate, and sorbitol; 5-mL dose applicator

P Ⓗ **Micralax Micro-Enema** (Medeva) *UK*
Sodium citrate 450 mg, sodium alkylsulphoacetate 45 mg, sorbic acid 5 mg/5 mL with glycerol and sorbitol; 5-mL dose applicator

P Ⓗ **Relaxit Micro-Enema** (Crawford) *UK*
Sodium citrate 450 mg, sodium lauryl sulphate 75 mg, sorbic acid 5mg/5 mL with glycerol and sorbitol; 5-mL dose applicator

SODIUM SULPHATE
(Glauber's salt)

UK
Indications. Constipation and impaction
Dose. *By mouth*.
Horses: 1–3 g/kg
Cattle: 60–120 g
Sheep: 10–15 g
Pigs: 15–30 g
Dogs: 0.5–2.0 g
Cats: 300–600 mg

3.6.4 Stimulant laxatives

In general, stimulant laxatives should not be used in the presence of severe constipation or obstructive lesions.
Bisacodyl and **phenolphthalein** are diphenylmethane stimulant laxatives, which produce their effect by stimulating colonic smooth muscle and the myenteric plexus to produce organised peristaltic contractions.
Bisacodyl is a useful adjunct to enemas for the treatment of mild to moderate constipation. Long-term treatment with bisacodyl can result in damage to the myenteric plexus.
Phenolphthalein has an initial effect of 4 to 6 hours but a proportion of the dose undergoes enterohepatic circulation. Therefore the action may be prolonged, although the circulating concentration may be too low to be effective.
Dantron is an anthraquinone laxative. Prolonged administration may cause degeneration of the myenteric plexus leading to loss of intestinal motility. Dantron is excreted into the milk and may affect offspring.
Docusate sodium probably acts both as a stimulant and as a softening agent.
Castor oil causes mucosal irritation and **linseed oil** can be toxic; they are infrequently used in veterinary medicine.

BISACODYL

UK
Indications. Constipation
Dose.
Dogs: (up to 5 kg body-weight) 5 mg daily; (5–25 kg body-weight) 10 mg daily; (more than 25 kg body-weight) 15–20 mg daily
Cats: 5 mg daily

GSL Ⓗ **Bisacodyl** (Non-proprietary) *UK*
Tablets, e/c, bisacodyl 5 mg

DANTRON
(Danthron)

Australia
Indications. Constipation
Contra-indications. Gastro-enteritis, diarrhoea, severe constipation, foreign body obstruction
Side-effects. Transient red-coloured urine

Warnings. Some dogs exhibit increased purgation and dose should be decreased

Dose. Dogs: by addition to feed, (10–20 kg body-weight) 1 g of powder; (25–35 kg body-weight) 2 g of powder

Bilex (Vetsearch) *Austral.*
Powder, dantron 300 mg, sodium lauryl sulphate 150 mg in 2 g powder, for *dogs*

DOCUSATE SODIUM
(Dioctyl sodium sulphosuccinate)

Australia

Indications. Constipation; pre-operative preparation (enema)

Warnings. Avoid inclusion of fats in the diet

Dose. See preparation details

Petese (Apex) *Austral.*
Enema, docusate sodium 21 mg with glycerol 0.9 mL/ 5 mL, for *cats, dogs*
Dose. Dogs, cats: 5 mL

Tympanyl (Intervet) *Austral.*
Liquid, docusate sodium 290 mg, carbomers 21 mg, soya bean oil 64.4 mL, triethanolamine 21 mg, polysorbate 80, 5.2 mL, sodium hydroxide 0.6 mg / 100 mL, for *cattle* (see section 3.2), *horses, sheep*
Dose. *Horses*: by mouth or stomach tube, 350 mL
Sheep: by mouth, 170 mL

USA

Indications. Constipation; pre-operative preparation (enema)

Dioctynate (Butler) *USA*
Enema/Oral solution, docusate sodium 5%, for *horses, dogs, cats*
Dose. *Horses*: by mouth, 240 mL in 3.785 litres water or mineral oil
Enema, 120–180 mL in 3.785 litres water
Dogs, cats: enema, 5 mL per 30 mL water. Give 60–90 mL of solution

Disposable Enema Syringe (Vedco) *USA*
Enema , docusate sodium 250 mg/syringe
Dose. 250 mg, may be repeated after 1 hour

Docusate Solution (Life Science) *USA*
Enema/Oral solution, docusate sodium 5%, for *horses, dogs, cats*
Withdrawal Periods. Should not be used in *horses* intended for human consumption
Dose. *Horses*: by mouth, 240 mL in 3.785 litres water or mineral oil
Enema, 120–180 mL in 3.785 litres water
Dogs, cats: enema, 5 mL per 30 mL water. Give 60–90 mL of solution

Enema-DSS (Butler) *USA*
Enema, docusate sodium 250 mg/syringe
Dose. 250 mg, may be repeated after 1 hour

Enema SA (Vetus) *USA*
Enema, docusate sodium 250 mg/12-mL syringe, for *dogs, cats*
Dose. 250 mg

Veterinary Surfactant (First Priority, Vedco) *USA*
Enema, Oral solution, docusate sodium 5%, for *horses, dogs, cats*
Dose. *Horses*: by mouth, 240 mL in 3.785 litres water or mineral oil
Enema, 120–180 mL in 3.785 litres water
Dogs, cats: enema, 10–15 mL in 60–90 mL water

LINSEED OIL

Australia

Indications. Constipation

Warnings. Rest horses for 48 hours after treatment

Pottie's Laxative Drench (Blue Cross) *Austral.*
Liquid, linseed oil 620 mL, turpentine oil 112 mL, ammonium carbonate solution 77 mL, tincture ginger 17 mL, tincture gentian 17 mL/L, for *horses*
Withdrawal Periods. *Horses*: slaughter withdrawal period nil
Dose. *Horses*: by mouth, 500 mL; *yearlings*: 250 mL

PHENOLPHTHALEIN

UK

Indications. Constipation

Warnings. See notes above

GSL **Laxative Tablets** (Bob Martin) *UK*
Tablets, phenolphthalein 100 mg, for *dogs*; 10

3.6.5 Bowel cleansers

Bowel cleansing solutions are used to evacuate the colon in preparation for colonoscopy, barium enema, and colon surgery. They are **not** treatments for constipation. When ingested, they produce a voluminous liquid stool with minimal changes in the patient's fluid and electrolyte balance. Bowel preparation is superior to that achieved by standard enema techniques.

In some patients vomiting may occur; this can be prevented by warming the lavage solution to body temperature or by giving parenteral metoclopramide (see section 3.4.1) before administration.

UK

Indications. See notes above

Contra-indications. Intestinal obstruction

Side-effects. Occasional vomiting, see notes above

P Ⓗ **Klean-Prep** (Norgine) *UK*
Oral solution, powder for reconstitution, anhydrous sodium sulphate 5.685 g, macrogol 3350 (polyethylene glycol 3350) 59 g, potassium chloride 743 mg, sodium bicarbonate 1.685 g, sodium chloride 1.465 g/sachet; 4
Reconstitute 1 sachet in 1 litre water
Dose. *Dogs*: by mouth, 12–18 hours before the procedure, administer 25–30 mL lavage solution/kg, repeat after 1 hour

3.7 Modulators of intestinal motility

Diphenoxylate and loperamide (see section 3.1.2) increase intestinal segmental (circular) contractions, decrease propulsive contractions, and are used for diarrhoea.

The antimuscarinics (anticholinergics), such as **atropine dimevamide**, **propantheline bromide**, and **hyoscine,** have antispasmodic activity. Propantheline bromide is less lipid soluble than atropine, and therefore less effectively absorbed and less likely to cross the blood-brain barrier. It has peripheral effects similar to atropine.

Hyoscine butylbromide in combination with metamizole (Buscopan Compositum, Spasmogesic) has been used in young calves for its antispasmodic effects in diarrhoea. However, the benefit of antispasmodics in diarrhoea is undetermined (see section 3.1.2). Buscopan Compositum is also used in equine colic both for its antispasmodic and analgesic properties. Buscopan Compositum is occasionally used in dogs as a long-acting gastro-intestinal antispasmodic. Side-effects in dogs include constipation and dysuria. It should not be used in cats.

Carbachol is a quaternary ammonium parasympathomimetic that increases intestinal motility. It is a very potent drug and can cause intestinal rupture. Conservative therapy, such as mineral oils for the treatment of intestinal blockage, is a safer alternative.

Metoclopramide (see section 3.4.1) stimulates gastric emptying and small intestinal transit, and enhances the strength of oesophageal sphincter contraction. In veterinary medicine, it is used to reduce vomiting in gastritis and following surgery, in the treatment of ruminal atony or abomasal atony and dilatation, for oesophageal reflux, and post-operative paralytic ileus in horses.

Cisapride is a motility stimulant that is believed to act by promoting release of acetycholine in the gut wall at the level of the myenteric plexus. Cisapride increases pressure of the lower oesophageal sphincter and thus assists in the treatment of reflux oesophagitis. Cisapride also promotes gastric emptying in animals with delayed voiding of gastric contents, and increases colonic motility in feline megacolon. Cisapride is reported to be an agonist at serotonin-4 (5-HT$_4$) receptors. Cisapride has been shown to increase gut motility in chronic cases of grass sickness in horses.

Ranitidine and **nizatidine** (see section 3.8.2) are H$_2$ receptor antagonists used to reduce gastric acidity. However at antisecretory dosages these drugs also inhibit acetylcholinesterase which leads to stimulation of gastric motility. They are therefore useful in treating delayed gastric emptying in dogs and cats.

Erythromycin (see section 1.1.4) is a macrolide antibacterial, which has prokinetic effects at microbially ineffective dosages through its action at motilin receptors in cats and 5HT$_3$ receptors in dogs. Erythromycin at a dose of 0.5 to 1.0 mg/kg can be used where there is delayed gastric emptying or intestinal pseudo-obstruction.

Many drugs have been tried for treatment of post operative ileus in horses. They include cisapride, lidocaine, neostigmine, metoclopramide, phenylephrine, domperidone, bethanecol, and erythromycin; none have shown consistant efficacy and some have undesirable side-effects.

ATROPINE SULPHATE

UK

Indications. Adjunct in gastro-intestinal disorders characterised by smooth muscle spasm; pre-anaesthetic medication (see section 6.6.1), antidote for organophosphorus poisoning (see Treatment of poisoning)
Contra-indications. Glaucoma, congestive heart failure, intestinal hypomotility
Side-effects. Dry mouth, dilatation of pupils and photophobia, constipation, urinary retention, tachycardia
Dose. *By subcutaneous injection.*
Horses, cattle: 10 micrograms/kg
Sheep: 80–160 micrograms/kg
Pigs: 20–40 micrograms/kg
Dogs, cats: 30–100 micrograms/kg

See section 6.6.1 for preparation details

CISAPRIDE

UK

Indications. Motility stimulant; reflux oesophagitis; feline megacolon
Side-effects. High dosage may cause vomiting, diarrhoea, abdominal cramp in dogs and cats and dosage should be reduced in these patients; initial transient worsening of clinical signs of colic in horses
Dose. *By mouth.*
Horses: 200–800 micrograms/kg twice daily for 7 days
Dogs, cats: 100–500 micrograms/kg 2–3 times daily

POM Ⓗ **Prepulsid** (Janssen-Cilag) *UK*
Note. Product licence recently suspended in the UK until further notice because product has been associated with serious cardiovascular side-effects in humans

DIMEVAMIDE

USA

Indications. Gastro-intestinal disorders characterised by smooth muscle spasm
Contra-indications. Glaucoma
Side-effects. Disturbances in urination, dryness of the mouth and eyes
Warnings. Use with caution in pyloric obstruction
Dose. *Dogs, cats*: *by subcutanous or intramuscular injection,* (<4.5 kg body-weight) 100 micrograms 2–3 times daily

Centrine (Fort Dodge) *USA*
Injection, dimevamide hydrogen sulphate 0.5 mg/mL, for *dogs, cats*

Centrine (Fort Dodge) *USA*
Tablets, dimevamide hydrogen sulphate 0.2 mg, for *dogs, cats*

PROPANTHELINE BROMIDE

UK

Indications. Adjunct in gastro-intestinal disorders characterised by smooth muscle spasm; urinary incontinence (see section 9.3)
Contra-indications. Glaucoma, urinary obstruction
Side-effects. Dry mouth, increased intra-ocular pressure, constipation, tachycardia
Dose. *Dogs*: *by mouth,* 15–30 mg 2–3 times daily (large dogs only)

See section 9 3 for preparation details

Australia

Indications. Spasmodic colic, choke, rectal palpation
Contra-indications. Dry choke
Side-effects. Tachycardia
Dose. *Horses*: acute spasmodic colic, *by intravenous injection,* 100–300 mg
Rectal palpation, *by intravenous injection,* 50–100 mg

Propan B (RWR) *Austral.*
Injection, powder for reconstitution, propantheline bromide 300 mg, for *horses*
Withdrawal Periods. *Horses*: slaughter 28 days

New Zealand

Indications. Spasmodic colic, rectal palpation
Dose. *Horses*: *by intramuscular or intravenous injection,*
60–750 micrograms/kg (doses vary)

Propan-B (Vetpharm) *NZ*
Injection, propantheline bromide 300 mg, for *horses*
Dose. *Horses*: by intramuscular or intravenous injection, 250–750 micro-
grams/kg

Relax (Virbac) *NZ*
Injection, propantheline bromide 300 mg, for *horses*
Withdrawal Periods. Slaughter 28 days
Dose. *Horses*: by intramuscular or intravenous injection, 60–600 micro-
grams/kg

COMPOUND ANTISPASMODICS

UK

Indications. Gastro-intestinal spasm, urogenital spasm
Contra-indications. Intramuscular injection in horses;
pregnant animals
Warnings. Drug Interactions – other anticholinergic or
analgesic drugs
Dose. See preparation details

POM **Buscopan Compositum** (Boehringer Ingelheim) *UK*
Injection, metamizole 500 mg/mL, hyoscine butylbromide 4 mg/mL, for
horses, cattle, dogs; 100 mL
Withdrawal Periods. *Horses*: slaughter 9 days. *Cattle*: slaughter 9 days
(intravenous injection), 15 days (single intramuscular injection), 18 days
(multiple intramuscular injections), should not be used in cattle producing
milk for human consumption
Dose. *Horses*: by intravenous injection, 5 mL/100 kg
Cattle: by intramuscular or intravenous injection, 5 mL/100 kg; *calves*: 5
mL/50 kg mL
Dogs: by intramuscular or intravenous injection, 0.1 mL/kg

Australia

Indications. Gastro-intestinal spasm, urogenital spasm
Contra-indications. Intramuscular injection in horses
Dose. See preparation details

Buscopan Compositum (Boehringer Ingelheim) *Austral.*
Injection, hyoscine butylbromide 4 mg/mL, metamizole 500 mg/mL, for
horses, dogs
Withdrawal Periods. *Horses*: slaughter 28 days
Dose. *Horses*: by intravenous injection, 20–30 mL; foals: 5–10 mL
Dogs: by subcutaneous or intravenous injection, 1.0–2.5 mL

Buscopan Compositum (Boehringer Ingelheim) *Austral.*
Tablets, hyoscine butylbromide 10 mg, metamizole 250 mg, for *dogs*
Dose. *Dogs*: by mouth, (<10 kg body-weight), 1 tablet twice daily; (10–20
kg body-weight), 2 tablets twice daily; (20–40 kg body-weight), 3 tablets
twice daily

Spasmogesic (Ilium) *Austral.*
Injection, hyoscine butylbromide 4 mg/mL, metamizole 500 mg/mL, for
horses, dogs
Withdrawal Periods. *Horses*: slaughter 28 days
Dose. *Horses*: by intravenous injection, 20–30 mL; foals: 5–10 mL
Dogs: by subcutaneous or intravenous injection, 1.0–2.5 mL

New Zealand

Indications. Gastro-intestinal spasm, urogenital spasm
Dose. See preparation details

Buscopan Compositum Solution (Boehringer Ingelheim) *NZ*
Injection, hyoscine butylbromide 4 mg/mL, metamizole sodium 500 mg/mL,
for *horses, cattle, pigs, dogs*
Withdrawal Periods. *Horses*: slaughter 2 days. *Cattle*: slaughter 14 days,
milk 12 hours. *Pigs*: slaughter 14 days
Dose. *Horses*: by intravenous injection, 20–30 mL
Cattle: by intramuscular or intravenous injection, 20–25 mL; *calves*: by
intramuscular injection, 5–10 mL
Pigs: by intramuscular injection, 5–10 mL; *piglets*: 1–2 mL
Dogs: by subcutaneous or intravenous injection, 1.0–2.5 mL

Buscopan Compositum Tablets (Boehringer Ingelheim) *NZ*
Tablets, hyoscine butylbromide 10 mg, metamizole sodium 250 mg, for *dogs*
Dose. *Dogs*: by mouth, (2–10 kg body-weight), 1 tablet twice daily; (10–20
kg body-weight), 2 tablets twice daily; (20–40 kg body-weight), 3 tablets
twice daily

3.8 Antacids and ulcer-healing drugs

3.8.1 Antacids
3.8.2 Ulcer-healing drugs

The treatment and prevention of gastric and duodenal ulceration includes antacids alone or in combination with ulcer-
healing drugs.

3.8.1 Antacids

Antacids are used in the therapy of gastric ulceration (see
section 3.8.2). They neutralise gastric acid and this helps
ulcers to heal.

Antacids are also used to prevent and treat mild ruminal acidosis. Ruminal acidosis is caused by excessive carbohydrate intake from grain engorgement or soluble
carbohydrate overload, which leads to the production of
large quantities of lactic acid in the rumen instead of the
normal volatile fatty acids. While antacids alone may be
sufficient in mild ruminal acidosis, more severe cases will
require the adminstration of intravenous sodium bicarbonate and isotonic fluids therapy. Rumenotomy should be
performed in very severe cases in patients that are recumbent.

Sodium bicarbonate is soluble and acts rapidly, producing
carbon dioxide. This carbon dioxide may worsen pre-existing bloat often encountered in severe ruminal acidosis or
may be released by eructation. Gas may accumulate if the
rumen is atonic and lead to free gas bloat (see section 3.2).
Bicarbonate may be absorbed systemically and produce
alkalosis.

Aluminium- and **magnesium-containing** antacids react
with gastric acid to form an insoluble colloid which is not
absorbed to a significant extent. They are therefore long-
acting if retained in the stomach. Aluminium salts tend to
cause constipation whereas magnesium-containing antacids
may act as laxatives. Aluminium hydroxide lines gastric
mucosa and acts as a mechanical barrier against excess
acid. Aluminium accumulation does not appear to be a risk.
Aluminium salts are potent intestinal phosphate binders and
are also used to reduce serum-phosphate concentrations in
patients with renal failure. Aluminium hydroxide is the
drug of choice for ruminal acidosis.

Antacids should be given at least six times daily because infrequent antacid administration results in rebound acid hypersecretion. Antacids are best administered between meals and at night-time to dogs and cats. The need for frequent administration often makes therapy impractical in small animal medicine.

ALUMINIUM HYDROXIDE

UK
Indications. Gastric acidosis, gastric ulceration
Side-effects. Constipation
Warnings. Reduces the absorption of other drugs, see Drug Interactions – Appendix 1 (antacids)

GSL Ⓗ **Aluminium Hydroxide** (Non-proprietary) *UK*
Tablets, dried aluminium hydroxide 500 mg
Mixture (gel), approximately 40 mg Al₂O₃/mL; 200 mL
Dose. *Dogs, cats*: *by mouth*, 0.25–0.5 mL/kg 4–6 times daily, see notes above

Oral powder, aluminium hydroxide, available from chemical suppliers
Dose. *By mouth*.
Cattle: 15–30 g 2–3 times daily
Sheep: 1–2 g 2–3 times daily

GSL Ⓗ **Maalox** (Rhône-Poulenc Rorer) *UK*
Oral suspension, magnesium hydroxide 195 mg/5 mL, dried aluminium hydroxide 220 mg/5 mL; 500 mL
Dose. *Dogs, cats*: *by mouth*, 0.25–0.5 mL/kg 4–6 times daily, see notes above
Note. A mixture of aluminium hydroxide and magnesium hydroxide with the proportions expressed in the form *x/y* where *x* and *y* are the strengths in milligrams per unit dose of magnesium hydroxide and aluminium hydroxide respectively is called co-magaldrox.

GSL **Anti Flatulence Tablets** (Bob Martin) *UK*
Tablets, dried aluminium hydroxide gel 120 mg, magnesium trisilicate 250 mg, for *dogs*; 32

MAGNESIUM CARBONATE

UK
Indications. Adjunct in the treatment of abomasal ulceration
Dose. *Cattle*: 16 g

MAGNESIUM HYDROXIDE

UK
Indications. Adjunct in the treatment of abomasal ulceration
Dose. *Cattle*: 400–450 g/450 kg 2–3 times daily
Sheep: 10–30 g 2–3 times daily

USA
Indications. Mild ruminal acidosis; constipation

See section 3.6.3 for preparation details

MAGNESIUM OXIDE

UK
Indications. Adjunct in the treatment of abomasal ulceration
Dose. *Cattle*: 1–2 mg/kg

USA
Indications. Mild ruminal acidosis; constipation

See section 3.6.3 for preparation details

MAGNESIUM TRISILICATE

UK
Indications. Adjunct in the treatment of abomasal ulceration
Dose. *Cattle*: up to 16 g

SODIUM BICARBONATE

UK
Indications. Ruminal acidosis
Warnings. See notes above
Dose. *Cattle*: 60–120 g 2–3 times daily
Sheep: 40–60 g 2–3 times daily

USA
Indications. Ruminal acidosis
Warnings. Allow free access to water; withhold grain and-feed good quality roughage

Neutalizer (RXV) *USA*
Oral paste, sodium bicarbonate 50% (227 g/454 g paste), for *cattle*
Dose. *Cattle*: by mouth, 113.5 g/227 kg body-weight

3.8.2 Ulcer-healing drugs

Gastric ulceration may occur in all species but most commonly occurs in foals, performance horses, and dogs. Mucosal damage may be caused by parasite invasion, incorrect diet, liver disease, neoplasia, uraemia, or prolonged use of anti-inflammatory drugs such as NSAIDs or corticosteroids. In foals, stress appears to be an important factor. Management of gastric ulceration is aimed at treatment of the primary cause (if identified), inhibition of gastric acid secretion, and, if necessary, control of gastric haemorrhage. The finding that much gastric ulceration in humans is associated with infection by *Helicobacter pylori* has directed veterinary attention towards this genus, particularly in dogs and cats. Ulcers in these species are increasingly being managed using antimicrobial therapy, especially after gastric biopsy has confirmed their involvement.

In pigs, oesophageal ulceration has been associated with feeding finely ground particulate food, whey feeding, high dietary concentration of copper, fungal spoiling of food, inadequate concentrations of vitamin E and selenium, and is predisposed by environmental stress. Primary management should be by avoidance of dietary factors. Inclusion of zinc carbonate at a dose of 110 g/tonne in the pig ration reduces the ulcerogenic effect of dietary copper. Susceptibility to stress is heritable in some breeds of pigs.

The treatment of abomasal ulceration in cattle is usually conservative and includes kaolin and pectin oral suspension (see section 3.1.1) and antacids such as magnesium carbonate, magnesium oxide, or magnesium trisilicate.

Adult horses suffering from gastric ulceration may exhibit non-specific clinical signs such as poor appetite, unthrifti-ness, and abdominal pain. The significance of ulcers detected gastroscopically is not always clear. Omeprazole or ranitidine are used for treatment.

Cimetidine, famotidine, nizatidine, and **ranitidine** block H_2-receptors and inhibit the secretion of gastric acid and reduce pepsin output. Reduced gastric acid secretion allows the ulcer to heal. These drugs block hepatic microsomal drug metabolism and should be used with caution in patients receiving concurrent drug therapy. Famotidine and ranitidine are more potent than cimetidine and do not share its drug metabolism inhibitory properties.

Cimetidine can be used as an adjunct in the treatment of exocrine pancreatic insufficiency to inhibit acid peptic breakdown of pancreatic enzyme supplements.

Sucralfate binds to proteins at an ulcer site thereby provid-ing a protective barrier against acid-pepsin attack. It is used in conjunction with other drugs for the treatment of gastric ulceration. It should be given on an empty stomach at least one hour before a meal to avoid the drug binding to the food rather than the ulcer site. Sucralfate should not be relied upon as the sole treatment for gastric ulceration in horses. It is thought to be ineffective for lesions confined to the squa-mous mucosa of the stomach.

Omeprazole inhibits the hydrogen-potassium adenosine triphosphatase enzyme system (the 'proton pump'), which is responsible for gastric acid production by the parietal cell. It is more potent and longer acting than the H_2-receptor antagonists, and is used in patients failing to respond to other treatment.

Misoprostol, a synthetic analogue of prostaglandin E_1 (alprostadil) increases mucosal blood flow and mucus secretion and inhibits gastric acid secretion thereby promot-ing gastric and duodenal ulcer healing. It can protect against NSAID-associated gastric and duodenal ulcers. The use of misoprostol in horses is not well documented.

CIMETIDINE

UK

Indications. Gastric and duodenal ulceration; reflux oesophagitis; uraemic gastritis (see section 3.4.1); adjunct in exocrine pancreatic insufficiency; equine melanoma (but see notes above)
Warnings. Drug Interactions – see Appendix 1
Dose.
Horses: (*foals*) gastric ulceration, **by mouth,** 20 mg/kg 1–3 times daily
by intravenous injection, 8–10 mg/kg 4–6 times daily
Dogs, cats: gastric ulceration, *by mouth or by intramuscular or intravenous injection,* 10 mg/kg 3–4 times daily
Uraemic gastritis, *by mouth or by intravenous injection,* 2.5–5.0 mg/kg 2–3 times daily

POM Ⓗ **Cimetidine** (Non-proprietary) *UK*
Tablets, cimetidine 200 mg, 400 mg, 800 mg; more than 14 tablets

POM Ⓗ **Dyspamet** (SmithKline Beecham) *UK*
Oral suspension, cimetidine 40 mg/mL; 600 mL

POM Ⓗ **Tagamet** (SmithKline Beecham) *UK*
Tablets, f/c, cimetidine 200 mg; 12, 24
Syrup, cimetidine 40 mg/mL; 600 mL
Injection, cimetidine 100 mg/mL; 2 mL

P Ⓗ **Tagamet 100** (SmithKline Beecham) *UK*
Tablets, cimetidine 100 mg; 12, 24

FAMOTIDINE

UK

Indications. Gastric and duodenal ulceration
Dose. *Dogs*: *by mouth,* 500 micrograms/kg 1–2 times daily

POM Ⓗ **Pepcid** (MSD) *UK*
Tablets, famotidine 20 mg, 40 mg; 28, 50

P Ⓗ **Pepcid AC** (MSD) *UK*
Tablets, famotidine 10 mg; 6, 12

MISOPROSTOL

UK

Indications. NSAID-associated gastric and duodenal ulceration
Contra-indications. Pregnant animals
Side-effects. Dose dependent and may include diarrhoea, abdominal pain, nausea, abortion in pregnant animals
Warnings. Pregnant women should avoid exposure to miso-prostol
Dose. *Dogs*: *by mouth,* 2–5 micrograms/kg 3 times daily

POM Ⓗ **Cytotec** (Searle) *UK*
Tablets, scored, misoprostol 200 micrograms; 60

NIZATIDINE

UK

Indications. Gastric and duodenal ulceration; motility dis-orders
Dose. *Dogs*: *by mouth,* 2.5–5.0 mg/kg daily

POM Ⓗ **Nizatidine** (Non-proprietary) *UK*
Capsules, nizatidine 150 mg, 300 mg

POM Ⓗ **Axid** (Lilly) *UK*
Capsules, nizatidine 150 mg, 300 mg

OMEPRAZOLE

UK

Indications. Gastric and duodenal ulceration, see notes above; Zollinger-Ellison syndrome; reflux oesophagitis
Warnings. Prolonged administration not recommended
Dose. *By mouth.*
Horses: 1–4 mg/kg once daily
Dogs: *by mouth,* 0.5–1.0 mg/kg once daily

POM Ⓗ **Losec** (Astra) *UK*
Capsules, omeprazole 10 mg, 20 mg, 40 mg
Note. Should be dispensed in original container which contains a dessicant

RANITIDINE

UK

Indications. Gastric and duodenal ulceration; reflux oesophagitis; motility disorders

Dose.

Horses: *by mouth*, 6.6 mg/kg 3 times daily
foals: *by mouth*, 4–6 mg/kg 2–3 times daily
by intravenous injection, 1–2 mg/kg 3 times daily
Dogs: *by mouth or by intravenous injection*, 2 mg/kg twice daily

POM Ⓗ **Ranitidine** (Non-proprietary) *UK*
Tablets, ranitidine (as hydrochloride) 150 mg, 300 mg

POM Ⓗ **Zantac** (GlaxoWellcome) *UK*
Tablets, f/c, ranitidine (as hydrochloride) 150 mg; 60
Tablets, dispersible, scored, ranitidine (as hydrochloride) 150 mg; 60. Dissolve or mix with water before administration
Syrup, ranitidine (as hydrochloride) 15 mg/mL; 300 mL
Injection, ranitidine (as hydrochloride) 25 mg/mL; 2 mL

P Ⓗ **Zantac 75** (GlaxoWellcome) *UK*
Tablets, ranitidine (as hydrochloride) 75 mg; 5, 10

SUCRALFATE

UK

Indications. Gastric and duodenal ulceration; uraemic gastritis (see section 3.4.1)
Warnings. May affect absorption of other drugs and other oral drug therapy should not be given within 2 hours of sucralfate
Dose. Give on an empty stomach 1 hour before a meal, *by mouth*.

Foals: 10–20 mg/kg 4 times daily
Dogs: 0.25–1.0 g 3 times daily
Cats: 250 mg 2–3 times daily

POM Ⓗ **Sucralfate** (Non-proprietary)
Tablets, sucralfate 1 g

POM Ⓗ **Antepsin** (Chugai)
Tablets, scored, sucralfate 1 g; 112
Oral suspension, sucralfate 200 mg/mL; 560 mL

3.9 Treatment of pancreatic disease

Acute pancreatitis occurs most commonly in dogs, but has recently also been recognised in cats. The basis for treatment is maintenance of fluid and electrolyte balance while the pancreas is rested by withholding food, therefore allowing it to recover from the acute inflammation. Severe cases of pancreatitis require aggressive intravenous fluid therapy given over several days with nil given by mouth. Parenteral antibacterial prophylaxis is usually administered during this period. Analgesic therapy such as butorphanol is given if abdominal pain is severe. Transfusion of plasma or whole blood may be life-saving in severely ill patients that continue to deteriorate despite supportive care. Once vomiting has ceased, small amounts of water and then food may be re-introduced. The diet should be high in carbohydrate and low in fat to minimise pancreatic stimulation. Recurrence may be prevented by avoiding high fat content foods and reducing obesity. A low fat maintenance diet should be fed to dogs that have multiple attacks.

Exocrine pancreatic insufficiency (EPI) in dogs, particularly German Shepherds, is usually due to pancreatic acinar atrophy, infrequently to chronic pancreatitis, and rarely to neoplasia. Exocrine pancreatic insufficiency is less common in cats. Most dogs and cats with this condition can be successfully managed by supplementing each meal with pancreatin supplements. These supplements contain enzymes having protease, lipase and amylase activity that are able to assist in the digestion of protein, fat, and starch, respectively. Pancreatin is inactivated by gastric acid. Enteric-coated tablets may be administered just before feeding; other preparations are given with or sprinkled onto the feed. Oral powder or granules are much more effective than capsules or tablets. Capsules may be opened and contents sprinkled on or mixed with food and tablets can be crushed and sprinkled on or mixed with food. However, caution should be exercised because the powder may be irritant to skin and the respiratory system.

In refractory cases, cimetidine (see section 3.8.2) may be used as an adjunct to pancreatin therapy. Cimetidine reduces gastric acid production thereby decreasing inactivation of pancreatin. Treatment of secondary bacterial overgrowth may be useful as adjunctive treatment in dogs with exocrine pancreatitic insufficiency.

Pancreatin dosage is adjusted according to response of the individual patient. For guidance, addition of two 5-mL spoonfuls of powdered non-enteric coated preparation with each meal per 20 kg body-weight is a good starting dose. Frequent small amounts of a diet containing low fat, low fibre, highly digestible carbohydrate, and high quality protein, or dietetic pet foods (see section 16.8) may aid in the management of pancreatic insufficiency. A strict diet should be maintained with any dietary changes introduced slowly.

Medium chain triglycerides can be used as a readily absorbed caloric supplement in dogs with severe fat malabsorption.

PANCREATIN

UK

Indications. Treatment of diarrhoea and weight loss due to exocrine pancreatic insufficiency
Warnings. May be irritant, wash hands after handling product and avoid inhalation

GSL **Pancrex-Vet** (Pharmacia & Upjohn) *UK*
Tablets, uncoated, amylase 5000 units, lipase 5600 units, protease 330 units, for *dogs, cats*; 500
Dose. *Dogs, cats*: *by mouth*, 2–4 tablets/100 g of feed consumed
Oral powder, amylase 30 000 units, lipase 25 000 units, protease 1400 units/g, for *dogs, cats*; 250 g
Dose. *Dogs, cats*: *by mouth*, ½ of 5-mL spoonful/100 g of feed consumed

GSL **Panzym** (Vet Plus) *UK*
Oral powder, amylase 32 500 units/g, lipase 36 000 units/g, protease 1850 units/g, for *dogs, cats*
Dose. *Dogs, cats*: *by mouth*, (<10 kg body-weight) 0.3–0.5 spoonful (0.8–1.25 g)/meal; (>10 kg body-weight) 0.5–1.0 spoonful (1.25–2.5 g)/meal

GSL **Tryplase** (Intervet) *UK*
Capsules, amylase 9000 units, lipase 13 000 units, protease 450 units, for *dogs, cats*; 100, 250
Dose. Mix contents of capsule with food
Dogs: *by mouth*, 2–5 capsules daily. (5 capsules for 500 g of feed consumed)
Cats: 1–2 capsules daily (2 capsules for 250 g of feed consumed)

Eire

Indications. Treatment of diarrhoea and weight loss due to exocrine pancreatic insufficiency
Warnings. May be irritant, wash hands after handling product

Tryplase (Intervet) *Eire*
Capsules, amylase 9000 units, lipase 13,000 units, protease 450 units, for *dogs, cats*
Dose. *Dogs*: *by mouth*, 2–5 capsules
Cats: 1–2 capsules daily

USA

Indications. Treatment of diarrhoea and weight loss due to exocrine pancreatic insufficiency
Contra-indications. Sensitivity to the product

Pancreatic Plus Powder (Butler) *USA*
Oral powder, lipase 71,400 units, protease 388,000 units, amylase 460, 000 units in 1 teaspoonful (2.8 g), for *dogs, cats*
Dose. *Dogs*: *by mouth*, 0.75–1 teaspoon/meal
Cats: *by mouth*, 0.25–0.75 teaspoon/meal

Pancreatic Plus Tablets (Butler) *USA*
Tablets, lipase 9000 units, protease 57,000 units, amylase 64,000 units in each tablet, for *dogs, cats*
Dose. *Dogs*: *by mouth*, 2–3 tablets/meal
Cats: *by mouth*, 0.5–1.0 tablet/meal

Pancrezyme (Daniels) *USA*
Oral powder, lipase 71,400 units, protease 388,000 units, amylase 460, 000 units in 1 teaspoonful (2.8 g), for *dogs, cats*
Dose. *Dogs*: *by mouth*, 0.75–1 teaspoon/meal
Cats: *by mouth*, 0.25–0.75 teaspoon/meal

Pancrezyme (Daniels) *USA*
Tablets, lipase 9000 units, protease 57,000 units, amylase 64,000 units in each tablet, for *dogs, cats*
Dose. *Dogs*: *by mouth*, 2–3 tablets/meal
Cats: *by mouth*, 0.5–1.0 tablet/meal

Viokase-V (Fort Dodge) *USA*
Tablets, lipase 9000 units, protease 57,000 units, amylase 64,000 units/ tablet, for *dogs, cats*
Dose. *Dogs*: *by mouth*, 2–3 tablets/meal
Cats: *by mouth*, 0.5–1.0 tablet/meal

Viokase-V (Fort Dodge) *USA*
Oral powder, lipase 71, 000 units, protease 388, 000 units, amylase 460,000 units/ 2.8 g powder (1 teaspoonful), for *dogs, cats*
Dose. *Dogs*: *by mouth*, 0.75–1 teaspoon/meal
Cats: *by mouth*, 0.25–0.75 teaspoon/meal

TRIGLYCERIDES

UK

Indications. Severe fat malabsorption
Dose. See preparation details

Ⓗ **MCT Oil** (Bristol-Myers) *UK*
Triglycerides from medium chain fatty acids
Dose. 0.4–4.0 5-mL spoonfuls daily, given with food

3.10 Drugs used in the treatment of hepatic disease

Acute hepatic disease may be caused by a wide variety of agents which differ from species to species. Causative agents include bacterial, viral, and parasitic infections. Foals will occasionally develop hepatic disease as a result of equine herpesvirus 1, *Rhodococcus equi* abcessation, *Parascaris equorum* larval migration, Tyzzer's disease, or neonatal septicaemia. In ruminants, migration by ascarids or liver fluke may be problematic and helminth migration may precipitate *Clostridium oedematiens* proliferation with acute toxaemia. Massive hepatic necrosis in dogs may be associated with canine infectious hepatitis virus infection and drugs such as mebendazole; in cats a similar syndrome may be seen with drug toxicity due to diazepam. Hepatotoxins, systemic or metabolic disorders, and ischaemic or hypoxic injury, may also cause acute liver disease. In some species, traumatic hepatitis is likely to result in localised abscessation. In many cases, the causative agent cannot be identified.

Chronic liver disease may result from a chronic exposure to toxicants such as copper, drugs including antiepileptics, plant toxins for example ragwort, or mycotoxins. Dietary deficiency may result in liver disease in some species, for example, vitamin E and selenium in pigs, fatty liver syndrome in high yielding dairy cows, and pregnancy toxaemia in sheep and goats. Chronic infection with liver fluke in ruminants results in cholangitis and hepatic fibrosis. Cholestasis or immunologic injury may be the apparent cause of chronic liver disease, or the disease may result from severe hepatic necrosis. Dogs are prone to develop chronic hepatitis; many forms are breed specific. Cats more commonly develop cholangiohepatitis, either lymphocytic (immune-mediated) or suppurative (bacterial). Cirrhosis is end stage liver disease.

In congenital portosystemic shunts, clinical signs are due to diversion of portal blood rather than actual liver disease.

Treatment of hepatic disease includes removal of the initiating cause if identified, and wherever possible, followed by management of the resulting hepatic insufficiency. In liver disease many drugs should be used with caution because the liver is the major site of drug metabolism. Antibacterials are specifically indicated for the treatment of suppurative cholangiohepatitis, cholecystitis, and hepatic abscesses. **Antibacterials** that are excreted in an active form and at therapeutic concentrations in bile, without being hepatotoxic, are most suitable for the treatment of hepatobiliary infections, for example ampicillin, amoxicillin with clavulanic acid, cephalosporins, or enrofloxacin.

Corticosteroids are used to modulate the inflammatory and fibrotic response in canine chronic hepatitis and feline lymphocytic cholangiohepatitis. They have the disadvantage of being catabolic and immunosuppressive, contra-indicating their use in animals with hepatoencephalopathy or infectious hepatitis, while high dosages may cause a reversible hepatopathy. For dogs with chronic hepatitis that fail to respond to corticosteroid therapy alone, or to decrease the severity of side-effects, prednisolone (1 to 2 mg/kg daily in dogs or 2 mg/kg daily in cats) may be combined with azathioprine (1 mg/kg daily). Alternate-day treatment is advised to minimise drug toxicity and can be considered once the animal shows a good clinical response to daily therapy.

Copper chelation therapy is indicated in Bedlington or West Highland White terriers with copper hepatotoxicosis. **Penicillamine** is used most commonly. The chelating agent **trientine** may be used in dogs that do not tolerate penicillamine; this drug has a similar potency but has few or no side-effects. Control of the condition includes restriction of copper intake and provision of a high fat diet to stimulate biliary secretion and copper excretion.

Ursodeoxycholic acid is used in the treatment of a variety of chronic hepatobiliary disorders in dogs and cats. It protects hepatocytes by displacing toxic hydrophobic bile acids, but it also has choleretic and immunomodulatory properties. It should be used in conjunction with other measures aimed at controlling the pathogenesis of the disease.

Menbutone is a choleretic agent which may increase appetite although efficacy is not proven.

Complications of hepatic disease such as ascites (see diuretics, section 4.2), gastro-intestinal bleeding, and hepatic encephalopathy should be managed. Photosensitised animals should be kept out of sunlight. Supportive measures such as fluid therapy should be initiated. Multivitamins are often administered.

Dietary modification in all species may include feeding a high energy, restricted high biological value protein diet. Nutritional therapy is important in dogs and cats with chronic liver disease. Adequate calories (1.25 to 1.5 MER) should be fed because these patients are often catabolic and in negative nitrogen balance. Frequent feeding of small meals is recommended in order to reduce fasting hypoglycaemia and to increase protein tolerance. Dietary protein should not be restricted unless the animal is encephalopathic because adequate protein is important for hepatocyte repair. Protein should be of high quality and digestibility. Restriction of dietary fat is only indicated in dogs with severe cholestasis and steatorrhoea. Maintenance requirements for water soluble vitamin B should be doubled because these frequently become deficient in liver disease. Zinc supplementation (zinc sulphate 2 mg/kg daily or zinc gluconate 3 mg/kg daily) is recommended.

Hepatic encephalopathy is a neurological syndrome that results from acute or chronic liver failure. The most common cause in dogs and cats is the presence of congenital portosystemic shunts that allow mesenteric blood to bypass the liver and directly enter the systemic circulation. It may also occur with acquired portosystemic shunting resulting from chronic liver disease and portal hypertension. Uncommonly, hepatic encephalopathy develops without shunting after severe acute hepatic necrosis. Clinical signs are associated with impaired hepatic removal of neuroactive metabolites (especially ammonia, derived from colonic bacterial protein metabolism) from the mesenteric blood. Neurological signs such as disorientation, ataxia, and behavioural changes are most common, and are often worse after a high-protein meal. Other signs include anorexia and vomiting, stunted growth, polyuria and polydipsia, and urate cystic calculi. Medical management of hepatic encephalopathy is directed towards reducing gut bacterial protein metabolism. This is achieved by limiting absorption of ammonia from the colon, suppressing urease-producing bacteria, and feeding a low-protein diet.

Lactulose (see section 3.6.3) produces an osmotic diarrhoea of low faecal pH, discourages the proliferation of ammonia-producing organisms, and reduces absorption of ammonia from the colon. It is thus useful in the treatment of hepatic encephalopathy. In acute cases of hepatic encephalopathy, lactulose can also be used as a retention enema.

Antibacterials that are not absorbed from the gastro-intestinal tract assist in reducing ammonia-producing bacteria. Oral neomycin (see section 1.1.3) at a dose of 20 mg/kg 3 times daily for dogs and 10 to 20 mg/kg twice daily for cats has been used. The dose of neomycin for horses is 50 to 100 mg/kg once daily. Oral amoxicillin (see section 1.1.1.3) may be given at a dose of 11 mg/kg twice daily in dogs. Metronidazole (see section 1.1.8) is active against urease-positive anaerobes that produce ammonia within the intestine, and is as effective as neomycin in controlling blood-ammonia concentrations. The dose for oral metronidazole is 10 to 15 mg/kg 2 to 3 times daily for dogs and 7.5 mg/kg twice daily for cats.

A high dose of **mineral oil** is used to aid removal of ammonia in horses. Horses with hepatic encephalopathy usually require sedatives but these should be administered at minimum dosage.

COLESTYRAMINE
(Cholestyramine)

Indications. See Prescribing for rabbits and rodents

POM Ⓗ **Questran** (Bristol-Myers) *UK*
Powder, colestyramine (anhydrous) 4 g/sachet

MENBUTONE

Eire

Indications. Stimulation of gastro-intestinal function
Contra-indications. Cardiac impairment; Do not mix with solutions of calcium salts, procaine pencillin, or vitamin B
Side-effects. Increased ruminal motility, salivation, and tear production; darkened faeces
Dose. *Horses, cattle, sheep, pigs*: *by slow intravenous injection*, 10 mg/kg. Repeat after 24 hours if necessary

Genebile (Boehringer Ingelheim) *Eire*
Injection, menbutone 100 mg/mL, for *horses, cattle, sheep, pigs*
Withdrawal Periods. *Horses, cattle, sheep, pigs*: slaughter 2 days. *Cattle, sheep*: milk 2 days

PENICILLAMINE

UK

Indications. Copper hepatotoxicosis; cystine calculi (see section 9.4); copper and lead poisoning (see Treatment of poisoning)
Side-effects. Anorexia, vomiting; pyrexia; nephrotic syndrome
Dose. *Dogs*: copper hepatotoxicosis, *by mouth*, 10–15 mg/kg daily, preferably given on an empty stomach. May be mixed with food or daily dose divided if vomiting occurs

See section 9.4 for preparation details

TRIENTINE DIHYDROCHLORIDE

UK

Indications. Copper hepatotoxicosis in dogs intolerant to penicillamine
Dose. *Dogs*: *by mouth*, 20 mg/kg twice daily

POM Ⓗ **Trientine Dihydrochloride** (Non-proprietary) *UK*
Capsules, trientine dihydrochloride 300 mg

URSODEOXYCHOLIC ACID
(Ursodiol)

UK

Indications. Chronic hepatic disease associated with cholestasis
Contra-indications. Extrahepatic biliary obstruction
Dose. *Dogs, cats*: *by mouth*, 10–15 mg/kg once daily

POM Ⓗ **Destolit** (Norgine)
Tablets, scored, ursodeoxycholic acid 150 mg; 60

3.11 Oral hygiene preparations

Tooth brushing with dentifrice is helpful in oral plaque control. Dentifrice is a dental cleaning preparation containing an inorganic abrasive, some also contain fluoride and chlorhexidine. Toothpaste specifically for dogs and cats should be used. Human toothpaste is indigestible and contains a foaming agent. Veterinary toothpastes are available in flavours palatable to animals. Proper toothbrushing technique is essential for plaque control.
Chlorhexidine is an effective antiplaque agent which has both immediate and sustained antimicrobial activity after oral application. Side-effects include an unpleasant taste. It is used in patients with periodontal disease usually as an oral rinse once or twice daily but may also be applied by swabbing the gums with a cotton swab soaked in solution or gel or by using a dental spray or sustained release oral patches.
A fibrous or dry diet is important in controlling build-up of plaque. Products aimed at encouraging chewing activity are also of benefit, by maximising the self cleansing effect of salivary flow and composition. However, tooth brushing remains the single most effective way of preventing plaque deposition.

UK

CET (Virbac) *UK*
Dental paste, glucose oxidase, lactoperoxidase, for *dogs*; 70 g, 125. Available in malt and poultry flavour

CET Forte (Virbac) *UK*
Dental paste, glucose oxidase, lactoperoxidase, for *cats*; 125 g

CHx (Virbac) *UK*
Dental solution, chlorhexidine gluconate 0.12%; 59 mL, 237 mL
Dental gel, chlorhexidine gluconate 0.12%; 32 g, 54 g, 320 g

CHx Guard (Virbac) *UK*
Dental gel, chlorhexidine gluconate, zinc gluconate; 240 mL

CHx Guard LA (Virbac) *UK*
Dental gel, chlorhexidine gluconate 0.12%, zinc gluconate; 13 mL, 32 mL

Dentagyl (Merial) *UK*
Dental paste, chlorhexidine, fine abrasives, fluoride, for *dogs, cats*; 60 g

Dentipet Premier (Arnolds) *UK*
Dental paste, chlorhexidine, fine abrasives, fluoride, for *dogs, cats*; 60 g

Doggyfrice (Vétoquinol) *UK*
Tablets, enzymatic complex, fluorine, for *dogs*

Logic Dental Gel (Ceva) *UK*
Dental gel, enzymatic complex, fine abrasives, for *dogs, cats*; 70 g

Nolvadent (Fort Dodge) *UK*
Dental solution, chlorhexidine acetate 0.1%, for *horses, dogs, cats*; 230 mL

Nolvadent (Fort Dodge) *UK*
Dental spray, chlorhexidine acetate 0.1%, for *horses, dogs, cats*; 115 mL, 230 mL

MaxiGuard (distributed by Millpledge) *UK*
Oral gel, zinc ascorbate cysteine, for *dogs, cats*

Stomadhex C100 (Vétoquinol) *UK*
Oral adhesive patch, chlorhexidine (as diacetate) 100 micrograms, nicotinamide 8.25 mg, for *dogs and cats less than 10 kg body-weight*; 200

Stomadhex C300 (Vétoquinol) *UK*
Oral adhesive patch, chlorhexidine (as diacetate) 300 micrograms, nicotinamide 25 mg, for *dogs more than 10 kg body-weight*; 200

4 Drugs used in the treatment of disorders of the
CARDIOVASCULAR SYSTEM

Contributor:
P G G Darke BVSc, PhD, DVR, DVC, DipECVIM, MRCVS

Congestive heart failure is usually a progressive disease despite treatment. Treatment of causative factors such as nutritional imbalance, bacterial endocarditis, or pericardial effusions may produce symptomatic improvement but frequently the pathological changes in valvular or myocardial tissues are irreversible. In sedentary dogs and cats, management of congestive heart failure can significantly improve life expectancy and the quality of life. However, for working animals, therapy is rarely economically viable.

4.1 Myocardial stimulants
4.2 Diuretics
4.3 Vasodilators
4.4 Antidysrhythmics
4.5 Adrenoceptor stimulants
4.6 Anticoagulants
4.7 Haemostatics

4.1 Myocardial stimulants

4.1.1 Cardiac glycosides
4.1.2 Methylxanthines

Few studies have demonstrated any sustained beneficial effect of myocardial stimulants in animals. Furthermore, even if inotropes are shown to be effective, until the arrival of inodilators there has been little proof of increased longevity in humans or animals. Studies in humans with systolic failure, for example dilated cardiomyopathy, suggest that, paradoxically, early intervention with a low dose of beta-adrenoceptor blocking drugs may prolong life. Nonetheless, in systolic failure cardiac function can be very poor, and most cardiologists would employ inotropes in all animals in cardiac failure when systolic function is very poor. Myocardial stimulants are indicated where myocardial failure is either a primary or secondary problem. Myocardial stimulants used in veterinary practice include cardiac glycosides, inodilators, and methylxanthines. Adrenoceptor stimulants such as dobutamine (see section 4.5) also act as potent myocardial stimulants.

4.1.1 Cardiac glycosides

Cardiac glycosides act as positive inotropes by increasing the force of myocardial contraction by mechanisms that enhance calcium influx into the myocardial cells. There is also an increase in the refractory period of the cells and a decrease in conductivity throughout the myocardium. This causes a reduction in the rate of contraction (negative chronotropy). The effect of cardiac glycosides on the auto-nomic nervous system also contributes to a slowed heart-rate. Parasympathomimetic effects cause slowing of the sino-atrial node rate and delayed conduction in the atrioventricular (A-V) node. Any increase in cardiac output resulting from digoxin treatment may lead to a reduction in sympathetic drive.

In dogs and cats a major indication for cardiac glycoside therapy is in the control of supraventricular tachycardias, especially atrial fibrillation. In horses, digoxin is occasionally used in cases of atrial fibrillation refractory to quinidine sulphate.

Cardiac glycosides also have a place in the management of congestive heart failure where it is associated with primary or secondary myocardial failure (notably in dilated cardiomyopathy). They are not primarily indicated for the treatment of congestive heart failure caused by valvular insufficiency or intracardiac shunts unless there is secondary myocardial failure or tachycardia.

Digoxin excretion is mainly via the kidney as unchanged drug. Therefore the dose should be decreased in patients with reduced renal perfusion. It is suggested that the dose may be reduced by 50% for every 50% increase in plasma-urea concentration, and then serum-digoxin concentration measured, with titration of subsequent doses. See also Prescribing in renal impairment for information on dosage adjustment. Digoxin has a plasma half-life of 20 to 55 hours in dogs and 12 to 48 hours in horses. **Digitoxin** undergoes hepatic metabolism and has a half-life of 8 to 12 hours in dogs; it is excreted in the faeces and urine as metabolites.

These drugs have a narrow therapeutic margin and doses should be titrated for each patient. Slow digitalisation is the method of choice. This relies on the plateau principle, which depends on the half-life of the drug. In dogs therapeutic plasma-drug concentrations, in the range 1.0 to 2.5 micrograms/litre, are achieved within 4 to 5 times the half-life, that is 3 to 5 days for digoxin and 1 to 2 days for digitoxin. Doubling the first dose results in the therapeutic concentration being reached more rapidly with minimal risk of toxic signs. Blood concentration of glycosides should be evaluated at about 8 hours after administration.

Authorities advise that the use of digitoxin in horses and cats is not recommended.

The bioavailability of digitalis glycosides varies with the gastro-intestinal flora and the lipid solubility of the particular preparation. These factors result in individual variation to specific doses and in variable clinical responses to different preparations. Ideally the digoxin oral dose form should not be altered, and when changing from a tablet to an elixir formulation the dose should be reduced by 25%. Any change in dose form during maintenance therapy will take 6 to 8 days for the effect to be evident.

A number of factors increase the animal's susceptibility to the toxic effects of cardiac glycosides including hypothyroidism, renal insufficiency, old age, obesity, and hypokalaemia resulting from prolonged diuretic therapy (see section 4.2). Adverse effects can include various types of dysrhythmia. Indications of toxicity include depression, with gastro-intestinal disturbances such as anorexia, vomiting, and diarrhoea. Clients should be warned to withdraw the drug if these signs are seen. Overdosage with cardiac glycosides may cause an excessively slow heart-rate, which reduces cardiac output and causes renal dysfunction as a result of hypoperfusion.

Phenytoin (see section 4.4.1) has been used in the treatment of ventricular tachycardias caused by cardiac glycoside toxicity.

Conversion tables from body-weight to surface area are included in Appendix 3.

DIGITOXIN

UK

Indications. Supraventricular arrhythmias; congestive heart failure

Contra-indications. Side-effects. Warnings. See under Digoxin; see also notes above

Dose. *Dogs*: *by mouth,* 20–30 micrograms/kg 2–3 times daily

POM (H) **Digitoxin** (Non-proprietary) *UK*
Tablets, digitoxin 100 micrograms

DIGOXIN

UK

Indications. Congestive heart failure with systolic failure; supraventricular tachycardias

Contra-indications. Hypertrophic myocardial disorders, severe dysrhythmias including bradycardia

Side-effects. Depression, anorexia, vomiting, diarrhoea, bradycardia, arrhythmias

Warnings. Reduce dose in renal impairment, see also notes above; higher rate of gastro-intestinal absorption of elixirs necessitates lower absolute doses, see notes above; use with care in cats; Drug Interactions – see Appendix 1 (cardiac glycosides)

Dose.

Horses: *by mouth,* initial dose 20 micrograms/kg then 20 micrograms/kg daily in 2 divided doses

by intravenous injection, 2.5–5.0 micrograms/kg twice daily

Dogs: *by mouth,* 220 micrograms/m^2 twice daily. This is achieved by (small dogs) 10 micrograms/kg twice daily; (large dogs) 5 micrograms/kg twice daily. Reduce dose further for Dobermanns

Cats: *by mouth,* 7–10 micrograms/kg on alternate days *or* 4 micrograms/kg daily. Elixir should be used for cats

POM (H) **Digoxin** (Non-proprietary) *UK*
Tablets, digoxin 62.5 micrograms, 125 micrograms, 250 micrograms
Injection, digoxin 100 micrograms/mL, digoxin 250 micrograms/mL; 2 mL

POM (H) **Lanoxin** (GlaxoWellcome) *UK*
Tablets, digoxin 125 micrograms, 250 micrograms (scored); 500
Injection, digoxin 250 micrograms/mL; 2 mL

POM (H) **Lanoxin-PG** (GlaxoWellcome) *UK*
Tablets, digoxin 62.5 micrograms; 500
Elixir, digoxin 50 micrograms/mL; 60 mL
Note. Elixir should not be diluted

USA

Indications. Supraventricular tachycardias; heart failure; atrial fibrillation; atrial flutter

Contra-indications. Ventricular premature contractions, ventricular tachycardia (except if secondary to decreased cardiac output), heart block greater then first degree

Side-effects. Depression, anorexia, vomiting, diarrhoea, bradycardia, arrhythmias

Warnings. Frequent monitoring of patient required; care in renal or hepatic impairment, hypothyroidism and hyperthyroidism; monitor serum-potassium concentration

Dose. *Dogs*: *by mouth,* (<9 kg body-weight) initial dose 11 micrograms/m^2-10%; (>9 kg body-weight) initial dose 22 micrograms/m^2-10%

Cardoxin (Evsco) *USA*
Elixir, digoxin 150 micrograms/mL, for *dogs*

Cardoxin LS (Evsco) *USA*
Elixir, digoxin 50 micrograms/mL, for *dogs*

4.1.2 Methylxanthines

The methylxanthines (see section 5.1.1) **aminophylline**, **etamiphylline**, and **theophylline** are mainly used as bronchodilators but also have a mild diuretic action and positive chronotropic and inotropic activity. They are also used to relieve coughing in congestive heart failure in dogs. Methylxanthines may cause tachycardia and vomiting.

4.2 Diuretics

4.2.1 Thiazides
4.2.2 Loop diuretics
4.2.3 Potassium-sparing diuretics
4.2.4 Potassium-sparing diuretics with thiazides
4.2.5 Osmotic diuretics

Diuretics are mainly used in veterinary medicine to reduce oedema in, for example, cases of heart failure, hepatic disease, cerebral oedema, hypoproteinaemia, and udder oedema. Most act by promoting sodium excretion, thus reducing the volume of extracellular fluid (ECF). Some also have vascular effects, for example furosemide administered intravenously is a venodilator. Diuretics reduce hypertension and furosemide is claimed to aid in the treatment of exercise induced pulmonary haemorrhage (EIPH) in horses. Diuretics are the mainstay of therapy for congestive heart failure where there is pulmonary or systemic fluid retention. However, diuretics are known to stimulate adverse humoral responses, such as angiotensin and aldosterone concentration. This effect may be minimised by combining therapy with an angiotensin-converting enzyme (ACE) inhibitor (see section 4.3.1) or an inodilator (see section 4.3.2) and by reducing the dosage of diuretic to the minimum required to suppress signs of oedema and heart failure.

Prolonged therapy with certain diuretics may lead to excessive loss of potassium and magnesium in urine. Hypokalaemia increases the animal's susceptibility to toxicity from cardiac glycosides (see section 4.1.1) and to cardiac dysrhythmias and may impair carbohydrate metabolism. The risk of hypokalaemia is increased by anorexia. To avoid potassium depletion, dietary supplementation may be used or diuretics may be combined with ACE inhibitors (see section 4.3.1), inodilators (see section 4.3.2), or with potassium-sparing agents (see section 4.2.4). Depletion of extracellular fluid volume without the loss of bicarbonate ions may lead to metabolic alkalosis. Excessive use of diuretics may also cause hypovolaemia and loss of cardiac output, leading to reduced renal blood flow and glomerular filtration-rate, thereby compromising renal function; care should be taken in animals with low cardiac output, especially cats.

Treatment of chronic left-sided congestive heart failure in dogs may also require therapy for coughing due to small airway disease and bronchial occlusion by the enlargened left atrium. Additional treatment which may be required includes bronchodilators such as methylxanthines (see section 5.1.1), antitussives such as opioids (see section 5.4), sedatives (see section 6.1), or corticosteroids (see section 7.2.1). Cardiac glycosides (see section 4.1.1) may be used to control heart rate.

Severe pulmonary (alveolar) oedema is often acute in onset and may be life-threatening in dogs, cats, and horses. Intensive therapy is required. A suitable regimen is intravenous furosemide, intramuscular morphine, and transcutaneous glyceryl trinitrate, with additional oxygen therapy (administered via a nasopharyngeal cannula in dogs and cats). Coupage (percussion of the thorax) may also be helpful to aid removal of secretions. This combination therapy is likely to reduce elevated pulmonary venous pressure in most cases. However, careful monitoring and maintenance treatment will also be required.

Attempts to mobilise oedema fluid with short periods of intensive diuresis will create phases during which the animal is predisposed to acute hypovolaemia followed by extended phases when its kidneys negate the effect of the diuretic. Therefore, over a 24-hour period, a short-acting potent diuretic may have poorer efficacy than a less potent but longer-acting diuretic.

Diuretics are usually classified according to their site of action because this affects their likely side-effects. For example, loop diuretics are much more potent than diuretics acting distally because the loop is the site of greater sodium reabsorption. However, the animal responds to the induced sodium depletion by producing more aldosterone, thus the distal tubule becomes an important site of potassium loss. Distally active potassium-sparing diuretics may be used, therefore, to reduce this unwanted potassium loss, alongside a more potent diuretic (see section 4.2.4). In animals in which oedema or ascites becomes resistant to treatment, combination therapy, using two or more diuretics from different groups, may prove valuable.

4.2.1 Thiazides

Thiazide diuretics, such as **bendroflumethiazide**, **chlorothiazide**, **hydrochlorothiazide**, and **trichlormethiazide**, inhibit sodium reabsorption in the early distal tubule. These drugs act proximal to the site of aldosterone-stimulated sodium and potassium exchange. The delivery of increased amounts of sodium to this area causes greater potassium loss, and potassium supplementation may be necessary when using thiazides for diuresis. Thiazides decrease urinary calcium excretion and they may also be used to reduce the formation of oxalate uroliths in dogs.

Thiazides are used to treat cardiac or hypoproteinaemic oedema. Paradoxically, thiazides have also been used in the treatment of diabetes insipidus because they cause sodium, chloride, and water loss leading to hypovolaemia. This increases absorption of sodium and water from the proximal tubule. As a result, sodium delivery to the loop is reduced and formation of fully dilute urine is prevented; hence, the diuretic reduces the polyuria observed in diabetes insipidus. Hydrochlorothiazide remains effective for up to 12 hours and is thus given in divided doses. Bendroflumethiazide, a more potent diuretic, is effective for up to 24 hours and is usually administered in the morning.

BENDROFLUMETHIAZIDE
(Bendrofluazide)

UK

Indications. Oedema
Contra-indications. Renal failure with anuria
Side-effects. Hypokalaemia (may require potassium supplementation)
Warnings. Drug Interactions – see Appendix 1 (diuretics)
Dose. *Dogs, cats*: *by mouth*, 125–250 micrograms/kg once daily in the morning

POM Ⓗ **Bendroflumethiazide** (Non-proprietary) *UK*
Tablets, bendroflumethiazide 2.5 mg, 5 mg

CHLOROTHIAZIDE

USA

Indications. Post-parturient udder oedema
Warnings. Patients should be monitored for signs of electrolyte and fluid imbalance
Dose. *Cattle: by mouth*, 2 g 1–2 times daily for 3–4 days

Diuril Boluses (Merial) *USA*
Tablets, chlorothiazide 2 g, for *cattle*
Withdrawal Periods. Milk 72 hours

HYDROCHLOROTHIAZIDE

UK

Indications. Oedema; diabetes insipidus
Contra-indications. Side-effects. Warnings. See under Bendroflumethiazide
Dose. *Dogs, cats*: *by mouth*, 2–4 mg/kg twice daily

POM Ⓗ **HydroSaluric** (MSD) *UK*
Tablets, scored, hydrochlorothiazide 25 mg, 50 mg; 100

Eire

Indications. Oedema

Warnings. Use with care in pregnant animals, diabetes mellitus, osteoporosis, glaucoma, senility, renal or cardiac impairment

Dose. See manufacturers' details

Diurizone Injectable Solution (Vetoquinol) *Eire*
Injection, hydrochlorothiazide 50 mg/mL dexamethasone 500 micrograms/mL, for **horses, cattle, sheep**

Diurizone Powder (Vetoquinol) *Eire*
Oral powder, hydrochlorothiazide 1.5 mg/20 g, dexamethasone 5 mg/20 g (1 pack = 20 g), for **horses, cattle, sheep**

USA

Indications. Oedema

Warnings. Patients should be monitored for signs of electrolyte and fluid imbalance

Dose. *Cattle*: *by intramuscular or intravenous injection*, 125–250 mg

Hydrozide Injection (Merial) *USA*
Injection, hydrochlorothiazide 25 mg/mL, for **cattle**
Withdrawal Periods. Milk 3 days

TRICHLORMETHIAZIDE

Australia

Indications. Oedema

Contra-indications. Use in last trimester of pregnancy in cattle

Dose. Expressed as trichlormethiazide

Horses, cattle: *by mouth*, initial dose 200–400 mg, then 100–200 mg for up to 3 days

Naquasone Bolus (Schering-Plough) *Austral.*
Tablets, trichlormethiazide 200 mg, dexamethasone 5 mg, for **horses, cattle**
Withdrawal Periods. *Cattle*: milk 48 hours

New Zealand

Indications. Udder oedema

Contra-indications. Use in last trimester of pregnancy except 5 days before parturition

Warnings. Patients with severe renal impairment should be monitored

Dose. Expressed as trichlormethiazide

Cattle: *by mouth*, initial dose 200–400 mg, then 100–200 mg for up to 3 days

Naquasone Bolus (Schering-Plough) *NZ*
Tablets, dexamethasone 5 mg, trichlormethiazide 200 mg, for **cattle**
Withdrawal Periods. Slaughter 21 days, milk 36 hours

USA

Indications. Udder oedema

Contra-indications. Use in last trimester of pregnancy

Warnings. Patients with severe renal impairment should be monitored

Dose. Expressed as trichlormethiazide

Cattle: *by mouth*, initial dose 200–400 mg, then 100–200 mg for up to 3 days

Naquasone (Schering-Plough) *USA*
Tablets, trichlormethiazide 200 mg, dexamethasone 5 mg, for **cattle**
Withdrawal Periods. Milk 72 hours

4.2.2 Loop diuretics

Loop diuretics are the most potent group of diuretics, with a rapid onset of effect but a short duration of action. These drugs block sodium reabsorption in the loop of Henle. Loop diuretics are potent and excessive doses can lead to hypovolaemia and decompensation of renal function. However, their potency allows them to remain effective even when urine delivery is poor, as in renal impairment. Loop diuretics increase magnesium excretion and, as with thiazides, may cause severe potassium loss. Hypomagnesaemia potentiates the cardiac effects of hypokalaemia. Loop diuretics may potentiate the ototoxic effects of aminoglycoside antibacterials.

Furosemide is used to decrease oedema in conditions such as cardiovascular and pulmonary oedema, hepatic and renal dysfunction, hydrothorax, ascites, and non-specific oedema. Furosemide may be used in the treatment of EIPH in horses. When administered intravenously, furosemide may be an effective venodilator in the initial treatment of pulmonary oedema. Furosemide is advocated by some clinicians in anuric renal failure if intensive fluid therapy replacement leads to subcutaneous or pulmonary oedema through persistent anuria. However, in these cases the prognosis is very guarded. Furosemide is detectable in milk for up to 30 hours after treatment.

FUROSEMIDE
(Frusemide)

UK

Indications. Oedema

Contra-indications. Severe hepatic impairment; acute glomerular nephritis; some manufacturers state contra-indicated for renal failure with anuria; electrolyte or fluid deficiency disorders; cardiac glycoside overdose; concurrent treatment with ACE inhibitors in dogs with functional renal insufficiency, aminoglycosides, or cephalosporins; hypersensitivity to sulphonamides

Side-effects. Hypokalaemia; allergic reactions with concurrent sulphonamides

Warnings. Hypokalaemia may potentiate the toxic effects of cardiac glycosides; Drug Interactions – see Appendix 1 (diuretics); plasma-potassium concentration should be monitored during prolonged treatment or concurrent treatment with cardiac glycosides. (Potassium supplementation may be required); renal function should be monitoring in patients on long-term NSAIDs

Dose.

Horses: *by mouth*♦ or *by intramuscular or intravenous injection*, 0.5–1.0 mg/kg 1–2 times daily

Cattle: *by intramuscular or intravenous injection*, 0.5–1.0 mg/kg

Dogs, cats: *by mouth*, up to 5 mg/kg 1–2 times daily. Should be reduced to 1–2 mg/kg 1–2 times daily for maintenance

by intramuscular or intravenous injection, 2.5–5.0 mg/kg 1–2 times daily

POM **Frusecare** (Animalcare) *UK*
Tablets, scored, furosemide 40 mg, for *dogs and cats more than 4 kg body-weight*; 1000

POM **Frusedale** (Arnolds) *UK*
Tablets, scored, furosemide 40 mg, for *dogs and cats more than 4 kg body-weight*

POM **Frusemide Tablets BP (Vet)** (Millpledge) *UK*
Tablets, furosemide 20 mg, 40 mg

POM **Lasix 5% Solution** (Intervet) *UK*
Injection, furosemide 50 mg/mL, for *horses, cattle, dogs, cats*; 10 mL
Withdrawal Periods. *Cattle*: milk 2 milkings after treatment

POM **Lasix Tablets** (Intervet) *UK*
Tablets, furosemide 10 mg, for *dogs, cats*
Tablets, scored, furosemide 40 mg, for *dogs and cats more than 4 kg body-weight*; 100

Australia
Indications. Oedema
Contra-indications. Renal or hepatic impairment; concurrent neomycin administration; anuria
Warnings. Electrolytes should be monitored during prolonged treatment
Dose. Dosages vary, consult manufacturers' information

Flusapex Drops (Apex) *Austral.*
Oral drops, furosemide 10 mg/mL, for *dogs, cats*

Flusapex Injection (Apex) *Austral.*
Injection, furosemide 50 mg/mL, for *small and large animals*
Withdrawal Periods. Slaughter withdrawal period nil, milk withdrawal period nil

Flusapex Tablets (Apex) *Austral.*
Tablets, furosemide 40 mg, for *small and large animals*
Withdrawal Periods. Slaughter withdrawal period nil, milk withdrawal period nil

Frudix Tablets (Jurox) *Austral.*
Tablets, furosemide 40 mg, for *horses, cattle, dogs, cats*

Frusemide (Ilium) *Austral.*
Injection, furosemide 50 mg/mL, for *dogs, cats, horses, cattle*
Withdrawal Periods. *Horses*: slaughter withdrawal period nil. *Cattle*: slaughter withdrawal period nil, milk withdrawal period nil

Eire
Indications. Oedema
Contra-indications. Renal failure with anuria; acute glomerular nephritis; electrolyte deficiency disease; cardiac glycoside overdosage; concurrent aminoglycosides
Side-effects. Hypokalaemia. Plasma-potassium concentration should be monitored during prolonged treatment or concurrent treatment with cardiac glycosides. (Potassium supplementation may be required)
Warnings. Drug Interactions – aminoglycosides, cephalosporins, sulphonamides
Dose.
Horses, cattle: *by intramuscular or intravenous injection*, 0.5–1.0 mg/kg
Dogs, cats: *by intramuscular or intravenous injection*, 2.5–5.0 mg/kg

Lasix 5% Solution (Hoechst Roussel Vet) *Eire*
Injection, furosemide 50 mg/mL, for *horses, cattle, dogs, cats*
Withdrawal Periods. Should not be used in *horses* intended for human consumption. *Cattle*: slaughter 24 hours, milk 2 milkings

New Zealand
Indications. Oedema
Contra-indications. Hyponatraemia; renal or hepatic impairment; concurrent neomycin administration; anuria
Dose. Dosages vary, consult manufacturers' information

Flusapex (Ethical) *NZ*
Oral solution, furosemide 10 mg/mL, for *dogs, cats*

Frudix (Jurox) *NZ*
Tablets, furosemide 40 mg, for *dogs, cats*

Lasix (Animal Health) *NZ*
Injection, furosemide 50 mg/mL, for *horses, cattle, dogs, cats*
Withdrawal Periods. *Horses*: slaughter 1 day. *Cattle*: slaughter 1 day, milk withdrawal period nil

USA
Indications. Oedema
Contra-indications. Renal or hepatic impairment; anuria; hypersensitivity to the drug; pregnant bitches, mares, and stallions at stud; electrolyte imbalances
Side-effects. Electrolyte imbalance
Warnings. Electrolytes, blood-urea, and CO_2 should be monitored during prolonged treatment; Drug Interactions – corticosteroids, cardiac glycosides, aminoglycosides, cephalosporins, polymixins, sulphonamides; discontinue treatment 1 day before surgery
Dose.
Horses: *by intramuscular or intravenous injection*, 0.25–1.0 mg/kg
Cattle: *by intramuscular or intravenous injection*, 0.25–0.5 mg/kg
Dogs, cats: *by mouth*, 2.5–5.5 mg/kg
by intramuscular or intravenous injection, 5.5 mg/kg

Disal Injection (Boehringer Ingelheim Vetmedica) *USA*
Injection, furosemide 50 mg/mL, for *horses, dogs*
Withdrawal Periods. Should not be used in *horses* intended for human consumption

Disal Tablets (Boehringer Ingelheim Vetmedica) *USA*
Tablets, furosemide 12.5 mg, 50 mg, for *dogs*

Diuride Injection (Anthony) *USA*
Injection, furosemide 50 mg/mL, for *horses*
Withdrawal Periods. Should not be used in *horses* intended for human consumption

Equi-Phar Furosemide Injection (Vedco) *USA*
Injection, furosemide (as diethanolamine salt) 50 mg/mL, for *horses*
Withdrawal Periods. Should not be used in *horses* intended for human consumption

Furoject Injection (Vetus) *USA*
Injection, furosemide (as monoethanolamine salt) 50 mg/mL , for *horses, dogs*
Withdrawal Periods. Should not be used in *horses* intended for human consumption

Furosemide Injection 5% (Butler, Pro Labs, VetTek) *USA*
Injection, furosemide (as diethanolamine salt) 50 mg/mL, for *horses*
Withdrawal Periods. Should not be used in *horses* intended for human consumption

Furosemide Tablets (Butler, Vedco, Western Veterinary Supplies) *USA*
Tablets, furosemide 12.5 mg, 50 mg, for *dogs*

Furotabs (Vetus) *USA*
Tablets, furosemide 12.5 mg, 50 mg, for *dogs*

Lasix (Hoechst-Roussel) *USA*
Tablets, 12.5 mg, 50 mg, for **dogs**, **cats**

Lasix (Hoechst-Roussel) *USA*
Oral syrup, furosemide 10 mg/mL, for **dogs**, **cats**

Lasix (Hoechst-Roussel) *USA*
Injection, furosemide 50 mg/mL, for **horses, cattle, dogs, cats,**
Withdrawal Periods. Should not be used in **horses** intended for human con-
sumption. **Cattle**: slaughter 2 days, milk 2 days.

4.2.3 Potassium-sparing diuretics

Potassium-sparing diuretics act in the late distal tubule and
increase the excretion of sodium and reduce the excretion of
potassium. They can thus ameliorate the excessive potassium loss sometimes caused by more potent diuretics and
are usually combined with them. In addition, potassium-
sparing diuretics may enhance the therapeutic effect of
potent diuretics especially in resistant oedema, for example
ascites. Potassium-sparing diuretics also reduce magnesium
loss. Angiotensin-converting enzyme (ACE) inhibitors (see
section 4.3.1) have similar but less potent activity.

Spironolactone acts by competitively antagonising aldosterone by blocking the same receptor in the distal renal
tubules. The action of spironolactone is self-limiting
because any consequent hyperkalaemia will further increase
aldosterone secretion, allowing it to compete with the drug.

Amiloride does not act by specifically antagonising aldosterone. It has a direct effect on ion transport across the lumi-
nal face of tubular cells. Therefore, amiloride is effective
when there is no aldosterone excess and is the drug of
choice for combination with thiazides.

Potassium-sparing diuretics should be avoided in conditions
predisposing to hyperkalaemia such as renal failure, metabolic acidosis, and diabetes mellitus. They should also be
avoided in combination with beta-adrenoceptor blocking
drugs which impair cellular uptake of potassium, or ACE
inhibitors, which may predispose to hyperkalaemia.

AMILORIDE HYDROCHLORIDE

UK

Indications. Resistant oedema; prevention of hypokalae-
mia in diuresis
Contra-indications. Renal impairment; metabolic acido-
sis; diabetes mellitus
Side-effects. Hyperkalaemia with prolonged administra-
tion
Warnings. Drug Interactions – see Appendix 1 (diuretics)
Dose. *Dogs, cats*: *by mouth, 1–2 mg/kg daily*

POM Ⓗ **Amiloride** (Non-proprietary) *UK*
Tablets, amiloride hydrochloride 5 mg
Oral solution, amiloride hydrochloride 1 mg/mL (available as 'Special
Order' from Rosemont)

SPIRONOLACTONE

UK

Indications. Resistant oedema; prevention of hypokalaemia in diuresis

Contra-indications. **Side-effects**. **Warnings**. See under
Amiloride hydrochloride
Dose. *Dogs, cats*: *by mouth, 2–4 mg/kg daily*

POM Ⓗ **Spironolactone** (Non-proprietary) *UK*
Tablets, spironolactone 25 mg, 50 mg, 100 mg
Oral suspension, spironolactone 1 mg/mL, 2 mg/mL, 5 mg/mL, 10 mg/mL
(available as 'Special Order' from Rosemont)

POM Ⓗ **Aldactone** (Searle) *UK*
Tablets, spironolactone 25 mg, 50 mg, 100 mg

4.2.4 Potassium-sparing diuretics with thiazides

Combination preparations of potassium-sparing diuretics
and other diuretics are used in patients with oedema or
ascites refractory to loop diuretics, hypokalaemia requiring
diuresis, or if high doses of loop diuretics are required,
which may cause hypokalaemia. Co-flumactone, a combination of **hydroflumethiazide** and **spironolactone**, has
been used in veterinary practice.

HYDROFLUMETHIAZIDE / SPIRONOLACTONE

(Co-flumactone: preparations of hydroflumethiazide and
spironolactone in equal proportions by weight)

UK

Indications. Congestive heart failure; oedema, see notes
above
Contra-indications. See under Amiloride hydrochloride
(section 4.2.3) and Bendroflumethiazide (section 4.2.1)
Side-effects. Rarely hyperkalaemia
Warnings. Avoid concurrent administration with ACE
inhibitors or other potassium-sparing diuretics
Dose. See preparation details

POM Ⓗ **Hydroflumethiazide and Spironolactone** (Co-flumactone)
(Non-proprietary) *UK*
Tablets, hydroflumethiazide 25 mg, spironolactone 25 mg
Dose. *Dogs*: *by mouth, 1 tablet/6–12 kg body-weight*
Tablets, hydroflumethiazide 50 mg, spironolactone 50 mg
Dose. *Dogs*: *by mouth, 1 tablet/12–25 kg body-weight*

4.2.5 Osmotic diuretics

Osmotic diuretics include hypertonic solutions of **mannitol**. Administration of mannitol causes water retention
within the nephron, which dilutes urinary sodium and
opposes its reabsorption especially in the proximal tubule
and loop of Henle.

Mannitol is used to promote urine output, as in acute renal
failure, or to reduce cellular oedema in cerebral trauma or
oedema. It is **not** suitable for the mobilisation of general or
local oedema, because it may lead to cardiac overload.
Excessive administration of mannitol can produce severe
hypovolaemia and maintenance of extracellular fluid volume may require administration of an electrolyte solution
such as compound sodium lactate intravenous infusion
(Hartmann's solution) (see section 16.1.2).

MANNITOL

UK

Indications. Cerebral oedema; forced osmotic diuresis; glaucoma (see section 12.5)

Contra-indications. Congestive heart failure; pulmonary oedema

Warnings. Extravasation causes inflammation and thrombophlebitis

Dose.

Horses: *by slow intravenous injection or intravenous infusion*, 0.25–1.0 g/kg test dose. Repeat as necessary if diuresis occurs

Dogs: *by slow intravenous injection*, 1 g/kg test dose. Repeat as necessary if diuresis occurs

Cats: *by slow intravenous injection*, 250–500 mg/kg test dose. Repeat as necessary if diuresis occurs

POM Ⓗ **Mannitol** (Non-proprietary) *UK*
Intravenous infusion, mannitol 10%, 20%

USA

Indications. Diuresis

Dose. *By intravenous infusion*, 1.65–2.2 g/kg

Mannitol (Butler, Vedco, Vetus) *USA*
Injection, mannitol 180 mg/mL

4.3 Vasodilators

4.3.1 ACE inhibitors
4.3.2 Inodilators
4.3.3 Vasodilators
4.3.4 Cerebral vasodilators

Vasodilators effectively decrease the myocardial workload by increasing blood vessel volume. Venodilators reduce the preload and arteriodilators reduce afterload. Arteriodilators may promote cardiac output by increasing the forward stroke volume. Some drugs act on both veins and arteries. Vascular tone and intravascular pressure may be elevated in heart failure because of increased sympathetic tone, activation of angiotensin, release of vasopressin, or increased vascular wall stiffness caused by salt and water retention. Arteriolar dilatation is especially useful in mitral insufficiency in which the regurgitant fraction may be significantly reduced by therapy and in systemic hypertension.

4.3.1 ACE inhibitors

Benazepril, enalapril, and **ramipril** are angiotensin-converting enzyme (ACE) inhibitors that block the conversion of angiotensin I to angiotensin II. Angiotensin II is a potent vasoconstrictor and has further deleterious effects such as myocardial remodelling. In addition, angiotensin II is involved in the production of aldosterone, which contributes to oedema in congestive heart failure. ACE inhibitors have been shown to prolong life and to improve the quality of life in most dogs with moderate to severe heart failure. The blood pressure and volume loading on the heart may be lowered. ACE inhibitors may also help to improve ventricular diastolic function in cardiomyopathies, especially in cats, probably by inhibiting the re-modelling effects of angiotensin II.

BENAZEPRIL HYDROCHLORIDE

UK

Indications. Congestive heart failure; systemic hypertension♦

Contra-indications. Animals at risk of hypotension; breeding dogs, pregnant or lactating bitches unless the benefit-risk ratio is considered justified; reduced cardiac output due to aortic stenosis

Side-effects. Rarely clinical signs of tiredness or dizziness

Warnings. Drug Interactions – see Appendix 1; plasma-potassium concentration should be monitored when used concurrently with potassium-sparing diuretics

Dose. *Dogs*: *by mouth*, 250–500 micrograms/kg once daily. May be increased to 0.5–1.0 mg/kg once daily if required

POM **Fortekor 5 and 20** (Novartis) *UK*
Tablets, f/c, scored, benazepril hydrochloride 5 mg, 20 mg, for *dogs*; 14

Australia

Indications. Congestive heart failure

Contra-indications. Pregnant or lactating bitches

Warnings. Monitor patients with renal impairment

Dose. *Dogs*: *by mouth*, 250–500 micrograms/kg

Fortekor (Novartis) *Austral.*
Tablets, benazepril hydrochloride 5 mg, 20mg, for *dogs*

Eire

Indications. Congestive heart failure

Contra-indications. Breeding dogs, pregnant or lactating bitches unless the benefit-risk ratio is considered justified; reduced cardiac output due to aortic stenosis

Side-effects. Rarely clinical signs of tiredness or dizziness

Warnings. Drug Interactions – spironolactone

Dose. *Dogs*: *by mouth*, 250–500 micrograms/kg

Fortekor 5 & 20 (Novartis) *Eire*
Tablets, benazepril hydrochloride 5 mg, 20 mg, for *dogs*

ENALAPRIL MALEATE

UK

Indications. Congestive heart failure; systemic hypertension♦

Contra-indications. Animals at risk of hypotension; pregnant bitches; cardiac output failure; concurrent potassium-sparing diuretics

Side-effects. Transient and mild azotaemia, lethargy, drowsiness, hypotension, incoordination

Warnings. Renal function should be monitored before and for 2–7 days after start of treatment; safety in breeding dogs has not been established; Drug Interactions – diuretics, ACE inhibitors; treatment with diuretics should start 1 day before enalapril treatment

Dose. *Dogs*: *by mouth*, 500 micrograms/kg once daily. May be increased to 500 micrograms/kg twice daily if required

Cats ♦ : *by mouth*, 250–500 micrograms/kg once or twice daily

POM Cardiovet (Intervet) *UK*
Tablets, enalapril maleate 1 mg, 2.5 mg, 5 mg, 10 mg, 20 mg, for *dogs*

POM Enacard (Merial) *UK*
Tablets, enalapril maleate 1 mg, 2.5 mg, 5 mg, 10 mg, 20 mg, for *dogs*

Australia
Indications. Congestive heart failure
Contra-indications. Animals at risk of hypotension; breeding animals
Warnings. Renal function should be monitored; Drug Interactions – diuretics
Dose. *Dogs*: *by mouth*, 500 micrograms/kg

Enalfor (Merial) *Austral.*
Tablets, enalapril maleate 1 mg, 2.5 mg, 5 mg, 10 mg, 20 mg, for *dogs*

Eire
Indications. Congestive heart failure
Contra-indications. Animals at risk of hypotension; pregnant bitches; aortic stenosis
Side-effects. Transient and mild azotaemia, lethargy, drowsiness, hypotension, incoordination
Warnings. Renal function should be monitored before and during treatment; Drug Interactions – diuretics, ACE inhibitors, potassium-sparing diuretics; safety in breeding dogs has not been established
Dose. *Dogs*: *by mouth*, 500 micrograms/kg

Cardiovet (Intervet) *Eire*
Tablets, enalapril maleate 1 mg, 2.5 mg, 5mg, 10 mg, 20 mg, for *dogs*

USA
Indications. Congestive heart failure
Contra-indications. Animals at risk of hypotension; pregnant bitches
Side-effects. Transient and mild azotaemia, lethargy, drowsiness, hypotension, incoordination
Warnings. Renal function should be monitored before and during treatment; Drug Interactions – diuretics, ACE inhibitors, potassium-sparing diuretics; safety in breeding dogs has not been established
Dose. *Dogs*: *by mouth*, 500 micrograms/kg

Enacard (Merial) *USA*
Tablets, enalapril maleate 1 mg, 2.5 mg, 5 mg, 10 mg, 20 mg, for *dogs*

RAMIPRIL

Indications. Congestive heart failure
Contra-indications. Pregnant and lactating bitches; cardiac output failure; obstructive hypertrophic cardiomyopathy; concurrent low-sodium diet; concurrent potassium-sparing diuretics or NSAIDs
Side-effects. Hypotension
Warnings. Care in patients at risk of hypotension; Drug Interactions – diuretics
Dose. *Dogs*: *by mouth*, 125 micrograms/kg once daily. May be increased to 250 micrograms/kg once daily after 2 weeks

POM Vasotop (Intervet)
Tablets, scored, ramipril 1.25 mg, 2.5 mg, 5 mg, for *dogs*

4.3.2 Inodilators

Pimobendan has positive inotrope and vasodilator activity. It inhibits phosphodiesterase thereby increasing intracellular cyclic AMP concentrations. This results in vasodilatation in peripheral and coronary vessels. Pimobendan also increases the calcium sensitivity of cardiac myofilaments thereby increasing the contractility of the myocardium. The bioavailability of pimobendan is reduced with food; animals should be treated approximately one hour before feeding.

Isoxsuprine is a vasodilator which also stimulates beta-adrenergic receptors. It causes direct relaxation of vascular and uterine smooth muscle (see section 8.5). It is used in the treatment of navicular disease (see section 10.7). Isoxsuprine is also a positive inotrope.

PIMOBENDAN

Indications. Congestive heart failure
Contra-indications. Cardiac output failure; hypertrophic cardiomyopathy
Side-effects. Rarely vomiting, moderate chronotropic effect
Warnings. Safety in pregnant and lactating animals has not been established; Drug Interactions – verapamil, propranolol
Dose. *Dogs*: *by mouth*, 0.2–0.6 mg/kg daily in 2 divided doses and given approx. 1 hour before feeding

POM Vetmedin Capsules (Boehringer Ingelheim)
Capsules, pimobendan 2.5 mg, 5 mg, for *dogs*

4.3.3 Vasodilators

Glyceryl trinitrate and other nitrates relax venous smooth muscle and can be useful preload reducers especially in severe pulmonary oedema. It is also used in acute and chronic laminitis in horses as a vasodilator to improve laminar perfusion. Topical ointment formulations are applied to provide slow transcutaneous absorption.

Hydralazine is an arteriodilator causing relaxation of arteriolar smooth muscle, probably by local mechanisms. Adequate monitoring should be provided because the initial dose may lead to a precipitous fall in blood pressure. Furthermore, prolonged use of this agent leads to undesirable catecholamine release.

Sodium nitroprusside is administered intravenously in severe congestive heart failure because it is a potent arterial and venous dilator. It is usually combined with a positive inotrope such as dobutamine (see section 4.5) for use under intensive care conditions for the management of severe acute congestive heart failure. Sodium nitroprusside improves cardiac output but may result in marked hypotension. The positive inotropic effect of dobutamine appears to mitigate this. Both drugs have short duration of action with a half-life of only 2 to 3 minutes. The dosages given are for guidance and should be adjusted for the individual patient in accordance with intensive care monitoring parameters.

GLYCERYL TRINITRATE

UK

Indications. Cardiogenic pulmonary oedema; acute laminitis
Contra-indications. Cardiogenic shock
Side-effects. Hypotension; decreased cardiac output
Warnings. Operators should wear gloves for application of ointment to patients
Dose.
Horses: *by topical application*, 2.5 cm of 2% ointment applied to each digital vessel of affected feet (maximum dose 2.5 cm/60 kg body-weight)
Dogs, cats: *by topical application*, 0.5–4.0 centimetres of a 2% ointment applied to inside of pinna or other area free of hair and inaccessible to the patient

P Ⓗ **Percutol** (Dominion) *UK*
Ointment, glyceryl trinitrate 2%; 30 g

HYDRALAZINE HYDROCHLORIDE

UK

Indications. Mitral regurgitation and left-sided congestive heart failure
Side-effects. Reflex tachycardia; hypotension; gastro-intestinal disturbances; depression; anorexia
Dose.
Dogs: *by mouth*, 0.5–2.0 mg/kg twice daily
Cats: *by mouth*, 2.5 mg twice daily, increasing to 5 mg twice daily if required

POM Ⓗ **Hydralazine** (Non-proprietary) *UK*
Tablets, hydralazine hydrochloride 25 mg, 50 mg

SODIUM NITROPRUSSIDE

UK

Indications. Life-threatening congestive heart failure
Side-effects. Hypotension
Warnings. Mean arterial blood pressure should be monitored; to avoid cyanide toxicity total dose should be no greater than 1.5 mg/kg per 2 hours. Solutions should be prepared immediately before use and protected from light during infusion by wrapping the container in aluminium foil or some other light-proof material.
Dose. *Dogs*: *by intravenous infusion*, 5–15 micrograms/kg per minute increasing gradually, maintaining a mean arterial blood pressure above 70 mmHg

POM Ⓗ **Sodium Nitroprusside** (Non-proprietary) *UK*
Intravenous infusion, for dilution, sodium nitroprusside 10 mg/mL; 5 mL. To be diluted before use

4.3.4 Cerebral vasodilators

These drugs are claimed to improve mental function in aged animals. It is important that patients are thoroughly exam-

ined and investigation and treatment of specific diseases is employed before using these drugs.

Nicergoline is an ergot derivative which acts specifically on the vascular system and cells of the brain. It is an alpha-adrenoceptor blocking drug acting primarily on alpha₁ and alpha₂ adrenoceptors. Nicergoline also blocks serotonin and dopamine receptors.

Propentofylline is a xanthine derivative which which alters the physical characteristics of the blood by increasing erythrocyte flexibility, preventing aggregation of erythrocytes and platelets, decreasing fibrinogen levels, and inhibiting the action of some inflammatory cytokines.

NICERGOLINE

UK

Indications. Improvement of age-related disorders, particularly behavioural problems
Contra-indications. Use within 24 hours of administration of alpha₂-adrenoceptor agonists; use before administration of vasodilators such as acepromazine and prazosin
Dose. *Dogs*: *by mouth*, 250–500 micrograms/kg daily, given in the morning

POM **Fitergol** (Merial) *UK*
Tablets, or to prepare an oral solution, nicergoline 5 mg, for *dogs*; 100
Note. Tablets should not be broken. To administer the correct dosage to dogs 5–10 kg body-weight, dissolve 1 tablet in 10 mL water and give 5 mL of solution immediately. Remaining solution should be discarded

New Zealand

Indications. Improvement of age-related behavioural disorders
Contra-indications. Concurrent use of vasodilators
Warnings. Discontinue treatment 24 hours before xylazine anaesthesia
Dose. *Dogs*: *by mouth*, 250–500 micrograms/kg

Fitergol (Merial) *NZ*
Tablets, nicergoline 5 mg, for *dogs*

PROPENTOFYLLINE

UK

Indications. Dullness, lethargy in older dogs; navicular disease in horses♦ (see section 10.6)
Contra-indications. Manufacturer does not recommend use in pregnant or breeding animals
Side-effects. CNS and cardiovascular over-stimulation
Dose. *By mouth*, given on an empty stomach 30 minutes before feeding
Dogs: (<5 kg body-weight) 12.5 mg twice daily; (5–8 kg body-weight) 25 mg twice daily; (9–15 kg body-weight) 50 mg twice daily; (16–25 kg body-weight) 75 mg twice daily; (26–33 kg body-weight) 100 mg twice daily; (34–49 kg body-weight) 150 mg twice daily; (50–66 mg/kg body-weight) 200 mg twice daily; (67–83 kg body-weight) 250 mg twice daily

POM **Vivitonin** (Intervet) *UK*
Tablets, scored, propentofylline 50 mg, 100 mg, for *dogs*; 60

New Zealand
Indications. Conditions associated with ageing
Contra-indications. Pregnant or breeding animals
Side-effects. Rarely allergic skin reactions
Dose. *Dogs: by mouth*, 25–150 mg depending on body-weight

Karsivan/Vivitonin (Agvet) *NZ*
Tablets, propentofylline 50 mg, for *dogs*

4.4 Antidysrhythmics

4.4.1 Drugs for tachydysrhythmias
4.4.2 Drugs for bradydysrhythmias

Abnormal heart rhythms may often be controlled by anti-arrhythmic drugs, even if caused by myocardial disease. However, many or most rhythm disturbances are associated with metabolic, toxic, or endocrine disturbances, for example trauma, gastric torsion, pancreatitis, renal failure, CNS disease, adrenal or thyroid disease, hypoxia, or electrolyte imbalance. If the primary disease is treated, the dysrhythmia may also resolve even in the absence of cardiac therapy. When rhythm disturbances are detected, the animal should be thoroughly examined for the presence of primary myocardial disease and for metabolic disturbances.

Many drugs used to treat tachydysrhythmias are pro-arrhythmic in that they may exacerbate the disturbance or cause some further rhythm complication. Therefore therapy should be considered only after an evaluation of the case, and reserved particularly for disturbances in which the rhythm is considered dangerous and those in which the disturbance is contributing to signs of heart failure particularly at heart rate of >160/minute or <60/minute in dogs and >220/minute in cats. Examples of such conditions include severe heart block or multiple and/or frequent very early ventricular premature beats, which may precede fibrillation. Antidysrhythmic therapy is rarely considered essential for occasional premature beats or for sinus bradycardias.

4.4.1 Drugs for tachydysrhythmias

4.4.1.1 Class I anti-arrhythmics
4.4.1.2 Class II anti-arrhythmics
4.4.1.3 Class III anti-arrhythmics
4.4.1.4 Class IV anti-arrhythmics

Effective drugs are frequently grouped according to the Vaughan Williams classification (see above). Drugs from the same group should not be administered simultaneously. However in patients that do not respond to treatment, a combination of drugs from different groups can sometimes prove to be helpful.

There is rarely definitive guidance on which drug is most likely to be effective, and even the successful suppression of a rhythm disturbance may not presage an improved survival of the animal.

Atrial fibrillation is rarely reversible in dogs and cats. This disturbance is usually associated with significant atrial disease or dilatation. However, in performance horses there is frequently no underlying cardiac abnormality and the animal may often return to normal work after therapy with quinidine sulphate. Nonetheless, treatment requires reasonably intensive monitoring.

Other supraventricular tachycardias in dogs and cats may respond to vagal reflexes such as carotid sinus pressure or ocular pressure but any benefit may only be transient. Alternatively, a Class II beta-adrenoceptor blocking drug such as esmolol or a Class IV calcium antagonist may control the tachycardia. Additionally digoxin may be administered in combination with a drug from Class II or Class IV in cases resistant to therapy. This combination may also be used to control the ventricular rate in atrial fibrillation in dogs.

The efficacy of any individual agent for treatment of ventricular tachydysrhythmias is unpredictable although lidocaine (without epinephrine) is usually effective. However, lidocaine may only be administered intravenously and is rapidly excreted; it is best reserved for emergency treatment. Lidocaine is ineffective in patients with hypokalaemia and may be toxic (especially in cats); therapy for seizures should be available. Authorities suggest that bretylium, a class 1B drug, may prove useful. Procainamide is frequently used for maintenance therapy for ventricular tachycardias and is sometimes given in combination with a Class II drug. Beta-adrenoceptor blocking drugs (Class II agents) are often used in combination with drugs from classes I or III (not class IV because the combination may result in severe heart block) .

4.4.1.1 Class I anti-arrhythmics

Drugs included in this class have a local anaesthetic action. They have a membrane-stabilising effect that results in a reduced rate of depolarisation. Although the subdivision of this class into A, B, and C is based on their varied effects on the action potential there is no clinical significance in these divisions. Only drugs in classes 1A (procainamide and quinidine) and 1B (lidocaine, tocainide, and phenytoin) are commonly used in veterinary medicine.

Quinidine is used mainly to reverse atrial fibrillation in horses. It prolongs the atrial refractory period, is vagolytic, and is a negative inotrope. It is less commonly used in dogs.
Procainamide is rapidly absorbed after oral administration in the dog and has a plasma half-life of 2.5 to 4 hours. Most preparations are formulated as modified-release dosage forms to overcome problems of frequent administration. Procainamide is the drug of choice for maintenance therapy of ventricular arrhythmias in dogs. In patients with reduced renal function, the dose should be reduced by 50% for every 50% increase in plasma-urea concentration. See also Prescribing in renal impairment for information on dosage adjustment. Disopyramide has a half-life of less than 2 hours and causes profound myocardial depression, which precludes its routine use.

Lidocaine (without epinephrine) is used intravenously for severe acute ventricular arrhythmias of any cause. Efficient first-pass metabolism in the liver precludes oral use. **Phenytoin** (see section 6.9.1) has similar cardiovascular effects to lidocaine. It is used to treat arrhythmias caused by cardiac glycoside toxicity♦ in dogs at a dose of 35 to 50 mg/kg by mouth 3 times daily. **Mexiletine** is administered by mouth and has a similar anti-arrhythmic action to lidocaine. It is likely to depress myocardial function less than Class A drugs and is more desirable for dogs with mild congestive heart failure.

LIDOCAINE HYDROCHLORIDE
(Lignocaine hydrochloride)

UK
Indications. Life-threatening ventricular tachyarrhythmias such as tachycardia
Contra-indications. Atrial fibrillation or flutter
Side-effects. Seizures; hypotension; CNS disturbances
Warnings. Not effective in the presence of hypokalaemia; doses should be reduced in congestive heart failure or hepatic disease; Drug Interactions – see Appendix 1
Dose. *Dogs*: *by slow intravenous injection (given over 3–5 minutes)*, initial dose 2–4 mg/kg, followed *by intravenous infusion* at a rate of 25–75 micrograms/kg per minute

POM Ⓗ **Lidocaine in Glucose Injection** (Non-proprietary) *UK*
Intravenous infusion, lidocaine hydrochloride 1 mg/mL and 2 mg/mL in glucose intravenous infusion 5%; 500 mL

POM Ⓗ **Min-I-Jet Lignocaine** (Medeva) *UK*
Injection, lidocaine hydrochloride 10 mg/mL, 20 mg/mL; 10-mg/mL syringe 10 mL, 20-mg/mL syringe 5 mL

POM Ⓗ **Xylocard** (Astra) *UK*
Injection, lidocaine hydrochloride (anhydrous) 20 mg/mL; 5 mL

MEXILETINE HYDROCHLORIDE

UK
Indications. Ventricular tachydysrhythmias, especially frequent ventricular premature beats or ventricular tachycardia, after conversion with lidocaine
Contra-indications. Hypotension, very low cardiac output, heart block, bradycardia, hepatic impairment
Side-effects. Gastro-intestinal disturbances, CNS disturbances such as seizures
Dose. *Dogs*: *by mouth*, 4–8 mg/kg 2–3 times daily

POM Ⓗ **Mexitil** (Boehringer Ingelheim) *UK*
Capsules, mexiletine hydrochloride 50 mg, 200 mg; 100

PROCAINAMIDE HYDROCHLORIDE

UK
Indications. Ventricular arrhythmias such as frequent ventricular premature depolarisations or ventricular tachycardia
Contra-indications. Untreated atrial fibrillation, conduction blocks, poor left ventricular function
Side-effects. Gastro-intestinal disturbances
Warnings. Reduce dose in patients with renal impairment, see notes above

Dose. *Dogs*: *by mouth*, 8–30 mg/kg 4 times daily
by intramuscular injection, 8–20 mg/kg 4 times daily
by slow intravenous injection (given over 5 minutes), initial dose 6–8 mg/kg, followed *by intravenous infusion* at a rate of 10–40 micrograms/kg per minute

POM Ⓗ **Pronestyl** (Squibb) *UK*
Tablets, scored, procainamide hydrochloride 250 mg; 100
Injection, procainamide hydrochloride 100 mg/mL; 10 mL

QUINIDINE

UK
Indications. Supraventricular arrhythmias especially atrial fibrillation
Contra-indications. Hepatic impairment
Side-effects. Anorexia, vomiting, diarrhoea, tachycardia, ventricular fibrillation, allergic responses, laminitis, ataxia, nasal mucosal swelling
Warnings. Increased toxicity in cases with hypoalbuminaemia, monitor the ECG in horses; Drug Interactions – see Appendix 1
Dose. Expressed as quinidine sulphate
Horses: *by stomach tube*, 20 mg/kg every 2 hours until arrhythmia is abolished or toxic side-effects are seen (maximum 60 g daily)
Dogs: *by mouth*, 6–16 mg/kg 3–4 times daily

Note. Quinidine sulphate 200 mg = quinidine bisulphate 250 mg

POM Ⓗ **Quinidine Sulphate** (Non-proprietary) *UK*
Tablets, quinidine sulphate 200 mg, 300 mg
Oral powder, quinidine sulphate is available from Loveridge

POM Ⓗ **Kinidin Durules** (Astra) *UK*
Tablets, m/r, f/c, quinidine bisulphate 250 mg; 100

4.4.1.2 Class II anti-arrhythmics

Drugs included in this class are beta-adrenoceptor blocking drugs (beta-blockers), which antagonise sympathetic activity. The heart-rate is decreased by a reduction in the sinus node rate and prolongation of atrioventricular (A-V) node conduction. These drugs prevent reflex tachycardia and decrease the occurrence of both atrial and ventricular premature depolarisations. In addition, beta-adrenoceptor blocking drugs may lower blood pressure in hypertension and may be used to suppress the deleterious effects of ventricular hypertrophy (for example in hypertrophic cardiomyopathy, hyperthyroidism, or aortic stenosis) and in systemic hypertension.

Propranolol is the most common beta-adrenoceptor blocking drug used in veterinary practice for atrial arrhythmias. It undergoes hepatic metabolism and has a plasma half-life of 1.5 hours. In heart failure, hepatic blood flow is reduced and propranolol metabolism is altered with prolonged administration, therefore the drug is given every 8 hours. Bronchial smooth muscle constriction is an important, undesirable side-effect of non-specific beta-adrenoceptor blocking drugs. Therefore, high doses should be gradually introduced over 3 to 5 days.

There are many other compounds in this group. **Atenolol** is beta$_1$-receptor selective and long acting and is often useful for long-term therapy for example in cats with hypertrophic cardiomyopathy or hypertension. **Metoprolol** is highly beta$_1$-receptor selective and has been used in dogs and cats in preference to atenolol. **Esmolol** is ultra-short acting and very useful for the investigation and immediate therapy of tachycardias. For all beta-adrenoceptor blocking drugs, doses should be gradually increased from the lowest recommended levels, and titrated on an individual patient basis.

Carvedilol, a beta-adrenoceptor blocking drug with vasodilator properties, has been shown to be particularly effective at prolonging life in humans with congestive heart failure; studies in dogs are not yet reported.

ATENOLOL

UK

Indications. Supraventricular arrhythmias; excessive ventricular hypertrophy
Contra-indications. Concurrent administration of quinidine, hepatic impairment with decreased blood flow, asthma, small airway disease, sick sinus syndrome, atrioventricular block
Side-effects. Bronchospasm, myocardial depression, bradycardia, hypotension
Warnings. Bronchospasm, negative inotropic properties may exacerbate congestive heart failure, reduce dose in renal impairment
Dose. *Dogs*: *by mouth,* 100–500 micrograms/kg 1–2 times daily
Cats: *by mouth,* 1–2 mg/kg 1–2 times daily

POM Ⓗ **Atenolol** (Non-proprietary) *UK*
Tablets, atenolol 25 mg, 50 mg, 100 mg

POM Ⓗ **Tenormin** (Stuart) *UK*
Tablets, atenolol 25 mg, 50 mg, 100 mg
Syrup, atenolol 5 mg/mL; 300 mL

ESMOLOL HYDROCHLORIDE

UK

Indications. Tachycardias, especially supraventricular tachycardias; investigation and acute treatment of tachycardias
Contra-indications. Bradycardia, heart block
Side-effects. Weakness, bradycardia
Dose. *Dogs*: *by intravenous injection,* 100–500 micrograms/kg
by intravenous infusion, 0.5–1.0 mg/kg given over 5 minutes

POM Ⓗ **Brevibloc** (Baxter) *UK*
Injection, esmolol hydrochloride 10 mg/mL; 10 mL
Injection, for dilution, esmolol hydrochloride 250 mg/mL; 10 mL. For dilution before use as intravenous infusion

METOPROLOL TARTRATE

UK

Indications. Supraventricular arrhythmias; excessive ventricular hypertrophy
Contra-indications. **Side-effects**. **Warnings**. See under Atenolol
Dose. *Dogs, cats*: *by mouth,* 0.5–1.0 mg/kg 3 times daily

POM Ⓗ **Metoprolol** (Non-proprietary) *UK*
Tablets, metoprolol tartrate 50 mg, 100 mg

POM Ⓗ **Betaloc** (Astra)
Tablets, metoprolol tartrate 50 mg, 100 mg

POM Ⓗ **Lopresor** (Novartis)
Tablets, scored, metoprolol tartrate 50 mg, 100 mg

PROPRANOLOL HYDROCHLORIDE

UK

Indications. Supraventricular tachycardia; hypertrophic cardiomyopathy; thyrotoxicosis (see section 7.1.2) especially in cats; atrial or ventricular premature depolarisations; behaviour modification (see section 6.11.6)
Contra-indications. **Side-effects**. **Warnings**. See under Atenolol; caution in hepatic impairment
Dose. Cardiac conditions, *by mouth.*
Dogs: 20–100 micrograms/kg 3 times daily, increasing over 3–5 days to a maximum of 1 mg/kg 3 times daily as necessary
Cats: 2.5 mg 3 times daily, increasing over 3–5 days to up to 10 mg 3 times daily as necessary

POM Ⓗ **Propranolol** (Non-proprietary) *UK*
Tablets, propranolol hydrochloride 10 mg, 40 mg, 80 mg, 160 mg
Oral solution, propranolol hydrochloride 1 mg/mL, 2 mg/mL, 10 mg/mL (available as 'Special Order' from Rosemont)

POM Ⓗ **Inderal** (Zeneca)
Tablets, propranolol hydrochloride 10 mg, 40 mg, 80 mg

4.4.1.3 Class III anti-arrhythmics

Drugs in this class prolong the action potential and hence the effective refractory period. They are mainly used in ventricular tachycardia resistant to other therapy and are sometimes combined with Class I agents. **Sotalol** combines Class III activity with beta-adrenoceptor blockade and has been used effectively in dogs.

AMIODARONE HYDROCHLORIDE

UK

Indications. Supraventricular and ventricular arrhythmias
Contra-indications. Thyrotoxicosis, bradycardia
Side-effects. Pulmonary fibrosis, gastro-intestinal disturbances, negative inotropic properties, corneal deposits, thyroid disturbances
Warnings. This drug should be used with caution
Dose. *Dogs*: *by mouth,* 10 mg/kg twice daily. Dose should be reduced for maintenance, if possible
by intravenous injection, 10–20 mg/kg

POM Ⓗ **Amiodarone Hydrochloride** (Non-proprietary) *UK*
Tablets, amiodarone hydrochloride 100 mg, 200 mg

POM Ⓗ **Cordarone X** (Sanofi Winthrop) *UK*
Tablets, scored, amiodarone hydrochloride 100 mg, 200 mg; 28
Injection, for dilution, amiodarone hydrochloride 50 mg/mL; 3 mL. For dilution before use as intravenous infusion

BRETYLIUM TOSILATE
(Bretylium tosylate)

UK

Indications. Ventricular arrhythmias refractory to routine therapy (intravenous injection); protection against ventricular tachyarrhythmias in pigs under general anaesthesia (intravenous bolus or intravenous infusion)
Side-effects. Rarely hypotension, arrhythmias; ataxia, vomiting
Dose. *Dogs*: *by intravenous injection*, 5–20 mg/kg
Pigs: *by intravenous infusion*, 20 micrograms/kg per minute

POM Ⓗ **Bretylate** (GlaxoWellcome) *UK*
Injection, bretylium tosilate 50 mg/mL; 10 mL

POM Ⓗ **Min-I-Jet Bretylium Tosylate** (Medeva) *UK*
Injection, bretylium tosilate 50 mg/mL; 10-mL syringe

SOTALOL HYDROCHLORIDE

UK

Indications. Ventricular tachydysrhythmias
Contra-indications. Atrio-ventricular block
Side-effects. Bradycardia, atrio-ventricular block, weakness
Warnings. Use with care in moderate to severe congestive heart failure
Dose. *Dogs*: *by mouth*, 1–5 mg/kg twice daily. Commence with low dose and increase for individual patient

POM Ⓗ **Sotalol** (Non-proprietary) *UK*
Tablets, sotalol hydrochloride 80 mg, 160 mg

POM Ⓗ **Beta-Cardone** (Medeva)
Tablets, scored, sotalol hydrochloride 40 mg, 80 mg, 200 mg

POM Ⓗ **Sotacor** (Bristol-Myers)
Tablets, sotalol hydrochloride 80 mg, 160 mg

4.4.1.4 Class IV anti-arrhythmics

Drugs in this class inhibit slow calcium channels and dilate capillaries. They have a profound depressant effect on atrio-ventricular nodal conduction and are the drugs of choice for severe acute supraventricular tachycardias. In addition, they are potent coronary artery dilators and cause hypotension. A negative inotropic effect may exacerbate congestive heart failure. However, these drugs may also be valuable for hypertrophic ventricular disorders including hyperthyroidism, hypertrophic cardiomyopathy, and aortic stenosis, and for systemic hypertension.

Cardiac glycosides (see section 4.1.1) are also used in the treatment of supraventricular arrhythmias and congestive heart failure. **Verapamil** can reverse atrial fibrillation in some dogs and is therefore an alternative to quinidine in such cases. Verapamil is the calcium channel blocker of choice for intravenous administration, while **diltiazem** is used for long-term oral therapy and is believed to be a less potent negative inotrope than verapamil. Diltiazem may be used in the treatment of unresponsive supraventricular tachycardias in combination with digoxin (at a reduced dosage) or beta-adrenoceptor blocking drugs. **Amlodipine** is now the drug of choice for hypertension in cats. It is sometimes used in combination wih ACE-inhibitors (see section 4.3.1). Beta-adrenoceptor blocking drugs are also used.

AMLODIPINE BESILATE
(Amlodipine besylate)

UK

Indications. Hypertension, especially in cats
Contra-indications. Low cardiac output, shock, hypotension
Side-effects. Possible ataxia and lethargy
Dose. *Cats*: *by mouth,* 200 micrograms/kg once daily

POM Ⓗ **Istin** (Pfizer) *UK*
Tablets, amlodipine (as besylate) 5 mg, 10 mg

DILTIAZEM HYDROCHLORIDE

UK

Indications. Supraventricular tachyarrhythmias; hypertension; excessive ventricular hypertrophy
Contra-indications. Sick sinus syndrome, cardiac glycoside toxicity, atrioventricular block, myocardial failure, bradycardia, severe congestive heart failure
Side-effects. Hypotension, bradycardia
Warnings. Care should be taken in case of untreated congestive heart failure
Dose. *By mouth.*
Dogs: 0.5–1.25 mg/kg 3–4 times daily
Cats: 1.5–2.0 mg/kg 2–3 times daily

Note. Although the formulation of these preparations has called for the strict designation 'modified-release', the duration of action corresponds to that of tablets requiring several doses per day. Longer-acting preparations are also available and to avoid confusion, prescribers should specify a brand name

POM Ⓗ **Diltiazem** (Non-proprietary) *UK*
Tablets, m/r (but see note above), f/c, diltiazem hydrochloride 60 mg; 100

POM Ⓗ **Tildiem** (Sanofi-Synthelabo) *UK*
Tablets, m/r (but see note above), diltiazem hydrochloride 60 mg; 90

VERAPAMIL HYDROCHLORIDE

UK

Indications. Supraventricular tachyarrhythmias; sustained and paroxysmal tachycardia; excessive ventricular hypertrophy
Contra-indications. See under Diltiazem hydrochloride
Side-effects. Hypotension, bradycardia, myocardial depression

Warnings. See under Diltiazem hydrochloride; Drug Interactions – see Appendix 1
Dose. *Dogs*: *by mouth*, 1–5 mg/kg 3 times daily
by intravenous injection, 500 micrograms/kg every 10–30 minutes according to the patient's response
Cats: *by mouth*, 1.1–2.9 mg/kg 3 times daily

POM Ⓗ **Verapamil** (Non-proprietary) *UK*
Tablets, coated, verapamil hydrochloride 40 mg, 80 mg, 120 mg, 160 mg
Oral solution, verapamil hydrochloride 8 mg/mL (available as 'Special Order' from Rosemont)

POM Ⓗ **Cordilox** (Baker Norton) *UK*
Tablets, verapamil hydrochloride 40 mg, 80 mg, 120 mg, 160 mg
Injection, verapamil hydrochloride 2.5 mg/mL; 2 mL

POM Ⓗ **Securon** (Knoll) *UK*
Tablets, verapamil hydrochloride 40 mg, 80 mg, 120 mg
Injection, verapamil hydrochloride 2.5 mg/mL; 2 mL

4.4.2 Drugs for bradydysrhythmias

Before prolonged treatment for bradydysrhythmias, an animal should be carefully evaluated for metabolic, endocrine, and other extraneous disease.

If bradycardia is vagally mediated, antimuscarinic drugs, such as atropine may be effective. However, side-effects are likely. Adrenoceptor stimulants are rarely very useful and may precipitate serious tachycardias. For serious and persistent disease, artificial pacemakers may be essential. These should prevent cardiac asystole and therefore reduce episodes of syncope and prevent sudden death.

Atropine sulphate and **glycopyrronium** (see section 6.6.1) are used for the treatment of bradycardia♦, incomplete A-V block♦, and sino-atrial arrest♦ in dogs and cats. The dose for atropine is 10 to 20 micrograms/kg by intramuscular or intravenous injection or 30 to 40 micrograms/kg subcutaneously. The dose for glycopyrronium is 5 to 10 micrograms/kg by subcutaneous, intramuscular, or intravenous injection.

4.5 Adrenoceptor stimulants (Sympathomimetics)

Adrenoceptor stimulants are used for cardiovascular support in the management of critically ill patients. These are usually cases under anaesthesia or recovering from major surgery. Patients in shock, especially cardiogenic in origin, may also benefit from this type of support. However, prolonged use of these agents in humans has led to decreased survival.

The properties of adrenoceptor stimulants vary according to whether they act on alpha- or beta-adrenergic receptors.

Epinephrine acts on both alpha- and beta-receptors and increases both the heart-rate and the contractility (beta$_1$ effects). It can cause peripheral vasodilation (a beta$_2$ effect) or vasoconstriction (an alpha effect). Epinephrine is used in the emergency treatment of acute allergic and anaphylactic reactions. The use of epinephrine by intracardiac adminis-

tration is not recommended. In cardiac arrest, the drug is best administered either intratracheally or via a central vein. The cardiac stimulant **dobutamine** acts on beta$_1$-receptors in cardiac muscle, with minimal effect on heart-rate or systemic vascular resistance. It has a positive inotropic effect and is used for cardiogenic shock. It is also used during equine anaesthesia to maintain mean blood pressure above approximately 70 mmHg in order to prevent hypotension-induced myopathy, a not uncommon complication of anaesthesia in horses.

Isoprenaline is less selective and increases both heart-rate and contractility. It has been used to increase heart rate in some bradycardias but cardiac pacemakers are usually more effective. Isoprenaline may also cause tachycardia or fibrillation.

DOBUTAMINE

UK
Indications. Cardiogenic shock; dilated cardiomyopathy with congestive heart failure; hypotension during equine anaesthesia
Side-effects. Tachyarrhythmias; seizures in cats
Warnings. Monitor ECG; Drug Interactions – see Appendix 1 (adrenoceptor stimulants)
Dose.
Horses: *by intravenous infusion*, up to 5 micrograms/kg per minute (doses of less than 1 microgram/kg per minute are often sufficient)
Dogs: *by intravenous infusion*, 2–7 micrograms/kg per minute (for up to 3 days in cases of cardiomyopathy)
Cats: *by intravenous infusion*, up to 4 micrograms/kg per minute

POM Ⓗ **Dobutrex** (Lilly) *UK*
Intravenous infusion, for dilution, dobutamine (as hydrochloride) 12.5 mg/mL; 20 mL. To be diluted before use

EPINEPHRINE
(Adrenaline)

UK
Indications. Anaphylaxis; cardiac arrest
Side-effects. Anxiety, fear, restlessness; tachycardia, ventricular arrhythmias
Warnings. Epinephrine solutions should be diluted to at least 1 in 10 000 (100 micrograms/mL) for all animal use; monitor ECG; Drug Interactions — see Appendix 1 (adrenoceptor stimulants)
Dose. *By subcutaneous or intravenous injection or intratracheal administration*, 20 micrograms/kg

POM Ⓗ **Epinephrine Injection BP** (Non-proprietary) *UK*
Injection, epinephrine (as acid tartrate) 1 mg/mL (1 in 1000); 0.5 mL, 1.0 mL

POM Ⓗ **Epinephrine Injection** (Non-proprietary) *UK*
Injection, epinephrine (as acid tartrate) 100 micrograms/mL (1 in 10 000); 10 mL

USA

Indications. Anaphylaxis
Dose. *Horses, cattle, sheep, pigs*: *by subcutaneous or intramuscular injection*, 22 micrograms/kg
Dogs, cats: *by subcutaneous or intramuscular injection*, 100–500 micrograms

Epinephrine 1:1000 (AgriLabs, AgriPharm, DurVet) *USA*
Injection, epinephrine 1 mg/mL, for *horses, cattle, sheep, pigs*

Epinephrine Injection (Vedco) *USA*
Injection, epinephrine 1 mg/mL, for *cattle, horses, sheep, pigs, dogs, cats*

Epinephrine Injection 1:1000 (RXV) *USA*
Injection, epinephrine 1 mg/mL, for *horses, cattle, sheep, pigs, dogs, cats*

Epinephrine Injection USP (Phoenix, VetTek) *USA*
Injection, epinephrine 1 mg/mL, for *horses, cattle, sheep, pigs*

Epinephrine Injection USP 1:1,000 (Butler) *USA*
Injection, epinephrine 1 mg/mL, for *horses, cattle, sheep, pigs*

Epinject (Vetus) *USA*
Injection, epinephrine 1 mg/mL, for *horses, cattle, sheep, pigs*

ISOPRENALINE HYDROCHLORIDE

UK

Indications. Heart block; bradycardia
Side-effects. Ventricular tachycardias
Warnings. Monitor ECG; Drug Interactions – see Appendix 1 (adrenoceptor stimulants)
Dose. *Dogs*: *by mouth*, 5–10 mg 3–4 times daily
by intravenous infusion, 10 nanograms/kg per minute

POM (H) **Min-I-Jet Isoprenaline** (Medeva) *UK*
Injection, isoprenaline hydrochloride 20 micrograms/mL; 10-mL syringe

POM (H) **Saventrine IV** (Pharmax) *UK*
Intravenous infusion, for dilution, isoprenaline hydrochloride 1 mg/mL; 2 mL. To be diluted before use

4.6 Anticoagulants

4.6.1 Parenteral anticoagulants
4.6.2 Oral anticoagulants
4.6.3 Protamine sulphate

Anticoagulant drugs are much less frequently used in veterinary medicine than in human patients because atherosclerotic disease and prolonged postoperative recumbency are not common veterinary problems. Anticoagulants are mainly used to maintain the patency of vascular catheters and are part of the management of disseminated intravascular coagulation (DIC). In DIC, administration of fresh blood, platelet rich plasma, or plasma may also be indicated.

The main use of anticoagulants is to prevent thrombus formation or the extension of an existing thrombus. These drugs act by affecting the clotting mechanisms. **Aspirin** (see section 10.1) is an antiplatelet drug used in cats with thrombo-embolism secondary to cardiomyopathy; the dose for antiplatelet action is up to 75 mg by mouth, once every 3 days. Aspirin acts by reducing platelet aggregation and inhibiting thrombus formation particularly in the arterial circulation.

4.6.1 Parenteral anticoagulants

The action of **heparin** inhibits thrombus formation but does not affect fibrin that is already present. Heparin is rapidly effective, which makes it suitable for emergency situations. It is metabolised in the liver and has a plasma half-life of 2 hours. Heparin has been used in cats with thromboembolism. For patients receiving treatment, the activated partial thromboplastin time, activated coagulation time, or kaolin-cephalin time should be monitored frequently and maintained at 1.5 to 2.5 times normal.

> Partial thromboplastin time, activated coagulation time, and kaolin-cephalin time results are highly variable and practitioners are advised to use the normal values supplied by the appropriate veterinary testing laboratory.

For maintaining catheter patency, sodium chloride intravenous infusion 0.9% is as effective as heparin flushes for up to 48 hours and is therefore recommended for cannulas intended to be in place for up to 2 days. Heparin flushes are recommended for cannulas intended to be in place for longer than 48 hours. Heparin injection diluted to 5 units/mL in sodium chloride intravenous infusion 0.9% may be used. Commercially available heparin flushes should not be used for therapeutic purposes.

If haemorrhage occurs it is usually sufficient to withdraw heparin, but if rapid reversal of the effects of heparin is required, protamine sulphate is a specific antidote (see section 4.6.3).

Heparin may be indicated in equine laminitis (see section 15.1) both for its anticoagulant effect and its potentially beneficial effect on the laminar basement membrane.

HEPARIN SODIUM

UK

Indications. Venous thrombosis; disseminated intravascular coagulation; pulmonary thrombo-embolism; laminitis in horses (see section 15.1)
Contra-indications. Hepatic impairment, haemorrhage; Drug Interactions – see Appendix 1
Side-effects. Haemorrhage
Dose.

Horses: laminitis, *by subcutaneous injection*, 40–100 units/kg 3 times daily; see also chapter 15
Dogs: *by subcutaneous injection*, 100–250 units/kg 3 times daily
by intravenous injection, initial dose 100–200 units/kg then 50 units/kg every 3 hours
Cats: *by subcutaneous injection*, 200 units/kg 3 times daily

POM (H) **Heparin Injection** (Non-proprietary) *UK*
Injection, heparin sodium 1000 units/mL; 1 mL, 5 mL
Injection, heparin sodium 5000 units/mL; 1 mL, 5 mL
Injection, heparin sodium 25 000 units/mL; 1 mL, 5 mL

Heparin catheter flushes (**Not for therapeutic use**)

POM Ⓗ **Canusal** (CP) *UK*
Solution, heparin sodium 100 units/mL; 2 mL

POM Ⓗ **Hep-Flush** (Leo) *UK*
Solution, heparin sodium 100 units/mL; 2 mL, 10 mL

POM Ⓗ **Heplok** (Leo) *UK*
Solution, heparin sodium 10 units/mL; 5 mL

POM Ⓗ **Hepsal** (CP) *UK*
Solution, heparin sodium 10 units/mL; 5 mL

4.6.2 Oral anticoagulants

Coumarin derivative anticoagulants inhibit the hepatic synthesis of vitamin K-dependent clotting factors and are thus more suitable than heparin where prolonged therapy is required. **Warfarin** is well absorbed from the intestine and is highly bound to plasma albumin. The onset of effect occurs after 6 to 12 hours, with full benefit realised after 2 to 3 days of repetitive administration. The effects of warfarin therapy should be monitored. Two blood samples should be taken on separate days before treatment is started to establish the baseline one stage prothrombin time (OSPT) for that particular animal. OSPT should be monitored daily, with samples taken at the same time each day for comparative purposes, until it reaches a steady state of 1.5 to 2.0 times the base level for a particular dose of warfarin. Thereafter twice weekly OSPT measurements are advised for several weeks and then once every 2 months for animals on long-term therapy.

Warfarin is used in cats with thromboembolism, and has been used for treatment of navicular disease (but see section 10.7).

Phytomenadione (vitamin K$_1$) is used in the treatment of overdose of coumarin anticoagulants (see Treatment of poisoning).

Many drugs are capable of displacing warfarin from plasma albumin, causing an increase in free warfarin and possible haemorrhage (Drug Interactions – see Appendix 1).

WARFARIN SODIUM

UK
Indications. Vascular thrombosis; navicular disease (see section 10.7)
Contra-indications. Purpura, malnutrition, haemorrhage, late pregnancy; Drug Interactions – see Appendix 1
Side-effects. Haemorrhage
Warnings. Monitor effects of Warfarin therapy, see notes above; Drug Interactions – see Appendix 1
Dose. *Horses: by mouth,* 20 micrograms/kg daily increasing gradually to desired effect (usual dose range: 16–170 micrograms/kg)
Cats: by mouth, 500 micrograms once daily

POM Ⓗ **Warfarin** (Non-proprietary) *UK*
Tablets, scored, warfarin sodium 0.5 mg, 1 mg, 3 mg, 5 mg

4.6.3 Protamine sulfate

Although protamine sulfate is used to counteract overdosage with heparin, if used in excess it has an anticoagulant effect.

PROTAMINE SULFATE
(Protamine sulphate)

UK
Indications. See notes above
Dose. *By slow intravenous injection,* 1 mg neutralises 100 units heparin. Decrease dose by 50% for every hour elapsed since heparin administration.

POM Ⓗ **Protamine Sulfate** (Non-proprietary) *UK*
Injection, protamine sulfate 10 mg/mL; 5 mL

POM Ⓗ **Prosulf** (CP)
Injection, protamine sulfate 10 mg/mL; 5 mL

4.7 Haemostatics

The use of **phytomenadione** (vitamin K$_1$) in the treatment of anticoagulant poisoning is described in Treatment of poisoning. **Tranexamic acid** is an antifibrinolytic drug which inhibits breakdown of fibrin clots. It is used to prevent and control surgical haemorrhage.

Epinephrine (see section 4.5) may be applied topically as a haemostatic. **Ferric chloride solution** has also been used topically to arrest bleeding from small wounds.

Dressings containing **calcium alginate** (see section 14.7.4) are available for control of wound haemorrhage during surgical procedures.

TRANEXAMIC ACID
Australia
Indications. Control of haemorrhage
Dose. *By subcutaneous, intramuscular, or intravenous injection.*
Horses, cattle: 5–25 mg/kg
Pigs, dogs, cats: 10–15 mg/kg

Vasolamin 5% (Ilium) *Austral.*
Injection, tranexamic acid 50 mg/mL, for *pigs, dogs, cats*
Withdrawal Periods. w.p not given

Vasolamin S 10% (Ilium) *Austral.*
Injection, tranexamic acid 100 mg/mL, for *cattle, horses*

New Zealand
Indications. Control of haemorrhage
Dose. *By subcutaneous, intramuscular, or intravenous injection.*
Horses, cattle: 5–25 mg/kg
Dogs, cats: 4–20 mg/kg

Vasolamin 5% (Ethical) *NZ*
Injection, tranexamic acid 50 mg/mL, for *dogs, cats*

Vasolamin S 10% (Ethical) *NZ*
Injection, tranexamic acid 100 mg/mL, for *horses, cattle*
Withdrawal Periods. *Horses*: slaughter 2 days. *Cattle*: slaughter 2 days, milk 48 hours

5 Drugs used in the treatment of disorders of the
RESPIRATORY SYSTEM

Contributors:
B M Corcoran MVB, DipPharm, PhD, MRCVS
D H Grove-White BVSc, DBR, FRCVS
T S Mair BVSc, PhD, DEIM, MRCVS
D J Taylor MA, VetMB, PhD, MRCVS

5.1 Treatment of respiratory infections
5.2 Bronchodilators
5.3 Drugs for allergic and inflammatory disorders
5.4 Mucolytics and expectorants
5.5 Antitussives
5.6 Respiratory stimulants
5.7 Nasal decongestants

5.1 Treatment of respiratory infections

Bacterial and viral infections are among the main causes of respiratory disease. Wherever possible, the identity of the causative organism should be sought and appropriate treatment initiated before commencing symptomatic therapy. Respiratory bacterial infections may be primary (*Mannheimia haemolytica* in cattle and sheep, *Bordetella bronchiseptica* in horses, dogs, and cats, *Actinobacillus pleuropneumoniae* in pigs) but are often secondary infections involving a wide range of micro-organisms found in the upper airways as normal bacterial flora such as *Burkholderia cepacia*, *Klebsiella*, *E. coli*, *Proteus*, *Pasteurella*, *Staphylococcus*, *Streptococcus*, and *Haemophilus*.

In general, antibacterials effective for treatment of respiratory tract infections include the potentiated sulphonamides (see section 1.1.6.2), tetracyclines (see section 1.1.2), fluoroquinolones (see section 1.1.9), macrolides (see section 1.1.4), pleuromutilins (see section 1.1.10), and cephalosporins (see section 1.1.1.5).

Adjunctive treatment including NSAIDs, fluid and nutritional support may aid recovery.

Preventitive measures include attention to the quality of housing (particularly for farm livestock), transportation of animals, and quality of nutrition. The use of vaccines to provide specific protection against pulmonary and upper respiratory tract infection is described in Chapter 18.

Species-specific conditions and treatment are discussed below.

Conditions affecting horses. Strangles is a bacterial infection caused by *Streptococcus equi* subspecies *equi* and characterised by purulent lymphadenitis of the submandibular and retropharyngeal lymph nodes. Although the organism is susceptible to penicillins, antibacterial treatment should be avoided once abscesses have formed because this may delay their maturation and rupture. Penicillins may be effectively used before abscesses have developed or after they have ruptured. However, if used early in the course of infection, antibacterials may prevent the horse developing a protective immune response.

Inflammatory lower airway disease with secondary bacterial infection by a variety of bacterial species such as *Streptococcus equi* subspecies *zooepidemicus*, *Pasteurella* spp., and *Bordetella bronchiseptica* is common following viral infections. Primary infections with these bacteria and *Streptococcus pneumoniae* and *Mycoplasma* spp. may also occur in young Throughbreds in race training. Treatment with broad-spectrum antibacterials is helpful in these cases, which may also benefit from the administration of mucolytics and bronchodilators.

Pneumonia and pleurisy are uncommon in adult horses but sometimes develop in animals stressed by long-distance travel. Mixed bacterial infections including anaerobes are usually present in these conditions and aggressive antibacterial therapy based on bacterial culture and sensitivity results is required for treatment; metronidazole is helpful in cases where anaerobic infections are present. Rifampicin is frequently used in combination with erythromycin for the treatment of some pneumonic conditions in foals, particularly those caused by *Rhodococcus equi* infection.

In horses, viral causes of respiratory disease include the equine influenza group of myxoviruses and equine herpesvirus 1 and 4; vaccination against these viruses is available (see section 18.1).

Donkeys can carry subclinical infections of the lungworm *Dictyocaulus arnfieldi*, and horses may become infected when grazing pasture that has been contaminated. In horses, lungworm infections rarely reach patency but may induce a clinical disease characterised by chronic coughing. Treatment with ivermectin, moxidectin, or some benzimidazoles is effective in eliminating the infection.

In the UK, further information on control of respiratory infections is provided in the National Trainers Federation *Code of practice for respiratory diseases affecting horses* and the Horserace Betting Levy Board *Guidelines on strangles.*

Conditions affecting cattle. The aetiology of calf pneumonia is complex involving both non-infectious factors such as housing, weather, nutrition, and general management in addition to infectious agents namely viruses, mycoplasma, and bacteria. Infection usually includes secondary bacterial infection and primary viral infection (often involving more than one virus). The major viruses involved are parainfluenza 3, infectious bovine rhinotracheitis, bovine respiratory syncytial virus, and bovine virus diarrhoea, while the main bacteria involved are *Mannheimia haemolytica*, *Pasteurella multocida*, *Haemophilus somnus*, *Mycoplasma bovis*, and *Arcanobacterium pyogenes*.

Antibacterials used for treatment include broad-spectrum penicillins such as amoxicillin, cephalosporins for example ceftiofur and cefquinome, macrolides such as tylosin and tilmicosin, quinolones such as enrofloxacin and dano-floxacin, potentiated sulphonamides, florfenicol, spectino-mycin, and tetracyclines. Antibacterials may be used in individual animals or on a group basis. They may also be administered prophylactically before expected risk of disease for example after transport.

NSAIDs (see section 10.1) such as flunixin, ketoprofen, and carprofen may be used as an adjunct to antibacterial therapy with beneficial effects on both mortality and future growth rates. Corticosteroids (see section 7.2) are generally contraindicated although soluble short acting corticosteroids may be of value in acutely dyspnoeic animals such as in peracute bovine respiratory syncytial virus infections.

Mucolytics for example, bromhexine may be used in some cases of pneumonia.

Vaccines are available for prevention of viral pneumonias and *M. haemolytica* infection (see section 18.2.2) and live vaccines given by intranasal administration may reduce morbidity in an expected outbreak if given early in the disease.

Infection of cattle with the lungworm *Dictyocaulus vivipa-rus* results in respiratory disease and is a condition of economic importance. Pasture management, anthelmintic therapy, and vaccination (see section 18.2.10) are used to control lungworm infection.

Conditions affecting sheep. The major acute pneumonic condition of sheep is pasteurellosis caused by *Mannheimia haemolytica* serotype A2 and infection with this organism is susceptible to the same antimicrobials used for its treatment in cattle. *Pasteurella trehalosi* infections may present as pneumonia and may be treated in the same way but are less sensitive to penicillin. New and effective vaccines against these two infections mean that passive protection of the lamb and active protection of the growing and adult sheep are now routine. These vaccines are available alone or in combination with vaccines for clostridial infections (see section 18.2).

Conditions affecting pigs. Respiratory conditions in pigs are usually the result of several respiratory pathogens combined with environmental factors. On farms with endemic respiratory disease, growing and finishing pigs are mainly affected. Bacteria involved include *Pasteurella multocida*, *Actinobacillus pleuropneumoniae*, *Haemophilus parasuis*, *Bordetella bronchiseptica*, *Mycoplasma hyopneumoniae*, and *Streptococcus suis*. Viral infections may include porcine reproductive and respiratory syndrome virus, inclusion body rhinitis virus, varying strains of swine influenza virus, and respiratory coronavirus. The herpesvirus of Aujeszky's disease will also produce lung pathology. *Mycoplasma hyopneumoniae* continues to be a major cause of lung disease in pigs.

Environmental factors affect the incidence of respiratory disease in pigs. The conditions under which the pigs are kept such as temperature, humidity, ventilation, airborne dust, gases, and bacteria are important. In addition, social factors such as age, genetics, herd size, and stocking density

should be considered. Also management factors such as purchase of pigs, method of production and manure systems, and amount of mixing and moving of pigs should be taken into account.

Antibacterials effective for the treatment of pigs with enzootic pneumonia include tiamulin, valnemulin, ceftiofur, lincomycin, tetracyclines, and tylosin. A combination of tiamulin and chlortetracycline has been successful in control of the disease on many farms. Enrofloxacin and tilmicosin have been used in the treatment and control of enzootic pneumonia and bacterial pneumonia. Infection caused by *Actinobacillus pleuropneumoniae* has been successfully treated with ceftiofur, enrofloxacin, tiamulin, and sulfadiazine with trimethoprim but the damage caused by the lesions may be irreversible and the prognosis for individual affected pigs may be poor.

Adjunctive treatment with the NSAID ketoprofen (see section 10.1) is useful in controlling pyrexia and respiratory distress.

Verminous pneumonia caused by *Ascaris suum* or *Metastrongylus* spp. occurs in pigs. Pigs kept on pasture are more likely to be infected with lungworm. Treatment of individual animals is by injection with levamisole or avermectins, such as ivermectin or doramectin. Growing or adult pigs are treated with benzimadazoles, ivermectin, or thiophanate by group medication in the feed.

Control of respiratory disease in pigs is important and preventative strategies are developing. Targeting specific antimicrobial therapy (based on examination of suitable samples) is combined with vaccination and reduction of adverse environmental factors. The increased availability of vaccines for respiratory disease means that progressive atrophic rhinitis (*Pasteurella multocida*) is now preventable by maternal vaccination. Enzootic pneumonia and pleuropneumonia caused by the major serotypes of *Actinobacillus pleuropneumoniae*, and Glasser's disease caused by serotypes 4 and 5 of *Haemophilus parasuis* are all preventable by vaccination in young pigs. In countries where Aujeszky's disease occurs, vaccination programmes can prevent pneumonia caused by this virus in finishing pigs. Influenza vaccines and the use of modern vaccines against porcine respiratory and reproductive syndrome virus may also reduce respiratory disease where available.

Management practices are changing from keeping of all breeding and finishing pigs to multi-site operations. By segregating breeding, weaner, and finishing pigs on to separate sites there is reduction in the usual spread of infectious agents from older to younger pigs. Multi-site production combined with specific medication in all young weaners after removal from the dam and while still protected by passive maternal immunity (previously modified medicated early weaning, now isowean) has been successful in reducing and even eliminating conditions on farms with previously intractable respiratory disease of multiple aetiology. Batch farrowing, and strict hygiene and disinfection protocols are important. The complete depopulation and restocking of farms with pigs free from all respiratory disease is increasingly being practised. On farms which purchase weaners for finishing, pigs with the same known respiratory micro-organism profile are often mixed if more than one source of weaner is used. This practice is of little value unless account is taken of the serotypes and antibiotic resistance patterns of the two populations of organism.

Conditions affecting dogs and cats. In small animals, the main respiratory infectious agents are *Bordetella bronchiseptica* and canine parainfluenza virus in dogs, and *Chlamydophila felis* (*Chlamydia psittaci*), feline herpesvirus (feline rhinotracheitis virus), calicivirus, *Bordetella bronchiseptica*, and *Mycoplasma* spp. in cats. Effective vaccines against most of these pathogens are available; *B. bronchiseptica* is susceptible to most broad-spectrum antibacterials and the mycoplasma to tylosin, lincomycin, and fluoroquinolones.

Treatment of severe bronchopneumonia in dogs with multiple antibacterial therapy appears to be more beneficial than single antibacterial treatment. Recommendations vary but a typical regimen would include a cephalosporin, fluoroquinolone, and clindamycin. Addition of potentiated sulphonamides may be beneficial in some instances. Treatment should be given for at least 8 weeks. Concerns have been raised about the use of multiple antibacterial therapy in canine bronchopneumonia using inappropriate antibiotic combinations. It is standard recommendation that bacteriocidal (for example cephalosporins, fluoroquinolones) and bacteriostatic (such as clindamycin, potentiated sulphonamides, tetracyclines) should not be used together in the treatment of bacterial infections. However, clinical experience suggests that the use of such combinations in dogs with severe fulminating bacterial bronchopneumonia rarely causes problems and that the use of a single antibiotic alone is less likely to effect a cure.

Aminoglycosides such as gentamicin may be administered to dogs by nebulisation. Gentamicin 50 mg is diluted in 4 mL sodium chloride 0.9% and administered 4 times daily. The procedure is well tolerated and there are minimal renal toxic effects.

Adjunctive treatment of respiratory infectious disease may be necessary. Nutritional support may be required and assisted feeding is often necessary in animals with severe respiratory disease. For dogs and cats, additional therapy such as oxygen supplementation (for example delivered by nasal catheter), chest physiotherapy to assist removal of airway secretions, and adequate fluid and nutritional support (intravenous or naso-gastric feeding) can be vital in the successful treatment of respiratory disease. Concurrent medication with NSAIDs such as phenylbutazone, ketoprofen (dogs), or tolfenamic acid may also be useful.

The principal endoparasites affecting the respiratory system of dogs are *Oslerus osleri* (*Filaroides osleri*) and *Crenosoma vulpis*, and in cats, *Aelurostrongylus abstrusus*. Migrating ascarid larvae may also cause respiratory disease. Benzimidazole anthelmintics (see section 2.1.1.2) are the drugs of choice in treating respiratory parasites in dogs and cats.

5.2 Bronchodilators

5.2.1 Methylxanthines
5.2.2 Adrenoceptor stimulants
5.2.3 Antimuscarinic bronchodilators

Bronchodilators are used where there is suspicion of bronchial narrowing due to bronchial secretion or bronchoconstriction or where improved alveolar ventilation is required. In veterinary medicine these drugs are used for disorders including mild tracheobronchitis and chronic obstructive pulmonary disease (COPD) in horses, and bronchopneumonia and chronic pulmonary interstitial disease in all species. They are often used, with or without concurrent corticosteroid therapy, for the control of chronic bronchitis in dogs and asthma syndrome in cats. Hypoxaemia is a possible complication of bronchodilator therapy caused by ventilation-perfusion mismatching; this may be an important consideration in severe pneumonia especially in young animals such as calves and foals.

The assessment of airway function, airway calibre, and bronchomotor tone is often subjective. The choice and use of a bronchodilator may be primarily on an empirical basis. In diseases where the airway obstruction mainly affects the bronchioles, bronchodilator therapy may be most effective if administered by aerosol.

5.2.1 Methylxanthines

Methylxanthines including **aminophylline**, **etamiphylline**, **diprophylline**, and **theophylline** induce bronchodilation of the smaller airways by inhibition of phosphodiesterase and antagonism of adenosine receptors; they have little effect on larger airways. These drugs may also increase tidal volume by stimulating the respiratory centre in the medulla oblongata.

Methylxanthines are more effective where there is reversible airway obstruction than in chronic respiratory disease. Their ability to induce bronchodilation is severely impaired by pathological changes both in the airway walls and pulmonary interstitium. This accounts for the wide variability of response seen with these drugs and individual animal treatment is often determined on a trial-and-error basis.

Methylxanthines are also CNS and myocardial stimulants and diuretics. The therapeutic index of methylthanxines is low and they are erratically absorbed from the gastro-intestinal tract; they are difficult to use effectively in practice. At therapeutic doses they cause increased alertness and activity. Signs of toxicity include restlessness, tachycardia, tachypnoea, and convulsions.

AMINOPHYLLINE

UK
Indications. Respiratory disease where bronchodilation may be beneficial; myocardial stimulation (see section 4.1.2)
Side-effects. See under Theophylline

Dose. *By mouth or by intramuscular or slow intravenous injection.*
Dogs, cats: 10 mg/kg 2–3 times daily

Ⓗ **Aminophylline** (Non-proprietary) *UK*
P *Tablets*, aminophylline 100 mg
POM *Injection*, aminophylline 25 mg/mL; 10 mL

Australia
Indications. Adjunctive bronchodilation in cardiac disease; acute pulmonary oedema with bronchospasm; cardiac asthma
Contra-indications. Pregnancy, tachydysrhythmias, gastro-intestinal ulceration
Side-effects. Tachyarrhythmias, tachypnoea, restlessness, insomnia, vomiting, anorexia, rarely seizures
Warnings. Caution in congestive heart failure, hepatic impairment, hyperthyroidism, diabetes mellitus; Drug Interactions – cimetidine, erythromycin, propranolol
Dose. *Dogs, cats*: *by mouth,* 10 mg/kg 2–4 times daily

Aminyllin (Mavlab) *Austral.*
Tablets, aminophylline 100 mg, 200 mg, for *dogs, cats*

ETAMIPHYLLINE CAMSILATE
(Etamiphylline camsylate)

UK
Indications. Respiratory disease where bronchodilation may be beneficial; respiratory stimulation of neonates (see section 5.5); myocardial stimulation (see section 4.1.2)
Contra-indications. Racehorses 7 days prior to racing (see Prescribing for animals used in competitions)
Side-effects. Occasional CNS stimulations
Warnings. Safety in pregnant animals has not been established
Dose. *Horses*: *by addition to feed or as an oral solution,* up to 300 mg/100 kg body-weight up to 3 times daily. Reduce to lowest effective dose after 2 weeks
by subcutaneous or intramuscular injection, 1.4 g repeated up to 3 times daily if required
Dogs, cats: *by mouth,* (3–10 kg body-weight) 100 mg; (11–20 kg body-weight) 200 mg; (21–30 kg body-weight) 300 mg; (31–40 kg body-weight) 400 mg. May be repeated up to 3 times daily if required. Reduce to lowest effective dose after 2 weeks
by subcutaneous or intramuscular injection, (3–5 kg body-weight) 70 mg; (6–10 kg body-weight) 140 mg; (11–20 kg body-weight) 280 mg; (21–30 kg body-weight) 420 mg; (31–40 kg body-weight) 700 mg. Dose may be repeated up to 3 times daily if required

Millophyline-V (Arnolds) *UK*
P *Tablets*, s/c, etamiphylline camsilate 100 mg, for *dogs and cats more than 3 kg body-weight*; 100, 500 *Note*. Tablets should not be divided
P *Tablets*, s/c, etamiphylline camsilate 200 mg, 300 mg, for *dogs more than 3 kg body-weight*; 28
Note. Tablets should not be divided
P *Oral powder*, for addition to feed or to prepare an oral solution, etamiphylline camsilate 300 mg/sachet, for *horses*; 12
Withdrawal Periods. Should not be used in *horses* intended for human consumption

Millophyline-V (Arnolds) *UK*
POM *Injection*, etamiphylline camsilate 140 mg/mL, for *horses, dogs and cats more than 3 kg body-weight*; 50 mL
Withdrawal Periods. Should not be used in *horses* intended for human consumption

Australia
Indications. Cardiac and respiratory stimulation; adjunct in treatment of pneumonia and upper respiratory tract infections
Dose. *Horses, cattle*: *by subcutaneous or intramuscular injection,* 4.6 mg/kg (max. 2.1 g) *or* 1.4 g total dose
Dogs: *by subcutaneous or intramuscular injection,* 5–25 mg/kg *or* 140–700 mg
by mouth, 5–20 mg/kg *or* 100–300 mg every 8 hours
Cats: *by subcutaneous or intramuscular injection,* 5–25 mg/kg *or* 140–280 mg
by mouth, 5–20 mg/kg *or* 100 mg every 8 hours

Delcam Injection (Delvet) *Austral.*
Injection, etamiphylline camsilate 140 mg/mL, for *horses, dogs, cats*

Delcam Tablets (Delvet) *Austral.*
Tablets, etamiphylline camsilate 100 mg, 200 mg, for *dogs*

Millophyline-V (Virbac) *Austral.*
Injection, etamiphylline camsilate 140 mg/mL, for *horses, cattle, dogs, cats*
Withdrawal Periods. *Cattle*: slaughter 28 days

Millophyline-V (Virbac) *Austral.*
Tablets, etamiphylline camsilate 100 mg, for *dogs, cats*

New Zealand
Indications. Cardiac and respiratory stimulation; adjunct in treatment of pneumonia and upper respiratory tract infections
Contra-indications. Racehorses 144 hours prior to racing
Side-effects. Restlessness, tachycardia, tachypnoea, and convulsions with high dosage
Dose. *Horses, cattle*: *by subcutaneous or intramuscular injection,* 3 mg/kg *or* 1.4 g total dose
Dogs: *by subcutaneous or intramuscular injection,* 3–25 mg/kg *or* 140–700 mg
by mouth, 5–20 mg/kg *or* 100–400 mg every 8 hours
Cats: *by subcutaneous or intramuscular injection,* 3–25 mg/kg *or* 140–280 mg
by mouth, 5–20 mg/kg *or* 100 mg every 8 hours

Delcam Forte Tabs (Ethical) *NZ*
Tablets, etamiphylline camsilate 200 mg, for *dogs more than 20 kg body-weight*

Delcam Injection (Ethical) *NZ*
Injection, etamiphylline camsilate 140 mg/mL, for *horses, cattle, dogs, cats*
Withdrawal Periods. *Horses*: slaughter 1 day. *Cattle*: slaughter 1 day, milk 1 day

Delcam Tablets (Ethical) *NZ*
Tablets, etamiphylline camsilate 100 mg, for *dogs, cats*

Millophyline V Injection (Bomac) *NZ*
Injection, etamiphylline camsilate 140 mg/mL, for *horses, cattle, dogs, cats*
Withdrawal Periods. Slaughter withdrawal period nil, milk withdrawal period nil
Note. Solution may be diluted with equal volume of water and given by slow intravenous injection

Millophyline V Tablets (Bomac) *NZ*
Tablets, etamiphylline camsilate 100 mg, for *dogs, cats*

PROPENTOFYLLINE

See section 4.3.4

THEOPHYLLINE

UK

Indications. Bronchitis; congestive heart failure
Contra-indications. Acute myocardial disease; patients with history of epileptiform seizures
Side-effects. Restlessness, agitation, excitement, vomiting, diarrhoea, polydipsia, sedation, reduced appetite, polyuria
Warnings. Caution in hepatic impairment. Assess risk/benefit before administration to pregnant bitches; Drug Interactions – see Appendix 1
Dose. *Dogs*: *by mouth,* 20 mg/kg once daily given in the morning

POM **Corvental-D Capsules** (Vericore VP) *UK*
Capsules, theophylline 100 mg, 200 mg, 500 mg, for *dogs*; 60

New Zealand

Indications. Aid in treatment of bronchitis
Side-effects. Restlessness, vomiting, diarrhoea, polydipsia, sedation, reduced appetite, polyuria
Warnings. Caution in hepatic impairment, pregnant animals; Drug Interactions – ketamine, halothane, epinephrine, macrolides, phenobarbital, phenytoin
Dose. *Dogs*: *by mouth,* 20 mg/kg daily

Corvental-D (Novartis) *NZ*
Capsules, theophylline 100 mg, 200 mg, 500 mg, for *dogs*

5.2.2 Adrenoceptor stimulants (Sympathomimetics)

Adrenoceptor stimulants cause bronchodilation by stimulation of beta$_2$-receptors in the large and small airways. Beta$_2$-receptors are also found in vascular beds and the uterus. Beta$_2$-adrenoceptor stimulants such as **clenbuterol**, **albuterol**, **pirbuterol**, and **terbutaline** are direct-acting sympathomimetic drugs. **Ephedrine** is a sympathomimetic agent with direct and indirect effects on adrenoreceptors. It has alpha- and beta-adrenergic activity and is rarely used clinically.

The cardiac effects of beta$_2$-adrenoceptor stimulants may be more pronounced in cats. Signs of toxicity include tachycardia, erythema of the nostrils and ear pinnae, and tremors and sweating in horses; therapy should be immediately withdrawn. Aerosol administration of these drugs reduces the cardiac effects but is impractical in most animals except horses. In addition to bronchodilation these drugs increase ciliary beating of the respiratory mucosal cells and have a mucolytic action, which may contribute to their therapeutic effect.

Terbutaline may have a greater cardiac stimulant effect than clenbuterol. An oral dose for terbutaline has not been estab-lished for horses and potential side-effects may limit its usefulness in this species.

Clenbuterol has been shown to reduce transpulmonary pressure fluctuations in horses with chronic obstructive pulmonary disease (COPD). It has been found that some horses will not respond to the standard dosage of clenbuterol but require higher dosages. These horses should be treated initially at the standard dose (see below) for 3 days. If there is no improvement, the dose may be increased in incremental doses (from 0.8–1.6 micrograms/kg to 2.4–3.2 micrograms/kg♦) providing each dose for 3 days and stabilising the dose on amelioration of the condition. Treatment should not start at the higher dosages because some horses may show excitement, tremors, and sweating.

Pirbuterol and albuterol have been shown to be effective bronchodilators in horses with COPD when administered by nebulisation or dry powder inhalation. However the duration of action of these agents is approximately only one hour.

CLENBUTEROL HYDROCHLORIDE

UK

Indications. Bronchodilation in allergic respiratory disease, respiratory infection and inflammation, chronic obstructive pulmonary disease
Contra-indications. Cardiac disease, late pregnancy; hypersensitivity to the drug
Side-effects. Transient vasodilation and tachycardia with sweating and muscle tremor in horses
Warnings. May abolish uterine contractions; Drug Interactions – see Appendix 1
Dose.
Horses: *by mouth or by slow intravenous injection,* 800 nanograms/kg twice daily; see also dose♦ above
Dogs♦: *by mouth or by slow intravenous injection,* 1–5 micrograms/kg twice daily
Cats♦: *by mouth or by slow intravenous injection,* 1 microgram/kg 1–2 times daily

POM **Ventipulmin** (Boehringer Ingelheim) *UK*
Oral granules, for addition to feed, clenbuterol hydrochloride 16 micrograms/g, for *horses*; 10 g, 500 g
Withdrawal Periods. Should not be used in *horses* intended for human consumption
Syrup, for addition to feed, clenbuterol hydrochloride 100 micrograms/unit dose, for *horses*; 355-mL dose applicator (1 unit dose = 4 mL)
Withdrawal Periods. Should not be used in *horses* intended for human consumption
Dose. *By mouth,* 1 unit dose/125 kg body-weight
Injection, clenbuterol hydrochloride 30 micrograms/mL, for *horses*; 50 mL
Withdrawal Periods. Should not be used in *horses* intended for human consumption

Australia

Indications. Bronchodilation for disorders characterised by airway obstruction
Contra-indications. Last 7–14 days of pregnancy; concurrent treatment with corticosteroids, beta-adrenoceptor blocking drugs, prostaglandins, oxytocin
Dose. *Horses*: *by mouth or by intramuscular or intravenous injection,* 800 nanograms/kg twice daily

Broncopulmin (Jurox) *Austral.*
Oral powder, clenbuterol 16 micrograms/g, for *horses*
Withdrawal Periods. *Horses*: should not be used in animals intended for human consumption

Claire Gel (Vetsearch) *Austral.*
Oral paste, clenbuterol 40 micrograms/mL, for *horses*
Withdrawal Periods. Should not be used in *horses* intended for human consumption

Ventipulmin Granules (Boehringer Ingelheim) *Austral.*
Oral granules, clenbuterol hydrochloride 16 micrograms/g, for *horses*
Withdrawal Periods. Should not be used in *horses* intended for human consumption

Ventipulmin Injection (Boehringer Ingelheim) *Austral.*
Injection, clenbuterol hydrochloride 30 micrograms/mL, for *horses*
Withdrawal Periods. Should not be used in *horses* intended for human consumption

Ventipulmin + TMP/S (Boehringer Ingelheim) *Austral.* (see section 1.1.6.2)

Eire

Indications. Bronchodilation for disorders characterised by airway obstruction
Contra-indications. Late pregnancy ; concurrent treatment with beta-adrenoceptor blocking drugs, prostaglandins
Warnings. May abolish uterine contractions
Dose. *Horses*: *by mouth or by slow intravenous injection*, 800 nanograms/kg twice daily

Ventipulmin Granules (Boehringer Ingelheim) *Eire*
Oral granules, for addition to feed, clenbuterol hydrochloride 16 micrograms/g, for *horses*
Withdrawal Periods. Slaughter 28 days

Ventipulmin Injection Solution (Boehringer Ingelheim) *Eire*
Injection, clenbuterol hydrochloride 30 micrograms/mL, for *horses*
Withdrawal Periods. Slaughter 28 days

Ventipulmin Syrup (Boehringer Ingelheim) *Eire*
Syrup, for addition to feed, clenbuterol hydrochloride 25 micrograms/mL, for *horses*
Withdrawal Periods. Slaughter 28 days

Ventipulmin + TMP/S (Boehringer Ingelheim) *Eire* (see section 1.1.6.2)

New Zealand

Indications. Bronchodilation for disorders characterised by airway obstruction
Contra-indications. Late pregnancy; concurrent treatment with beta-adrenoceptor blocking drugs, prostaglandins, oxytocin
Warnings. May abolish uterine contractions
Dose. *Horses*: *by mouth or by intramuscular or intravenous injection*, 800 nanograms/kg twice daily

Ventipulmin Granules (Boehringer Ingelheim) *NZ*
Oral granules, clenbuterol hydrochloride 16 micrograms/g, for *horses*
Withdrawal Periods. Slaughter 28 days

Ventipulmin Injection (Boehringer Ingelheim) *NZ*
Injection, clenbuterol hydrochloride 0.03 mg/mL, for *horses*
Withdrawal Periods. Slaughter 28 days

Ventipulmin Syrup (Boehringer Ingelheim) *NZ*
Syrup, clenbuterol hydrochloride 25 micrograms/mL, for *horses*
Withdrawal Periods. Slaughter 28 days

Ventipulmin TMP/S (Boehringer Ingelheim) *NZ* (see section 1.1.6.2)

USA

Indications. Bronchodilation for disorders characterised by airway obstruction
Contra-indications. Late pregnancy; concurrent treatment with prostaglandins, oxytocin; cardiovascular impairment
Side-effects. Initial mild tachycardia, sweating, muscle tremors, restlessness, and urticaria; ataxia
Warnings. Safety in breeding animals has not been established
Dose. *Horses*: *by mouth*, 800 nanograms/kg twice daily

Ventipulmin Syrup (Boehringer Ingelheim Vetmedica) *USA*
Oral syrup, clenbuterol hydrochloride 72.5 micrograms/mL, for *horses*
Withdrawal Periods. Should not be used in *horses* intended for human consumption

TERBUTALINE SULPHATE

UK

Indications. Respiratory disease where bronchodilation may be beneficial
Dose. *Dogs*: *by mouth*, 1.25–5.0 mg 2–3 times daily
Cats: *by mouth*, 1.25 mg 2–3 times daily

POM Ⓗ **Bricanyl** (Astra) *UK*
Tablets, scored, terbutaline sulphate 5 mg; 100, 500
Syrup, terbutaline sulphate 300 micrograms/mL; 300 mL

5.2.3 Antimuscarinic bronchodilators

Smooth muscle contraction is an important cause of airway obstruction in horses with COPD, and is partly the result of activation of muscarinic receptors. The antimuscarinic drug **atropine** may be used for bronchodilation in COPD. However it causes significant side-effects including decreased mucociliary clearance, tachycardia, mydriasis, ileus, and excitement that limit its routine use. Although atropine may be administered by aerosol, it is rapidly absorbed and has systemic effects.

The antimuscarinic bronchodilator **ipratropium** has a quaternary ammonium structure, and little of the compound is absorbed from the respiratory tract after aerosol administration. Ipratropium does not inhibit mucociliary clearance. It can provide effective bronchodilation in horses with COPD for 4 to 6 hours.

IPRATROPIUM BROMIDE

UK

Indications. Reversible airways obstruction due to bronchospasm in COPD
Dose. *Horses*: *by inhalation*, (75 micrograms/mL solution) 2–3 micrograms/kg up to 4 times daily

POM Ⓗ **Atrovent** (Boehringer Ingelheim) *UK*
Nebuliser solution, ipratropium bromide 250 micrograms/mL; 1 mL, 2 mL
For use in horses, dilute to 75 micrograms/mL in sterile sodium chloride 0.9% solution

5.3 Drugs for allergic and inflammatory disorders

5.3.1 Antihistamines
5.3.2 Sodium cromoglicate
5.3.3 Leukotriene receptor antagonists

Respiratory diseases with a possible allergic aetiology are a poorly defined group of conditions in animals, and include pulmonary infiltration with eosinophilia (PIE) in dogs, feline asthma syndrome, acute bovine pulmonary emphysema and oedema (atypical interstitial pneumonia, fog fever) in cattle, and COPD and SPAOPD in horses. All are believed to involve an allergic reaction to either inhaled allergens (see below) or migrating pulmonary parasites.

Inflammatory lung disease has been recorded in pigs and other species following inhalation of irritant gases.

Allergic pulmonary disease may involve neutrophilic or eosinophilic migration into the lung parenchyma and airways, and mast-cell degranulation with release of inflammatory mediators such as histamine. Airway mucosal inflammatory mechanisms may be activated leading to the release of prostaglandins and leukotrienes. The symptoms of allergic pulmonary disease can vary from mild intractable coughing to severe respiratory distress and death.

Corticosteroids (see section 7.2.1) are the drugs of choice in the treatment of canine and feline allergic respiratory disease and have also been used in cattle and horses. Corticosteroids counteract the symptoms of respiratory disease in a variety of ways. They reduce airway inflammation due to histamine and prostaglandin release, prevent inflammatory mediator-induced bronchoconstriction, and may stabilise mast cell and lysosomal membranes. Reduction of inflammatory mediator release and mucus secretion improves mucociliary clearance of airway debris and reduces eosinophil migration into lung tissue. Corticosteroids also increase beta-receptor numbers and activity. In emergency situations intravenous corticosteroids such as dexamethasone or betamethasone should be used, followed by oral prednisolone for long-term maintenance.

Potential side effects of corticosteroids include immunosuppression, Cushings-like signs, and laminitis. Laminitis is probably the commonest side-effect of corticosteroid therapy seen in practice in horses, however immunosuppression and bacterial infections, including pneumonia, occur occasionally.

The **NSAIDs** (see section 10.1), flunixin meglumine and ketoprofen, may be used in the treatment of acute bovine pulmonary emphysema and oedema, and may significantly reduce the mortality due to this condition.

Allergens causing *chronic obstructive pulmonary disease* (COPD) in horses include mould spores from hay and bedding. Poor quality and 'heated' hay and straw carry the greatest concentration of these spores. Control of COPD is effected by avoiding these allergens, which is best achieved by keeping susceptible animals permanently at pasture. If affected horses need to be stabled, an alternative to straw,

such as shredded paper or shavings, should be used for bedding. Adequate ventilation of the stable is essential and each horse should be housed separately. Good quality hay should be fed and should be soaked before feeding to dampen down any dust. Better alternatives to feeding hay include the use of vacuum-packed haylage, silage, or hydroponic grass. Summer pasture-associated obstructive pulmonary disease (SPAOPD) is similar to COPD except that it occurs in pastured horses and is probably caused by pollen allergens. Treatment of COPD and SPAOPD should ideally be directed at preventing further exposure to the allergens rather than the use of long-term therapy. However, short-term therapy may be helpful when clinical signs are severe, and long-term treatment may be necessary when management changes are ineffective at controlling the disease.

Drugs that may be usefully employed include bronchodilators such as clenbuterol or ipratropium; mucolytics such as dembrexine; and sodium cromoglicate. Corticosteroids are also used. To reduce the risk of side effects, corticosteroids are administered by mouth or nebulisation. Oral prednisolone on an alternate day regime is advised. An initial dose of 1 to 2 mg/kg is administered every other morning. After two weeks of therapy, response to treatment should be assessed and the dosage reduced until the minimum effective dose is reached. Corticosteroid therapy should eventually be discontinued if possible.

In severe cases and in horses with acute exacerbations of disease, dexamethasone therapy may be necessary, but this drug carries a greater risk of undesirable side effects. An initial dose of intravenous dexamethasone (40 micrograms/kg) may be administered twice daily for 2 to 3 days, followed by a reducing dosage over the next 7 to 10 days (depending on the clinical response).

Inhaled corticosteroid therapy is becoming a more popular form of treatment for COPD in the horse. However, to date, inhalational therapy with corticosteroids has been insufficiently studied. Aerosol administration of beclomethasone (1320 micrograms twice daily) has recently been shown to improve respiratory function in horses with COPD.

Acute bovine pulmonary emphysema and oedema is probably initiated by ingestion of large quantities of DL-tryptophan in grass aftermath, although some cases have occurred due to migrating lungworms or inhalation of toxic gases. Fibrosing alveolitis involves a chronic allergic reaction to mould spores.

The most common allergens implicated in *feline asthma syndrome* have not been definitively identified but may include human and equine dander (epithelium) and house dust mite. In cats presented in status asthmaticus emergency therapy is required. Cats in respiratory distress often resent restraint making oxygen suplementation difficult. Reversal of severe bronchoconstriction can be achieved with intravenous aminophylline (2 to 5 mg/kg), intravenous atropine (20 to 40 micrograms/kg), or epinephrine 20 micrograms/kg by subcutaneous, intramuscular, or intravenous injection using epinephrine 100 micrograms/mL. The intravenous injection should be given with extreme caution. Corticosteroids have limited use in status asthmaticus.

For cats presented with acute bronchospasm associated with feline asthma, therapy may include intravenous aminophylline, atropine (15 micrograms/kg by intravenous injection or 40 micrograms/kg by intramuscular injection), or dexamethasone (0.2 to 1.0 mg/kg by slow intravenous injection). These drugs should give a rapid response and reversal of bronchospasm. The rapidity of the response can assist in making a diagnosis of this condition.

Routine management of feline asthma is effected by oral prednisolone. Initial treatment is 1 mg/kg once daily and then reduced over the subsequent 3 weeks to 200 micrograms/kg on alternate days, or to a dose sufficient to control the symptoms. Medication may be withdrawn at 6 to 8 weeks and re-introduced as required. Continuous medication may be necessary, particularly if the suspected airborne allergen cannot be identified or avoided. The potential long-term effects of corticosteroids should be considered (see section 7.2). Zafirlukast (see section 5.2.3) is reported to be a beneficial adjunct to standard feline asthma prophylactic therapy. Cyproheptadine (see section 5.2.1) may be used prophylactically in asthmatic cats. However, cyproheptadine should only be used if other control methods have failed.

5.3.1 Antihistamines

Antihistamines, such as **diphenhydramine** and **promethazine**, are antagonists of the histamine H_1 receptor and diminish or abolish the main actions of histamine in the body by competitive, reversible blockade of histamine receptor sites. Histamine is only one of many autacoids involved in hypersensitivity reactions and so antihistamines have limited use in the treatment of allergic respiratory disorders in animals.

Certain drugs are useful in the control of allergic rhinitis in the cat, but sedation often precludes long-term use. Nasal decongestants, such as pseudoephedrine (see section 5.6), are more effective therapy.

Cyproheptadine is an antihistamine with serotonin-antagonist and calcium-channel blocking properties. Cyproheptadine may be used for prophylaxis in feline asthma but should only be used if other control methods have failed.

CYPROHEPTADINE HYDROCHLORIDE

UK

Indications. Feline asthma; pituitary-dependent hyperadrenocorticism (see section 7.6)
Side-effects. Polyphagia
Dose. *By mouth.*
Horses: head shaking syndrome, 300 micrograms/kg twice daily
Hyperadrenocorticism, 0.6 mg/kg$^{0.75}$ increasing to 1.2 mg/kg$^{0.75}$ daily
Dogs: hyperadrenocorticism, 0.3 mg/kg increasing to 3.0 mg/kg daily
Cats: asthma, 300–500 micrograms/kg 3 times daily

P (H) **Periactin** (MSD) *UK*
Tablets, scored, cyproheptadine hydrochloride 4 mg; 100

DIPHENHYDRAMINE HYDROCHLORIDE

UK

Indications. Allergic respiratory disease; relief of coughing; pruritus in allergic skin disorders (see section 14.2); mild sedation (see section 6.11.10); motion sickness (see section 3.4.2)
Contra-indications. Urine retention, glaucoma, hyperthyroidism
Side-effects. CNS depression; drowsiness
Dose. *By mouth.*
Coughing, see preparation details

P (H) **Benylin Chesty Cough** (Warner Lambert) *UK*
Linctus, diphenhydramine hydrochloride 14 mg, menthol 1.1 mg/5 mL; 125 mL, 300 mL
Dose. *Coughing, by mouth.*
Horses, cattle: 60 mL as necessary; *foals, calves*: 10–20 mL 2–3 times daily
Dogs: 15–20 mL every 2–3 hours

PROMETHAZINE HYDROCHLORIDE

UK

Indications. Allergic respiratory disease
Side-effects. CNS depression; drowsiness
Dose. *By mouth or by subcutaneous injection.*
Dogs: 0.2–1.0 mg/kg 2–3 times daily

(H) **Phenergan** (Rhône-Poulenc Rorer) *UK*
P *Tablets*, f/c, promethazine hydrochloride 10 mg, 25 mg; 56
P *Elixir*, promethazine hydrochloride 1 mg/mL; 100 mL
POM *Injection*, promethazine hydrochloride 25 mg/mL; 1 mL

5.3.2 Sodium cromoglicate

Sodium cromoglicate inhibits mast-cell degranulation on antigen challenge and may also have membrane-stabilising properties, but its precise mode of action is unclear. It is used for prophylaxis of COPD in the horse. Sodium cromoglicate should not be administered during an allergic attack, but may be delivered by inhalation, using a face mask, prior to expected exposure to an allergen. The length of protection is dependent on the number of consecutive days that the drug is administered. Four days of sodium cromoglicate administration will protect the horse for up to 20 days.

SODIUM CROMOGLICATE
(Sodium cromoglycate)

Eire

Indications. Prophylactic therapy of allergic respiratory disease
Contra-indications. Manufacturer does not recommend use during the first part of pregnancy
Dose. *Horses*: *by inhalation*, 80 mg once daily

Cromovet (Schering-Plough) *Eire*
Nebuliser solution, sodium cromoglicate 20 mg/mL, for **horses**

5.3.3 Leukotriene receptor antagonists

The leukotriene receptor antagonists such as **zafirlukast** block the effects of cysteinyl leukotrienes in the airways. They are beneficial in terms of smooth muscle relaxation, chemotaxis for inflammatory cells, and vascular permeability. In cats, current advice is that they should be used to compliment glucocorticoid or bronchodilator therapy, but should not be used on their own. Anecdotal reports suggest that they are beneficial as adjunctive therapy for asthma where standard therapy is only partially effective. They should not be used to treat acute asthmatic attacks.

ZAFIRLUKAST

UK

Indications. Feline asthma prophylaxis in combination with standard therapy
Contra-indications. Acute asthmatic attacks; as sole therapy
Dose. *Cats*: *by mouth*, 1–2 mg/kg 1–2 times daily

POM Ⓗ **Accolate** (Zeneca) *UK*
Tablets, zafirlukast 20 mg

5.4 Mucolytics and expectorants

5.4.1 Mucolytics
5.4.2 Expectorants

Mucolytics alter the structure of mucus to decrease its viscosity and therefore facilitate its removal by ciliary action and expectoration. Expectorants increase the volume of secretions in the respiratory tract and therefore assist in removal by ciliary action and coughing.

5.4.1 Mucolytics

Mucolytic agents such as **bromhexine** and **dembrexine** reduce mucus viscosity in the tracheobronchial tree and are often prescribed for chronic bronchitis in dogs, bronchopneumonia in cattle, and chronic coughing in horses. The rationale for their use is that mucus of lower viscosity is more easily expectorated during coughing and is more easily carried up the tracheobronchial tree by the mucociliary clearance mechanism. **Ambroxol** is a metabolite of bromhexine and has similar actions.

Acetylcysteine is a mucolytic agent that reduces the viscosity of secretions probably by the splitting of disulphide bonds in mucoproteins. It is also used to detoxify an intermediate paracetamol metabolite that is present in paracetamol overdosage (see Treatment of poisoning).

In small animals inhalation of water vapour and chest physiotherapy are effective methods of mucus removal.

AMBROXOL

Australia

Indications. Respiratory disease where excess tenacious mucus is present

Dose. *By intravenous injection.*
Horses: 300 micrograms twice daily
Dogs: 600 micrograms twice daily

Ambroxol (RWR) *Austral.*
Injection, ambroxol hydrochloride 6 mg/mL, for **dogs, horses**
Withdrawal Periods. **Horses**: slaughter 28 days

BROMHEXINE

UK

Indications. Respiratory disease where excess tenacious mucus is present
Dose.
Horses: *by mouth*, 200–400 micrograms/kg once daily
Cattle: *by mouth or by intramuscular injection*, 500 micrograms/kg once daily
Pigs: *by mouth or by intramuscular injection*, 200–500 micrograms/kg once daily
Dogs: *by mouth*, 2 mg/kg twice daily
Cats: *by mouth*, 1 mg/kg once daily

POM **Bisolvon** (Boehringer Ingelheim) *UK*
Oral powder, for addition to feed or drinking water, bromhexine hydrochloride 10 mg/g, for **horses, cattle, pigs, dogs, cats**; 5 g, 100 g, 500 g
Withdrawal Periods. Should not be used in **horses** intended for human consumption. **Cattle**: slaughter 1 day, should not be used in cattle producing milk for human consumption. **Pigs**: slaughter withdrawal period nil
Injection, bromhexine hydrochloride 3 mg/mL, for **cattle, pigs**; 100 mL
Withdrawal Periods. **Cattle**: slaughter 1 day, should not be used in cattle producing milk for human consumption. **Pigs**: slaugher withdrawal period nil

Australia

Indications. Respiratory disease where excess tenacious mucus is present
Dose. *Dogs, cats*: *by mouth*, 2 mg/kg twice daily for 5–7 days, then 1 mg/kg twice daily

Bromotrimidine (Parnell) *Austral.* (see section 1.1.6.2)

Bisolvon Tablets (Boehringer Ingelheim) *Austral..*
Tablets, bromhexine hydrochloride 8 mg, for **dogs, cats**

Mucodine Tablets (Delvet) *Austral.*
Tablets, bromhexine hydrochloride 8 mg, for **dogs, cats**

Mucohexine Mucolytic Tablets (Apex) *Austral.*
Tablets, bromhexine hydrochloride 8 mg, for **dogs, cats**

Tridexine-S (Bioceuticals) *Austral* (see section 1.1.6.2)

Eire

Indications. Respiratory disease where excess tenacious mucus is present
Dose.
Horses: *by mouth or by intramuscular injection*, 200–400 micrograms/kg daily
Cattle: *by mouth or by intramuscular injection*, 500 micrograms/kg daily
Pigs: *by mouth or by intramuscular injection*, 200–500 micrograms/kg daily
Dogs: *by mouth*, 2 mg/kg twice daily
Cats: *by mouth*, 1 mg/kg daily

Bisolvomycin (Boehringer Ingelheim) *Eire*
See under Oxytetracycline section 1.1.2 for preparation details

Bisolvon Injection (Boehringer Ingelheim) *Eire*
Injection, bromhexine hydrochloride 3 mg/mL, for *horses, cattle, pigs*
Withdrawal Periods. *Horses*: slaughter 3 days. *Cattle*: slaughter withdrawal period 3 days, should not be used in cattle producing milk for human consumption. *Pigs*: slaughter withdrawal period nil

Bisolvon Powder (Boehringer Ingelheim) *Eire*
Oral powder, bromhexine hydrochloride 10 mg/g powder, for *horses, cattle, pigs, dogs, cats*
Withdrawal Periods. *Cattle*: slaughter withdrawal period nil, should not be used in cattle producing milk for human consumption. *Horses, pigs*: slaughter withdrawal period nil

New Zealand

Indications. Respiratory disease where excess tenacious mucus is present
Dose. *By mouth.*
Horses: 100–250 micrograms/kg daily
Cattle, pigs: 200–500 micrograms/kg daily
Dogs, cats: 0.3–1.0 mg/kg daily

Bisolvomycin Vet (Boehringer Ingelheim) *NZ* (see section 1.1.2)

Bisolvon (Boehringer Ingelheim) *NZ*
Oral powder, bromhexine hydrochloride 10 mg/g, for *horses, cattle, pigs, dogs, cats*
Withdrawal Periods. *Horses*: slaughter 28 days. *Cattle*: slaughter 7 days. *Pigs*: slaughter 5 days

Bromotrimidine (Parnell) *NZ* (see section 1.1.6.2)

Bromtrimsulp (Phoenix) *NZ* (see section 1.1.6.2)

Trizine Plus (Ethical) *NZ* (see section 1.1.6.2)

DEMBREXINE HYDROCHLORIDE

UK

Indications. Respiratory disease where excess or tenacious mucus is present in the airways
Dose. *Horses*: *by mouth*, 300 micrograms/kg twice daily

POM **Sputolosin** (Boehringer Ingelheim) *UK*
Oral powder, for addition to feed, dembrexine hydrochloride 5 mg/g, for *horses*; 420 g
Withdrawal Periods. Should not be used in *horses* intended for human consumption

Australia

Indications. Respiratory disease where excess or tenacious mucus is present in the airways
Dose. *Horses*: *by mouth*, 300 micrograms/kg twice daily

Sputolysin (Boehringer Ingelheim) *Austral.*
Powder, dembrexine 5 mg/g powder, for *horses*
Withdrawal Periods. *Horses*: slaughter 28 days

Eire

Indications. Respiratory disease where excess or tenacious mucus is present in the airways
Warnings. Safety in pregnant mares has not been established
Dose. *Horses*: *by mouth*, 300 micrograms/kg twice daily

Sputolosin Powder (Boehringer Ingelheim) *Eire*
Oral powder, dembrexine 5 mg/g, for *horses*
Withdrawal Periods. Should not be used in *horses* intended for human consumption

New Zealand

Indications. Respiratory disease where excess or tenacious mucus is present in the airways
Dose. *Horses*: *by mouth or intravenous injection*, 300 micrograms/kg twice daily

Sputolysin Injection (Boehringer Ingelheim) *NZ*
Injection, dembrexine hydrochloride 5 mg/mL, for *horses*
Withdrawal Periods. *Horses*: slaughter 5 days

Sputolysin Powder (Boehringer Ingelheim) *NZ*
Oral powder, dembrexine hydrochloride 5 mg/g, for *horses*
Withdrawal Periods. *Horses*: slaughter 5 days

5.4.2 Expectorants

Expectorants containing small doses of ipecacuanha, squill, and ammoniumn salts are claimed to aid removal of mucus from the airways by a mild irritant effect on the mucous membrane; their efficacy is unproven. Guaiacol has disinfectant properties and has been used as an expectorant for productive cough.

COMPOUND EXPECTORANTS

UK

GSL **Cold Mixture** (Johnson's) *UK*
Mixture, squill syrup BP 200 mg, ipecacuanha tincture BP 50 mg/mL, for *caged birds*; 15 mL

GSL **Cough & Cold Mixture** (Johnson's) *UK*
Mixture, squill syrup BP 200 mg, ipecacuanha tincture BP 50 mg/mL, for *dogs, cats*; 50 mL

Australia

Kofeze Cough Paste (Joseph Lyddy) *Austral.*
Oral paste, camphor 2.7 g/kg, aniseed oil 0.7 g/kg, squill tinctur concentrate 2.5 g/kg, glycyrrhiza extract 37.5 g/kg, for *horses*
Contra-indications. Use within 2 days prior to racing

Kof-Kontrol (Vetsearch) *Austral.*
Oral solution, ammonium chloride 34 mg/mL, liquorice liquid extract 80 mg/mL, tincture of squill 30 mg/mL, iodine 0.2 mg/mL, for *horses*
Withdrawal Periods. *Horses*: slaughter withdrawal period nil

Respireze (RWR) *Austral.*
Injection, ether 0.1 mL/mL, camphor 200 mg/mL, guaiacol 0.8 mL/mL, for *horses, cattle, sheep, pigs, dogs*
Withdrawal Periods. *Horses*: slaughter 28 days

Pottie's Cough Mixture (Blue Cross) *Austral.*
Oral solution, ammonium chloride 107 g/L, extract liquorice 80 g/L, tincture squill 27 mL/L, tincture ginger 27 mL/L, for *horses, cattle*
Withdrawal Periods. *Cattle, horses*: slaughter withdrawal period nil

Ranlixa (Ranvet) *Austral.*
Oral solution, diphenhydramine hydrochloride 84.74 mg, ammonium chloride 816 mg, sodium citrate 336 mg, chloroform 135.87 mg, menthol crystals 6.53 mg; all /30 mL, for *horses*
Withdrawal Periods. *Horses*: slaughter 7 days
Contra-indications. Use within 72 hours prior to racing

Throateze (Action Chemical) *Austral.*
Oral solution, potassium citrate 45.58 g/L, tincture ipecac 45.58 g/L, ammonium acetate 249.92 mg/L, for *dogs*

USA

Cough Syrup (Life Science) *USA*
Oral syrup, guaifenesin 8 g, ammonium chloride 8 g, sodium citrate 8 g, pyrilamine maleate 50 mg, phenylephrine hydrochloride 50 mg in 30 ml syrup, for *horses, dogs, cats*
Withdrawal Periods. Should not be used in *horses* intended for human consumption

Tri-Tussin (Life Science) *USA*
Oral powder, for addition to drinking water, guaifenesin 7%, ammonium chloride 75%, potassium iodide 2%, for *horses, cattle, pigs, chickens*

5.5 Antitussives

Cough suppressants are only beneficial where coughing is persistent and unproductive, interferes with the animal's sleep and rest, or causes muscular fatigue and exhaustion. They should not be used where there are excess secretions in the tracheobronchial tree, as in chronic bronchitis or bronchopneumonia. In general, the use of antitussives is restricted to dogs.

Antitussive drugs are selected to exploit the cough suppressant effects of opioid drugs, while minimising the sedative and drug dependency characteristics.

Butorphanol is the most effective antitussive and is also a potent opioid analgesic. **Codeine phosphate** is an opioid analgesic but has little analgesic activity and can induce constipation. All opioid drugs should be used with caution in cats. **Dextromethorphan** is used for relief of non-productive cough; it has a central action on the cough centre in the medulla. It is structually similar to opioids but has no analgesic and limited sedative properties. **Guaifenesin** is reported to increase the volume and reduce the viscosity of tenacious sputum.

BUTORPHANOL

UK
Indications. Non-productive cough; analgesia (see section 6.3)
Contra-indications. Chronic bronchitis, bronchiectasis, bronchopneumonia, or any other condition in which there is excess airway secretion; conditions causing CNS depression; hepatic impairment; cats
Side-effects. Mild sedation; rarely transient ataxia, anorexia and diarrhoea; respiratory depression
Dose. *Dogs*: *by mouth*, 500 micrograms/kg 2–4 times daily for up to 14 days

POM **Torbutrol** (Fort Dodge) *UK*
Tablets, butorphanol (as tartrate) 1 mg, 5 mg, 10 mg, for *dogs*

CODEINE PHOSPHATE

UK
Indications. Non-productive cough; analgesia (see section 6.3); non-specific diarrhoea (see section 3.1.2)
Contra-indications. See under Butorphanol
Side-effects. Sedation, ataxia; respiratory depression; constipation
Dose. *Dogs*: *by mouth*, 0.5–2.0 mg/kg twice daily

POM Ⓗ **Codeine Phosphate** (Non-proprietary) *UK*
Tablets, codeine phosphate 15 mg, 30 mg, 60 mg
Syrup, codeine phosphate 5 mg/mL; 100 mL

POM Ⓗ **Codeine Linctus** (Non-proprietary) *UK*
Linctus, codeine phosphate 3 mg/mL; 100 mL
Note. Codeine linctus is categorised as P when a single dose is 5 mL or less

POM Ⓗ **Codeine Linctus Paediatric** (Non-proprietary) *UK*
Linctus, codeine phosphate 3 mg/5 mL; 100 mL

DEXTROMETHORPHAN HYDROBROMIDE

UK
Indications. Non-productive cough
Contra-indications. See under Butorphanol
Side-effects. See under Codeine phosphate
Dose. *Dogs*: *by mouth*, up to 5 mg 3–4 times daily

P Ⓗ **Robitussin Dry Cough** (Whitehall) *UK*
Oral solution, dextromethorphan hydrobromide 1.5 mg/mL; 100 mL

P Ⓗ **Robitussin Junior Persistant Cough** (Whitehall) *UK*
Oral solution, dextromethorphan hydrobromide 750 micrograms/ mL; 100 mL

USA
Indications. Non-productive cough

Cough Tablets (Life Science) *USA*
Tablets, guaifenesin 100 mg, dextromethorphan hydrobromide 10 mg, for *dogs, cats*
Dose. *Dogs*: 0.5–1.0 tablet every four hours
Cats: 0.5 tablet every four hours

5.6 Respiratory stimulants

Respiratory stimulants are administered, at doses below the convulsive threshold, to stimulate respiration. Their main uses are to promote respiration in apnoeic newborn and pre-term animals and to reverse respiratory depression associated with general anaesthetic, sedative, or hypnotic drugs.

These drugs should not be used as an alternative to patient management. In drug-induced respiratory depression maintenance of an adequate airway and airflow by intubation and positive-pressure ventilation are the recognised methods of treatment. While analeptic drugs will temporarily increase tidal and minute volume, the oxygen gain may be partly offset by increased brain oxygen consumption.

All analeptics are CNS stimulants and may induce convulsions. **Doxapram** is selective as a respiratory stimulant. The principal mechanism of action of doxapram involves stimulation of the peripheral aortic and carotid body chemoreceptors rather than a central action.

The methylxanthines such as **diprophylline** and **etamiphylline,** in addition to their bronchodilatory action are also non-specific CNS stimulants. They increase respiratory drive by altering the respiratory centre's sensitivity to carbon dioxide.

DIPROPHYLLINE

Eire

Indications. Respiratory stimulation of calves; reversal of respiratory depression associated with overdose of general anaesthetic, hypnotic, and sedative drugs

Frecardyl Solution (Vetoquinol) *Eire*
Injection, heptaminol (as hydrochloride) 5 g/100 mL, diprophylline 5 g/100 mL, for *horses, cattle, pigs, dogs, cats*
Dose. *Horses, cattle, pigs, dogs, cats*: by mouth, intramuscular, intraperitoneal, or intravenous injection, 2 mL/10 kg

DOXAPRAM HYDROCHLORIDE

UK

Indications. Respiratory stimulation of neonates; reversal of respiratory depression associated with overdose of general anaesthetic, hypnotic, and sedative drugs
Contra-indications. Convulsions, renal or hepatic disease, hypocalcaemia
Side-effects. Convulsions
Warnings. Airway should be patent; overdosage may produce hyperventilation which may be followed by reduced carbon dioxide tension in blood, cerebral vasoconstriction, hypoxia, and possible brain damage; use with extreme caution in dogs that have been sedated with morphine; see also Drug Interactions – Appendix 1
Dose. Neonatal use.
Foals ♦, calves: by subcutaneous, intramuscular or intravenous injection, or by sublingual application, 40–100 mg
Lambs: by subcutaneous or intravenous injection, or by sublingual application, 5–10 mg
Puppies: by subcutaneous or intravenous injection, or by sublingual application, 1–5 mg
Kittens: by subcutaneous or intravenous injection, or by sublingual application, 1–2 mg

Post-anaesthetic use.
Horses: by intravenous injection, 0.5–1.0 mg/kg
Dogs, cats: by intravenous injection, 1–2 mg/kg following inhalational anaesthetic; 2–5 mg/kg following intravenous anaesthetic

Dopram-V (Fort Dodge) *UK*
PML *Oral drops*, doxapram hydrochloride 20 mg/mL, for *calves, lambs, puppies, kittens*; 5 mL
Withdrawal Periods. Should not be used in animals intended for human consumption except neonates. *Calves, lambs*: slaughter 28 days
POM *Injection*, doxapram hydrochloride 20 mg/mL, for *horses, calves, lambs, dogs, cats*; 20 mL
Withdrawal Periods. Should not be used in animals intended for human consumption except neonates. *Calves, lambs*: slaughter 28 days

Australia

Indications. Respiratory stimulation of neonates; reversal of respiratory depression associated with overdose of general anaesthetic drugs
Side-effects. Convulsions, hyperventilation
Warnings. Airway should be patent
Dose. Neonatal use.

Puppies: by subcutaneous or intravenous (umbilical vein) injection, or by sublingual application, 1–5 mg
Kittens: by subcutaneous or intravenous (umbilical vein) injection, or by sublingual application, 1–2 mg

Post-anaesthetic use.
Horses: by intravenous injection, 440–550 micrograms/kg
Dogs, cats: by intravenous injection, 1.1 mg/kg following inhalational anaesthetic; 5.5–11.0 mg/kg following barbiturate anaesthetic

Dopram-V (Pharmtech) *Austral.*
Injection, doxapram hydrochloride 20 mg/mL, for *horses, dogs, cats*

Eire

Indications. Respiratory stimulation of neonates; reversal of respiratory depression associated with overdose of general anaesthetic, hypnotic, and sedative drugs
Contra-indications. Convulsions, renal or hepatic disease, hypocalcaemia
Side-effects. Convulsions
Warnings. Airway should be patent; overdosage may produce hyperventilation which may be followed by reduced carbon dioxide tension in blood, cerebral vasoconstriction, hypoxia, and possible brain damage; use with extreme caution in dogs that have been sedated with morphine; see also Drug Interactions – Appendix 1
Dose. Neonatal use.
Calves: by subcutaneous, intramuscular or intravenous injection, or by sublingual application, 40–100 mg
Lambs: by subcutaneous or intravenous injection, or by sublingual application, 5–10 mg
Puppies: by subcutaneous or intravenous injection, or by sublingual application, 1–5 mg
Kittens: by subcutaneous or intravenous injection, or by sublingual application, 1–2 mg

Post-anaesthetic use.
Horses: by intravenous injection, 0.5–1.0 mg/kg
Dogs, cats: by intravenous injection, 1–2 mg/kg following inhalational anaesthetic; 2–5 mg/kg following intravenous anaesthetic

Dopram-V (Fort Dodge) *Eire*
Injection, doxapram hydrochloride 20 mg/mL, for *horses, calves, lambs, dogs, cats*
Withdrawal Periods. Should not be used in horses intended for human consumption. *Calves, lambs*: slaughter 28 days

Dopram-V Drops (Fort Dodge) *Eire*
Oral drops, doxapram hydrochloride 20 mg/mL, for *calves, lambs, puppies, kittens*
Withdrawal Periods. *Calves, lambs*: slaughter 28 days

New Zealand

Indications. Respiratory stimulation of neonates; reversal of respiratory depression associated with overdose of general anaesthetic drugs
Side-effects. Convulsions, hyperventilation
Warnings. Airway should be patent
Dose. Neonatal use.

Puppies: *by subcutaneous or intravenous (umbilical vein) injection, or by sublingual application*, 1–5 mg
Kittens: *by subcutaneous or intravenous (umbilical vein) injection, or by sublingual application*, 1–2 mg

Post-anaesthetic use.
Horses: *by intravenous injection*, 440–550 micrograms/kg
Dogs, cats: *by intravenous injection*, 1.1 mg/kg following inhalational anaesthetic; 5.5–11.0 mg/kg following barbiturate anaesthetic

Dopram (Bomac) *NZ*
Injection, doxapram hydrochloride 20 mg/mL, for ***horses, dogs, cats***

USA
Indications. Respiratory stimulation of neonates; reversal of respiratory depression associated with overdose of general anaesthetic
Side-effects. Convulsions, hyperventilation
Warnings. Airway should be patent
Dose. Neonatal use.
Puppies: *by subcutaneous or intravenous injection, or by sublingual application*, 1–5 mg
Kittens: *by subcutaneous or by sublingual application*, 1–2 mg

Post-anaesthetic use.
Horses: *by intravenous injection*, 0.5–1.0 mg/kg
Dogs, cats: *by intravenous injection*, 1.1 mg/kg following inhalational anaesthetic; 5.5–11.0 mg/kg following intravenous anaesthetic

Dopram-V Injectable (Fort Dodge) *USA*
Injection, doxapram hydrochloride 20 mg/mL, for ***dogs, cats, horses***

ETAMIPHYLLINE CAMSILATE
(Etamiphylline camsylate)

UK
Indications. Respiratory stimulation of neonates; respiratory disease where bronchodilation may be beneficial (see section 5.1); myocardial stimulation (see section 4.1.2)
Dose. *By mouth*.
Calves: 700 mg repeated after 3–4 hours if required
Lambs: (<2.5 kg body-weight) 140 mg; (>2.5 kg body-weight) up to 280 mg. Dose may be repeated after 3–4 hours if required
Piglets ♦: 70–140 mg

PML **Dalophylline** (Arnolds) *UK*
Oral gel, etamiphylline camsilate 140 mg/unit dose, for ***calves, lambs***; 32-mL metered-dose applicator (1 unit dose = 3.2 mL)
Withdrawal Periods. ***Calves, lambs***: slaughter 7 days
Dose. *Calves*: 5 unit doses. May be repeated after 3–4 hours
Lambs: 1–2 unit doses. May be repeated after 3–4 hours
Piglets ♦: ½–1 unit dose

5.7 Nasal decongestants

Nasal decongestants contain alpha-adrenoceptor stimulants to provide symptomatic relief in upper respiratory tract problems associated with profuse secretion; they should be used with caution. **Pseudoephedrine** may be of use in cats with allergic rhinitis.

UK

P Ⓗ **Sudafed** (Warner Lambert) *UK*
Elixir, pseudoephedrine hydrochloride 6 mg/mL; 100 mL
Dose. *Cats*: *by mouth*, 2–4 mg/kg twice daily

6 Drugs acting on the
NERVOUS SYSTEM

Contributors:
J C Brearley MA, VetMB, PhD, DVA, DipECVA, MRCVS
S E Heath BVSc, MRCVS
Professor R S Jones OBE, MVSc, DrMedVet, DVSc, DVA, MRCA, DipECVA, FIBiol, FRCVS
G C Skerritt BVSc, DipECVN, CBiol, MIBiol, FRCVS

6.1 Sedatives
6.2 Sedative antagonists
6.3 Analgesics
6.4 Neuroleptanalgesics
6.5 Opioid antagonists
6.6 General anaesthetics
6.7 Drugs modifying neuromuscular transmission
6.8 Local anaesthetics
6.9 Antiepileptics
6.10 Drugs used for euthanasia
6.11 Drugs used to modify behaviour

6.1 Sedatives

6.1.1 Phenothiazines
6.1.2 Butyrophenones
6.1.3 Alpha$_2$-adrenoceptor stimulants
6.1.4 Benzodiazepines

Sedatives produce calmness, drowsiness, and indifference to the surroundings. The difference between sedatives and tranquillisers is indistinct but, in general, tranquillisers produce a state of calmness with less drowsiness.

Sedatives are commonly included in pre-anaesthetic medication, and enable a 20 to 75% reduction in the dose of the general anaesthetic depending on the drug and species to which it is administered. Generally, sedatives are used for restraint, to facilitate handling and transport of animals, and to modify behaviour (see section 6.11). They are also used to facilitate minor surgery and X-ray examination.

There is a continuous gradation of levels of sedation from light sedation to a depth approaching anaesthesia. The level of sedation is determined by the drug, dosage, route of administration, the interacting effect of any other drugs that are being used to treat the animal at the time of administration, and the initial degree of excitement of the animal. In general, sedatives should be administered before an animal becomes excited. Once unsettled, the animal may require a much higher dose of sedative or the sedative may not have an appreciable calming effect. The doses given in each monograph below range from the lowest figure for light sedation to the highest amount appropriate for deep sedation. Deeply sedated animals require standards of monitoring equal to anaesthetised animals. If the procedure is more painful and the sedative does not have analgesic properties, administration of an opioid analgesic or local anaesthesia is essential.

The combination of an opioid analgesic with a sedative will produce greater sedation than seen with the sedative alone. This is termed neuroleptanalgesia (see sections 6.3.1 and 6.4 for further information and dosages).

6.1.1 Phenothiazines

Phenothiazine derivatives are neuroleptics that are effective sedatives commonly used in veterinary practice. They have a wide range of activity arising from their depressant actions on the CNS, dopamine inhibitory, alpha-adrenoceptor blocking, and weaker antimuscarinic activities.

Acepromazine produces mild to moderate sedation, but has no analgesic properties. Its effect is variable and may be unpredictable, with some excitable animals failing to show an observable response. Oral administration particularly produces unreliable results, especially in dogs and cats. While some effect may be seen after 15 minutes, maximal effect is generally only achieved after one hour following administration. Likewise, absorption following subcutaneous injection is variable and hence intramuscular or intravenous administration is preferred. Peak effect after intravenous injection is generally within 5 minutes. Duration of action of acepromazine can range from approximately 4 hours, with a low dose in a fit animal, to over 24 hours at higher doses or in debilitated animals. Doses greater than 100 micrograms/kg will not produce a deeper sedation, but lead to increased duration of action and side-effects. High doses may result in excitement and extrapyramidal side-effects in some animals. In the majority of animals doses♦ of 20 to 50 micrograms/kg will produce adequate moderate sedation to allow venous catheterisation or intravenous injection. Increased sedation may be achieved by the concomitant administration of an opioid analgesic rather than increasing the dose of acepromazine.

Contra-indications for the use of phenothiazine derivatives include premedication for procedures that may promote epileptiform seizures, such as myelography, premedication of known epileptic animals, and treatment of status epilepticus, because these drugs decrease the seizure threshold. Sedation of post-trauma patients is also contra-indicated because acepromazine causes hypotension, which may be fatal in a hypovolaemic animal. In the male horse the drug can cause priapism, paraphimosis, and paralysis of the retractor penis muscle. Although not totally contra-indicated in stallions, acepromazine should be used at the lower dose rates and the condition treated at once if it occurs, to prevent trauma to the penis.

The extrapyramidal side-effects observed with phenothiazines such as tremor, rigidity, and catalepsy are generally only seen at high doses. However the piperazine derivatives, for example prochlorperazine and perphenazine, are particularly prone to producing these effects hence they have largely been superseded by acepromazine.

Chlorpromazine (see section 3.4.1) is still used to treat non-specific vomiting and prevent motion sickness. Chlorpromazine may induce hepatic microsomal enzymes.

The effects of **propionylpromazine** and **promazine** are very similar to those of acepromazine. Propionylpromazine is widely used in Europe for sedation and premedication of both large and small animals. Promazine is reported to cause hepatic microsomal enzyme induction and so prolonged use of this drug could be expected to result in reduced pharmacological effects of other drugs which undergo biotransformation in the liver.

ACEPROMAZINE
(Acetylpromazine)

UK

Indications. Pre-anaesthetic medication; sedation; motion sickness (see section 3.4.2); behaviour modification (see section 6.11.1)

Contra-indications. Manufacturer does not recommend use in breeding stallions; pregnant female animals; epileptics; concurrent use with organophosphorus compounds or procaine hydrochloride in horses; horses should not be ridden within 36 hours of treatment; equine colic; hypovolaemia

Side-effects. See notes above; hypotension; thrombocytopenia; platelet dysfunction; protrusion of nictitating membrane in dogs and cats; ataxia; muscle tremors; hypothermia

Warnings. Care in male horses, see notes above; may cause syncope in canine brachycephalic breeds; caution in renal impairment, large breed dogs; some authorities recommend care when using for car travel especially in hot weather

Dose. Horses: *by mouth,* 130–260 micrograms/kg

by intramuscular or slow intravenous injection, 30–100 micrograms/kg

Dogs, cats: pre-anaesthetic medication, sedation, *by mouth,* 0.25–3.0 mg/kg

by subcutaneous, intramuscular or slow intravenous injection, 30–125 micrograms/kg (maximum 4 mg)

Motions sickness, *by mouth,* 0.5–1.0 mg/kg 15–30 minutes before a light meal

POM **ACP** (Vericore VP) *UK*
Tablets, acepromazine (as maleate) 10 mg, 25 mg, for *dogs, cats*; 500

POM **ACP** (Vericore VP) *UK*
Injection, acepromazine (as maleate) 2 mg/mL, for *dogs, cats*; 20 mL
Injection, acepromazine (as maleate) 10 mg/mL, for *horses*; 20 mL
Withdrawal Periods. Should not be used in *horses* intended for human consumption

POM **Oralject Sedazine-Acepromazine** (Vetsearch; distributed by Millpledge) *UK*
Oral paste, acepromazine (as maleate) 8.9 mg/mL, for *horses*; 30-mL metered dose applicator
Withdrawal Periods. Should not be used in *horses* intended for human consumption
Dose. Horses: *by mouth,* 4–10 mL/450 kg body-weight

Australia

Indications. Pre-anaesthetic medication; sedation; motion sickness

Contra-indications. Breeding stallions; concurrent use with organophosphorus compounds or procaine hydrochloride; canine epilepsy

Side-effects. Hypotension; penile prolapse in male horses

Warnings. Safety in pregnant animals not established; use with care in patients with low blood pressure, poor cardiac output, shock, male horses, and Boxer dogs; Drug Interactions – organophosphorus compounds, procaine hydrochloride

Dose.

Horses, cattle: by mouth, 120–240 micrograms/kg

by subcutaneous, intramuscular, or slow intravenous injection, 50–100 micrograms/kg

Sheep, pigs: *by subcutaneous, intramuscular, or slow intravenous injection,* 50–100 micrograms/kg

Dogs, cats: *by mouth,* 1–3 mg/kg

by intramuscular or slow intravenous injection, 100–200 micrograms/kg

Acemav (Mavlab) *Austral.*
Injection, acepromazine (as maleate) 10 mg/mL, for *horses, cattle, pigs, sheep*

Acepril 10 (Ilium) *Austral.*
Injection, acepromazine (as maleate) 10 mg/mL, for *horses, cattle, sheep, pigs*

ACP 2 (Delvet) *Austral.*
Injection, acepromazine (as maleate) 2 mg/mL, for *dogs, cats*

ACP 10 (Delvet) *Austral.*
Injection, acepromazine (as maleate) 10 mg/mL, for *horses, cattle, sheep, pigs*

ACP 10, 25 (Delvet) *Austral.*
Tablets, acepromazine (as maleate) 10 mg, 25 mg, for *small animals*

Anamav Injection (Mavlab) *Austral.*
Injection, acepromazine 10 mg/mL, atropine sulphate 1 mg/mL, for *dogs, cats, pigs, horses*
Dose. *By subcutaneous, intramuscular, or intravenous injection.*
Horses, pigs: 0.025–0.05 mL/kg
Dogs, cats: 0.05–0.1 mL/kg

Calmivet (Vetoquinol) *Austral.*
Injection, acepromazine (as maleate) 5 mg/mL, for *horses, cattle, sheep, goats, pigs, cats, dogs*
Withdrawal Periods. *Cattle*: slaughter 2 days, milk 2 days. *Horses, pigs, sheep, goats*: slaughter 2 days

Promex 2 Injection (Apex) *Austral.*
Injection, acepromazine 2 mg/mL, for *dogs, cats*

Promex 10 Injection (Apex) *Austral.*
Injection, acepromazine 10 mg/mL, for *horses, cattle, sheep, pigs*
Withdrawal Periods. *Cattle*: slaughter 28 days, milk 72 hours. *Horses, sheep, pigs*: slaughter 28 days

Promex 10 Tablets (Apex) *Austral.*
Tablets, acepromazine 10 mg, 25 mg, for *dogs, cats*

Sedazine-ACP (Vetsearch) *Austral.*
Oral paste, acepromazine maleate 12 mg/mL, for *horses, cattle*
Withdrawal Periods. *Cattle*: slaughter 3 days, should not be used in cattle producing milk for human consumption. *Horses*: slaughter 28 days

Eire

Indications. Pre-anaesthetic medication; sedation; motion sickness

Contra-indications. Breeding stallions; pregnant mares; concurrent use with organophosphorus compounds or procaine hydrochloride; horses should not be ridden within 36 hours of treatment

Side-effects. Hypotension

Warnings. Care in male horses; may cause syncope in canine brachycephalic breeds; Drug Interactions – organophosphorus compounds, procaine hydrochloride

Dose. *Horses*: *by intramuscular or intravenous injection, 30–100 micrograms/kg*

Dogs, cats: *subcutaneous, intramuscular or intravenous injection, 30–125 micrograms/kg*

by mouth, 0.25–3.0 mg/kg

ACP Injection 2mg/mL (Cypharm) *Eire*
Injection, acepromazine 2 mg/mL, for *dogs, cats*

ACP Injection 10mg/mL (Cypharm) *Eire*
Injection, acepromazine 10 mg/mL, for *horses*
Withdrawal Periods. Slaughter 28 days

ACP Tablets (Cypharm) *Eire*
Tablets, acepromazine 10 mg, 25 mg, for *dogs, cats*

New Zealand

Indications. Pre-anaesthetic medication; sedation; motion sickness

Contra-indications. Breeding stallions; epileptics; concurrent use with organophosphorus compounds or procaine hydrochloride; shock, severe hepatic or lung damage; hypovolaemia

Side-effects. Hypotension; hyperexcitability in horses at high dose

Warnings. Care in male horses; may cause syncope in canine brachycephalic breeds; caution in debilitated animals, aged animals, or cardiovascular disease; Drug Interactions – organophosphorus compounds, procaine hydrochloride

Dose. *Horses, cattle, sheep, pigs*: *by intramuscular or intravenous injection*, doses vary, 50–500 micrograms/kg

Dogs, cats: *by mouth*, 1–3 mg/kg

by intramuscular or intravenous injection, doses vary, 125–250 micrograms/kg

Ace 2 (Virbac) *NZ*
Injection, acepromazine (as maleate) 2 mg/mL, for *dogs, cats*

Ace 10 (Virbac) *NZ*
Injection, acepromazine (as maleate) 10 mg/mL, for *large animals*
Withdrawal Periods. Slaughter 7 days, milk 7 hours

Acezine 2 (Ethical) *NZ*
Injection, acepromazine (as maleate) 2 mg/mL, for *dogs, cats*

Acezine 10 (Ethical) *NZ*
Injection, acepromazine (as maleate) 10 mg/mL, for *horses, cattle, sheep, pigs*
Withdrawal Periods. *Horses, pigs*: slaughter 1 day. *Cattle, sheep*: slaughter 1 day, milk 24 hours

ACP Injection (Novartis) *NZ*
Injection, acepromazine (as maleate) 2 mg/mL, for *dogs, cats*

ACP Injection (Novartis) *NZ*
Injection, acepromazine (as maleate) 10 mg/mL, for *large animals*
Withdrawal Periods. Slaughter 7 days, milk 168 hours

ACP Tablets (Novartis) *NZ*
Tablets, acepromazine (as maleate) 10 mg or 25 mg, for *dogs, cats*

Combistress (Phoenix) *NZ*
Injection, acepromazine maleate 20 mg/mL, for *horses, dogs, cats*
Withdrawal Periods. *Horses*: slaughter 28 days

Oralject Sedazine (Bomac) *NZ*
Oral paste, acepromazine maleate 12 mg/mL, for *horses, cattle*
Withdrawal Periods. *Horses*: slaughter 28 days. *Cattle*: slaughter 3 days, milk 72 hours

USA

Indications. Pre-anaesthetic medication; sedation

Contra-indications. Breeding stallions; epileptics; concurrent use with organophosphorus compounds or procaine hydrochloride; shock, severe hepatic or lung damage; hypovolaemia

Side-effects. Hypotension

Warnings. Care in male horses; caution in debilitated animals, aged animals, or cardiovascular disease; Drug Interactions – organophosphorus compounds, procaine hydrochloride

Dose. *Horses*: *by subcutaneous, intramuscular or intravenous injection, 44–88 micrograms/kg*

Dogs: *by mouth, or subcutaneous, intramuscular or intravenous injection, 0.55–1.1 mg/kg*

Cats: *by mouth, or subcutaneous, intramuscular or intravenous injection, 1.1–2.2 mg/kg*

Aceproject (Vetus) *USA*
Injection, acepromazine maleate 10mg/mL, for *dogs*

Aceprotabs (Vetus) *USA*
Tablets, acepromazine maleate 10mg, 25mg, for *dogs*

Acepromazine Maleate (Butler, Vedco, Western Veterinary Supply) *USA*
Injection, acepromazine maleate 10 mg/mL , for *dogs*
Tablets, acepromazine maleate 10mg, 25mg, for *dogs*

Acepromazine Maleate Injection (Boehringer Ingelheim Vetmedica) *USA*
Injection, acepromazine maleate 10 mg/mL, for *dogs*

Acepromazine Maleate Tablets (Boehringer Ingelheim Vetmedica) *USA*
Tablets, acepromazine maleate 10 mg, 25 mg, for *dogs*

Promace (Fort Dodge) *USA*
Injection, acepromazine maleate 10 mg/mL, for *dogs, cats, horses*
Withdrawal Periods. Should not be used in *horses* intended for human consumption

Promace (Fort Dodge) *USA*
Tablets, acepromazine maleate 5mg, 10 mg, 25 mg, for *cats, dogs*

PROMAZINE

USA

Indications. Pre-anaesthetic medication; sedation; behaviour modification

Contra-indications. Concurrent use with organophosphorus compounds or procaine hydrochloride

Warnings. Caution in debilitation, cardiac impairment, sympathetic blockage, hypovolaemia, shock

Dose. *Horses*: *by mouth*, 1–2 mg/kg

Promazine Granules (Fort Dodge) *USA*
Oral granules, promazine hydrochloride 8 g/290 g granules, for *horses*

Tranquazine Injection (Anthony) *USA*
Injection, promazine hydrochloride 50 mg/mL, for *horses*
Withdrawal Periods. *Horses*: should not be used in horses intended for human consumption

6.1.2 Butyrophenones

Butyrophenones used in veterinary medicine include **azaperone, droperidol,** and **fluanisone**. Fluanisone is available in combination with fentanyl in a neuroleptic combination (see section 6.4). Azaperone is primarily used in pigs to control fighting, reduce stress, prevent maternal rejection of piglets, and sedation for obstetric procedures. Animals should be left alone in a quiet environment during the induction period. The long duration of action of azaperone results in prolonged anaesthetic recovery when it is used as a premedicant. Azaperone may cause violent reactions in horses and is not recommended in this species.

Droperidol may be used for pre-anaesthetic medication and also sedation for motion sickness and restlessness.

AZAPERONE

UK

Indications. Pre-anaesthetic medication; behaviour modification (see section 6.11.1)
Contra-indications. Dose of 1 mg/kg should not be exceeded in boars
Side-effects. Transient salivation or panting; extrapyramidal effects; hypotension; respiratory stimulation
Warnings. Avoid use of azaperone in very cold conditions
Dose. *Pigs*: pre-anaesthetic medication, *by intramuscular injection*, 1–2 mg/kg

POM **Stresnil** (Janssen) *UK*
Injection, azaperone 40 mg/mL, for *pigs*; 100 mL
Withdrawal Periods. *Pigs*: slaughter 10 days

Australia

Indications. Pre-anaesthetic medication; behaviour modification
Side-effects. Transient salivation or panting
Warnings. Avoid use of azaperone in wet or dusty conditions
Dose. *Pigs*: *by intramuscular injection*, 1–2 mg/kg

Stresnil (Boehringer Ingelheim) *Austral.*
Injection, azaperone 40 mg/mL, for *pigs*
Withdrawal Periods. *Pigs*: slaughter 6 hours

Eire

Indications. Pre-anaesthetic medication; behaviour modification
Contra-indications. Dose of 1 mg/kg should not be exceeded in boars
Side-effects. Transient salivation or panting
Warnings. Avoid use of azaperone in very cold conditions
Dose. *Pigs*: pre-anaesthetic medication, *by intramuscular injection*, 1–2 mg/kg

Stresnil (Janssen) *Eire*
Injection, azaperone 40 mg/mL, for *pigs*
Withdrawal Periods. *Pigs*: slaughter 7 days

New Zealand

Indications. Pre-anaesthetic medication; behaviour modification

Side-effects. Transient salivation or panting
Warnings. Avoid use of azaperone in wet or dusty conditions
Dose. *Pigs*: *by intramuscular injection*, 1–2 mg/kg

Fentazin (Parnell) *NZ* (see section 6.4)

Stresnil (Boehringer Ingelheim) *NZ*
Injection, azaperone 40 mg/mL, for *pigs*
Withdrawal Periods. *Pigs*: slaughter 1 day

6.1.3 Alpha$_2$-adrenoceptor stimulants

Xylazine, medetomidine, romifidine, and detomidine, are all alpha$_2$-adrenoceptor stimulants, with marked sedative, muscle relaxant, and analgesic properties. Sedation is dose dependent for the recommended range for all the drugs, but at higher doses there is an increased incidence of side-effects. Characteristic of the group is the marked bradycardia produced at even moderate doses. The bradycardia results from sino-atrial and atrioventricular heart block, partially produced in reflex response to an initial drug-induced hypertension. There is a subsequent moderate hypotension with all drugs in this group. Hyperglycaemia and polyuria also occur with all drugs in this group, again due to alpha$_2$-adrenoceptor stimulation. The hyperglycaemia can be sufficient to result in glucosuria. The specific alpha$_2$-adrenoceptor antagonist, atipamezole (see section 6.2.1) has been used to reverse all of these drugs, although specifically authorised to reverse medetomidine.

Xylazine is used in cats, dogs, horses, and cattle as a sedative to allow minor procedures (with local anaesthesia) and to facilitate handling. It is also used as a premedicant in these species. In dogs and cats, vomiting frequently occurs after administration of xylazine. Therefore it is contra-indicated in animals with gastro-intestinal obstruction. Vomiting may be advantageous in animals not starved for at least the preceding 6 hours. The amount of induction agent should be reduced by 50–75% in animals premedicated with xylazine to avoid fatal overdose. Concurrent administration of atropine (see section 6.6.1) in dogs and cats may be advantageous to reduce salivation and the bradycardic effects of xylazine. The bradycardia associated with the alpha$_2$-agonists is primarily a physiological response to the initial hypertension associated with the use of these drugs and should not be viewed as pathological. Although the bradycardia can be prevented by the concurrent use of anticholinergics such as atropine, this is controversal as the resultant increase in myocardial oxygen consumption may not be met by supply and so a hypoxic myocardium will result. This may produce malignant cardiac arrhythmias. Care should be exercised if administration to elderly or debilitated animals is contemplated, due to the profound cardiovascular changes the drug induces.

Xylazine is a useful sedative in horses. Approximately twice as much drug is required to achieve comparable sedation if given intramuscularly rather than intravenously. Xylazine may initially cause bradycardia and second degree heart block, which resolve after approximately 10 minutes. Arterial blood pressure will rise sharply after intravenous injection, then fall to a level slightly below normal. Horses sedated with xylazine usually remain standing although they will sway if given high doses. Care must be exercised when using xylazine because an animal that appears deeply sedated can still kick accurately in response to a stimulus.

The depth and reliability of sedation can be increased by administering an opioid analgesic concomitantly, and drugs such as pethidine, morphine, methadone, or butorphanol have been used in combination with xylazine for standing sedation in horses. The duration of action of many opioid analgesics is longer than that of xylazine in the horse, and acepromazine is often included in combinations of xylazine and opioid analgesics, to provide continued sedation. This is particularly important when pure opioid agonists such as morphine or methadone are used.

As a premedicant in horses, xylazine may be followed by thiopental, methohexital, or ketamine. With ketamine, a premedicant dose of xylazine 1.1 mg/kg is required to an induction dose of 2.2 mg/kg ketamine. The dose of xylazine should not be reduced below this because ketamine, without adequate sedation, will cause muscle rigidity and tremors in horses. The induction agent should be given a few minutes after the xylazine when sedation has reached its peak level.

Cattle are approximately 10 times more sensitive to xylazine than horses. Low doses of xylazine in cattle will produce sedation, while high doses will cause recumbency. Xylazine is useful for sedating animals before surgery under local anaesthesia. Before general anaesthesia, xylazine can be used to produce recumbency and permit endotracheal intubation with the laryngeal reflexes intact, thereby reducing the occurrence of inhalation of rumen contents.

The onset and duration of action of xylazine is species-dependent. In cattle, the onset is usually within 5 minutes with peak effect 15 minutes following administration. In horses, peak action is achieved within 5 minutes following intravenous administration and lasts for 15 minutes; the sedative effect has a duration of action between 40 and 60 minutes. In dogs and cats, xylazine analgesia lasts between 15 and 30 minutes and sedation for 1 to 2 hours. The dose of xylazine should not be repeated in the event of an unsatisfactory response. Instead the entire procedure should be repeated the following day with a higher dose of xylazine.

In ruminants, specific precautions are essential in recumbent animals (see section 6.6).

Xylazine may also be used in the growth hormone stimulation test♦ (see section 7.5.1) at a dose of 100 micrograms/kg administered by intravenous injection.

Detomidine is specifically produced for use in horses. Deep sedation lasts for about 40 minutes after detomidine and its effects may persist for hours. Detomidine is more potent than xylazine. Fatal arrhythmias have been reported when detomidine has been administered in conjunction with potentiated sulphonamides.

As a premedicant, detomidine can be followed by thiopental, methohexital, or ketamine. Maximum sedation should be allowed to develop before administration of the induction agent and this may take approximately 5 minutes.

Detomidine, romifidine, and xylazine increase the circulation time, and loss of consciousness after intravenous injection of thiopental or methohexital will be approximately one minute longer than with other premedicants.

Detomidine has been used in combination with opioid analgesics to produce deeper and more reliable sedation in horses. Many opioid analgesics may be used but butorphanol has proved to be particularly useful. Ataxia is increased when opioid analgesics are used with detomidine in standing horses.

Medetomidine is structurally similar to xylazine and detomidine, and has similar side-effects when used in dogs and cats. It is more potent than xylazine. As a premedicant, medetomidine may be followed by thiopental or propofol in dogs. In cats, medetomidine may be used in combination with ketamine for the induction of general anaesthesia. The effects of medetomidine can be reversed by the specific antagonist atipamezole (see section 6.2.1) and the two drugs may be useful for procedures such as radiography in healthy animals.

Romifidine is used for sedation and premedication in horses. It is reported to cause less ataxia than detomidine or xylazine and is therefore a useful sedative for farriery and radiography. Animals sedated with romifidine can be walked, making it useful for loading, transportation, and turning out animals that have been stabled for a period.

Romifidine can also be administered in combination with butorphanol. Romifidine has been used as a premedicant prior to induction of anaesthesia with ketamine or thiopental with good success.

DETOMIDINE HYDROCHLORIDE

UK

Indications. Sedation; sedation in combination with Butorphanol; general anaesthesia in combination with Ketamine (see section 6.6.2.4)

Contra-indications. Concurrent administration of adrenoceptor stimulants or potentiated sulphonamides; last month of pregnancy in animals except at parturition; detomidine and butorphanol combination in hepatic impairment, pregnancy, colic, or pre-existing cardic disease

Side-effects. Cardiac arrhythmias; sweating; ataxia; hyperglycaemia; polyuria

Warnings. Drug Interactions – see Appendix 1

Dose.

Sedation.

Horses: *by intramuscular or slow intravenous injection*, 10–80 micrograms/kg

Sedation, in combination with Butorphanol.

Horses: (200 kg body-weight or less) detomidine, *by slow intravenous injection*, 12 micrograms/kg, followed not more than 5 minutes later by butorphanol, *by intravenous injection*, 25 micrograms/kg; (> 200 kg body-weight), detomidine, *by slow intravenous injection*, 5 mg, followed by butorphanol, *by intravenous injection*, 10 mg

POM **Domosedan** (Pfizer) *UK*
Injection, detomidine hydrochloride 10 mg/mL, for *horses*; 5 mL, 20 mL
Withdrawal Periods. Should not be used in *horses* intended for human consumption

Australia

Indications. Sedation
Contra-indications. Last trimester of pregnancy in animals
Side-effects. Piloerection, sweating, diuresis, occasional slight tremor, transient cardiac arrhythmias, penile relaxation
Warnings. Use with caution in male horses, particularly stallions during the breeding season
Dose. *Horses*: *by intramuscular or slow intravenous injection*, 10–80 micrograms/kg

Dormosedan (Ranvet) *Austral.*
Injection, detomidine hydrochloride 10 mg/mL, for *horses*
Withdrawal Periods. Slaughter 72 hours but should not be used in *horses* intended for human consumption

Eire

Indications. Sedation
Contra-indications. Concurrent administration of adrenoceptor stimulants or potentiated sulphonamides; pregnant animals; pre-existing atrio-ventricular or sino-atrial block; severe cardiac insufficiency; cerebro-vascular disease; chronic renal failure
Side-effects. Cardiac arrhythmias; sweating; ataxia; slight tremor
Warnings. Drug Interactions – adrenoceptor stimulants, potentiated sulphonamides
Dose. *Horses*: *by intramuscular or slow intravenous injection*, 10–80 micrograms/kg

Domosedan (Pfizer) *Eire*
Injection, detomidine hydrochloride 10 mg/mL, for *horses*
Withdrawal Periods. Should not be used in *horses* intended for human consumption

New Zealand

Indications. Sedation; analgesia
Contra-indications. Last trimester of pregnancy in animals
Side-effects. Transient sweating and piloerection
Warnings. Drug Interactions – potentiated sulphonamides
Dose. *Horses, cattle*: *by intramuscular or slow intravenous injection*, 10–150 micrograms/kg

Dormosedan (Novartis) *NZ*
Injection, detomidine hydrochloride 10 mg/mL, for *horses, cattle*
Withdrawal Periods. Slaughter 2 days

USA

Indications. Sedation; analgesia
Contra-indications. Concurrent administration of potentiated sulphonamides; pre-existing atrio-ventricular or sino-atrial block, severe cardiac insufficiency, cerebro-vascular disease, respiratory disease, or chronic renal failure
Side-effects. Sweating; ataxia; excitation; hypertension; piloerection; tremors; salivation; penile prolapse
Warnings. Not recommended for use in breeding animals; avoid extremes of temperature; Drug Interactions – potentiated sulphonamides

Dose. *Horses*: *by intramuscular or slow intravenous injection*, 20–40 micrograms/kg

Dormosedan (Pfizer) *USA*
Injection, detomidine hydrochloride 10 mg/mL, for *horses*
Withdrawal Periods. Should not be used in *horses* intended for human consumption

MEDETOMIDINE HYDROCHLORIDE

UK

Indications. Sedation; sedation in combination with Butorphanol; pre-anaesthetic medication; general anaesthesia in combination with Butorphanol and Ketamine (see section 6.6.2.4)
Contra-indications. Concurrent administration of adrenoceptor stimulants; pregnant animals
Side-effects. Hypothermia; polyuria; occasional vomiting
Warnings. Caution in cardiovascular disease and debilitated animals
Dose.
Sedation.
Dogs: *by subcutaneous, intramuscular, or intravenous injection*, 10–80 micrograms/kg
Cats: *by subcutaneous or intramuscular injection*, 50–150 micrograms/kg

Sedation, in combination with Butorphanol.
Dogs: *by intramuscular or intravenous injection*, butorphanol 100 micrograms/kg in combination with medetomidine 10–25 micrograms/kg
Cats: *by subcutaneous or intramuscular injection*, butorphanol 400 micrograms/kg in combination with medetomidine 50 micrograms/kg

Pre-anaesthetic medication.
Dogs: *by subcutaneous, intramuscular, or intravenous injection*, 10–40 micrograms/kg
Cats: *by subcutaneous or intramuscular injection*, 80 micrograms/kg

POM **Domitor** (Pfizer) *UK*
Injection, medetomidine hydrochloride 1 mg/mL, for *dogs, cats*; 10 mL

Australia

Indications. Sedation
Contra-indications. Concurrent administration of adrenoceptor stimulants; pregnant animals
Side-effects. Hypothermia; bradycardia; muscle jerking; occasional vomiting
Warnings. Caution in cardiovascular, respiratory, renal, or hepatic disease and debilitated animals; Drug Interactions – adrenoceptor stimulants, other CNS depressants, antimuscarinics
Dose. *Dogs*: *by intramuscular or intravenous injection*, 10–80 micrograms/kg
Cats: *by intramuscular injection*, 50–150 micrograms/kg

Domitor (Novartis) *Austral.*.
Injection, medetomidine hydrochloride 1 mg/mL, for *dogs, cats*

Eire

Indications. Sedation

Contra-indications. Concurrent administration of adrenoceptor stimulants; pregnant animals

Side-effects. Hypothermia; bradycardia; muscle jerking; occasional vomiting; hypotension

Warnings. Caution in cardiovascular disease and debilitated animals; Drug Interactions – adrenoceptor stimulants, other CNS depressants

Dose. *Dogs*: *by subcutaneous, intramuscular, or intravenous injection*, 10–80 micrograms/kg

Cats: *by subcutaneous or intramuscular injection*, 50–150 micrograms/kg

Domitor (Pfizer) *Eire*
Injection, medetomidine hydrochloride 1.0 mg/mL, for *dogs, cats*

New Zealand

Indications. Sedation

Contra-indications. Pregnant animals

Side-effects. Hypothermia; bradycardia; decreased respiratory rate; occasional vomiting

Dose. *Dogs*: *by intramuscular or intravenous injection*, 10–80 micrograms/kg

Cats: *by intramuscular injection*, 50–100 micrograms/kg

Domitor (Novartis) *NZ*
Injection, medetomidine 1 mg/mL, for *dogs, cats*

USA

Indications. Sedation

Contra-indications. Cardiovascular, respiratory, renal, or hepatic disease and debilitated animals; shock

Side-effects. Hypothermia; bradycardia; decreased respiratory rate; hyperglycaemia; occasional vomiting;

Dose. *Dogs*: *by intramuscular injection*, 1000 micrograms/m^2

by intravenous injection, 750 micrograms/m^2

Domitor (Pfizer) *USA*
Injection, medetomidine hydrochloride 1 mg/mL, for *dogs*

ROMIFIDINE

UK

Indications. Sedation; sedation in combination with Butorphanol; pre-anaesthetic medication; general anaesthesia in combination with Ketamine (see section 6.6.2.4)

Contra-indications. Last month of pregnancy in animals, concurrent administration of potentiated sulphonamides

Side-effects. Cardiac arrhythmias, bradycardia, incoordination, sweating, hyperglycaemia, diuresis

Warnings. Drug Interactions – see Appendix 1

Dose.
Sedation.
Horses: *by intravenous injection*, 40–120 micrograms/kg

Sedation, in combination with Butorphanol.
Horses: *by intravenous injection*, romifidine 40–120 micrograms/kg, followed 5 minutes later by butorphanol 20 micrograms/kg

POM **Sedivet** (Boehringer Ingelheim) *UK*
Injection, romifidine 10 mg/mL, for *horses*; 20 mL
Withdrawal Periods. Should not be used in *horses* intended for human consumption

Australia

Indications. Sedation

Side-effects. Hypotension, bradycardia, AV block, increased skin sensitivity of the hindlimbs

Warnings. Safety in pregnant animals has not been established

Dose. *Horses*: *by intravenous injection*, 40–120 micrograms/kg

Sedivet Injectable Sedative for Horses (Boehringer Ingelheim) *Austral.*
Injection, romifidine 10 mg/mL, for *horses*
Withdrawal Periods. *Horses*: slaughter 6 days

Eire

Indications. Sedation

Contra-indications. Last month of pregnancy in animals, concurrent administration of potentiated sulphonamides

Side-effects. Cardiac arrhythmias, bradycardia, heart block, hypotension, incoordination, sweating, hyperglycaemia, diuresis

Warnings. Drug Interactions – potentiated sulphonamides

Dose. *Horses*: *by intravenous injection*, 40–120 micrograms/kg

Sedivet (Boehringer Ingelheim) *Eire*
Injection, romifidine 10 mg, for *horses*
Withdrawal Periods. *Horses*: slaughter 6 days

New Zealand

Indications. Sedation

Contra-indications. Concurrent administration of potentiated sulphonamides

Side-effects. Cardiac arrhythmias, bradycardia, heart block, hypotension, incoordination, sweating, hyperglycaemia, diuresis, increased skin sensitivity of the hindlimbs

Warnings. Safety in pregnant animals has not been established, Drug Interactions – potentiated sulphonamides

Dose. *Horses*: *by intravenous injection*, 40–120 micrograms/kg

Sedivet (Boehringer Ingelheim) *NZ*
Injection, romifidine 10 mg/mL, for *horses*
Withdrawal Periods. *Horses*: slaughter 6 days

XYLAZINE

UK

Indications. Sedation; pre-anaesthetic medication; general anaesthesia in combination with Ketamine (see section 6.6.2.4); epidural injection♦ (see section 6.8)

Contra-indications. Later stages of pregnancy in animals, except parturition; mechanical obstruction of the gastrointestinal tract in dogs and cats; concurrent administration of adrenoceptor stimulants

Side-effects. Vomiting in dogs and cats; cardiac arrhythmias; bradycardia; polyuria; hypoxaemia; transient hyperglycaemia; profuse salivation and bloat in cattle

Warnings. Caution when pulmonary disease is present or suspected; transient rise followed by fall in blood pressure in horses; safety during first month of pregnancy in animals not established; avoid tympany in recumbant cattle by maintaining animal insternal recumbancy; see notes above

Dose.

Sedation.

Horses: by intramuscular injection, 2.2–3.0 mg/kg
by slow intravenous injection, 0.6–1.1 mg/kg
Cattle: by intramuscular injection, 50–300 micrograms/kg
Dogs: by subcutaneous, intramuscular (preferred), or intravenous injection, 1–3 mg/kg
Cats: by intramuscular injection, 3 mg/kg
Deer, zoo animals: information on dose available from manufacturers

POM **Chanazine 2%** (Chanelle) *UK*
Injection, xylazine 20 mg/mL, for *horses, cattle, dogs, cats*; 25 mL
Withdrawal Periods. Should not be used in *horses* intended for human consumption. *Cattle*: slaughter 14 days, milk 2 days

POM **Chanazine 10%** (Chanelle) *UK*
Injection, xylazine 100 mg/mL, for *horses*; 50 mL
Withdrawal Periods. Should not be used in *horses* intended for human consumption

POM **Rompun 2%** (Bayer) *UK*
Injection, xylazine (as hydrochloride) 20 mg/mL, for *horses, cattle, dogs, cats*; 25 mL
Withdrawal Periods. Should not be used in *horses* intended for human consumption. *Cattle*: slaughter 14 days, milk 2 days

POM **Rompun Dry Substance** (Bayer) *UK*
Injection, powder for reconstitution, xylazine (as hydrochloride) 500 mg, for *horses, zoo animals including deer*
Withdrawal Periods. Should not be used in *horses, deer, zoo animals* intended for human consumption

POM **Virbaxyl 2%** (Virbac) *UK*
Injection, xylazine 20 mg/mL, for *horses, cattle, dogs, cats*; 25 mL
Withdrawal Periods. Should not be used in *horses* intended for human consumption. *Cattle*: slaughter 14 days, should not be used in cattle producing milk for human consumption

POM **Virbaxyl 10%** (Virbac) *UK*
Injection, xylazine 100 mg/mL, for *horses*; 50 mL
Withdrawal Periods. Should not be used in *horses* intended for human consumption

POM **Xylazine 2%** (Millpledge)
Injection, xylazine 20 mg/mL, for *horses, cattle, dogs, cats*; 25 mL
Withdrawal Periods. Should not be used in *horses* intended for human consumption. *Cattle*: slaughter 14 days

Australia

Indications. Sedation; pre-anaesthetic medication
Contra-indications. Cardiovascular disease, shock, late pregnancy; mechanical obstruction of the gastro-intestinal tract
Side-effects. Cardiac dysrhythmias and second degree A-V block; decreased respiratory rate, transient hypotension; profuse salivation in cattle; ruminal atony, bloating, regurgitation, and aspiration pneumonia with prolonged recumbancy in cattle; hyperthermia in cattle; intestinal stasis in cattle; vomiting in dogs and cats;
Warnings. Protect cattle from direct sunlight
Dose. *Horses*: by intramuscular injection, 1.0–2.5 mg/kg
by slow intravenous injection, 0.5–1.1 mg/kg

Cattle: by intramuscular injection, 100–350 micrograms/kg
by intravascular injection, 50–175 micrograms/kg
Sheep, goats: by intramuscular injection, 10–220 micrograms/kg
Dogs, cats: by intravenous injection, 0.5–1.0 mg/kg
by intramuscular injection, 1–2 mg/kg

Anased Injection (Novartis) *Austral.*
Injection, xylazine 100 mg/mL, for *horses, cattle*

Bomazine 20 (Pharmtech) *Austral.*
Injection, xylazine 20 mg/mL, for *cattle, dogs, cats*
Withdrawal Periods. *Cattle*: slaughter 3 days, milk withdrawal period nil

Bomazine 100 (Pharmtech) *Austral.*
Injection, xylazine 100 mg/mL, for *horses, cattle*
Withdrawal Periods. Should not be used in *horses* intended for human consumption. Cattle: slaughter 3 days, milk withdrawal period nil

Romazine 20 (Jurox) *Austral.*
Injection, xylazine (as hydrochloride) 20 mg/mL, for *cattle, horses, dogs, cats*
Withdrawal Periods. *Cattle*: slughter 3 days. *Deer*: slaughter 28 days

Romazine 100 (Jurox) *Austral.*
Injection, xylazine (as hydrochloride) 100 mg/mL, for *horses*
Withdrawal Periods. *Horses, deer*: slaughter 28 days

Rompun (Bayer) *Austral.*
Injection, xylazine hydrochloride 20 mg/mL, for *cattle, horses, dogs, cats*
Withdrawal Periods. Should not be used in *horses* intended for human consumption. *Cattle*: slaughter 3 days

Rompun 100 (Bayer) *Austral.*
Injection, xylazine hydrochloride 100 mg/mL, for *cattle, horses, dogs, cats*
Withdrawal Periods. Should not be used in *horses* intended for human consumption. *Cattle*: slaughter 3 days

Xyla-Sed (Fort Dodge) *Austral.*
Injection, xylazine (as hydrochloride) 100 mg/mL, for *horses, deer*
Withdrawal Periods. *Horses, deer*: slaughter 28 days

Thiazine 50 (RWR) *Austral.*
Injection, xylazine (as hydrochloride) 50 mg/mL, for *horses*
Withdrawal Periods. *Horses*: slaughter 28 days

Xylaze 100 Injection (Parnell) *Austral.*
Injection, xylazine (as hydrochloride) 100 mg/mL, for *horses, deer*
Withdrawal Periods. *Horses, deer*: slaughter 28 days

Xylazil-20 (Ilium) *Austral.*
Injection, xylazine 20 mg/mL, for *cattle, sheep, goats, cats, dogs*
Withdrawal Periods. *Cattle, sheep, goats*: slaughter 28 days

Xylazil-100 (Ilium) *Austral.*
Injection, xylazine 100 mg/mL, for *horses*
Withdrawal Periods. *Horses*: slaughter 28 days

Eire

Indications. Sedation; pre-anaesthetic medication
Contra-indications. Later stages of pregnancy in animals, mechanical obstruction of the gastro-intestinal tract; diabetes mellitus; renal or hepatic impairment; concurrent administration of adrenoceptor stimulants
Side-effects. Vomiting in dogs and cats; cardiac arrhythmias; bradycardia; polyuria; profuse salivation in cattle; ruminal atony, bloating
Warnings. Transient rise followed by fall in blood pressure in horses; safety during first month of pregnancy in animals not established; caution when pulmonary disease is present or suspected and in caesarian section in larger animals

Dose. *Horses*: *by intramuscular injection*, 1.0–2.0 mg/kg
by slow intravenous injection, 0.5–1.0 mg/kg
Cattle: *by intramuscular injection*, 50–300 micrograms/kg
Sheep: *by intramuscular injection*, 200–500 micrograms/kg
Dogs: *by intramuscular injection*, 1–3 mg/kg
Cats: *by intramuscular injection*, 3 mg/kg

Chanazine 2% (Chanelle) *Eire*
Injection, xylazine 20 mg/mL, for *horses, cattle, sheep, dogs, cats*
Withdrawal Periods. *Horses*: slaughter 5 days. Cattle: slaughter 5 days, milk 24 hours. Sheep: slaughter 5 day; should not be used in sheep producing ,ilk for human consu,ption

Chanazine 10% (Chanelle) *Eire*
Injection, xylazine 100 mg/mL, for *horses*
Withdrawal Periods. Slaughter 5 days

Rompun 2% Solution (Bayer) *Eire*
Injection, xylazine 20 mg/mL, for *cattle, horses, dogs, cats*
Withdrawal Periods. *Horses*: slaughter 28 days. *Cattle*: slaughter 14 days, milk 48 hours

New Zealand

Indications. Sedation; pre-anaesthetic medication
Contra-indications. Last trimester of pregnancy; cardiovascular disease; respiratory depression; renal or hepatic impairment; shock; concurrent administration of adrenoceptor stimulants
Side-effects. Vomiting in dogs and cats; cardiac arrhythmias; bradycardia; profuse salivation, ruminal atony, bloat, intestinal stasis, and regurgitation in cattle; hypothermia or hyperthermia; anxiety; tremors
Dose. *Horses*: *by intramuscular injection*, 1.0–2.5 mg/kg
by slow intravenous injection, 0.5–1.1 mg/kg
Cattle: *by intramuscular injection*, 50–350 micrograms/kg
by intravascular injection, 50–150 micrograms/kg
Sheep, goats: *by intramuscular injection*, 50–200 micrograms/kg
Dogs, cats: *by intramuscular injection*, 1–3 mg/kg
by intravenous injection, 25–50 micrograms/kg

Anased 2% (Lloyd) *NZ*
Injection, xylazine 20 mg/mL, for *horses, cattle, sheep, goats, deer, dogs, cats*
Withdrawal Periods. *Horses, deer*: slaughter 3 days. *Cattle, sheep, goats*: slaughter 3 days, should not be used in cattle, sheep or goats producing milk for human consumption

Anased 10% (Lloyd) *NZ*
Injection, xylazine 100 mg/mL, for *horses, deer*
Withdrawal Periods. Slaughter 3 days

Bomazine 2% (Bomac) *NZ*
Injection, xylazine (as hydrochloride) 20 mg/mL, for *cattle, sheep, deer, dogs, cats*

Bomazine 10% (Bomac) *NZ*
Injection, xylazine (as hydrochloride) 100 mg/mL, for *horses, cattle, deer, zoo animals*

Romazine 20 (Jurox) *NZ*
Injection, xylazine (as hydrochloride) 20 mg/mL, for *horses, cattle, deer, dogs, cats*
Withdrawal Periods. *Horses, deer*: slaughter 3 days. *Cattle*: slaughter 3 days, should not be used in cattle producing milk for human consumption

Romazine 50 (Jurox) *NZ*
Injection, xylazine (as hydrochloride) 50 mg/mL, for *horses, cattle, deer*
Withdrawal Periods. *Horses, deer*: slaughter 3 days. *Cattle*: slaughter 3 days, should not be used in cattle producing milk for human consumption

Romazine 100 (Jurox) *NZ*
Injection, xylazine (as hydrochloride) 100 mg/mL, for *horses, deer*
Withdrawal Periods. Slaughter 3 days

Rompun 2% (Bayer) *NZ*
Injection, xylazine 20 mg/mL, for *horses, cattle, sheep, goats, deer, dogs, cats*
Withdrawal Periods. Horses, cattle, sheep, goats, deer: slaughter 2 days

Rompun 10% (Bayer) *NZ*
Injection, xylazine 100 mg/mL, for *horses, deer*
Withdrawal Periods. Slaughter 2 days

Rompun Dry Substance (Bayer) *NZ*
Injection, xylazine (as hydrochloride) 500 mg, for *horses, wild animals*
Withdrawal Periods. Slaughter 2 days

Thiazine 20 (Vetpharm) *NZ*
Injection, xylazine (as hydrochloride) 20 mg/mL, for *horses, deer, dogs, cats*
Withdrawal Periods. *Horses, deer*: slaughter 3 days

Thiazine 50 (Vetpharm) *NZ*
Injection, xylazine (as hydrochloride) 50 mg/mL, for *horses, deer*
Withdrawal Periods. Slaughter 3 days

Virbazine 2 (Virbac) *NZ*
Injection, xylazine (as hydrochloride) 20 mg/mL, for *horses, deer, dogs, cats*
Withdrawal Periods. *Horses, deer*: slaughter 3 days

Virbazine 5 (Virbac) *NZ*
Injection, xylazine(as hydrochloride) 50 mg/mL, for *horses, deer*
Withdrawal Periods. Slaughter 3 days

Virbazine 10 (Virbac) *NZ*
Injection, xylazine (as hydrochloride) 100 mg/mL, for *horses, cattle, deer*
Withdrawal Periods. Slaughter 3 days

Xylaze (Parnell) *NZ*
Injection, xylazine 20 mg/mL, for *horses, cattle, deer, dogs, cats*
Withdrawal Periods. *Horses, deer*: slaughter 3 days. *Cattle*: slaughter 3 days, milk 168 hours

Xylaze 100 (Parnell) *NZ*
Injection, xylazine 100 mg/mL, for *horses, deer*
Withdrawal Periods. Slaughter 3 days

Xylaze Forte (Parnell) *NZ*
Injection, xylazine 50 mg/mL, for *horses, cattle, deer*
Withdrawal Periods. *Horses, deer*: slaughter 3 days. *Cattle*: slaughter 3 days, milk 168 hours

Xylazine 2% Injection (Phoenix) *NZ*
Injection, xylazine 20 mg/mL, for *horses, cattle, deer, dogs, cats*
Withdrawal Periods. *Horses, cattle, deer*: slaughter 3 days

Xylazine 5% Injection (Phoenix) *NZ*
Injection, xylazine 50 mg/mL, for *horses, cattle, deer*
Withdrawal Periods. Slaughter 3 days

Xylazine 10% Injection (Phoenix) *NZ*
Injection, xylazine 100 mg/mL, for *horses, deer*
Withdrawal Periods. Slaughter 3 days

USA

Indications. Sedation; pre-anaesthetic medication
Contra-indications. Pregnancy
Side-effects. Vomiting in dogs and cats; cardiac arrhythmias; bradycardia; bloat; sweating; polyuria; hyperthermia
Warnings. Caution in cardiovascular disease, respiratory depression, renal or hepatic impairment, or shock
Dose. *Horses*: *by intramuscular injection*, 2.2 mg/kg
by slow intravenous injection, 1.1 mg/kg
Dogs, cats: *by subcutaneous or intramuscular injection*, 2.2 mg/kg; *by intravenous injection*, 1.1 mg/kg

Anased Injectable (Lloyd) *USA*
Injection, xylazine 100 mg/mL, for *horses, deer*
Withdrawal Periods. Should not be used in *horses or deer* intended for human consumption

Anased Injection (Lloyd) *USA*
Injection, xylazine 20 mg/mL, for *dogs, cats*

Rompun (Bayer) *USA*
Injection, xylazine (as hydrochloride) 100 mg/mL, for *horses*
Withdrawal Periods. Should not be used in *horses* intended for human consumption
Injection, xylazine (as hydrochloride) 20 mg/mL, for *dogs, cats*

Sedazine (Fort Dodge) *USA*
Injection, xylazine 100 mg/mL, for *horses, deer, elk*
Withdrawal Periods. Should not be used in *horses* intended for human consumption

Tranquived Injectable (Vedco) *USA*
Injection, xylazine (as hydrochloride) 20 mg/mL, for *dogs, cats*

Tranquived Injectable (Vedco) *USA*
Injection, xylazine (as hydrochloride) 100 mg/mL, for *horses*
Withdrawal Periods. Should not be used in *horses* intended for human consumption

X-Ject E (Vetus) *USA*
Injection, xylazine 100 mg/mL, for *horses, cervidae*
Withdrawal Periods. Should not be used in animals intended for human consumption

Xyla-Ject (Phoenix) *USA*
Injection, xylazine 20 mg/mL, for *dogs, cats*

Xyla-Ject (Phoenix) *USA*
Injection, xylazine 100 mg/mL, for *horses, cervidae*
Withdrawal Periods. Should not be used in animals intended for human consumption

Xylazine-20 Injection (Butler) *USA*
Injection, xylazine 20 mg/mL, for *dogs*

Xylazine HCL Injection (Boehringer Ingelheim Vetmedica) *USA*
Injection, xylazine 100 mg/mL, for *horses*
Withdrawal Periods. Should not be used in *horses* intended for human consumption

Xylazine HCL Injection (VetTek) *USA*
Injection, xylazine 100 mg/mL, for *horses, cervidae*
Withdrawal Periods. Should not be used in animals intended for human consumption

6.1.4 Benzodiazepines

Benzodiazepines can be useful premedicants in elderly, debilitated animals, epileptics, or before procedures such as myelography that may induce epileptiform seizures. They are also used in intensive care, in conjunction with opioid analgesics to sedate animals requiring invasive monitoring. Sedation for intensive care (to control restlessness and allow nursing procedures to be undertaken) in combination with sufficient analgesia can be provided by diazepam (up to 1 mg/kg per hour). The analgesia can be provided by morphine (100–500 micrograms/kg) or any of the pure opioids at routine dose rates (see section 6.3.1).
Intravenous administration of these drugs to normal healthy animals can result in marked excitation.
Diazepam is the most commonly used representative of the benzodiazepines. The shorter-acting **midazolam** may also be used. Midazolam produces less sedation than diazepam.
Zolazepam is used in combination with tiletamine.

At clinical doses, the cardiovascular effects are minimal as are the respiratory effects in healthy animals. In debilitated animals respiratory depression may become clinically significant and necessitate ventilatory support. Muscle relaxation may be marked and is probably central in origin. In conscious horses, this property results in ataxia and may cause panic reactions. In dogs and cats, muscle relaxation is not a problem. In combination with fentanyl or morphine, profound sedation is achieved with minimal disturbance to the cardiovascular system and allows smaller doses of induction agent, such as propofol, to be used to achieve endotracheal intubation. This may be of considerable importance in animals with compromised circulatory systems.
Benzodiazepines are used in combination with ketamine after antimuscarinic premedication to produce chemical restraint in dogs and cats for radiography. Premedication is not essential but may control hypersalivation which may occur with ketamine administration.

DIAZEPAM

UK

Indications. Sedation in intensive care; pre-anaesthetic medication for foals under one month of age, epileptics, before myelography, high risk cardiac patients, and geriatric dogs and cats; status epilepticus (see section 6.9.2); behaviour modification (see section 6.11.3)
Contra-indications. Severe hepatic disease; normal animals
Side-effects. See notes above
Dose. Sedation.
Horses: *by intravenous injection*, 0.05–2.0 mg/kg
Dogs: *by intravenous injection*, 100–500 micrograms/kg
by intramuscular injection, 300–500 micrograms/kg
Cats: *by intravenous injection*, 100–500 micrograms/kg
by intramuscular injection, 0.3–1.0 mg/kg
Sedation, in combination with ketamine.
Dogs, cats: diazepam *by intravenous injection*, 200 micrograms/kg with ketamine 5–10 mg/kg

See section 6.9.2 for preparation details

MIDAZOLAM

UK

Indications. Sedation in intensive care; pre-anaesthetic medication for foals under one month of age, epileptics, before myelography, high risk cardiac patients, and geriatric dogs and cats
Contra-indications. Side-effects. See under Diazepam and notes above
Dose. Sedation.
Dogs: *by intravenous injection*, 100–200 micrograms/kg

Sedation, in combination with ketamine.
Dogs, cats: midazolam *by intravenous injection*, 500 micrograms/kg with ketamine 10 mg/kg

POM (H) **Hypnovel** (Roche) *UK*
Injection, midazolam (as hydrochloride) 2 mg/mL, 5 mg/mL

POM (H) **Midazolam** (Non-proprietary)
Injection, midazolam (as hydrochloride) 1 mg/mL

6.2 Sedative antagonists

6.2.1 Alpha$_2$-adrenoceptor antagonists
6.2.2 Benzodiazepine antagonists

6.2.1 Alpha$_2$-adrenoceptor antagonists

Atipamezole and **yohimbine** are alpha$_2$-adrenoceptor blocking drugs. Atipamezole is authorised to reverse the effects of medetomidine. However, it also effectively reverses the effects of detomidine and xylazine in various species. Care must be taken if the adrenoceptor stimulant is reversed within a short period of time after its administration because re-sedation may occur after the effect of atipamezole subsides, such as in the case of the longer-acting detomidine. Provided 15 to 40 minutes is allowed to lapse between the administration of medetomidine and that of atipamezole, re-sedation is very rare.

Atipamezole will not reverse the sedative action of other classes of sedative or anaesthetic drugs. Therefore care should be exercised if, for example, ketamine has also been previously administered to a dog as this drug is unsuitable as a sole anaesthetic agent in this species.

Yohimbine is widely used in North America to reverse the effects of the alpha$_2$-receptor agonist agents. It is a much less alpha$_2$-receptor specific antagonist than atipamezole and so has significant alpha-1 antagonistic actions.

Fampridine facilitates the release of neurotransmitter from nerve endings and hence aids in the competitive reversal of alpha$_2$-receptor agonist agents by enhancing the synaptic concentration of norepinephrine (the natural neurotransmitter). However it has mainly been used in conjunction with yohimbine and is unlikely to enhance the effect of the more specific alpha$_2$-receptor antagonist atipamezole.

ATIPAMEZOLE HYDROCHLORIDE

UK
Indications. Reversal of sedative effects of medetomidine
Contra-indications. Manufacturer does not recommend use in pregnant animals; see notes above
Side-effects. Transient over-alertness and tachycardia with high dosage; transient hypotension; hypothermia; rarely vomiting, defecation, panting, and muscle tremors
Warnings. Operator should wear impervious gloves
Dose. In micrograms/kg, *by intramuscular injection.*
Horses ♦: 150 micrograms/kg
Dogs: 5 times the previously administered medetomidine dose (= same volume of medetomidine previously administered)
Cats: 2.5 times the previously administered medetomidine dose (= ½ volume of medetomidine previously administered)

POM **Antisedan** (Pfizer) *UK*
Injection, atipamezole hydrochloride 5 mg/mL, for *dogs, cats*; 10 mL

Australia
Indications. Reversal of sedative effects of medetomidine
Contra-indications. Pregnant animals
Side-effects. Transient over-alertness and tachycardia with overdosage; transient hypotension; rarely vomiting and panting
Dose. In micrograms/kg, *by intramuscular injection.*
Dogs: 5 times the previously administered medetomidine dose (= same volume of medetomidine previously administered)
Cats: 2.5 times the previously administered medetomidine dose (= ½ volume of medetomidine previously administered)

Antisedan (Novartis) *Austral.*
Injection, atipamezole hydrochloride 5 mg/mL, for *dogs, cats*

Eire
Indications. Reversal of sedative effects of medetomidine
Contra-indications. Pregnant animals
Side-effects. Transient over-alertness and tachycardia with overdosage; transient hypotension and diuresis; rarely vomiting, panting, muscle tremors, defecation; hypothermia in cats
Warnings. Caution in hepatic impairment
Dose. In micrograms/kg, *by intramuscular injection.*
Dogs: 5 times the previously administered medetomidine dose (= same volume of medetomidine previously administered)
Cats: 2.5 times the previously administered medetomidine dose (= ½ volume of medetomidine previously administered)

Antisedan (Pfizer) *Eire*
Injection, atipamezole hydrochloride 5 mg/mL, for *dogs, cats*

New Zealand
Indications. Reversal of sedative effects of medetomidine
Contra-indications. Pregnant animals
Side-effects. Transient over-alertness and tachycardia with overdosage; transient hypotension; rarely vomiting, panting
Dose. In micrograms/kg, *by intramuscular injection.*
Dogs: 5 times the previously administered medetomidine dose (= same volume of medetomidine previously administered)
Cats: 2–4 times the previously administered medetomidine dose

Antisedan (Novartis) *NZ*
Injection, atipamezole 5 mg/mL, for *dogs, cats*

USA
Indications. Reversal of sedative effects of medetomidine
Contra-indications. Pregnant, lactating, or breeding animals
Side-effects. Excitment or apprehensiveness; occasional vomiting; hypersalivation; muscle tremors; diarrhoea
Dose. In micrograms/kg, *by intramuscular injection.*

Dogs: 5 times the previously administered medetomidine dose (= same volume of medetomidine previously administered)

Antisedan (Pfizer) *USA*
Injection, atipamezole hydrochloride 5 mg/mL, for *dogs*

FAMPRIDINE
(4-Aminopyridine)

Australia
Indications. Reversal of sedative effects of xylazine (in combination with yohimbine)
Contra-indications. Cardiovascular, renal, or hepatic impairment; deer; patients in which recovery from xylazine has substantially progressed
Dose. *Cattle: by intravenous injection*, 300 micrograms/kg in combination with yohimbine 125 micrograms/kg

Antagozil SA (Ilium) *Austral.* (see under Yohimbine)

Reverzine SA (Parnell) *Austral.* (see under Yohimbine)

Xylex (Parnell) *Austral.*
Injection, fampridine 24 mg/mL, for *cattle*
Withdrawal Periods. *Cattle*: slaughter 28 days, should not be used in cattle producing milk for human consumption

TOLAZOLINE
Indications. Reversal of sedative effects of xylazine
Contra-indications. Gastro-intestinal ulceration
Side-effects. Hypotension, gastro-intestinal haemorrhage, nausea, vomiting diarrhoea, hepatitis
Dose. *By intravenous injection*, 2–4 mg/kg

Tolazine (Lloyd) *NZ*
Injection, tolazoline (as hydrochloride) 100 mg/mL, for *horses, cattle, sheep, goats, deer, dogs, cats*
Withdrawal Periods. *Horses, deer*: slaughter 30 days. *Cattle, sheep, goats*: slaughter 30 days, should not be used in cattle, sheep or goats producing milk for human consumption

USA
Indications. Reversal of sedative effects of xylazine
Contra-indications. Debilitation, cardiac impairment, stress, sympatheticblockage, hypovolaemia, shock
Side-effects. Transient hypertension, tachycardia, peripheral vasodilatation, hyperalgesia of the lips, piloerection, lacrimal and nasal secretions, muscle tremors, apprehensiveness
Warnings. Safety in pregnant, lactating, or breeding animals has not been established
Dose. *Horses*: *by intravenous injection*, 4 mg/kg

Tolazine Injection (Lloyd) *USA*
Injection, tolazoline 100 mg/mL, for *horses*
Withdrawal Periods. *Horses*: should not be used in horses intended for human consumption

YOHIMBINE

Australia
Indications. Reversal of sedative effects of xylazine

Contra-indications. Cardiovascular, renal, or hepatic impairment; patients in which recovery from xylazine has substantially progressed
Side-effects. Occasional anxiety and mild tremor in dogs and cats
Warnings. Avoid intra-arterial injection
Dose. *By intravenous injection.*
Cattle: 125 micrograms/kg in combination with fampridine
Deer: 250 mg/kg
Dogs, cats: see preparation details

Antagozil SA (Ilium) *Austral.*
Injection, yohimbine hydrochloride 1.25 mg/mL, fampridine 2 mg/mL, for *dogs, cats*
Dose. *By intravenous injection.*
Dogs: 0.05-0.25 mL/kg
Cats: 0.1-0.25 mL/kg

Reverzine (Parnell) *Austral.*
Injection, yohimbine hydrochloride 10 mg/mL, for *deer, cattle*
Withdrawal Periods. *Deer, cattle*: slaughter 28 days

Reverzine SA (Parnell) *Austral.*
Injection, yohimbine hydrochloride 1.25 mg/mL, fampridine 2 mg/mL, for *dogs, cats*
Dose. *By intravenous injection.*
Dogs: 0.1 mL/kg
Cats: 0.25 mL/kg

New Zealand
Indications. Reversal of sedative effects of xylazine
Contra-indications. Cardiovascular, renal, or hepatic impairment
Side-effects. Transient CNS stimulation, hyperaesthesia, anxiety, blood pressure fluctuations, anorexia in deer
Warnings. Avoid intra-arterial injection
Dose. *Deer: by intravenous injection*, 200–250 mg/kg

Contran-H (Parnell) *NZ* (see section 6.5)

Himbine (Virbac) *NZ*
Injection, yohimbine hydrochloride 10 mg/mL, for *deer*
Withdrawal Periods. *Deer*: slaughter 6 hours

Reversal (Phoenix) *NZ*
Injection, yohimbine hydrochloride 10 mg/mL, for *deer*
Withdrawal Periods. *Deer*: slaughter 1 day

Reverzine (Parnell) *NZ*
Injection, yohimbine hydrochloride 10 mg/mL, for *deer*
Withdrawal Periods. *Deer*: slaughter 1 day

Contran-H (Parnell) *NZ* (see section 6.5)

USA
Indications. Reversal of sedative effects of xylazine
Contra-indications. Use 30 days before or during the hunting season
Side-effects. Hypotension, transient excitement in deer; transient apprehensiveness in dogs
Warnings. Safety in pregnant or breeding dogs has not been established; caution with use in dogs prone to epilepsy
Dose. *Deer, elk: by intravenous injection*, 200–300 mg/kg
Dogs: by intravenous injection, 110 mg/kg

Antagonil (Wildlife Pharm) *USA*
Injection, yohimbine hydrochloride 5 mg/mL, for *deer, elk*

Withdrawal Periods. Should not be used in animals intended for human consumption

Yobine Injection (Lloyd) *USA*
Injection, yohimbine (as hydrochloride) 2 mg/mL, for *dogs*

6.2.2 Benzodiazepine antagonists

Flumazenil is a benzodiazepine antagonist used for reversal of the central sedative effects of benzodiazepine overdosage. Flumazenil has a shorter half-life than diazepam or midazolam in humans and there is a risk that patients may become re-sedated.

FLUMAZENIL

UK

Indications. Reversal of benzodiazepine overdosage
Warnings. May see overstimulation, not commonly used in animals
Dose. By *intravenous injection*, 100 micrograms/kg given at 1 minute intervals until signs of consciousness return

POM (H) **Anexate** (Roche) *UK*
Injection, flumazenil 100 micrograms/mL; 5 mL

6.3 Analgesics

6.3.1 Opioid analgesics
6.3.2 Non-opioid analgesics
6.3.3 Compound analgesics

Analgesic drugs are used for the relief of pain. They have many indications, ranging from their use in the first aid situations to the relief of severe visceral pain. Analgesics are also used routinely as part of the pre-operative medication and, combined with a sedative drug, provide analgesia for minor surgery.

During recent years there has been a greater understanding and appreciation of pain perception in animals. Alongside this development there has been an increase in the number and variety of analgesic drugs available to the veterinary profession. There is now little excuse for any animal to suffer pain during and after veterinary procedures. Even routine surgery such as ovariohysterectomy results in a degree of post-operative discomfort that can be prevented by the use of appropriate analgesic drugs.

The opioid analgesics are the most potent drugs for the control of pain. The NSAIDs (see section 10.1) also have analgesic activity. Although this property of NSAIDs is largely through their anti-inflammatory action, recent studies have shown that they also act at the spinal level. NSAIDs are widely used perioperatively.

6.3.1 Opioid analgesics

Opioid analgesics interact at opioid receptor sites in the CNS and other tissues. There are 3 main receptor types: μ (mu), κ (kappa), and δ (delta). Stimulation of μ receptors results in analgesia (mainly at supraspinal sites), respiratory depression, miosis, reduced gastro-intestinal motility, and euphoria. Stimulation of κ receptors gives analgesia (mainly in the spinal cord) and less intense miosis and respiratory depression. Stimulation of δ receptors probably provides analgesia.

Opioid analgesics act at one or more of these receptors as agonists, antagonists, or a combination of both (partial agonists). Morphine, etorphine, and fentanyl are examples of potent agonists; they act primarily at μ and perhaps κ and δ receptors. Codeine and pethidine are less potent agonists. Pentazocine, buprenorphine, and butorphanol are regarded as mixed agonist-antagonists (partial agonists). Pentazocine appears to act as a κ agonist and μ antagonist whereas buprenorphine is a partial agonist at μ receptors with some antagonist activity at κ receptors. Diprenorphine and nalorphine are also partial agonists but closer to pure antagonists, reversing all of the effects of the agonist but retaining a degree of intrinsic activity that is expressed at higher doses. Naloxone is a pure antagonist having no sedative or analgesic action at recommended doses but capable of reversing the effects of an agonist.

There are major species differences in the responses elicited by opioid analgesics. In the CNS, opioid analgesics modify pain perception and behavioural reaction to pain. They also relieve anxiety and distress but may induce drowsiness from which the animal can usually be aroused. Cats, horses, cattle, sheep, goats, and pigs often become hyperexcited at high doses. **Excitement is less likely in animals in pain than in pain-free animals**.

Due to their misuse potential, opioid analgesics are subject to the *Misuse of Drugs Regulations 1985*. It is recommended, therefore, that they should only be used when there is no non-opioid alternative for moderate to severe pain, and that the newer, less addictive drugs should be used, where appropriate, rather than morphine or methadone.

Opioid analgesics are contra-indicated in head injury because they induce an increase in cerebrospinal fluid and raise intracranial pressure, which may interfere with neurological examination.

Morphine provides the standard against which the analgesic potency and actions of other opioid analgesics are compared (see Table 6.1). Morphine remains the drug of choice for severe pain as in injury sustained in road traffic accidents. Side-effects of morphine include constriction of pupils (dilation in species that show excitability at moderate to high doses), peripheral vasodilation, respiratory depression, vomiting, exaggerated spinal cord reflexes, initially defecation followed by constipation, transient hypotension, urinary retention, sweating in horses, and bradycardia, but high doses can cause tachycardia in horses and dogs, and respiratory depression in neonates if used in pregnant animals before birth. Morphine is commonly used only in dogs; in cats, low doses produce analgesia without excitement, although high doses induce *profound excitement*. In horses, morphine is not recommended because of the excitement it produces.

Oxymorphone has actions similar to morphine. It causes less sedation than morphine, and is not antitussive. It is used for perioperative pain and pre-anaesthesia in dogs.

Methadone is a synthetic opioid that has the same analgesic potency as morphine. Side-effects and contra-indications are similar to those of morphine, although it causes less sedation.

Pethidine is a synthetic opioid analgesic that is structurally unlike morphine. It produces a prompt but short-acting analgesia. In cats, rapid detoxification of pethidine results in unpredictable effects. The recommended dose produces satisfactory analgesia for more than 2 hours; doses of more than 6 mg/kg are unnecessarily high and may result in excitation. Side-effects and contra-indications are similar to those of morphine, although it is less likely to cause vomiting; it also causes less respiratory depression, which makes it more suitable for pregnant animals before parturition.

In dogs the maximum analgesic effect of pethidine is reached about 45 minutes after oral administration, or about 20 minutes after subcutaneous injection.

Pethidine has significant antimuscarinic activity and therefore has an antispasmodic action on the smooth muscle of the large intestine and it is frequently used in the treatment of equine colic.

Table 6.1 Relative analgesic potencies of opioid analgesics

Drug	Equivalent analgesic potency
Buprenorphine	10–20
Butorphanol	4–7
Etorphine	at least 1000
Fentanyl	80–100
Methadone	1
Morphine	1
Oxymorphone	10
Pentazocine	0.33–0.5
Pethidine	0.1

Pentazocine is a partial agonist with similar side-effects and contra-indications to morphine, although it has little sedative effect, does not induce excitement, has little action on the gastro-intestinal tract, and does not cause vomiting. The respiratory depression produced by pentazocine is less than with morphine. Pentazocine is a useful analgesic in the dog for both musculoskeletal and visceral pain, and it is helpful in the control of colic pain in horses. *Although pentazocine has been used in cats, its use is not recommended in this species.*

Buprenorphine is a partial agonist with similar side-effects and contra-indications to morphine, although it causes less respiratory depression, only mild sedation, rarely vomiting, and does not cause constipation or excitement.

The analgesic effects of buprenorphine are slow in onset, occurring after approximately 15 minutes even when administered intravenously. This, together with the long duration of action (up to 12 hours), may give rise to toxicity if repeated doses are administered. The effects of buprenorphine are only partially reversed by naloxone, more of the latter being needed than to reverse a pure agonist.

Butorphanol is a synthetic opioid analgesic with similar side-effects and contra-indications to morphine, although it causes less intense sedation, slight respiratory depression, and minimal cardiovascular effects. It is particularly useful for the relief of visceral pain in horses and may be combined with detomidine hydrochloride in this species (see section 6.1.3). Butorphanol is used as an antitussive in dogs (see section 5.4). In both dogs and cats butorphanol is used as an analgesic and may be combined with medetomidine to give profound sedation.

Combinations of opioid analgesics and sedatives are used to provide neuroleptanalgesia (see section 6.4).

In cats, the combined use of butorphanol, medetomidine, and ketamine by either intramuscular or intravenous injection provides anaesthesia for at least 30 minutes.

Carfentanil is an opioid analgesic related to fentanyl (see section 6.4) but it is very much more potent. It is approximately 10 000 times more potent than morphine and can be dangerous to the user. This drug should not be used by the operator alone, and an opioid antagonist (for example diprenorphine) should be readily available.

BUPRENORPHINE

UK

Indications. Moderate to severe post-operative pain; sedation

Contra-indications. See under Morphine sulphate; impaired respiratory function; concurrent use of other opioid-type analgesics

Side-effects. Less sedation than morphine and does not cause excitement or constipation; rarely may cause vomiting

Warnings. Repeated doses may cause overdosage, see notes above; caution in hepatic impairment or pregnant animals; Drug Interactions – see Appendix 1

Dose.

Dogs: post-operative analgesia, *by intramuscular injection*, 10–20 micrograms/kg. May be repeated after 12 hours

Sedation, *by intramuscular injection*, 10 micrograms/kg. May be repeated after 12 hours

Cats◆: *by subcutaneous or intramuscular injection*, 5–10 micrograms/kg

Neuroleptanaesthesia◆, in combination with Acepromazine.

Dogs, cats: *by intramuscular injection*, acepromazine 30 micrograms/kg, and buprenorphine, 10 micrograms/kg

CD **Vetergesic** (Alstoe) *UK*

Injection, buprenorphine (as hydrochloride) 300 micrograms/mL, for *dogs*; 1 mL

BUTORPHANOL

UK

Indications. Moderate to severe pain; sedation in dogs and cats in combination with Medetomidine (see section 6.1.3); sedation in horses in combination with Detomidine and Romifidine (see section 6.1.3); general anaesthesia in dogs and cats in combination with Medetomidine and Ketamine (see section 6.6.2.4); non-productive cough in dogs (see section 5.4)

Contra-indications. See under Morphine sulphate; hepatic impairment; horses with pre-existing cardiac dysrhythmias; butorphanol and detomidine combination in pregnancy or colic; butorphanol and romifidine combination in last month of pregnancy

Side-effects. Less intense sedation than morphine; ataxia; transient diarrhoea, anorexia in dogs, mydriasis in cats

Warnings. If respiratory depression occurs, naloxone may be used as an antidote. In dogs transient ataxia, anorexia, and diarrhoea have been reported as occurring rarely

Dose. Analgesia.

Horses: *by intravenous injection*, 100 micrograms/kg

Dogs: *by subcutaneous, intramuscular, or intravenous injection*, 200–300 micrograms/kg

Cats: pre-operative analgesia, *by subcutaneous or intramuscular injection*, 400 micrograms/kg

Post-operative analgesia, *by subcutaneous or intramuscular injection*, 400 micrograms/kg

by intravenous injection, 100 micrograms/kg

Pre-anaesthetic medication.

Dogs: *by subcutaneous or intramuscular injection*, 100–200 micrograms/kg

Neuroleptanaesthesia♦, in combination with Medetomidine.

Dogs, cats: *by intramuscular injection*, medetomidine 10 micrograms/kg, and butorphanol 200 micrograms/kg

POM **Torbugesic** (Fort Dodge) *UK*
Injection, butorphanol (as tartrate) 10 mg/mL, for **horses, dogs, cats**
Withdrawal Periods. Should not be used in **horses** intended for human consumption

Australia

Indications. Moderate to severe pain

Contra-indications. Geriatric animals, lower respiratory infection, hepatic impairment

Side-effects. Sedation; ataxia

Warnings. Safety in breeding animals or dogs with heartworm has not been established

Dose. Analgesia.

Horses: *by intravenous injection*, 100 micrograms/kg

Dogs: *by subcutaneous or intramuscular injection*, 200–400 micrograms/kg

by intravenous injection, 100–200 micrograms/kg

Cats: *by subcutaneous or intramuscular injection*, 400 micrograms/kg

Dolorex (Intervet) *Austral.*
Injection, butorphanol tartrate 10 mg/mL, for **horses, dogs, cats**
Withdrawal Periods. **Horses**: slaughter 28 days
May begiven by intravenous injection to cats

Torbugesic (Fort Dodge) *Austral.*
Injection, butorphanol (as tartrate) 10 mg/mL, for **horses, dogs, cats**
Withdrawal Periods. **Horses**: slaughter 28 days

Eire

Indications. Moderate to severe pain

Contra-indications. Geriatric animals, lower respiratory infection, hepatic impairment

Side-effects. Sedation; ataxia

Dose. Analgesia.

Horses: *by intravenous injection*, 100 micrograms/kg

Dogs: *by subcutaneous, intramuscular, or intravenous injection*, 200–300 micrograms/kg

Cats: *by subcutaneous or intramuscular injection*, 400 micrograms/kg

Torbugesic Injection (Fort Dodge) *Eire*
Injection, butorphanol (as tartrate) 10 mg/mL, for **horses, dogs, cats**
Withdrawal Periods. Should not be used in **horses** intended for human consumption

New Zealand

Indications. Moderate to severe pain; coughing

Contra-indications. Hepatic impairment

Side-effects. Sedation; ataxia; mild CNS stimulation

Dose. *Horses*: analgesia, *by intramuscular or intravenous injection*, 100 micrograms/kg

Dogs: analgesia, *by subcutaneous or intramuscular injection*, 400–800 micrograms/kg

Coughing, by subcutaneous or intramuscular injection, 50–100 micrograms/kg

Butorphic (Lloyd) *NZ*
Injection, butorphanol (as tartrate) 10 mg/mL, for **horses, dogs**
Withdrawal Periods. **Horses**: slaughter 28 days

Dolorex (Chemavet) *NZ*
Injection, butorphanol tartrate 10 mg/mL, for **horses**
Withdrawal Periods. **Horses**: Slaughter 24 hours

USA

Indications. Moderate to severe pain; coughing

Contra-indications. Hepatic impairment; lower respiratory tract disorders

Side-effects. Sedation; ataxia; rarely anorexia and diarrhoea in dogs

Warnings. Safety in breeding animals or dogs with heartworm has not been established

Dose. *Horses*: analgesia, *by intravenous injection*, 100 micrograms/kg

Dogs: coughing, *by mouth or subcutaneous injection*, 55 micrograms/kg

Cats: analgesia, *by subcutaneous injection*, 400 micrograms/k

Coughing, by subcutaneous or intramuscular injection, 50–100 micrograms/kg

Torbugesic (Fort Dodge) *USA*
Injection, butorphanol (as tartrate) 10 mg/mL, for **horses**
Withdrawal Periods. **Horses**: should not be used in horses intended for human consumption

Torbugesic-SA (Fort Dodge) *USA*
Injection, butorphanol (as tartrate) 2 mg/mL, for *cats*

Torbutrol (Fort Dodge) *USA*
Injection, butorphanol (as tartrate) 0.5 mg/mL, for *dogs*

Torbutrol (Fort Dodge) *USA*
Tablets, butorphanol (as tartrate) 5 mg or 10 mg, for *dogs*

CARFENTANIL

USA
Indications. Immobilisation of wild species
Contra-indications. Use 45 days before or during the hunting season
Warnings. See above and under Etorphine (section 6.4)

Wildnil (Wildlife Pharm) *USA*
Injection, carfentanil (as citrate) 3 mg/mL, for *deer, elk, moose*
Withdrawal Periods. Should not be used in animals intended for human consumption

METHADONE HYDROCHLORIDE

UK
Indications. Severe pain
Contra-indications. Side-effects. Warnings. See under Morphine sulphate; less sedation than morphine
Dose. Analgesia.
Horses, dogs: *by intramuscular injection*, 200 micrograms/kg
by intravenous injection, 100 micrograms/kg

Neuroleptanaesthesia, in combination with Acepromazine.
Dogs, cats: *by intramuscular injection*, acepromazine 20 micrograms/kg, and methadone 200 micrograms/kg

CD (H) **Methadone** (Non-proprietary) *UK*
Injection, methadone hydrochloride 10 mg/mL

Australia
Indications. Pain; pre-anaesthetic medication
Contra-indications. Parturition, severe respiratory depression, cats
Warnings. Caution in hypothyroidism, adrenocortical insufficiency, renal and hepatic impairment, shock
Dose. *Horses*: analgesia, *by subcutaneous or intramuscular injection*, 220 micrograms/kg
Restraint, *by intravenous injection*, 110 micrograms/kg with acepromazine 55 micrograms/kg
Dogs: analgesia, *by subcutaneous or intramuscular injection*, 110–550 micrograms/kg
Pre-anaesthetic medication, *by subcutaneous injection*, 1.1 mg/kg

Methone Injection (Parnell) *Austral.*
Injection, methadone hydrochloride 10 mg/mL, for *horses, dogs*
Withdrawal Periods. *Horses*: slaughter 28 days

MORPHINE SULPHATE

UK
Indications. Severe pain

Contra-indications. Head injury and raised intracranial pressure; see notes above
Side-effects. See notes above; constriction of pupils (dilation in species that show excitability at moderate to high doses); peripheral vasodilation; respiratory depression; vomiting; exaggerated spinal cord reflexes; initially defaecation followed by constipation; transient hypotension; urinary retention; sweating in horses; bradycardia but high doses can cause tachycardia in horses and dogs; respiratory depression in neonates if used in pregnant animals prior to birth
Warnings. Hyperexcitability in cats, see notes above
Dose.
Dogs: *by subcutaneous or intramuscular injection*, 200 micrograms/kg
Cats: *by subcutaneous injection*, 100 micrograms/kg

Neuroleptanaesthesia, in combination with Acepromazine.
Dogs, cats: *by intramuscular injection*, acepromazine 20 micrograms/kg, and morphine, 200 micrograms/kg

CD (H) **Morphine Sulphate** (Non-proprietary)
Injection, morphine sulphate 10 mg/mL, 15 mg/mL, 20 mg/mL, 30 mg/mL

NALBUPHINE HYDROCHLORIDE

UK
Indications. Moderate to severe pain
Dose. See Prescribing for rabbits and rodents

POM (H) **Nubain** (Du Pont)
Injection, nalbuphine hydrochloride 10 mg/mL; 1 mL, 2 mL

OXYMORPHONE

USA
Indications. Moderate to severe pain
Contra-indications. Side-effects. Warnings. See under Morphine sulphate
Dose. *Dogs*: *by subcutaneous, intramuscular, or intravenous injection*, 0.75–4.0 mg/kg
Cats: *by subcutaneous, intramuscular, or intravenous injection*, 0.4–1.5 mg/kg

P/M Oxymorphone HCL Injection (Schering-Plough) *USA*
Injection, oxymorphone hydrochloride 1.5 mg/mL, for *dogs, cats*

PENTAZOCINE

UK
Indications. Moderate to severe pain
Contra-indications. Should not be used in cats; see under Morphine sulphate
Side-effects. See under Morphine sulphate; less sedation and respiratory depression than morphine; does not cause excitement and vomiting
Dose. *Horses*: *by intramuscular or slow intravenous injection*, 330 micrograms/kg, repeat after 15 minutes if required
Dogs: *by intramuscular injection*, 2 mg/kg

CD Ⓗ **Pentazocine** (Non-proprietary) *UK*
Injection, pentazocine (as lactate) 30 mg/mL; 1 mL, 2 mL

PETHIDINE HYDROCHLORIDE
(Meperidine hydrochloride)

UK
Indications. Moderate to severe pain; sedation
Contra-indications. Renal impairment; obstructive equine colic; concurrent use of detomidine; see under Morphine sulphate
Side-effects. See under Morphine sulphate; less respiratory depression and vomiting than morphine
Warnings. Hyperexcitability in cats, see notes above; overdosage may cause excitement in horses; safety in pregnant animals has not been established
Dose.
Analgesia
By intramuscular injection.
Horses: spasmodic colic, 2 mg/kg
Dogs, cats: pre-anaesthetic medication, analgesia, 3.3 mg/kg

Neuroleptanaesthesia♦, in combination with Acepromazine.
Dogs, cats: *by intramuscular injection*, acepromazine 20 micrograms/kg, and pethidine, 4 mg/kg

Neuroleptanaesthesia♦, in combination with Medetomidine.
Dogs, cats: *by intramuscular injection*, medetomidine 10 micrograms/kg, and pethidine, 4 mg/kg

CD **Pethidine Injection 50 mg/ml** (Arnolds) *UK*
Injection, pethidine hydrochloride 50 mg/mL, for *horses, dogs, cats*; 50 mL
Withdrawal Periods. Should not be used in *horses* intended for human consumption

Australia
Indications. Pain; spasmodic colic in horses; coughing in dogs
Contra-indications. Renal impairment; pregnant animals; obstructive equine colic; concurrent use of detomidine; see under Morphine sulphate
Side-effects. Severe hypotension with rapid intravenous administration; profuse sweating, hyperpnoea, and tachycardia in horses; bronchoconstriction in dogs
Warnings. Hyperexcitability in horses and cats; caution in inflammatory respiratory disease, acute respiratory dysfunction, severe renal insufficiency
Dose. *Horses, cattle*: spasmodic colic, *by intramuscular or slow intravenous injection*, 1–2 mg/kg
Dogs, cats: pre-anaesthetic medication, analgesia, *by subcutaneous or intramuscular injection*, 1–5 mg/kg

Pethidine Injection (Parnell) *Austral.*
Injection, pethidine hydrochloride 50 mg/mL, for *horses, cattle, dogs, cats*
Withdrawal Periods. Slaughter withdrawal period nil, milk withdrawal period nil

6.3.2 Non-opioid analgesics

Paracetamol (acetaminophen) is an analgesic with relatively weak anti-inflammatory activity. It should not be administered to cats. Cats have a reduced capacity for glucuronide conjugation and the drug is converted to a reactive electrophilic metabolite in this species. Clinical signs of toxicity include anaemia, methaemoglobinaemia, and liver failure (see Treatment of poisoning).
Non-steroidal anti-inflammatory drugs (NSAIDs) are described in section 10.1. They are used for musculoskeletal pain and perioperative pain.

6.3.3 Compound analgesics

Compound analgesic preparations are relatively infrequently used in veterinary practice compared with human medicine. They combine a non-opioid analgesic such as paracetamol, with an opioid analgesic such as codeine, which is related to morphine and has similar but less potent actions.

UK
Indications. Mild to moderate pain
Contra-indications. Patients with cardiac, renal, or hepatic disease, where there is the possibility of gastro-intestinal ulceration or bleeding, where there is evidence of a blood dyscrasia or hypersensitivity to the drug; treatment with other NSAIDs concurrently or within 24 hours; cats
Side-effects. Occasional constipation
Warnings. Caution with use in animals less than 6 weeks of age, or aged animals; avoid use in dehydrated, hypovolaemic, or hypotensive patients; avoid concurrent administration of potentially nephrotoxic drugs

P **Pardale-V Tablets** (Arnolds) *UK*
Tablets, scored, codeine phosphate 9 mg, paracetamol 400 mg, for *dogs*
Dose. *Dogs: by mouth*, (up to 6 kg body-weight) ½ tablet 3 times daily; (6–18 kg body-weight) ½–1½ tablets 3 times daily; (18–42 kg body-weight) 1½–3½ tablets 3 times daily. Treatment course should not exceed 5 days

6.4 Neuroleptanalgesics

Neuroleptanalgesia is defined as a state of quiescence, reduced awareness and analgesia. It is a state of sedation combined with analgesia, which is similar, although not equal, to a light plane of anaesthesia. The animal no longer responds to surroundings or to pain but is not totally unconscious. Therefore, handling and minor surgical procedures may be carried out painlessly without having to resort to full anaesthesia. This technique has the advantage of increased sedation without increasing the dose of sedative, thus reducing sedative related side-effects as well as providing a degree of analgesia. The latter is extremely useful if the combination is used prior to anaesthesia for an invasive procedure. By providing analgesia before pain is experienced the amount of analgesia required after the procedure is reduced (pre-emptive analgesia) because sensitisation of the central nervous system by pain is either reduced or prevented.

In dogs and cats, acepromazine has been combined with a variety of opioid analgesics including pethidine and buprenorphine to produce deep sedation. Butorphanol may be combined with medetomidine in dogs and cats to produce sedation. In cats, butorphanol, medetomidine, and ketamine may be combined to provide general anaesthesia. Acepromazine, detomidine, and xylazine are often combined with opioid analgesics, especially butorphanol, in horses to produce deep sedation.

Opioid antagonists (see section 6.5) may be used to reverse the sedation of neuroleptanalgesia, such that recovery is rapid and relatively safe. Dogs may be left alone to recover, which usually takes between 1.5 and 2 hours, although close supervision during this period is essential.

Etorphine is a derivative of thebaine and at least 1000 times more potent than morphine (see Table 6.1). In combination with a phenothiazine such as acepromazine, neuroleptanalgesia is induced that is suitable for minor surgical procedures. Only a small volume of the drug is required, therefore it is useful for darting, as in zoo practice and deer farming. Horses should be stabled and protected from extremes of temperature and supervised for at least 24 hours after administration.

Fentanyl is a synthetic opioid analgesic similar in structure to pethidine. Its analgesic potency is 80 to 100 times that of morphine. Fentanyl is used in combination with fluanisone or xylazine. The fentanyl and fluanisone neuroleptanalgesic combination is indicated for use in rabbits and rodents such as guinea pigs, rats, and mice.

ETORPHINE HYDROCHLORIDE and PHENOTHIAZINES

UK

Indications. Neuroleptanalgesia
Contra-indications. Horses with cardiac arrhythmias, endocarditis, or hepatic impairment; fallow deer; cats
Side-effects. Tachycardia in horses, or bradycardia in dogs, hypertension or hypotension; mild residual sedation; priapism leading to paraphimosis in horses; respiratory depression; transient muscle tremor in horses; enterohepatic recirculation may cause excitement 6–8 hours after remobilisation
Warnings. Caution in elderly animals and pregnant animals (respiratory depression in newborn if used during birth); protect horses' eyes from bright light; animals must be kept stabled, protected from extremes of temperature, and under close supervision for at least 24 hours after administration; care must be taken to avoid hypothermia or hyperthermia
Etorphine and phenothiazine combination is a very potent neuroleptanalgesic, which is highly toxic to humans; it causes dizziness, nausea, and pin-point pupils, followed by respiratory depression, hypotension, cyanosis, and in severe cases, loss of consciousness and cardiac arrest. Operators should wear surgical gloves. Immobilon should not be used without an assistant, capable of administering the reversing agent to the operator, being present and a stock of Narcan and Revivon being available

CD Large Animal Immobilon (Vericore VP) *UK*
Injection, etorphine (as hydrochloride) 2.25 mg, acepromazine maleate (as maleate) 7.38 mg/mL, for *horses, deer*; 10.5 mL
Withdrawal Periods. Must not be used in animals intended for human or animal consumption
Dose. *Horses: by intravenous injection,* 0.5 mL/50 kg. May be given by intramuscular injection if intravenous injection not possible
Deer. Tame deer: by intramuscular injection, 0.5 mL/50 kg (reduce dose by 30% in pregnant hinds)
Rutting or wild deer: by intramuscular injection, up to 1 mL/50 kg
Note. Reversal, see section 6.5

If there is any danger that a human may have absorbed or self-injected Immobilon, the following steps should be taken IMMEDIATELY. Before calling medical assistance, inject reversing agent such as 0.8–1.2 mg naloxone (2–3 mL Narcan) intravenously or intramuscularly (see section 6.5). Revivon may be used in humans in extreme emergencies. Repeat dose every 2 to 3 minutes until symptoms are reversed. Wash area with water. MAINTAIN RESPIRATION AND HEARTBEAT UNTIL MEDICAL ASSISTANCE ARRIVES. The data sheet or pack leaflet should be handed to the attending doctor.

Eire

Indications. Neuroleptanalgesia
Contra-indications. Horses with cardiac arrhythmias, endocarditis, or hepatic impairment; pregnant animals
Side-effects. Muscular tremor, tacycardia, hypertension, mild sedation, hyperthermia, hypothermia, paraphimosis
Warnings. Caution in geriatrics; protect eyes from sun or bright light; animals must be stabled and kept under supervision for 24 hours after treatment; extreme care should be taken to avoid accidental self-innoculation (see box)

Large Animal Immobilon (Cypharm) *Eire*
Injection, etorphine hydrochloride 2.45 mg/mL, acepromazine maleate 10 mg/mL, for *horses*
Withdrawal Periods. Should not be used in *horses* intended for human consumption
Dose. *Horses: by intravenous injection,* 0.01 mL/kg

Small Animal Immobilon (Cypharm) *Eire*
Injection, etorphine hydrochloride 0.074 mg/mL, methotrimeprazine 18 mg/mL, for *dogs*
Dose. *Dogs: by intramuscular injection,* 0.1 mL/kg

FENTANYL CITRATE and FLUANISONE

UK

Indications. Neuroleptanalgesia
Side-effects. Bradycardia, hypotension, respiratory depression, salivation, defaecation, hypersensitivity
Warnings. Involuntary movements sometimes occur, especially in response to stimulation. If respiratory depression occurs, administration of a reversing agent and oxygen may be required
Dose. See preparation details and Prescribing for rabbits and rodents

CD **Hypnorm** (Janssen) *UK*
Injection, fentanyl citrate 315 micrograms, fluanisone 10 mg/mL, for *rabbits, mice, rats, guinea pigs*; 10 mL
Withdrawal Periods. Should not be used in animals intended for human consumption
Dose. Sedation.
Rabbits: *by intramuscular injection*, 0.5 mL/kg
Guinea pigs: *by intramuscular injection*, 1 mL/kg
Rats: *by intramuscular or intraperitoneal injection*, 0.4 mL/kg
Mice: *by intraperitoneal injection*, 0.01 mL/30 g

FENTANYL, AZAPERONE, and XYLAZINE

New Zealand
Indications. Neuroleptanalgesia
Contra-indications. Late pregnancy, severe respiratory depression, cardiac insufficiency
Warnings. Extreme care should be taken to avoid accidental self-innoculation (see box)

Fentazin 5 (Parnell) *NZ*
Injection, azaperone 3.2 mg/mL, fentanyl citrate 0.4 mg/mL, xylazine hydrochloride 58.3 mg/mL, for *deer*
Withdrawal Periods. Slaughter 3 days

Fentazin 10 (Parnell) *NZ*
Injection, azaperone 6.4 mg/mL, fentanyl citrate 0.8 mg/mL, xylazine hydrochloride 116.6 mg/mL, for *deer*
Withdrawal Periods. Slaughter 3 days

6.5 Opioid antagonists

These drugs are used to reverse the effects of opioid analgesics (see section 6.3), especially in neuroleptanalgesia (see section 6.4). They are chemically related to opioid analgesics and are able to reverse all their actions, including analgesia and respiratory depression.

Nalorphine was the first drug to be used as an opioid antagonist but has now been superseded by naloxone. **Naloxone** is a pure antagonist so there is minimal danger of overdose. However, the short duration of action in dogs means that the antagonistic effect may cease before the action of the opioid, previously administered, has been eliminated, and sedation may recur. Naloxone is recommended in the event of self-administration of etorphine (see Warnings under Etorphine hydrochloride, section 6.4).

Diprenorphine is structurally similar to etorphine and is used as an antagonist to that drug.

DIPRENORPHINE

UK
Indications. Reversing agent for etorphine

POM **Large Animal Revivon** (Vericore VP) *UK*
Injection, diprenorphine (as hydrochloride) 3 mg/mL, for *horses, deer*; 10.5 mL
Withdrawal Periods. Slaughter 28 days
Dose. *Horses, deer*: *by intravenous injection*, a volume equal to the total volume of Large Animal Immobilon (Etorphine hydrochloride, see section 6.4) previously administered

Eire
Indications. Reversing agent for etorphine

Large Animal Revivon (Cypharm) *Eire*
Injection, diprenorphine hydrochloride 3.26 mg/mL, for *horses*
Withdrawal Periods. Should not be used in *horses* intended for human consumption
Dose. *Horses*: *by intravenous injection*, a volume equal to the total volume of Large Animal Immobilon (Etorphine hydrochloride, see section 6.4) previously administered

Small Animal Revivon (Cypharm) *Eire*
Injection, diprenorphine hydrochloride 0.295 mg/mL, for *dogs*
Dose. *dogs*: *by intravenous injection*, a volume equal to the total volume of Small Animal Immobilon (Etorphine hydrochloride, see section 6.4) previously administered

NALOXONE HYDROCHLORIDE

UK
Indications. Reversing agent for opioid analgesics; reversal of accidental etorphine poisoning in humans (see Warnings under Etorphine hydrochloride, section 6.4); behaviour modification (see section 6.11.8)
Warnings. Short acting, possibility of relapse (see notes above)
Dose. *Dogs*: reversal of opioid analgesia, *by subcutaneous, intramuscular, or intravenous injection*, 0.04–1.0 mg/kg

POM Ⓗ **Naloxone** (Non-proprietary) *UK*
Injection, naloxone hydrochloride 20 micrograms/mL; 2 mL
Injection, naloxone hydrochloride 400 micrograms/mL; 1 mL

POM Ⓗ **Narcan** (Du Pont) *UK*
Injection, naloxone hydrochloride 400 micrograms/mL; 1 mL, 10 mL

New Zealand
Indications. Reversing agent for fentanyl and xylazine (Fentazin)
Dose. See preparation details

Contran-H (Parnell) *NZ*
Injection, naloxone hydrochloride 0.1 mg/mL, yohimbine hydrochloride 10 mg/mL, for *deer*
Withdrawal Periods. *Deer*: slaughter 1 day
Dose. *Deer*: *by intravenous injection*, 2.0–2.5 mL/100 kg

USA
Indications. Reversing agent for opioid analgesics
Dose. *Dogs*: *by subcutaneous, intramuscular, or intravenous injection*, 40 micrograms/kg

P/M Naloxone HCL Injection (Schering-Plough) *USA*
Injection, naloxone hydrochloride 400 micrograms/mL, for *dogs*

NALTREXONE

Indications. Reversing agent for carfentanil
Contra-indications. During or for 45 days before hunting season

Trexonil (Wildlife Pharm) *USA*
Injection, naltrexone hydrochloride 50 mg/mL, for *elk, moose*
Withdrawal Periods. Should not be used in animals intended for human consumption

6.6 General anaesthetics

6.6.1 Antimuscarinic pre-anaesthetic medication

6.6.2 Injectable anaesthetics

6.6.3 Inhalational anaesthetics

The main aims of general anaesthesia are to produce unconsciousness, immobility, and muscle relaxation so that surgical or other procedures may be performed painlessly. Most anaesthetic drugs also cause profound alterations in the function of vital body systems, in particular the cardiovascular and respiratory systems. Careful technique with attention to basic principles such as airway management, constant patient monitoring, and the use of properly maintained equipment, all contribute to good anaesthetic practice with minimal complications.

Most anaesthetic drugs have a narrow therapeutic index and careful attention to dose rates is required. A common source of error is inaccurate weight estimation and all patients should be weighed as part of their preparation for anaesthesia.

Anaesthetic drugs cause respiratory depression and, in general, during anaesthesia the inspired oxygen concentration should not be less than 30% and in horses, particularly in dorsal recumbancy, should be 100%. This necessitates supplementary oxygen in all cases. This can be provided via a nasal tube or face mask but in most cases it is convenient to intubate the animal and connect the patient to a suitable circuit and anaesthetic machine, which also allows the use of inhalational anaesthetic agents. In cats, young goats♦, and pigs♦, intubation may be facilitated by the use of lidocaine administered as a spray to avoid laryngospasm.

The majority of patients undergo elective surgery and can be prepared for general anaesthesia under optimal conditions. Cats, dogs, and horses should be starved for at least 6 hours so that the stomach is empty. Overnight starvation is convenient. Water should be allowed until premedication or one hour before anaesthesia if the animal is not to be premedicated. In general, very young and very small animals have high metabolic rates and food should be withheld for shorter periods.

Sick and debilitated animals require individual pre-anaesthetic regimens. The health status of patients must be assessed before general anaesthesia in order to identify potential complications that may occur during or after the operation. The presence of underlying disease and concurrent medication increases the risks of general anaesthesia.

If possible, pre-existing disease should be treated and the animal stabilised before undergoing elective anaesthesia.

The commonest problems of profound sedation and general anaesthesia in ruminants are regurgitation, inhalational pneumonia, and bloat, all of which relate to ruminal filling, fermentation, and fluidity of ruminal contents. While it would take days to significantly reduce the volume of rumenal contents, it is advisable to minimise the risk of regurgitation and bloat by withholding fermentable foodstuffs for 24 hours and water for 12 hours. Periods of starvation longer than 48 hours are associated with acid-base disturbances (in particular ketoacidosis).

During general anaesthesia further precautions include endotracheal intubation with a cuffed endotracheal tube to safeguard the airway against regurgitated material. A larynx-high nose-down position in lateral recumbency and head-down position in dorsal recumbency allows drainage of any regurgitated material and the copious amounts of saliva ruminants continue to produce during anaesthesia. The placement of a ruminal tube will allow relief of increased ruminal pressure from gas production caused by fermentation.

In horses, size in combination with variations in blood pressure predispose the recumbent animal to nerve and muscle injury. The nerve injury is generally due to direct pressure on a superficial nerve while the muscle injury may result from ischaemia due to hypoxia and hypotension leading to decreased oxygen delivery to muscle masses. The result is that animals may exhibit postoperative signs ranging from limb stiffness to total inability to stand. Current attempts at prevention include careful positioning, maintaining oxygenation, and support of blood pressure with dobutamine and intravenous fluid therapy. There have been reports of post anaesthesia spinal injury in horses positioned in dorsal recumbency during anaesthesia. Although the cause of injury may be multifactorial, prevention may include tilting the animal from the dorsal position if practicable for surgery.

Pre-anaesthetic medication is appropriate in most patients. The main aims are to calm the patient, provide analgesia if needed, reduce the dose of anaesthetic agent, reduce or counteract the side-effects of anaesthetic drugs, and to provide a smooth anaesthetic induction and recovery. These aims are generally achieved by using sedatives, opioid analgesics, and antimuscarinic drugs either alone or in combination. The dose of barbiturate for induction can be reduced by a third to a half (except in the horse) if a light pre-anaesthetic medication such as acepromazine is used. When heavier premedication is produced by drugs such as xylazine or medetomidine, the dose of barbiturate may need to be reduced further (or halved in the horse). In horses, the dose of barbiturate for induction may only be reduced when heavier premedication is used. Doses of other induction agents are also reduced if pre-anaesthetic medication is given (see Dose under drug monographs).

Patients should be closely monitored during recovery to ensure safe return to normal; analgesics may be required during this period.

6.6.1 Antimuscarinic pre-anaesthetic medication

Antimuscarinic drugs are used to reduce salivation and bronchial secretion and to prevent and treat vagally-mediated cardiac arrhythmias caused by the procedure or anaesthetic drugs. Their routine use in anaesthesia is declining because halogenated inhalational agents are less irritant to the airways than ether. Premedicants may be indicated in cats and small dogs in which a small amount of saliva can block the airway but their routine use in larger dogs is controversial.

Atropine and **hyoscine** are not recommended as premedicants in horses because the central excitation and mydriasis that these drugs produce can be unpleasant, and gastrointestinal motility will be reduced. **Glycopyrronium** may be better for use in horses, if required, because it does not cross the blood-brain barrier and so does not produce central effects. Administration of antimuscarinic drugs to ruminants does not inhibit salivation but results in production of a more viscid saliva and is therefore generally contra-indicated in these species. In horses, atropine or preferably glycopyrronium is used intra-operatively for ocular and head and neck surgery to block the vagal reflexes stimulated by manipulation of the eye and vago-sympathetic nerve trunk. Glycopyrronium causes reduced intensity of tachycardias compared to atropine. Glycopyrronium is also preferred in caesarean section because it does not cross the placenta.

Atropine and other antimuscarinic drugs prevent the muscarinic side-effects of anticholinesterases, which are used to reverse the effects of competitive non-depolarising neuromuscular blocking drugs.

Antimuscarinic drugs continue to be important for the treatment of bradycardia. Atropine is the most commonly used. It produces a more stable heart rate during anaesthesia than hyoscine. The latter also has greater central effects, which are generally undesirable.

ATROPINE SULPHATE

UK

Indications. Drying secretions; adjunct in gastro-intestinal disorders characterised by smooth muscle spasm (see section 3.7); antidote for organophosphorus compound poisoning (see Treatment of poisoning); in combination with anticholinesterases (see section 6.7.4); vagally-mediated cardiac arrhythmias

Contra-indications. Glaucoma; pre-existing tachycardia; ventricular arrhythmias; known myocardial ischaemia

Side-effects. Tachycardia; constipation; urinary retention; dilation of pupils and photophobia

Warnings. Intravenous injection may initially increase bradyarrhythmias due to central vagal stimulation

Dose. Antimuscarinic use, *by subcutaneous injection.*

Horses, cattle: 30–60 micrograms/kg

Sheep: 80–160 micrograms/kg

Pigs: 20–40 micrograms/kg

Dogs, cats: 30–50 micrograms/kg

Organophosphorus poisoning.

By subcutaneous injection, 25–200 micrograms/kg at approximately 3–4 hour intervals until clinical signs of poisoning relieved. In severe cases, a quarter of the dose may be given by intramuscular or slow intravenous injection and the remainder by subcutaneous injection

POM **Atrocare** (Animalcare) *UK*

Injection, atropine sulphate 600 micrograms/mL, for *horses, cattle, sheep, pigs, dogs, cats*; 25 mL

Withdrawal Periods. *Cattle*: slaughter 14 days (antimuscarinic use), 28 days (antidote use); milk 3 days (antimuscarinic use), 6 days (antidote use). *Sheep, pigs*: slaughter 14 days (antimuscarinic use), 28 days (antidote use)

Australia

Indications. Pre-anaesthetic medication; treatment of organophosphorus compound poisoning

Contra-indications. Glaucoma; pyloric stenosis; cardiac impairment; paralytic ileus; constipation

Dose. Antimuscarinic use, *by subcutaneous, intramuscular, or intravenous injection,* 50 micrograms/kg

Organophosphorus poisoning, 0.1–2.0 mg/kg. One quarter to half of the dose is given by intravenous injection and the remainder by subcutaneous or intramuscular injection

Atropine Injection (Apex) *Austral.*

Injection, atropine sulphate 600 micrograms/mL

Withdrawal Periods. Slaughter withdrawal period nil, milk withdrawal period nil

Atrosite (Ilium) *Austral.*

Injection, atropine sulphate 650 micrograms/mL, for *dogs, cats*

New Zealand

Indications. Pre-anaesthetic medication; treatment of organophosphorus compound poisoning

Contra-indications. Glaucoma; cardiac insufficiency or failure

Side-effects. Dry mouth, dilation of pupils

Dose. *Dogs*: *by subcutaneous or intramuscular injection,* 0.325–1.3 mg

Cats: *by subcutaneous or intramuscular injection,* 0.13–0.39 mg

Atropine Injection (Phoenix) *NZ*

Injection, atropine sulphate 650 micrograms/mL, for *dogs, cats*

USA

Indications. Pre-anaesthetic medication; treatment of organophosphorus compound poisoning

Contra-indications. Glaucoma; tachycardia

Dose. *Dogs, cats*: antimuscarinic use, *by subcutaneous, intramuscular, or intravenous injection,* 40–59 micrograms/kg

Organophosphorus poisoning. One-quarter to one-third of the dose is given by intravenous injection and the remainder by subcutaneous or intramuscular injection

Horses: 143 micrograms/kg

Cattle: 660 micrograms/kg

Sheep: 1.1 mg/kg

Dogs, cats: doses vary: 120–480 (usual dose 158 micrograms/kg)

Atroject (Vetus) *USA*

Injection, atropine sulphate 0.54 mg/mL, for *dogs, cats*

Atropine Injection Large Animal (Vedco) *USA*

Injection, atropine sulphate 15 mg/mL, for *horses, cattle, sheep*

Atropine Injection Small Animal (Vedco) *USA*
Injection, atropine sulphate 0.54 mg/mL, for *dogs*, *cats*

Atropine L.A. (Butler) *USA*
Injection, atropine sulphate 15 mg/mL, for *cattle*, *horses*, *sheep*

Atropine S.A. (Butler) *USA*
Injection, atropine sulphate 0.54 mg/mL, for *dogs*, *cats*

Atropine Sulfate 1/120 (VetTek) *USA*
Injection, atropine sulphate 0.54 mg/mL, for *dogs*, *cats*

Atropine Sulfate Injection (Phoenix) *USA*
Injection, atropine sulphate 0.54 mg/mL, for *dogs*, *cats*

Atropine Sulfate Injection 1/120 Grain (Western Veterinary Supply) *USA*
Injection, atropine sulphate 0.54 mg/mL, for *dogs*, *cats*

Atropine Sulfate Injection 15 mg/mL L.A. (RXV, Western Veterinary Supply) *USA*
Injection, atropine sulphate 15 mg/mL, for *horses*, *cattle*, *sheep*

GLYCOPYRRONIUM BROMIDE
(Glycopyrrolate bromide)

UK
Indications. Treatment of vagally induced bradycardia; drying secretions; in combination with anticholinesterases (see section 6.7.4)
Side-effects. See under Atropine sulphate
Warnings. Concurrent administration of adrenoceptor stimulants may cause tachycardia and fatal dysrhythmias in horses
Dose. *Horses*: by intravenous injection, 1–3 micrograms/kg
Dogs: by intramuscular or intravenous injection, 2–8 micrograms/kg

POM (H) **Robinul** (Anpharm) *UK*
Injection, glycopyrronium bromide 200 micrograms/mL; 1 mL, 3 mL

Australia
Indications. Pre-anaesthetic medication
Contra-indications. Pregnant animals
Dose. *By intramuscular or intravenous injection.*
Horses: 2.8–5.6 micrograms/kg
Dogs, *cats*: 11 micrograms/kg

Glycosate Vet (RWR) *Austral.*
Injection, glycopyrronium bromide 280 micrograms/mL, for *horses*, *dogs*, *cats*
Withdrawal Periods. *Horses*: slaughter 28 days

USA
Indications. Pre-anaesthetic medication
Contra-indications. Pregnant animals
Side-effects. Mild mydriasis, xerostomia, tachycardia
Warnings. Drug excretion may be prolonged in renal impairment or impaired gastro-intestinal function
Dose. *Dogs*: by subcutaneous, intramuscular, or intravenous injection, 11 micrograms/kg
Dogs: by intramuscular injection, 11 micrograms/kg

Robinul-V Injectable (Fort Dodge) *USA*
Injection, glycopyronnium bromide 200 micrograms/mL, for *dogs*, *cats*

HYOSCINE HYDROBROMIDE
(Scopolamine hydrobromide)

UK
Indications. Drying secretions
Contra-indications. **Side-effects**. See under Atropine sulphate and notes above
Dose. *Dogs*, *cats*: by intramuscular injection, 10–20 micrograms/kg

POM (H) **Hyoscine** (Non-proprietary) *UK*
Injection, hyoscine hydrobromide 400 micrograms/mL, 600 micrograms/mL; 1 mL

6.6.2 Injectable anaesthetics

6.6.2.1 Barbiturates
6.6.2.2 Propofol
6.6.2.3 Steroid anaesthetics
6.6.2.4 Dissociative anaesthetics
6.6.2.5 Metomidate

Injectable anaesthetics have a rapid onset of action and are commonly used as induction agents to effect rapid passage through the light planes of anaesthesia during which the patient may struggle. These drugs are eliminated by metabolism and excretion and there is no way of increasing the rate of removal from the body to compensate for overdosage. Urinary pH may be altered to increase drug excretion but this is usually only employed for barbiturate poisoning. Most injectable anaesthetics cause respiratory depression; periods of apnoea commonly occur, but are not hazardous provided the patient is monitored closely and intermittent positive pressure ventilation (IPPV) can be provided if necessary. Other effects of injectable anaesthetics include hypotension and tachycardia.

The doses indicated in the monographs below represent a guide. There is inter-individual variation to a given dose. Therefore the entire calculated dose should not be administered but the drug given until the required depth of anaesthesia is achieved. This method of administration ensures an appropriate depth of anaesthesia and avoids overdosage.

6.6.2.1 Barbiturates

Thiopental is the standard drug for induction with which others are compared. It is administered intravenously as an aqueous solution of the sodium salt, which is alkaline and highly irritant. Extravascular injection may lead to tissue necrosis. If extravascular injection occurs, the area should be infiltrated with sodium chloride 0.9%, containing lidocaine 2% or procaine 5% if required, to reduce the local alkalinity by dilution and minimise irritation. Intra-arterial injection may lead to gangrene of an extremity and injection into the carotid artery may cause death. Solutions should be as dilute as possible, using a 1.25% solution for neonates and cats, and a 2.5% solution for dogs. Horses, ruminants, and pigs require more concentrated solutions, to minimise the volume required, and this should always be given via an intravenous catheter.

The initial dose of thiopental rapidly reaches the brain, and is then redistributed to the viscera, muscles, and fat, and slowly metabolised in the liver. Therefore, recovery from a single dose of thiopental is not dependent upon immediate excretion or metabolism. In general, when the animal recovers consciousness, the full dose of thiopental is still present in its body. For this reason, minimal doses of thiopental should be used wherever possible to achieve the desired effect. If high doses are required (for example 25–30 mg/kg) a very prolonged recovery should be anticipated and precautions taken to maintain fluid and thermal balance. Pre-anaesthetic medication should be given wherever possible in order to reduce the dose of thiopental administered. If repeated doses of thiopental are administered, the tissues may become saturated with thiopental and recovery will be prolonged for many hours. Therefore, thiopental is not generally suitable for maintenance of anaesthesia of more than 15 to 20 minutes.

Recovery from thiopental may be prolonged in Greyhounds and hounds of similar physique; some authorities state that use of thiopental is contra-indicated in these breeds. Methohexital has been used for many years in breeds with little body fat but use of propofol is becoming popular due to the smoother induction and recovery observed with this drug. Thiopental should be used with a sedative pre-anaesthetic medicant in dogs and horses. If used alone the recovery may be violent in these species. When a phenothiazine premedicant is used in horses the dose of thiopental should not be reduced.

Methohexital is shorter acting than thiopental, but causes greater respiratory depression. Induction and recovery are generally more excitable than with thiopental. The solution is irritant and care should be taken to avoid extravasation. Methohexital is more rapidly metabolised than thiopental although recovery from a single dose is still mainly dependent on redistribution.

Pentobarbital is mainly used for the treatment of status epilepticus (see section 6.9.2), control of muscle rigidity and convulsions as a result of poisoning (see Treatment of poisoning), and euthanasia (see section 6.10). As an anaesthetic, excitement may occur during induction because pentobarbital is slow to cross the blood-brain barrier. Respiratory and cardiovascular depression are marked and hypothermia is common as a result of the long recovery period. In the majority of species, onset of action, duration of action, and recovery from pentobarbital are protracted and as an anaesthetic it has been superseded by other agents such as thiopental and propofol. However, small ruminants metabolise the drug more rapidly than other species and in anaesthesia of these species, pentobarbital still has a role. In sheep and goats, pentobarbital produces 15 to 30 minutes of surgical anaesthesia, with a quiet recovery time of approximately 30 minutes.

PENTOBARBITAL SODIUM
(Pentobarbitone sodium)

UK
Indications. General anaesthesia; convulsions and muscle rigidity in poisoning (see Treatment of poisoning); status epilepticus (see section 6.9.2); euthanasia (see section 6.10)

Contra-indications. Hepatic impairment

Warnings. Respiratory depression may be enhanced; extravascular injection may cause local irritation and slough

Dose. Status epilepticus

Dogs: *by rapid intravenous injection (bolus)*, 13 mg/kg followed *by intravenous infusion*, 13 mg/kg given according to the patient's response

Sedation.

Dogs, cats, rabbits, guinea pigs: *by slow intravenous injection*, 13 mg/kg

General anaesthesia (without pre-anaesthetic medication).

Sheep ♦, goats ♦: *by slow intravenous injection*, 24 mg/kg

Dogs, cats, rabbits, guinea pigs: *by slow intravenous injection*, 26 mg/kg, see also Prescribing for rabbits and rodents

POM **Sagatal** (Merial) *UK*
Injection, pentobarbital sodium 60 mg/mL, for *dogs, cats, guinea pigs, rabbits*; 100 mL
Withdrawal Periods. Should not be used in *rabbits* intended for human consumption

Australia
Indications. General anaesthesia

Contra-indications. Severe renal or hepatic impairment; caesarian section

Side-effects. Voluminous salivation in cattle; excitement on induction or recovery; rearing and falling backwards in horses if used as sole anaesthetic agent

Warnings. Caution in pug nosed dogs, Greyhounds and similar breeds, debilitated animals, anaemia

Dose. *By slow intravenous injection.*

Horses: 16.8 mg/kg

Cattle, sheep, pigs: 24 mg/kg

Dogs: 27.6 mg/kg

Cats: 22.8 mg/kg

Nembutal (Merial) *Austral.*
Injection, pentobarbital sodium 60 mg/mL, for *horses, cattle, sheep, pigs, dogs, cats*
Withdrawal Periods. *Horses, cattle, pigs, sheep*: slaughter 28 days

Eire
Indications. Sedation, general anaesthesia

Warnings. Caution in hepatic impairment, thin animals, debilitated animals, severe tissue reaction if administered extravascularly

Dose. Sedation, *by intravenous injection*, 13 mg/kg
General anaesthesia, *by intravenous injection*, 26 mg/kg

Sagatal (Merial) *Eire*
Injection, pentobarbital sodium 60 g/mL, for *dogs, cats, rabbits, guinea pigs*
Withdrawal Periods. Should not be used in *rabbits* intended for human consumption

New Zealand

Indications. General anaesthesia

Contra-indications. Severe renal or hepatic impairment; caesarian section

Warnings. Caution in debilitated animals and anaemia, severe tissue reaction if administered extravascularly

Dose. *By intravenous injection,* 24–30 mg/kg

Nembutal (Virbac) *NZ*
Injection, pentobarbital sodium 60 mg/mL, for **horses, cattle, sheep, pigs, dogs, cats**

USA

Indications. General anaesthesia

Contra-indications. Severe renal or hepatic impairment; severe respiratory depression

Side-effects. Delayed recovery in hypothermia and thin animals

Warnings. Caution in anaemia, hypovolaemia, cardiac or respiratory disorders

Dose. *Dogs, cats: by intravenous injection,* 24.2–28.6 mg/kg

Sodium Pentobarbital Injection (Butler) *USA*
Injection, sodium pentobarbital 65 mg/mL, for **dogs, cats**

THIOPENTAL SODIUM
(Thiopentone sodium)

UK

Indications. Induction of general anaesthesia

Contra-indications. Foals less than 2 months of age, puppies and kittens less than 2–3 months of age; conditions causing diminished cardiac output

Side-effects. Respiratory depression; transient apnoea; hypotension; tachycardia; reduction in pain threshold at sub-anaesthetic doses

Warnings. Extravasation may cause local irritation and slough; caution in hepatic impairment, cardiovascular disease, and hypoproteinaemia and hypovolaemia associated with shock; care in pregnant animals; Drug Interactions – see Appendix 1; slight limb movement or respiratory irregularities may not be abolished during surgery

Dose.

General anaesthetic induction (without pre-anaesthetic medication).

Dogs, cats: by intravenous injection, 25–30 mg/kg (maximum 1.25 g) of 1.25% or 2.5% solution; see notes above

General anaesthetic induction (*with* pre-anaesthetic medication).

Horses: by intravenous injection, 5.5–10.0 mg/kg of 5% solution

Dogs, cats: by intravenous injection, 8–12 mg/kg

POM Intraval Sodium (Merial) *UK*
Injection, powder for reconstitution, thiopental sodium 2.5 g, 5 g, for **horses, dogs, cats**
Withdrawal Periods. Should not be used in **horses** intended for human consumption

POM Thiovet (Vericore VP) *UK*
Injection, powder for reconstitution, thiopental sodium 2.5 g, 5 g, for **horses, dogs, cats**
Withdrawal Periods. Should not be used in **horses** intended for human consumption

Australia

Indications. General anaesthesia

Side-effects. Respiratory depression

Warnings. Caution in hepatic or renal impairment, anaemia, shock; Drug Interactions – pre-anaesthetic agents, analgesics, some tranquilisers, corticosteroids, sulphonamides

Dose. General anaesthetic, *by intravenous injection.*

Horses, cattle: 8.8–15.4 mg/kg; **calves**: 6.6 mg/kg

Sheep: 9.9–14.0 mg/kg

Pigs: 5.5–11.0 mg/kg

Dogs: 15–17 mg/kg

Cats: 9–11 mg/kg

Pentothal (Merial) *Austral.*
Injection, powder for reconstitution, thiopental sodium 5 g, for **horses, cattle, sheep, pigs, dogs, cats,**
Withdrawal Periods. Slaughter 28 days

Eire

Indications. General anaesthesia

Contra-indications. Foals less than 2–3 months of age, puppies and kittens less than 2–3 months of age; conditions causing diminished cardiac output

Warnings. Extravasation may cause local irritation and slough; caution in hepatic impairment, cardiovascular disease, and hypoglycaemia associated with shock; care in administration to pregnant animals; Drug Interactions – streptomycin, chloramphenicol, kanamycin

Dose. General anaesthetic, *by intravenous injection.*

Horses: 10–11 mg/kg (*with* pre-anaesthetic medication)

Dogs: 10–25 mg/kg (without pre-anaesthetic medication)

Cats: 20–25 mg/kg (without pre-anaesthetic medication)

Thiovet 2.5 g & 5 g (Cypharm) *Eire*
Injection, powder for reconstitution, thiopentone sodium, for **horses, dogs, cats**
Withdrawal Periods. Should not be used in **horses** intended for human consumption; slaughter 28 days

Intraval Sodium (Merial) *Eire*
Injection, powder for reconstitution, thiopental sodium, for **horses, dogs, cats**
Withdrawal Periods. Should not be used in **horses** intended for human consumption; slaughter 28 days

New Zealand

Indications. General anaesthesia

Contra-indications. Foals and calves less than 2–3 months of age, puppies and kittens less than 2–3 months of age; intra-arterial injection; conditions causing diminished cardiac output

Warnings. Extravasation may cause local irritation and slough; caution in hepatic impairment, cardiovascular disease, and hypoglycaemia associated with shock; care in administration to pregnant animals; Drug Interactions – streptomycin, chloramphenicol, kanamycin

Dose. General anaesthetic, *by intravenous injection.*
Large animals: 10–16 mg/kg
Dogs, cats: 13–26 mg/kg

Bomathal (Bomac) *NZ*
Injection, thiopental sodium 5 g, for *large and small animals*

Intraval Sodium (Merial) *NZ*
Injection, thiopental sodium 5 g, for *large and small animals*

Pentothal (Virbac) *NZ*
Injection, thiopental sodium 5 g, for *large and small animals*

Thiovet (Novartis) *NZ*
Injection, thiopental sodium 2.5 g, 5.0 g, for *horses, dogs, cats*
Withdrawal Periods. Should not be used in *horses* intended for human consumption

USA

Indications. General anaesthesia
Side-effects. Respiratory depression
Warnings. Caution in hepatic or renal impairment, anaemia, shock; Drug Interactions – pre-anaesthetic agents, analgesics, some tranquilisers, corticosteroids, sulphonamides
Dose. General anaesthetic, *by intravenous injection.*
Horses, cattle: 8.8–15.4 mg/kg
Sheep: 9.9–14.0 mg/kg
Pigs: 5.5–11.0 mg/kg
Dogs: 13–26 mg/kg
Cats: 17–26 mg/kg

Veterinary Pentothal (Merial) *USA*
Injection, thiopental sodium 2.5 g for reconstitution, for *horses, cattle, sheep, pigs, dogs, cats,*

6.6.2.2 Propofol

Propofol produces anaesthesia after intravenous injection in a similar manner to thiopental, although cardiovascular depression is slightly greater. The incidence of transient apnoea seen during and immediately after induction may be reduced by injecting the drug over a period of 20 to 30 seconds rather than by bolus administration. This may also reduce the dose necessary for intubation.

The recovery from propofol is rapid and generally smooth, even when no sedative premedication has been given. Therefore, the drug is useful for minor out-patient procedures and caesarian section. Recovery from propofol is by metabolism rather than redistribution so that repeated doses can be given with little increase in recovery time. Cats do not metabolise propofol as efficiently as dogs.

Propofol is not irritant to tissues and extravasation does not cause problems, but pain on injection occurs in humans and may be observed in some animals.

PROPOFOL

UK

Indications. Induction and maintenance of general anaesthesia
Side-effects. During the recovery phase vomiting and evidence of excitation may occur; if panting is evident before induction, this may continue through anaesthesia and recovery; transient apnoea during induction; paw and face licking during recovery in cats
Warnings. Caution in patients with cardiac, hepatic, respiratory, or renal impairment
Dose.
General anaesthetic induction (without pre-anaesthetic medication).
Dogs: *by intravenous injection*, 6.5 mg/kg
Cats: *by intravenous injection*, 8 mg/kg

General anaesthetic induction (*with* pre-anaesthetic medication).
Dogs: *by intravenous injection*, 4 mg/kg
Cats: *by intravenous injection*, 6 mg/kg

General anaesthetic maintenance.
Dogs, cats: *by intravenous injection*, 2.5–5.0 mg/kg given according to the patient's response

POM **Rapinovet** (Schering-Plough) *UK*
Injection, propofol 10 mg/mL, for *dogs, cats*; 20 mL

Australia

Indications. General anaesthesia
Side-effects. During the recovery phase vomiting and evidence of excitation may occur; if panting is evident before induction, this may continue through anaesthesia and recovery; transient apnoea and hypertension during induction; paw and face licking during recovery in cats
Warnings. Caution in cardiac, hepatic, respiratory, or renal impairment; hypovolaemia; debilitated animals
Dose. General anaesthetic induction (without pre-anaesthetic medication).
Dogs: *by intravenous injection*, 6.5 mg/kg
Cats: *by intravenous injection*, 8 mg/kg

Rapinovet (Schering-Plough) *Austral.*
Injection, propofol 10 mg/mL, for *dogs, cats*

Eire

Indications. General anaesthesia
Side-effects. During the recovery phase vomiting and evidence of excitation may occur; if panting is evident before induction, this may continue through anaesthesia and recovery; transient apnoea during induction; paw and face licking during recovery in cats
Warnings. Caution in cardiac, hepatic, respiratory, or renal impairment; hypovolaemia; debilitated animals
Dose. General anaesthetic induction (without pre-anaesthetic medication).
Dogs: *by intravenous injection*, 6.5 mg/kg
Cats: *by intravenous injection*, 8 mg/kg

Rapinovet (Schering-Plough) *Eire*
Injection, propofol 10 mg/mL, for *dogs, cats*

New Zealand

Indications. General anaesthesia
Warnings. Caution in cardiac, hepatic, respiratory, or renal impairment; hypovolaemia; debilitated animals

Dose. General anaesthetic induction (without pre-anaesthetic medication).

Dogs, cats: *by intravenous injection*, according to response

Rapinovet (Schering-Plough) *NZ*
Injection, propofol 10 mg/mL, for ***dogs, cats***

USA

Indications. General anaesthesia
Side-effects. Vomiting, excitation, transient tachypnoea and apnoea during induction, hypotension, paddling during recovery, sneezing
Warnings. Safety in pregnant animals or animals less than 10 weeks of age has not been established
Dose. General anaesthetic induction (without pre-anaesthetic medication).

Dogs: *by intravenous injection*, 5.5 mg/kg

Propoflo (Abbott) *USA*
Injection, propofol 10 mg/mL, for ***dogs***

Rapinovet (Schering-Plough) *USA*
Injection, propofol 10 mg/mL, for ***dogs***

6.6.2.3 Steroid anaesthetics

Alfadolone and **alfaxalone** in combination are insoluble in water and are solubilised in polyoxyl 35 castor oil (Cremophor EL). This vehicle may cause histamine release, which is usually mild in cats but can be severe in dogs. The drug combination is not irritant and may be given by intravenous or deep intramuscular injection. Recovery from alfaxalone and alfadolone anaesthesia is by metabolism and may be prolonged by repeated administration or continuous infusion.

ALFADOLONE ACETATE and ALFAXALONE
(Alphadolone and Alphaxalone)

UK

Indications. Induction and maintenance of general anaesthesia
Contra-indications. Dogs, see notes above
Side-effects. Transient unilateral or bilateral erythema and oedema of paws, pinnae, or both; sneezing during induction and recovery in cats; excessive salivation in monkeys
Warnings. Rarely oedema of larynx; rarely necrotic lesions of the extremities
Dose. Expressed as alfadolone acetate + alfaxalone (total steroids).
General anaesthesia (without pre-anaesthetic medication).
Cats: *by intramuscular injection*, 18 mg/kg
by intravenous injection, initial dose 9 mg/kg, followed by 3 mg/kg increments if required

POM **Saffan** (Schering-Plough) *UK*
Injection, alfadolone acetate 3 mg, alfaxalone 9 mg/mL (12 mg total steroids/mL), for ***cats***; 5 mL, 10 mL

Australia

Indications. General anaesthesia
Contra-indications. Dogs

Side-effects. Transient unilateral or bilateral erythema and oedema of paws, pinnae, or both; sneezing during induction and recovery in cats
Warnings. Caution in geriatrics, stressed animals, shock, caesarian section
Dose. Expressed as alfadolone acetate + alfaxalone (total steroids).
Cats: *by intramuscular injection*, 9–18 mg/kg
by intravenous injection, 9 mg/kg

Alfaxan (Jurox) *Austral.*
Injection, alfaxalone 9 mg/mL, alfadolone acetate 3 mg/mL, for ***cats, monkeys***

Saffan (Schering-Plough) *Austral.*
Injection, alfaxalone 9 mg/mL, alfadolone acetate 3 mg/mL, for ***cats, monkeys***

Eire

Indications. General anaesthesia
Contra-indications. Dogs
Side-effects. Transient unilateral or bilateral erythema and oedema of paws, pinnae, or both; sneezing during induction and recovery in cats
Warnings. Rarely oedema of larynx; rarely necrotic lesions of the extremities
Dose. Expressed as alfadolone acetate + alfaxalone (total steroids).
Cats: *by intramuscular injection*, 4–18 mg/kg
by intravenous injection, 9 mg/kg

Saffan (Schering-Plough) *Eire*
Injection, alfadolone acetate 3 mg/mL, alfaxalone 9 mg, for ***cats***

New Zealand

Indications. General anaesthesia
Contra-indications. Dogs
Side-effects. Rarely anaphylactoid reactions, muscular tremors during recovery
Warnings. Caution in respiratory disease, anaemia
Dose. Expressed as alfadolone acetate + alfaxalone (total steroids).
Cattle: *by intravenous injection*, 3 mg/kg
Sheep, goats: *by intravenous injection*, 3 mg/kg; ***young sheep and goats***: *by intravenous injection*, 6 mg/kg; ***lambs***: *by intramuscular injection*, 9–12 mg/kg; ***kids***: *by intramuscular injection*, 9 mg/kg
Cats: *by intramuscular injection*, 4–18 mg/kg
by intravenous injection, 9 mg/kg

Alfaxan (Jurox) *NZ*
Injection, alfadolone acetate 3 mg/mL, alfaxalone 9 mg/mL, for ***cattle less than 200 kg body-weight, sheep, goats, cats***
Withdrawal Periods. ***Cattle, sheep, goats***: slaughter 30 days, should not be used in lactating dairy animals producing milk for human consumption

Saffan (Schering-Plough) *NZ*
Injection, alfadolone acetate 3 mg/mL, alfaxalone 9 mg/mL, for ***cattle less than 200 kg body-weight, sheep, goats, cats***

6.6.2.4 Dissociative anaesthetics

Ketamine and tiletamine are phencyclidine derivatives and have antagonistic actions at the N-methyl d-aspartate

(NMDA) receptors in the brain and spinal cord. They interrupt the cerebral association between the limbic and cortical systems. The animal may appear to be in a light plane of anaesthesia but is insensitive to surgical stimulation. Muscle relaxation may be poor when these drugs are used alone and the addition of either an alpha$_2$-adrenoceptor stimulant such as xylazine, or a benzodiazepine such as diazepam will increase muscle relaxation.

Ketamine may be used as a sole anaesthetic in cats and primates. In cats, the eyes remain open during ketamine anaesthesia and a bland eye ointment may be used to protect the cornea. Ketamine may be given intramuscularly or intravenously, although intramuscular injection is painful. Ketamine should be given to horses and donkeys only after deep sedative premedication with xylazine, romifidine, or detomidine. Induction of anaesthesia in horses with ketamine is generally calm, but quiet surroundings and handling are important. There are a few reports of failure of ketamine to induce anaesthesia in horses and this potential problem should be remembered. Ketamine may produce convulsions in dogs when used as the sole anaesthetic.

Tiletamine is used in combination with the benzodiazepine zolazepam. When used as a sole anaesthetic agent, tiletamine has a long duration of action, provides no muscle relaxation, and causes profuse salivation, lacrimation, and mydriasis. Combination with zolazepam allows the effective dose of tiletamine to be reduced and affords reasonable muscle relaxation. However, recovery can still be prolonged. Cardiovascular and respiratory effects of tiletamine are similar to those of ketamine.

KETAMINE

UK
Indications. General anaesthesia, in combination with Butorphanol, Detomidine, Medetomidine, Romifidine, or Xylazine

Contra-indications. Sole anaesthetic in horses, donkeys, or dogs; hepatic or renal impairment; latter stages of pregnancy in animals

Side-effects. Excessive salivation in cats; hypotension; increased cardiac output; tachycardia; muscle twitching and mild tonic convulsions in cats

Warnings. A small proportion of animals are reported to be unresponsive to ketamine at normal doses

Dose.

General anaesthesia (without pre-anaesthetic medication).

Cats: *by subcutaneous, intramuscular (preferred), or intravenous injection*, 11–33 mg/kg

Primates: information on dose available from manufacturers

General anaesthesia, in combination with Detomidine.

Horses: *by intravenous injection*, detomidine 20 micrograms/kg, followed 5 minutes later by ketamine 2.2 mg/kg

Sedation or general anaesthesia, in combination with Diazepam.

Dogs: *by intravenous injection*, diazepam 200–300 micrograms/kg, and ketamine 5–6 mg/kg (provide sedative premedication)

Cats: *by intramuscular or slow intravenous injection*, diazepam 200 micrograms/kg, and ketamine 10 mg/kg

General anaesthesia, in combination with Medetomidine.

Dogs: *by intramuscular injection*, medetomidine 40 micrograms/kg, followed by ketamine, 5.0–7.5 mg/kg

Cats: *by intramuscular injection*, medetomidine 80 micrograms/kg, followed by ketamine, 2.5–7.5 mg/kg

by intravenous injection, medetomidine 40 micrograms/kg with ketamine 1.25 mg/kg

General anaesthesia, in combination with Butorphanol and Medetomidine.

Dogs: *by intramuscular injection*, butorphaonol 100 micrograms/kg with medetomidine 25 micrograms/kg, followed 15 minutes later by ketamine 5 mg/kg

Cats: *by intramuscular injection*, butorphanol 400 micrograms/kg and medetomidine 80 micrograms/kg and ketamine 5 mg/kg

by intravenous injection, butorphanol 100 micrograms/kg and medetomidine 40 micrograms/kg and ketamine 1.25–2.5 mg/kg

Sedation or general anaesthesia, in combination with Midazolam.

Dogs: *by intravenous injection*, midazolam 500 micrograms/kg, and ketamine 10 mg/kg

Cats: *by intramuscular injection*, midazolam 200 micrograms/kg, and ketamine 10 mg/kg

by intravenous injection, midazolam 200 micrograms/kg, and ketamine 5 mg/kg

General anaesthesia, in combination with Romifidine.

Horses: *by intravenous injection*, romifidine 100 micrograms/kg, followed 5–10 minutes later by ketamine 2.2 mg/kg

General anaesthesia, in combination with Xylazine.

Horses: xylazine, *by slow intravenous injection*, 1.1 mg/kg, followed 2 minutes later by ketamine, *by intravenous injection*, 2.2 mg/kg

Dogs: *by intramuscular injection*, xylazine 1–2 mg/kg, followed 10 minutes later by ketamine 10–15 mg/kg

Cats: *by intramuscular injection*, xylazine 1.1 mg/kg, followed by ketamine 22 mg/kg

Donkeys♦, primates, exotic animals♦: contact manufacturer for further information

POM **Ketaset** (Fort Dodge) *UK*
Injection, ketamine (as hydrochloride) 100 mg/mL, for **horses, dogs, cats, primates**; 10 mL, 50 mL
Withdrawal Periods. Should not be used in **horses** intended for human consumption

POM **Vetalar-V** (Pharmacia & Upjohn) *UK*
Injection, ketamine (as hydrochloride) 100 mg/mL, for *horses, dogs, cats, primates*; 10 mL, 20 mL
Withdrawal Periods. Should not be used in *horses* intended for human consumption

Australia

Indications. General anaesthesia
Contra-indications. Hepatic or severe renal impairment, cerebral trauma, hypovolaemia, cardiovascular insufficiency, myocardial damage, epilepsy
Side-effects. Salivation, vocalisation, emesis, muscle twitching, dyspnoea, respiratory depression
Warnings. Use low dosage in cats with renal impairment; cat's eyes remain open during anaesthesia; care with use for caesarian section
Dose. *Horses:* by intravenous injection, xylazine 1.1 mg/kg, followed by ketamine 2.2 mg/kg
Cattle: by intravenous injection, 2 mg/kg with xylazine
Sheep: by intramuscular injection, 22 mg/kg with xylazine
Pigs: by intramuscular injection, 10–15 mg/kg with xylazine
Dogs: by intravenous injection, 11 mg/kg with xylazine
Cats: by intramuscular injection, 11–44 mg/kg
Other species: contact manufacturer for further information

Ketamav 100 (Mavlab) *Austral.*
Injection, ketamine (as hydrochloride) 100 mg/mL, for *horses, cats, birds, echidnas, marsupials, reptiles , zoo felidae*
Withdrawal Periods. Should not be used in *horses* intended for human consumption

Ketamil (Ilium) *Austral.*
Injection, ketamine (as hydrochloride) 100 mg/mL, for *cats, turtles, tortoises, ferrets*

Ketamine Injection (Parnell) *Austral.*
Injection, ketamine (as hydrochloride) 100 mg/mL, for *horses, cattle, pigs, sheep, dogs, cats, goats, reptiles, birds, wombat, koala, camel, deer*
Withdrawal Periods. *Cattle, sheep, pigs*: slaughter 28 days. *Poultry*: should not be used in poultry intended for human consumption, should not be used in poultry producing eggs for human consumption

Ketapex (Apex) *Austral.*
Injection, ketamine hydrochloride 100 mg/mL, for *cats*

Ketaset (Fort Dodge) *Austral.*
Injection, ketamine (as hydrochloride) 100 mg/mL, for , *horses, cats, birds, echidnas, marsupials, reptiles , zoo felidae*
Withdrawal Periods. Should not be used in *horses* intended for human consumption.

Ketavet 100 (Delvet) *Austral.*
Injection, ketamine (as hydrochloride) 100 mg/mL, for *cats*

Eire

Indications. General anaesthesia
Contra-indications. Ophthalmic surgery, hypertension, hepatic or renal impairment, cardiovascular insufficiency
Side-effects. Salivation, vocalisation, emesis, muscle twitching, dyspnoea, respiratory depression
Warnings. Eyes remain open during anaesthesia; caution in pulmonary disease
Horses: by intravenous injection, xylazine 1.1 mg/kg, followed by ketamine 2.2 mg/kg
Dogs: by intramuscular injection, 10–20 mg/kg with xylazine

by intravenous injection, 5–8 mg/kg with xylazine
Cats: by intramuscular injection, 11–33 mg/kg
Other species: contact manufacturer for further information

Clorketam Injectable Solution (Vetoquinol) *Eire*
Injection, ketamine 10 g/100 mL, ketamine 5 g/100 mL, for *dogs, cats, laboratory animals*

Ketaset Injection (Fort Dodge) *Eire*
Injection, ketamine hydrochloride 100 mg/mL, for *horses, dogs, cats*
Withdrawal Periods. Should not be used in *horses* intended for human consumption

Velalar V (Pharmacia & Upjohn) *Eire*
Injection, ketamine (as hydrochloride) 100 mg/mL, for *horses, dogs, cats, primates*
Withdrawal Periods. *Horses*: slaughter 28 days

New Zealand

Indications. General anaesthesia
Contra-indications. Hepatic or renal impairment, cardiovascular insufficiency
Side-effects. Salivation, cardiovascular stimulation, pupillary dilation, muscle twitching, respiratory depression
Horses: by intravenous injection, xylazine 1.1 mg/kg, followed by ketamine 2.2 mg/kg
Dogs: by intravenous injection, 11 mg/kg with xylazine
Cats: by intramuscular injection, 15–20 mg/kg
by intravenous injection, 5–6 mg/kg
Other species: contact manufacturer for further information

Ketamine Injection (Parnell) *NZ*
Injection, ketamine 100 mg/mL, for *horses, dogs, cats*
Withdrawal Periods. *Horses*: slaughter 28 days

Ketamine Injection (Phoenix) *NZ*
Injection, ketamine hydrochloride 100 mg/mL, for *cats*

Xylaket 15/5 (Phoenix) *NZ*
Injection, xylazine 150 mg/mL (as hydrochloride), ketamine hydrochloride 50 mg/mL, for *deer*
Withdrawal Periods. Slaughter 5 days

USA

Indications. General anaesthesia
Contra-indications. Hepatic or renal impairment, cardiovascular insufficiency
Side-effects. Salivation, emesis, vocalisation, cardiovascular stimulation, muscle twitching, respiratory depression
Warnings. Eyes remain open during anaesthesia
Dose. *Cats: by intramuscular injection*, 11–33 mg/kg
Other species: contact manufacturer for further information

Ketaject (Phoenix) *USA*
Injection, ketamine (as hydrochloride) 100 mg/mL, for *cats, primates*

Keta-Sthetic (Western Veterinary Supply) *USA*
Injection, ketamine (as hydrochloride) 100 mg/mL, for *cats, primates*

Ketamine Hydrochloride Injection (Boehringer Ingelheim Vetmedica, VetTek) *USA*
Injection, ketamine (as hydrochloride) 100 mg/mL, for *cats, primates*

Ketaset (Fort Dodge) *USA*
Injection, ketamine (as hydrochloride) 100 mg/mL, for *cats, primates*

Ketaved (Vedco) *USA*
Injection, ketamine (as hydrochloride) 100 mg/mL, for *cats, primates*

Vetaket Injection (Lloyd) *USA*
Injection, ketamine (as hydrochloride) 100 mg/mL, for *cats, primates*

Vetalar (Fort Dodge) *USA*
Injection, ketamine (as hydrochloride) 100 mg/mL, for *cats, primates*

Vetamine (Schering-Plough) *USA*
Injection, ketamine (as hydrochloride) 100 mg/mL, for *cats, primates*

TILETAMINE with ZOLAZEPAM

Australia

Indications. General anaesthesia
Contra-indications. Pancreatic disease, renal or hepatic impairment, severe cardiac or pulmonary dysfunction, severe hypertension, pregnant animals, caesarian section
Side-effects. Hypothermia, athetoid movements, eye remain open during anaesthesia
Warnings. Reduce dose in renal impairment, debilitated and geriatric animals; Drug Interactions – chloramphenicol in cats
Dose. Expressed as tiletamine + zolazepam
Dogs: *by intramuscular injection*, 6.5–15 mg/kg
by intravenous injection, 5–10 mg/kg
Cats: *by intramuscular injection*, 10–16 mg/kg
by intravenous injection, 5.0–7.5 mg/kg

Telazol (Fort Dodge) *Austral.*
Injection, powder for reconstitution, tiletamine 50 mg/mL, zolazepam 50 mg/mL, for *dogs, cats*

Zoletil 50 (Virbac) *Austral.*
Injection, powder for reconstitution, tiletamine 50 mg/mL, zolazepam 50 mg/mL, for *dogs, cats, wild and zoo animals*

Zoletil 100 (Virbac) *Austral.*
Injection, powder for reconstitution, tiletamine 100 mg/mL, zolazepam 100 mg/mL, for *dogs, cats, wild and zoo animals*

New Zealand

Indications. General anaesthesia
Contra-indications. Pancreatic disease, severe renal or hepatic impairment, cardiac or pulmonary dysfunction, pregnant animals
Side-effects. Salivation with high dosage
Dose. Expressed as tiletamine + zolazepam
Dogs: *by intramuscular injection*, 7–25 mg/kg
Cats: *by intramuscular injection*, 10–15 mg/kg

Zoletil 50 (Virbac) *NZ*
Injection, powder for reconstitution, tiletamine 50 mg/mL, zolazepam 50 mg/mL, for *dogs, cats*

Zoletil 100 (Virbac) *NZ*
Injection, powder for reconstitution, tiletamine 100 mg/mL, zolazepam 100 mg/mL, for *dogs, cats*

USA

Indications. General anaesthesia
Contra-indications. Pancreatic disease, renal impairment, severe cardiac or pulmonary dysfunction, pregnant animals, caesarian section
Side-effects. Hypothermia, athetoid movements, eye remain open during anaesthesia, pain on injection

Warnings. Reduce dose in renal impairment, debilitated and geriatric animals; Drug Interactions – chloramphenicol in cats; phenothiazine derivatives
Dose. Expressed as tiletamine + zolazepam
Dogs: *by intramuscular injection*, 6.6–13.2 mg/kg
Cats: *by intramuscular injection*, 9.7–15.8 mg/kg

Telazol (Fort Dodge) *USA*
Injection, powder for reconstitution, tiletamine 50 mg/mL, zolazepam 50 mg/mL, for *dogs, cats*

6.6.2.5 Metomidate

Metomidate is the methyl analogue of etomidate. Metomidate is not particularly good as a sole anaesthetic agent because analgesia is limited and the animal will respond to stimuli. It is used in combination with azaperone.

6.6.3 Inhalational anaesthetics

Inhalational anaesthetics may be gases or volatile liquids. They can be used for induction and maintenance of anaesthesia, and may be used following induction with an injectable anaesthetic (see section 6.6.2). Halogenated inhalational anaesthetics such as halothane, enflurane, and isoflurane, are the most commonly used agents.

Inhalational anaesthetics are absorbed and excreted unchanged via the lungs although some metabolism does occur for most agents. However, recovery does not depend upon drug metabolism and therefore these agents are useful in species for which there is little information on use of general anaesthetics, because their action will be similar in all mammals. Removal of an overdose of inhalational anaesthetic can be hastened by mechanical ventilation of the lungs.

Humans should not be exposed to inhalational anaesthetics for long periods, even in small doses, and some form of waste gas scavenging is essential when these agents are used. The inhalational anaesthetics should always be administered using an appropriate precision vaporiser.

Halothane is the most commonly used halogenated inhalational anaesthetic. It is a potent agent and the vapour is non-irritant; induction is smooth with little, if any, excitement, although restraint is difficult while holding the mask in position. Halothane provides moderate to good analgesia and muscle relaxation. Adverse effects associated with the use of halothane include vasodilation, hypotension, cardiac arrhythmias, and shivering and tremor on recovery; malignant hyperthermia has been reported in pigs, horses, and dogs. Halothane, enflurane, and isoflurane concentrations in the brain and myocardium can rise quickly if high inspired concentrations are given, producing severe cardiorespiratory depression and cardiac arrest. These adverse effects caused by halothane are dose-dependent and the horse is particularly susceptible. To avoid very high concentrations of halothane, it should be vaporised in a mixture of oxygen and nitrous oxide, which accelerates induction.

Enflurane produces more rapid induction and recovery than halothane because of its lower blood solubility. Cardiovascular depression is greater than that produced by halothane. Enflurane may produce seizure-like electroencephalogram (EEG) activity and should be avoided in epileptic patients. Enflurane is not recommended for horses because cardiovascular depression is severe and recovery is rapid but violent.

Isoflurane has similar physical properties to halothane, but is slightly less soluble in blood and so induction and recovery are more rapid than with halothane or enflurane. In addition less isoflurane is metabolised in the liver (0.2%) than halothane (20%), the vast majority being excreted unchanged via the lungs. Although changes in peripheral arterial blood pressure are similar with both anaesthetic agents, the fall in blood pressure observed with isoflurane is primarily due to vasodilation rather than myocardial depression as is found with halothane. This property, in association with less sensitisation of the myocardium to epinephrine, makes isoflurane the agent of choice in high risk cardiac cases. It does not produce seizure-like changes in EEG activity. Isoflurane may be used in horses; it is not certain whether it offers any real advantages over halothane and there have been reports that recovery may be more violent than with halothane.

Methoxyflurane induction is slow because of its high blood solubility and low saturated vapour pressure. Recovery is also prolonged. The effects of methoxyflurane are similar to halothane. However, it is contra-indicated in animals with renal or hepatic impairment.

Nitrous oxide is a weak anaesthetic and is incapable of producing general anaesthesia when used alone in animals. It is used to supplement other drugs, especially inhalational anaesthetics allowing a significant reduction in their dosage, and provides analgesia and anaesthesia with relatively few adverse effects. It is usually used at the highest possible inspired concentration, between 50% and 70%, with oxygen and an inhalational anaesthetic drug. Induction and recovery with nitrous oxide are rapid.

The main danger when using nitrous oxide is hypoxia. Modern anaesthetic machines have interlocks to shut off the nitrous oxide if the oxygen supply fails. If nitrous oxide is used in rebreathing circuits then an oxygen meter is needed to check that the inspired oxygen concentration does not fall below 30%. Diffusion hypoxia may occur at the end of nitrous oxide anaesthesia and the patient should be allowed to breathe 100% oxygen for 2 to 10 minutes depending on the duration of exposure to nitrous oxide.

In animals anaesthetised via a circle breathing system, nitrous oxide should not be used unless inspiratory oxygen concentration can be measured. In animals with large ventilation:perfusion differences, nitrous oxide should not be used due to the risk of hypoxia.

ENFLURANE

UK

Indications. Inhalational anaesthesia
Contra-indications. Horses (see notes above); animals prone to seizures

Side-effects. See under Halothane and notes above; seizures
Dose. Maintenance of anaesthesia, inspired concentration of 1.5–2.5%

P (H) **Enflurane** (Abbott) *UK*
Enflurane; 250 mL

HALOTHANE

UK

Indications. Inhalational anaesthesia
Contra-indications. Concurrent administration of epinephrine
Side-effects. Cardiovascular and respiratory depression, cardiac arrhythmias, hypotension, vasodilation; see also notes above
Warnings. When anaesthetising an animal with head injury, artificial ventilation may be required to maintain normal carbon dioxide concentration to avoid increase in cerebral blood flow
Dose. Induction of anaesthesia, inspired concentration of 1–7%
Maintenance of anaesthesia, inspired concentration of 0.5–2.0%

P **Fluothane** (Schering-Plough) *UK*
Halothane, for *horses, dogs, cats*; 250 mL
Withdrawal Periods. Should not be used in *horses* intended for human consumption

P **Halothane Vet** (Merial) *UK*
Halothane, for *non food-producing animals, non domesticated mammals, reptiles, and birds*; 250 mL
Withdrawal Periods. Slaughter withdrawal period 28 days, milk withdrawal period 7 days

P **Vetothane** (Virbac) *UK*
Withdrawal Periods. Should not be used in *horses* intended for human consumption

Australia

Indications. Inhalational anaesthesia
Warnings. Drug Interactions – gallamine, tubocurarine, epinephrine; can induce hepatic damage
Dose. Induction of anaesthesia, inspired concentration of 2–4% (small animals), 5–8% (large animals)
Maintenance of anaesthesia, inspired concentration of 0.5–2.0%

Halothane M&B (Merial) *Austral.*
Liquid, halothane, thymol 0.01% (stabilising agent), for *domestic and farm animals and birds, and wild mammals, birds, reptiles*

VCA Halothane (Veterinary Companies of Australia) *Austral.*
Solution, halothane, thymol 0.01% (stabilising agent), for *large and small animals*
Withdrawal Periods. Should not be used in animals producing food for human consumption

Eire

Indications. Inhalational anaesthesia
Side-effects. Cardiovascular and respiratory depression, rarely malignant hyperthermia, delayed uterine involution followng caesarian

Warnings. Drug Interactions – gallamine, tubocurarine, epinephrine
Dose. Induction of anaesthesia, inspired concentration of 2–4%
Maintenance of anaesthesia, inspired concentration of 0.5–2.0%

Halothane-Vet (Merial) *Eire*
Volatile liquid, halothane, for *mammals, birds, reptiles*
Withdrawal Periods. Should not be used in animals intended for human consumption.

USA

Indications. Inhalational anaesthesia
Contra-indications. Obstetrical anaesthesia unless relaxation required
Side-effects. Cardiovascular and respiratory depression, hypothermia, pyrexia, mild hepatic impairment, hypotension, rarely malignant hyperthermia
Warnings. Drug Interactions – aminoglycosides; safety in pregnant animals has not been established
Dose. Induction of anaesthesia, inspired concentration of 2–5%
Maintenance of anaesthesia, inspired concentration of 0.5–2.0%

Halothane, USP (Fort Dodge) *USA*
Inhalational anaesthetic, halothane 250 mL
Withdrawal Periods. Should not be used in animals intended for human consumption

ISOFLURANE

UK

Indications. Inhalational anaesthesia
Contra-indications. Susceptibility to malignant hyperthermia
Side-effects. Cardiovascular and respiratory depression, cardiac arrhythmias, hypotension, vasodilation; see also notes above
Warnings. When anaesthetising an animal with head injury, artificial ventilation may be required to maintain normal carbon dioxide concentration to avoid increase in cerebral blood flow; manufactuer recommends arterial blood pressure be monitored throughout anaesthesia
Dose. Induction of anaesthesia, inspired concentration of 2–5%
Maintenance of anaesthesia, inspired concentration of 0.25–3.0%

POM Isofane (Vericore VP) *UK*
Isoflurane 100%, for *horses, dogs, cats, ornamental birds, reptiles, small mammals*
Withdrawal Periods. Should not be used in *animals* intended for human consumption

POM IsoFlo Vet (Schering-Plough) *UK*
Isoflurane 100%, for *horses, dogs, cats, ornamental birds, reptiles, small mammals*; 100 mL, 250 mL
Withdrawal Periods. Should not be used in *animals* intended for human consumption

POM Isoflurane Vet (Merial) *UK*
Isoflurane 99.9%, for *horses, dogs, cats, ornamental birds*; 100 mL, 250 mL
Withdrawal Periods. Should not be used in *horses* intended for human consumption

USA

Indications. Inhalational anaesthesia
Side-effects. Cardiovascular and respiratory depression, hypotension
Warnings. Drug Interactions – non-depolarising muscle relaxants
Dose. Induction of anaesthesia, inspired concentration of 3–5% (horses); 2–2.5% (dogs)
Maintenance of anaesthesia, inspired concentration of 1.5–1.8%

Aerrane (Fort Dodge) *USA*
Inhalational anaesthetic, isoflurane 99.9%, for *horses, dogs*
Withdrawal Periods. Should not be used in *horses* intended for human consumption

Isoflo (Abbott) *USA*
Inhalational anaesthetic, isoflurane 99.9%, for *horses, dogs*
Withdrawal Periods. Should not be used in *horses* intended for human consumption

Iso-Thesia (Vetus) *USA*
Inhalational anaesthetic, isoflurane 99.9%, for *horses, dogs*
Withdrawal Periods. Should not be used in *horses* intended for human consumption

METHOXYFLURANE

USA

Indications. Inhalational anaesthesia
Side-effects. Occasional mild vomiting
Warnings. Use with caution in hepatic impairment and toxaemia

Metofane (Schering-Plough) *USA*
Inhalational anaesthetic, methoxyflurane 100%, for *wide variety of species*

NITROUS OXIDE

UK

Indications. Inhalational anaesthesia in combination with other inhalational drugs
Warnings. The amount of oxygen used with nitrous oxide should not fall below 30% to prevent hypoxia
Dose. Inspired concentration of 50–70%
Note. Cylinders are painted blue

6.7 Drugs modifying neuromuscular transmission

6.7.1 Non-depolarising muscle relaxants
6.7.2 Depolarising muscle relaxants
6.7.3 Centrally-acting muscle relaxants
6.7.4 Muscle relaxant antagonists

Muscle relaxants are also known as neuromuscular blocking drugs or myoneural blocking drugs. These drugs interfere with transmission at the neuromuscular junction, thereby causing voluntary muscle paralysis or relaxation. Non-depolarising and depolarising muscle relaxants should not be administered together.

In veterinary anaesthesia muscle relaxants facilitate endotracheal intubation and endoscopy, and cause relaxation of skeletal muscle for easier surgical access and reduction of joint dislocation and bone fractures. They allow lighter levels of general anaesthesia to be employed, and are also used to facilitate artificial respiration and reduce movement of horses during induction.

Respiration should always be controlled in animals that have received a muscle relaxant until the drug has either been metabolised or antagonised. On humane grounds, muscle relaxants should given only to animals that are already unconscious.

> Muscle relaxants should only be used by veterinary anaesthetists familiar with their use and where facilities for endotracheal intubation, intermittent positive pressure ventilation, and resuscitation are available

6.7.1 Non-depolarising muscle relaxants

These drugs, also known as competitive muscle relaxants, block neuromuscular transmission by competing with acetylcholine for receptor sites at the neuromuscular junction. The postsynaptic receptors are occupied but the membrane is not depolarised. The action of non-depolarising muscle relaxants may be reversed by anticholinesterases such as neostigmine (see section 6.7.4).

In veterinary anaesthetic practice, these drugs are used mainly for orthopaedic or intrathoracic surgical procedures. **Atracurium** has a duration of action of 30 to 40 minutes in horses, sheep, dogs, and cats, which may be prolonged by hypothermia. The drug has minimal vagolytic or sympatholytic properties. It can be administered to animals with hepatic or renal failure, and is non-cumulative after repeated doses.

Gallamine has a duration of action which varies between the species (see below). Gallamine causes an undesirable tachycardia as a result of its vagolytic action. The drug is excreted unchanged in urine.

Pancuronium has an initial duration of action of 30 to 45 minutes in horses, cattle, sheep, goats, pigs, and cats. Although it does not cause histamine release or significant changes in blood pressure, pancuronium may produce tachycardia, especially in dogs and cats, as a result of its vagolytic properties. Pancuronium is excreted partly unchanged in urine and partly metabolised by the liver.

Vecuronium has a duration of action of approximately 30 minutes in dogs and horses, and 15 minutes in sheep. It does not cause histamine release, sympathetic blockade, or vagolytic actions and therefore has minimal cardiovascular effects. The drug is relatively non-cumulative and is excreted mainly by the liver.

One-fifth to one-tenth of the usual dosage of atracurium or vecuronium may be used to provide muscle relaxation during anaesthesia in dogs suffering from myasthenia gravis;

adequate monitoring of neuromuscular transmission is essential.

ATRACURIUM BESILATE
(Atracurium besylate)

UK

Indications. Non-depolarising muscle relaxant of medium duration

Side-effects. See notes above

Warnings. Inactivated by thiopental and other alkaline solutions; Drug Interactions – see Appendix 1 (muscle relaxants)

Dose. *By slow intravenous injection.*

Horses: initial dose 150 micrograms/kg then increments of 60 micrograms/kg

Sheep, dogs, cats: initial dose 500 micrograms/kg then increments of 200 micrograms/kg

POM (H) **Tracrium** (GlaxoWellcome) *UK*
Injection, atracurium besilate 10 mg/mL; 2.5 mL, 5 mL, 25 mL

CISATRACURIUM

UK

Indications. Non-depolarising muscle relaxant of medium duration

Warnings. Drug Interactions – see Appendix 1 (muscle relaxants)

Dose. *By slow intravenous injection.*

Dogs: 100 micrograms/kg, followed by increments of 20 micrograms/kg

POM (H) **Nimbex** (GlaxoWellcome) *UK*
Injection, cisatracurium (as besilate) 2 mg/mL, 5 mg/mL

GALLAMINE TRIETHIODIDE

UK

Indications. Non-depolarising muscle relaxant of medium duration

Contra-indications. Renal impairment

Side-effects. Tachycardia

Warnings. Drug Interactions – see Appendix 1 (muscle relaxants)

Dose. *By slow intravenous injection.*

Horses: 1 mg/kg, which has an initial duration of action of 20–25 minutes, followed by increments of 200 micrograms/kg

Cattle: 500 micrograms/kg, which has an initial duration of action of 30–40 minutes, followed by increments of 100 micrograms/kg; *calves*: 400 micrograms/kg, which has an initial duration of 4 hours

Sheep: 400 micrograms/kg, which has an initial duration of action of more than 2 hours

Pigs: 4 mg/kg, which has an initial duration of action of 20 minutes, followed by increments of 800 micrograms/kg

Dogs: 1 mg/kg, which has an initial duration of action of 30 minutes, followed by increments of 200 micrograms/kg

Cats: 1 mg/kg, which has an initial duration of action of 15–20 minutes, followed by increments of 200 micrograms/kg

POM (H) **Flaxedil** (Concord) *UK*
Injection, gallamine triethiodide 40 mg/mL; 2 mL

MIVACURIUM

UK

Indications. Non-depolarising muscle relaxant of short duration
Warnings. Drug Interactions – see Appendix 1 (muscle relaxants)
Dose. *By slow intravenous injection.*
Dogs, cats: 30 micrograms/kg, followed by increments of 10 micrograms/kg

POM (H) **Mivacron** (GlaxoWellcome) *UK*
Injection, mivacurium (as chloride) 2 mg/mL

PANCURONIUM BROMIDE

UK

Indications. Non-depolarising muscle relaxant of medium duration
Contra-indications. Hepatic or renal impairment; obesity
Side-effects. See notes above
Warnings. Drug Interactions – see Appendix 1 (muscle relaxants)
Dose. *By slow intravenous injection.*
Horses: initial dose 60 micrograms/kg then increments of 10 micrograms/kg
Cattle: initial dose 40 micrograms/kg then increments of 8 micrograms/kg
Sheep, goats: initial dose 25 micrograms/kg then increments of 5 micrograms/kg
Pigs: initial dose 100 micrograms/kg then increments of 20 micrograms/kg
Dogs: initial dose 60 micrograms/kg then increments of 10 micrograms/kg
Cats: initial dose 80 micrograms/kg then increments of 20 micrograms/kg

POM (H) **Pavulon** (Organon-Teknika) *UK*
Injection, pancuronium bromide 2 mg/mL; 2 mL

ROCURONIUM BROMIDE

UK

Indications. Non-depolarising muscle relaxant of short duration
Contra-indications. Hepatic or renal impairment
Warnings. Drug Interactions – see Appendix 1 (muscle relaxants)
Dose. *By slow intravenous injection.*
Dogs, cats: 500 micrograms/kg, followed by increments of 200 micrograms/kg

POM (H) **Esmeron** (Organon-Teknika) *UK*
Injection, rocuronium bromide 10 mg/mL

VECURONIUM BROMIDE

UK

Indications. Non-depolarising muscle relaxant of medium duration
Contra-indications. Hepatic impairment
Side-effects. See notes above
Warnings. Drug Interactions – see Appendix 1 (muscle relaxants)
Dose. *By slow intravenous injection.*
Horses: initial dose 100 micrograms/kg then increments of 20 micrograms/kg
Sheep: initial dose 40 micrograms/kg then increments of 10 micrograms/kg
Dogs, cats: initial dose 100 micrograms/kg then increments of 20 micrograms/kg

POM (H) **Norcuron** (Organon-Teknika) *UK*
Injection, powder for reconstitution, vecuronium bromide 10 mg

6.7.2 Depolarising muscle relaxants

The depolarising muscle relaxant **suxamethonium** produces a neuromuscular blockade by depolarising the end-plates at the neuromuscular junction similarly to the action of acetylcholine. Depolarisation is prolonged since disengagement from the receptor site and subsequent breakdown is slower than for acetylcholine. The initial depolarisation causes transient muscular spasm, which may be painful, and is followed by paralysis.

Paralysis is rapid, complete, and predictable, and recovery is spontaneous. Unlike non-depolarising muscle relaxants, the action of suxamethonium cannot be reversed by anticholinesterases.

In veterinary anaesthesia, suxamethonium is used to facilitate endotracheal intubation especially in pigs, cats, and primates. It may also be used by repeated injection for longer surgical procedures and is occasionally administered by infusion.

Suxamethonium is metabolised in the liver. It has a rapid onset and relatively short duration of action. The duration of action may be prolonged with concomitant administration of anticholinesterases (see section 6.7.4), or in animals that have received organophosphorus compounds within the preceding month.

> Muscle relaxants should only be used by veterinary anaesthetists familiar with their use and where facilities for endotracheal intubation, intermittent positive pressure ventilation, and resuscitation are available

SUXAMETHONIUM CHLORIDE
(Succinylcholine chloride)

UK

Indications. Depolarising muscle relaxant of short duration

Contra-indications. Hepatic impairment
Side-effects. See notes above
Warnings. Drug Interactions – see Appendix 1 (muscle relaxants) and notes above
Dose. *By slow intravenous injection.*
Horses: 100 micrograms/kg produces paralysis for up to 5 minutes
Cattle, sheep: 20 micrograms/kg produces paralysis for 6–8 minutes
Pigs: 2 mg/kg produces paralysis for 2–3 minutes
Dogs: 300 micrograms/kg produces paralysis for 25–30 minutes
Cats: 1.5 mg/kg produces paralysis for 5 minutes
Primates: 1 mg/kg produces paralysis for 5 minutes

POM Ⓗ **Anectine** (GlaxoWellcome) *UK*
Injection, suxamethonium chloride 50 mg/mL; 2 mL

POM Ⓗ **Suxamethonium Chloride** (Non-proprietary) *UK*
Injection, suxamethonium chloride 50 mg/mL; 2 mL

6.7.3 Centrally-acting muscle relaxants

Guaifenesin is a centrally-acting muscle relaxant which acts by blocking the internuncial neurones within the brain stem and the spinal cord. Relaxation of skeletal muscle and sedation are seen. Solutions containing guaifenesin greater than 150 mg/mL may cause haemolysis, although it may not be of clinical significance.

Methocarbamol is a centrally acting skeletal muscle relaxant which acts on the internuncial neurones of the spinal cord resulting in reduced skeletal muscle hyperactivity without alteration in muscle tone.

GUAIFENESIN
(Guaiphenesin)

Australia
Indications. Muscle relaxation in intravenous anaesthesia
Contra-indications. Pregnant animals unless fetal viability is not of importance
Side-effects. Thrombophlebitis; carbonate crystalluria with high dosage; subclinical haemolysis
Warnings. Avoid extravascular injection
Dose. *Horses: by slow intravenous injection,* 80–100 mg/kg

Giafen (Parnell) *Austral.*
Injection, guaifenesin 100 mg/mL, for *horses*
Withdrawal Periods. *Horses*: should not be used in horses intended for human consumption

New Zealand
Indications. Muscle relaxation
Warnings. Avoid extravascular injection
Dose. *Horses: by slow intravenous injection,* 80–100 mg/kg

Giafen (Parnell) *NZ*
Injection, guaifenesin 100 mg/mL, for *horses*

USA
Indications. Muscle relaxation in intravenous anaesthesia
Contra-Indications. Use without facilities for endotracheal intubation, intermittent positive pressure ventilation, and resuscitation available
Warnings. Drug Interactions – physostigmine; avoid extravascular injection; use with care in anaemia, hypovolaemia, cardiac or respiratory impairment
Dose. *Horses: by slow intravenous injection,* 110 mg/kg

Guaifenesin Injection (Butler) *USA*
Injection, guaifenesin 50 mg/mL, for *horses*
Withdrawal Periods. Should not be used in *horses* intended for human consumption

Guailaxin (Fort Dodge) *USA*
Injection, powder for reconstitution, guaifenesin 50 mg/mL, for *horses*
Withdrawal Periods. Should not be used in *horses* intended for human consumption

METHOCARBAMOL

Australia
Indications. Muscle relaxation
Contra-indications. Renal impairment
Side-effects. Salivation, vomiting, ataxia, muscle weakness with high dosage
Warnings. Safety in pregnant animals has not been established; avoid extravascular injection
Dose. *Horses*: by intravenous injection, 4.4–55 mg/kg
Dogs, cats: by mouth, initial dose, 132 mg/kg then 55–132 mg/kg daily
by intravenous injection, 44–220 mg/kg

Robaxin (Pharmtech) *Austral.*
Injection, methocarbamol 100 mg/mL, for *horses, cats, dogs*
Withdrawal Periods. *Horses*: should not be used in horses intended for human consumption.

Robaxin (Pharmtech) *Austral.*
Tablets, methocarbamol 500 mg, for *cats, dogs*

New Zealand
Indications. Muscle relaxation
Contra-indications. Renal impairment
Side-effects. Salivation, vomiting, ataxia, muscle weakness with high dosage
Dose. *Horses*: by intravenous injection, 4.4–55 mg/kg
Dogs, cats: by mouth, initial dose, 132 mg/kg then 55–132 mg/kg daily
by intravenous injection, 44–220 mg/kg

Robaxin Injectable (Bomac) *NZ*
Injection, methocarbamol 100 mg/mL, for *horses, dogs, cats*
Withdrawal Periods. *Horses*: slaughter 28 days

Robaxin Tablets (Bomac) *NZ*
Tablets, methocarbamol 500 mg, for *dogs, cats*

USA
Indications. Muscle relaxation
Contra-indications. Renal impairment
Side-effects. Salivation, vomiting, ataxia, muscle weakness with high dosage

Warnings. Safety in pregnant animals has not been established; avoid extravascular injection
Dose. *Horses*: *by intravenous injection*, 4.4–55 mg/kg
Dogs, cats: *by mouth*, initial dose, 132 mg/kg then 66–132 mg/kg daily
by intravenous injection, 44–330 mg/kg

Robaxin-V (Fort Dodge) *USA*
Injection, methocarbamol 100 mg/mL, for *dogs, cats, horses*
Withdrawal Periods. *Horses*: should not be used in horses intended for human consumption

Robaxin-V (Fort Dodge) *USA*
Tablets, methocarbamol 500 mg, for *dogs, cats*

6.7.4 Muscle relaxant antagonists (Anticholinesterases)

Anticholinesterases inhibit the hydrolysis of acetylcholine by cholinesterases. Consequently, acetylcholine accumulates and its action is prolonged. Anticholinesterase drugs reverse the effects of the non-depolarising muscle relaxant drugs, but they prolong the duration of action of the depolarising muscle relaxants.

These drugs are used to antagonise the neuromuscular block of non-depolarising muscle relaxants (see section 6.7.1), and are preferably administered only on the return of muscular activity as determined by a nerve stimulator. Clinical signs such as discernible diaphragmatic movement or an increase in jaw tone may also be used to indicate the return of neuromuscular activity. Before administration of an anticholinesterase, an antimuscarinic drug (see section 6.6.1) should be given to prevent excessive salivation, bradycardia, vomiting, and diarrhoea. Glycopyrronium, at a dose of 10 micrograms/kg, or atropine, at a dose of 44 micrograms/kg, for all species, are the drugs commonly used. Glycopyrronium causes reduced intensity of tachycardias compared to atropine. Glycopyrronium is also preferred in caesarean section because it does not cross the placenta. If the initial dose of anticholinesterase is repeated, then the dose of atropine or glycopyrronium should also be repeated. However, it would appear that there are species variations and antimuscarinics are not required before edrophonium administration in horses. Antimuscarinics must always be readily available to treat severe cholinergic effects should they occur.

Neostigmine is commonly used for the reversal of non-depolarising neuromuscular block. It acts within 2 minutes of intravenous injection and has a duration of action of at least 30 minutes. **Edrophonium** has a rapid onset and a relatively short duration of action.

Myasthenia gravis is a disease of dogs which is classified as either congenital or acquired. In the congenital form of the disease there is deficiency of the acetylcholine receptor in the post-synaptic membrane. The acquired disease is caused by an immune-mediated disorder of muscle. There is an antibody-mediated autoimmune response directed against nicotinic acetylcholine receptors in skeletal muscle. The disease is characterised by muscle weakness which is exacerbated by exercise and alleviated by rest. Megaoesophagus is commonly present in these animals.

Diagnosis is made on clinical signs and confirmed by the intravenous administration of edrophonium: an improvement of short duration occurs. Electromyography or radioimmunoassay may also be used to confirm the diagnosis. The condition may be treated by thymectomy and by drug therapy. Oral therapy with neostigmine bromide is the treatment of choice. Alternatively pyridostigmine may be used. However it is essential that the dosage should be modified in the light of the response to therapy. Prednisolone (see section 7.2.1) may also be used in relatively high doses♦ of 2 to 5 mg/kg in daily divided doses. The dose of prednisolone is reduced to alternate day therapy if response to treatment is observed. Owner compliance and dedication is important because treatment may need to be continued for 6 to 8 months.

EDROPHONIUM CHLORIDE

UK

Indications. Reversal of non-depolarising muscle relaxants; diagnosis of myasthenia gravis
Side-effects. See notes above
Warnings. Should be administered with an antimuscarinic agent (see notes above)
Dose.
Horses, cattle, sheep, pigs: reversal of muscle relaxant, *by slow intravenous injection*, 0.5–1.0 mg/kg, repeat after 5 minutes if required
Dogs: reversal of muscle relaxant, *by slow intravenous injection*, 0.5–1.0 mg/kg, repeat after 5 minutes if required
Diagnosis of myasthenia gravis, *by intravenous injection*, 100–500 micrograms
Cats: reversal of muscle relaxant, *by slow intravenous injection*, 0.5–1.0 mg/kg, repeat after 5 minutes if required

POM Ⓗ **Edrophonium** (Non-proprietary) *UK*
Injection, edrophonium chloride 10 mg/mL; 1 mL

NEOSTIGMINE

UK

Indications. Reversal of non-depolarising neuromuscular block; treatment of myasthenia gravis
Side-effects. See notes above
Warnings. Should be administered with an antimuscarinic agent (see notes above)
Dose.
Horses, cattle, sheep, pigs: reversal of muscle relaxant, *by slow intravenous injection*, 50 micrograms/kg, repeat after 5 minutes if required
Dogs: reversal of muscle relaxant, *by intravenous injection*, 100 micrograms/kg, repeat after 5 minutes if required
Treatment of myasthenia gravis, *by mouth*, 500 micrograms/kg 3 times daily. Reduce dose according to individual response
Cats: reversal of muscle relaxant, *by intravenous injection*, 100 micrograms/kg, repeat after 5 minutes if required

POM Ⓗ **Neostigmine** (Non-proprietary) *UK*
Tablets, scored, neostigmine bromide 15 mg
Injection, neostigmine metilsulfate 2.5 mg/mL; 1 mL

PYRIDOSTIGMINE BROMIDE

UK
Indications. Treatment of myasthenia gravis
Side-effects. See notes above
Dose. *Dogs*: treatment of myasthenia gravis, *by mouth*, 2 mg/kg 3 times daily. Reduce dose according to individual response

POM Ⓗ **Mestinon** (ICN) *UK*
Tablets, scored, pyridostigmine bromide 60 mg; 200

6.8 Local anaesthetics

Local anaesthetics act by blocking conduction in nerve fibres and other conduction pathways such as myocardial cells. Conduction block in nerves results in muscle paralysis, loss of sensation, or both depending on the type of fibre involved. If sympathetic nerves are blocked, vasodilation and other effects will be observed. The slowing of conduction in myocardial cells after intravenous administration is classified as a toxic effect if the local anaesthetic was intended for intravenous regional anaesthesia, but can be desirable in the treatment of ventricular tachycardias (see section 4.4.1).

Local anaesthetics are often used to block conduction in pain fibres, producing complete analgesia. This may be required for diagnostic purposes or to permit minor surgery. The use of local anaesthetics for the control of traumatic or postoperative pain is limited by anatomical considerations, but they are useful in certain circumstances, such as intercostal nerve blockade.

There are several ways in which local anaesthetics can be used to produce local analgesia.

Perineural injection is the technique used when the precise anatomical position of the nerve supplying the area or region to be anaesthetised is known. A solution of a local anaesthetic is injected as closely as possible to the nerve and conduction in the nerve is blocked as the drug diffuses into the nerve trunk. For example, cornual anaesthesia or cornual nerve block in cattle is produced when the drug is injected subcutaneously about 2.5 cm below the base of the horn or horn bud. In general, only small quantities of drug are needed for perineural blocks.

A *field block* occurs when a solution of a local anaesthetic is injected along a line, blocking conduction in the nerves that pass through the tissue. All regions supplied by the distal sections of these nerves will be anaesthetised. Much more local anaesthetic is required than for perineural injection.

Both perineural injection and field blocks may produce regional anaesthesia.

Epidural and *spinal injections* of local anaesthetics around the spinal cord will block conduction in spinal nerves or the entire spinal cord. Large areas of the body can be anaesthe-tised with small amounts of drug. Anterior epidural anaesthesia is used for surgery on the recumbent animal or extrusion of the penis in bulls. A caudal epidural injection is used mainly to anaesthetise the perineal region because of the problems of producing limb paralysis with higher blocks. It is useful for obstetric operations, surgery on the anal and peri-anal areas, and administering enemas to horses. Xylazine (see section 6.1.3) may be administered by epidural injection♦ in horses to provide sensory anaesthesia with little ataxia. A dose of 170 micrograms/kg bodyweight is administered. For a 500 kg horse the required dose would be 85 mg. The appropriate volume for injection is achieved by using the following dilution: 0.85 mL of a solution containing xylazine 100 mg/mL is diluted to 10 mL in sodium chloride 0.9%. The onset of anaesthesia occurs after 30 to 45 minutes and lasts for at least 3.5 hours.

Intra-articular injection is mainly used as a diagnostic aid in horses to confirm the presence of joint pain. Strict aseptic technique is essential. Excess joint fluid is aspirated before instilling the local anaesthetic and lameness is re-assessed after 5 to 45 minutes. The volume of the solution required depends on the joint size; the equine fetlock (metacarpo- and metatarsophalangeal joint) requires about 10 mL, the coffin joint (distal interphalangeal joint) 6 mL, and the stifle joint (femorotibial and femoropatellar joint) 50 mL.

Intravenous regional anaesthesia (IVRA) is produced when a local anaesthetic is injected intravenously distal to a tourniquet applied to isolate the blood supply to a limb. All sensation in the limb is lost until the tourniquet is released. Prilocaine is recommended for this technique because of its low toxicity.

Surface anaesthesia is application of local anaesthetics directly to the cornea or mucous membranes, producing anaesthesia of the surface layer of tissue. Normal skin is too thick and impervious for most preparations of local anaesthetics to have much effect if applied topically. However, a cream containing lidocaine and prilocaine is available that will anaesthetise skin in about 60 minutes and allow painless venepuncture. An occlusive dressing should be applied over the cream.

The speed of onset of neuronal blockade produced by local anaesthetic drugs is determined by the drug, its concentration, the accuracy of injection, and the size of the nerve. Drugs that are more lipid soluble diffuse more readily through the tissues and nerve trunk. The duration of the block is determined by the type of drug, the amount used, the site of injection, and whether or not a vasoconstrictor has been added. The duration of action of local anaesthetics is increased by adding a vasoconstrictor, usually epinephrine, which decreases the rate of absorption. Potential toxicity from the more slowly metabolised local anaesthetics is also reduced.

Vasoconstrictors such as epinephrine should not be added to solutions used for intra-articular, intravenous, epidural, or intradigital anaesthesia as tissue necrosis and cardiac arrhythmias may occur. Vasoconstrictors should be used with caution in horses because they may cause digital ischaemia when used for lower limb nerve blocks, and the coat colour at the site of injection may turn permanently white.

Local anaesthetics will cause systemic toxicity if excess amounts are used or if absorption is too rapid, which may occur if injected into infected or inflamed tissues. The signs of toxicity seen in animals are convulsions followed by CNS depression.

Inadvertent intravenous injection of local anaesthetics may produce toxic plasma-drug concentrations. If intravenous regional anaesthesia is used, toxicity caused by early tourniquet removal (less than 20 minutes) may be avoided if the tourniquet is loosened for 10 to 15 seconds, retightened for 2 minutes, and the procedure repeated several times before complete removal. Tourniquet application for more than 2 hours is associated with tissue necrosis and lameness.

Bupivacaine has a long duration of action of up to 8 hours. It is therefore useful for spinal or epidural blocks where a prolonged action is required. It is also indicated when local anaesthetics are used for pain relief, for example in intercostal nerve blocks following rib trauma. Bupivacaine has a similar therapeutic index as lidocaine, but with its longer duration of action, blocks should not be repeated within 4 to 6 hours to avoid accumulation and hence toxicity.

Lidocaine is widely used for most applications. It diffuses readily through the tissues and has a rapid onset of action. Duration of action is about 45 minutes without epinephrine and 90 minutes with epinephrine at a concentration of 1 in 200 000 (5 micro-grams/mL). The use of epinephrine is limited as indicated previously and is contra-indicated if lidocaine is used in the treatment of ventricular arrhythmias (see section 4.4.1).

Mepivacaine produces less tissue irritation than lidocaine and has been recommended when intra-articular anaesthesia is required. Its duration of action is similar to that of lidocaine. Mepivacaine does not cause vasodilation and epinephrine is not required to prolong its effect.

Prilocaine is similar to lidocaine but of low toxicity and is preferred for intravenous regional anaesthesia. **Procaine** spreads through tissues less readily than lidocaine and is now rarely used. **Proxymetacaine** and **tetracaine** are used for topical analgesia of the cornea. They produce less initial stinging than other agents (see section 12.7).

BUPIVACAINE HYDROCHLORIDE

UK
Indications. Epidural, field block, and perineural anaesthesia
Contra-indications. Warnings. Should not be used for intravenous regional anaesthesia; care should be taken to avoid intravenous or intra-arterial injection; maximum dose should not exceed 2 mg/kg
Dose. Expressed as bupivacaine hydrochloride 0.5% (5 mg/mL).
Horses, cattle: by perineural injection, 1–2 mL/site
Dogs, cats: by epidural injection, 1 mL/5 kg

POM Ⓗ **Marcain 0.5%** (Astra) *UK*
Injection, bupivacaine hydrochloride 5 mg/mL; 10 mL

LIDOCAINE HYDROCHLORIDE
(Lignocaine hydrochloride)

UK
Indications. Local anaesthesia; arrhythmias (see section 4.4.1)
Warnings. Safety in pregnant animals has not been established; caution in patients with cardiac or hepatic impairment

POM **Intubeaze** (Arnolds) *UK*
Laryngeal spray, lidocaine 2–4 mg/spray, for *cats*; 10 mL
Contra-indications. Hypovolaemia, heart block
Dose. *Cats*: apply 1–2 sprays to back of throat. Allow 30–90 seconds to elapse before attempting intubation

Australia
Indications. Local anaesthesia; arrhythmias
Warnings. Some manufacturers advise use with caution in pregnant animals, patients with cardiac or hepatic impairment
Dose. Expressed as lidocaine 2% (20 mg/mL).
Dosages vary, consult manufactuer's data sheet

Ban-Itch Spray (Apex) *Austral.*
Spray (pump), lidocaine hydrochloride 40 mg/mL, denatonium benzoate 0.1 mg/mL, for *dogs, cats, horses*
Contra-indications. Use within 3 days before racing in horses and dogs

Lignocaine 2% (Delvet) *Austral.*
Injection, lidocaine hydrochloride 20 mg/mL, for *dogs, cats, cattle , horses*

Lignocaine 2% (Ilium) *Austral.*
Injection, lidocaine hydrochloride 20 mg/mL, for *horses, cattle, sheep, dogs, cats*
Withdrawal Periods. Slaughter withdrawal period nil, milk withdrawal period nil

Lignomav (Mavlab) *Austral.*
Injection, lidocaine hydrochloride 20 mg/mL,, for *horses, cattle, dogs, cats*

Eire
Indications. Local anaesthesia
Dose. Expressed as lidocaine 2% (20 mg/mL).
Dosages vary, consult manufactuer's data sheet

Lignavet Injection (Cypharm) *Eire*
Injection, lignocaine hydrochloride 20 mg/mL, for *cattle*
Withdrawal Periods. Slaughter 28 days, milk 7 days

New Zealand
Indications. Local anaesthesia
Dose. Expressed as lidocaine 2% (20 mg/mL).
Dosages vary, consult manufactuer's data sheet

Bomacaine (Bomac) *NZ*
Injection, lidocaine hydrochloride 20 mg/mL, for *horses, cattle, sheep, goats, deer, pigs, dogs, cats*

Lignavet (Novartis) *NZ*
Injection, lidocaine hydrochloride 20 mg/mL, for *large and small animals*

Local (Virbac) *NZ*
Injection, lidocaine hydrochloride 20 mg/mL, for *large and small animals*

Lopaine 2% (Ethical) *NZ*
Injection, lidocaine hydrochloride 20 mg/mL, for *horses, cattle, sheep, goats, pigs, dogs, cats*

Nopaine 2% (Phoenix) *NZ*
Injection, lidocaine hydrochloride 20 mg/mL, for *horses, cattle, deer, dogs*

USA

Indications. Local anaesthesia
Dose. Expressed as lidocaine 2% (20 mg/mL).
Dosages vary, consult manufactuer's data sheet

Lidocaine 2% Injectable (Butler) *USA*
Injection, lidocaine hydrochloride 20 mg/mL, for *cattle, horses, dogs, cats*

Lidocaine HCL 2% (Western Veterinary Supply) *USA*
Injection, lidocaine hydrochloride 20 mg/mL, for *cattle, dogs, horses*

Lidocaine HCL Injectable 2% (Aspen) *USA*
Injection, lidocaine hydrochloride 20 mg/mL, for *cattle, horses, dogs, cats*

Lidocaine HCL Injection 2% (RXV) *USA*
Injection, lidocaine hydrochloride 20 mg/mL, for *horses, cattle, dogs, cats*

Lidocaine Hydrochloride 2% (VetTek) *USA*
Injection, lidocaine hydrochloride 20 mg/mL, for *cattle, horses, dogs*

Lidocaine Hydrochloride Injectable-2% (Phoenix) *USA*
Injection, lidocaine hydrochloride 20 mg/mL, for *cattle, horses, dogs, cats*

Lidocaine Hydrochloride Injection 2% (Pro Labs) *USA*
Injection, lidocaine hydrochloride 20 mg/mL, for *cattle, horses, dogs, cats*

Lidocaine Injectable 2% (Vedco) *USA*
Injection, lidocaine hydrochloride 20 mg/mL, for *cattle, horses, dogs, cats*

Lidoject (Vetus) *USA*
Injection, lidocaine hydrochloride 20 mg/mL, for *cattle, horses, dogs, cats*

LIDOCAINE with EPINEPHRINE
(Lignocaine with adrenaline)

UK

Indications. Field block and perineural anaesthesia, see notes above
Contra-indications. Intra-articular, intravenous, epidural, or intradigital administration
Warnings. Some manufacturers advise do not use or use with caution in pregnant or lactating animals, patients with cardiac or hepatic impairment
Dose. Expressed as lidocaine 2% (20 mg/mL).
Horses: *by field block injection*, maximum 200 mL
Dogs: *by field block injection*, 25–50 mL
by perineural injection, 2–4 mL/site
Cats: *by field block injection*, 5–20 mL

PML Lignavet Plus (Vericore VP) *UK*
Injection, lidocaine hydrochloride 20 mg, epinephrine 11 micrograms/mL, for *horses, dogs, cats*; 100 mL
Withdrawal Periods. Should not be used in *horses* intended for human consumption

POM Lignadrin (Vétoquinol) *UK*
Injection, lidocaine hydrochloride 30 mg, epinephrine (as acid tartrate) 12.5 micrograms/mL, for *horses, dogs, cats*; 100 mL
Withdrawal Periods. Should not be used in *horses* intended for human consumption

PML Lignocaine and Adrenaline (Norbrook) *UK*
Injection, lidocaine hydrochloride 20 mg, epinephrine 12.5 micrograms/mL, for *horses*; 100 mL
Withdrawal Periods. Should not be used in *horses* intended for human consumption

PML Lignol (Arnolds) *UK*
Injection, lidocaine hydrochloride 20 mg, epinephrine 10 micrograms/mL, for *horses, dogs, cats*; 100 mL
Withdrawal Periods. Should not be used in *horses* intended for human consumption

PML Locaine 2% (Animalcare) *UK*
Injection, lidocaine hydrochloride 20 mg, epinephrine 11 micrograms/mL, for *horses, dogs, cats*; 100 mL
Withdrawal Periods. Should not be used in *horses* intended for human consumption

POM Locovetic (Bimeda) *UK*
Injection, lidocaine hydrochloride 30 mg, epinephrine (as bitartrate) 12.5 micrograms/mL, for *horses, dogs, cats*; 100 mL
Withdrawal Periods. Should not be used in *horses* intended for human consumption

Australia

Indications. Local anaesthesia

Lignocaine 2% with Adrenaline 1-100,000 (Ilium) *Austral.*
Injection, lidocaine hydrochloride 20 mg/mL, epinephrine tartrate 0.0182 mg/mL, for *horses, cattle, sheep, dog cats*
Withdrawal Periods. Slaughter withdrawal period nil, milk withdrawal period nil

Eire

Indications. Local anaesthesia
Dosages vary, consult manufactuer's data sheet

Lignavet Plus Injection (Cypharm) *Eire*
Injection, lignocaine hydrochloride 20 mg/mL, adrenaline 0.011 mg/mL, for *horses, cattle, sheep, pigs, dogs, cats*
Withdrawal Periods. *Horses, pigs*: slaughter 28 days. *Cattle, sheep*: slaughter 28 days, milk 7 days

Lignocaine & Adrenaline Injection (Interpharm) *Eire*
Injection, lidocaine hydrochloride 20 mg/mL, epinephrine 0.0125 mg/mL, for *cattle*

Norocaine Injection (Norbrook) *Eire*
Injection, lidocaine hydrochloride 20 mg/mL, epinephrine (as acid tartrate) 0.0125 mg/mL, for *horses, cattle, sheep, pigs*
Withdrawal Periods. *Horses, pigs*: slaughter 28 days. *Cattle, sheep*: slaughter 28 days, milk 7 days

New Zealand

Indications. Local anaesthesia

Anecaine 2 (Phoenix) *NZ*
Injection, lidocaine hydrochloride 20 mg/mL, epinephrine bitartrate 0.036 mg/mL, for *horses, cattle, sheep, goats, pigs, dogs, cats*

USA

Indications. Local anaesthesia

Lidocaine With Epinephrine Injection (Life Science) *USA*
Injection, lidocaine hydrochloride 20 mg/mL, epinephrine 0.01 mg/mL

MEPIVACAINE HYDROCHLORIDE

UK

Indications. Epidural, field block, intra-articular, and perineural anaesthesia
Dose. Expressed as mepivacaine hydrochloride 2% (20 mg/mL). *Horses*: *by field block injection*, 2–5 mL
by intra-articular injection, 4–10 mL
by perineural injection, 2–10 mL depending on site of nerve

POM **Intra-Epicaine** (Arnolds) *UK*
Injection, mepivacaine hydrochloride 20 mg/mL, for *horses*; 10 mL
Withdrawal Periods. Should not be used in *horses* intended for human consumption

Australia
Indications. Epidural anaesthesia
Dose. Expressed as mepivacaine hydrochloride 2% (20 mg/mL).
Horses: *by epidural injection*, 5–20 mL
by intra-articular injection, 10–15 mL
by perineural injection, 3–15 mL

Mepivacaine (RWR) *Austral.*
Injection, mepivacaine hydrochloride 20 mg/mL, for *horses, other species*
Withdrawal Periods. *Horses*: slaughter 28 days

Vetacaine (Ilium) *Austral.*
Injection, mepivacaine hydrochloride 20 mg/mL, for *horses, other species*

USA
Indications. Epidural, field block, intra-articular, and perineural anaesthesia
Dose. Expressed as mepivacaine hydrochloride 2% (20 mg/mL).
Horses: *by field block injection*, 20–50 mL
by epidural injection, 5–20 mL
by intra-articular injection, 10–15 mL
by perineural injection, 3–15 mL
by topical application (spray) to larynx, 25–40 mL

Carbocaine-V (Pharmacia & Upjohn) *USA*
Injection, mepivacaine hydrochloride 2 mg/mL, for *horses*
Withdrawal Periods. Should not be used in *horses* intended for human consumption

---

PRILOCAINE HYDROCHLORIDE

UK
Indications. Caudal epidural, field block, and intravenous regional anaesthesia
Dose. Expressed as prilocaine hydrochloride 0.5% (5 mg/mL).
Cattle: *for intravenous regional anaesthesia*, 20–30 mL
by epidural and field block injection, a suitable volume
Dogs: *for intravenous regional anaesthesia*, 2–3 mL

POM (H) **Citanest 0.5%** (Astra) *UK*
Injection, prilocaine hydrochloride 5 mg/mL; 20 mL, 50 mL

Australia
Indications. Epidural and field block anaesthesia
Dose. Expressed as prilocaine hydrochloride 2% (20 mg/mL).
Horses, cattle: *field block anaesthesia*, up to 20 mL
by epidural injection, 12–150 mL
Dogs, cats: *by field block anaesthesia*, up to 5 mL
by epidural injection, 1 mL/5 kg

Prilocaine (Parnell) *Austral.*
Injection, prilocaine hydrochloride 20 mg/mL, for *dogs, cats, cattle, horses*
Withdrawal Periods. Slaughter withdrawal period nil, milk withdrawal period nil

Prilocaine 2% (Delvet) *Austral.*
Injection, prilocaine hydrochloride 20 mg/mL, for *dogs, cats, cattle, horses*

PROCAINE HYDROCHLORIDE

UK
Indications. Field block and perineural anaesthesia
Contra-indications. Intravenous, intra-articular, or epidural administration; concurrent sulphonamides
Dose. Expressed as procaine hydrochloride 5% (50 mg/mL).
Cattle: *by field block or perineural injection*, 2–5 mL
Dogs, cats: *by field block or perineural injection*, 0.25–1.0 mL

PML **Willcain** (Arnolds) *UK*
Injection, procaine hydrochloride 50 mg, epinephrine 2 micrograms/mL; 100 mL
For field block and perineural injection, including cornual injection

USA
Indications. Epidural anaesthesia
Dose. Expressed as procaine hydrochloride 2.5% (25 mg/mL).
Horses, cattle: *by epidural injection*, 10–50 mL
Dogs, cats: *by epidural injection*, 1.5–6.0 mL

Epidural Injection (Vedco) *USA*
Injection, procaine hydrochloride 25 mg/mL , for *dogs, cats, cattle, horses*

COMPOUND LOCAL ANAESTHETICS

UK
POM (H) **Emla** (Astra) *UK*
Cream, lidocaine 2.5%, prilocaine 2.5%; 5 g, 30 g
For topical anaesthesia; will anaesthetise skin in about 60 minutes. An occlusive dressing should be applied over the cream.

6.9 Antiepileptics

6.9.1 Drugs used in control of epilepsy
6.9.2 Drugs used in status epilepticus

6.9.1 Drugs used in control of epilepsy

Except in certain large breeds of dog, therapy for epilepsy should not be commenced in any animal in which a single isolated seizure has occurred unless it develops into status epilepticus. In all cases, a thorough investigation should be carried out to determine any underlying cause, such as poisoning, hepatic encephalopathy, or hypoglycaemia before diagnosis of epilepsy can be confirmed. Therapy should be directed towards the disorder rather than routine use of antiepileptic drugs. Long-term therapy in horses involves expense, commitment, and a horse which has suffered seizures is unsafe to ride until seizure-free for 6 months without the administration of antiepileptics.

Epilepsy is most common in dogs, although cases do occur in cats, horses, and cattle. In foals, seizures may be associated with neonatal maladjustment syndrome. Some dogs, usually of the large breeds such as Golden Retrievers and

German Shepherds suffer from cluster seizures, that is 3 to 15 seizures in close succession over 24 to 48 hours, followed by an interval of 1 to 3 weeks. In those breeds in which cluster seizures occur, it is advisable to commence therapy with antiepileptic drugs at an early stage for example after one or two seizures.

In dogs it is often difficult to distinguish between generalised (grand mal) and partial (focal) seizures. Primary epilepsy is characterised by seizures that are generalised at the outset. Partial seizures may yield localising signs but often undergo rapid secondary generalisation. Epileptogenic foci within the temporal lobe of the cerebrum may result in psychomotor or behavioural seizures.

Partial seizures are more difficult to control than those that are generalised. There is no clear evidence that any of the antiepileptic drugs have a specific indication for a particular type of seizure in dogs.

The object of treatment is to suppress seizures by maintaining an effective concentration of the drug in plasma and brain tissue and minimising side-effects. Therapy should be started in any dog having seizures at a frequency greater than once every 6 weeks, clusters of seizures more than once every 8 weeks, or recurrent seizures accompanied by aggression. Therapy should also be commenced in any dog suffering from epilepsy in which the seizures, although infrequent, are severe, generalised, and of concern to the owner. Successful control may not mean complete abolition of seizures. Some control is being achieved if there is a significant increase in the time interval between fits.

The dose and the frequency of administration vary with the absorption, metabolism, and half-life of the drug and the species to which it is administered. Absorption is more rapid from an empty stomach. Antiepileptic drugs are mainly lipid soluble and are distributed readily to all tissues, including the nervous system, such that plasma-drug concentrations accurately reflect tissue concentrations.

Control is ideally achieved by the administration of a single drug. Multiple antiepileptic drug therapy does not necessarily give an additive therapeutic effect, but the combination of two drugs with different pharmacological actions may be beneficial. Most antiepileptic drugs are potent liver enzyme inducers, enhancing their own metabolism and the metabolism of other drugs.

Sudden withdrawal of therapy may precipitate severe rebound seizures and should be avoided. In a dog that has not suffered a seizure for 6 to 12 months, a very gradual reduction in dosage may be attempted. Any change to another drug should be made with similar caution, withdrawing the first drug only when the new regimen has largely been established.

Patients should be monitored regularly during therapy to allow early detection of hepatotoxicity. The determination of plasma-drug concentrations is the only way to assess whether the administration regimen is appropriate. Routine assays of some antiepileptics including phenobarbital, primidone, potassium bromide, and phenytoin are commercially available.

Apparent failure of therapy may be caused by drug tolerance or by concurrent disease affecting drug absorption. Care is needed when prescribing drugs to epileptics for conditions unrelated to the seizures because they may alter the absorption or metabolism of the antiepileptic drugs. Alternatively, owner non-compliance or inadequate prescribing may affect therapeutic efficacy. Incorrect diagnosis or the existence of refractory epilepsy will also lead to apparent failure of treatment.

Agents such as acepromazine and evening primrose oil, which lower the seizure threshold should not be administered to epileptic patients.

Phenobarbital is the drug of choice for the treatment of canine epilepsy and is both effective and safe to use in cats, cattle, and horses. The half-life of phenobarbital in dogs varies from 47 to 74 hours so that therapy for 2 to 3 weeks is required to achieve a steady state plasma-drug concentration; the therapeutic plasma-phenobarbital concentration is within the range 15 to 45 micrograms/mL, although it is advisable to aim for 25 to 35 micrograms/mL initially and increase the dose, if required, according to response.

In suckling and weanling foals, phenobarbital may be used to control seizures and then continued as maintenance therapy for 3 to 6 months. Without changing the amount administered, the dose in mg/kg is slowly reduced as the foal grows and gains weight.

Methylphenobarbital may be administered as an alternative to phenobarbital. It is less sedative and appears to have better anticonvulsant activity than phenobarbital. It can be substituted for phenobarbital in rare cases of paradoxical hyperactivity occuring with phenobarbital therapy.

Pentobarbital 200 mg/mL has been used in large animals for sedation in the treatment of tetany caused by hypomagnesaemia. Preparations intended for euthanasia (see section 6.10) have been used but may not be sterile; if used, the veterinarian must take full responsibility.

Primidone is commonly used in dogs. Approximately 85% of the antiepileptic activity of primidone is achieved by its phenobarbital metabolite, and it is therefore illogical to give primidone and phenobarbital together. The half-life of primidone in dogs is between 5 and 10 hours. The rate of metabolic conversion increases after 14 days of treatment and results in lower plasma-drug concentrations. Initially, primidone therapy may cause temporary ataxia and depression. Thus it is recommended that therapy be commenced at low doses and then gradually increased over several weeks. Primidone is more hepatotoxic than phenobarbital.

Phenytoin has a half-life of only 3 to 4 hours in the dog, but 24 to 100 hours in the cat and can cause toxicity in this species. Absorption and metabolism of phenytoin are variable, and it is difficult to achieve therapeutic plasma-drug concentrations in dogs because of its rapid metabolism. Absorption of phenytoin is enhanced and gastro-intestinal disturbances minimised if the drug is given with food.

Diazepam (see section 6.9.2) has antiepileptic effects but its short half-life renders it unsuitable for maintenance therapy in canine epilepsy. Oral administration of diazepam has a bioavailability of only 2 to 3%. Its metabolites have only about one-third the anticonvulsant activity of unchanged diazepam. In cats the half-life of diazepam is 15 to 20 hours so that in this species it may be used for oral therapy; it is used at a dose of 1 to 5 mg 2 to 3 times daily increasing or decreasing the dose by 0.5 to 2.0 mg increments according to response.

Clonazepam (see section 6.9.2) is more useful than diazepam for oral therapy in canine epilepsy because its half-life is dose-dependent and increases with the duration of drug administration. It is used at a dose of 100 to 500 micrograms/kg 3 times daily. Many dogs develop tolerance to clonazepam after about 6 weeks.

Sodium valproate also has a short half-life in the dog making it impossible to maintain therapeutic plasma concentrations. However, clinical trials have indicated that it may be effective in animals refractory to other medication, particularly when it is given in conjunction with another antiepileptic drug such as phenobarbital.

Ethosuximide is an antiepileptic suitable for use in dogs. Its primary indication is in the treatment of petit mal episodes, or absence seizures, which are rare in dogs. Some success is also reported for the use of ethosuximide in the control of the flexor spasms (often called myoclonus) of distemper virus infection in dogs.

Potassium bromide may be used as an adjunct to phenobarbital therapy when full control has not been achieved. Oral administration is well tolerated and in dogs the therapeutic serum concentration is 500 to 2000 mg/litre, although the steady state plasma-drug concentration is not reached until 4 to 5 months after the start of therapy. In some dogs, a dose of 15 mg/kg may give rise to brominism which may occur some months after treatment because of the very long half-life of potassium bromide. Careful clinical observation and regular monitoring of serum-bromide concentration is essential. Potassium bromide is also occasionally used in horses.

ETHOSUXIMIDE

UK
Indications. Petit mal in dogs; flexor spasms associated with canine distemper
Contra-indications. Pregnant animals
Warnings. Abrupt cessation of therapy may precipitate seizures or status epilepticus
Dose. *Dogs*: *by mouth,* initial dose 40 mg/kg once then 15–25 mg/kg 3 times daily

POM (H) **Emeside** (LAB) *UK*
Capsules, ethosuximide 250 mg; 112
Syrup, ethosuximide 50 mg/mL; 200 mL

POM (H) **Zarontin** (Parke-Davis) *UK*
Capsules, ethosuximide 250 mg; 50, 500
Syrup, ethosuximide 50 mg/mL; 300 mL

METHYLPHENOBARBITAL
(Methylphenobarbitone)

UK
Indications. Epilepsy
Contra-indications. Hepatic impairment
Side-effects. Transient sedation; polyphagia, polydipsia, and polyuria; weight gain; paradoxical hyperactivity may occur
Warnings. Abrupt cessation of therapy may precipitate seizures or status epilepticus
Dose. *Dogs: by mouth,* 1–5 mg/kg twice daily

CD (H) **Prominal** (Sanofi-Synthelabo) *UK*
Tablets, methylphenobarbital 30 mg, 60 mg, 200 mg; 100

PHENOBARBITAL
(Phenobarbitone)

UK
Indications. Epilepsy; status epilepticus◆ (see section 6.9.2); behaviour modification◆ (see section 6.11.7)
Contra-indications. Pregnant animals, nursing bitches, hepatic impairment
Side-effects. Occasionally transient polyphagia, polyuria, polydipsia, sedation, paradoxical hyperactivity
Warnings. Drug Interactions – see Appendix 1. Hepatic function should be monitored before and during treatment. Abrupt cessation of therapy may precipitate seizures or status epilepticus
Dose. Epilepsy, *by mouth.*
Horses◆: 4–10 mg/kg twice daily
Dogs: initial dose, 2–5 mg/kg daily in 2 divided doses
Cats◆: 1.5–5.0 mg/kg twice daily

Note. For therapeutic purposes phenobarbital and phenobarbital sodium may be considered equivalent in effect

CD **Epiphen** (Vétoquinol) *UK*
Tablets, phenobarbital 30 mg, 60 mg, for *dogs*; 1000

CD (H) **Phenobarbital** (Non-proprietary) *UK*
Tablets, phenobarbital 15 mg, 30 mg, 60 mg
Elixir, phenobarbital 3 mg/mL in a vehicle containing alcohol 38%; 100 mL

CD (H) **Phenobarbital Sodium** (Non-proprietary) *UK*
Injection, phenobarbital sodium 200 mg/mL; 1 mL
Note. phenobarbital injection 200 mg/mL must be diluted 1 in 10 with water for injection before intravenous injection

Australia
Indications. Epilepsy
Side-effects. Sedation, ataxia, polyphagia, polyuria, polydipsia, prolonged administration may cause hepatic impairment
Warnings. Use with caution in pregnancy and hepatic impairment; reduce dose in geriatric patients with severe respiratory insufficiency; drug tolerance may develop; Drug Interactions – drugs metabolised by hepatic microsomal enzymes
Dose. *Dogs: by mouth,* 5–10 mg/kg daily

Epiphen (Hi-Perform) *Austral.*
Tablets, phenobarbital 100 mg, for *dogs*

Phenomav (Mavlab) *Austral.*
Tablets, phenobarbital 100 mg, for *dogs*

PHENYTOIN SODIUM

UK

Indications. Epilepsy
Contra-indications. Cats, see notes above; hepatic impairment; pregnant animals
Side-effects. Transient ataxia, gastro-intestinal disturbance, peripheral neuropathy, hepatotoxicity
Warnings. Abrupt cessation of therapy may precipitate seizures or status epilepticus; Drug Interactions – see Appendix 1
Dose. *Dogs: by mouth,* 10–35 mg/kg 3 times daily given with food; adjust dose according to the patient's response and serum-phenytoin concentration

POM (H) **Phenytoin** (Non-proprietary) *UK*
Tablets, coated, phenytoin sodium 50 mg, 100 mg
Capsules, phenytoin sodium 50 mg, 100 mg

POM (H) **Epanutin** (Parke-Davis) *UK*
Capsules, phenytoin sodium 25 mg, 50 mg, 100 mg, 300 mg; 20

Australia

Indications. Tying-up syndrome
Side-effects. Sedation, ataxia, rarely seizures
Warnings. Safety in pregnant animals has not been established; use with caution in hepatic impairment; Drug Interactions – highly-protein bound drugs
Dose. *Horses: by mouth,* 6 mg/kg twice daily for 2 days, then 4 mg/kg twice daily for 8 days

Rexin Oral Paste for Horses (Parnell) *Austral.*
Oral paste, phenytoin 184 mg/mL, for *horses*
Withdrawal Periods. *Horses:* slaughter 28 days

POTASSIUM BROMIDE

UK

Indications. Epilepsy, used as an adjunct to phenobarbital
Side-effects. Somnolence; ataxia; polyphagia; polydipsia; gastro-intestinal irritation (give with food)
Warnings. Abrupt cessation of therapy may precipitate seizures or status epilepticus; rarely potassium bromide may contribute to the development of pancreatitis
Dose. See preparation details

Epilease (Vet Plus)
Capsules, potassium bromide 985 mg, for *dogs, cats*
Dose. *By mouth,* 50–80 mg/kg once daily
Adjunct to phenobarbital, 20–40 mg/kg

KBr Tablets (Genitrix)
Tablets, scored, potassium bromide 325 mg
Dose. *Dogs: by mouth,* (20 kg body-weight) 325 mg twice daily

Potassium Bromide Powder
Oral solution, prepared from Potassium Bromide BP powder 250 mg/mL syrup
Dose. *Horses: by mouth,* 10–15 mg/kg twice daily

Australia

Indications. Epilepsy, used as an adjunct to phenobarbital
Contra-indications. Seizures due to cerebral ischaemia, hysteria, neoplasia, toxaemia, hypothermia, hypoglycaemia, hypocalcaemia; renal impairment; pregnant animals
Side-effects. Sedation; ataxia; hindlimb weakness, aggression or hyperactivity; shivering; vomiting; diarrhoea; skin eruptions; polyphagia; polydipsia; polyuria; rarely hypothyroidism; rarely pancreatitis
Warnings. Abrupt cessation of therapy may precipitate seizures or status epilepticus; reduce dose of phenobarbital by 50% 2 days before starting treatment
Dose. *Dogs: by mouth,* 20–40 mg/kg daily

Bromapex (Apex) *Austral.*
Oral liquid, potassium bromide 250 mg/mL, for *dogs*

Epibrom (Hi-Perform) *Austral.*
Tablets, potassium bromide 200 mg, for *dogs*

PRIMIDONE

USA

Indications. Epilepsy
Contra-indications. Cats
Side-effects. Transient ataxia, polydipsia, polyuria, polyphagia
Warnings. Abrupt cessation of therapy may precipitate seizures or status epilepticus; chronic treatment may cause hepatotoxicity; megaloblastic anaemia
Dose. *Dogs: by mouth,* 55 mg/kg daily

Neurosyn (Boehringer Ingelheim Vetmedica) *USA*
Tablets, primidone 250 mg, for *dogs*

Primidone (Butler, Vedco, Western Veterinary Supplies) *USA*
Tablets, primidone 250 mg, for *dogs*

Primidone (Fort Dodge) *USA*
Tablets, primidone 50 mg, 250 mg, for *dogs*

Primitabs (Vetus) *USA*
Tablets, primidone 250 mg, for *dogs*

SODIUM VALPROATE

UK

Indications. Epilepsy
Side-effects. Sedation, hepatopathy
Warnings. Abrupt cessation of therapy may precipitate seizures or status epilepticus
Dose. *Dogs: by mouth,* 60 mg/kg 3 times daily
When sodium valproate and phenobarbital are used in combination, the dose of each drug should be reduced by 33–50% depending on plasma-drug concentrations and clinical signs

POM (H) **Sodium Valproate** (Non-proprietary) *UK*
Tablets, e/c, sodium valproate 200 mg, 500 mg
Oral solution, sodium valproate 40 mg/mL; 100 mL

POM (H) **Epilim** (Sanofi-Synthelabo) *UK*
Tablets, (crushable) scored, sodium valproate 100 mg; 100

6.9.2 Drugs used in status epilepticus

The occurrence of repeated seizures without intervening periods of consciousness is called status epilepticus. Animals that suffer from cluster seizures are at particular risk of developing status epilepticus. This is an emergency situation that requires prompt and appropriate therapy to avoid serious brain damage and death. If the cause of seizures is known or suspected to be due to hypoglycaemia, hypocalcaemia, or thiamine deficiency, then appropriate therapy should be instituted. Once the seizures are controlled, adequate ventilation must be maintained.

If the cause is unknown, the first priority is to administer an antiepileptic drug. **Diazepam** and **clonazepam** cross the blood-brain barrier more quickly than other antiepileptics, hence their value in treating status epilepticus. Diazepam, given intravenously, is the drug of choice (although clonazepam is more potent). It is available in a solvent-based preparation and as an oil-in-water emulsion. The solvent-based preparation may be painful on intravenous injection and cause damage to vessel intima resulting in thrombophlebitis. The solvent-based preparation is even more painful on intramuscular injection with slow absorption and therefore should not be used by this route. The emulsion preparation is less irritant by intravenous injection but is not suitable for intramuscular injection. Diazepam is only slightly soluble and it is important to avoid crystallisation in intravenous infusions (see preparation details).

Neither diazepam nor clonazepam are authorised for veterinary use in the UK but, nethertheless, they are the most suitable drugs to administer in the first instance in any case of status epilepticus in dogs or cats.

If diazepam is not effective then **pentobarbital sodium** (see section 6.6.2.1) should be administered intravenously. A dose of 13 mg/kg may be administered to dogs. Overmedication should be avoided, and only enough drug administered to suppress the seizures.

Phenobarbital sodium (see section 6.9.1) is slower in its action than pentobarbital but has been used intravenously subsequent to the initial control. In a dog that has not previously received oral phenobarbital, 3 to 6 mg per hour, as a diluted solution, should be administered intravenously. If the patient is on long-term oral phenobarbital therapy before the onset of status epilepticus, the drug may be administered by intravenous injection at a dose equivalent to the oral dose routinely given. Thereafter, the dose of phenobarbital should be administered according to the patient's response.

CLONAZEPAM

UK

Indications. Status epilepticus; epilepsy (see section 6.9.1)
Contra-indications. Pregnant animals
Side-effects. Sedation at high doses
Dose. *Dogs*: status epilepticus, *by intravenous injection*, 50–200 micrograms/kg

POM Ⓗ **Rivotril** (Roche) *UK*
Tablets, scored, clonazepam 500 micrograms, 2 mg; 100, 500
Injection, for dilution, clonazepam 1 mg/mL; 1 mL. To be diluted immediately before use

DIAZEPAM

UK

Indications. Status epilepticus; epilepsy (see section 6.9.1); convulsions caused by poisoning (see Treatment of poisoning); urinary retention (see section 9.3); behaviour modification (see section 6.11.3)
Contra-indications. Hepatic impairment
Side-effects. Respiratory depression at high doses
Warnings. Diazepam potentiates phenobarbital and may precipitate respiratory and cardiovascular collapse; Drug Interactions – see Appendix 1
Dose. Status epilepticus.

Horses, cattle: *by slow intravenous injection*, 25–100 mg doses according to response, followed by phenobarbital, *by intravenous injection*, 5 mg/kg

foals: *by slow intravenous injection*, 5–10 mg doses according to response, followed by phenobarbital, *by intravenous injection*, 9 mg/kg

Dogs, cats: *by intravenous injection*, 5–50 mg given in 5–10 mg doses, followed *by slow intravenous infusion*, 2–5 mg/hour in glucose 5% intravenous infusion

POM Ⓗ **Diazepam** (Non-proprietary) *UK*
Tablets, scored, diazepam 2 mg, 5 mg, 10 mg
Oral solution, diazepam 400 micrograms/mL; 100 mL

POM Ⓗ **Diazemuls** (Dumex) *UK*
Injection (emulsion), diazepam 5 mg/mL; 2 mL
Note. If used for intravenous infusion, dilute to a maximum concentration of 200 mg in 500 mL of glucose 5% or 10% intravenous infusion. Allow not more than 6 hours between addition and completion of administration.

POM Ⓗ **Valium** (Roche) *UK*
Injection (solution), diazepam 5 mg/mL; 2 mL
Note. If used for intravenous infusion, dilute to a maximum concentration of 40 mg in 500 mL of glucose 5% intravenous infusion or sodium chloride 0.9% intravenous infusion. Allow not more than 6 hours between addition and completion of administration.

Australia

Indications. Status epilepticus; epilepsy; convulsions caused by poisoning; pre-anaesthetic medication
Contra-indications. Pregnant animals
Warnings. Avoid injection into small veins and intra-arterial injection
Dose. *Horses*: pre-anaesthetic medication, *by slow intravenous injection*, 10 micrograms/kg, followed by xylazine and ketamine
Foals: convulsions in neonatal foals, *by slow intravenous injection*, 100–400 micrograms/kg
Dogs: pre-anaesthetic medication, *by intravenous injection*, 200–600 micrograms/kg
Status epilepticus, *by slow intravenous infusion*, 5 mg, followed by pentobarbital if required
Strychnine poisoning, *by slow intravenous infusion*, 1 mg/kg, followed by the same dose given by intramuscular injection

Pamlin Injection (Parnell) *Austral.*
Injection, diazepam 5 mg/mL, for *horses, dogs*
Withdrawal Periods. *Horses*: slaughter 28 days

New Zealand

Indications. Status epilepticus; epilepsy; convulsions caused by poisoning; pre-anaesthetic medication; appetite stimulation
Contra-indications. Pregnant animals;
Warnings. Avoid injection into small veins and intra-arterial injection
Dose. *Horses*: pre-anaesthetic medication, *by intramuscular injection*, 10 micrograms/kg, followed by xylazine and ketamine
Foals: convulsions in neonatal foals, *by slow intravenous injection*, 100–400 micrograms/kg
Dogs: pre-anaesthetic medication, *by intramuscular or slow intravenous injection*, 200–600 micrograms/kg
Epilepsy, *by slow intravenous infusion*, 1 mg/kg

Pamlin (Parnell) *NZ*
Injection, diazepam 5 mg/mL, for *horses, dogs*
Withdrawal Periods. *Horses*: slaughter 28 days

6.10 Drugs used for euthanasia

Euthanasia of animals is carried out in veterinary practice. Whatever the reason for euthanasia, once the veterinarian is satisfied that this is the only option, and that the client fully understands the situation and gives written consent, an agent for euthanasia is chosen to satisfy several criteria. Euthanasia should be as painless as possible and the procedure should not cause undue anxiety or fear. Prior sedation or tranquilisation may be necessary.

Barbiturates are the most suitable drugs to comply with the criteria for acceptable agents. Preparations are in injectable form and not necessarily sterile. Intravenous injection of **pentobarbital sodium for euthanasia** produces a smooth and rapid loss of consciousness in many species. Euthanasia may be delayed in animals with severe cardiac or respiratory impairment. It can also be administered by the intraperitoneal route; intracardiac injection is painful and should not be used in conscious animals, although it can be used in unconscious animals. Overdosage of barbiturates causes death by depression of medullary respiratory and vasomotor centres. In horses, pentobarbital may cause excitement and a short-acting barbiturate or sedative such as an alpha$_2$-adrenoceptor stimulant should be administered initially or an alternative method of euthanasia should be used.

Other methods of euthanasia of animals and useful guidance is given in *Humane Killing of Animals*. 4th ed. England: UFAW, 1989 and *The humane killing of livestock using firearms*. England: HSA, 1999.

PENTOBARBITAL SODIUM for euthanasia

UK

Indications. Euthanasia only
Warnings. Preparations are not suitable for general anaesthesia
Dose. *By rapid intravenous (preferred), intraperitoneal, or intracardiac injection*, 120–200 mg/kg as necessary

---

Animals given pentobarbital sodium for euthanasia should not be used for animal or human consumption. In addition, the VMD provides the following warning: **Carcasses of chemically euthanased animals must be incinerated and not sent to the knackers yard**.

CD **Dolethal** (Vétoquinol) *UK*
Injection, pentobarbital sodium 200 mg/mL, for *cattle, dogs, cats*; 100 mL, 250 mL

CD **Euthatal** (Merial) *UK*
Injection, pentobarbital sodium 200 mg/mL, for *dogs, cats, other small animals*; 100 mL

CD **Lethobarb** (Fort Dodge) *UK*
Injection, pentobarbital sodium 200 mg/mL, for *small farm animals, domestic pets*; 100 mL

CD **Pentobarbital Solution 20% for Euthanasia** (Loveridge) *UK*
Injection, pentobarbital sodium 200 mg/mL; 100 mL, 500 mL

CD **Pentoject** (Animalcare) *UK*
Injection, pentobarbital sodium 200 mg/mL, for *dogs, cats, other small animals, mink*; 100 mL, 500 mL

Accidental contact through skin, eyes, or ingestion or self-injection may be fatal in humans. Contact area should be washed or irrigated with water and medical aid obtained. In case of accidental self-injection seek urgent medical attention, advising medical services of barbiturate poisoning. Do not leave patient unattended. Maintain airways and give symptomatic and supportive treatment.

Australia

Indications. Euthanasia only
Contra-indications. Animals intended for human or animal consumption
Warnings. Preparations are not suitable for general anaesthesia
Dose. *By rapid intravenous (preferred), intraperitoneal, or intracardiac injection*, 150–300 mg/kg as necessary

Euthanasia Fort Solution (Apex) *Austral.*
Injection, pentobarbital sodium 400 mg/mL with muscle relaxant, for *dogs, cats, horses*
Withdrawal Periods. *Horses*: should not be used in horses intended for human consumption

Euthanasia Solution (Apex) *Austral.*
Injection, pentobarbital sodium 320 mg/mL, for *dogs, cats*

Lethabarb (Virbac) *Austral.*
Injection, pentobarbital sodium 325 mg/mL, for *small animals*

Valabarb (Jurox) *Austral.*
Injection, pentobarbital sodium 300 mg/mL
Withdrawal Periods. Should not be used in animals intended for human consumption.

Eire
Indications. Euthanasia only
Contra-indications. Animals intended for human or animal consumption
Warnings. Preparations are not suitable for general anaesthesia
Dose. *By rapid intravenous (preferred), intraperitoneal, or intracardiac injection*, 150–300 mg/kg as necessary

Euthatal (Merial) *Eire*
Injection, pentobarbitone sodium 200 mg/mL, for *dogs, cats, other small animals*
Withdrawal Periods. Should not be used in animals intended for human consumption

Dolethal Solution for Injection (Vetoquinol) *Eire*
Injection, pentobarbital (as sodium) 182.2 mg/ mL, for *dogs, cats*

New Zealand
Indications. Euthanasia only
Contra-indications. Animals intended for human or animal consumption
Warnings. Preparations are not suitable for general anaesthesia
Dose. *By rapid intravenous (preferred), intraperitoneal, or intracardiac injection*, 125–150 mg/kg as necessary

Pentobarb 300 (NZVet) *NZ*
Injection, pentobarbital sodium 300 mg/mL, for *dogs, cats*

Pentobarb 500 (NZVet) *NZ*
Injection, pentobarbital sodium 500 mg/mL, for *horses, cattle*

USA
Indications. Euthanasia only
Contra-indications. Animals intended for human or animal consumption
Warnings. Preparations are not suitable for general anaesthesia
Dose. *By rapid intravenous (preferred), intraperitoneal, or intracardiac injection*, 80–115 mg/kg as necessary

Pentosol Injection (Med-Pharmex) *USA*
Injection, pentobarbital sodium 360 mg/mL, for *horses*

Sleepaway (Fort Dodge) *USA*
Injection, pentobarbital sodium 260 mg/mL, for *dogs, cats*

Socumb-6 GR (Butler) *USA*
Injection, pentobarbital sodium 389 mg/mL, for *dogs, cats*

COMPOUND PREPARATIONS FOR EUTHANASIA

A compound preparation for euthanasia is available in the UK containing secobarbital (quinalbarbitone) and cinchocaine. It is claimed that the cardiotoxic properties of cinchocaine result in rapid cardiac arrest and generally gasping does not occur. However, it is recommended that the injection is given slowly (25 mL in 10 to 15 seconds) to mini-

mise the risk of premature cardiac arrest. There is debate over the benefit of prior sedation to reduce agonal gasping. Some authorities suggest that horses are sedated with detomidine and cattle with xylazine. Other authorities indicate that sedation increases the risk of agonal gasping and muscle tremors.

In other countries, preparations containing pentobarbital and phenytoin are available; the effect of pentobarbital is potentiated by phenytoin resulting in faster cessation of cardiac electrical activity. Embutramide has a strong narcotic action and paralyses the respiratory centre. Mebezonium iodide has a curariform paralytic action on striated muscle and respiratory muscle.

UK
Indications. Euthanasia only
Contra-indications. Animals intended for human or animal consumption
Warnings. Preparations are not suitable for general anaesthesia
Dose. See preparation details

CD **Somulose** (Arnolds) *UK*
Injection, cinchocaine hydrochloride 25 mg, secobarbital sodium 400 mg/ mL, for *horses, cattle, dogs, cats*; 25 mL
Withdrawal periods. Should not be used in animals intended for animal or human consumption
Dose. *By intravenous injection.*
Horses, cattle: 0.1 mL/kg
Dogs, cats: 0.25 mL/kg

Australia
Indications. Euthanasia only
Contra-indications. Animals intended for human or animal consumption
Warnings. Preparations are not suitable for general anaesthesia
Dose. See preparation details

Euthal (Delvet) *Austral.*
Injection, pentobarbital sodium 170 mg/mL, phenytoin sodium 25 mg/mL, for *dogs, cats*
Dose. *By intravenous injection.*
Dogs, cats: 0.5 mL/kg

New Zealand
Indications. Euthanasia only
Contra-indications. Animals intended for human or animal consumption
Warnings. Preparations are not suitable for general anaesthesia

Euthal (Ethical) *NZ*
Injection, ethanol 180 mg/mL, pentobarbital sodium 170 mg/mL, phenytoin sodium 25 mg/mL, for *dogs, cats*
Dose. *By intravenous injection.*
Dogs, cats: 0.5 mL/kg

T 61 (Animal Health) *NZ*
Injection, amethocaine hydrochloride 5 mg/mL, embutramide 200 mg/mL, mebezonium iodide 50 mg/mL, for *large and small animals*
Warnings. Handle this preparation with caution
Dose. *By intravenous injection.*
Large animals: 4–6 mL/50 kg
Dogs, cats: 0.3 mL/kg

USA

Indications. Euthanasia only
Contra-indications. Animals intended for human or animal consumption
Warnings. Preparations are not suitable for general anaesthesia

Beuthanasia-D Special (Schering-Plough) *USA*
Injection, pentobarbital sodium 390 mg/mL, phenytoin sodium 50 mg/mL, for *dogs*
Dose. *By intravenous injection.*
Dogs: 0.22 mL/kg

Euthasol (Delmarva) *USA*
Injection, pentobarbital sodium 390 mg/mL, phenytoin sodium 50 mg/mL, for *dogs*
Dose. *By intravenous injection.*
Dogs: 0.22 mL/kg

6.11 Drugs used to modify behaviour

The use of drugs to treat animal behavioural problems is a relatively new field of veterinary medicine. A wide range of drugs from different pharmacological classes is employed, many of which have other indications for use in veterinary medicine. Readers should also consult monographs in other sections of the book where indicated. The drugs listed below are not intended to be comprehensive but represent drugs that are commonly used for behaviour modification. The recommended dose ranges given are compiled from a variety of sources and represent current information available but due to the dynamic nature of the subject this information is constantly under review.

When using drugs in this field, it is important to consider the limitations of medical treatment. Drug therapy alone is unlikely to be effective in dealing with behavioural problems and it is important to also institute appropriate behavioural modification programmes. Also, it is well recognised that behavioural symptoms may be seen in conjunction with medical conditions and these should be addressed.

There are many non-veterinary behavioural counsellors involved in the treatment of behavioural problems and veterinarians are reminded that the animal must be 'under his/her care' to enable drug prescribing. In addition, many of the drugs prescribed for behaviour modification in animals have potential for human abuse and it is important that their use is under adequate control.

6.11.1 Neuroleptics
6.11.2 Azapirones
6.11.3 Benzodiazepines
6.11.4 Antidepressants
6.11.5 Monoamine oxidase inhibitors
6.11.6 Beta-adrenoceptor blocking drugs
6.11.7 Antiepileptics
6.11.8 Opioid antagonists
6.11.9 Central nervous system stimulants
6.11.10 Antihistamines
6.11.11 Hormonal preparations
6.11.12 Adrenoceptor stimulants
6.11.13 Cerebral vasodilators
6.11.14 Artificial 'pheromones'

6.11.1 Neuroleptics

Neuroleptics (also known as antipsychotics in human medicine) include the butyrophenones, the phenothiazines, and the thioxanthenes. These drugs cause varying degrees of sedation, antimuscarinic effects, alpha-adrenoceptor blocking activity, and extrapyramidal effects. They are commonly used in veterinary medicine for sedation and restraint.

Butyrophenones such as **haloperidol** and **azaperone** may be classified as high potency neuroleptics. They have the least sedative, least hypotensive, and the least antimuscarinic effects of the neuroleptics. However, they are nonspecific in their action and are more likely to produce extrapyramidal effects. Some authorities advocate these drugs for compulsive and aggressive states in dogs. However their use is controversial and they are not commonly used for therapy in companion animals other than exotic birds. Haloperidol is contra-indicated for use in horses. Azaperone is used to control aggression and fighting and to decrease excitement in pigs.

Phenothiazines, for example **acepromazine**, are characterised by pronounced sedative effects and moderate antimuscarinic and extrapyramidal side-effects. They are nonspecific in their action and can affect aspects of the animal's behaviour other than those being targeted. They decrease motor function and reduce awareness of external stimuli. Animals treated with phenothiazines should be assessed carefully because some may become more reactive to noises and can be easily startled. The level of sedation associated with doses used to control behavioural clinical signs may limit the usefulness of these drugs. In addition, sedation and general indifference to the environment can affect the ability of the animal to learn and thereby jeopardise behavioural modification and this, together with doubts over the anxiolytic properties of phenothiazines and concerns over their sometimes unpredictable effects, has led to a decrease in their use in behavioural cases.

ACEPROMAZINE

UK

Indications. Sedation, decrease response to stimuli, fears, and phobias but see notes above; pre-anaesthetic medication (see section 6.1.1); motion sickness (see section 3.4.2)
Contra-indications. See section 6.1.1
Side-effects. See section 6.1.1; reduced social and exploratory behaviour
Warnings. Noise startle effect can lead to unpredictable behaviour; see also section 6.1.1
Dose. Behaviour modification♦, *by mouth.*
Dogs: 0.1–2.0 mg/kg 1–4 times daily
Cats: 0.5–2.2 mg/kg daily

See section 6.1.1 for preparation details

AZAPERONE

UK

Indications. Behaviour modification; pre-anaesthetic medication (see section 6.1.2)
Contra-indications. Side-effects. Warnings. See section 6.1.2
Dose. *Pigs*: aggression, stress, *by intramuscular injection*, 0.4–2.0 mg/kg

See section 6.1.2 for preparation details

HALOPERIDOL DECANOATE

UK

Indications. Behaviour modification
Dose. Prescribing for exotic birds

POM Ⓗ **Dozic** (Rosemount) *UK*
Oral liquid, haloperidol 1 mg/mL; 100 mL

POM Ⓗ **Haldol** (Janssen-Cilag) *UK*
Oral liquid, haloperidol 2 mg/mL; 100 mL

POM Ⓗ **Serenace** (Baker Norton) *UK*
Oral liquid, haloperidol 2 mg/mL; 100 mL

6.11.2 Azapirones

Drugs in this class have specific anxiolytic action and are reported to have minimal side-effects. The exact mode of action is unknown but their primary action appears to be as serotonin agonists, although they are also thought to interact with norepinephrine, acetylcholine, and dopamine systems.
Buspirone is considered to be safe, does not interfere with learning, and has been shown to cause minimal problems on withdrawal. It is theoretically ideal for the treatment of anxiety related problems and its use in the treatment of indoor urine spraying in cats is well documented. It has also been used in cases of aggression, including fear related aggression, in dogs and cats but caution is advised because buspirone may cause a paradoxical increase in aggression in some cats. Alternatively, some cats may show an increase in friendliness and attention seeking behaviour and this side-effect has been used to advantage in aiding the introduction of semi-feral animals into a domestic environment. Its use is limited in treatment of fears and phobias because, although effective for low grade anxieties, it is ineffective when the animal is exposed to intense fear inducing stimuli. The onset of the effects of buspirone is gradual and full effects may not be seen for up to four weeks.

BUSPIRONE HYDROCHLORIDE

UK

Indications. Feline urine marking, anxiety related behavioural problems, (stereotypies), feline bonding problems
Contra-indications. Severe renal or hepatic impairment; epileptics
Side-effects. Disinhibition, increased friendliness

Warnings. Paradoxical increase in aggression in some cats; response to treatment may take 2 weeks
Dose. *By mouth.*
Dogs: mild anxiety, 1 mg/kg 2–3 times daily
Cats: indoor urine spraying, 5 mg/cat twice daily for 1 week. If patient responds, continue treatment for 8 weeks, than gradually withdraw treatment
Anxiety, 0.5–1.0 mg/kg 2–3 times daily for 6–8 weeks

POM Ⓗ **Buspar** (Bristol-Myers) *UK*
Tablets, buspirone hydrochloride 5 mg, 10 mg; 100

POM Ⓗ **Buspirone Hydrochloride** (Non-proprietary)
Tablets, buspirone hydrochloride 5 mg, 10 mg

6.11.3 Benzodiazepines

Benzodiazepines such as **diazepam, clorazepate,** and **alprazolam** are used as anxiolytics in behavioural medicine. **Brotizolam** is used as an appetite stimulant in cattle. When used as anxiolytics, benzodiazepines are found to produce adverse effects and induce physical dependence. These drugs are often associated with some degree of psychomotor impairment and also an impairment of memory (particularly short term) and consequently learning ability.
Benzodiazepines are contra-indicated in patients with impaired liver function and the long-term use of these drugs in cats is believed to be associated with hepatic damage. In cats, benzodiazepines may have diabetogenic effects. They may also affect depth perception and render cats unable to judge distances between objects or proximity of approaching cars; a serious concern for cats that have access to outdoors.
Diazepam has an extremely short half-life in the dog and frequent administration can seriously limit its usefulness. Clorazepate has a longer duration of action in dogs and is advocated as more effective but has been associated with liver failure. Alprazolam is a short acting highly potent benzodiazepine.
One major limitation of the use of benzodiazepines in canine aggression is the risk of disinhibition, which can lead to a paradoxical escalation in the level of aggression.
Physical dependence is well recognised in conjunction with benzodiazepine use in humans and a distinctive withdrawal syndrome associated with resurgence of anxiety is well documented. Animals also show an anxiety withdrawal response after the use of benzodiazepines and this accounts for the high recurrence rate for urine spraying in cats when treated with diazepam. Guidance for prescribing benzodiazepines as anxiolytics in humans includes use for as short a time as possible and at the lowest effective dose. Gradual reduction in plasma-drug concentration is essential and withdrawal of therapy over a period of weeks is recommended. These principles apply equally to the use of benzodiazepines in the veterinary field.

ALPRAZOLAM

UK

Indications. Acute fears, refractory feline elimination problems, feline anxiety related conditions, appetite stimulation

Contra-indications. See under Diazepam

Side-effects. Warnings. See under Diazepam, paradoxical excitement

Dose. *Dogs*: *by mouth,* 100–125 micrograms/kg twice daily

Cats: *by mouth,* 100 micrograms/kg 3 times daily

POM Ⓗ **Xanax** (Pharmacia & Upjohn) *UK*
Tablets, scored, alprazolam 250 micrograms, 500 micrograms; 60

BROTIZOLAM

Eire

Indications. Appetite stimulation in cattle

Dose. *Cattle*: *by intravenous injection,* 2 micrograms/kg

Mederantil (Boehringer Ingelheim) *Eire*
Injection, brotizolam 200 micrograms/mL, for *cattle*
Withdrawal Periods. Slaughter 6 hours, milk 6 hours

CLORAZEPATE DIPOTASSIUM

UK

Indications. Anxiety related behaviours, noise phobias, thunderstorm phobias

Contra-indications. See under Diazepam

Side-effects. See under Diazepam; sedation, hepatic damage

Warnings. See under Diazepam

Dose. *Dogs*: *by mouth,* 0.55–2.2 mg/kg daily

POM Ⓗ **Tranxene** (Boehringer Ingelheim) *UK*
Capsules, clorazepate dipotassium 7.5 mg, 15 mg; 20

DIAZEPAM

UK

Indications. Anxiety related behaviour problems, feline urine spraying, fear of thunder, some forms of feline aggression, appetite stimulation; epilepsy (see section 6.9); urine retention (see section 9.3)

Contra-indications. Hepatic impairment

Side-effects. Disinhibition, interference with learning and memory, ataxia or depression but paradoxical increase in activity possible

Warnings. Dependence and consequent problems of withdrawal, see notes above

Dose. *Dogs*: behaviour modification, *by mouth,* 0.55–2.2 mg/kg as required

Cats: behaviour modification, *by mouth,* 200–400 micrograms/kg 1–2 times daily

Appetite stimulation, 0.5–1.0 mg/kg

See section 6.9.2 for preparation details

6.11.4 Antidepressants

Antidepressants used in veterinary medicine include tricyclic antidepressants (TCAs), selective serotonin re-uptake inhibitors (SSRIs), and the tetracyclic antidepressant mianserin. Depending on the drug used there may be inhibition of norepinephrine re-uptake, serotonin re-uptake, or both.

Other atypical antidepressants include monoamine oxidase inhibitors (see section 6.11.5) and **lithium**. The use of lithium as a mood stabilising compound is well established in human medicine but its narrow margin of safety precludes its use in veterinary medicine.

Amitriptyline, clomipramine, desipramine, and **doxepin** are TCAs. Clomipramine inhibits the re-uptake of serotonin and also inhibits the re-uptake of norepinephrine through the action of the active metabolite desmethylclomipramine. Desipramine primarily inhibits norepinephrine re-uptake and has little effect on serotonin re-uptake.

Antidepressants produce varying degrees of sedation depending on the antimuscarinic and antihistaminic effects seen. Alpha-adrenergic side-effects are seen with clomipramine and amitriptyline and may be useful in cases where incontinence is a feature.

TCAs are used frequently in veterinary behavioural medicine and are the subject of extensive research. They are indicated for a wide range of behavioural disorders when used in association with behavioural therapy. In addition to their antidepressant effects, they have noticeable anxiolytic properties and their blocking action on the re-uptake of serotonin makes them useful in the treatment of stereotypic conditions. TCAs are reported to be potentially cardiotoxic with reference made to causing tachycardia, arrhythmias, and hypotension. In clinical use these side-effects are found to be infrequent but it is recommended that treatment should start at a low dose and gradually be increased to optimal level over several weeks. A delay in the onset of action of antidepressants, which varies from one to four weeks, is often quoted as a disadvantage of their usage. Certainly this potential delay precludes the use of serotonergic antidepressants on an 'as needed' basis.

The non-tricyclic antidepressant **fluoxetine** is a selective serotonin re-uptake inhibitor (SSRI) which has been advocated for the treatment of compulsive behaviours in dogs. Fluoxetine has also been suggested for its mood stabilising effects for some cases of affective aggression in dogs and cats. Other SSRI's have attracted interest in the field of behavioural medicine. **Fluvoxamine** has been advocated for the treatment of compulsive behaviours and shares many of the indications of fluoxetine. **Sertraline**, a potent and specific inhibitor of serotonin re-uptake, has been used in the treatment of panic associated with sound phobias and other fearful states.

Another antidepressant which has been discussed within the context of veterinary behavioural medicine is **mianserin**. It belongs to the piperazino-azepine group of compounds which are chemically unrelated to the tricyclic antidepressants. It lacks antimuscarinic side-effects and is thought to have its action primarily on serotonergic pathways. It also blocks central and peripheral H_1-receptors and blocks pre-synaptic alpha$_2$-receptors, which enhances norepinephrine secretion and thus increases the turnover of this neurotransmitter. In human psychiatry, mianserin is widely used for its antidepressant, anxiolytic, and sleep improving effects and there have been reports of its successful use in the treatment of depressive states associated with anorexia, apathy, and excessive sleeping in both cats and dogs.

AMITRIPTYLINE HYDROCHLORIDE

UK

Indications. Generalised anxiety, separation problems, excessive grooming
Contra-indications. Side-effects. See under Clomipramine; also antihistaminic effects
Dose. *By mouth.*
Dogs: 1–2 mg/kg 1–2 times daily. (May be increased to 4 mg/kg 1–2 times daily)
Cats: 0.5–1.0 mg/kg once daily

POM Ⓗ **Amitriptyline** (Non-proprietary) *UK*
Tablets, coated, amitriptyline hydrochloride 10 mg, 25 mg, 50 mg
Oral solution, amitriptyline (as hydrochloride), 5 mg/mL, 10 mg/mL; 200 mL

CLOMIPRAMINE HYDROCHLORIDE

UK

Indications. Separation-related anxiety, generalised anxiety♦, feline urine spraying♦, stereotypies♦ (including acral lick dermatitis)
Contra-indications. Male breeding dogs; hypersensitivity to the drug
Side-effects. Occasional vomiting, changes in appetitie or lethargy, antimuscarinic effects
Warnings. Use with caution in patients with cardiovascular dysfunction, epilepsy, narrow angle glaucoma, reduced gastro-intestinal motility, or urinary retention; safety in pregnant or lactating dogs has not been established; Drug Interactions – see Appendix 1
Dose. *By mouth.*
Dogs: 1–2 mg/kg twice daily in combination with behavioral modification techniques. May be given with small amount of food to reduce vomiting
Treatment of stereotypies♦, 1 mg/kg twice daily for 2 weeks, then 2 mg/kg twice daily for 2 weeks, then 3 mg/kg twice daily to effect, then gradually withdraw therapy
Cats ♦: 0.5–1.0 mg/kg once daily

POM **Clomicalm** (Novartis) *UK*
Tablets, scored, clomipramine hydrochloride 5 mg, 20 mg, 80 mg, for *dogs more than 1.25 kg body-weight and 6 months of age*; 30

Eire

Indications. Separation-related anxiety
Contra-indications. Male breeding dogs
Side-effects. Occasional vomiting, changes in appetite or lethargy, antimuscarinic effects
Warnings. Use with caution in patients with cardiovascular dysfunction, epilepsy, narrow angle glaucoma, reduced gas-

tro-intestinal motility, or urinary retention; safety in pregnant and lactating dogs and dogs <1.25 kg and 6 months of age has not been established; Drug Interactions – see Appendix 1
Dose. *Dogs*: *by mouth,* 1–2 mg/kg twice daily in combination with behavioral modification techniques

Clomicalm (Novartis) *Eire*
Tablets, clomipramine hydrochloride 5 mg, 20 mg, for *dogs*

DOXEPIN

UK

Indications. Acral lick dermatitis, compulsive stereotypic behaviours
Contra-indications. Side-effects. Warnings. See under Clomipramine, moderate sedation, potent antihistaminic effects
Dose. *By mouth.*
Dogs: 3–5 mg/kg 2–3 times daily
Cats: 0.5–1.0 mg/kg 1–2 times daily

POM Ⓗ **Sinequan** (Pfizer) *UK*
Capsules, doxepin (as hydrochloride) 10 mg, 25 mg, 50 mg, 75 mg

FLUOXETINE

UK

Indications. Stereotypies, 'depression', generalised and recurrent fears and anxieties, aggression
Contra-indications. Severe hepatic or renal impairment
Warnings. Caution in diabetes mellitus, epilepsy; response to treatment may take from 8 days to 4 weeks
Dose. *By mouth.*
Dogs: 1 mg/kg once daily
Cats: 0.5–1.0 mg/kg once daily

POM Ⓗ **Fluoxetine** (Non-proprietary)
Capsules, fluoxetine (as hydrochloride) 20 mg

POM Ⓗ **Prozac** (Dista)
Capsules, fluoxetine (as hydrochloride) 20 mg, 60 mg; 30, 98
Oral liquid, fluoxetine (as hydrochloride) 4 mg/mL; 70 mL

6.11.5 Monoamine oxidase inhibitors

Conventional monoamine oxidase inhibitors (MAOIs), which inhibit both monoamine oxidase-A and monoamine oxidase-B enzymes, are not commonly used in veterinary practice due to the potentially fatal toxic reaction that can occur when these drugs are used in combination with certain foods. However, **selegiline** which is a selective monoamine oxidase-B inhibitor does not have such effects. Selegiline is believed to have three main types of activity on the CNS which result in its application within the behavioural field. Synaptic transmission is enhanced via the inhibitory effects on monoamine oxidase-B and is also affected by inhibition of the re-uptake of certain neurotransmitters, in particular dopamine and secondarily norepinephrine. A modulatory effect on transmission by catecholamines (dopamine and norepinephrine) is also effected through the action of selegiline on phenylethylamine concentration. Selegiline has a neuroprotective action via its activation of superoxide dismutase and catalase, two enzymes which are responsible for removing free radicals, and has been shown to antagonise the effects of exogenous neurotoxic substances.

Behavioural indications for selegiline include age related behavioural disorders, where decreased dopamine concentration is believed to cause problems of memory loss, disorientation, and disruptions to the sleep-wake cycle. Also behavioural problems of an emotional origin such as fears, phobias, depression, and anxiety. As with any psychoactive medication, the drug should always be used in combination with behavioural therapy. Concurrent administration of monoamine oxidase inhibitors and tricyclic antidepressants should be avoided and a drug free period of two weeks between therapy with these two groups is recommended.

SELEGILINE

UK
Indications. Behavioural problems of an emotional origin such as depression, anxiety, fears♦, phobias♦; age related behavioural problems♦; aggression; pituitary-dependent hyperadrenocorticism♦ (see section 7.6)
Contra-indications. Concurrent or treatment within 1 day of administration of alpha₂-adrenoceptor stimulants; concurrent administration of pethidine, fluoxetine, phenothiazines, or TCAs
Warnings. Safety in pregnant and lactating bitches has not been established; Drug Interactions – see Appendix 1
Dose. *By mouth.*
Dogs: behaviour modification, 500 micrograms/kg daily for a minimum of 2 months

POM **Selgian 8 kg** (Ceva) *UK*
*Tablets, f/c, scored, selegiline hydrochloride 4 mg, for **dogs less than 8 kg body-weight***

POM **Selgian 20 kg** (Ceva) *UK*
*Tablets, f/c, scored, selegiline hydrochloride 10 mg, for **dogs***

6.11.6 Beta-adrenoceptor blocking drugs

Beta-adrenoceptor blocking drugs (beta blockers) are used in behavioural therapy to reduce anxiety and decrease the somatic symptoms such as tremors and palpitations which are associated with an anxious state. Without these somatic signals, the fear response can be significantly reduced and the use of medication can thus vastly improve the success of concomitant behavioural therapy. Since stress, anxiety, and high levels of arousal predispose patients to aggressive incidents, these drugs may also have a role in anti-aggressive therapy. It is thought that propanolol may inhibit aggression through an elevation of serotonin at the synaptic level.

Propranolol may be used as a sole agent in cases of situational anxieties. It has also been suggested by some authorities for use in combination with other drugs for the treatment of fears, phobias, and separation related problems. Propranolol and phenobarbital combination has been suggested by some authorities as a treatment for wide range of fear-based conditions including fear related separation problems and specific phobias. Its use in combination with TCAs has been advocated in cases of separation related anxiety and combined administration of propanolol and buspirone has been suggested for the treatment of certain fears and phobias. Withdrawal of propranolol should be gradual in order to avoid a norepinephrine rush which can trigger a reaction of intense fear.

PROPRANOLOL

UK
Indications. Decrease somatic signs of anxiety; used in combination with phenobarbital in fears, phobias, and fear-related separation problems; arrhythmias (see section 4.4.2)
Contra-indications. Side-effects. See under Propranolol, section 4.4.2
Warnings. Gradual withdrawal required
Dose. Behaviour modification, *by mouth.*
Dogs: 0.5–3.0 mg/kg 2 times daily (sole use); 2–3 mg/kg twice daily (in combination with phenobarbital)
Cats: 0.2–1.0 mg/kg 3 times daily (sole use); 5 mg/cat twice daily (in combination with phenobarbital)

See section 4.4.2 for preparation details

6.11.7 Antiepileptics

Where behavioural symptoms are related to seizure activity, antiepileptic therapy (see section 6.9) is specifically indicated.

Psychomotor epilepsy is a form of epilepsy particularly important in a behavioural context. In human medicine, antiepileptics have also been used in the treatment of aggressive patients where violent mood swings are involved, when they are believed to have a nonspecific mood stabilising effect. Diazepam has been described in the treatment of seizure related aggression but the short half-life in dogs effectively limits its use. In behavioural medicine, barbiturates can be of value in controlling acute anxiety states due to their anxiolytic properties. The use of phenobarbital in conjunction with propranolol is suggested by some authorities as therapy in cases of fear related problems and phobic responses. However, with increasing research into psychoactive medication in the veterinary field and availability of newer medications, the indications for the use of barbiturates is decreasing. Care must be taken when administering phenobarbital due to risks of disinhibition. Gradual withdrawal is required and when using phenobarbital in combination with other medication, the possibility of an effect on the hepatic metabolism of these other drugs must be considered.

Carbamazepine, a tricyclic compound, is used in humans for the treatment of implosive aggression, temporal lobe epilepsy, and acute mania. In dogs it has been suggested for the treatment of psychomotor epilepsy, anxiety conditions and 'compulsive behaviours'. In cats, carbamazepine has been used for treatment of aggression with a fear basis and has been reported to increase affection toward people in some cats. Carbamazepine is slightly sedating, mildly antimuscarinic, and does not cause significant muscle relaxation in animals, however disinhibition is a potential side-effects of its use.

CARBAMAZEPINE

UK
Indications. Psychomotor epilepsy; 'compulsive disorders'; fear based aggression in cats
Contra-indications. Renal, hepatic, cardiovascular, and haematological disorders; breeding animals
Side-effects. Ataxia, gastro-intestinal disturbances, locomotor disturbances
Warnings. Disinhibition may lead to paradoxical increases in aggression and careful monitoring is required
Dose. *By mouth*.
Dogs: 4–10 mg/kg given in 3 divided doses
Cats: 4–8 mg/kg twice daily

POM Ⓗ **Carbamazepine** (Non-proprietary) *UK*
Tablets, carbamazepine 100 mg, 200 mg, 400 mg

POM Ⓗ **Tegretol** (Novartis) *UK*
Tablets, scored, carbamazepine 100 mg, 200 mg, 400 mg

PHENOBARBITAL

UK
Indications. Psychomotor epilepsy♦; feline excessive vocalisation♦; used in combination with propanolol in fears♦, phobias♦, and fear related separation problems♦; epilepsy (see section 6.9)
Contra-indications. Side-effects. Warnings. See under Phenobarbital, section 6.9.2
Dose. Behaviour modification, *by mouth*.
Dogs: 2–3 mg/kg twice daily (sole use or in combination with propranolol)
Cats: 1–3 mg/kg 1–2 times daily (sole use); 7.5 mg/cat twice daily (in combination with propranolol)

See section 6.9.2 for preparation details

6.11.8 Opioid antagonists

Opioid antagonists such as naloxone and naltrexone have been used in the treatment of stereotypic behaviours such as self-mutilation, tail-chasing, flank- sucking, and acral lick dermatitis. It is believed that the release of endogenous opiates is an integral part of the mechanisms of stereotypic behaviour, although current knowledge of the dynamics of endorphins within stereotypic and non-stereotypic animals is limited. Some researchers have expressed concern over the effects that the blocking of opioid pathways may have on other aspects of the animal's behaviour and on the total quality of life. **Naloxone** has a short half-life and is only available in injectable form, therefore its usefulness is limited. **Naltrexone** is the opioid antagonist most likely to be used. However, its application is usually limited to research situations.

NALOXONE HYDROCHLORIDE

UK
Indications. Stereotypic behaviours including self-mutilation; reversal of opioid analgesia (see section 6.5)
Side-effects. Sedation
Dose. *Dogs*: behaviour modification, *by subcutaneous, intramuscular, or intravenous injection*, 11–12 micrograms/kg

See section 6.5 for preparation details

NALTREXONE HYDROCHLORIDE

UK
Indications. Stereotypic behaviours including self-mutilation
Side-effects. Sedation
Dose. *By mouth*.
Dogs: 2.2 mg/kg 1–2 times daily
Cats: 2–4 mg/kg once daily (up to 25–50 mg/cat)

POM Ⓗ **Nalorex** (Du Pont) *UK*
Tablets, f/c, scored, naltrexone hydrochloride 50 mg; 50

6.11.9 Central nervous system stimulants

Hyperactive is a term often used by owners when describing their 'problem' dog when, in the majority of cases, overactive would be a more accurate term. In fact, true hyperkinesis, a recognised medical condition, is extremely rare. Overactivity is treated using a combination of owner education and alterations in management along with recognised behavioural modification techniques, whereas hyperkinesis does require medical treatment. It is essential that the diagnosis is confirmed before therapy is instituted; **dexamfetamine** results in a paradoxical decrease in heart rate and activity in hyperkinetic individuals. Treatment can then be instituted with **methylphenidate**. Narcolepsy, a very rare behavioural condition, may also be treated with stimulants.

DEXAMFETAMINE SULPHATE
(Dexamphetamine sulphate)

UK
Indications. Diagnosis of hyperkinesis
Contra-indications. Side-effects. Warnings. See under Methylphenidate
Dose. *Dogs*: *by mouth*, 0.2–1.3 mg/kg

CD Ⓗ **Dexedrine** (Medeva) *UK*
Tablets, scored, dexamfetamine sulphate 5 mg; 28

METHYLPHENIDATE HYDROCHLORIDE

UK
Indications. Hyperkinesis; narcolepsy
Contra-indications. Cardiovascular disease, glaucoma, hyperthyroidism

Side-effects. Increased heart rate and respiratory rate; anorexia; tremors; aggression; insomnia; hyperthermia
Warnings. Potential for human abuse
Dose. *By mouth.*
Dogs: hyperkinesis, 2–4 mg/kg 2–3 times daily
Narcolepsy, 250 micrograms/kg

CD Ⓗ **Ritalin** (Novartis) *UK*
Tablets, scored, methylphenidate hydrochloride 10 mg; 30

6.11.10 Antihistamines

Antihistamines such as **chlorphenamine** and **diphenhydramine** are primarily used for behavioural conditions relating to car travel where mild sedation is required due to apprehension on the part of the animal, and cases involving pruritus and self-trauma. These effects should be considered as side-effects of the drugs. Owners should be made aware of the antimuscarinic properties of these drugs.

CHLORPHENAMINE MALEATE
(Chlorpheniramine maleate)

UK
Indications. Mild sedation (for example car travel), compulsive scratching; premedication for drugs that may induce an anaphylactic reaction (see section 5.2.1); pruritus in allergic skin disorders (see section 14.2)
Contra-indications. Urine retention, glaucoma, hyperthyroidism
Side-effects. Mild CNS depression, constipation, dry mouth
Dose. Behaviour modification, *by mouth.*
Dogs: 220 micrograms/kg 3 times daily (maximum 1 mg/kg daily)
Cats: 1–2 mg/cat 2–3 times daily (low dose), 2–4 mg/cat twice daily (high dose)

See section 14.2.2 for preparation details

DIPHENHYDRAMINE HYDROCHLORIDE

UK
Indications. Mild sedation (for example car travel), late night activity patterns, behavioural cases involving pruritus and self mutilation; allergic respiratory disease and relief of coughing (see section 5.2.1); pruritus in allergic skin disorders (see section 14.2)
Contra-indications. Side-effects. Warnings. See Chlorphenamine
Dose. *By mouth.*
Dogs, cats: 2–4 mg/kg 2–3 times daily

See section 14.2.2 for preparation details

6.11.11 Hormonal preparations

In the past, hormonal preparations such as the progestogens and oestrogens have been commonly used to treat behaviours that are believed to have a dimorphic component such

as canine aggression and feline marking. There is little doubt that these drugs can have a role to play in behavioural modification but there has been a tendency in the past to view them as a cure-all for behavioural problems and this is not the case. Behavioural patterns are complex in their aetiology and it important that comprehensive behavioural histories are taken before prescribing these drugs. In addition, progestogens have many potential side-effects and it is essential that owners are informed of adverse effects before long-term usage is considered.

In the case of feline marking it is true that the behaviour is sexually dimorphic to an extent but there are many other components such as anxiety and social conflict involved, and it is recognised that hormonal preparations do not work uniformly in spraying cats. The beneficial effect observed in some individuals may not be limited to the hormonal action of the drug, and in the case of progestogen therapy some of the therapeutic value stems from the nonspecific calming and sedative effect of the progestogen.

In canine aggression, the progestogens are believed to have an effect via their anti-androgenic properties and also nonspecific CNS depression. The use of low doses of progestogens as a short-term measure in the treatment of behavioural cases may be considered acceptable, but modern psychoactive drugs have largely superseded their use.

Progestogen therapy is used in male dogs when the behavioural problem is believed to have a strong sexual component and to be under hormonal control. Reversible chemical castration is often seen as the first step in assessment for surgical castration. **Delmadinone** competes with androgens for receptor sites and can be a useful indicator of the potential effects of surgical castration. However it also acts upon the limbic system to give behavioural effects and although administration of delmadinone may markedly reduce aggression in some male dogs, it is not a guarantee that surgical castration will have the same effect. Delmadinone is used extensively in the treatment of hypersexual behaviour in male dogs. It is imperative that an accurate behavioural history is taken since the behaviour must be sexually motivated if this course of treatment is to be effective. In some cases delmadinone may result in increased aggression due to a behavioural side-effect of disinhibition.

The extensive list of potential side-effects is a major limiting factor in the use of progestogens such as **megestrol** and **medroxyprogesterone** (see section 8.2.2), especially when long-term use is being considered.

Oestrogens such as **diethylstilbestrol** have been shown to be effective in the control of aggression in bitches after spaying although potential side-effects such as bone marrow suppression must be considered and may limit their use. Blood parameters should be monitored regularly.

DELMADINONE ACETATE

UK
Indications. Sexually dimorphic male behaviours including roaming, mounting, dog to dog aggression

Contra-indications. Side-effects. Warnings. See section 8.2.2

Dose. *Dogs, cats*: *by subcutaneous or intramuscular injection,* 1–2 mg/kg depending on the severity of the condition, repeat dose after 8 days if no improvement. Repeat dose every 3–4 weeks in animals showing improvement

See section 8.2.2 for preparation details

MEDROXYPROGESTERONE ACETATE

UK

Indications. See Megestrol acetate
Contra-indications. Side-effects. Warnings. See section 8.2.2
Dose. *Dogs. Males♦*: *by subcutaneous or intramuscular injection,* 5–11 mg/kg 3 times a year
Cats. Males♦: *by subcutaneous or intramuscular injection,* 5–20 mg/kg 3 times a year

See section 8.2.2 for preparation details

MEGESTROL ACETATE

UK

Indications. Calming effect, feline urinary marking, aggression, suppression of male species-typical behaviour; oestrus control (see section 8.2.2)
Contra-indications. Side-effects. Warnings. See section 8.2.2
Dose. Behaviour modification, *by mouth.*
Dogs. Males: 2 mg/kg daily for 7 days then 4 mg/kg for 7 days if no improvement in behaviour, followed by 1 mg/kg daily for 14 days if some improvement in behaviour *or* 2 mg/kg daily for 7 days then 1 mg/kg daily for 14 days if some improvement in behaviour. A low weekly maintenance dose or repeated short courses may be necessary
Cats. Males♦: 2.5–10.0 mg for 7 days, then reduce dose every 2 weeks to lowest effective dose

See section 8.2.2 for preparation details

DIETHYLSTILBESTROL
(Stilboestrol)

UK

Indications. Urinary incontinence leading to house soiling, aggression in bitches post spaying; prostate hyperplasia (see section 8.2.1)
Contra-indications. Side-effects. Warnings. See section 8.2.1
Dose. *Dogs*: *by mouth,* up to 1.0 mg/dog for 3–5 days, than decrease to lowest effective dose given 1–2 times weekly

See section 8.2.1 for preparation details

6.11.12 Adrenoceptor stimulants

Alpha-adrenoceptor stimulants (sympathomimetics) such as **phenylpropanolamine** may be used to help increase urethral sphincter tone in cases of submissive or excitement related urine leaking. Its use is also indicated in house soiling problems which result from urinary incontinence. The adverse side-effects are minimal but in a behavioural context one possible side-effect is increased aggression and owners should be made aware of this before treatment is started.

PHENYLPROPANOLAMINE HYDROCHLORIDE

UK

Indications. Urinary incontinence leading to house soiling, submissive urination
Contra-indications. Side-effects. Warnings. See section 9.3
Dose. Behavioural modification♦, *by mouth.*
Dogs: 1.1–4.4 mg/kg 2–3 times daily
Cats: 1.0–1.5 mg/kg twice daily

See section 9.3 for preparation details

6.11.13 Cerebral vasodilators

Nicergoline is an alpha-adrenoceptor antagonist (alpha blocker). One of the most important clinical actions of nicergoline is thought to be cerebral vasodilation resulting in increased blood supply to the brain and a reversal of chronic hypoxia which has been indicated ad one of the factors underlying age related behavioural disorders. Nicergoline also exerts a neuroprotective action on neural cells which limits the damage caused by chronic hypoxia and anoxic attack, and increases the rate of recovery following damage due to hypoxia.

Propentofylline is a xanthine derivative and has been suggested for treatment of dullness and lethargy in older dogs. Age-related behavioural disorders can be divided into those involving a general loss of activity and interest and those with more specific signs of cognitive decline such as disorientation and alteration in sleep-wake cycle. In the latter cases, treatment with a monamine oxidase B inhibitor is recommended (see section 6.11.5).

NICERGOLINE

UK

Indications. Improvement of age-related changes for example diminished vigour and vigilance, fatigue, sleep disorders, loss of house training, reduced appetite, and psychomotor disturbances such as episodes of ataxia
Contra-indications. Use within 24 hours of administration of alpha$_2$-adrenoceptor stimulants; use before administration of vasodilators such as acepromazine and prazosin
Dose. *Dogs*: *by mouth,* 250–500 micrograms/kg once daily, given in the morning

See section 4.3.4 for preparation details

6.11.14 Artificial 'pheromones'

Pheromonatherapy is a relatively new therapeutic approach to behavioural disorders. Social odours are the olfactory signals by which animals communicates and they are detected in the cat by the use of the vomeronasal or Jacobson's organ. Feline territorial social odours are classified into three groups. Firstly there are those contained in urine spots and those associated with scratching, secondly there are the so called alarm marks which consist of the scent signals contained in anal gland secretions and paw pad sweat gland secretions and finally the identification marks which are produced in the facial skin and consist of the so called 'facial pheromones'. Preparations are available that contain the third type 'pheromones'. These products are marketed for use in conjunction with behavioural modification programmes for a number of behavioural problems and although they are not strictly classed as medication they are only available through a veterinary practice and they should only be provided for clients in association with suitable behavioural advice.

Feliway (Ceva) is known as the 'familiarisation pheromone' and it is believed to provide a feeling of security for cats in unfamiliar or stressful situations. It is a synthetic analogue of the F3 fraction of the so called 'feline facial pheromone'. Its applications reflect this belief although the exact mode of action is as yet unclear. The major applications are indoor urine marking, inappropriate scratching, and stress during transportation but Feliway is also extremely useful in decreasing stress for cats in confinement both in veterinary hospital cages and in cattery conditions. It has also been shown to decrease stress in cats during handling for anaesthesia induction and during other medical examination when it is applied to the consulting or preparation table. Feliway is an environmental product and needs to be applied 15 to 30 minutes before cats are allowed access to treated areas.

The cleaning regime for soiled areas must be modified when the product is used for cases of indoor urine marking. Either a combination of biological washing powder followed by an application of surgical spirit is used, followed by application of the product after 24 hours or the biological washing powder is omitted, the area is washed with boiling water and surgical spirit is applied before waiting 30 minutes and application of the product.

Felifriend (Ceva) is a synthetic analogue of the F4 fraction of the so called 'feline facial pheromone' and is believed to assist in the development of an atmosphere of confidence between cats and unfamiliar people. Felifriend is applied to the palms of each hand and is rubbed over the hands and wrists of the handler. It is marketed specifically for use in the veterinary consulting room where it is believed to reduce the cat's anxiety. It has been advocated for use with particularly fractious cats during consultation and at other times of restraint. In studies the use of Felifriend has significantly reduced the major signs of aggression during consultations including attempts to bite and scratch the handler. In France, Felifriend is also marketed for use in cases of aggression between cats in the same household and in these cases it is applied to the neck and flank region of each cat. The spray must not be applied near to the cat's eyes or directly onto the head.

In some cases Felifriend has been found to induce what appears to be a panic reaction and it is suggested that this is most likely to occur when the cat is faced with a human or feline who is already strongly associated with hostility and therefore the visual signal of threat is in direct contradiction to the appeasing scent signal. The best results are obtained when the person is totally unknown or where intercat aggression is in its early stages.

7 Drugs used in the treatment of disorders of the ENDOCRINE SYSTEM

Contributor:
M E Herrtage BVSc, MA, DVR, DVD, DSAM, DipECVIM, DipECVDI, MRCVS

7.1 Thyroid and antithyroid drugs

7.1.1 Thyroid drugs
7.1.2 Antithyroid drugs

Hypothyroidism is one of the most common endocrine disorders of the dog, but is diagnosed uncommonly in other domestic animals. In dogs, the most frequent causes of hypothyroidism are related to impaired production and secretion of the thyroid hormones, thyroxine (T_4) and tri-iodothyronine (T_3), which usually result from destruction of the thyroid gland (primary hypothyroidism). However, hypothyroidism may also result from pituitary disorders (secondary hypothyroidism) or hypothalamic dysfunction (tertiary hypothyroidism). Clinical signs are variable and may include lethargy, poor exercise tolerance, obesity, hair loss, and skin disease.

Hyperthyroidism is recognised most commonly in older cats, but has been reported rarely in dogs. Feline hyperthyroidism is associated with increased circulating levels of thyroxine and tri-iodothyronine and is usually caused by nodular hyperplasia of the thyroid or thyroid adenomas. Hyperthyroidism is characterised by weight loss despite polyphagia, restlessness, nervousness, polydipsia, polyuria, tachycardia, heat intolerance, and a poor matted or unkempt hair coat.

Thyrotrophin (thyroid-stimulating hormone, TSH) or thyrotrophin-releasing hormone (TRH) may be used in the assessment of thyroid function (see sections 7.5.1 and 7.5.3).

7.1.1 Thyroid drugs

Thyroid hormones are used in the treatment of hypothyroidism regardless of the cause. Congenital hypothyroidism requires prompt treatment if normal development is to be attained.

Levothyroxine sodium is commonly used for maintenance therapy because thyroxine is the main secretory product of the thyroid gland. Part of the absorbed dose of levothyroxine is de-iodinated in peripheral tissues, to the more active

tri-iodothyronine. The clinical effects of levothyroxine sodium may not be apparent for several days and resolution of all the clinical signs may take several months. Although rare, thyrotoxicosis may develop while receiving levothyroxine treatment. Clinical signs include polyuria, polydipsia, nervousness, panting, tachycardia, weight loss, diarrhoea, and increase in appetite.

Liothyronine sodium is an exogenous source of tri-iodothyronine. It has a similar action to levothyroxine, but is more rapidly metabolised and thus has a shorter duration of activity. Although tri-iodothyronine is the active intracellular hormone, liothyronine is only indicated when levothyroxine therapy has failed to achieve a response in dogs with confirmed hypothyroidism. The dose should be adjusted for the individual patient. Liothyronine is also used in the tri-iodothyronine (T_3) suppression test for the diagnosis of mild hyperthyroidism in cats.

The dog is relatively resistant to thyrotoxicosis from over-supplementation with thyroid drugs because of the animal's efficient metabolism and excretion of thyroid hormone. However, patients with pre-existing cardiac disorders should initially receive lower doses of thyroid drug.

Dried thyroid gland preparations should not be used because their potency varies and their effects are unpredictable.

LIOTHYRONINE SODIUM
(L-Tri-iodothyronine sodium)

UK
Indications. Hypothyroidism; tri-iodothyronine suppression test in cats
Side-effects. Rarely thyrotoxicosis, see notes above
Dose. *By mouth.*
Dogs: initially 2–3 micrograms/kg 3 times daily. Adjust dose for each individual animal. May be increased to 4–6 micrograms/kg if required
Cats: tri-iodothyronine suppression test, 25 micrograms every 8 hours for a total of 7 doses

POM (H) **Tertroxin** (Goldshield) *UK*
Tablets, scored, liothyronine sodium 20 micrograms; 100

LEVOTHYROXINE SODIUM
(Thyroxine sodium)

UK
Indications. Hypothyroidism
Contra-indications. Thyrotoxicosis, uncorrected adrenal insufficiency
Side-effects. Rarely thyrotoxicosis, see notes above
Warnings. Care in administration to patients with clinically significant cardiac disease or hypertension
Dose. *By mouth.*

Dogs: initially 22–44 micrograms/kg once daily. Adjust dose for each individual animal after approximately 8 weeks of therapy. Occasionally divided doses are required to maintain adequate blood concentrations. Measurement of serum-thyroxine concentrations before and 4–6 hours after administration can be used to assess the adequacy of the dosage.

Cats ◆: 10–20 micrograms/kg daily in divided doses

POM Soloxine (Arnolds) *UK*
Tablets, scored, levothyroxine sodium 100 micrograms, 200 micrograms, 300 micrograms, 500 micrograms, 800 micrograms, for *dogs*; 250

Australia
Indications. Hypothyroidism
Contra-indications. Hyperthyroid animals, acute myocardial infarction, uncorrected hypoadrenocorticism
Warnings. Care in administration to patients with cardiac disease, hypertension, or increased metabolic rate; Drug Interactions – insulin, oral anticoagulants
Dose. *By mouth.*
Dogs: 20 micrograms/kg twice daily
Cats: 50–200 micrograms once daily

Thyroxine (Apex) *Austral.*
Tablets, levothyroxine sodium 400 micrograms, for *dogs, cats*

USA
Indications. Hypothyroidism
Contra-indications. Thyrotoxicocis; acute myocardial infarction; uncorrected hypoadrenocorticism
Warnings. Safety in pregnant animals has not been evaluated; care in administration to patients with cardiac disease, hypertension, or increased metabolic rate
Dose. Dosages vary, consult manufacturer's information

Heska Chewable Thyroid Supplement For Dogs (Heska) *USA*
Tablets, levothyroxine 0.1 mg, 0.2 mg, 0.3 mg, 0.4 mg, 0.5 mg, 0.6 mg, 0.7 mg, 0.8 mg, for *dogs*

Levo-Powder (Vetus) *USA*
Oral powder, levothyroxine sodium 2.2 mg/g, for *horses*
Withdrawal Periods. Should not be used in *horses* intended for human consumption

Levotabs (Vetus) *USA*
Tablets, levothyroxine sodium 0.1 mg, 0.2 mg, 0.3 mg, 0.4 mg, 0.5 mg, 0.6 mg, 0.7 mg, 0.8 mg, for *dogs*

Nutrived T-4 Chewables (Vedco) *USA*
Tablets, levothyroxine sodium 0.2 mg, 0.3 mg, 0.5 mg and 0.8 mg, for *dogs*

Soloxine (Daniels) *USA*
Tablets, levothyroxine sodium 0.1 mg, 0.2 mg, 0.3 mg, 0.4 mg, 0.5 mg, 0.6 mg, 0.7 mg, 0.8 mg, for *dogs*

Thyro-Form (Vet-A-Mix) *USA*
Tablets, levothyroxine sodium 0.2 mg, 0.5 mg, 0.8 mg, for *dogs*

Thyro-L (Vet-A-Mix) *USA*
Oral powder, levothyroxine sodium 220 mg/g, for *horses*

Thyrosyn (Vedco) *USA*
Tablets, levothyroxine sodium 0.1 mg, 0.2 mg, 0.3 mg, 0.5 mg, 0.8 mg, for *dogs*

Thyro-Tabs (Vet-A-Mix) *USA*
Tablets, levothyroxine sodium 0.1 mg, 0.2 mg, 0.3 mg, 0.4 mg, 0.5 mg, 0.6 mg, 0.7 mg, 0.8 mg, for *dogs*

Thyrozine (Phoenix, Western Veterinary Supplies) *USA*
Tablets, levothyroxine sodium 0.1 mg, 0.2 mg, 0.3 mg, 0.4 mg, 0.5 mg, 0.6 mg, 0.7 mg, 0.8 mg, for *dogs*

Thyroxine-L Tablets (Butler) *USA*
Tablets, levothyroxine sodium 0.1 mg, 0.2 mg, 0.3 mg, 0.4 mg, 0.5 mg, 0.6 mg, 0.7 mg, 0.8 mg, for *dogs*

7.1.2 Antithyroid drugs

Antithyroid drugs are used in the pre-operative preparation of hyperthyroid patients for thyroidectomy or for long-term management of hyperthyroidism.

Carbimazole is the drug of choice and is used for palliative treatment before surgery or radiotherapy, or following recurrence after surgery, chemotherapy, or radioactive iodine treatment. Carbimazole should be used in preference to **propylthiouracil**, which has a much higher incidence of side-effects. Thiamazole (methimazole) is the active metabolite of carbimazole. These antithyroid drugs act primarily by interfering with the synthesis of thyroid hormones.

Iodine and **iodide** are used before thyroidectomy to block the release of thyroxine and tri-iodothyronine and to reduce the vascularity of the thyroid gland. Iodine should not be used for long-term treatment because its antithyroid action tends to diminish and patients may not achieve the euthyroid state.

Radioactive iodine (^{131}I) has been used successfully in the management of feline hyperthyroidism. Indications for ^{131}I include intolerance to or owner non-compliance with drug treatment, recurrence following surgery, or surgery is contra-indicated due to location of the tumour or the condition of the individual patient. The lowest dose required to restore euthyroidism should be employed. In practice, doses between 37 and 370 MBq have been used. Isolation facilities are required when radioactive iodine is used as indicated in the *Ionising Radiations Regulations 1999* (SI 1999/3232).

Propranolol (see section 4.4.2) is given in hyperthyroidism to prevent many of the cardiovascular and neuromuscular effects and control the associated tachycardia, tachyarrhythmias, and hyperexcitability. It is generally considered to have no effect on serum concentrations of thyroid hormones and has been used with antithyroid drugs in the pre-operative management of hyperthyroid patients. The dose of propranolol for cats is 2.5 to 5.0 mg 3 times daily before surgery and for 2 days post surgery.

Hypocalcaemia may be encountered after bilateral thyroidectomy, due to damage to the parathyroid glands, and monitoring of serum-calcium concentration is recommended. Treatment includes calcium (see section 16.5.1), by intravenous injection, followed by oral calcium and vitamin D supplementation (see section 16.6.4).

CARBIMAZOLE

UK
Indications. Hyperthyroidism
Side-effects. Anorexia, vomiting, lethargy, pruritus, bleeding disorders, jaundice

Dose. *By mouth*.

Dogs: 10–15 mg daily in divided doses increasing dose as required to control clinical signs and maintain the serum-thyroxine concentration within the normal range.

Cats: 10–15 mg daily in divided doses for 1 to 3 weeks will produce a euthyroid state in most patients. Then adjust dose for each individual animal to the lowest effective dosage using measurement of serum-thyroxine concentrations. At least once-daily administration is required to control thyroid hormone synthesis.

POM Ⓗ **Neo-Mercazole** (Roche) *UK*
Tablets, carbimazole 5 mg, 20 mg; 100

IODINE and IODIDE

UK

Indications. Hyperthyroidism (pre-operative management)
Side-effects. Hypersalivation, anorexia, vomiting
Dose. *Cats*: *by mouth*, Aqueous Iodine Oral Solution, 3 to 5 drops daily for 7–14 days before surgery

Ⓗ **Aqueous Iodine Oral Solution** (Lugol's Solution) *UK*
Iodine 5 g, potassium iodide 10 g, water to 100 mL. Total iodine (free and combined) 130 mg/mL

PROPYLTHIOURACIL

UK

Indications. Hyperthyroidism
Side-effects. See under Carbimazole, immune-mediated haemolytic anaemia, development of serum antinuclear antibodies, lupus-like syndrome
Dose. *Cats*: *by mouth*, 50 mg 3 times daily. Adjust dose as described under Carbimazole

POM Ⓗ **Propylthiouracil** (Non-proprietary) *UK*
Tablets, propylthiouracil 50 mg

7.2 Corticosteroids

7.2.1 Glucocorticoids
7.2.2 Treatment of hypoadrenocorticism

The corticosteroids secreted by the adrenal cortex are the glucocorticoids and the mineralocorticoids. Glucocorticoids alter glucose, protein, and calcium metabolism and possess anti-inflammatory activity; and mineralocorticoids affect water and electrolyte balance.

7.2.1 Glucocorticoids

The action of glucocorticoids in suppressing inflammatory reactions may be useful in a wide variety of conditions: respiratory disease such as chronic obstructive pulmonary disease and feline asthma syndrome (section 5.2); gastro-intestinal disease including colitis in the dog (section 3.1.3); and inflammatory lesions of the eye (section 12.3.1), ear (section 14.8), and skin (section 14.2.1). The use of glucocorticoids in the treatment of mastitis is described in section

11.1.1. Glucocorticoids are capable of producing symptomatic improvement in many conditions, but without treatment of the underlying disease.

In musculoskeletal disorders (section 10.2) the benefits of suppression of the disease process are weighed against the protective effects of reduced mobility if therapy is withheld. Glucocorticoids are not indicated where only mild analgesia is required.

Clinical signs of hypersensitivity disorders including allergic dermatitis and urticaria, and auto-immune diseases such as haemolytic anaemia, thrombocytopenia, systemic lupus erythematosus, myasthenia gravis, and pemphigus variants may be reduced by glucocorticoid administration.

Glucocorticoids may also be used as adjunctive therapy in the management of mast cell and lymphoid neoplasia (see section 13.2).

Early administration of large doses of intravenous corticosteroids such as betamethasone, dexamethasone, hydrocortisone, or methylprednisolone may be of benefit in acute circulatory failure or shock irrespective of the cause; intravenous fluid therapy should also be administered.

Glucocorticoids have been used in the management of acute spinal cord injury. Methylprednisolone sodium succinate is the glucocorticoid of choice because it also has free radical scavenging properties when used at very high dosages. Methylprednisolone sodium succinate has a neuroprotective effect when given at the time of, or soon after, spinal cord injury. The aim of treatment is to maintain therapeutic concentrations for up to 24 to 48 hours after lesion development. The protective effect is lost after 48 hours and the use of glucocorticoids at this stage may be detrimental and worsen the outcome.

The use of large doses of dexamethasone with the aim of reducing post traumatic swelling is widespread. However, experimental trials examining the efficacy of dexamethasone have failed to show a beneficial effect and their use may even be detrimental to the patient's recovery. The use of high doses of dexamethasone in the treatment of acute spinal cord injuries should be avoided. Anti-inflammatory doses of prednisolone have been used for dogs with thoracolumbar and cervical spinal pain usually resulting from a protrusion of an intervertebral disc. However, such patients are at increased risk of gastro-intestinal haemorrhage and care should be taken to ensure enforced confinement (cage rest) whilst animals are receiving prednisolone.

Glucocorticoids are used for the induction of parturition in cattle and sheep♦ in late pregnancy; dexamethasone may be administered. This practice is sometimes suggested in cases of possible fetal oversize and periparturient oedema of the udder in cattle, and in sheep to aid in the treatment of pregnancy toxaemia or when it is necessary to compress or shorten the lambing season.

Glucocorticoids should be given after day 260 of gestation in cattle and after day 138 in sheep to avoid production of premature offspring.

Glucocorticoids are commonly used in the treatment of ketosis (see section 16.4) in cattle and goats♦ and also for pregnancy toxaemia♦ in sheep and goats, but are contra-indicated for the treatment of the related condition of equine hyperlipaemia.

Administration of glucocorticoids. Acceptable doses of glucocorticoids vary widely depending upon the potency of the drug employed, its formulation, rate and route of administration; the nature and severity of the condition being managed; and the goals of therapy. **Betamethasone, dexamethasone, flumetasone, isoflupredone, methylprednisolone, prednisolone,** and **triamcinolone** are commonly used for their anti-inflammatory activity. The anti-inflammatory effect of a corticosteroid parallels its gluconeogenic potency. Relative anti-inflammatory potencies of glucocorticoids are listed in Table 7.1.

Table 7.1 Relative anti-inflammatory potencies of glucocorticoids

Drug	Equivalent anti-inflammatory potency
Hydrocortisone	1
Prednisolone	4
Methylprednisolone	5
Triamcinolone	5
Betamethasone	30
Dexamethasone	30

Sodium phosphate salts and succinate esters are soluble, readily absorbed, and eliminated within 8 to 24 hours. They can be administered intravenously and are used when high plasma or tissue concentrations are required rapidly such as in cases of shock or allergic reactions; intravenous fluid therapy is also required. Despite the rapid elimination of some of these corticosteroid formulations, suppression of the hypothalamic-pituitary-adrenal (HPA) axis may be prolonged.

Other esters including acetate, adamantoate, dipropionate, isonicotinate, phenylpropionate, pivalate, and trioxa-undecanoate are insoluble and should not be given intravenously. They are less rapidly absorbed and metabolised. Insoluble esters of dexamethasone are usually intermediate-acting and effective for 4 to 14 days.

Depot or long-acting corticosteroids such as insoluble esters of methylprednisolone or triamcinolone may be effective for 3 to 6 weeks. These preparations are used for sustained therapy including intra-articular injection. Alternatively, continued treatment may be effected by oral administration. In courses of therapy lasting longer than 2 weeks, the dose of prednisolone should be tapered to the lowest clinically acceptable maintenance level with a gradual transition to administration of twice this maintenance dose on alternate days. This regimen, combined with morning medication in dogs may minimise HPA axis suppression. Evening medication in cats is suggested although the diurnal rhythm in cats is uncertain. If treatment is to be discontinued, the dose should be gradually reduced.

The use of injectable combination preparations containing a corticosteroid and an antimicrobial is not generally justified.

Side-effects of glucocorticoids. Prolonged corticosteroid treatment with either rapidly eliminated formulations or depot preparations may have suppressive effects on the HPA axis and lead to adrenal atrophy. Unnecessarily prolonged therapy should be avoided in order to minimise the possibility of precipitating signs of adrenal insufficiency during superimposed stress or when glucocorticoid treatment is finally withdrawn.

Corticosteroids should be used with caution in pregnant animals because they may cause abortion and fetal abnormalities. The use of glucocorticoids to induce parturition is associated with an increased incidence of retained placenta in cattle, although subsequent fertility may not necessarily be affected. Fetal abnormalities have been observed in laboratory animals, particularly when the drug is given during the first third of pregnancy. In breeding mares, administration in late dioestrus or pro-oestrus may affect normal oestrous behaviour and ovulation. Corticosteroids may induce a temporary fall in milk yield when given to lactating animals.

Catabolic effects of glucocorticoids include muscle wasting, cutaneous atrophy, telogen arrest of hair follicles, and delayed wound healing. In cases of corneal ulceration, repair of corneal stroma and epithelium is suppressed. Corticosteroids should not be used for the treatment of laminitis in horses. In addition, corticosteroids may induce laminitis when they are used to treat other conditions. Chronic use of exogenous glucocorticoids may lead to iatrogenic hyperadrenocorticism (iatrogenic Cushing's syndrome). Administration of corticosteroids may result in hepatomegaly with concurrent raised serum-hepatic enzyme concentrations.

Diabetes mellitus may be unmasked by glucocorticoid therapy and alteration of insulin requirements in established diabetics may occur. Gastric and colonic ulceration, sometimes with perforation, may occur in patients given glucocorticoid treatment particularly when used in conjunction with certain NSAIDs.

Immunosuppressive effects and modification of inflammatory reactions by glucocorticoids may facilitate the progression of concurrent infectious disease. In pre-existing infections, an appropriate antimicrobial drug should be administered at the same time if glucocorticoids are used. Corticosteroids should not be administered in conjunction with a vaccine.

BETAMETHASONE

UK

Indications. Shock; inflammatory and allergic disorders

Contra-indications. Renal impairment; diabetes mellitus; pregnant animals

Side-effects. Polydipsia, polyuria, polyphagia, calcinosis cutis, immunosuppression, delayed wound healing, gastrointestinal ulceration

Warnings. May cause Cushingoid syndrome

Dose.

Horses: inflammatory disorders, shock, *by intramuscular or intravenous injection*, 40–80 micrograms/kg

Cattle: inflammatory disorders, shock, *by intramuscular or intravenous injection*, 40–80 micrograms/kg

Pigs: inflammatory disorders, shock, *by intramuscular or intravenous injection*, 40–80 micrograms/kg

Dogs, cats: inflammatory disorders, initial dose, *by mouth*, 25 micrograms/kg daily. Adjust dose for each individual animal

Inflammatory disorders, shock, *by intramuscular or intravenous injection*, 40–80 micrograms/kg

POM **Betsolan Tablets** (Schering-Plough) *UK*
Tablets, scored, betamethasone 250 micrograms, for *dogs, cats excluding young kittens*; 1000

POM **Betsolan Injection** (Schering-Plough) *UK*
Injection, betamethasone 2 mg/mL, for *horses, dogs, cats*; 50 mL
Withdrawal Periods. Should not be used in *horses* intended for human consumption
For intramuscular injection

POM **Betsolan Soluble** (Schering-Plough) *UK*
Injection, betamethasone (as sodium phosphate) 2 mg/mL, for *horses, cattle, pigs, dogs, cats*; 50 mL
Withdrawal Periods. Should not be used in *horses* intended for human consumption. *Cattle*: slaughter 28 days, milk 7 days. *Pigs*: slaughter 28 days
For intramuscular or intravenous injection

POM **Norbet** (Norbrook) *UK*
Tablets, betamethasone 250 micrograms, for *dogs*; 200, 1000

Australia
Indications. Inflammatory and allergic disorders; ketosis
Contra-indications. Side-effects. Warnings. See notes above
Dose.

Horses: *by intramuscular injection*, 10–30 mg
Cattle: ketosis, *by intramuscular*, 20–30 mg
other indications, *by intramuscular injection*, 10–30 mg
Dogs, cats: *by intramuscular injection*, 50 micrograms/kg

Betsolan (Jurox) *Austral.*
Injection, betamethasone 2 mg/mL, for *horses, cattle, dogs, cats*
Withdrawal Periods. *Cattle, horses*: slaughter 28 days

Eire
Indications. Inflammatory and allergic disorders; ketosis; induction of parturition in cattle
Contra-indications. Side-effects. Warnings. See notes above
Dose.

Horses, cattle, sheep, pigs: *by intramuscular injection*, 40–80 micrograms/kg
Dogs, cats: *by mouth*, 25 micrograms/kg
by intramuscular injection, 40–80 micrograms/kg

Betsolan Injection (Schering-Plough) *Eire*
Injection, betamethasone 2 mg/mL, for *horses, cattle, sheep, goats, pigs, dogs, cats*
Withdrawal Periods. *Cattle*: slaughter 28 days, milk 7 days. *Sheep*: slaughter 7 days. *Pigs*: slaughter 28 days

Betsolan Tablets (Schering-Plough) *Eire*
Tablets, betamethasone 0.25 mg, for *dogs, cats*

New Zealand
Indications. Inflammatory and allergic disorders
Contra-indications. Side-effects. Warnings. See notes above
Dose. *Dogs, cats*: *by mouth*, 50 micrograms/kg

Betsolan (Schering-Plough) *NZ*
Tablets, betamethasone 0.25 mg, for *dogs, cats*

USA
Indications. Inflammatory and allergic disorders
Contra-indications. Side-effects. Warnings. See notes above
Dose. *Dogs*: *by intramuscular injection*, 190–385 micrograms/kg

Betasone (Schering-Plough) *USA*
Injection, betamethasone (as dipropionate and diphosphate) 7 mg/mL , for *dogs*

DEXAMETHASONE

UK
Indications. Shock; inflammatory and allergic disorders; ketosis; induction of parturition in cattle; hypoadrenocorticism (see section 7.2.2); chronic granulomatous enteritis in horses (see section 3.1.3)
Contra-indications. Except in emergencies: renal impairment; diabetes mellitus; chronic nephritis, congestive heart failure, osteoporosis, viral infections during viraemic stage, pregnant animals except in cattle to induce parturition; laminitis
Side-effects. Polydipsia, polyuria, polyphagia, hypokalaemia, calcinosis cutis, immunosuppression, delayed wound healing, gastro-intestinal ulceration, decreased milk yield in lactating cows
Warnings. May cause Cushingoid syndrome
Dose. See under preparation details

Note. Dexamethasone 1 mg = dexamethasone acetate 1.1 mg = dexamethasone isonicotinate 1.3 mg = dexamethasone sodium phosphate 1.3 mg = dexamethasone trioxaundecanoate 1.4 mg (approximately)

POM **Colvasone** (Norbrook) *UK*
Injection, dexamethasone sodium phosphate 2 mg/mL, for *horses, cattle dogs, cats*; 50 mL
Withdrawal Periods. Should not be used in *horses* intended for human consumption. *Cattle*: slaughter 21 days, milk 2 days
Dose. *By intramuscular or intravenous injection.*
Horses, cattle: 80 micrograms/kg
Dogs, cats: 200 micrograms/kg

POM **Dexadreson** (Intervet) *UK*
Injection, dexamethasone (as sodium phosphate) 2 mg/mL, for *horses, cattle, pigs, dogs, cats*; 50 mL
Withdrawal Periods. Should not be used in *horses* intended for human consumption. *Cattle*: slaughter 21 days, milk 3 days. *Pigs*: slaughter 21 days
Dose.
Horses: inflammatory disorders, *by intramuscular or intravenous injection*, 60 micrograms/kg daily
Shock, *by intravenous injection*, 4–6 mg/kg
Cattle: *by intramuscular injection.*
Inflammatory disorders, 60 micrograms/kg daily
Ketosis, 10–20 mg, may be repeated after 2 days

Induction of parturition, 20 mg

Pigs: inflammatory disorders, *by intramuscular injection*, 60 micrograms/kg daily

Dogs, cats: inflammatory disorders, *by intramuscular injection*, 100 micrograms/kg daily

Note. May also be administered by intra-articular injection (see section 10.2)

POM **Dexafort** (Intervet) *UK*

Injection, dexamethasone (as phenylpropionate) 2 mg, dexamethasone (as sodium phosphate) 1 mg/mL, for *horses, cattle, pigs, dogs, cats*; 50 mL
Withdrawal Periods. Should not be used in *horses* intended for human consumption. *Cattle*: slaughter 36 days, milk 6 days. *Pigs*: slaughter 36 days
Dose. *By intramuscular injection.*
Horses: 0.02 mL/kg
Cattle: inflammatory disorders, 0.02 mL/kg
Ketosis, 5–10 mL
Induction of parturition, 10 mL
Pigs: 0.02 mL/kg
Dogs, cats: 0.05 mL/kg

POM **Duphacort Q** (Fort Dodge) *UK*

Injection, dexamethasone sodium phosphate 2 mg/mL, for *horses, cattle, dogs, cats*; 50 mL
Withdrawal Periods. Should not be used in *horses* intended for human consumption. *Cattle*: slaughter 21 days, milk 2 days
Dose. *By intramuscular or intravenous injection.*
Horses, cattle: 80 micrograms/kg
Dogs, cats: 200 micrograms/kg

POM **Opticorten** (Novartis) *UK*

Tablets, scored, dexamethasone 250 micrograms, for *dogs and cats more than 5 kg body-weight*; 1000, 5000
Dose. **Dogs, cats**: *by mouth*, 25–100 micrograms/kg daily in divided doses
Tablets, or to prepare an oral solution, scored, dexamethasone 5 mg, for *horses*; 20
Withdrawal Periods. Should not be used in *horses* intended for human consumption
Dose. **Horses**: *by mouth*, 5 mg/100 kg body-weight. May be repeated after 2 days

POM **Voren** (Boehringer Ingelheim) *UK*

Injection, dexamethasone isonicotinate 1 mg/mL, for *horses, cattle, pigs, dogs, cats*; 50 mL
Withdrawal Periods. Should not be used in *horses* intended for human consumption. *Cattle*: slaughter 36 days, milk 2 days. *Pigs*: slaughter 36 days
Dose.
Horses, cattle, pigs: *by intramuscular or intravenous injection*, 20 micrograms/kg; *piglets*: 100 micrograms/kg
Dogs, cats: *by subcutaneous, intramuscular, or intravenous injection*, 100 micrograms/kg

POM **Voren 14** (Boehringer Ingelheim) *UK*

Depot injection, dexamethasone isonicotinate 3 mg/mL, for *horses, dogs, cats*; 50 mL
Withdrawal Periods. Should not be used in *horses* intended for human consumption
Dose. *By intramuscular injection.*
Horses: 3 mg/50 kg, repeat after 14 days
Dogs, cats: 225–300 micrograms/kg, repeat after 14 days

Australia

Indications. Shock; inflammatory and allergic disorders; ketosis; induction of parturition
Contra-indications. Side-effects. Warnings. See notes above
Dose. Dosages vary, see manufacturer's information

Colvasone Injection (Novartis) *Austral.*

Injection, dexamethasone sodium phosphate 2 mg/mL, for *horses, cattle, pigs, sheep, dogs, cats*

Dexadreson (Intervet) *Austral.*

Injection, dexamethasone sodium phosphate 2 mg/mL, for *horses, cattle, sheep, goats, pigs, cats, dogs*
Withdrawal Periods. *Horses, cattle, sheep, pigs, goats*: slaughter 2 days

Dexadreson V (Intervet) *Austral.*

Injection, dexamethasone sodium phosphate 5 mg/mL, for *horses, cattle, sheep, goats, pigs*
Withdrawal Periods. *Horses, cattle, sheep, pigs, goats*: slaughter 2 days

Dexafort (Intervet) *Austral.*

Injection, dexamethasone (as phenpropionate) 2 mg/mL, dexamethasone (as sodium phosphate) 1 mg/mL, for *horses, cattle, sheep, goats, pigs, dogs, cats*
Withdrawal Periods. *Horses, cattle, goats, sheep, pigs*: slaughter 7 days

Dexapent (Ilium) *Austral.*

Injection, dexamethasone sodium phosphate 5 mg/mL, for *horses, cattle*
Withdrawal Periods. *Horses*: slaughter 10 days. *Cattle*: slaughter 10 days, milk 72 hours

Dexaphos 5 (Jurox) *Austral.*

Injection, dexamethasone (as sodium phosphate) 5 mg/mL, for *horses, cattle, dogs, cats*
Withdrawal Periods. Horses: slaughter 14 days. Cattle: slaughter 14 days, milk withdrawal period nil

Dexason (Ilium) *Austral.*

Injection, dexamethasone (as sodium phosphate) 2 mg/mL, for *horses, cattle, pigs, dogs, cats*

Dexol-5 (Pharmtech) *Austral.*

Injection, dexamethasone sodium phosphate 5 mg/mL, for *horses, cattle*
Withdrawal Periods. *Horses*: slaughter 10 days. *Cattle*: slaughter 10 days, milk 72 hours

Dexone-5 (Virbac) *Austral.*

Injection, dexamethasone sodium phosphate 5 mg/mL, for *horses, cattle*

Methasone (Apex) *Austral.*

Tablets, dexamethasone 0.5 mg, for *dogs, cats*
Injection, dexamethasone sodium phosphate 2 mg/mL, for *horses, dogs, cats*
Withdrawal Periods. *Horses*: slaughter 60 days

Trimedexil (Ilium) *Austral.*

Injection, dexamethasone trimethylacetate 5 mg/mL, for *horses, cattle, pigs, dogs*
Withdrawal Periods. *Horses, pigs*: slaughter withdrawal period nil. *Cattle*: slaughter withdrawal period nil, milk withdrawal period nil

Voren (Boehringer Ingelheim) *Austral.*

Injection, dexamethasone 21-isonicotinate 1 mg/mL, for *cattle, horses, sheep, pigs*
Withdrawal Periods. *Cattle, horses, sheep, pigs*: slaughter 28 days

Voren Depot (Boehringer Ingelheim) *Austral.*

Injection, dexamethasone 21-isonicotinate 3 mg/mL in a microcrystalline suspension, for *cattle, horses, dogs, cats*
Withdrawal Periods. *Horses, cattle*: slaughter 28 days

Eire

Indications. Inflammatory and allergic disorders
Contra-indications. Side-effects. Warnings. See notes above
Dose. Dosages vary, see manufacturer's information

Colvasone (Norbrook) *Eire*

Injection, dexamethasone sodium phosphate 2 mg/mL, for *horse, cattle, dogs, cats*
Withdrawal Periods. *Cattle*: slaughter 21 days, milk 72 hours

Dexa Tad (Whelehan) *Eire*

Injection, dexamethasone (as disodium phosphate) 2 mg/mL, for *horses, cattle, sheep, goats, pigs, dogs, cats*
Withdrawal Periods. *Horses, cattle, sheep, goats, pigs*: slaughter 3 days. *Cattle, sheep*: milk 24 hours

Dexadreson (Intervet) *Eire*

Injection, dexamethasone (as sodium phosphate) 2 mg/mL, for *horses, cattle, pigs, dogs, cats*
Withdrawal Periods. Should not be used in *horses* intended for human consumption. *Cattle*: slaughter 21 days, milk 72 hours. *Pigs*: slaughter 21 days

Dexafort (Intervet) *Eire*
Injection, dexamethasone (as sodium phosphate) 2 mg/mL, dexamethasone (as sodium phosphate) 1 mg/mL, for *horses, cattle, pigs, dogs, cats*
Withdrawal Periods. Should not be used in *horses* intended for human consumption. *Cattle*: slaughter 36 days, milk 6 days. *Pigs*: slaughter 36 days

Dexameth Injection (Interpharm) *Eire*
Injection, dexamethasone sodium phosphate 2 mg/mL, for *horses, cattle, sheep, goats, pigs, dogs, cats*

Duphacort Q (Interchem) *Eire*
Injection, dexamethasone sodium phosphate 2 mg/mL, for *horses, cattle, dogs, cats*
Withdrawal Periods. Should not be used in *horses* intended for human consumption. *Cattle*: slaughter 21 days, milk 48 hours

Voren 14 (Boehringer Ingelheim) *Eire*
Injection, dexamethasone-21-isonicotinate 3 mg/mL, for *horses, dogs, cats*
Withdrawal Periods. *Horses*: slaughter 42 days.

Voren Suspension (Boehringer Ingelheim) *Eire*
Injection, dexamethasone-21-isonicotinate 2 mg/mL, for *horses, cattle, pigs, dogs, cats*
Withdrawal Periods. *Horses*: slaughter 21 days. *Cattle*: slaughter 28 days, milk 56 hours. *Pigs*: slaughter 16 days

New Zealand

Indications. Shock; inflammatory and allergic disorders; ketosis; induction of parturition in cattle
Contra-indications. **Side-effects**. **Warnings**. See notes above
Dose. Dosages vary, see manufacturer's information

Dexa 0.2 (Phoenix) *NZ*
Injection, dexamethasone sodium phosphate 2.64 mg/mL, for *horses, cattle, sheep, goats, pigs, dogs, cats*
Withdrawal Periods. *Horses, pigs*: slaughter withdrawal period nil. *Cattle, sheep, goats*: slaughter withdrawal period nil, milk withdrawal period nil

Dex 5 (Virbac) *NZ*
Injection, dexamethasone phosphate (as sodium salt) 5 mg/mL, for *horses, cattle, sheep, dogs*
Withdrawal Periods. *Horses*: slaughter withdrawal period nil. *Cattle, sheep*: slaughter withdrawal period nil, milk withdrawal period nil

Dexadreson (Chemavet) *NZ*
Injection, dexamethasone sodium phosphate 2 mg/mL, for *horses, cattle, sheep, goats, pigs, dogs, cats*

Dexadreson V (Chemavet) *NZ*
Injection, dexamethasone sodium phosphate 5 mg/mL, for *horses, cattle, sheep, goats, pigs*

Dexafort (Chemavet) *NZ*
Injection, dexamethasone (as phenylpropionate) 2 mg/mL, dexamethasone (as sodium phosphate) 1 mg/mL, for *horses, cattle, sheep, goats, pigs, dogs, cats*
Withdrawal Periods. *Horses, pigs*: slaughter 30 days. *Cattle, sheep, goats*: slaughter 30 days, milk 96 hours

Dexavet A.P. (Bomac) *NZ*
Injection, dexamethasone trimethylacetate 5 mg/mL, for *cattle*
Withdrawal Periods. Slaughter 8 days, milk 24 hours

Dexol 5 (Bomac) *NZ*
Injection, dexamethasone sodium phosphate 5 mg/mL, for *horses, cattle*
Withdrawal Periods. *Horses*: slaughter 28 days. *Cattle*: slaughter withdrawal period nil, milk withdrawal period nil

Dexone-5 (Bomac) *NZ*
Injection, dexamethasone sodium phosphate 5 mg/mL, for *horses, cattle*
Withdrawal Periods. *Horses*: slaughter 28 days. *Cattle*: slaughter withdrawal period nil, milk withdrawal period nil

Opticortenol 0.5% (Bomac) *NZ*
Injection, dexamethasone trimethylacetate 5 mg/mL, for *horses, cattle, pigs, dogs*
Withdrawal Periods. *Horses*: slaughter 8 days. *Cattle*: slaughter 8 days, milk 24 hours. *Pigs*: slaughter 6 days

Voren (Boehringer Ingelheim) *NZ*
Injection, dexamethasone isonicotinate 1 mg/mL, for *horses, cattle, pigs, dogs, cats*
Withdrawal Periods. *Horses, pigs*: slaughter 14 days. *Cattle*: slaughter 14 days, milk 96 hours

Voren A.P. (Boehringer Ingelheim) *NZ*
Injection, dexamethasone isonicotinate 3 mg/mL, for *horses, cattle, dogs, cats*
Withdrawal Periods. *Horses*: slaughter 28 days. *Cattle*: slaughter 14 days, milk 96 hours

USA

Indications. Shock; inflammatory and allergic disorders; ketosis
Contra-indications. **Side-effects**. **Warnings**. See notes above
Dose. Dosages vary, see manufacturer's information

Azium (Schering-Plough) *USA*
Oral powder, dexamethasone 10mg, for *horses, cattle*
Withdrawal Periods. Should not be used in *horses* intended for human consumption. *Cattle*: should not be used in calves intended for veal production
Injection, dexamethasone 2 mg/mL, for *horses, cattle*

Dexaject (Vetus) *USA*
Injection, dexamethasone 2 mg/mL, for *horses, cattle*
Withdrawal Periods. Should not be used in *calves* intended for veal production

Dexaject SP (Vetus) *USA*
Injection, dexamethasone (as sodium phosphate) 3 mg/mL, for *horses*
Withdrawal Periods. Should not be used in *horses* intended for human consumption

Dexamethasone Injection (Butler, Pro Labs) *USA*
Injection, dexamethasone 2 mg/mL, for *horses*
Withdrawal Periods. Should not be used in *horses* intended for human consumption

Dexamethasone Injection (Vetus) *USA*
Injection, dexamethasone 2 mg/mL, for *horses, cattle, dogs*
Withdrawal Periods. Should not be used in *horses* intended for human consumption

Dexamethasone 2mg/mL Injection (RXV) *USA*
Injection, dexamethasone 2 mg/mL, for *horses*
Withdrawal Periods. Should not be used in *horses* intended for human consumption

Dexamethasone Sodium Phosphate Injection (Butler, Steris, Vedco) *USA*
Injection, dexamethasone sodium phosphate 4 mg/mL, for *horses*
Withdrawal Periods. Should not be used in *horses* intended for human consumption

Dexamethasone Sodium Phosphate Injection 4mg/mL (VetTek) *USA*
Injection, dexamethasone sodium phosphate 4 mg/mL, for *horses*
Withdrawal Periods. Should not be used in *horses* intended for human consumption

Dexamethasone Solution (Butler, VetTek) *USA*
Injection, dexamethasone 2 mg/mL, for *horses, cattle, dogs, cats*
Withdrawal Periods. Should not be used in *calves* intended for veal production

Dexamethasone Solution (Phoenix) *USA*
Injection, dexamethasone 2 mg/mL, for *horses, cattle*
Withdrawal Periods. Should not be used in *calves* intended for veal production

Dexamethasone Solution 2mg/mL (Aspen) *USA*
Injection, dexamethasone 2 mg/mL, for ***horses, cattle, dogs, cats***
Withdrawal Periods. Should not be used in *calves* intended for veal production

Dexameth-A-Vet Injection (Anthony) *USA*
Injection, dexamethasone 2 mg/mL, for ***horses***
Withdrawal Periods. Should not be used in *horses* intended for human consumption

Dex-A-Vet Injection (Anthony) *USA*
Injection, dexamethasone 4 mg/mL, for ***horses***
Withdrawal Periods. Should not be used in *horses* intended for human consumption

Voren Sterile Suspension (Bio-Ceutic) *USA*
Injection, dexamethasone-21-isonicotinate 1 mg/mL, for ***horses***
Withdrawal Periods. Should not be used in *horses* intended for human consumption

FLUMETASONE
(Flumethasone)

USA

Indications. Inflammatory and allergic disorders
Contra-indications. Side-effects. Warnings. See   notes
above
Dose. See manufacturer's information

Flucort Solution (Fort Dodge) *USA*
Injection, flumetasone 0.5 mg/mL, for ***horses, dogs, cats***

ISOFLUPREDONE

New Zealand

Indications. Shock; inflammatory and allergic disorders; ketosis
Contra-indications. Side-effects. Warnings. See   notes
above
Dose. See manufacturer's information

Predef 2X (Pharmacia & Upjohn) *NZ*
Injection, isoflupredone acetate 2 mg/mL, for ***cattle, pigs***
Withdrawal Periods. *Cattle*: slaughter 7 days, milk withdrawal period nil.
Pigs: slaughter 7 days

USA

Indications. Inflammatory and allergic disorders
Contra-indications. Side-effects. Warnings. See   notes
above
Dose. See manufacturer's information

Predef 2X (Pharmacia & Upjohn) *USA*
Injection, isoflupredone acetate 2 mg/mL, for ***horses, cattle, pigs***
Withdrawal Periods. *Cattle*: slaughter 7 days, should not be used in calves intended for veal production

METHYLPREDNISOLONE

UK

Indications. Shock; inflammatory and allergic disorders
Contra-indications. Side-effects. Warnings. See   notes
above
Dose. *Horses*: by depot intramuscular injection, 200 mg
Dogs: *by mouth*, (dependent on individual clinical circumstances and body-weight) initially 1–8 mg in divided doses

by intramuscular, slow intravenous injection or by intravenous infusion, 20–30 mg/kg 4–6 times daily for 1–2 days as necessary
by depot intramuscular injection, 1–2 mg/kg
Spinal injury, *by intravenous injection*, 30 mg/kg as a single dose, then♦ *by intravenous infusion*, 5.4 mg/kg/hour for 24 hours
Cats: *by mouth*, (dependent on individual clinical circumstances and body-weight) initially 1–8 mg in divided doses
by intramuscular, slow intravenous injection or by intravenous infusion, 20–30 mg/kg 4–6 times daily for 1–2 days as necessary
by depot intramuscular injection, 1–2 mg/kg
Spinal injury, *by intravenous injection*, 30 mg/kg, then♦ at 2 and 6 hours *by intravenous injection* 15 mg/kg, then by intravenous infusion 2.5 mg/kg/hour for 42 hours

POM **Depo-Medrone V** (Pharmacia & Upjohn) *UK*
Depot injection, methylprednisolone acetate 40 mg/mL, ***horses, dogs, cats***; 5 mL
Withdrawal Periods. Should not be used in *horses* intended for human consumption
For depot intramuscular injection
Note. May also be administered by intrasynovial or intratendinous injection (see section 10.2)

POM **Medrone V Tablets** (Pharmacia & Upjohn) *UK*
Tablets, scored, methylprednisolone 2 mg, 4 mg, for ***dogs, cats***; 1000

POM **Solu-Medrone V** (Pharmacia & Upjohn) *UK*
Injection, powder for reconstitution, methylprednisolone (as sodium succinate) 125 mg, 500 mg, for ***dogs, cats***
For intramuscular or intravenous injection or intravenous infusion
For intravenous infusion, dilute in glucose 5% in water, glucose 5% in sodium chloride 0.9%, or sodium chloride 0.9%

Australia

Indications. Inflammatory and allergic disorders
Contra-indications. Side-effects. Warnings. See   notes
above
Dose. See manufacturer's information

Depo Medrol Aqueous Suspension (Pharmacia & Upjohn) *Austral.*
Injection, methylprednisolone 40 mg/ mL, 20 mg/mL, for ***horses, dogs, cats***

Depredil (Ilium) *Austral.*
Injection, methylprednisolone acetate 40 mg/mL, for ***horses, dogs, cats***

Depredone (Jurox) *Austral.*
Injection, methylprednisolone acetate 40 mg/mL, for ***horses, dogs, cats***
Withdrawal Periods. *Horses*: slaughter 28 days

Vetacortyl (Vetoquinol) *Austral.*
Injection, methylprednisolone acetate 40 mg/mL, for ***dogs, cats***

Eire

Indications. Inflammatory and allergic disorders
Contra-indications. Side-effects. Warnings. See   notes
above
Dose. See manufacturer's information

Depo-Medrone V (Pharmacia & Upjohn) *Eire*
Injection, methylprednisolone acetate 40 mg/mL, for ***horses, dogs, cats***
Withdrawal Periods. Should not be used in *horses* intended for human consumption

New Zealand

Indications. Inflammatory and allergic disorders
Contra-indications. **Side-effects**. **Warnings**. See   notes above
Dose. See manufacturer's information

Vetacortyl (Vetoquinol) *Austral.*
Injection, methylprednisolone acetate 40 mg/mL, for **horses, dogs, cats**

USA

Indications. Inflammatory and allergic disorders
Contra-indications. **Side-effects**. **Warnings**. See   notes above
Dose. See manufacturer's information

Depo-Medrol (Pharmacia & Upjohn) *USA*
Injection, methylprednisolone acetate 20 mg/mL or 40 mg/mL, for **horses, dogs, cats**

Medrol (Pharmacia & Upjohn) *USA*
Tablets, methylprednisolone 4 mg, for **dogs, cats**

Methylprednisolone Tablets (Boehringer Ingelheim Vetmedica, Vedco) *USA*
Tablets, methylprednisolone 2 mg, for **dogs, cats**

PREDNISOLONE

UK

Indications. Inflammatory and allergic disorders; adreno-cortical insufficiency (see section 7.2.2); myasthenia gravis (see section 6.7.4), cancer therapy (see section 13.2); Inflammatory bowel disease (see section 3.1.3)
Contra-indications. **Side-effects**. **Warnings**. See   notes above
Dose. **Dogs, cats**: inflammatory disorders, *by mouth,* 0.1–2.0 mg/kg daily. For prolonged treatment, gradually reduce to lowest effective dose and give alternate day administration in the morning for dogs, in the evening for cats

POM Prednicare (Animalcare) *UK*
Tablets, prednisolone 1 mg, 5 mg, for **dogs, cats**

POM Prednidale 5 (Arnolds) *UK*
Tablets, scored, prednisolone 5 mg, for **dogs, cats**

POM Prednisolone Tablets BP (Vet) (Millpledge) *UK*
Tablets, scored, prednisolone 1 mg, 5 mg

Australia

Indications. Shock; inflammatory and allergic disorders
Contra-indications. **Side-effects**. **Warnings**. See   notes above
Dose. See manufacturer's information

Delta Cortef Tablets (Pharmacia & Upjohn) *Austral.*
Tablets, prednisolone 5 mg, for **dogs**

Macrolone 20 Tablets (Mavlab) *Austral.*
Tablets, prednisolone 5 mg, for **dogs, cats**

Macrolone Granules (Mavlab) *Austral.*
Oral granules, prednisolone 20 mg/g granules, for **horses**
Withdrawal Periods. **Horses**: slaughter 28 days

Microlone (Mavlab) *Austral.*
Tablets, prednisolone 5 mg, for **dogs, cats**

Preddy Granules (Vetsearch) *Austral.*
Oral granules, prednisolone 200 mg/5 g granules, for **horses**
Withdrawal Periods. **Horses**: slaughter 28 days

Prednisolone Tablets (Jurox) *Austral.*
Tablets, prednisolone 5 mg, for **dogs**

Pred-X Injection (Apex) *Austral.*
Injection, prednisolone acetate 10 mg/mL, for **horses, dogs, cats**
Withdrawal Periods. **Horses**: should not be used in horses intended for human consumption

Pred-X 5 Tablets (Apex) *Austral.*
Tablets, prednisolone 5 mg, for **dogs, cats**

Pred-X 20 Tablets (Apex) *Austral.*
Tablets, prednisolone 20 mg, for **horses, dogs**
Withdrawal Periods. **Horses**: slaughter 7 days

Solu-Delta-Cortef Solution (Pharmacia & Upjohn) *Austral.*
Injection, prednisolone (as sodium succinate) 10 mg/mL, for **horses, dogs, cats**

New Zealand

Indications. Shock; inflammatory and allergic disorders
Contra-indications. **Side-effects**. **Warnings**. See   notes above
Dose. See manufacturer's information

Preddy Granules (Bomac) *NZ*
Oral granules, prednisolone 200 mg/sachet, for **horses**
Withdrawal Periods. Slaughter 28 days

Solu-Delta-Cortef (Pharmacia & Upjohn) *NZ*
Injection, prednisolone sodium succinate 10 mg/mL, for **horses, dogs, cats**

USA

Indications. Shock; inflammatory and allergic disorders; adrenocortical insufficiency
Contra-indications. **Side-effects**. **Warnings**. See   notes above
Dose. See manufacturer's information

Prednistab (Vedco, Vet-A-Mix) *USA*
Tablets, prednisolone 5 mg, for **dogs**

Prednistab (Vet-A-Mix) *USA*
Tablets, prednisolone 20 mg, for **dogs**

Solu-Delta-Cortef (Pharmacia & Upjohn) *USA*
Injection, prednisolone sodium succinate 100 mg/10 mL, 500 mg/10 mL, for **horses, dogs, cats**

Sterisol-20 Injection (Anthony) *USA*
Injection, prednisolone sodium phosphate 20 mg/mL, for **dogs**

PREDNISONE

USA

Indications. Inflammatory and allergic disorders
Contra-indications. **Side-effects**. **Warnings**. See   notes above
Dose. See manufacturer's information

Meticorten (Schering-Plough) *USA*
Injection, prednisone 10 mg/mL, 40 mg/mL, for **horses, dogs, cats**
Withdrawal Periods. Should not be used in **horses** intended for human consumption

TRIAMCINOLONE

Australia

Indications. Inflammatory and allergic disorders
Contra-indications. Side-effects. Warnings. See notes above
Dose. See manufacturer's information

Triamolone Forte (Jurox) *Austral.*
Injection, triamcinolone acetonide 6 mg/mL, for *horses, dogs, cats*
Withdrawal Periods. *Horses*: slaughter 28 days

USA

Indications. Inflammatory and allergic disorders
Contra-indications. Side-effects. Warnings. See notes above
Dose. See manufacturer's information

Cortalone (Vedco) *USA*
Tablets, triamcinolone (as acetonide) 0.5 mg, 1.5 mg, for *dogs, cats*

Triamcinolone Acetonide Tablets (Boehringer Ingelheim Vetmedica) *USA*
Tablets, triamcinolone acetonide 0.5 mg, 1.5 mg, for *dogs, cats*

Triamtabs (Vetus) *USA*
Tablets, triamcinolone acetonide 0.5 mg, 1.5 mg, for *dogs, cats*

Vetalog Parenteral (Fort Dodge) *USA*
Injection, triamcinolone acetonide 2 mg/mL or 6 mg/mL, for *horses, dogs, cats*
Withdrawal Periods. Should not be used in *horses* intended for human consumption

Vetalog Tablets (Fort Dodge) *USA*
Tablets, triamcinolone acetonide 0.5 mg, 1.5 mg, for *dogs, cats*

7.2.2 Treatment of hypoadrenocorticism

Hypoadrenocorticism is a deficiency of both glucocorticoid and mineralocorticoid secretion from the adrenal cortices. Destruction of both adrenal cortices is termed primary hypoadrenocorticism (Addison's disease). Secondary hypoadrenocorticism is caused by a deficiency of corticotropin (ACTH) that leads to atrophy of the zona fasciculata of the adrenal cortices and impaired secretion of glucocorticoids. The production of mineralocorticoids from the zona glomerulosa, however, usually remains adequate. Primary hypoadrenocorticism is seen in dogs and cats. Clinical signs include anorexia, lethargy, depression, weakness (usually episodic), waxing and waning illness, dehydration, intermittent vomiting and diarrhoea.

In acute primary hypoadrenocorticism, sodium chloride 0.9% intravenous infusion and glucocorticoid therapy should be given. **Hydrocortisone sodium succinate** and **dexamethasone sodium phosphate** are suitable for intravenous glucocorticoid therapy. However, if plasma-cortisol concentrations are to be measured for diagnosis, then dexamethasone should be used to avoid interference with the assay. Dexamethasone 0.5 to 1.0 mg/kg twice daily by intravenous injection should be administered until oral therapy can be tolerated. Once the animal has improved, maintenance therapy with mineralocorticoids can be instigated. Chronic primary hypoadrenocorticism requires supplementation with **fludrocortisone acetate**, an oral synthetic adrenocortical steroid with mineralocorticoid activity. The dose should be adjusted until the plasma-sodium concentration and plasma-potassium concentration are within the normal range. The majority of cases do not require continuous daily glucocorticoid supplementation after initial stabilisation. However, owners should be given a supply of **prednisolone** or **hydrocortisone** tablets and clear instructions for their appropriate use in animals requiring additional glucocorticoid treatment. Either prednisolone at a dose of 100 to 200 micrograms/kg daily or hydrocortisone at a dose of 500 micrograms/kg twice daily can be used for replacement therapy.

Salt supplementation is required initially to correct hyponatraemia but is not usually required long term. Dogs requiring unusually high doses of fludrocortisone may respond to lower doses with salt supplementation.

It is advisable to administer prednisolone or hydrocortisone at replacement dosages (see above) to patients with adrenocortical insufficiency before situations that may be stressful such as general anaesthesia and surgery.

CORTICOTROPIN
(Corticotrophin)

Australia

Indications. Adrenocortical insufficiency following prolonged cortisone use
Contra-indications. Pregnant animals, congestive heart failure, renal impairment, oedema
Dose. *Horses*: *by subcutaneous or intramuscular injection*, 200 units

ACTH (Virbac) *Austral.*
Injection, corticotropin 200 units/5 mL, for *horses*

USA

Indications. Corticotropin deficiency; diagnosis of adrenal dysfunction in dogs
Contra-indications. Ineffective where atrophy of adrenal glands has occurred
Side-effects. Prolonged administration may induce hyperplasia and hypertrophy of the adrenal cortex
Dose. *Dogs, cats*: *by subcutaneous or intramuscular injection*, 2.2 units/kg

ACTH Gel (Butler, Vedco) *USA*
Injection, corticotropin 40, 80 units, for *dogs, cats*

ACTH Gel Injection (Anthony) *USA*
Injection, corticotropin 40, 80 units, for *dogs, cats*

DESOXYCORTONE PIVALATE
(Deoxycortone pivalate, Deoxycorticosterone pivalate)

USA

Indications. Adrenocortical insufficiency
Contra-indications. Pregnant animals, congestive heart failure, renal impairment, oedema
Dose. *Dogs*: *by intramuscular injection*, 1.65–2.2 mg/kg

Percorten-V (Novartis) *USA*
Injection, desoxycortone pivalate 25 mg/mL, for *dogs*

FLUDROCORTISONE ACETATE

UK

Indications. Mineralocorticoid replacement in adrenocortical insufficiency
Dose. *Dogs, cats*: *by mouth*, 15–20 micrograms/kg daily. The dose may need to be increased during the first 6 to 18 months of therapy and may be required twice daily in a few cases.

POM Ⓗ **Florinef** (Squibb) *UK*
Tablets, scored, fludrocortisone acetate 100 micrograms; 56

HYDROCORTISONE

UK

Indications. Glucocorticoid replacement in adrenocortical insufficiency; shock
Contra-indications. Side-effects. Warnings. See section 7.2.1
Dose. *Dogs*: adrenocortical insufficiency, *by mouth*, 500 micrograms/kg twice daily
by intramuscular injection, 5–10 mg/kg
by intravenous injection, 1–10 mg/kg
Shock, *by intravenous injection*, 50 mg/kg, repeat after 3–6 hours if required

POM Ⓗ **Efcortesol** (Sovereign) *UK*
Injection, hydrocortisone (as sodium phosphate) 100 mg/mL; 1 mL, 5 mL

POM Ⓗ **Hydrocortone** (MSD) *UK*
Tablets, scored, hydrocortisone 10 mg, 20 mg; 30

POM Ⓗ **Solu-Cortef** (Pharmacia & Upjohn) *UK*
Injection, powder for reconstitution, hydrocortisone (as sodium succinate) 100 mg

7.3 Anabolic steroids

Anabolic steroids are synthetic derivatives of testosterone. They have some androgenic activity but less virilising effects. In some countries, including the UK, the use of anabolic steroids is prohibited in animals used in competitions, and animals intended for human consumption (*Animals and Animal Products (Examination for Residues and Maximum Residue Limits) Regulations 1997*).
Anabolic steroids are indicated to promote nitrogen retention in animals with catabolic diseases. They also cause retention of sodium, calcium, potassium, chloride, sulphate, and phosphate.
Anabolic steroids stimulate appetite, increase muscle mass, retain intracellular water, increase skin thickness, increase skeletal mass, close growth plates prematurely, and increase production of erythrocytes. **Despite potential benefits, the clinical efficacy of anabolic steroids is unproven.** Anabolic steroids may be used as an adjunct to the treatment of chronic renal failure, in debilitating diseases and convalescence, and to promote tissue repair.

Anabolic steroids are also indicated in the management of hypoplastic anaemia and anaemia due to uraemia and neoplasia. The erythropoietic effects result partly from increased erythropoietin production and partly from direct stimulatory effect on bone marrow stem cells. Danazol (see section 13.2) has been used as part of the immunosuppressive therapy in immune-mediated thrombocytopenia and immune-mediated haemolytic anaemia.
Injectable anabolic steroid products contain esters in oil to prolong absorption. Phenylpropionate esters allow absorption over about one week, whereas laurate and undecenoate esters prolong absorption for 3 to 4 weeks.
Anabolic steroids, particularly the alkylated compounds, including ethylestrenol and methyltestosterone (see section 8.2.3) must be administered with care because of potential hepatotoxicity.

BOLDENONE

Australia

Indications. Aid in debility
Contra-indications. Pregnancy, circulatory failure, renal impairment
Side-effects. Transient masculising effects

Boldebal-H (Ilium) *Austral.*
Injection, boldenone undecylenate 50 mg/mL, for *horses, cattle, pigs*

Boldenone 50 (Jurox) *Austral.*
Injection, boldenone undecylenate 50 mg/mL, for *horses, cattle, dogs, cats*
Withdrawal Periods. Should not be used in *horses* intended for human consumption

Sybolin (Ranvet) *Austral.*
Injection, boldenone undecylenate 25 mg/mL, for *horses*
Withdrawal Periods. *Horses*: slaughter 70 days

USA

Indications. Aid in debility
Contra-indications. Pregnant animals and stallions
Side-effects. Over-aggressiveness

Equipoise (Fort Dodge) *USA*
Injection, boldenone (as undecylenate) 25 or 50 mg/mL, for *horses*
Withdrawal Periods. Should not be used in *horses* intended for human consumption

ETHYLESTRENOL
(Ethyloestrenol)

UK

Indications. Supportive management of chronic renal failure
Contra-indications. Androgen-dependent neoplasia, pregnant animals
Side-effects. Virilism with high doses, hepatopathy, possible production of very odorous urine in cats
Warnings. Caution in hepatic impairment
Dose. *Dogs, cats*: *by mouth,* 50 micrograms/kg daily in divided doses if possible

POM **Nandoral** (Intervet) *UK*
Tablets, scored, ethylestrenol 500 micrograms, for *dogs, cats*; 500

Australia

Indications. Aid in debility
Warnings. Drug Interactions – anticoagulants; monitor hepatic function during prolonged treatment

Nandoral (Intervet) *Austral.*
Tablets, ethylestrenol 0.5 mg, for **horses, dogs, cats**
Withdrawal Periods. Should not be used in **horses** intended for human consumption

Nitrotain (Biochemical Veterinary Research) *Austral.*
Oral paste, ethylestrenol 15 mg/4 g paste, for **horses**
Withdrawal Periods. Should not be used in **horses** intended for human consumption

Eire

Indications. Supportive management of chronic renal failure, debility, anorexia
Contra-indications. Pregnant animals
Side-effects. Possible production of very odorous urine in cats
Warnings. Caution in hepatic impairment

Nandoral Tablets (Intervet) *Eire*
Tablets, ethylestrenol 0.5 mg, for **dogs, cats**

New Zealand

Indications. Aid in debility; anaemia
Warnings. Monitor hepatic function during prolonged treatment

Nandoral (Chemavet) *NZ*
Tablets, ethylestrenol 0.5 mg, for **dogs, cats**

Nitrotain (Parnell) *NZ*
Oral paste, ethylestrenol 15 mg/4 g, for **horses**
Withdrawal Periods. Slaughter 180 days

METHANDRIOL

Australia

Indications. Aid in debility
Contra-indications. Hepatic impairment; concurrent coumarin or indanedione anticoagulants; stallions at stud; pregnant or lactating mares
Side-effects. Androgenic effects and impaired liver function with prolonged treatment
Warnings. Caution in growing animals; caution in horses less than 18 months of age

Anadiol Depot (Ilium) *Austral.*
Injection, methandiol dipropionate 75 mg/mL, for **horses, dogs, cats**

Anadocalin (Ranvet) *Austral.*
Injection, methandriol dipropionate 40 mg, deoxycortone enanthate 20 mg, testosterone enanthate 25 mg/mL, for **horses**
Withdrawal Periods. Slaughter 70 days

Anavite (RWR) *Austral.*
Powder, methandriol dipropionate 1.2 g/kg powder (also contains yeast, vitamins, glucose), for **horses, dogs**
Withdrawal Periods. Should not be used in **horses** intended for human consumption

Orabol H Paste (Vetsearch) *Austral.*
Oral paste, methandriol dipropionate 100 mg/5 mL, for **horses**
Withdrawal Periods. Should not be used in **horses** intended for human consumption

Protabol (RWR) *Austral.*
Injection, methandriol dipropionate 75 mg/mL, for **horses**
Withdrawal Periods. Should not be used in **horses** intended for human consumption

Superbolin (Vetsearch) *Austral.*
Injection, methandriol dipropionate 75 mg/mL, for **horses, dogs**
Withdrawal Periods. Should not be used in **horses** intended for human consumption

New Zealand

Indications. Aid in debility
Contra-indications. Pregnant or lactating mares, stallions; renal impairment
Side-effects. Androgenic effect or liver function impairment with prolonged treatment

Oralject Orabol-H (Bomac) *NZ*
Oral paste, methandriol dipropionate 20 mg/mL, for **horses**
Withdrawal Periods. Slaughter 60 days

NANDROLONE

UK

Indications. Supportive management of chronic renal failure; some cases of anaemia♦
Contra-indications. Side-effects. Warnings. See under Ethylestrenol; use in prepubertal animals may result in early epiphyseal closure
Dose. See preparation details

POM **Laurabolin** (Intervet) *UK*
Depot injection (oily), nandrolone laurate 25 mg/mL, 50 mg/mL, for **dogs, cats**; 10 mL
Dose. Dogs, cats: *by subcutaneous or intramuscular injection*, 2–5 mg/kg. Repeat every 21 days if required

POM **Nandrolin** (Intervet) *UK*
Depot injection (oily), nandrolone phenylpropionate 25 mg/mL, 50 mg/mL, for **dogs, cats**; 25-mg/mL vial 10 mL; 50-mg/mL vial 25 mL
Dose. Dogs, cats: *by subcutaneous or intramuscular injection*, 2–5 mg/kg. Repeat every 6–7 days if required

POM **Retarbolin** (Vericore VP) *UK*
Depot injection (oily), nandrolone cyclohexylpropionate 10 mg/mL, for **dogs, cats**; 10 mL
Contra-indications. Breeding bitches or queens
Dose. Dogs, cats: *by intramuscular injection*, 1 mg/kg. Repeat after 21 days if required

Australia

Indications. Aid in debility
Side-effects. Androgenic effects with prolonged treatment

Deca 50 (RWR) *Austral.*
Injection, nandrolone decanoate 50 mg/mL, for **horses**
Withdrawal Periods. Should not be used in **horses** intended for human consumption

Dynabol 50 (Jurox) *Austral.*
Injection, nandrolone cypionate 50 mg/mL, for **horses, dogs, cats**
Withdrawal Periods. Should not be used in **horses** intended for human consumption

Laurabolin (Intervet) *Austral.*
Injection, nandrolone laurate 25 mg/mL, 50 mg/mL, for **horses, dogs, cats**
Withdrawal Periods. Should not be used in **horses** intended for human consumption

Nandrolin (Intervet) *Austral.*
Injection, nandrolone phenylpropionate 20 mg/mL, 50 mg/mL, for *horses, dogs, cats*
Withdrawal Periods. Should not be used in *horses* intended for human consumption

Reepair (Jurox) *Austral.*
Injection, nandrolone undecylenate 80 mg, propionylestradiol 2 mg, hydroxyprogesterone hexanoate 80 mg), for *horses, dogs*
Withdrawal Periods. Should not be used in *horses* intended for human consumption
Contra-indications. Pregnant animals, teat or prostate neoplasia, circulatory failure, renal impairment

Eire
Indications. Aid in debility; anaemia
Contra-indications. Pregnant animals
Side-effects. Possible production of very odorous urine in cats

Laurabolin (Intervet) *Eire*
Injection (oily), nandrolone laurate 25 mg/mL, 50 mg/mL, for *dogs, cats*

Nandrolin Injection (Intervet) *Eire*
Injection, nandrolone phenylproprionate 25 mg/mL, 50 mg/mL, for *dogs, cats*

New Zealand
Indications. Aid in debility

Laurabolin (Chemavet) *NZ*
Injection, nandrolone laurate 25 mg/mL, 50 mg/mL, for *horses, dogs, cats*

NORETHANDROLONE

Australia
Indications. Aid in debility

Anaplex (Jurox) *Austral.*
Tablets, norethandrolone 5 mg (with di-isopropylamine dichloroacetate, vitamins, minerals, amino acids), for *dogs, cats*

Eire
Indications. Aid in debility

Nandrolin (Chemavet) *NZ*
Injection, norandrostenolone phenylpropionate 25 mg/mL, for *horses, dogs, cats*

STANOZOLOL

Australia
Indications. Aid in debility
Contra-indications. Renal impairment
Warnings. Care in renal impairment and congestive heart failure

Stanabolic (Ilium) *Austral.*
Injection, stanozolol 50 mg/mL, for *horses, dogs, cats*
Withdrawal Periods. *Horses*: slaughter 28 days

Stanazol (RWR) *Austral.*
Injection, stanozolol 50 mg/mL, for *horses, dogs, cats*
Withdrawal Periods. Should not be used in *horses* intended for human consumption

Stanosus 50 (Jurox) *Austral.*
Injection, stanozolol 50 mg/mL, for *horses, dogs*
Withdrawal Periods. Should not be used in *horses* intended for human consumption

New Zealand
Indications. Aid in debility
Contra-indications. Pregnant animals
Warnings. Caution in congestive heart failure and renal impairment; mild androgenic effects with prolonged treatment

Stanabolic (Ethical) *NZ*
Injection, stanozolol 50 mg/mL, for *horses, dogs, cats*
Withdrawal Periods. Slaughter 60 days

Stanazol (Vetpharm) *NZ*
Injection, stanozolol 50 mg/mL, for *horses, dogs, cats*
Withdrawal Periods. Slaughter 28 days

Stanol (Virbac) *NZ*
Injection, stanozolol 50 mg/mL, for *horses, dogs, cats*
Withdrawal Periods. Slaughter 60 days

USA
Indications. Aid in debility
Contra-indications. Pregnant animals
Warnings. Caution in congestive heart failure, renal impairment, aged animals with chronic interstitial nephritis; mild androgenic effects with prolonged treatment

Winstrol-V (Pharmacia & Upjohn) *USA*
Tablets, stanozolol 2 mg, for *dogs, cats*

COMPOUND ANABOLIC STEROIDS

Australia
Drive (RWR) *Austral.*
Injection, boldenone undecylenate 25 mg/mL, methandriol dipropionate 30 mg/mL, to aid in debility in *horses*
Withdrawal Periods. Should not be used in *horses* intended for human consumption

Tribolin 75 (Ranvet) *Austral.*
Injection, methandriol dipropionate 40 mg/mL, nandrolone decanoate 35 mg/mL, to aid in debility in *horses*
Withdrawal Periods. Slaughter 70 days

New Zealand
Filybol Forte (Vetpharm) *NZ*
Injection, methandriol dipropionate 40 mg/mL, nandrolone decanoate 30 mg/mL, for *horses*

Tribolin 75 (Vetpharm) *NZ*
Injection, methandriol dipropionate 40 mg/mL, nandrolone decanoate 35 mg/mL, for *horses*

7.4 Drugs used in diabetes mellitus

7.4.1 Insulin
7.4.2 Oral antidiabetic drugs
7.4.3 Treatment of diabetic ketoacidosis
7.4.4 Treatment of hypoglycaemia

Insulin-dependent diabetes mellitus occurs because of a deficiency of insulin and is recognised mainly in dogs and cats. Non-insulin dependent diabetes mellitus arises following a resistance to the effects of insulin and is more typical of equine cases.

7.4.1 Insulin

7.4.1.1 Short-acting insulin
7.4.1.2 Intermediate-and long-acting insulins

Insulin plays a key role in the regulation of carbohydrate, fat, and protein metabolism. A relative or absolute deficiency of insulin results in a decreased utilisation of glucose, amino acids, and fatty acids by peripheral tissues, including the liver, muscle, and adipose cells. The majority of animals with diabetes mellitus require exogenous insulin to maintain satisfactory control.

Insulin is a polypeptide hormone of complex structure. It is extracted mainly from beef or pork pancreas and purified by crystallisation. Human insulins can be made biosynthetically by recombinant DNA technology using *Escherichia coli* (prb or crb depending on the precise technique) or yeast (pyr). They may also be prepared semisynthetically by enzymatic modification of porcine insulin and are termed emp. All insulin preparations are likely to be immunogenic in animals to a greater or lesser extent, but resistance to exogenous insulin action is uncommon.

Insulin is inactivated by gastro-intestinal enzymes and therefore must be given by injection. The subcutaneous route is ideal in most circumstances. However, when treating diabetic ketoacidosis (see section 7.4.3), insulin should be given by the intravenous or intramuscular route because absorption from subcutaneous depots may be slow and erratic. Insulin is usually administered using a specific 0.5 mL or 1 mL syringe calibrated in units (100 units/mL or 40 units/mL). Insulin preparations should be stored in a refrigerator at 2°C to 8°C because they are adversely affected by heat or freezing. Preparations should be shaken gently to resuspend before use.

Management of diabetes mellitus. The aim of the treatment is to achieve the best possible control of plasma-glucose concentration throughout the day in order to maintain the patient's ideal body-weight with normal water consumption and urine output while avoiding periods of hypoglycaemia. Intermediate- or long-acting insulins are usually used in doses of 0.5 to 1.0 unit/kg body-weight when initiating treatment. The dose is then tailored to the individual requirements of the patient. It is recommended that the maximum daily dose change, either increase or decrease, is 2 units.

An animal will usually require 3 to 4 days to equilibrate to changes in insulin dosage or preparation. The dose should be increased gradually until optimal control of blood glucose is reached without periods of hypoglycaemia. Thereafter the animal's condition should be monitored regularly by the owner by recording details of urine-glucose concentration, time and amount of insulin administered, daily water intake, and time and amount of feed consumed. Measurement of glycated proteins such as fructosamine and glycosylated haemoglobin are used to monitor the response to treatment and reflect the average blood-glucose concentration over the preceding few weeks.

Stabilisation requires understanding on behalf of the owner and a regular fixed daily routine for the patient. Intermediate-acting insulin is usually given subcutaneously once daily followed by two or more small meals of a constant and measured diet to minimise postprandial hyperglycaemia. The meals should be timed to coincide with the activity of the insulin preparation used. Increased dietary fibre intake is believed to improve control of blood glucose. A regular and constant pattern of exercise is also essential because the amount of exercise will affect the daily insulin requirement.

Insulin requirements will be increased by infection, oestrus, pregnancy, glucocorticoid therapy, and ketoacidosis. Obesity must be avoided because this will increase insulin resistance.

The duration of action of different insulin preparations varies considerably from one patient to another and needs to be assessed for each individual. The times indicated below are only approximations.

The range of authorised veterinary insulin preparations available in the UK provides a short-acting insulin suitable for the management of diabetic emergencies and an intermediate- and a long-acting insulin preparation suitable for stabilisation of the majority of dogs and cats with diabetes mellitus. These authorised veterinary insulin preparations should be used in the first instance, although it is recognised that some diabetic patients will require authorised human insulin preparations to provide adequate glycaemic control.

Insulin is also indicated in the management of equine hyperlipaemia♦ although its effects are limited by the insulin-resistance existing in hyperlipaemic patients.

7.4.1.1 Short-acting insulin

Soluble Insulin is a short-acting form of insulin. It is the only appropriate insulin for use in diabetic emergencies (see section 7.4.3) and may be used at the time of surgical operations. It is the only form of insulin that can be administered intravenously, and also intramuscularly and subcutaneously.

When injected subcutaneously or intramuscularly, soluble insulin has a rapid onset of action of 15 to 30 minutes, peak activity between 2 and 4 hours, and a duration of action of up to 8 hours. When injected intravenously, soluble insulin has a very short half-life and its effect disappears within 2 to 4 hours.

SOLUBLE INSULIN
(Insulin Injection; Neutral Insulin)

UK

Indications. Diabetes mellitus; diabetic ketoacidosis (see section 7.4.3)

Contra-indications. Hypoglycaemia

Side-effects. See notes above; overdosage causes hypoglycaemia

Warnings. Dosage requirements may change with glucocorticoids, hyperadrenocorticism, oestrus, pregnancy, or chronic infections

Dose. *Dogs, cats*: *by subcutaneous, intramuscular, or intravenous injection, or intravenous infusion*, according to patient's requirements; see notes above

POM **Insuvet Neutral** (Schering-Plough) *UK*
Injection, soluble insulin (bovine, highly purified) 100 units/mL, for *dogs, cats*; 10 mL

7.4.1.2 Intermediate- and long-acting insulins

When given by subcutaneous injection, intermediate-acting insulin has an onset of activity of approximately 1 to 2 hours, peak activity at 6 to 12 hours, and a duration of action of 18 to 26 hours in the dog. The times for peak activity and duration of action are often shorter in the cat. Intermediate-acting insulins are usually administered once daily.

Insulin Zinc Suspension (30% amorphous, 70% crystalline) is a mixture of **Insulin Zinc Suspension (Amorphous)**, which has an intermediate duration of action and **Insulin Zinc Suspension (Crystalline)**, which has a more prolonged duration of action. It has proved a useful preparation in the long-term management of diabetes mellitus in the dog and cat. **Isophane Insulin** is a suspension of insulin with protamine but is shorter acting and needs to be administered twice daily in most patients to achieve blood glucose control. **Biphasic Insulins** are ready-mixed combinations of an intermediate-acting insulin with soluble insulin and may require twice daily injection.

Protamine Zinc Insulin and **Insulin Zinc Suspension (Crystalline)** are long-acting insulins. When injected subcutaneously they have an onset of activity of 4 to 6 hours, peak action around 14 to 24 hours and duration of activity 32 to 36 hours. These insulin preparations are particularly useful in the long-term management of diabetes mellitus in cats and hyperlipaemia in ponies♦.

All types of insulin are used in veterinary practice, although Insulin Zinc Suspension, Isophane Insulin, and Protamine Zinc Insulins are used most commonly.

INSULIN ZINC SUSPENSION
(Insulin Zinc Suspension (Mixed); I.Z.S.)

UK
Indications. Diabetes mellitus
Side-effects. See notes above; overdosage causes hypoglycaemia
Dose. *Dogs, cats*: *by subcutaneous or intramuscular injection*, according to patient's requirements; see notes above

POM **Caninsulin** (Intervet) *UK*
Injection, insulin zinc suspension (porcine, highly purified) 40 units/mL, for *dogs*; 2.5 mL, 10 mL

POM **Insuvet Lente** (Schering-Plough) *UK*
Injection, insulin zinc suspension (bovine, highly purified) 100 units/mL, for *dogs, cats*; 10 mL

Australia
Indications. Diabetes mellitus
Contra-indications. Hypoglycaemia
Side-effects. Hypoglycaemia with overdosage

Caninsulin (Intervet) *Austral.*
Injection, insulin zinc suspension 40 units/mL, for *dogs, cats*

Eire
Indications. Diabetes mellitus
Contra-indications. Hypoglycaemia
Side-effects. Hypoglycaemia with overdosage

Caninsulin (Intervet) *Eire*
Injection, insulin 40 i.u./mL, for *dogs*

New Zealand
Indications. Diabetes mellitus
Contra-indications. Hypoglycaemia
Side-effects. Hypoglycaemia with overdosage

Caninsulin (Chemavet) *NZ*
Injection, insulin zinc suspension (porcine, highly purified) 40 units/mL, for *dogs, cats*

INSULIN ZINC SUSPENSION (CRYSTALLINE)
(Cryst. I.Z.S.)

A sterile neutral suspension of bovine insulin or of human insulin in the form of a complex obtained by the addition of a suitable zinc salt

UK
Indications. Diabetes mellitus
Side-effects. See under Insulin Zinc Suspension
Dose. *Dogs, cats*: *by subcutaneous injection*, according to patient's requirements; see notes above

POM Ⓗ **Human Ultratard** (Novo Nordisk) *UK*
Injection, insulin zinc suspension, crystalline (human, pyr) 100 units/mL; 10 mL
Note. Long-acting

POM Ⓗ **Humulin Zn** (Lilly) *UK*
Injection, insulin zinc suspension, crystalline (human, prb) 100 units/mL; 10 mL
Note. Intermediate-acting

ISOPHANE INSULIN
(Isophane Insulin Injection; Isophane Protamine Insulin Injection; Isophane Insulin (NPH))

A sterile suspension of bovine or porcine insulin or of human insulin in the form of a complex obtained by the addition of protamine sulphate or another suitable protamine

UK
Indications. Diabetes mellitus
Side-effects. See under Insulin Zinc Suspension
Dose. *Dogs, cats*: *by subcutaneous injection*, according to patient's requirements; see notes above

Highly purified animal insulin

POM (H) **Hypurin Bovine Isophane** (CP) *UK*
Injection, isophane insulin (bovine, highly purified) 100 units/mL; 10 mL

POM (H) **Pork Insulatard** (Novo Nordisk) *UK*
Injection, isophane insulin (porcine, highly purified) 100 units/mL; 10 mL

Human sequence insulin

POM (H) **Human Insulatard ge** (Novo Nordisk) *UK*
Injection, isophane insulin (human, pyr) 100 units/mL; 10 mL

POM (H) **Humulin I** (Lilly) *UK*
Injection, isophane insulin (human, prb) 100 units/mL; 10 mL

PROTAMINE ZINC INSULIN
(Protamine Zinc Insulin Injection)

UK

Indications. Diabetes mellitus in dogs and cats; hyperlipaemia in horses ◆
Side-effects. See under Insulin Zinc Suspension
Dose. *Ponies* ◆: *by subcutaneous injection,* 0.15 units/kg twice daily in combination with carbohydrate treatment
Dogs, cats: *by subcutaneous injection,* according to patient's requirements; see notes above

POM **Insuvet Protamine Zinc** (Schering-Plough) *UK*
Injection, protamine zinc insulin (bovine, highly purified) 100 units/mL, for *dogs, cats*; 10 mL

BIPHASIC ISOPHANE INSULIN
(Biphasic Isophane Insulin Injection)

A sterile buffered suspension of porcine insulin complexed with protamine sulphate (or another suitable protamine) in a solution of porcine insulin *or* a sterile buffered suspension of human insulin complexed with protamine sulphate (or another suitable protamine) in a solution of human insulin

UK

Indications. Diabetes mellitus
Side-effects. See under Insulin Zinc Suspension
Dose. *Dogs, cats*: *by subcutaneous injection,* according to patient's requirements; see notes above

Highly purified animal insulin

POM (H) **Mixtard 30/70** (Novo Nordisk) *UK*
Injection, biphasic isophane insulin (porcine, highly purified), 30% soluble, 70% isophane, 100 units/mL; 10 mL

Human sequence insulin

POM (H) **Human Mixtard 30 ge** (Novo Nordisk) *UK*
Injection, biphasic isophane insulin (human, pyr), 30% soluble, 70% isophane, 100 units/mL; 10 mL

POM (H) **Humulin M1** (Lilly) *UK*
Injection, biphasic isophane insulin (human, prb), 10% soluble, 90% isophane, 100 units/mL; 10 mL

POM (H) **Humulin M2** (Lilly) *UK*
Injection, biphasic isophane insulin (human, prb), 20% soluble, 80% isophane, 100 units/mL; 10 mL

POM (H) **Humulin M3** (Lilly) *UK*
Injection, biphasic isophane insulin (human, prb), 30% soluble, 70% isophane, 100 units/mL; 10 mL

POM (H) **Humulin M4** (Lilly) *UK*
Injection, biphasic isophane insulin (human, prb), 40% soluble, 60% isophane, 100 units/mL; 10 mL

POM (H) **Humulin M5** (Lilly) *UK*
Injection, biphasic isophane insulin (human, prb), 50% soluble, 50% isophane, 100 units/mL; 10 mL

7.4.2 Oral antidiabetic drugs

Treatment with oral antidiabetic drugs is rarely successful since most cases of diabetes mellitus in dogs and cats require insulin for control. Non-insulin-dependent diabetes can only rarely be controlled by diet alone. The two major groups of oral antidiabetic drugs are the sulphonylureas and the biguanides.

The sulphonylureas, which include **chlorpropamide, glipizide, glibenclamide**, and **tolbutamide**, act mainly by augmenting insulin secretion and consequently are only effective when some residual pancreatic beta-cell activity is present. These drugs have been used occasionally in dogs and cats. Chlorpropamide may also enhance the secretion of antidiuretic hormone and has been used in the treatment of partial cranial diabetes insipidus (see section 7.5.2).

The biguanides act mainly by decreasing gluconeogenesis and increasing peripheral utilisation of glucose and are again only effective with some residual functioning pancreatic islet cells. The biguanide, **metformin** has also been used for the treatment of non-insulin dependent diabetes mellitus.

CHLORPROPAMIDE

UK

Indications. Non-insulin-dependent diabetes mellitus, diabetes insipidus (see section 7.5.2)
Side-effects. Overdosage causes hypoglycaemia, vomiting, hepatic enzyme induction
Warnings. Use with caution in patients with hepatic or renal impairment
Dose. *Dogs*: *by mouth,* 10–40 mg/kg daily in divided doses. Adjust dose as necessary to produce normoglycaemia

POM (H) **Chlorpropamide** (Non-proprietary) *UK*
Tablets, chlorpropamide 100 mg, 250 mg

GLIBENCLAMIDE

UK

Indications. Non-insulin-dependent diabetes mellitus
Side-effects. Overdosage causes hypoglycaemia, vomiting, hepatic enzyme induction
Warnings. Use with caution in patients with hepatic or renal impairment
Dose. *Dogs*: *by mouth,* 200 micrograms/kg daily. Adjust dose as necessary to produce normoglycaemia

POM (H) **Glibenclamide** (Non-proprietary) *UK*
Tablets, glibenclamide 2.5 mg, 5 mg

POM (H) **Semi-Daonil** (Hoechst Marion Roussel) *UK*
Tablets, scored, glibenclamide 2.5 mg; 28

GLIPIZIDE

UK

Indications. Non-insulin-dependent diabetes mellitus
Side-effects. Overdosage causes hypoglycaemia, vomiting, hepatic enzyme induction
Warnings. Use with caution in patients with hepatic or renal impairment
Dose. *Dogs, cats*: *by mouth*, 250–500 micrograms/kg twice daily. Adjust dose as necessary to produce normoglycaemia

POM Ⓗ **Glipizide** (Non-proprietary) *UK*
Tablets, glipizide 2.5 mg, 5 mg; 56

POM Ⓗ **Glibenese** (Pfizer) *UK*
Tablets, scored, glipizide 5 mg; 56

POM Ⓗ **Minodiab** (Pharmacia & Upjohn) *UK*
Tablets, glipizide 2.5 mg, 5 mg (scored); 60

METFORMIN HYDROCHLORIDE

UK

Indications. Non-insulin-dependent diabetes mellitus
Side-effects. Overdosage causes hypoglycaemia; vomiting; hepatic enzyme induction
Warnings. Use with caution in patients with hepatic or renal impairment
Dose. *Dogs*: *by mouth*, 250–500 mg twice daily with food. Adjust dose as necessary to produce normoglycaemia

POM Ⓗ **Metformin** (Non-proprietary) *UK*
Tablets, coated, metformin hydrochloride 500 mg, 850 mg

TOLBUTAMIDE

UK

Indications. Non-insulin-dependent diabetes mellitus
Side-effects. Hepatopathy, overdosage causes hypoglycaemia, vomiting
Warnings. Use with caution in patients with hepatic or renal impairment
Dose. *Dogs*: *by mouth*, 20–100 mg/kg daily. Adjust dose as necessary to produce normoglycaemia

POM Ⓗ **Tolbutamide** (Non-proprietary) *UK*
Tablets, tolbutamide 500 mg

7.4.3 Treatment of diabetic ketoacidosis

Clinical signs of diabetic ketoacidosis include anorexia, vomiting, diarrhoea, lethargy, weakness, dehydration, and increased depth and rate of respiration.

Soluble insulin may be used in the management of diabetic ketoacidosis and hyperosmolar non-ketotic coma in dogs and cats. It is the only form of insulin that may be given intravenously. It is necessary to achieve and maintain an adequate plasma-insulin concentration until the metabolic disturbance is brought under control.

Soluble insulin is best given by intravenous infusion because a single bolus dose will achieve an adequate concentration for only a short period of time. Plasma concen-

trations are effectively maintained with infusion rates of 0.1 unit/kg per hour (5 units/100 mL electrolyte infusion and given at a rate of 50 to 100 mL electrolyte infusion/hour in dogs and 50 mL electrolyte infusion/hour in cats). Insulin is diluted in the replacement fluids taking care to ensure the insulin is not injected into the 'dead space' of the injection port of the infusion bag and is thoroughly mixed with the replacement fluid. The infusion should be continued until the blood-glucose concentration has fallen to 10 mmol/litre and the patient is willing to eat. Subcutaneous administration of an intermediate- or long-acting preparation can then be started.

If facilities for administering insulin by continuous infusion are inadequate, 0.25 unit/kg of soluble insulin may be given intravenously and 0.75 unit/kg intramuscularly. The dose should be repeated every 4 to 6 hours until the blood-glucose concentration reaches 10 mmol/litre. Some clinicians consider this is more likely to result in hypokalaemia than the infusion technique.

Intravenous replacement of fluid and electrolytes with sodium chloride 0.9% infusion is an essential part of the management of ketoacidosis. Potassium chloride should be included in the infusion as appropriate to prevent hypokalaemia induced by the insulin. The rate of potassium administration should not exceed 0.5 mmol/kg body-weight per hour. Sodium bicarbonate 2.74% infusion is only used in life-threatening acidosis because the acid-base disturbance is normally corrected by insulin and fluid therapy.

7.4.4 Treatment of hypoglycaemia

7.4.4.1 Acute hypoglycaemia
7.4.4.2 Chronic hypoglycaemia

Signs of hypoglycaemia include disorientation, weakness, hunger, shaking, ataxia, convulsions and coma. The occurrence of clinical signs is thought to be dependent on the rate of decline of plasma-glucose concentration as well as on the severity of hypoglycaemia.

7.4.4.1 Acute hypoglycaemia

Acute hypoglycaemia occurs most commonly when a diabetic animal is given too much insulin or exercises too strenuously. If mild signs of hypoglycaemia are seen, the animal should be fed its normal food. Alternatively, glucose or sugar dissolved in a little water may be given and repeated, if necessary, after 10 to 15 minutes. If severe signs are observed, **glucose** (see section 16.1.2) should be given intravenously. A dose of 1 mL/kg of 50% glucose intravenous infusion should be adequate to correct the hypoglycaemia. The dose of insulin should be adjusted to prevent further episodes.

Glucagon may be used as an alternative to parenteral glucose in acute hypoglycaemia. It is a polypeptide hormone produced by the alpha cells of the islets of Langerhans. Its action is to increase plasma-glucose concentration by mobilising glycogen stores in the liver. Glucagon may be given by subcutaneous, intramuscular, or intravenous injection and a response to treatment will usually be observed within 10 minutes. If glucagon therapy is not effective within 15 minutes, intravenous glucose should be administered.

GLUCAGON

UK
Indications. Acute hypoglycaemia; insulin overdose
Contra-indications. Insulinoma, phaeochromocytoma, glucagonoma
Side-effects. Nausea, vomiting, diarrhoea, and hypokalaemia reported in human patients
Dose. *Dogs, cats*: *by subcutaneous, intramuscular, or intravenous injection,* 20–30 micrograms/kg. Repeat as necessary. If no response after 15 minutes, intravenous glucose should be given

POM (H) **GlucaGen** (Novo Nordisk) *UK*
Injection, powder for reconstitution, glucagon (as hydrochloride); 1 mg (1 mg = 1 unit)

7.4.4.1 Chronic hypoglycaemia

Chronic hypoglycaemia usually results from excess endogenous insulin secretion from an islet cell tumour (insulinoma). Islet cell tumours in dogs are generally malignant, but slow growing. Surgical excision is the treatment of choice, although virtually all islet cell tumours recur after excision. The median survival time following excision is about one year. If surgical treatment is not possible or not successful, or if hypoglycaemic episodes return after surgery, medical therapy is indicated.

Initial medical management for chronic hypoglycaemia should include giving small frequent meals high in proteins, fats, and complex carbohydrates. Glucocorticoids are also recommended. **Prednisolone** (see section 7.2.1) at a dose of 0.5 to 1.0 mg/kg daily in divided doses is used most frequently.

Diazoxide is a non-diuretic benzothiadiazine antihypertensive drug, which acts primarily by suppressing insulin secretion by the pancreas. It is useful in treating hypoglycaemia due to islet cell tumours, but is of no value in the management of acute hypoglycaemia.

Octreotide is a long-acting somatostatin analogue, which inhibits insulin synthesis and secretion. It has been effective in some but not all dogs with insulinoma. An attempt should be made to withdraw octreotide after amelioration of clinical signs while maintaining dietary control and glucocorticoid therapy.

DIAZOXIDE

UK
Indications. Chronic hypoglycaemia
Side-effects. Anorexia, vomiting, cataract formation
Dose. *Dogs*: *by mouth,* 10 mg/kg daily in divided doses increasing up to 60 mg/kg daily if necessary. Usually used

in combination with frequent feeding and prednisolone (see notes above).

POM (H) **Eudemine** (Medeva) *UK*
Tablets, diazoxide 50 mg; 100

OCTREOTIDE

UK
Indications. Uncontrollable clinical signs due to islet cell tumour (insulinoma)
Side-effects. Anorexia, vomiting, diarrhoea
Warnings. May increase depth and duration of hypoglycaemia, patient should be monitored closely
Dose. *Dogs*: *by subcutaneous injection,* 10–20 micrograms/animal 2–3 times daily

POM (H) **Sandostatin** (Novartis) *UK*
Injection, octreotide (as acetate) 50 micrograms/mL, 100 micrograms/mL, 200 micrograms/mL, 500 micrograms/mL

7.5 Pituitary and hypothalamic hormones

7.5.1 Anterior pituitary hormones
7.5.2 Posterior pituitary hormones
7.5.3 Hypothalamic hormones

7.5.1 Anterior pituitary hormones

The anterior lobe of the pituitary gland produces and releases a number of trophic hormones of which thyrotrophin (TSH), corticotropin (ACTH), growth hormone (GH), follicle-stimulating hormone (FSH), luteinising hormone (LH), and prolactin are the most important.

Protirelin (thyrotrophin-releasing hormone, TRH) (see section 7.5.3) is used as a diagnostic agent to confirm the presence of hypothyroidism and to distinguish between primary and secondary forms of the disease.

Tetracosactide (an active fragment of ACTH) is used mainly as a diagnostic agent to assess adrenocortical function. Failure of the plasma-cortisol concentration to increase after administration of tetracosactide indicates adrenocortical insufficiency due to either hypoadrenocorticism (Addison's disease) or the exogenous administration of glucocorticoids. An excessive elevation of plasma-cortisol concentration following administration of tetracosactide indicates hyperadrenocorticism (Cushing's syndrome). An exaggerated response may also result from uncontrolled diabetes mellitus, pyometra, or chronic renal disease.

GH (somatropin) has been used in the treatment of panhypopituitarism (pituitary dwarfism) and growth hormone-responsive alopecia. Although GH assays are available for the dog, a GH stimulation test is often required for diagnosis of deficiency. Clonidine (see section 7.8) 10 micrograms/kg, given by intravenous injection, or xylazine (see section 6.1.3) 100 micrograms/kg, administered by intravenous injection, are used for stimulation. It is important to eliminate possible hypothyroidism or hyperadrenocorticism because these conditions may induce a reversible GH deficiency. The use of GH preparations in food-producing animals is prohibited in the UK. Potential side-effects to GH therapy include hypersensitivity reactions and diabetes mellitus.

Prolactin secretion may be decreased with the use of dopamine agonists (see section 8.6). In theory, prolactin secretion may be increased with the use of dopamine antagonists such as metoclopramide, although this drug is used clinically to inhibit the side-effects of bromocriptine treatment.

SOMATROPIN
(Synthetic human growth hormone)

UK
Indications. Growth-hormone responsive alopecia
Side-effects. Hypersensitivity reactions, diabetes mellitus
Warnings. Treatment should cease if glycosuria occurs
Dose. *Dogs*: *by subcutaneous injection*, 0.1 unit/kg 3 times weekly for up to 6 weeks

POM Ⓗ **Genotropin** (Pharmacia & Upjohn) *UK*
Injection, powder for reconstitution, somatropin (rbe) 16 units

POM Ⓗ **Humatrope** (Lilly) *UK*
Injection, powder for reconstitution, somatropin (rbe) 4 units, 16 units

TETRACOSACTIDE
(Tetracosactrin)

UK
Indications. Diagnostic use; see notes above
Side-effects. See under Glucocorticoids (see section 7.2.1)
Dose. *Horses*: *by intravenous injection*, 1 mg
Dogs: *by intramuscular or intravenous injection*, (< 5 kg body-weight) 125 micrograms; (>5 kg body-weight) 250 micrograms
Cats: *by intravenous injection*, 125 micrograms

POM Ⓗ **Synacthen** (Alliance) *UK*
Injection, tetracosactide (as acetate) 250 micrograms/mL; 1 mL

7.5.2 Posterior pituitary hormones

The posterior lobe of the pituitary gland releases stored vasopressin (antidiuretic hormone, ADH) and oxytocin, which are synthesised in the hypothalamus. The domestic species, like man, store arginine-vasopressin (argipressin) except for the pig, which has lysine-vasopressin (lypressin). Oxytocin (see section 8.4) is used mainly in obstetrics.

Diabetes insipidus is a syndrome caused by an absolute or relative deficiency of vasopressin. It may result from a partial or total failure to synthesise or release vasopressin (cranial diabetes insipidus) or from a failure of the kidney to respond to vasopressin (nephrogenic diabetes insipidus). **Desmopressin**, a vasopressin analogue, has been used in the treatment of cranial diabetes insipidus and is particularly indicated when the disease is severe. The dose should be adjusted to the requirements of the individual patient.

Desmopressin is considered to have a longer duration of action than vasopressin and does not possess its vasoconstrictor activity. The intranasal solution is effective if placed in the conjunctival sac. This route of administration is preferred because repeated intranasal use may prove difficult. Desmopressin may be given orally using tablets but this regimen appears to be less effective than by using the intranasal or injectable solutions. The maximal effect of the drug occurs from 2 to 8 hours after administration and its duration of action varies from 8 to 24 hours.

Desmopressin injection is also used to boost von Willebrand factor antigen concentrations and thus reduce the bleeding time in von Willebrand's disease.

Excessive desmopressin medication can lead to hyponatraemia and water intoxication. Clinical signs may include depression, salivation, vomiting, ataxia, muscle tremors, convulsions, and coma.

Aqueous **vasopressin** is not suitable for long-term management of cranial diabetes insipidus because its duration of action is only a few hours.

Desmopressin injection and vasopressin are used in the differential diagnosis of diabetes insipidus to distinguish the cranial form of the disease from the nephrogenic form. This test (ADH response test) is performed after a water-deprivation test has confirmed that the animal cannot concentrate its urine. Restoration of the ability to concentrate urine confirms a diagnosis of cranial diabetes insipidus. Failure to respond is indicative of nephrogenic diabetes insipidus.

In dogs or cats with nephrogenic or partial cranial diabetes insipidus, thiazides (see section 4.2.1) may have a paradoxical effect in reducing urinary output. **Hydrochlorothiazide** at a dose of 2 to 4 mg/kg twice daily by mouth and **chlorothiazide** 20 to 40 mg/kg twice daily by mouth have been used in conjunction with low-sodium diets. Plasma-electrolyte concentrations should be monitored so that changes, particularly hypokalaemia, can be corrected.

Chlorpropamide (see section 7.4.2) has also been used in the treatment of partial cranial diabetes insipidus and is thought to act by potentiating the renal tubular effects of remaining endogenous vasopressin. A suggested dose for dogs is 10 to 40 mg/kg daily and cats 50 mg per day. Results are inconsistent and it may take 1 to 2 weeks of trial medication to obtain an effect. Hypoglycaemia is a potential side-effect.

DESMOPRESSIN

UK
Indications. Cranial diabetes insipidus; von Willebrand's disease; see notes above
Side-effects. See notes above
Dose. *Dogs, cats*:
Cranial diabetes insipidus, *by instillation into the conjunctival sac*, 2–4 drops (of intranasal solution desmopressin 100 micrograms/mL) 1–2 times daily
by mouth, 200 micrograms 1–3 times daily (but see note above)
by intramuscular injection, 1–4 micrograms 1–2 times daily

Vasopressin (ADH) response test, *by intramuscular injection*, (<15 kg body-weight) 2 micrograms; (dogs >15 kg body-weight) 4 micrograms. Urine samples should be collected 2-hourly following the injection until maximum concentration is achieved

Von Willebrand's disease, *by intravenous injection*, 1 microgram/kg if the patient is bleeding

POM Ⓗ **DDAVP** (Ferring) *UK*
Tablets, scored, desmopressin acetate 100 micrograms, 200 micrograms; 90
Injection, desmopressin 4 micrograms/mL; 1 mL
Intranasal solution, desmopressin acetate 100 micrograms/mL; 2.5 mL

VASOPRESSIN

UK
Indications. See notes above
Side-effects. Vasoconstriction and hypersensitivity reactions; see notes above
Dose. *Dogs, cats*: vasopressin (ADH) response test, *by intramuscular injection*, 0.5 unit/kg (maximum 5 units). Urine samples should be collected 2-hourly following the injection until maximum concentration is achieved.

POM Ⓗ **Pitressin** (Goldshield) *UK*
Injection, argipressin (synthetic vasopressin) 20 units/mL; 1 mL
Note. Preparations of argipressin are not generally available. A written order, stating case details, should be sent to the manufacturer to obtain a supply of the preparation.

7.5.3 Hypothalamic hormones

Protirelin (thyrotrophin-releasing hormone, TRH) is used mainly for diagnostic purposes in the evaluation of hypothyroidism and equine pituitary adenoma. Thyroid hormone concentrations are measured before and after intravenous administration of protirelin. Failure to respond adequately, as defined by the laboratory undertaking the thyroid estimations, suggests primary or secondary hypothyroidism. In dogs, serum-thyrophin concentrations can be measured before and 30 minutes after injection of protirelin to differentiate primary and secondary hypothyroidism.

Doses of protirelin greater than 100 micrograms/kg may produce salivation, vomiting, miosis, tachycardia, and tachypnoea.

PROTIRELIN
(Thyrotrophin-releasing hormone, TRH)

UK
Indications. Diagnostic use in hypothyroidism in dogs and cats; diagnostic use in hyperthyroidism in cats; diagnostic use in equine pituitary adenoma
Side-effects. See notes above
Dose. *Horses*: *by intravenous injection*, 1 mg/horse. Blood samples should be taken for cortisol estimations before and at 15 to 30 minutes after injection
Dogs, cats: *by intravenous injection*, 200 mg *or* 100 micrograms/kg according to the protocol used. Blood samples

should be taken for thyroid hormone estimations before and at 4 or 6 hours after injection.

POM Ⓗ **Protirelin** (Non-proprietary) *UK*
Injection, protirelin 100 micrograms/mL; 2 mL
Note. Preparations of protirelin are not generally available. A written order, stating case details, should be sent to the manufacturer to obtain a supply of the preparation.

7.6 Drugs used in hyperadrenocorticism

Hyperadrenocorticism (Cushing's syndrome) is associated with abnormal production or prolonged administration of glucocorticoids and is one of the most commonly diagnosed endocrinopathies affecting dogs and horses. Clinical signs in dogs include polydipsia, polyuria, polyphagia, muscle wasting and weakness, abdominal distension, poor exercise tolerance, and skin and hair coat changes. Hyperadrenocorticism is seen rarely in cats. Clinical signs in horses include hirsutism, laminitis, polydipsia, polyuria, and hyperhidrosis.

Hyperadrenocorticism can be spontaneous or iatrogenic. Spontaneously occurring hyperadrenocorticism may be associated with inappropriate secretion of corticotropin by the pituitary gland (pituitary-dependent hyperadrenocorticism) or associated with an adrenal tumour (adrenal-dependent hyperadrenocorticism). Pituitary-dependent hyperadrenocorticism accounts for most cases in dogs and all cases in horses with naturally occurring hyperadrenocorticism.

Diagnosis is usually made using either an ACTH stimulation test or a low-dose dexamethasone suppression test for screening in dogs. A high-dose dexamethasone suppression test may then be employed to differentiate pituitary-dependent hyperadrenocorticism from adrenal-dependent hyperadrenocorticism. A combined dexamethasone suppression/ ACTH stimulation test, although controversial, has been used as a screening test in dogs and horses. In addition, urinary cortisol:creatinine ratios may be used for screening in dogs and TRH-stimulation tests for diagnosis in horses.

Although pituitary-dependent hyperadrenocorticism has been managed surgically by hypophysectomy or bilateral adrenalectomy, medical management using mitotane is the treatment of choice in dogs. **Mitotane** is a cytotoxic drug that selectively destroys the zona fasciculata and zona reticularis of the adrenal cortex while tending to preserve the zona glomerulosa. Although considerable care is required in its use, many cases have been successfully managed with this drug in the long term. Some clinicians recommend routine replacement of glucocorticoids at the start of mitotane therapy. However, most patients do not exhibit signs of glucocorticoid deficiency and do not require replacement therapy. Higher doses (up to 75 mg/kg) may be necessary to treat cases of adrenal-dependent hyperadrenocorticism.

Selegiline (see section 6.11.5) is a monoamine oxidase inhibitor that inhibits ACTH secretion by increasing dopaminergic tone to the hypothalmic-pituitary axis. The use of selegiline has been evaluated in dogs for the treatment of pituitary-dependent hyperadrenocorticism. Although the effectiveness of treatment is variable, severe side-effects including iatrogenic hypoadrenocorticism are not seen.

Ketoconazole (see section 1.2), an imidazole derivative used primarily for its antifungal properties, is an alternative to mitotane in dogs. It has a reversible inhibitory effect on glucocorticoid synthesis whilst having negligible effects on mineralocorticoid production. Hepatotoxicity may occur in some patients.

Cyproheptadine is an antihistamine with serotonin-antagonist and calcium-channel blocking properties. The action of cyproheptadine in endocrine disorders is unclear, although antagonism of serotonin has been suggested. Cyproheptadine and **bromocriptine** (see section 8.6) may decrease the secretion of corticotropin in some animals with pituitary-dependent hyperadrenocorticism. However, both appear to have limited usefulness because of the small percentage of cases that do respond and the frequency with which relapses occur. **Pergolide** is more potent than bromocriptine and has been used in the treatment of pituitary-dependent hyperadrenocorticism in horses with variable results.

Surgical adrenalectomy is considered the treatment of choice for adrenal-dependent hyperadrenocorticism, although mitotane therapy is also recommended. Presurgical treatment with ketoconazole may reduce the relatively high morbidity and mortality associated with surgical extirpation of the adrenal glands.

BROMOCRIPTINE

UK
Indications. Pituitary-dependent hyperadrenocorticism; pseudopregnancy (see section 8.6)
Side-effects. Vomiting, anorexia, depression, and behavioural changes
Dose. *By mouth.*
Horses: 100 micrograms/kg twice daily
Dogs: hyperadrenocorticism, up to 100 micrograms/kg daily in divided doses given in gradually increasing amounts
Pseudopregnancy, 10 micrograms/kg twice daily for 10 days *or* 30 micrograms/kg once daily for 16 days

See section 8.6 for preparation details

CYPROHEPTADINE HYDROCHLORIDE

UK
Indications. Pituitary-dependent hyperadrenocorticism; feline asthma (see section 5.2.1)
Side-effects. Polyphagia
Dose. *By mouth.*
Horses: hyperadrenocorticism, 0.6 mg/kg$^{0.75}$ increasing to 1.2 mg/kg$^{0.75}$ daily
Dogs: hyperadrenocorticism, 0.3 mg/kg increasing to 3.0 mg/kg daily

See section 5.2.1 for preparation details

KETOCONAZOLE

UK
Indications. Pituitary-dependent hyperadrenocorticism, adrenal-dependent hyperadrenocorticism (presurgery)
Side-effects. Anorexia, vomiting, diarrhoea, hepatopathy, and jaundice
Dose. *Dogs*: *by mouth,* 5 mg/kg twice daily for 7 days increasing to 10 mg/kg twice daily for 7 to 14 days, then 15 mg/kg twice daily. Monitor response using the ACTH stimulation test

See section 1.2 for preparation details

MITOTANE
(*o,p′* DDD)

UK
Indications. Pituitary-dependent hyperadrenocorticism, adrenal-dependent hyperadrenocorticism
Side-effects. Lethargy, anorexia, vomiting, weakness, diarrhoea, and neurological signs such as ataxia, incoordination, circling, blindness, facial paralysis, and seizures
Dose. *Dogs*: *by mouth,* 50 mg/kg daily until thirst returns to normal (usually 7 to 10 days). Then 50 mg/kg every 1–2 weeks to prevent recurrence of clinical signs (**but see notes above**). Treatment should be monitored using the ACTH stimulation test. Mitotane should be given with food to improve absorption.

Mitotane (Available from IDIS, *UK*)
Mitotane preparations are not available in the UK. To obtain a supply, the veterinarian should obtain a Special Treatment Authorisation from the VMD

PERGOLIDE

UK
Indications. Pituitary-dependent hyperadrenocorticism
Side-effects. Anorexia, depression, sweating, dyspnoea, behavioural changes
Dose. *By mouth.*
Horses: 500 micrograms once daily increasing gradually to 3 mg once daily
Ponies: 250 micrograms once daily increasing gradually until euglycaemia is re-established

POM Ⓗ **Celance** (Lilly) *UK*
Tablets, scored, pergolide (as mesilate) 50 micrograms, 250 micrograms, 1 mg

SELEGILINE HYDROCHLORIDE

UK
Indications. Pituitary-dependent hyperadrenocorticism♦; behaviour modification (see section 6.11.5)
Contra-indications. Concurrent diabetes mellitus, pancreatitis, cardiac impairment, renal impairment, or other severe illness
Warnings. Over 50% of dogs may fail to respond adequately to treatment; Drug Interactions – see Appendix 1

Dose. *Dogs*: pituitary-dependent hyperadrenocorticism♦, *by mouth*, 1 mg/kg daily. If inadequate response after 2 months, increase to 2 mg/kg daily. If ineffective, alternative treatment is necessary

See section 6.11.5 for preparation details

USA
Indications. Pituitary-dependent hyperadrenocorticism
Contra-indications. Hypersensitivity to the drug
Warnings. Not recommended for Cushing's syndrome not of pituitary origin; Drug Interactions – ephedrine, amitraz
Dose. *Dogs*: *by mouth*, 1 mg/kg

Anipryl (Pfizer) *USA*
Tablets, selegiline hydrochloride 2 mg, 5 mg, 10 mg, 15 mg, 30mg, for *dogs*

7.7 Calcium regulating drugs

7.7.1 Calcitonin
7.7.2 Bisphosphonates

See also calcium (section 16.5.1), phosphorus (section 16.5.3), and vitamin D (section 16.6.4).

7.7.1 Calcitonin

Calcitonin is involved with parathyroid hormone in the regulation of bone turnover and hence in the maintenance of calcium balance and homeostasis. It is used to reduce bone resorption in poisoning due to rodenticides containing ergocalciferol (see also Treatment of poisoning).

CALCITONIN (SALMON)
(Salcatonin)

UK
Indications. Hypercalcaemia due to ergocalciferol poisoning
Side-effects. Vomiting, anorexia
Dose. *By subcutaneous or intramuscular injection.*
Dogs, cats: 8–18 units/kg daily in divided doses

POM Ⓗ **Calsynar** (Rhône-Poulenc Rorer) *UK*
Injection, calcitonin (salmon) 100 units/mL, 200 units/mL

POM Ⓗ **Forcaltonin** (Straken) *UK*
Injection, calcitonin (salmon) 100 units/mL

POM Ⓗ **Miacalcic** (Novartis) *UK*
Injection, calcitonin (salmon) 50 units/mL, 100 units/mL, 200 units/mL

7.7.2 Bisphosphonates

Sodium clodronate and **disodium etidronate** are osteoclast inhibitors, which have been used in dogs as a palliative treatment for primary hyperparathyroidism and hypervita-minosis D. Although treatment of hypercalcaemia is based on identification and management of the underlying disease, during investigation symptomatic therapy to lower the serum-calcium concentration may be required to reduce renal toxicity.

DISODIUM ETIDRONATE
Indications. Reduction of serum-calcium concentration in primary hyperparathyroidism and hypervitaminosis D
Contra-indications. Moderate to severe renal impairment
Side-effects. Nausea, diarrhoea, asymptomatic hypocalaemia, and skin reactions reported in humans
Dose. *Dogs*: *by mouth*, 5 mg/kg daily

POM Ⓗ **Didronel** (Procter & Gamble Pharm.) *UK*
Tablets, disodium etidronate 200 mg

SODIUM CLODRONATE
(Dichloromethylene diphosphonate)

UK
Indications. Reduction of serum-calcium concentration in primary hyperparathyroidism and hypervitaminosis D
Contra-indications. Moderate to severe renal impairment
Side-effects. Nausea, diarrhoea, asymptomatic hypocalaemia, and skin reactions reported in humans
Dose. *Dogs*: *by intravenous infusion*, 20–25 mg/kg diluted in 500 mL sodium chloride 0.9% and given as a single infusion over 4 hours

POM Ⓗ **Bonefos** (Boehringer Ingelheim) *UK*
Concentrate, for dilution and use as intravenous infusion, sodium clodronate 60 mg/mL; 5 mL

POM Ⓗ **Loron for Infusion** (Roche) *UK*
Intravenous solution, for dilution and use as intravenous infusion, sodium clodronate 30 mg/mL; 10 mL

7.8 Clonidine

Clonidine is an alpha$_2$-adrenoceptor stimulant used for the diagnosis of growth hormone (GH) deficiency. The drug induces production of endogenous growth hormone releasing factor thereby stimulating the release of GH.

CLONIDINE HYDROCHLORIDE

UK
Indications. Diagnostic use, see notes above
Side-effects. Transient sedation, bradycardia
Dose. *Dogs*: *by intravenous injection*, 10 micrograms/kg (maximum 300 micrograms)

POM Ⓗ **Catapres** (Boehringer Ingelheim) *UK*
Injection, clonidine hydrochloride 150 micrograms/mL; 1 mL

8   Drugs acting on the
REPRODUCTIVE SYSTEM

Contributor:
Professor D E Noakes BVetMed, PhD, DVRep, FRCVS

8.1 Drugs used to promote gonadal function
8.2 Sex hormones
8.3 Prostaglandins
8.4 Myometrial stimulants
8.5 Myometrial relaxants
8.6 Prolactin antagonists
8.7 Non-hormonal abortificants
8.8 Drugs for uterine infections

Many drugs are used at different stages of the oestrous cycle to manage the response of the reproductive system; these are summarised in Table 8.1.

8.1 Drugs used to promote gonadal function

8.1.1 Gonadotrophins
8.1.2 Gonadotrophin-releasing hormones
8.1.3 Melatonin

8.1.1 Gonadotrophins

Chorionic gonadotrophin (human chorionic gonadotrophin, hCG) is a complex glycoprotein excreted in the urine of women during pregnancy. It has a similar effect to luteinising hormone (LH) secreted by the anterior pituitary gland in both males and females.

In veterinary practice, it is used to supplement or replace luteinising hormone in cases of ovulation failure or delay or to help predict timing of ovulation. In mares, chorionic gonadotrophin (hCG) is used to induce ovulation in animals with prolonged oestrus during the transitional phase from winter anoestrus to the onset of normal cyclical ovarian activity, and before mating or AI.

In males, chorionic gonadotrophin (hCG) stimulates the secretion of testosterone by interstitial testicular cells. It is used to improve libido, with variable results, and also to identify the presence of a retained testis in cryptorchids. Detection of a cryptorchid is most frequently employed in horses. Two blood samples are taken: one before and the second 30 to 120 minutes after an injection of chorionic gonadotrophin (6000 units♦ given by intravenous injection). A serum-testosterone concentration greater than 100 pg/mL, a rise in serum-testosterone concentration in response to chorionic gonadotrophin, or preferably both, confirms the presence of testicular tissue. This is known as the hCG stimulation test. It can also be used in other species

using a similar regimen but with different dosages (for example 50 units/kg♦ is used in dogs).

Serum gonadotrophin (equine chorionic gonadotrophin, eCG) is also a complex glycoprotein. It is extracted from mares' serum during the first trimester of pregnancy. The effects of serum gonadotrophin (eCG) in animals are similar to both luteinising hormone and, more predominantly, follicle-stimulating hormone (FSH) secreted by the anterior pituitary gland.

Serum gonadotrophin (eCG) is used to advance the onset of follicular growth and ovulation, in combination with progestogen-impregnated intravaginal sponges, in sheep and goats♦ (see section 8.2.2). In general, the earlier the time of the onset of the breeding season is advanced and the lower the normal prolificacy of the flock, the higher the dose of serum gonadotrophin (equine chorionic gonadotrophin) required. Therefore it is recommended that accurate flock records are kept including breed, date and dose of drug administered, and lambs produced so that the drug dose may be adjusted in future seasons to provide optimal results. Serum gonadotrophin (eCG) is sometimes used in conjunction with a progesterone-releasing intravaginal device (Prid, see section 8.2.4) to stimulate cyclical activity in acyclical cows. In combination with chorionic gonadotrophin (hCG), serum gonadotrophin (eCG) can induce oestrus in bitches in anoestrus.

Serum gonadotrophin (eCG) is employed to induce superovulation in cattle used as donors in embryo transfer. The general procedure is as follows. Serum gonadotrophin (eCG) is given on day 9 to 13 of a normal oestrous cycle. Luteolysis is induced 48 hours later by administration of a prostaglandin $F_{2\alpha}$ or analogue, given at 1.5 times the normal dose. Oestrus will be evident within 48 hours. Artificial insemination is carried out at 60 and 72 hours after prostaglandin administration. Fertilised embryos are collected 6 to 8 days after insemination and transferred to suitable synchronised recipients. The efficacy of this procedure is very variable and an exaggerated response may occur due to the long half-life of serum gonadotrophin.

Follicle stimulating hormone is used to induce superovulation. Porcine or ovine follicle stimulating hormone is used for superovulation of cattle in preference to serum gonadotrophin, which has a longer half-life and produces an excessive superovulatory response. The superovulatory response and the quality of recovered embryos can be influenced by the relative amounts of FSH and LH in the product.

In males, serum gonadotrophin (eCG) promotes spermatogenesis. Individuals may show a variable response to serum gonadotrophin (eCG) and the degree of efficacy is low. Recommended doses♦ are as follows: stallions and bulls 1000 to 3000 units, rams and boars 500 to 700 units, and dogs 400 to 800 units. The drug is administered by intramuscular injection weekly for 4 to 6 weeks.

Table 8.1 Drugs affecting the reproductive system[1]

Indications	Drug	Species	Comments
Synchronisation and regulation of the oestrous cycle	Prostaglandins: alfaprostol[1] Cloprostenol, dinoprost, luprostiol	horses, cattle	contra-indicated in pregnant animals; improved synchronisation in cows if used in conjunction with GnRH
	Etiproston[1]	cattle	
	Progesterone + estradiol benzoate (Prid)	cattle	better synchronisation if combined with prostaglandin
	Progestogens: Altrenogest Flugestone acetate Medroxyprogesterone acetate	horses, pigs sheep, goats♦ sheep, goats♦	
	Norgestomet + estradiol valerate (Crestar)	cattle	
	Progestone (Eazi-Breed CIDR)	cattle	improved synchronisation if used in conjunction with GnRH or estradiol
Stimulation of the onset of cyclical ovarian activity	Progesterone + estradiol benzoate (Prid)	cattle	may be used in conjunction with a low dose of serum gonadotrophin
	Progestogens: chlormadinone Flugestone acetate Medroxyprogesterone acetate Altrenogest	sheep, goats♦ sheep, goats♦ horses, pigs	used in conjunction with serum gonadotrophin
	Synthetic gonadotrophin-releasing hormones: deslorelin[1], fertirelin[1], lecirelin[1] Buserelin Gonadorelin	horses, cattle, rabbits cattle	
	Chorionic gonadotrophin + serum gonadotrophin (PG600)	pigs	
	Melatonin	sheep	
Superovulation	Chorionic gonadotrophin, serum gonadotrophin, follicle stimulating hormone (ovine)[1], follicle stimulating hormone (porcine), menotrophin[1]	cattle	

Table 8.1 Drugs affecting the reproductive system[1]

Indications	Drug	Species	Comments
Misalliance and pregnancy termination	Estradiol benzoate	dogs	use within 7 days of mating
	Prostaglandins: Cloprostenol, luprostiol	horses, cattle	will only be effective when corpus luteum is responsive to prostaglandin and before other sources of progesterone synthesis become dominant
	Dinoprost	horses, cattle, pigs	
	Etiproston	cattle	
	Aglepristone[1]	dogs	
	Lotrifen[1]	dogs	
Induction of parturition	Corticosteroids: (see section 7.2.1)		administer after day 260 of gestation in cattle, after day 138 of gestation in sheep
	Dexamethasone	cattle, sheep♦	
	Prostaglandins: Cloprostenol, luprostiol	cattle, pigs	administer within 7 days of full term in cattle, within 3 days of full term in pigs
	Dinoprost, etiproston	cattle	
	Tiaprost	pigs	
	Luprostiol	horses	
	Alfaprostol[1]		
Overt pseudopregnancy	Prolactin antagonists: Bromocriptine[1],	dogs	side-effects occur
	Cabergoline, metergoline[1]	dogs	
	Androgens: Methyltestosterone, testosterone esters	dogs	
	Ethinylestradiol + methyltesto-sterone (Sesoral)		
Suppression of ovarian activity	Medroxyprogesterone acetate	dogs, cats	must be used at the correct stage of the oestrous cycle
	Megestrol acetate	dogs, cats	
	Proligesterone	dogs, cats	
	Mibolerone[1]	dogs	
	Methyltestosterone	dogs	
	Altrenogest	horses	

[1]drug or indications not authorised in the UK

Menotrophin contains human menopausal gonadotrophins extracted from the urine of postmenopausal women. It has both luteinising and follicle-stimulating hormone activity in equal amounts. It is an effective method of inducing super-ovulation.

CHORIONIC GONADOTROPHIN
(Human chorionic gonadotrophin, hCG)

UK

Indications. See Dose under preparation details
Warnings. Immune-mediated reduced effect after repeated doses, occasional anaphylactic reactions; ensure that mares are not pregnant before treatment
Dose. See preparation details and notes above

POM **Chorulon** (Intervet) *UK*
Injection, powder for reconstitution, chorionic gonadotrophin 1500 units, for *horses, cattle, dogs*
Withdrawal Periods. Slaughter withdrawal period nil, milk withdrawal period nil
Dose.
Horses: induction of ovulation, *by intramuscular or intravenous injection*, 1500–3000 units 24 hours before mating or AI
Cattle: repeated failure of conception, *by intramuscular or intravenous injection*, 1500 units at mating or AI
Cystic ovarian disease, *by intravenous injection*, 3000 units
Dogs. Females: anoestrus, *by intramuscular or intravenous injection*, 500 units on first day of oestrus after pretreatment with serum gonadotrophin *by subcutaneous injection*, 20 units/kg daily for 10 days
Ovulation failure♦, *by intramuscular injection*, 100–500 units on day of mating
Delayed ovulation, prolonged pro-oestrus, *by intramuscular injection*, 100–800 units daily *or* 20 units/kg♦ until vaginal bleeding ceases. Mate on behavioural oestrus
Males: deficient libido, *by intramuscular injection*, 100–500 units twice weekly for up to 6 weeks *or* 6–12 hours before mating (temporary effect)

Australia
Indications. Fertility disorders, see notes above
Warnings. Immune-mediated reduced effect after repeated doses, occasional anaphylactic reactions
Dose. *Horses*: *by subcutaneous, intramuscular, or intravenous injection*, 1500–5000 units
Cattle: *by subcutaneous, intramuscular, or intravenous injection*, 1500–3000 units
Dogs: *by intramuscular injection*, 100–500 units

Chorulon (Intervet) *Austral.*
Injection, powder for reconstitution, chorionic gonadotrophin 1500 units, 5000 units, for *cattle, horses, dogs, fish*

Eire
Indications. Fertility disorders, see notes above
Warnings. Immune-mediated reduced effect after repeated doses, occasional anaphylactic reactions
Dose. *Horses, cattle*: *by intramuscular or intravenous injection*, 1500 or 3000 units (depending on indication)
Dogs: *by intramuscular injection*, 100–800 units (depending on indication

Chorulon (Intervet) *Eire*
Injection, chorionic gonadotrophin 1500 units, for *horses, cattle, dogs*
Withdrawal Periods. *Horses*: slaughter withdrawal period nil. *Cattle*: slaughter withdrawal period nil, milk withdrawal period nil

New Zealand
Indications. Fertility disorders, see notes above
Warnings. Immune-mediated reduced effect after repeated doses, occasional anaphylactic reactions
Dose. *Horses*: *by subcutaneous or intramuscular injection*, 1500–5000 units (depending on indication)
Cattle: *by subcutaneous or intramuscular injection*, 1000–3000 units (depending on indication)
Pigs: *by intramuscular injection*, 500–1000 (depending on indication)
Dogs: *by intramuscular injection*, 500 units

Chorulon (Chemavet) *NZ*
Injection, chorionic gonadotrophin 300 units/mL, 1000 units/mL, for *horses, cattle, sheep, goats, pigs, dogs*

USA
Indications. Frequent or constant oestrus due to cystic ovaries
Warnings. Immune-mediated reduced effect after repeated doses, occasional anaphylactic reactions
Dose. *Cattle*: *by intramuscular injection*, 10 000 units
by intravenous injection, 2500–5000
by intrafollicular injection, 500–2500 units

Chorionic Gonadotropin (Butler) *USA*
Injection, powder for reconstitution, chorionic gonadotrophin 1000 units/mL, for *cattle*

Chorionic Gonadotropin for Injection (Steris) *USA*
Injection, chorionic gonadotropin 500 units/mL, 1000 units/mL, for *cattle*

Chorulon (Intervet) *USA*
Injection, chorionic gonadotropin 1000 units/mL, for *cattle*

FOLLICLE STIMULATING HORMONE (OVINE)

Australia
Indications. Induction of superovulation
Dose. Dosages vary, consult manufacturer's information

Embryo S (Jurox) *Austral.*
Injection, follicle stimulating hormone (ovine) 50 units, for *cattle, sheep, goats*
Withdrawal Periods. Slaughter withdrawal period nil

Ovagen (Pacific Vet) *Austral.*
Injection, follicle stimulating hormone (ovine) 18 mg, for *cattle, sheep, goats*

New Zealand
Indications. Induction of superovulation
Side-effects. Occasional local reaction at injection site
Dose. *By intramuscular injection.*
Cattle: 25 units/250 kg (maximum 50 units/500 kg)
Sheep, goats: 25 units

Embryo S (Jurox) *NZ*
Injection, follicle stimulating hormone (ovine) 25 units, 50 units, for *cattle, sheep, goats*

FOLLICLE STIMULATING HORMONE (PORCINE)

UK
Indications. Superovulation in cattle
Warnings. Immune-mediated reduced effect after repeated doses, occasional anaphylactic reactions
Dose. See preparation details

POM **Super-Ov** (Global Genetics) *UK*
Injection, powder for reconstitution, follicle stimulating hormone (porcine) 75 units, for *cattle*
Withdrawal Periods. *Cattle:* slaughter 28 days, milk should not be taken for human consumption within 24 hours of embryo collection
Dose. Cattle: by intramuscular injection, 25 units daily for 3 days. Prostaglandin $F_{2\alpha}$ is administered at time of 3rd injection. Embryos are recovered from donor cows 6–8 days after AI. Prostaglandin $F_{2\alpha}$ is administered immediately after embryo recovery

Australia
Indications. Induction of superovulation
Contra-indications. Pigs
Dose. *By intramuscular injection.*
Cattle: 400 mg

Folltropin-V (Vetrepharm) *Austral.*
Injection, follicle stimulating hormone (porcine) 400 mg, for *cattle*
Withdrawal Periods. Slaughter withdrawal period nil

New Zealand
Indications. Induction of superovulation; supplemental source of FSH
Contra-indications. Pigs
Dose. Dosages vary, consult manufacturer's information

Folltropin V (Virbac) *NZ*
Injection, follicle stimulating hormone (porcine) 20 mg/mL, for *horses, cattle, sheep, goats, dogs*

Ovagen (Immuno-Chemical) *NZ*
Injection, follicle stimulating hormone (porcine), for *cattle, sheep, goats, deer*

SERUM GONADOTROPHIN
(Equine chorionic gonadotrophin, eCG)

UK
Indications. See Dose under preparation details
Warnings. Immune-mediated reduced effect after repeated doses, occasional anaphylactic reactions
Dose. See preparation details

POM **Folligon** (Intervet) *UK*
Injection, powder for reconstitution, serum gonadotrophin 1000 units, for *cattle, sheep, pigs, dogs*
Withdrawal Periods. *Cattle:* (superovulation) slaughter 28 days, milk 48 hours after second prostaglandin treatment at time of embryo collection; (other conditions) slaughter withdrawal period nil, milk withdrawal period nil. *Sheep, pigs:* slaughter withdrawal period nil, milk withdrawal period nil
Dose. *Cattle:* oestrus control in acyclical maiden dairy heifers, *by subcutaneous or intramuscular injection,* 400–700 units, following treatment with progestogen (Crestar, Prid, see section 8.2.4)
Superovulation, *by subcutaneous or intramuscular injection,* 1500–4000 units, see notes above
Sheep: induction of oestrus outside normal breeding season, *by subcutaneous or intramuscular injection,* up to 500 units at time of progestogen–impregnated sponge removal

Pigs: anoestrus post weaning, *by subcutaneous or intramuscular injection,* 1000 units. *Note.* Fertile oestrus usually follows in 3–7 days
Dogs: oestrus induction (subnormal oestrus with non-acceptance), *by subcutaneous injection,* 20 units/kg daily for 10 days, followed *by intramuscular or intravenous injection,* 500 units chorionic gonadotrophin on day 10

POM **Fostim 6000** (Pharmacia & Upjohn) *UK*
Injection, powder for reconstitution, serum gonadotrophin 6000 units, for *cattle, sheep, goats, pigs*
Withdrawal Periods. Slaughter withdrawal period nil, milk withdrawal period nil
Dose. *By subcutaneous or intramuscular injection.*
Cattle: induction of oestrus in acyclic animals, anoestrus, 300–1500 units
Sheep: induction of oestrus outside normal breeding season, for synchronised mating, 300–800 units
Goats: induction of oestrus outside normal breeding season, for synchronised mating, 400–600 units
Pigs: anoestrus, 1000–1500 units

POM **PMSG-Intervet** (Intervet) *UK*
Injection, powder for reconstitution, serum gonadotrophin 5000 units, for *cattle, sheep, pigs, dogs*
Withdrawal Periods. *Cattle:* (superovulation) slaughter 28 days, milk 48 hours after prostaglandin treatment at time of embryo collection; (other conditions) slaughter withdrawal period nil, milk withdrawal period nil. *Sheep, pigs:* slaughter withdrawal period nil, milk withdrawal period nil
Dose. See under Folligon above

Australia
Indications. Fertility disorders; induction of superovulation
Warnings. Rarely anaphylactic reactions
Dose. Dosages vary, see manufacturer's information

Folligon (Intervet) *Austral.*
Injection, powder for reconstitution, serum gonadotrophin 1000 units, 5000 units, 20 000 units, for *horses, cattle, pigs, sheep, goats, dogs*

Pregnecol Injection (Novartis) *Austral.*
Injection, powder for reconstitution, serum gonadotrophin 1000 units, 6000 units, 20 000 units, for *sheep, goats, cattle, pigs, dogs*

Eire
Indications. Fertility disorders; induction of superovulation
Warnings. Rarely anaphylactic reactions
Dose. See manufacturer's information

Folligon PMSG 1000 (Intervet) *Eire*
Injection, serum gonadotrophin 1000 units, 5000 units, for *cattle, sheep, pigs, dogs*
Withdrawal Periods. *Cattle* : (superovulation) slaughter 28 days, milk 48 hours after 2nd prostaglandin treatment. Other indications: slaughter withdrawal period nil, milk withdrawal period nil

New Zealand
Indications. Fertility disorders
Warnings. Rarely anaphylactic reactions
Dose. See manufacturer's information

Folligon (Chemavet) *NZ*
Injection, serum gonadotrophin 200 units/mL, for *horses, cattle, sheep, goats, pigs, dogs*

Pregnecol (Pastoral) *NZ*
Injection, serum gonadotrophin 6000 units, 20 000 units, for *cattle, sheep, goats, pigs, dogs*

8.1.2 Gonadotrophin-releasing hormones

Endogenous gonadotrophin-releasing hormone (GnRH) is a decapeptide secreted by the hypothalamus. Gonadotrophin releasing-hormone causes release of both LH and FSH from the anterior pituitary gland. **Fertirelin** and **gonadorelin** are synthetic forms of GnRH. **Buserelin** and **lecirelin** are synthetic analogues of GnRH in which specific amino acid substitutions have been made in their molecular structure resulting in reduced susceptibility to proteolytic enzymes and greater affinity for binding to GnRH receptors; a tenfold increase in potency is claimed. **Deslorelin** is a synthetic analogue of gonadorelin with more than 100 times greater potency than naturally occurring GnRH.

The increase in LH concentration that follows treatment with GnRH can be used to induce ovulation in horses, cattle, and rabbits. In mares, ovulation is induced in animals with prolonged oestrus during the transitional phase from winter anoestrus to the onset of normal cyclical ovarian activity, and also after mating. These drugs are used for treatment in cattle with follicular cysts. Administration at the time of service or insemination may improve conception rates in mares and cows. In cows, administration 11 or 12 days post service may increase pregnancy rates. GnRHs are also used in conjunction with progestogens and prostaglandin $F_{2\alpha}$ in oestrus synchronisation treatment regimens to control follicular growth in cows thereby improving pregnancy rates. Buserelin is also used in the fish farming industry.

BUSERELIN

UK

Indications. See under Dose
Warnings. Avoid contamination of product with traces of disinfectant or alcohol
Dose.
Horses: *by subcutaneous, intramuscular (preferred), or intravenous injection.*
Induction of ovulation (see notes above), 40 micrograms 6 hours before insemination, repeat after 1 day if required
Cattle: *by subcutaneous, intramuscular (preferred), or intravenous injection.*
Anoestrus, 20 micrograms, repeat after 8–22 days if required
Delayed ovulation, 10 micrograms 6–8 hours before or at time of insemination
Improvement in pregnancy rate, 10 micrograms 6–8 hours before or at time of insemination or 11–12 days after insemination
Follicular cysts, 20 micrograms, repeat after 10–14 days if required
Rabbits: *by subcutaneous injection.*
Induction of ovulation post partum, 800 nanograms (0.2 mL) 24 hours after parturition, and followed by insemination
Improvement of conception rate, 800 nanograms at time of insemination

Rainbow trout: *by intramuscular injection.*
To facilitate stripping and to reduce mortality due to egg binding, 3–4 micrograms/kg

POM **Receptal** (Intervet) *UK*
Injection, buserelin 4 micrograms/mL, for *horses, cattle, rabbits, rainbow trout*; 10 mL
Withdrawal Periods. *Horses, cattle, rabbits*: slaughter withdrawal period nil, milk withdrawal period nil. Should not be used in *fish* intended for human consumption

Australia

Indications. Anoestrus; cystic ovarian disorders
Dose. *Horses, cattle*: 20 micrograms

Receptal (Hoechst Roussel Vet) *Austral.*
Injection, buserelin acetate 4 micrograms/mL, for *cattle, horses*

Eire

Indications. Infertility disorders
Dose. *Horses*: *by intramuscular injection*, 40 micrograms
Cattle: *by intramuscular injection,* 10 or 20 micrograms (depending on indication)

Receptal (Hoechst Roussel Vet) *Eire*
Injection, buserelin 4 micrograms/mL, for *horses, cattle, rabbits, rainbow trout*
Withdrawal Periods. *Horses, cattle, rabbits*: slaughter withdrawal period nil. *Cattle*: milk withdrawal period nil. *Trout*: not to be used in trout intended for human consumption.

New Zealand

Indications. Fertility disorders; increase conception rate
Dose. *By subcutaneous, intramuscular, or intravenous injection.*
Horses: 20 micrograms
Cattle: 10 or 20 micrograms (depending on indication)

Receptal (Animal Health) *NZ*
Injection, buserelin acetate 4 micrograms/mL, for *horses, cattle, rabbits*
Withdrawal Periods. *Horses, rabbits*: slaughter withdrawal period nil. *Cattle*: slaughter withdrawal period nil, milk withdrawal period nil

DESLORELIN

Australia

Indications. Induction of ovulation
Warnings. Care with handling of preparations of the drug by women of child-bearing age
Dose. *Horses*: *by subcutaneous administration,* one implant

Ovuplant (Peptech) *Austral.*
Implant, deslorelin (as acetate) 2.1 mg, for *horses*
Withdrawal Periods. Slaughter withdrawal period nil

New Zealand

Indications. Induction of ovulation
Warnings. Care with handling of preparations of the drug by women of child-bearing age
Dose. *Horses*: *by administration,* one implant

Ovuplant (Peptech) *NZ*
Implant, deslorelin (as acetate) 2.1 mg, for *horses*
Withdrawal Periods. Slaughter 60 days

GONADORELIN

UK
Indications. See under Dose
Contra-indications. Hypersensitivity to the drug
Warnings. See under Buserelin
Dose. *Cattle*: *by intramuscular injection*.
In conjunction with artificial insemination, 250 micrograms on day of insemination
Cystic ovaries, 500 micrograms, repeat if required
Anoestrus post partum, 250 micrograms less than 40 days post partum *or* 500 micrograms ♦ after 40 days post partum, repeat after 1–3 weeks

POM **Fertagyl** (Intervet) *UK*
Injection, gonadorelin 100 micrograms/mL, for *cattle*; 5 mL
Withdrawal Periods. *Cattle*: slaughter withdrawal period nil, milk withdrawal period nil

Australia
Indications. Fertility disorders; induction of ovulation
Dose. *Cattle*: *by intramuscular injection*.
Cystic ovaries, 100–500 micrograms
Other indications, 250 micrograms

Fertagyl (Intervet) *Austral.*
Injection, gonadorelin 100 micrograms/mL, for *cattle, rabbits*

Eire
Indications. Fertility disorders; induction of ovulation
Dose. *Cattle*: *by intramuscular injection*.
Cystic ovaries, 500 micrograms
Other indications, 250 micrograms

Fertagyl (Intervet) *Eire*
Injection, gonadorelin 100 micrograms/ml, for *cattle*
Withdrawal Periods. Slaughter withdrawal period nil, milk withdrawal period nil

New Zealand
Indications. Fertility disorders; induction of ovulation
Dose. *Cattle*: *by intramuscular injection*.
Cystic ovaries, 500 micrograms

Fertagyl (Chemavet) *NZ*
Injection, gonadorelin 100 micrograms/mL, for *cattle, rabbits*

USA
Indications. Cystic ovaries
Dose. *Cattle*: *by intramuscular injection*.
Cystic ovaries, 100 micrograms

Factrel (Fort Dodge) *USA*
Injection, gonadorelin (as hydrochloride) 50 micrograms/mL, for *cattle*
Withdrawal Periods. Slaughter withdrawal period nil, milk withdrawal period nil

Fertagyl (Intervet) *USA*
Injection, gonadorelin (as diacetate tetrahydrate) 43 micrograms/mL, for *cattle*

8.1.3 Melatonin

Melatonin advances the time of onset of cyclical ovarian activity in the ewe by mimicking the natural production of melatonin by the pineal gland. This gives improved reproductive performance of flocks mated early in the season. A single dose of 18 mg, in a modified-release formulation, is implanted behind the ear. This is carried out 30 to 40 days before the introduction of the ram. It is important that ewes are completely separated from rams and also male goats for no less than 30 days after implantation.

In the UK, for Suffolk and Suffolk cross-breeds, the drug should be administered from mid-May to late June, for ram introduction in late June and July. For Mule and Half-bred flocks, melatonin should be administered from early June to late July, for ram introduction from mid-July to late August. In New Zealand, for Merinos, Merino cross-breds, and Corriedales, use in October to January. In British breeds, the drug is effective only in flocks joined after 10 January to end of February. Angora goats should be treated in November or December.

MELATONIN

UK
Indications. Induction of ovulation
Contra-indications. Sexually immature animals
Warnings. Use of drug in ewes suckling lambs at foot may not give optimum results. The drug should not be used at times other than recommended, see notes above
Dose. *Sheep*: *by subcutaneous administration*, 1 implant

POM **Regulin** (Ceva) *UK*
Implant, m/r, melatonin 18 mg, for *sheep*; 100
Withdrawal Periods. *Sheep*: slaughter withdrawal period nil, milk withdrawal period nil

New Zealand
Indications. Improved early breeding and ovulation rates
Contra-indications. Sexually immature animals; pregnant animals
Warnings. The drug should not be used at times other than recommended, see notes above; goats should be shorn about 120 days after implantation
Dose. *Sheep, goats*: *by subcutaneous administration*, 1 implant

Regulin Sheep (Novartis) *NZ*
Implant, melatonin 18 mg, for *sheep, goats*

8.2 Sex hormones

8.2.1 Oestrogens
8.2.2 Progestogens
8.2.3 Antiprogestogens
8.2.4 Androgens
8.2.5 Compound hormonal preparations

8.2.1 Oestrogens

Oestrogens are responsible physiologically for initiating behavioural signs of oestrus, preparing the female reproductive tract for fertilisation and developing the secretory tissue of the mammary gland. They also have anabolic activity.

In cattle, oestrogens are used to treat chronic endometritis and appear to be effective at low dosages. These drugs increase the natural uterine defence mechanisms to infection. They must not be used in acute uterine infections because they enhance the absorption of bacterial toxins. Oestrogens are used in the treatment of misalliance in the bitch. They act by inhibiting the transport of the fertilised ova down the oviducts in addition to causing hypertrophy of the uterine mucosa. Urinary incontinence in the spayed or entire bitch may also be controlled with oestrogens (see section 9.3).

In males, oestrogens are used in the treatment of excess libido, anal adenoma, and, with caution, for prostate hyperplasia.

The use of stilbenes, such as diethylstilbestrol (with the following exception) is prohibited in food-producing animals because they have been found to be carcinogenic in humans under some circumstances. Administration is allowed, if **prior** steps are taken to ensure that the treated animal and its products are not available for human or animal consumption. This exemption allows the administration of authorised-human products to farm animals for research purposes and also to companion and laboratory animals.

Oestrogens may cause aplastic anaemia in dogs and cats and cystic endometrial hyperplasia in bitches, and overdosage can cause severe inhibition of pituitary function and cystic ovaries particularly in cattle and pigs.

DIETHYLSTILBESTROL
(Stilboestrol)

UK

Indications. See under Dose; urinary incontinence (see section 9.3); behavioural modification (see section 6.11.11)
Contra-indications. See notes above
Warnings. See under Ethinylestradiol
Dose. *Dogs*: prostatic hyperplasia, anal adenoma, *by mouth*, up to 1 mg daily, reducing to maintenance dose

POM Ⓗ **Diethylstilbestrol** (Non-proprietary) *UK*
Tablets, diethylstilbestrol 1 mg, 5 mg

Australia

Indications. Suppression of lactation; hormone-responsive urinary incontinence; prostate neoplasia
Dose. *Dogs*: *by mouth*, 200–500 micrograms
incontinence, 0.1–1.0 mg daily for 3–5 days, then 1 mg weekly

Stilboestrol (Apex) *Austral.*
Tablets, diethylstilbestrol 1 mg, for *dogs*

ESTRADIOL
(Oestradiol)

UK

Indications. See Dose under preparation details; urinary incontinence (see section 9.3)
Contra-indications. Cats
Warnings. Oestrogens, particularly if used repeatedly, may cause aplastic anaemia and increased risk of cystic endometrial hyperplasia and pyometra in bitches
Dose. *Cattle*: endometritis, pyometra, *by intramuscular injection*, 3 mg/500 kg body-weight. Repeat at 7-day intervals if required

Dogs: misalliance, *by subcutaneous or intramuscular injection*, 10 micrograms/kg administered on day 3, day 5, and (if required) day 7 after mating (**but see Warnings**)

POM **Mesalin** (Intervet) *UK*
Injection (oily), estradiol benzoate 200 micrograms/mL, for *dogs*; 5 mL

POM **Oestradiol Benzoate** (Intervet) *UK*
Injection (oily), estradiol benzoate 5 mg/mL, for *cattle*; 10 mL
Withdrawal Periods. *Cattle*: slaughter 15 days, milk withdrawal period nil
Contra-indication. Should not be used in dogs

Australia

Indications. Fertility disorders; hormone-responsive urinary incontinence; metritis; pyometra; prostatehyperplasia, circumanal neoplasia
Warnings. Care in cattle and cats
Dose. *By subcutaneous or intramuscular injection*.
Horses, cattle: 10 micrograms/kg
Dogs: *females*, 10 micrograms/kg
males, 30 micrograms/kg
Cats: 30 micrograms/kg

Oestradiol Benzoate (Intervet) *Austral.*
Injection, estradiol benzoate 5 mg/mL, for *horses, cattle, dogs, cats*
Withdrawal Periods. Horses, cattle: slaughter withdrawal period nil

Oestradiol Benzoate SA (Intervet) *Austral.*
Injection, estradiol benzoate 200 micrograms/mL, for *dogs, cats*

Eire

Indications. **Dose**. Consult manufacturer's information

Oestradiol Benzoate Injection (Intervet) *Eire*
Injection (oily), estradiol benzoate 5 mg/mL, for *horses, cattle, dogs*
Withdrawal Periods. *Horses*: slaughter 5 days. *Cattle*: slaughter 5 days, milk 2 days

New Zealand

Indications. Indications vary, consult manufacturer's information
Contra-indications. Oestrogen-dependent neoplasia; where desired pregnancy exists
Dose. Dosages vary, consult manufacturer's information

Cidirol Capsules (Livestock Improvement) *NZ*
Intravaginal device, estradiol benzoate 10 mg, for *cattle*
Withdrawal Periods. Slaughter withdrawal period nil, milk withdrawal period nil

Cidirol Injection (Livestock Improvement) *NZ*
Injection, estradiol benzoate 0.5 mg/mL, for *cattle*
Withdrawal Periods. Slaughter withdrawal period nil, milk withdrawal period nil

E.C.P (Pharmacia & Upjohn) *NZ*
Injection, estradiol cypionate 2 mg/mL, for *cattle*
Withdrawal Periods. Slaughter 30 days, milk 96 hours

Oestradiol Benzoate (Chemavet) *NZ*
Injection, estradiol benzoate 0.2 mg/mL or 5 mg/mL, for *horses, cattle, sheep, goats, pigs, dogs*

USA

Indications. Fertility disorders; pyometra
Dose. *By intramuscular injection.*
Cattle: 3–10 mg (depending on indication)

ECP (Pharmacia & Upjohn) *USA*
Injection, estradiol cypionate 2 mg/mL, for *cattle*

ETHINYLESTRADIOL
(Ethinyloestradiol)

UK

Indications. See notes above and under Dose
Side-effects. Feminisation
Warnings. Overdosage may cause severe inhibition of pituitary function, anaemia and thrombocytopaenia, squamous metaplasia of the prostate, cystic endometrial hyperplasia in bitches
Dose. *By mouth.*
Dogs. Males: prostatic hyperplasia, anal adenoma, 50–100 micrograms daily. If feminisation occurs, cease treatment. Recommence therapy at half original dose

POM Ⓗ **Ethinylestradiol** (Non-proprietary) *UK*
Tablets, ethinylestradiol 10 micrograms, 50 micrograms, 1 mg

8.2.2 Progestogens

Progestogens are steroids that mimic the effects of progesterone and thus prepare and maintain the female reproductive tract for implantation and pregnancy. They cause development of the mammary glands to the point of lactation. Progestogens inhibit oestrus and ovulation by supressing the production of hormones from the anterior pituitary gland, and consequently, the development of ovarian follicles. In male animals, progestogens reduce testosterone production by the same action.

In mares, cows, ewes, does♦, and sows, progestogens are used to synchronise oestrus in groups of animals or enable the occurrence of oestrus to be predicted. Administration of a progestogen for 10 to 14 days will suppress oestrus. Longer periods of administration may cause decreased fertility. On removal of the progestogen source, the negative feedback on the pituitary and the hypothalamus is removed and oestrus is initiated. This facilitates the use of artificial insemination and stud males. This treatment may also be used in individual animals.

Altrenogest is administered in the feed to mares, gilts, and sows. **Flugestone** and **medroxyprogesterone** are administered as intravaginal sponges in ewes and does♦. On withdrawal of the sponge, serum gonadotrophin may be administered as a single dose, the dose varying according to breed of sheep and times of administration. This method is used to advance the time of onset of cyclical ovarian activity. **Progesterone** is administered to cattle by using a progesterone-releasing intravaginal device (Eazi-Breed CIDR, see also Prid section 8.2.4). Prostaglandin $F_{2\alpha}$ or analogue may be administered before removal of the progesterone device to improve the accuracy of synchronisation. **Norgestomet** is used in combination with estradiol valerate (Crestar, see section 8.2.4) to synchronise oestrus in beef cattle and dairy heifers. Progestogens may be used to stimulate the onset of cyclical ovarian activity in anoestrus mares, cows, ewes, does♦, and sows. Their effect is evident following withdrawal.

Animals are usually mated at synchronised oestrus, although ewes may be mated at the second oestrus after removal of a progestogen-impregnated sponge.

In dogs and cats, **medroxyprogesterone, megestrol, progesterone,** and **proligestone** are used to postpone or suppress oestrus. Guidelines for medical oestrus prevention include use in animals for which breeding or whelping involves a high degree of risk for the animal's life, animals which are poor surgical risks for ovariohysterectomy, and animals from which litters are not desired.

In cats, eosinophilic granuloma and 'miliary dermatitis' (crusting dermatosis) are responsive to progestogens because they have a glucocorticoid-like anti-inflammatory effect, although their use for dermatitis is contra-indicated (see section 14.2). Prolonged administration of megestrol acetate may lead to side-effects (see below) and oral corticosteroids or preferably elimination of the causative agent are recommended for the treatment of 'miliary dermatitis'.

Megestrol and medroxyprogesterone♦ may be given for behavioural problems in dogs (see section 6.11.11).

Delmadinone is used in the treatment of prostatic hypertrophy, prostatic carcinoma, and perianal tumours. It improves behaviour in some forms of aggression, nervousness, and hypersexuality.

Hydroxyprogesterone has actions similar to other progestogens and has been used to prevent recurrent abortion.

Progestogens should be used with caution. All synthetic progestogens differ in their pharmacological profile and their capacity to produce side-effects in different animal species. For example, although some progestogens may be used to inhibit or retard the growth of certain oestrogen-dependent mammary tumours and treat pseudopregnancy in bitches, it is known that other progestogens can cause or aggravate these conditions.

Progestogens stimulate the proliferative and secretory activity of the uterine endometrium leading to cystic endometrial hyperplasia, mucometra, or pyometra. Therefore, progestogens should not be administered to animals with a history of vaginal discharge or reproductive abnormalities, sexually immature animals, or dogs and cats intended for breeding. When used for suppression of oestrus in dogs and cats, animals should be allowed to have a normal cycle every 18 to 24 months.

Progestogens antagonise the hypoglycaemic effects of insulin and therefore should not be given to diabetic animals. The possibility of pre-existing disease should be considered when treating patients requiring long-term progestogen therapy. Some progestogens such as megestrol acetate may induce profound adrenal cortical suppression and possibly hypoadrenacortical syndrome on rapid withdrawal. Progestogens may induce acromegaly in entire bitches.

Subcutaneous injection of progestogens may cause hair discoloration and localised alopecia and thinning of the skin.Injection should be given in an inconspicuous area such as the inner fold of the flank or medial aspect of the thigh.

Some patients given progestogens may develop a tendency for obesity or a change in temperament.

Preparations containing progestogens should be handled with care, particularly by women of child-bearing age. Impervious gloves and suitable protective overalls should be worn when in contact with such preparations.

ALTRENOGEST

UK

Indications. See under Dose

Contra-indications. Male animals, immature animals, animals with uterine infection, see notes above

Side-effects. See notes above

Warnings. Partly consumed medicated feed should be safely destroyed and not given to any other animal. Care must be taken to avoid any contact between preparations of the drug and women of child-bearing age; the manufacturer recommends that women of child-bearing age should not be associated with the use of these preparations; woman with irregular menstrual periods after exposure to these preparations should consult their doctor; operators should wear protective clothing when handling the product

Dose. *By mouth.*

Horses: anoestrus (not deep anoestrus), suppression of prolonged oestrus during the transitional phase before the resumption of normal cyclical ovarian activity, 44 micrograms/kg daily for 10 days

Suppression and control of oestrus in cycling mares, 44 micrograms/kg daily for 15 days

Pigs: (gilts) synchronisation of oestrus, 20 mg daily for 18 days; (sows) synchronisation of oestrus, 20 mg daily for 3 days, starting on day of weaning

POM **Regumate Equine** (Intervet) *UK*
Oral solution, for addition to feed, altrenogest 2.2 mg/mL, for *horses*; 250 mL
Withdrawal Periods. Should not be used in *horses* intended for human consumption

POM **Regumate Porcine** (Intervet) *UK*
Oral suspension, for addition to feed, altrenogest 20 mg/unit dose, for *pigs*; 360-mL metered-dose applicator (1 unit dose = 5 mL)
Withdrawal Periods. *Pigs*: slaughter 15 days

Australia

Indications. Control of oestrus

Dose. *Horses*: *by mouth,* 27.5 mg

Regumate for Horses (Hoechst Roussel Vet) *Austral.*
Oral liquid, altrenogest 2.2 mg/mL, for *horses*
Withdrawal Periods. Slaughter 28 days

Eire

Indications. Control of oestrus

Contra-indications. Male animals, mares suffering from uterine infection

Dose. *Horses*: *by mouth,* 44 micrograms/kg

Regumate Equine (Hoechst Roussel Vet) *Eire*
Oral solution, to mix with feed, altrenogest 2.2 mg/mL, for *horses*
Withdrawal Periods. Slaughter 15 days

New Zealand

Indications. Control of oestrus

Contra-indications. Male animals, mares suffering from uterine infection

Dose. *Horses*: *by mouth,* 27.5 mg

Regumate (Agvet) *NZ*
Oral solution, altrenogest 2.2 mg/mL, for *horses*

USA

Indications. Suppression of oestrus

Contra-indications. Mares suffering from uterine infection,

Dose. *Horses*: *by mouth,* 44 micrograms/kg

Regu-Mate (Hoechst-Roussel) *USA*
Oral solution , altrenogest 0.22% (2.2 mg/mL), for *horses*
Withdrawal Periods. Should not be used in *horses* intended for human consumption

DELMADINONE ACETATE

UK

Indications. Treatment of hypersexuality, relief of prostatic hypertrophy, perianal (circumanal, hepatoid) gland tumours; certain behavioural problems (see section 6.11.11)

Contra-indications. Concurrent administration of other progestogens

Side-effects. Transient reduction in fertility and libido; transient increased appetite, polydipsia and polyuria; change of hair colour at site of injection

Warnings. Clinical response to treatment is 2–4 days

Dose. *Dogs, cats*: *by subcutaneous or intramuscular injection,* 1–2 mg/kg depending on the weight of the animal and severity of the condition, repeat dose after 8 days if no improvement. Repeat dose every 3–4 weeks in animals showing improvement

POM **Tardak** (Pfizer) *UK*
Injection, delmadinone acetate 10 mg/mL, for *dogs, cats*; 10 mL

Australia

Indications. Treatment of hypersexuality, relief of prostatic hypertrophy, perianal gland tumours

Contra-indications. Use in dogs with history of poor fertility or lack of libido if such animals are to be subsequently used at stud

Warnings. Care in dogs receiving additional steroid treatment

Dose. *Dogs*: *by subcutaneous or intramuscular injection,* 1–2 mg/kg depending on body-weight

Tardak (Jurox) *Austral.*
Injection, delmadinone acetate 10 mg/mL, for *dogs*

New Zealand

Indications. Treatment of hypersexuality, relief of prostatic hypertrophy, circumanal gland tumours
Contra-indications. Use in dogs with history of poor fertility or lack of libido if such animals are to be subsequently used at stud
Warnings. Care in dogs receiving additional steroid treatment
Dose. *Dogs*: *by subcutaneous or intramuscular injection*, 1–2 mg/kg depending on body-weight

Tardak (Jurox) *NZ*
Injection, delmadinone acetate 10 mg/mL, for *dogs*

FLUGESTONE ACETATE
(Flurogestone acetate)

UK

Indications. See under Dose
Contra-indications. Ewe lambs, ewes not previously bred; see notes above
Side-effects. See notes above
Warnings. Operators must wear protective gloves when handling sponges
Dose. *Sheep, goats* ♦: synchronisation of oestrus, induction of oestrus and ovulation during non-breeding season, *by intravaginal administration*, one 30-mg sponge. Remove after 12–14 days
May be followed within 6 hours in the non-breeding season by serum gonadotrophin, *by subcutaneous or intramuscular injection*, 500 units

POM **Chronogest** (Intervet) *UK*
Vaginal sponge, flugestone acetate 30 mg, for *sheep*; 25, 50, 100
Disinfectant
Liquid concentrate, benzalkonium bromide 5%. To be diluted before use
Dilute 1 volume in 90 volumes water
Withdrawal Periods. *Sheep*: slaughter 14 days after removal of sponge, should not be used in sheep producing milk for human consumption
Note. After each application, the sponge applicator should be wiped clean and placed in the supplied disinfectant. Do not use alcohols, cresols, phenols, sheep dip or other disinfectants

Australia

Indications. Controlled breeding
Side-effects. Slight decrease in milk production for several days after sponge removal
Warnings. Care in administration to goats
Dose. *Sheep, goats*: *by intravaginal administration*, one sponge

Chrono-gest (Intervet) *Austral.*
Vaginal sponge, flugestone acetate 30 mg, 40 mg and 45 mg/intravaginal sponge, for *sheep, goats*
Withdrawal Periods. Sheep, goats: slaughter 14 days, milk 14 days (after removal)

Ovakron Intravaginal Sponge (Novartis) *Austral*
Vaginal sponge, flugestone acetate 30 mg, for *sheep*
Withdrawal Periods. Slaughter 14 days, milk 14 days

Eire

Indications. Controlled breeding
Contra-indications. Ewe lambs, ewes not previously bred
Warnings. Operators must wear protective gloves when handling sponges
Dose. *Sheep*: *by intravaginal administration*, one sponge. Remove after 12–14 days

Chronogest (Intervet) *Eire*
Vaginal sponge, flugestone acetate 30 mg/sponge, for *sheep*
Withdrawal Periods. Slaughter 5 days after sponge removal, milk withdrawal period nil

New Zealand

Indications. Controlled breeding
Warnings. Operators must wear protective gloves when handling sponges; will not improve fertility in barren ewes
Dose. *Sheep*: *by intravaginal administration*, one sponge. Remove after 12–14 days

Chronogest 40 for Sheep (Chemavet) *NZ*
Intravaginal device, flugestone acetate 40 mg, for *sheep*
Withdrawal Periods. Slaughter 16 days, milk 48 hours (after removal of device)

HYDROXYPROGESTERONE CAPROATE
(Hydroxyprogesterone hexanoate)

Australia

Indications. Recurrent or threatened abortion
Dose. Dosages vary, consult manufacturer's information

Depoluteine 100 (Jurox) *Austral.*
Injection, hydroxyprogesterone caproate 100 mg/mL, for *horses, cattle*
Withdrawal Periods. Horses, cattle: slaughter 60 days

Gesteron-500 (Ilium) *Austral.*
Injection, hydroxyprogesterone caproate 100 mg/mL, for *horses, dogs, cats*

Hydroxy P 500 (Ranvet) *Austral.*
Injection, hydroxyprogesterone caproate 100 mg/mL, for *horses*
Withdrawal Periods. Slaughter 7 days

Lutogeston (Jurox) *Austral*
Injection, hydroxyprogesterone caproate 250 mg/mL, for *horses, dogs*
Withdrawal Periods. Slaughter 60 days

Procyte Depo (RWR) *Austral*
Injection, hydroxyprogesterone caproate 100 mg/mL, for *horses*
Withdrawal Periods. Should not be used in horses intended for human consumption

New Zealand

Indications. Recurrent or threatened abortion
Dose. Dosages vary, consult manufacturer's information

Gesteron-500 (Ethical) *NZ*
Injection, hydroxyprogesterone caproate 100 mg/mL, for *horses*
Withdrawal Periods. Slaughter 60 days

Hydroxy P 500 (Vetpharm) *NZ*
Injection, hydroxyprogesterone 1 mg/mL, for *horses*

Lutogeston (Jurox) *NZ*
Injection, hydroxyprogesterone caproate 250 mg/mL, for *horses*

MEDROXYPROGESTERONE ACETATE

UK

Indications. See under Dose; behaviour modification♦ (see section 6.11.11)
Contra-indications. Bitches primarily intended for breeding purposes; see notes above
Side-effects. See notes above
Dose.

Sheep, goats ♦: synchronisation of oestrus, *by intravaginal administration*, one 60-mg sponge. Remove after 13–17 days

Advancement of breeding season, in combination with serum gonadotrophin, *by subcutaneous or intramuscular injection*, 300–750 units, given at time of sponge removal (dose dependent on breed and time interval to normal breeding)

Dogs: prevention of oestrus, by subcutaneous injection, 50 mg given in anoestrus. Repeat after 6 months

Suppression (interruption) of oestrus, *by mouth*, (<15 kg body-weight) 10 mg daily for 4 days then 5 mg daily for 12 days; (>15 kg body-weight) 20 mg daily for 4 days then 10 mg daily for 12 days, given when pro-oestral bleeding evident

Cats: long-term prevention of oestrus, *by mouth*, 5 mg once weekly, given in dioestrus or anoestrus

POM **Perlutex** (Leo) *UK*
Tablets, scored, medroxyprogesterone acetate 5 mg, for *dogs, cats*; 20

POM **Promone-E** (Pharmacia & Upjohn) *UK*
Injection, medroxyprogesterone acetate 50 mg/mL, for *dogs*; 1 mL

POM **Veramix Sheep Sponge** (Pharmacia & Upjohn) *UK*
Vaginal sponge, medroxyprogesterone acetate 60 mg, for *sheep*; 20, 100
Withdrawal Periods. *Sheep*: slaughter 14 days after removal of sponge, should not be used in sheep producing milk for human consumption
Note. After each application, the sponge applicator should be wiped clean and washed in water containing a suitable disinfectant such as cetrimide 0.5–1.0%. Do not use alcohols, cresols, phenols, or similar disinfectants

Australia

Indications. Fertility disorders; behaviour modification; control of oestrus
Dose. Dosages vary, consult manufacturer's information

MPA-50 (Ilium) *Austral.*
Injection, medroxyprogesterone acetate 50 mg/mL, for *dogs, cats*

Perlutex Leo Injection (Boehringer Ingelheim) *Austral.*
Injection, medroxyprogesterone acetate 25 mg/mL, for *horses, dogs, cats*

Perlutex Leo Tablets (Boehringer Ingelheim) *Austral.*
Tablets, medroxyprogesterone acetate 5 mg, for *dogs, cats*

Promone E Aqueous Suspension (Pharmacia & Upjohn) *Austral.*
Injection, medroxyprogesterone acetate 50 mg/mL, for *dogs, cats*

Suprestral Injectable (Vetoquinol) *Austral.*
Injection, medroxyprogesterone acetate 50 mg/mL, for *dogs, cats*

Suprestral Tablets (Vetoquinol) *Austral.*
Tablets, medroxyprogesterone acetate 10 mg, for *dogs*

Eire

Indications. Prevention of oestrus; control of oestrus
Contra-indications. Sexually immature animals; pregnant animals; animals with reproductive abnormalities; diabetes mellitus, acromegaly
Side-effects. Increased appetite; mammary enlargement; possible changes in temperament
Dose. Dosages vary, consult manufacturer's information

Perlutex Injection (Leo) *Eire*
Injection, medroxprogesterone acetate 25 mg/mL, for *dogs*

Promone E (Pharmacia & Upjohn) *Eire*
Injection, medroxyprogesterone acetate 50 mg/mL, for *dogs*

Veramix Sheep Sponge (Pharmacia & Upjohn) *Eire*
Vaginal sponge, medroxyprogesterone acetate 60 mg, for *sheep*
Withdrawal Periods. Slaughter withdrawal period nil, milk withdrawal period nil

New Zealand

Indications. Prevention of oestrus; behaviour modification
Dose. Dosages vary, consult manufacturer's information

Perlutex for Injection (Boehringer Ingelheim) *NZ*
Injection, medroxyprogesterone acetate 25 mg/mL, for *dogs, cats*

Perlutex Tablets (Boehringer Ingelheim) *NZ*
Tablets, medroxyprogesterone acetate 5 mg, for *dogs, cats*

Promone E (Pharmacia & Upjohn) *NZ*
Injection, medroxyprogesterone acetate 50 mg/mL, for *dogs, cats*

Suprestral (Ethical) *NZ*
Injection, medroxyprogesterone acetate 50 mg/mL, for *dogs, cats*

MEGESTROL ACETATE

UK

Indications. See notes above and under Dose; behaviour modification (see section 6.11.11)
Contra-indications. Side-effects. See notes above. Progestogens may inhibit parturition. If used in pregnant cats, drug should be withdrawn 2–3 weeks before parturition
Warnings. Do not give more than 2 courses of treatment for postponement of oestrus/12 months in bitches
Dose. *By mouth.*

Dogs. Females: prevention of oestrus, 2 mg/kg daily for 8 days *or* 2 mg/kg daily for 4 days then 500 micrograms/kg daily for 16 days, given at pro-oestrus

Postponement of oestrus, 500 micrograms/kg daily for up to 40 days given in anoestrus and 7–14 days before postponement is required

Males: behavioural problems, see section 6.11.11

Cats. miliary dermatitis, eosinophilic granuloma, 2.5–5.0 mg every 2–3 days until lesions regress then once weekly until satisfactory response. Then maintenance dose of 2.5 mg every 7–14 days if required (**but see section 14.2**)

Females: prevention of oestrus, 5 mg daily for 3 days given in pro-oestrus

Postponement of oestrus, 2.5 mg once weekly for up to 30 weeks and given in anoestrus

POM **Ovarid** (Schering-Plough) *UK*
Tablets, scored, megestrol acetate 5 mg, 20 mg, for *dogs, cats*; 200

Australia

Indications. Prevention and control of oestrus; miliary dermatitis

Contra-indications. Diabetes; pregnancy; disorders of the reproductive tract; immature females

Side-effects. Increased appetite and weight gain

Dose. Dosages vary, consult manufacturer's information

Megecat (Vetoquinol) *Austral.*
Tablets, megestrol acetate 5 mg, for *cats*

Ovarid (Jurox) *Austral.*
Tablets, megestrol acetate 5 mg, 20 mg, for *dogs, cats*

Suppress (Jurox) *Austral.*
Tablets, megestrol acetate 5mg , 20 mg, for *dogs, cats*

Eire

Indications. Control of oestrus; behaviour modification

Contra-indications. Diabetes; pregnancy; disorders of the reproductive tract; immature females; male dogs intended for breeding

Side-effects. Increased appetite and weight gain; cystic endometrial hyperplasia; lethargy; mammary hyperplasia

Dose. Consult manufacturer's information

Ovarid (Schering-Plough) *Eire*
Tablets, megestrol acetate 5 mg, 20 mg, for *dogs, cats*

New Zealand

Indications. Prevention of oestrus; miliary dermatitis; eosinophilic granuloma

Contra-indications. Diabetes; pregnancy; disorders of the reproductive tract; immature females; male dogs intended for breeding

Side-effects. Increased appetite and weight gain; cystic endometrial hyperplasia

Dose. Consult manufacturer's information

Ovarid (Schering-Plough) *NZ*
Tablets, megestrol acetate 5 mg, 20 mg, for *dogs, cats*

Suppress (Jurox) *NZ*
Tablets, megestrol acetate 5 mg, 20 mg, for *dogs, cats*

USA

Indications. Control of oestrus; pseudopregnancy

Contra-indications. Diabetes; pregnancy; disorders of the reproductive tract; immature females; mammary tumours

Side-effects. Increased appetite; pyometra; mammary enlargement; lactation; lethargy

Dose. *Dogs*: by mouth, 2.2 mg/kg

Ovaban (Schering-Plough) *USA*
Tablets, megestrol acetate 5mg, 20 mg, for *dogs*

PROGESTERONE

UK

Indications. See under Dose

Contra-indications. Side-effects. See notes above; when used to maintain pregnancy, occasionally delayed parturition with fetal death, to masculinisation of female puppies may occur

Dose. *Cattle*: synchronisation of oestrus, induction of ovulation in anoestrus, *by intravaginal administration,* 1 device. Remove after 7–12 days. Administer prostaglandin at time of removal or at any time from 6 days after insertion
Dogs: progesterone treatment of short duration, *by subcutaneous or intramuscular injection,* 1–3 mg/kg
Cats: progesterone treatment of short duration, *by subcutaneous or intramuscular injection,* 0.2–2.0 mg/kg

POM Eazi-Breed CIDR (ART) *UK*
Intravaginal device, progesterone 1.9 g, for *cattle*; 10
Withdrawal Periods. *Cattle*: slaughter 6 hours after removal of device, milk withdrawal period nil

POM Progesterone Injectable (Intervet) *UK*
Injection (oily), progesterone 25 mg/mL, for *dogs, cats*; 50 mL

Australia

Indications. Control of oestrus; habitual and threatened abortion

Contra-indications. Intravaginal device in animals with vaginal abnormalities

Warnings. Operators should wear rubber gloves when handling intravaginal device

Dose. Dosages vary, consult manufacturer's information

Eazi-Breed CIDR-G (Novartis) *Austral.*
Intravaginal device, progesterone 0.3 g, for *sheep, goats*
Withdrawal Periods. Slaughter 1 day

Progesterone (Jurox) *Austral.*
Injection, progesterone 25 mg/mL, for *horses, cattle, dogs, cats*
Withdrawal Periods. *Horses*: slaughter 60 days. *Cattle*: slaughter 28 days

Progestin (Intervet) *Austral.*
Injection, progesterone 25 mg/mL in oily solution, for *cattle, horses, sheep, dogs, cats*
Withdrawal Periods. *Horses, cattle, sheep*: slaughter 2 days

Eire

Indications. Control of oestrus; habitual and threatened abortion

Contra-indications. Diabetes mellitus

Side-effects. Uterine changes; masculinisation of female puppies

Dose. Consult manufacturer's information

Progesterone Injection (Intervet) *Eire*
Injection, progesterone 25 mg/mL, for *cattle, dogs, cats*
Withdrawal Periods. *Cattle*: slaughter 5 days, milk 2 days

New Zealand

Indications. Control of oestrus; habitual and threatened abortion

Contra-indications. Intravaginal device in animals with vaginal abnormalities

Warnings. Operators should wear rubber gloves when handling intravaginal device

Dose. Dosages vary, consult manufacturer's information

CIDR Cattle Insert (Livestock Improvement) *NZ*
Intravaginal device, progesterone 1.38 g, for *cattle*
Withdrawal Periods. Slaughter withdrawal period nil, milk withdrawal period nil

CIDR Sheep & Goat Insert (Livestock Improvement) *NZ*
Intravaginal device, progesterone 0.3 g, for *sheep, goats*
Withdrawal Periods. Slaughter withdrawal period nil, milk withdrawal period nil

Progestin (Chemavet) *NZ*
Injection, progesterone 25 mg/mL, for *horses, cattle, sheep, goats, dogs, cats*

PROLIGESTONE

UK

Indications. See notes above and under Dose
Contra-indications. See notes above
Side-effects. Occasional anaphylactic reactions; see notes above
Dose. *By subcutaneous injection.*
Dogs: permanent postponement of oestrus, 10–33 mg/kg (larger animals receive proportionally lower doses), repeat after 3, 4, and 5 months
Temporary postponement of oestrus (<1 month before effect required), suppression of oestrus at onset of pro-oestrus, 10–33 mg/kg as a single dose
Pseudopregnancy, 10–33 mg/kg. May repeat after 1 month if required
Cats: postponement and suppression of oestrus, 100 mg
Miliary dermatitis, 33–50 mg/kg, repeat every 4 months, or more frequently depending on response (**but see section 14.2**)
Ferrets: to prevent problems associated with prolonged oestrus, 50 mg/animal

POM **Delvosteron** (Intervet) *UK*
Injection, proligestone 100 mg/mL, for *dogs, cats, ferrets*; 20 mL

Australia

Indications. Control of oestrus; miliary dermatitis; pseudopregnancy
Side-effects. Increased appetite; endometritis; lethargy; occasional pain at injection site; hair loss or discolouration at injection site
Dose. *By subcutaneous injection.*
Dogs: 10–33 mg/kg
Cats: 100 mg

Covinan (Intervet) *Austral.*
Injection, proligestone 100 mg/mL, for *dogs, cats*

Eire

Indications. Control of oestrus
Side-effects. Increased appetite; endometritis; lethargy; occasional pain at injection site; hair loss or discolouration at injection site
Dose. *By subcutaneous injection.*
Dogs: 10–33 mg/kg
Cats: 33–50 mg/kg

Delvosteron (Intervet) *Eire*
Injection, proligestone 100 mg/mL, for *dogs, cats, ferrets*

New Zealand

Indications. Control of oestrus; miliary dermatitis; pseudopregnancy

Side-effects. Endometritis; occasional pain at injection site; hair loss or discolouration at injection site
Warnings. Breeding capacity may be affected
Dose. *By subcutaneous injection.*
Dogs: 100–600 mg depending on body-weight
Cats: 100 mg

Delvosteron (Chemavet) *NZ*
Injection, proligestone 100 mg/mL, for *dogs, cats*

8.2.3 Antiprogestogens

Antiprogestogens such as aglepristone are used to terminate pregnancy in dogs. These act as competitive progesterone receptor antagonists. They interfere with the ability of progesterone derived from the corpora lutea to maintain pregnancy.

8.2.4 Androgens

Testosterone esters and methyltestosterone promote and maintain primary and secondary anatomical, physical, and psychological male sexual characteristics. Anabolic steroids (see section 7.3) are synthetic derivatives of testosterone. In the female, they can be used to exert a negative feedback effect on the pituitary thereby reducing gonadotrophin secretion.

Although androgens are used in the treatment of deficient libido in males, the results are generally unreliable and may depress spermatogenesis. Androgens are administered for the treatment of hormonal alopecia in dogs and cats and for mammary tumours and pseudopregnancy with lactation in bitches. These drugs may also be used for suppression of oestrus.

Care should be taken to avoid inducing excess virilism. Androgen therapy should not be given to animals suffering from conditions known to be aggravated by testosterone such as prostatic hypertrophy in dogs.

The effects of **methyltestosterone** last for 1 to 3 days, while oily injections of **testosterone phenylpropionate** are effective for 14 days.

Mibolerone is a synthetic androgen-derived steroid with no progestagenic or oestrogenic activity. It selectively inhibits luteinising hormone thereby preventing oestral activity. It will not postpone pro-oestrus or oestrus once these have begun. It should not be used for more than 2 years.

METHYLTESTOSTERONE

UK

Indications. See notes above and under Dose
Contra-indications. Pregnant animals, hepatic impairment, congestive heart failure
Side-effects. Virilisation with overdosage, masculisation in female animals
Warnings. Use with caution in female animals intended for breeding, early epiphyseal closure may occur in young animals

Dose. Treat according to individual response, gradual reduction of dose rather than abrupt cessation of treatment, *by mouth*.

Dogs. Females: treatment of oestrogen-dependent mammary tumours (**but see section 13.3**), suppression of oestrus, pseudopregnancy, certain hormonal alopecias, 500 micrograms/kg daily

Males: deficient libido, reversion of feminisation after removal of testicular tumour, certain hormonal alopecias, 500 micrograms/kg daily

Cats. Females: certain hormonal alopecias, 500 micrograms/kg daily

Males: deficient libido, certain hormonal alopecias, 500 micrograms/kg daily

POM **Orandrone** (Intervet) *UK*
Tablets, methyltestosterone 5 mg, for *dogs, cats*; 500

MIBOLERONE

USA

Indications. Oestrus prevention
Contra-indications. Hepatic or renal impairment; immature bitches, male dogs, puppies, cats
Warnings. Use with caution in younger mature bitch (7 months of age or less)
Dose. *Dogs*: *by mouth*, 30–180 micrograms(depending on body-weight)

Cheque Drops (Pharmacia & Upjohn) *USA*
Oral solution, mibolerone 100 micrograms /mL, for *dogs*

TESTOSTERONE ESTERS

UK

Indications. See notes above and preparation details
Contra-indications. Pregnant animals, hepatic impairment, renal impairment, congestive heart failure, dogs with prostatic hypertrophy or androgen-dependent neoplasia
Side-effects. Virilisation in females with overdosage; possible spraying in male cats
Warnings. Early epiphyseal closure may occur in young animals
Dose. See preparation details

POM **Durateston** (Intervet) *UK*
Depot injection (oily), testosterone decanoate 20 mg, testosterone isocaproate 12 mg, testosterone phenylpropionate 12 mg, testosterone propionate 6 mg/mL, for *dogs, cats*; 5 mL
Dose. *By subcutaneous or intramuscular injection*. Repeat dose after 28 days, if required
Dogs. Females: suppression of oestrus, pseudopregnancy, 0.05–0.1 mL/kg
Males: reversion of feminisation due to Sertoli cell tumour, certain hormonal alopecias, 0.05–0.1 mL/kg
Cats: 0.05–0.1 mL/kg

Australia

Indications. Lack of libido; hormonal-responsive alopecia; pseudopregnancy; oestrogen-dependent mammary tumours; sheath rot in sheep
Contra-indications. Prostate carcinoma or hyperplasia; circulatory failure; renal impairment

Dose. *Horses, dogs, cats*: dosages vary, consult manufacturer's information
Sheep: *by subcutaneous injection*, 75–150 mg
by implant administration, 1 implant

Durateston (Intervet) *Austral.*
Injection, testosterone propionate 6 mg, testosterone phenylpropionate 12 mg, testosterone isocaproate 12 mg, testosterone decanoate 20 mg/ mL, for *dogs, cats*
Withdrawal Periods. Should not be used in animals intended for human consumption.

Ropel Liquid Testosterone (Dover) *Austral.*
Injection, testosterone enanthate 75 mg/mL, for *sheep*
Withdrawal Periods. Slaughter 21 days

Ropel Testosterone Pellets (Dover) *Austral.*
Implants, testosterone propionate 23.5 mg, for *sheep*
Withdrawal Periods. Slaughter 21 days

Supertest (Vetsearch) *Austral.*
Injection, testosterone propionate 50 mg/mL, for *horses*
Withdrawal Periods. Should not be used in *horses* intended for human consumption

Tepro Hormone Injection (Virbac) *Austral.*
Injection, testosterone propionate 100 mg/mL, for *sheep*
Withdrawal Periods. Slaughter 21 days

Testo LA (Jurox) *Austral.*
Injection, testosterone cypionate 100 mg/mL, for *horses, cattle, dogs*
Withdrawal Periods. Horses, cattle: slaughter 60 days

Testoprop (Jurox) *Austral.*
Injection, testosterone propionate 50 mg/mL, for *horses, cattle, dogs*
Withdrawal Periods. *Horses*: slaughter 60 days. *Cattle*: slaughter 21 days.

Testosus 100 (Jurox) *Austral.*
Injection, testosterone 100 mg/mL (suspension), for *horses, dogs*
Withdrawal Periods. Slaughter 28 days

Eire

Indications. Lack of libido; hormonal-responsive alopecia; pseudopregnancy; oestrogen-dependent mammary tumours
Contra-indications. Cardiac insufficiency, renal or hepatic impairment; pregnant animals; prostate hypertrophy
Side-effects. Spraying in cats; virilism with overdosage
Dose. *Dogs, cats*: 0.5–1.0 mg/10 kg

Durateston (Intervet) *Eire*
Injection (oily), testosterone proprionate 6 mg/mL, testosterone phenylproprionate 12 mg/mL, testosterone isocaproate 12 mg/mL, testosterone decanoate, 20 mg/mL, for *dogs, cats*

New Zealand

Indications. Lack of libido; hormonal-responsive alopecia; pseudopregnancy; oestrogen-dependent mammary tumours
Contra-indications. Prostate carcinoma or hyperplasia
Dose. Consult manufacturer's information

Durateston (Chemavet) *NZ*
Depot injection, testosterone decanoate 20 mg/mL, testosterone isocaproate 12 mg/mL, testosterone phenylpropionate 12 mg/mL, testosterone propionate 6 mg/mL, for *horses, cattle, sheep, dogs, cats*

8.2.5 Compound hormonal preparations

A combination of hormones is used to induce a preseasonal ovulation, synchronise oestrus in a group of animals, or enable prediction of the time of oestrus. Some compound preparations are also used in the treatment of ovarian cysts or for the control of clinical signs of pseudopregnancy.

Their use is unlikely to produce satisfactory results in animals in deep anoestrus, immature animals, animals with genital-tract abnormalities, or when breeding problems have resulted from severe nutritional deficiency or other stresses.

UK

POM **Crestar** (Intervet) *UK*
Injection, norgestomet 1.5 mg, estradiol valerate 2.5 mg/mL, for *beef cattle, maiden dairy heifers*; 2 mL
Implant, norgestomet 3 mg, for *beef cattle, maiden dairy heifers*
Withdrawal Periods. *Cattle*: slaughter 14 days after removal of implant, should not be used in cattle producing milk for human consumption
Contra-indications. Treatment of cows before 45 days after calving; treatment of heifers less than 65–70% adult weight and less than 15–20 months of age; pregnant cattle
Dose. *Cattle*: synchronisation of oestrus, *by subcutaneous implantation*, 1 implant, followed immediately *by intramuscular injection*, by 2 mL of Crestar Injection. Remove implant after at least 9 days, and follow by insemination. PMSG required if animals not cycling at time of treatment
Artificial insemination is carried out at the following times, according to type of cattle: beef and dairy heifers, at 2 days after removal of implant; nursing beef cattle, at 56 hours, after removal of implant
Note. The injection and implant are supplied as a single pack by the manufacturer

POM **Nymfalon** (Intervet) *UK*
Injection, powder for reconstitution, chorionic gonadotrophin 3000 units, progesterone 125 mg, for *horses* (see note below*), cattle*; 5 mL after reconstitution
Side-effects. Rarely multiple ovulation with haemorrhage in mares
Dose. *Horses*: delayed ovulation, nymphomania, *by slow intravenous injection*, 5 mL of reconstituted solution. Repeat after 10–14 days if required **but note** that nymphomania in the mare may be due to granulosa cell tumour or may be a behavioural problem unrelated to any endocrine factors
Cattle: cystic ovaries, nymphomania, *by slow intravenous injection*, 5 mL of reconstituted solution. Repeat after 7 days if required

POM **PG 600** (Intervet) *UK*
Injection, powder for reconstitution, chorionic gonadotrophin 200 units, serum gonadotrophin 400 units, for *pigs more than 5 months of age*; 5 mL when reconstituted
Withdrawal Periods. *Pigs*: slaughter withdrawal period nil
Dose. *Sows, gilts*: anoestrus, suboestrus, *by intramuscular injection*, 5 mL of reconstituted solution
Sows, post weaning: to promote early postpartum oestrus, *by intramuscular injection*, 5 mL of reconstituted solution within 2 days of weaning
Note. Gilts more than 5 months of age, a single dose normally results in fertile oestrus within 5 days

POM **Prid** (Ceva) *UK*
Intravaginal device, progesterone 1.55 g, estradiol benzoate 10 mg, for *cows, mature heifers*; 6
Withdrawal Periods. *Cattle*: milk withdrawal period nil
Note. For 24 hours after insertion, animals must not be sent for slaughter and at all times the intravaginal device should be removed at least 6 hours before slaughter
Contra-indications. Immature heifers; cows calved less than 30 days except when using at 21 days onwards for late calving herds where, in healthy cows, early service is required; pregnant cattle; genital tract infections
Dose. *Cattle*: anoestrus, suboestrus, synchronisation of oestrus, *by intravaginal administration*, 1 device. Remove after 12 days, and follow by insemination either 2 times, at 48 hours and 72 hours, *or* once at 56 hours, after removal

POM **Sesoral** (Intervet) *UK*
Tablets, scored, ethinylestradiol 5 micrograms, methyltestosterone 4 mg, for *dogs*; 500

Contra-indications. Renal impairment, hepatic impairment, chronic congestive heart failure, pregnant animals
Dose. *Dogs*: pseudopregnancy, *by mouth,* initial dose, 1 tablet/6 kg then 1 tablet/6 kg daily in divided doses and given for 5-10 days (depending on severity of clinical signs)

Australia

Crestar (Intervet) *Austral.*
Implant/Injection, norgestomet 3 mg/implant, norgestomet 1.5 mg/mL, estradiol valerate 2.5 mg/mL injection, for synchronisation of oestrus and oestrus control in *cattle*
Withdrawal Periods. Slaughter 51 days, should not be used in cattle producing milk for human consumption

Nymfalon (Intervet) *Austral.*
Injection, powder for reconstitution, chorionic gonadotrophin 3000 units, progesterone 125 mg/5 mL after reconstitution, for cystic ovaries in cattle; oestrus cycle irregularities in *horses, cattle*
Withdrawal Periods. Horses: slaughter 1 day. Cattle: slaughter 1 day, milk withdrawal period nil

P.G. 600 (Intervet) *Austral.*
Injection, powder for reconstitution, serum gonadotrophin 400 units, chorionic gonadotrophin 200 units, to promote oestrus in *pigs*

Sesoral (Intervet) *Austral.*
Tablets, ethinylestradiol 5 micrograms, methyltestosterone 4 mg, for pseudopregnancy in *dogs, cats*

Eire

Crestar (Intervet) *Eire*
Injection; Implant, norgestomet 3 mg/2 mL, estradiol valerate 5 mg/2 mL; norgestomet 3 mg, for control of oestrus in *beef cattle, dairy heifers*
Withdrawal Periods. Slaughter 14 days, should not used in cattle producing milk for human consumption

Nymfalon (Intervet) *Eire*
Injection, powder for reconstitution, chorionic gonadotrophin 3000 iu, progesterone 125 mg, for mature follicle ovulation, cystic ovaries in *cattle*
Withdrawal Periods. Slaughter 3 days, milk 1 day

PG 600 (Intervet) *Eire*
Injection, powder for reconstitution, serum gonadotrophin 400 units/5 mL, chorionic gonadotrophin 200 units/5 mL, for oestrus induction in *pigs*
Withdrawal Periods. Slaughter withdrawal period nil

Prid (Interpharm) *Eire*
Intravaginal device, progesterone 1.55 g, estradiol benzoate 10 mg, for stimulation of ovarian activity, follicular cysts in *cattle*
Withdrawal Periods. Slaughter withdrawal period nil, milk withdrawal period nil

Sesoral Tablets (Intervet) *Eire*
Tablets, ethinylestradiol 0.005 mg, methyltestosterone 4.0 mg, for pseudopregnancy in *dogs*

New Zealand

CIDR Plus Cattle Insert (Livestock Improvement) *NZ*
Intravaginal device, estradiol benzoate 10 mg, progesterone 1.38 g, for controlled breeding programmes in *cattle*
Withdrawal Periods. Slaughter withdrawal period nil, milk withdrawal period nil

Crestar (Chemavet) *NZ*
Implant and injection, implant: norgestomet 3 mg, injection: estradiol valerate 5 mg/2 mL, norgestomet 3 mg/2 mL, for controlled breeding programmes in *cattle*
Withdrawal Periods. Slaughter 30 days

P.G. 600 (Chemavet) *NZ*
Injection, chorionic gonadotrophin 40 units/mL, serum gonadotrophin 80 units/mL, for ovarian stimulation in *pigs*

Sesoral (Chemavet) *NZ*
Tablets, ethinylestradiol 0.005 mg, methyltestosterone 4 mg, for pseudopregnancy in *dogs*

USA

P.G. 600 (Intervet) *USA*
Injection, chorionic gonadotrophin 200 units/ 5 mL, serum gonadotrphin 400 units/ 5 mL, for oestrus control in *pigs*

Syncro-Mate-B (Merial) *USA*
Implant and Injection, norgestomet 6 mg/ implant; norgestomet 3 mg and estradiol valerate 5 mg/2 mL injection, for synchronised oestrus in *cattle*
Withdrawal Periods. Should not be used in *cattle* producing milk for human consumption

8.3 Prostaglandins

Alfaprostol, cloprostenol, dinoprost, luprostiol, etiproston, and **tiaprost** are synthetic prostaglandin $F_{2\alpha}$ or analogues available for use in veterinary practice. Prostaglandins, which are derivatives of arachidonic acid, are ubiquitous substances and have an important role in many physiological and pathological processes.

Their primary effect on the reproductive system is regression of the corpus luteum. In veterinary practice they are used to control cyclical ovarian activity in polyoestrous species, for termination of pregnancy, or for induction of parturition. In addition, prostaglandins are used to treat a number of pathological conditions including mummified fetus, pyometra, and luteal cysts in cattle, and pseudopregnancy in goats♦.

The corpus luteum is refractory to the action of prostaglandin $F_{2\alpha}$ or analogues for at least 5 days post ovulation in mares, cows, ewes, and does; in sows the refractory period is up to 11 days; in bitches and queens the corpus luteum is generally unresponsive at any time after ovulation unless subject to repeated doses.

Prostaglandin $F_{2\alpha}$ also has an ecbolic effect and is sometimes used to treat 'open' pyometra in bitches♦. It, or one of the analogues, has been used to terminate pregnancy♦ in bitches in combination with cabergoline.

Side-effects such as transient sweating and mild colic with or without diarrhoea occasionally follow the use of prostaglandins in mares. On occasion some prostaglandins may produce severe reactions at the site of intramuscular injections, severe cellulitis, and systemic reactions sometimes leading to death.

Prostaglandins of the $F_{2\alpha}$ type can be absorbed through the skin and may cause bronchospasm or miscarriage. Care should be taken when handling the product to avoid self-injection or skin contact. In the event of accidental administration to a person, medical advice should be sought promptly. Women of child-bearing age, asthmatics, and persons with bronchial or other respiratory problems should avoid contact with, or wear disposable gloves when administering, the product. Accidental spillage on the skin should be washed off immediately with soap and water.

In general, treatment and administration of prostaglandins should be by the veterinarian but, for pigs, for induction of farrowing, the preparations may have to be dispensed for use by the farmer. When used for induction on farrowing in pigs, prostaglandins must not be given more than 2 days before expected parturition. The average gestation length should be calculated for each farm and prostaglandins used only where accurate service records are kept. Prostaglandin preparations are POM and should be issued by a veterinarian only to a farmer who is a bona fide client, on the basis that the named person(s) signs a receipt for the consignment and is responsible for its proper storage, use, and accountability. The veterinarian must advise the farmer that the product issued must be kept in a secure locked place except when required for administration. The veterinarian should issue only sufficient of the product for immediate foreseeable use on the farm, and periodic checks of the farmer's stock and amounts used should be carried out by the veterinarian. The farmer should be instructed on the safe handling of the product as indicated above. Prostaglandins should not be dispensed to lay persons except under these very carefully controlled circumstances (see also *British Veterinary Association Code of Practice on Medicines*).

CLOPROSTENOL

UK

Indications. See notes above and under Dose
Contra-indications. Pregnant animals unless termination required
Side-effects. See notes above
Warnings. Women of child-bearing age, asthmatics, and persons with bronchial or other respiratory problems should avoid contact with, or wear disposable gloves when administering the product. Accidental spillage on the skin should be washed off immediately with soap and water.
Dose. *By intramuscular injection.*
Horses: induction of oestrus in mares with persistent luteal function (prolonged dioestrus), type I pseudopregnancy♦ (associated with persistent luteal function in the absence of endometrial cups), pregnancy termination before 35 days, induction of oestrus for service management, 250–500 micrograms
Ponies, donkeys: 125–250 micrograms
Cattle: induction of oestrus, pregnancy termination before 150 days, endometritis, pyometra, luteal cysts, fetal mummification, synchronisation of oestrus, induction of parturition, 500 micrograms
Goats♦: pseudopregnancy, 500 micrograms
Pigs: induction of parturition, 175 micrograms

POM **Estrumate** (Schering-Plough) *UK*
Injection, cloprostenol (as sodium salt) 250 micrograms/mL, for *horses, ponies, donkeys, cattle*; 10 mL, 20 mL
Withdrawal Periods. Should not be used in *horses* intended for human consumption. *Cattle*: slaughter 1 day, milk withdrawal period nil

POM **Planate** (Schering-Plough) *UK*
Injection, cloprostenol (as sodium salt) 87.5 micrograms/mL, for *pigs*; 10 mL, 20 mL
Withdrawal Periods. *Pigs*: slaughter 4 days

Australia

Indications. Control of oestrus; induction of parturition; pregnancy termination; fertility disorders

Contra-indications. Pregnant animals unless termination required; patients with acute or subacute disorders of the gastro-intestinal tract or respiratory system

Warnings. Women of child-bearing age, asthmatics, and persons with bronchial or other respiratory problems should use extreme care when handling the product

Dose. *By intramuscular injection.*

Horses: 250–500 micrograms

Cattle: 500 micrograms

Estroplan (Parnell) *Austral.*
Injection, cloprostenol (as sodium) 250 micrograms/mL, for *cattle, horses*
Withdrawal Periods. *Horses*: slaughter 1 day. *Cattle*: slaughter 1 day, milk withdrawal period nil

Estrumate (Schering-Plough) *Austral.*
Injection, cloprostenol (as sodium) 250 micrograms/mL, for *cattle, horses*
Withdrawal Periods. *Horses*: slaughter 1 day. *Cattle*: slaughter 1 day, milk withdrawal period nil

Juramate (Jurox) *Austral.*
Injection, cloprostenol (as sodium) 250 micrograms/mL, for *cattle, horses*
Withdrawal Periods. *Horses*: slaughter 1 day. *Cattle*: slaughter 1 day, milk withdrawal period nil

Eire

Indications. Control of oestrus; induction of parturition; pregnancy termination; fertility disorders

Contra-indications. Pregnant animals unless termination required; patients with acute or subacute disorders of the gastro-intestinal tract or respiratory system

Side-effects. Transient sweating, decreased rectal temperature, increased heart rate, increased respiratory rate, and some abdominal discomfort in horses; transient increased body temperature, respiratory rate, salivation, defecation, urination, erythema, and restlessness in pigs; transient salivation, tremor, restlessness, and mild diarrhoea in cattle

Warnings. Women of child-bearing age, asthmatics, and persons with bronchial or other respiratory problems should use extreme care when handling the product

Dose. *By intramuscular injection.*

Horses: 250–500 micrograms

Cattle: 500 micrograms

Pigs: 175 micrograms

Estrumate (Schering-Plough) *Eire*
Injection, cloprostenol sodium 263 micrograms/mL (cloprostenol 250 micrograms/mL), for *horses, donkeys, cattle*
Withdrawal Periods. Should not be used in *horses* intended for human consumption. *Cattle*: slaughter 24 hours, milk withdrawal period nil

Planate (Schering-Plough) *Eire*
Injection, cloprostenol (as sodium) 175 micrograms/2 mL, for *pigs*
Withdrawal Periods. Slaughter 24 hours

New Zealand

Indications. Control of oestrus; induction of parturition; pregnancy termination; fertility disorders

Contra-indications. Pregnant animals unless termination required; patients with acute or subacute disorders of the gastro-intestinal tract or respiratory system

Side-effects. Transient sweating, decreased rectal temperature, increased heart rate, increased respiratory rate, and some abdominal discomfort in horses; transient increased body temperature, respiratory rate, salivation, defecation, urination, erythema, and restlessness in pigs; transient salivation, tremor, restlessness, and mild diarrhoea in cattle

Warnings. Women of child-bearing age, asthmatics, and persons with bronchial or other respiratory problems should use extreme care when handling the product

Dose. *By intramuscular injection.*

Horses: 250–500 micrograms

Cattle: 500 micrograms

Pigs: 175 micrograms

Estroplan (Parnell) *NZ*
Injection, cloprostenol (as sodium) 250 micrograms/mL, for *horses, cattle, pigs*
Withdrawal Periods. *Horses, pigs*: slaughter 1 day. *Cattle*: slaughter 1 day, milk withdrawal period nil

Estrumate (Schering-Plough) *NZ*
Injection, cloprostenol sodium 263 micrograms/mL, for *horses, cattle, pigs*
Withdrawal Periods. *Horses*: slaughter 28 days. *Cattle, pigs*: slaughter 1 day

Juramate (Jurox) *NZ*
Injection, cloprostenol (as sodium) 250 micrograms/mL, for *horses, cattle*
Withdrawal Periods. *Horses*: slaughter 1 day. *Cattle*: slaughter 1 day, milk withdrawal period nil

USA

Indications. Control of oestrus

Contra-indications. Pregnant animals unless termination required

Warnings. Women of child-bearing age, asthmatics, and persons with bronchial or other respiratory problems should use extreme care when handling the product

Dose. *Cattle*: *by intramuscular injection,* 500 micrograms

Estrumate (Schering-Plough) *USA*
Injection, cloprostenol (as sodium) 250 micrograms/mL, for *cattle*

DINOPROST

UK

Indications. See under Dose

Contra-indications. Pregnant animals unless termination required; patients with acute or subacute disorders of the vascular system, gastro-intestinal tract, or respiratory system

Side-effects. Transient sweating, decreased rectal temperature, increased heart rate, increased respiratory rate, and some abdominal discomfort in horses; transient increased body temperature, respiratory rate, salivation, defecation, urination, erythema, and restlessness in pigs; increased rectal temperature, transient salivation, tremor, restlessness, and mild diarrhoea in cattle

Warnings. Women of child-bearing age, asthmatics, and persons with bronchial or other respiratory problems should avoid contact with, or wear disposable gloves when administering the product. Accidental spillage on the skin should be washed off immediately with soap and water.

Dose. *By intramuscular injection*.

Horses: induction of oestrus in mares with persistent luteal function (persistent dioestrus), type I pseudopregnancy♦ (associated with persistent luteal function in the absence of endometrial cups), pregnancy termination before 35 days, synchronisation of oestrus for service management, 5 mg
Cattle: induction of oestrus, luteal cysts, chronic metritis and pyometra, pregnancy termination before 150 days, induction of parturition on or after 270 days, 25 mg. May be repeated after 10–12 days
Synchronisation of recipient cattle for embryo transplantation, 25 mg, repeat after 10–12 days
Pigs: induction of parturition within 3 days of farrowing, 10 mg
Stimulation of uterine contractions postpartum, 10 mg 1–2 days after parturition
Dogs♦: 'open' pyometra, 250 micrograms/kg daily for at least 5 days

POM **Enzaprost** (Ceva) *UK*
Injection, dinoprost 5 mg/mL, for *cattle*; 30 mL
Withdrawal Periods. *Cattle*: slaughter 1 day, milk withdrawal period nil

POM **Lutalyse** (Pharmacia & Upjohn) *UK*
Injection, dinoprost (as tromethamine) 5 mg/mL, for *horses, cattle, pigs*; 10 mL, 30 mL
Withdrawal Periods. *Horses*: slaughter 1 day. *Cattle*: slaughter 1 day, milk withdrawal period nil. *Pigs*: slaughter 1 day

POM **Noroprost** (Norbrook) *UK*
Injection, dinoprost 5 mg/mL, for *cattle*
Withdrawal Periods. *Cattle*: slaughter 1 day, milk withdrawal period nil

Australia
Indications. Control of oestrus; pregnancy termination; induction ofparturition; pseudopregnancy
Contra-indications. Pregnant animals unless termination required; patients with acute or subacute disorders of the vascular system, gastro-intestinal tract, reproductive tract, or respiratory system
Side-effects. Transient sweating, decreased rectal temperature, increased heart rate, increased respiratory rate, and some abdominal discomfort in horses; transient increased respiratory rate, salivation, defecation, urination, restlessness, and erythema in pigs; transient increased rectal temperature, salivation, in cattle
Warnings. Women of child-bearing age, asthmatics, and persons with bronchial or other respiratory problems should notadminister the product
Dose. *By intramuscular injection*.
Horses: 5 mg
Cattle: 25–35 mg
Pigs: 10 mg

Lutalyse Solution (Pharmacia & Upjohn) *Austral.*
Injection, dinoprost (as trometamol) 5 mg/mL, for *horses, cattle, pigs*
Withdrawal Periods. *Horses*: slaughter 3 days. *Cattle*: slaughter 3 days, milk withdrawal period nil. *Pigs*: slaughter 1 day

Eire
Indications. Control of oestrus; pregnancy termination; induction ofparturition

Contra-indications. Pregnant animals unless termination required; patients with acute or subacute disorders of the vascular system, gastro-intestinal tract, reproductive tract, or respiratory system
Side-effects. Transient sweating, decreased rectal temperature, increased heart rate, increased respiratory rate, and some abdominal discomfort in horses; transient increased body temperature, respiratory rate, salivation, defecation, urination, restlessness, and erythema in pigs; transient increased rectal temperature, salivation, in cattle
Warnings. Women of child-bearing age, asthmatics, and persons with bronchial or other respiratory problems should notadminister the product
Dose. *By intramuscular injection*.
Horses: 5 mg
Cattle: 25 mg
Pigs: 10 mg

Glandin (Whelehan) *Eire*
Injection, dinoprost 5 mg/mL, for *cattle*
Withdrawal Periods. Slaughter 2 days

Lutalyse (Pharmacia & Upjohn) *Eire*
Injection, dinoprost (as tromethamine) 5 mg/mL, for *horses, cattle, pigs*
Withdrawal Periods. *Horses, cattle, pigs*: slaughter 24 hours. *Cattle*: milk withdrawal period nil

New Zealand
Indications. Control of oestrus; pregnancy termination; induction ofparturition
Contra-indications. Pregnant animals unless termination required; patients with acute or subacute disorders of the vascular system, gastro-intestinal tract, reproductive tract, or respiratory system
Side-effects. Transient sweating, decreased rectal temperature, increased heart rate, increased respiratory rate, and some abdominal discomfort in horses; transient increased body temperature, respiratory rate, salivation, defecation, urination, restlessness, and erythema in pigs; transient increased rectal temperature, salivation, in cattle
Warnings. Women of child-bearing age, asthmatics, and persons with bronchial or other respiratory problems should notadminister the product
Dose. *By intramuscular injection*.
Horses: 5 mg
Cattle: 15–25 mg
Sheep: 5–10 mg
Pigs: 10–20 mg

Glandin N (Ethical) *NZ*
Injection, dinoprost 5 mg/mL, for *cattle, sheep, pigs*
Withdrawal Periods. Slaughter 24 hours

Lutalyse (Pharmacia & Upjohn) *NZ*
Injection, dinoprost (as tromethamine) 5 mg/mL, for *horses, cattle, pigs*
Withdrawal Periods. Slaughter 24 hours

USA
Indications. Control of oestrus; pregnancy termination; induction of parturition
Contra-indications. Pregnant animals unless termination required; patients with acute or subacute disorders of the

vascular system, gastro-intestinal tract, reproductive tract, or respiratory system

Side-effects. Transient sweating, decreased rectal temperature, increased heart rate, increased respiratory rate, and some abdominal discomfort in horses; transient increased body temperature, respiratory rate, salivation, defecation, urination, restlessness, and erythema in pigs; transient increased rectal temperature, salivation, in cattle

Warnings. Women of child-bearing age, asthmatics, and persons with bronchial or other respiratory problems should notadminister the product

Dose. *By intramuscular injection.*

Horses: 1 mg/45.5 kg

Cattle: 25 mg

Pigs: 10 mg

Lutalyse (Pharmacia & Upjohn) *USA*
Injection, dinoprost (as tromethamine), for *horses, cattle, pigs*
Withdrawal Periods. Should not be used in *horses* intended for human consumption *Cattle*: slaughter withdrawal period nil, milk withdrawal period nil. *Pigs*: slaughter withdrawal period nil.

ETIPROSTON TROMETHAMINE

Eire

Indications. Fertility disorders; control of oestrus

Contra-indications. Pregnant animals unless termination required

Warnings. Women of child-bearing age, asthmatics, and persons with bronchial or other respiratory problems should take care when handling the product. Accidental spillage on the skin should be washed off immediately with soap and water

Dose. *Cattle*: *by intramuscular injection*, 5 mg

Prostavet Injectable Solution (Virbac) *Eire*
Injection, etiproston tromethamine 2.5 mg/mL, for *cattle*
Withdrawal Periods. Slaughter 24 hours, milk withdrawal period nil

New Zealand

Indications. Fertility disorders; control of oestrus

Contra-indications. Pregnant animals unless termination required

Warnings. Women of child-bearing age, asthmatics, and persons with bronchial or other respiratory problems should take care when handling the product

Dose. *Cattle*: *by intramuscular injection*, 5 mg

Prostavet (Virbac) *NZ*
Injection, etiproston 2.5 mg/mL, for *cattle*
Withdrawal Periods. Slaughter 36 hours, milk withdrawal period nil

LUPROSTIOL

UK

Indications. See notes above and under Dose

Contra-indications. Pregnant animals unless termination required

Side-effects. Transient sweating and diarrhoea in horses, abdominal discomfort in cattle

Warnings. Women of child-bearing age, asthmatics, and persons with bronchial or other respiratory problems should avoid contact with, or wear disposable gloves when administering the product. Accidental spillage on the skin should be washed off immediately with soap and water.

Dose. *By intramuscular injection.*

Horses: induction of oestrus in mares with persistent luteal function (prolonged dioestrus), induction of parturition after day 330, pregnancy termination before 150 days, induction of oestrus for service management, 7.5 mg

Cattle: induction of oestrus, synchronisation of oestrus, pregnancy termination before 150 days, induction of parturition after day 270, endometritis, pyometra, *cows*: 15 mg; *heifers*: 7.5 mg

Pigs: induction of parturition not earlier than 48 hours before expected farrowing, see preparation details

POM **Prosolvin** (Intervet) *UK*
Injection, luprostiol 7.5 mg/mL, for *horses, cattle, pigs*; 10 mL, 20 mL
Withdrawal Periods. Should not be used in *horses* intended for human consumption. *Cattle:* slaughter 4 days, milk 6 hours. *Pigs:* slaughter 4 days
Dose. *Pigs*: *by intramuscular injection*, 7.5 mg

POM **Prostapar** (Intervet) *UK*
Injection, luprostiol 1.5 mg/mL, for *pigs*
Withdrawal Periods. Slaughter 24 hours
Dose. *Pigs*: *by intramuscular injection*, 3 mg

Australia

Indications. Control of oestrus; induction of parturition; pregnancy termination; pyometra

Contra-indications. Pregnant animals unless termination required

Warnings. Women of child-bearing age, asthmatics, and persons with bronchial or other respiratory problems should take care when handling the product

Dose. *By intramuscular injection.*

Horses: 7.5 mg

Cattle: *cows*: 15 mg; *heifers*: 7.5 mg

Pigs: 3 mg

Prosolvin (Intervet) *Austral.*
Injection, luprostiol 7.5 mg/mL, for *horses, cattle*
Withdrawal Periods. Slaughter 1 day

Prostapar (Intervet) *Austral.*
Injection, luprostiol 1.5 mg/mL, for *horses, cattle, pigs*

Eire

Indications. Control of oestrus; induction of parturition; pregnancy termination

Contra-indications. Pregnant animals unless termination required

Side-effects. Transient sweating and diarrhoea in horses, abdominal discomfort in cattle

Warnings. Women of child-bearing age, asthmatics, and persons with bronchial or other respiratory problems should avoid contact with, or wear disposable gloves when administering the product. Accidental spillage on the skin should be washed off immediately with soap and water

Dose. *By intramuscular injection.*

Horses: 7.5 mg

Cattle: *cows*: 15 mg; *heifers*: 7.5 mg

Pigs: 7.5 mg

Prosolvin (Intervet) *Eire*
Injection, luprostiol 7.5 mg/mL, for *horses, cattle, pigs*
Withdrawal Periods. Should not be used in *horses* intended for human consumption. *Cattle, pigs*: slaughter 24 hours

New Zealand
Indications. Control of oestrus; induction of parturition; pregnancy termination
Contra-indications. Pregnant animals unless termination required
Warnings. Women of child-bearing age, asthmatics, and persons with bronchial or other respiratory problems should take care when handling the product
Dose. *By intramuscular injection.*
Horses: 7.5 mg
Cattle: *cows*: 15 mg; *heifers*: 7.5 mg
Pigs: 7.5 mg

Prosolvin (Chemavet) *NZ*
Injection, luprostiol 7.5 mg/mL, for *horses, cattle, pigs*
Withdrawal Periods. Slaughter 24 hours

TIAPROST

UK
Indications. See under Dose
Contra-indications. Pregnant animals unless termination required. Should not be administered before day 111 of pregnancy or 2 days before farrowing as calculated from farm records
Side-effects. Transient increased urination and defaecation and slight signs of unrest
Warnings. Women of child-bearing age, asthmatics, and persons with bronchial or other respiratory problems should avoid contact with, or wear disposable gloves when administering the product. Accidental spillage on the skin should be washed off immediately with soap and water.
Dose. *Pigs*: induction of parturition, *by intramuscular injection*, 300–600 micrograms

POM **Iliren** (Intervet) *UK*
Injection, tiaprost 150 micrograms/mL, for *pigs*; 10 mL
Withdrawal Periods. *Pigs*: slaughter 4 days

8.4 Myometrial stimulants

This group includes extracts of mammalian **posterior pituitary gland**, which will contain all posterior pituitary hormones, or synthetic preparations of **oxytocin**. Carbotocin is a synthetic analogue of oxytocin, which has a much longer half-life than oxytocin. These agents stimulate contraction of the oestrogen-sensitised myometrium and mammary myoepithelial cells. This activity may be of benefit in dystocia due to secondary uterine inertia. Myometrial stimulants should not be used when dystocia is related to faulty fetal disposition or feto-maternal disproportion.

Myometrial stimulants are also used in the control of postpartum haemorrhage, to hasten uterine involution immediately after parturition in all species, to aid clearance of uterine discharge in mares, and to remove retained placenta in mares, sows, bitches, and queens; they have no effect on separation of the placenta in ruminant species. Oxytocin is also used to reduce the size of a previously prolapsed uterus♦ after replacement in cattle and occasionally mares. Myometrial stimulants are used for agalactia due to failure of milk 'let down' in all species.

OXYTOCIN

UK
Indications. See notes above and under Dose
Contra-indications. Dystocia due to obstruction, closed pyometra
Side-effects. Swelling or sloughing at injection site

POM **Oxytocin** (Leo) *UK*
Injection, oxytocin 10 units/mL, for *horses, cattle, sheep, pigs*; 20 mL
Withdrawal Periods. Slaughter withdrawal period nil, milk withdrawal period nil
Dose. *Horses*: uterine inertia, *by intramuscular injection*, 20–40 units; *by slow intravenous injection*, 5–10 units
Agalactia due to failure of 'let down', uterine involution, *by intramuscular injection*, 20–40 units; *by slow intravenous injection*, 5–10 units of diluted solution
Retained fetal membranes♦, *by intramuscular injection*, 20–40 units; *by intravenous infusion*, 50 units in sodium chloride 0.9% given over 1 hour
Expulsion of uterine fluid♦, *by intramuscular injection*, 25 units
Uterine prolapse♦, *by intramuscular injection*, 2.5–10.0 units
by intravenous infusion, 2.5–10.0 units in sodium chloride 0.9%, or sodium chloride 0.18% + glucose 4% infusion
Cattle: uterine inertia, *by intramuscular injection*, 10–40 units; *by slow intravenous injection*, 2.5–10.0 units of diluted solution
Agalactia due to failure of 'let down', uterine involution, *by intramuscular injection*, 20–80 units; *by slow intravenous injection*, 5–20 units of diluted solution
Uterine prolapse♦, *by intramuscular injection*, 2.5–10 units
Sheep, pigs: uterine inertia, *by intramuscular injection*, 2–10 units; *by slow intravenous injection*, 0.5–2.5 units of diluted solution
Agalactia due to failure of 'let down', uterine involution, *by intramuscular injection*, 4–20 units; *by slow intravenous injection*, 1–5 units of diluted solution

POM **Oxytocin-S** (Intervet) *UK*
Injection, oxytocin 10 units/mL, for *horses, cattle, sheep, goats, pigs, dogs, cats*; 25 mL
For intravenous injection dilute 1 volume with 9 volumes water for injection
Withdrawal Periods. Slaughter withdrawal period nil, milk withdrawal period nil
Dose. *Horses*: uterine inertia, agalactia due to failure of 'let down', promote uterine involution, *by subcutaneous or intramuscular (preferred) injection*, 10–40 units; *by slow intravenous injection*, 2.5–10.0 units of diluted solution
Retained fetal membranes♦, *by intramuscular injection*, 20–40 units; *by intravenous infusion*, 50 units in sodium chloride 0.9% given over 1 hour
Expulsion of uterine fluid♦, *by intramuscular injection*, 25 units
Uterine prolapse♦, *by intravenous infusion*, 2.5–10.0 units in sodium chloride 0.9%, or sodium chloride 0.18% + glucose 4% infusion
Cattle: uterine inertia, agalactia due to failure of 'let down', promote uterine involution, *by subcutaneous or intramuscular (preferred) injection*, 10–40 units; *by slow intravenous injection*, 2.5–10.0 units of diluted solution
Mastitis, *by subcutaneous or intramuscular (preferred) injection*, initial dose 80 units before stripping out and initial intramammary treatment, then 20 units before each stripping out and concurrent intramammary treatment
Uterine prolapse♦, *by intramuscular injection*, 2.5–10 units
Sheep, goats, pigs, dogs: uterine inertia, agalactia due to failure of 'let down', promote uterine involution, *by subcutaneous or intramuscular (preferred) injection*, 2–10 units; *by slow intravenous injection*, 0.5–2.5 units of diluted solution
Cats: uterine inertia, agalactia due to failure of 'let down', promote uterine involution, *by subcutaneous or intramuscular (preferred) injection*, 2–5 units; *by slow intravenous injection*, 0.5–1.25 units of diluted solution

Australia

Indications. Acceleration of parturition and expulsion of placenta; uterine contraction after caesarian section; milk 'let down'

Contra-indications. Dystocia due to obstruction, undilated cervix

Dose. Dosages vary, consult manufacturer's information

Butocin Oxytocin Injection (Pharmtech) *Austral.*
Injection, oxytocin 20 units/mL, for *horses, cattle, pigs, sheep, dogs, cats*
Withdrawal Periods. Slaughter withdrawal period nil, milk withdrawal period nil

Oxytocin Injection (Novartis) *Austral.*
Injection, oxytocin 10 units/mL

Oxytocin -S (Intervet) *Austral.*
Injection, synthetic oxytocin, equivalent to oxytocin 10 units/mL, for *horses, cattle, sheep, goats, pigs, dogs, cats*

Syntocin (Ilium) *Austral.*
Injection, oxytocin 10 units/mL, for *cattle, sheep, pigs, horses, dogs, cats*
Withdrawal Periods. Slaughter withdrawal period nil, milk withdrawal period nil

Eire

Indications. Acceleration of parturition and expulsion of placenta; uterine contraction after caesarian section; milk 'let down'

Contra-indications. Dystocia due to obstruction, undilated cervix

Dose. Dosages vary, consult manufacturer's information

Oxytocin Leo (Leo) *Eire*
Injection, oxytocin 10 units/mL, for *horses, cattle, sheep, pigs*
Withdrawal Periods. Slaughter withdrawal period nil

Pitry Injection (Interpharm) *Eire*
Injection, oxytocin 10 units/mL, for *horses, cattle, sheep, pigs*

Oxytocin-S (Intervet) *Eire*
Injection, oxytocin 10 units/mL, for *horses, cattle, sheep, goats, pigs, dogs, cats*
Withdrawal Periods. *Horses, cattle, sheep, goats, pigs*: slaughter withdrawal period nil. *Cattle, sheep*: milk withdrawal period nil

Oxytocin-Tad (Whelehan) *Eire*
Injection, oxytocin 10 units/mL, for *horses, cattle, sheep, goats, pigs, dogs, cats*

New Zealand

Indications. Acceleration of parturition and expulsion of placenta; uterine contraction after caesarian section; milk 'let down'

Contra-indications. Dystocia due to obstruction, undilated cervix

Dose. Dosages vary, consult manufacturer's information

Butocin (Bomac) *NZ*
Injection, oxytocin 20 units/mL, for *horses, cattle, sheep, pigs, dogs, cats*
Withdrawal Periods. *Horses, pigs*: slaughter withdrawal period nil. *Cattle, sheep*: slaughter withdrawal period nil, milk withdrawal period nil

Leotocin (Boehringer Ingelheim) *NZ*
Injection, oxytocin 10 units/mL, for *horses, cattle, sheep, pigs, dogs, cats*
Withdrawal Periods. *Horses, pigs*: slaughter withdrawal period nil. *Cattle, sheep*: slaughter withdrawal period nil, milk withdrawal period nil

Oxytocin EA (Ethical) *NZ*
Injection, oxytocin 10 units/mL, for *horses, cattle, sheep, goats, pigs, dogs, cats*

Oxytocin TAD (Ethical) *NZ*
Injection, oxytocin 10 units/mL, for *horses, cattle, sheep, goats, pigs, dogs, cats*

Oxytocin-S (Chemavet) *NZ*
Injection, oxytocin 10 units/mL, for *horses, cattle, sheep, goats, pigs, dogs, cats*

Oxytocin-V (Vetpharm) *NZ*
Injection, oxytocin 10 units/mL, for *horses, cattle, sheep, deer, pigs, dogs, cats*
Withdrawal Periods. *Horses, deer, pigs*: slaughter withdrawal period nil. *Cattle, sheep*: slaughter withdrawal period nil, milk withdrawal period nil

USA

Indications. Acceleration of parturition and expulsion of placenta; uterine contraction after caesarian section; milk 'let down'

Contra-indications. Dystocia due to obstruction, undilated cervix

Dose. Dosages vary, consult manufacturer's information

Oxoject (Vetus) *USA*
Injection, oxytocin 20 units/mL, for *horses, cattle, pigs, sheep,*

Oxytocin Injection (Aspen, Phoenix, Pro Labs, Vet Tek) *USA*
Injection, oxytocin 20 units/mL, for *cattle, horses, pigs, sheep, dogs, cats*

Oxytocin Injection (Osborn, RXV) *USA*
Injection, oxytocin 20 units/mL, for *cattle, horses, sheep, pigs*

Oxytocin Injection (Anthony, Vedco, Western Veterinary Supplies) *USA*
Injection, oxytocin 20 units/mL, for *cattle, horses*

Oxytocin Injection (Anthony) *USA*
Injection, oxytocin 20 units/mL, for *pigs, sheep*

PITUITARY EXTRACT (POSTERIOR LOBE)

UK

Indications. See notes above and Dose under preparation details

Contra-indications. Dystocia due to obstruction, closed pyometra; intestinal tympany in horses

Side-effects. Occasionally swelling and sloughing at the site of injection

Dose. Expressed as units of oxytocic activity, see preparation details

POM Hyposton (Pharmacia & Upjohn) *UK*
Injection, oxytocic activity (porcine origin) 10 units/mL, for *horses, cattle, sheep, goats, pigs, dogs, cats*; 50 mL
Withdrawal Periods. Slaughter withdrawal period nil, milk withdrawal period nil

Dose. *By subcutaneous or intramuscular injection.*
Horses: uterine inertia, uterine involution , 30–100 units
Cattle: uterine inertia, facilitate replacement of prolapsed uterus, control of uterine haemorrhage, agalactia due to failure of 'let down', 30–100 units
Sheep, goats: facilitate replacement of prolapsed uterus, 20–50 units
Pigs: uterine inertia, uterine involution, control of uterine haemorrhage, aid expulsion of retained fetal membranes and uterine debris, agalactia due to failure of 'let down', 10–30 units
Dogs: uterine inertia, uterine involution, control of uterine haemorrhage, aid expulsion of retained fetal membranes and uterine debris, 2.5–20.0 units
Cats: uterine inertia, uterine involution, control of uterine haemorrhage, aid expulsion of retained fetal membranes and uterine debris, 2.5–5.0 units

POM **Pituitary Extract (Synthetic)** (Animalcare) *UK*
Injection, oxytocic activity 10 units/mL, for *horses, cattle, sheep, goats, pigs, dogs, cats*; 25 mL
Withdrawal Periods. Slaughter withdrawal period nil, milk withdrawal period nil
For intravenous injection dilute 1 volume with 9 volumes water for injections
Dose. Uterine inertia, agalactia due to failure of 'let down', control of post-partum haemorrhage, uterine involution and aid expulsion of retained placenta
Horses, cattle: by subcutaneous or intramuscular (preferred) injection, 10–40 units; by slow intravenous injection, 2.5–10 units
Sheep, goats, pigs: by subcutaneous or intramuscular (preferred) injection, 2–10 units; by slow intravenous injection, 0.5–2.5 units
Dogs: by subcutaneous or intramuscular (preferred) injection, 2–10 units; by slow intravenous injection, 0.5–2.5 units
Cats: by subcutaneous or intramuscular (preferred) injection, 2–5 units; by slow intravenous injection, 0.5–1.25 units

8.5 Myometrial relaxants

These drugs cause relaxation of the uterus and are used to aid obstetrical manoeuvres during dystocias and to facilitate handling of the uterus during caesarean section. They are sometimes used to facilitate the recovery of embryos from donors for embryo transfer, and to facilitate replacement of a prolapsed uterus. They can be used to delay parturition so that it may occur when greater observation and care are available. In addition, when used in heifers, calving can be delayed sufficiently to allow better relaxation of the birth canal and perineum. Myometrial relaxants are sometimes used in the treatment of incomplete cervical dilation (ring-womb) in sheep, although their effect is questionable.

Clenbuterol is a beta$_2$-adrenoceptor stimulant and therefore is antagonistic to the effects of oxytocin and prostaglandins. It relaxes and coordinates contractions in all species except cats. When using clenbuterol, it is important to avoid ingestion by refraining from eating, drinking, or smoking. Skin contamination should be washed off immediately. Accidental self-injection may result in tachycardia and tremor and hence immediate medical treatment should be sought.

Vetrabutine is a papaverine-like drug. It interrupts the contractions caused by oxytocin with periods of relaxation; if used concurrently with oxytocin a lower than usual dose of oxytocin should be administered. Vetrabutine is not as effective as clenbuterol but can be used for ringwomb in sheep. It should not be used in cats.

Isoxsuprine is a vasodilator which also stimulates beta-adrenergic receptors. It causes direct relaxation of vascular (see section 4.3.1) and uterine smooth muscle.

CLENBUTEROL HYDROCHLORIDE

UK

Indications. Facilitating obstetrical manoeuvres
Contra-indications. Concurrent administration of atropine, adrenoceptor stimulants, vasodilators, or general anaesthetics, oxytocin, prostaglandins
Side-effects. Transient vasodilation and tachycardia with sweating and muscle tremors with high dosage
Warnings. Drug Interactions – see Appendix 1

Dose. *Cattle*: by intramuscular or slow intravenous injection, 300 micrograms as a single dose

POM **Planipart** (Boehringer Ingelheim) *UK*
Injection, clenbuterol hydrochloride 30 micrograms/mL, for *cattle*; 50 mL
Withdrawal Periods. *Cattle*: slaughter 6 days, milk 5 days

Australia

Indications. Facilitating obstetrical manoeuvres; postponement of parturition
Contra-indications. Concurrent administration of adrenoceptor stimulants, vasodilators, atropine, general anaesthesia
Dose. *By intramuscular or slow intravenous injection.*
Cattle: 60 micrograms/100 kg body-weight
Sheep: 210 micrograms/100 kg body-weight

Planipart (Boehringer Ingelheim) *Austral.*
Injection, clenbuterol hydrochloride 30 micrograms/mL, for *cattle, sheep*
Withdrawal Periods. *Cattle*: slaughter 6 days, milk 6 days. *Sheep*: slaughter 6 days

Eire

Indications. Facilitating obstetrical manoeuvres
Contra-indications. Concurrent administration of atropine, adrenoceptor stimulants, vasodilators, or general anaesthetics, oxytocin, prostaglandins
Dose. *Cattle*: by intramuscular or slow intravenous injection, 300 micrograms as a single dose

Planipart (Boehringer Ingelheim) *Eire*
Injection, clenbuterol hydrochloride 30 micrograms/mL, for *cattle*
Withdrawal Periods. Slaughter 6 days, milk 5 days

New Zealand

Indications. Facilitating obstetrical manoeuvres
Contra-indications. Concurrent administration of adrenoceptor stimulants
Dose. *Cattle*: by intramuscular or slow intravenous injection, 300 micrograms

Planipart (Boehringer Ingelheim) *NZ*
Injection, clenbuterol hydrochloride 30 micrograms/mL, for *cattle*
Withdrawal Periods. Slaughter 12 days, milk 5 days

ISOXSUPRINE

Indications. Facilitating obstetrical manoeuvres

Australia

Indications. Facilitating obstetrical manoeuvres
Contra-indications. Equine colic; undilated cervix
Dose. *By intramuscular injection.*
Cattle: 115–230 mg
Sheep, goats, pigs: 46 mg
Dogs: 4.6–23 mg
Cats: 2.3 mg

Duphaspasmin Injection (Novartis) *Austral.*
Injection, isoxsuprine lactate 11.58 mg/mL, for *cattle, sheep, goats, pigs, dogs, cats*

Eire

Indications. Facilitating obstetrical manoeuvres

Dose. *By intramuscular injection.*
Horses, cattle: 230 mg
Sheep, goats: 46 mg
Pigs: 46–92 mg
Dogs: 4.6–23 mg
Cats: 2.3 mg

Duphaspasmin (Interchem) *Eire*
Injection, isoxsuprine lactate 11.58 mg/mL, for *horses, cattle, sheep, goats, pigs, dogs, cats*

New Zealand
Indications. Facilitating obstetrical manoeuvres
Side-effects. Occasional transient signs of tachycardia and muscle spasms
Dose. *By intramuscular injection.*
Horses, cattle: 46 mg/100 kg
Sheep, goats: 7 mg/10 kg
Pigs: 3.5 mg/10 kg
Dogs: 4.6–5.7 mg/10 kg
Cats: 0.5 mg/kg

Fort Dodge Duphaspasmin (Pacificvet) *NZ*
Injection, isoxsuprine lactate 11.58 mg/mL, for *horses, cattle, sheep, goats, pigs, dogs, cats*

VETRABUTINE HYDROCHLORIDE
(Dimophebumine hydrochloride)

UK
Indications. Facilitating obstetrical manoeuvres
Contra-indications. Should not be used in cats
Warnings. Pregnant women and women of child-bearing age should exercise extreme caution to avoid self-injection
Dose. *By intramuscular injection.*
Cattle: 2.5 mg/kg as a single dose
Sheep: 3 mg/kg as a single dose
Pigs: 2 mg/kg as a single dose
Dogs: 2 mg/kg. May be repeated at 30–60 minute intervals for up to 3 doses

POM **Monzaldon** (Boehringer Ingelheim) *UK*
Injection, vetrabutine hydrochloride 100 mg/mL, for *cattle, sheep, pigs, dogs*; 50 mL
Withdrawal Periods. *Cattle*: slaughter 28 days, milk 7 days. *Sheep, pigs*: slaughter 28 days

Eire
Indications. Facilitating obstetrical manoeuvres
Contra-indications. Should not be used in cats
Warnings. Pregnant women and women of child-bearing age should exercise extreme caution to avoid self-injection
Dose. *Pigs*: *by intramuscular injection*, 5 g

Monzaldon (Boehringer Ingelheim) *Eire*
Injection, vetrabutine hydrochloride 100 mg/mL, for *pigs*
Withdrawal Periods. Slaughter 28 days

8.6 Prolactin antagonists

The corpus luteum of bitches is probably dependent upon the luteotrophic support of pituitary-derived prolactin dur-

ing the second half of the luteal phase of metoestrus and pregnancy. Pregnancy in this species is maintained by the presence of corpora lutea; if they regress, pregnancy will be terminated. Prolactin inhibitors, such as bromocriptine have been used to terminate pregnancy in bitches but the results have been unreliable and side-effects occur.

The prolactin inhibitor **cabergoline** exerts its effect by inhibiting prolactin release by direct stimulation of dopamine receptors in dopamine releasing cells in the anterior pituitary. As a consequence the corpora lutea regress and pregnancy is terminated. Towards the end of metoestrus as the corpora lutea regress, there is a concommitant rise in prolactin which is responsible for the overt signs of pseudopregnancy such as behavioural signs and mammary development and lactation. Cabergoline reduces prolactin release and is used for the treatment of overt pseudopregnancy in the bitch.

Bromocriptine is a potent dopamine receptor agonist (dopamine receptor stimulant). It inhibits prolactin release from the anterior pituitary gland. Bromocriptine is used in the treatment of pseudopregnancy in bitches. It should be reserved for cases where other methods fail because side-effects of bromocriptine are common and may be severe. Metoclopramide (see section 3.4.1) can be used concurrently as an anti-emetic even though it has dopamine receptor blocking properties.

Metergoline is a serotonin agonist with actions similar to bromocriptine; it is used to suppress lactation.

BROMOCRIPTINE

UK
Indications. Pseudopregnancy; pituitary-dependent hyperadrenocorticism (see section 7.6)
Side-effects. Vomiting, anorexia, depression, and behavioural changes
Dose. *By mouth.*
Horses: 100 micrograms/kg twice daily
Dogs: hyperadrenocorticism, up to 100 micrograms/kg daily in divided doses given in gradually increasing amounts
Pseudopregnancy, 10 micrograms/kg twice daily for 10 days *or* 30 micrograms/kg once daily for 16 days

POM Ⓗ **Bromocriptine** (Non-proprietary) *UK*
Tablets, bromocriptine (as mesilate) 2.5 mg

POM Ⓗ **Parlodel** (Novartis) *UK*
Tablets, scored, bromocriptine (as mesilate) 1 mg, 2.5 mg; 1-mg tablets 100; 2.5-mg tablets 30, 100
Capsules, bromocriptine (as mesilate) 5 mg, 10 mg; 100

CABERGOLINE

UK
Indications. Pseudopregnancy; suppression of lactation; termination of pregnancy ◆
Contra-indications. Pregnant animals; lactating animals unless suppression of lactation required; use directly after surgery while animal still recovering from anaesthesia

Side-effects. Transient hypotension, occasionally vomiting or anorexia, transient drowsiness

Warnings. Drug Interactions – see Appendix 1

Dose. *Doe goats*♦, to suppress lactation, *by mouth,* 5 micrograms/kg

Dogs: by mouth, 5 micrograms/kg once daily for 4–6 days. May be mixed with food

POM **Galastop** (Boehringer Ingelheim) *UK*
Oral solution, cabergoline 50 micrograms/mL, for *dogs*; 7 mL, 15 mL (3 drops = cabergoline 5 micrograms)

METERGOLINE

Australia
Indications. Pseudopregnancy; suppression of lactation
Dose. *Dogs: by mouth,* 100 micrograms/kg twice daily

Contralac 2.0 Metergoline (Virbac) *Austral.*
Tablets, metergoline 2 mg, for *dogs*

New Zealand
Indications. Pseudopregnancy; suppression of lactation
Side-effects. Vomiting, mild diarrhoea, agitated behaviour
Dose. *Dogs: by mouth,* 200 micrograms/kg daily in 2 divided doses

Contralac 20 (Virbac) *NZ*
Tablets, metergoline 2 mg, for *dogs*

8.7 Non-hormonal abortificants

Lotrifen is a phenyltriazole isoquinoline which causes embryopathy and abortion in many species such as rats, hamsters, gunea pigs, and dogs. It is most effective in dogs when administered around 20 days of gestation and it is used as in dogs for pregnancy termination. The mode of action is unclear: the drug may be embryotoxic, it may reduce blood supply to the gravid uterus, or modify the animal's immune response.

8.8 Drugs for uterine infections

Bacteria will contaminate the uterus of most individuals after normal parturition. However these micro-organisms will soon be eliminated by natural defence mechanisms. The bacteria may originate from the environment and are opportunist pathogens or may be specific venereal pathogens; failure to eliminate them due to impaired defence mechanisms will result in infection. In addition, trauma associated with dystocia and heavy bacterial contamination are also likely to predispose to infection. Uterine infection may be acute, frequently involving all layers of the uterine wall (metritis) or chronic, usually involving the endometrium (endometritis). The former may be fatal.

Treatment of metritis includes the use of systemic antimicrobials (see section 1.1) and supportive therapy. Chronic infection involving the endometrium can be treated by the intra-uterine infusion of broad-spectrum antimicrobials,

administered at the usual therapeutic dosage. In the cow, if a corpus luteum is present, endometritis is best treated by administration of prostaglandin $F_{2\alpha}$ or an analogue. Alternatively, in the absence of a corpus luteum up to 5 mg of estradiol benzoate♦ may be administered. Estradiol benzoate must not be used in cows with acute metritis.

In bitches endometritis and pyometra most commonly occur in the luteal phase of the oestrus cycle (metoestrus). In animals with 'open' pyometra with dilated cervix and vaginal discharge, dinoprost♦ (see section 8.3) is administered at a dose of 250 micrograms/kg for at least 5 days. It is contraindicated in bitches with very enlarged uteri, animals with heart conditions, and patients with 'closed' pyometra. Side-effects occur within 15 minutes of administration and include panting, salivation, vomiting, and whimpering. These symptoms are transient and cease within one hour.

In the UK, the Horserace Betting Levy Board publishes *Codes of Practice on contagious equine metritis (CEM) Klebsiella pneumoniae, Pseudomonas aeruginosa; equine viral arteritis (EVA); and equid herpesvirus-1 (EHV-1),* which include recommendations for disease prevention and control.

UK
POM **Metrijet 1500** (Intervet) *UK*
Intra-uterine solution, oxytetracycline (as hydrochloride) 100 mg/mL, for *cattle*; 15-mL dose applicator
Withdrawal Periods. *Cattle*: slaughter 5 days, milk withdrawal period nil
Dose. *Cattle: by intra-uterine administration*, the contents of 1 applicator, repeat after 7 days if required

POM **Utocyl** (Novartis) *UK*
Pessaries, benzylpenicillin 62.7 mg, formosulphathiazole 1.75 g, streptomycin (as sulphate) 50 mg, for *cattle*; 18
Withdrawal Periods. *Cattle*: slaughter 2 days, milk withdrawal period nil
Dose. *Cattle: by intra-uterine administration*, 6 pessaries for prophylaxis only

Australia
Metrijet (Intervet) *Austral.*
Intr-uterine solution, oxytetracycline hydrochloride 24 mg, clioquinol 25 mg, ethinyloestradiol 0.025 mg, dl-alpha-tocopheryl 10 mg/g, for *cattle*
Withdrawal Periods. Slaughter 21 days, milk 7 days

Oblicarmine Intra-Uterine Tablets (Boehringer Ingelheim) *Austral.*
Intra-uterine tablets, tetracycline hydrochloride 500 mg, for *horses, cattle, sheep, goats, pigs*
Withdrawal Periods. *Cattle*: slaughter 14 days, milk 36 hours (single dose) or 72 hours (multiple dose). *Horses, sheep, goats, pigs*: slaughter 14 days

Tribactral Duals (Jurox) *Austral.*
Pessary/Tablet, sulfadiazine 1000 mg, trimethoprim 200 mg/ pessary, for *horses, cattle, sheep*
Withdrawal Periods. *Cattle*: slaughter 14 days, milk 36 hour (single dose) or 72 hours (multiple dose). *Horses, sheep*: slaughter 14 days

Tribrissen Bolus/Pessary (Jurox) *Austral.*
Pessary/Tablet, sulfadiazine 1000 mg, trimethoprim 200 mg/ pessary, for *cattle, horses, sheep, pigs*
Withdrawal Periods. *Cattle*: slaughter 14 days, milk 36 hours (single dose) or 72 hours (multiple dose). *Horses, sheep, pigs*: slaughter 14 days

Utozyme Foaming Pessaries (Jurox) *Austral.*
Pessaries, oxytetracycline (as hydrochloride) 500 mg, bacterial proteinase 200 mg, for *cattle, sheep, pigs, goats*
Withdrawal Periods. *Cattle*: slaughter 14 days, milk 36 hours (single dose) or 72 hours (multiple dose). *Sheep, goats, pigs*: slaughter 14 days

Eire

Metrijet 1500 (Intervet) *Eire*
Injection, oxytetracycline (as hydrochloride) 100 mg/mL, for **cattle**
Withdrawal Periods. Slaughter 5 days, milk withdrawal period nil

Chlortetracycline Uterine Boluses (Vetoquinol) *Eire*
Intrauterine boluses, chlortetracycline hydrochloride 500 mg, for **cattle**
Withdrawal Periods. Slaughter 10 days, milk 5 days

New Zealand

Metricure (Chemavet) *NZ*
Intra-uterine injection, per syringe: cefapirin 500 mg, for **cattle**
Withdrawal Periods. Slaughter 4 days, milk withdrawal period nil

Oxyfoam Forte (Virbac) *NZ*
Intravaginal device, oxytetracycline hydrochloride 1 g, for **cattle**
Withdrawal Periods. Slaughter 7 days, milk 96 hours

Tetravet Foaming Pessary (Bomac) *NZ*
Pessary, oxytetracycline hydrochloride 1 g, for **horses, cattle, sheep, goats, deer, pigs**
Withdrawal Periods. **Horses, deer, pigs**: slaughter 7 days. **Cattle, sheep, goats**: slaughter 7 days, milk 96 hours

Tetracycline Hydrochloride 0.5 g Intra-uterine Oblets (Phoenix) *NZ*
Intra-uterine device, tetracycline hydrochloride 500 mg, for **cattle, sheep, goats**
Withdrawal Periods. Slaughter 7 days, milk 96 hours

USA

Amifuse (Vetus) *USA*
Intra-uterine solution, amikacin sulphate 250 mg/mL, for **horses**
Withdrawal Periods. Should not be used in **horses** intended for human consumption

Amiglyde-V Intrauterine Solution (Fort Dodge) *USA*
Intra-uterine solution, amikacin sulphate 250 mg/mL, for **horses**
Withdrawal Periods. Should not be used in **horses** intended for human consumption

Amikacin E Solution (Phoenix) *USA*
Intra-uterine solution, amikacin (as sulphate) 250 mg/mL, for **horses**
Withdrawal Periods. Should not be used in **horses** intended for human consumption

Amikacin Sulfate Solution (VetTek) *USA*
Intra-uterine solution, amikacin (as sulphate) 250 mg/mL, for **horses**
Withdrawal Periods. Should not be used in **horses** intended for human consumption

Genta-Fuse (Vetus) *USA*
Intra-uterine solution, gentamicin (as sulphate) 100 mg/mL, for **horses**
Withdrawal Periods. Should not be used in **horses** intended for human consumption

Gentaglyde (Fort Dodge) *USA*
Intra-uterine solution, gentamicin (as sulphate) 100 mg/mL, for **horses**
Withdrawal Periods. Should not be used in **horses** intended for human consumption

Gentamax (Phoenix) *USA*
Intra-uterine solution, gentamicin (as sulphate) 100 mg/mL, for **horses**
Withdrawal Periods. Should not be used in **horses** intended for human consumption

Gentamicin Sulfate Solution (Anthony, Aspen, Boehringer Ingelheim Vetmedica, Butler, VetTek, Western Veterinary Supply) *USA*
Intra-uterine solution, gentamicin (as sulphate) 100 mg/mL, for **horses**
Withdrawal Periods. Should not be used in **horses** intended for human consumption

Gentaved 100 (Vedco) *USA*
Intra-uterine solution, gentamicin (as sulphate) 100 mg/mL, for **horses**
Withdrawal Periods. Should not be used in **horses** intended for human consumption

Gentocin (Schering-Plough) *USA*
Intra-uterine solution, gentamicin (as sulphate) 50 mg/mL, 100 mg/mL, for **horses**
Withdrawal Periods. Should not be used in **horses** intended for human consumption

Intrauterine Bolus (AgriLabs) *USA*
Intra-uterine Tablets, urea 13.4 g, for **cattle, sheep**

Legacy (Pro Labs) *USA*
Intra-uterine solution, gentamicin (as sulphate) 100 mg/mL, for **horses**
Withdrawal Periods. Should not be used in **horses** intended for human consumption

Ticillin (Pfizer) *USA*
Intra-uterine powder, for reconstitution, ticarcillin 6 g/vial, for **horses**
Withdrawal Periods. Should not be used in **horses** intended for human consumption

Uterine Bolus (DurVet, Phoenix) *USA*
Intra-uterine tablet, urea 13.4 g/ bolus, for **cattle, sheep**

9 Drugs used in the treatment of disorders of the URINARY SYSTEM

Contributor:
Professor A S Nash BVMS, PhD, CBiol, FIBiol, DipECVIM, MRCVS

9.1 Drugs used in the treatment of renal failure
9.2 Drugs for cystitis
9.3 Drugs for urinary retention and incontinence
9.4 Drugs for urolithiasis

9.1 Drugs used in the treatment of renal failure

The kidneys play a central role in maintaining and regulating fluid, acid-base, and electrolyte balance. They excrete waste products of protein metabolism and are active in the production of erythropoietin and hydroxylation of vitamin D. In renal impairment the kidneys are unable to maintain normal function and the consequences of reduced renal function are seen in many body systems.

Acute renal failure may result from severe cardiac and circulatory failure, extremes of temperature (heatstroke), hypovolaemic and septic shock, prolonged anaesthesia, bacterial infection, and drug or chemical induced toxicity. The clinical signs of acute renal failure are dependent on the cause of dysfunction and may include oliguria, polydipsia, abdominal pain, shock, pyrexia, dehydration, vomiting, diarrhoea, constipation, uraemic signs, convulsions, and possibly sudden death.

The biochemical changes seen with acute renal failure include azotaemia, hyperphosphataemia, metabolic acidosis, and sodium, potassium, and chloride imbalances.

If possible, management should be aimed at identifying and eliminating the causative problem, which may include the following: cardiac disease, nephrotoxins, bacterial infections, or urinary calculi. Treatment including fluid therapy may be employed. Diuretics are used to promote urine production if the patient is well hydrated and producing some urine.

Chronic renal failure results from primary glomerular, tubular and interstitial diseases or combinations of these. Generalised renal neoplasia and chronic urinary outflow obstructions may also lead to chronic renal failure. The condition may be characterised by reduced vitality, loss of body and coat condition, anorexia, polydipsia, polyuria, vomiting, uraemia, dehydration, oral ulceration, diarrhoea, secondary hyperparathyroidism, and anaemia. Hypertension may develop in some cases.

In dogs and cats, the biochemical changes seen with chronic renal failure include azotaemia, hypoalbuminaemia, hyperphosphataemia, metabolic acidosis, and changes in plasma sodium, potassium, and calcium concentrations. In horses, plasma-calcium concentration can be markedly elevated. Phosphate concentrations often vary inversely with the calcium concentration, except in renal dysfunction resulting

from vitamin D intoxication. The aim of treatment is to minimise the clinical and biochemical consequences of reduced renal function.

Non-regenerative anaemia is mainly caused by reduced renal production of erythropoietin. Epoetin (recombinant human erythropoietin) may be used for treatment although limited data is available on the use of this drug in animals. If hypertension is confirmed, epoetin should not be used until the hypertension has been controlled. The clinical efficacy of epoetin alfa and epoetin beta is similar and they can be used interchangeably. Other factors which contribute to anaemia of chronic renal failure such as iron or folate deficiency should also be corrected. Anabolic steroids (see section 7.3) may also be administered but their effectiveness in respect of anaemia caused by chronic renal failure is doubtful.

The diet (see section 16.8 for dietetic pet foods for dogs and cats) should be assessed and changed according to the individual patient's needs. Azotaemic or uraemic animals require a diet containing low protein of high biological value, whereas others may benefit from normal protein concentration because of loss due to proteinuria or haemorrhage. The content of sodium and potassium in the diet should also be assessed on an individual patient basis. Oral potassium supplements (see section 16.5.10) may be administered if necessary but should be used with care. Angiotensin-converting enzyme (ACE) inhibitors and potassium-sparing diuretics may potentiate the risk of hyperkalaemia.

Hyperphosphataemia in dogs and cats leads to hypocalcaemia and parathyroid hyperplasia resulting in increased production of parathyroid hormone. Resorption of bone may result (renal osteodystrophy, secondary hyperparathyroidism). Reduced dietary phosphorus is essential and special diets may be given (see section 16.8). If necessary hyperphosphataemia may also be controlled by the use of antacids such as aluminium hydroxide (see section 3.8.1) that bind intestinal phosphorus.

If hypertension is confirmed, treatment with ACE inhibitors or other hypotensive drugs (see section 4.3.1) may be instituted.

Renal dysfunction also affects the ability of the kidney to metabolise vitamin D_3 to its active form leading to reduced absorption of intestinal calcium. After hyperphosphataemia has been controlled, oral calcium (see section 16.5.1) or vitamin D supplements (see section 16.6.4) may be administered. Multivitamin preparations containing B vitamins may be required to compensate urinary loss of water-soluble vitamins.

Initial treatment for vomiting and diarrhoea may require intravenous fluid therapy (see section 16.1.2). Thereafter vomiting may be controlled with cimetidine or sucralfate (see section 3.8.2) and diarrhoea with antidiarrhoeals (see section 3.1). Alkalinisers (see section 16.1.2) are used to control metabolic acidosis.

Patients should be kept warm and comfortable and allowed unrestricted access to water (unless repeatedly vomiting). Prescribers should avoid administration of drugs that may cause nephrotoxicity or that are excreted through the kidneys (see Prescribing in renal impairment).

Primary glomerulonephropathies may result in persistent severe proteinuria and resultant hypoalbuminaemia, with possible development of *nephrotic syndrome*, characterised by peripheral and body cavity fluid retention. When fluid retention occurs, diuretic therapy should be instituted using furosemide (see section 4.2.2) and maintained until after the oedema and ascites have resolved.

Immune-mediated glomerulonephropathies have been treated with corticosteroids, such as prednisolone (see section 7.2.1) but there is no convincing evidence of their efficacy in this respect in domestic animals. Moreover, renal amyloidosis, which can lead to protein losing nephropathy in dogs, cats, and cattle, is exacerbated by the use of corticosteroids.

Examination of renal biopsy material is required for diagnostic confirmation of underlying glomerulonephropathies.

EPOETIN ALFA and BETA
(Recombinant human erythropoietin)

UK

Indications. Anaemia associated with chronic renal failure
Contra-indications. Hypertension
Side-effects. Some animals may develop an immune-mediated response to the drug which may reduce its efficacy
Warnings. Regular haematological monitoring is required to ensure that the PCV does not rise above normal
Dose. *Dogs, cats*: *by subcutaneous injection*, 50–100 units/kg 3 times weekly until packed cell volume is within normal range. Then reduce to lowest effective dose or widen dosage interval

Note. The clinical efficacy of epoetin alfa and epoetin beta is similar and they can be used interchangeably

POM Ⓗ **Eprex** (Janssen-Cilag) *UK*
Injection, epoetin alfa 2000 units/mL; 0.5 mL, 1 mL
Injection, epoetin alfa 4000 units/mL; 0.5 mL, 1 mL
Injection, epoetin alfa 10 000 units/mL; 0.3 mL, 0.4 mL, 1 mL
Note. May be difficult to obtain a supply of this preparation

POM Ⓗ **NeoRecormon** (Roche) *UK*
Injection, powder for reconstitution, epoetin beta 500 units, 1000 units, 2000 units, 5000 units, 10 000 units
Multidose injection, powder for reconstitution, epoetin beta 50 000 units, 100 000 units
Note. May be difficult to obtain a supply of this preparation

9.2 Drugs for cystitis

9.2.1 Acidifiers
9.2.2 Alkalinisers

Cystitis is commonly caused by *Escherichia coli* and other coliforms, *Proteus*, *Pseudomonas aeruginosa*, *Corynebacterium suis* (pigs), *Corynebacterium renale* (cattle), staphylococci, and streptococci. Chronic cystitis may be complicated by urinary calculi or neoplasia and ascending infection may result in pyelonephritis.

Treatment for acute cystitis usually requires a 10 to 14 day course of a systemic antibacterial (see section 1.1) that is excreted unchanged by the kidneys. Chronic cystitis may require therapy for at least 3 weeks and possibly up to 6 weeks. Effective drugs include amoxicillin, nitrofurantoin, cefalexin, amoxicillin with clavulanic acid, sulfadiazine and trimethoprim, and fluoroquinolones.

The urinary pH may affect the efficacy of antibacterials. Erythromycin, streptomycin, sulfadiazine and trimethoprim, and fluoroquinolones are more effective at pH 8, whereas penicillin, tetracycline, and nitrofurantoin are more active at pH 5.5.

9.2.1 Acidifiers

Ascorbic acid, ammonium chloride, ammonium sulphate, ethylenediamine, methionine, or **sodium acid phosphate** may be used to acidify the urine, which is useful in the treatment of cystitis. In cases of infection appropriate antimicrobials should be given (see above). Acidifiers are also used in control of struvite calculi (see section 9.4).

Ascorbic acid is inconsistent in lowering urinary pH and is usually unpalatable at the recommended dosages. In horses, ammonium chloride has been shown to be ineffective in lowering urinary pH at low doses (20 mg/kg daily). It has also been given at doses of 100 to 500 mg/kg daily but is unpalatable. Ammonium sulphate is more palatable and has proved effective at the recommended dose.

The antimicrobial action of methenamine (hexamine) is due to formaldehyde, which is liberated during acid hydrolysis; low urinary pH is required.

ASCORBIC ACID

UK

Indications. Urine acidification; adjunct in the treatment of paracetamol poisoning (see Treatment of poisoning)
Dose. *By mouth.*
Horses: 2 g/kg daily
Dogs: 100–500 mg 3 times daily
Cats: 100 mg 3 times daily

See section 16.6.3 for preparation details

AMMONIUM CHLORIDE

UK

Indications. Urine acidification
Dose. See preparation details

Ammonium Chloride *UK*
Dose. By mouth.
Horses: see notes above
Dogs: 100 mg/kg 1–2 times daily
Cats: ¼ of 5-mL spoonful with food

Uroeze (Arnolds) *UK*
Oral powder, for addition to feed, ammonium chloride 400 mg/650 mg of powder, for *cats*; 113 g. (650 mg of powder = ¼ 5-mL spoonful)
Contra-indications. Kittens; severe hepatic or renal impairment; acidosis
Side-effects. May cause gastric irritation
Dose. *Cats*: *by mouth*, 400 mg/4.5 kg body-weight twice daily with food. Adjust dose until desired urinary pH change achieved

Australia
Indications. Urine acidification
Warnings. Some manufacturers state risk of crystalluria if used in conjunction with sulphonamides
Dose. *Dogs, cats*: *by mouth*, 20 mg/kg 1–2 times daily (up to 800 mg daily in cats)

Acidurin Tablets (Apex) *Austral*
Tablets, ammonium chloride 100 mg, for *dogs, cats*

Urimav 100 mg Urinary Acidifier Tablets (Mavlab) *Austral*
Tablets, ammonium chloride 100 mg, for *dogs, cats*

Urimav 400 mg Urinary Acidifier Tablets (Mavlab) *Austral*
Tablets, ammonium chloride 400 mg, for *dogs, cats*

USA
Indications. Urine acidification
Contra-indications. Severe hepatic or renal impairment, acidosis
Side-effects. Gastric mucosa irritation
Dose. *Dogs, cats*: *by mouth*, 200–400 mg/4.5 kg body-weight twice daily

Uroeze 200 (Daniels) *USA*
Oral powder, ammonium chloride 200 mg/0.65 g powder, for *cats, dogs*

Uroeze 200 (Daniels) *USA*
Tablets, ammonium chloride 200 mg, for *cats, dogs*

Uroeze Powder (Daniels) *USA*
Oral powder, ammonium chloride 400 mg/0.65 g powder, for *cats, dogs*

Uroeze Tablets (Daniels) *USA*
Tablets, ammonium chloride 400 mg, for *cats, dogs*

AMMONIUM SULPHATE

UK
Indications. Urine acidification
Dose. *By mouth.*
Horses: 175 mg/kg 2 times daily

ETHYLENEDIAMINE

UK
Indications. Urine acidification
Contra-indications. Acidotic or azotaemic animals
Side-effects. Occasionally vomiting. Tablets should not be broken or crushed but administered whole
Dose. *By mouth.* Adjust dose according to urinary pH.
Dogs, cats: (<10 kg body-weight) 1 tablet 3 times daily, (10–25 kg body-weight) 2 tablets 3 times daily, (>25 kg body-weight) 3 tablets 3 times daily

POM Chlorethamine (Intervet) *UK*
Tablets, ethylenediamine dihydrochloride 90 mg, for *dogs, cats*; 500

METHIONINE

Australia
Indications. Urine acidification; prevention of struvite calculi
Contra-indications. Severe hepatic or renal impairment or pancreatic disease; administration to animals with an empty stomach; acidotic animals
Warnings. High dosage may cause gastro-intestinal disturbances
Dose. *Dogs, cats*: *by mouth*, 50 mg/kg in 2 divided doses

Deltameth '500' Tablets (Delvet) *Austral*
Tablets, methionine 500 mg, for *dogs, cats*

Methapex (Apex) *Austral*
Tablets, methionine 500 mg, for *cats, dogs*

Methigel (Apex) *Austral*
Oral paste, methionine 80 mg/g, for *cats, dogs*

Methio-Form Chewable Tablets (Novartis) *Austral*
Tablets, methionine 500 mg, for *cats, dogs*

Methionine 500 (Apex) *Austral*
Tablets, methionine 500 mg, for *cats, dogs*

Methnine 90 (Vetsearch) *Austral*
Tablets, methionine 500 mg, for *cats, dogs*

USA
Indications. Urine acidification
Contra-indications. Severe hepatic or renal impairment or pancreatic disease; acidotic animals; some manufacturers state pregnant or nursing animals and animals less than 1 year of age
Warnings. High dosage may cause gastro-intestinal disturbances when given on an empty stomach
Dose. Dosages vary, see manufacturer's information. For guidance.
Dogs: *by mouth*, 400–1000 mg daily in divided doses
Cats: *by mouth*, 200–400 mg daily in divided doses

Ammonil Tablets (Daniels) *USA*
Tablets, methionine 200 mg, 500 mg, for *cats, dogs*

d-l-m Tablets (Butler) *USA*
Tablets, methionine 200mg or 500mg, for *dogs, cats*

d-l-Methionine Powder (Butler) *USA*
Oral powder, methionine 100%, for *dogs, cats*

D-L-Methionine Powder (First Priority) *USA*
Oral powder, methionine , for *dogs, cats*

Methigel (Evsco) *USA*
Oral gel, methionine 400 mg/ 5g gel, for *dogs, cats*

Methio-Form (Vet-A-Mix) *USA*
Tablets, methionine 500 mg (6.7 mEq), for *dogs, cats*

Methio-Tab (Vet-A-Mix) *USA*
Tablets, methionine 200mg (2.68 mEq) and 500 mg (6.7 mEq), for *dogs, cats*

SODIUM ACID PHOSPHATE

UK
Indications. Urine acidification
Dose. *Dogs*: *by mouth*, 1–2 tablets daily

POM **Hexamine and Sodium Acid Phosphate Tablets** (Arnolds) *UK*
Tablets, methenamine (hexamine) 150 mg, anhydrous mono sodium phosphate 116 mg, for *dogs*; 250

9.2.2 Alkalinisers

Sodium bicarbonate, sodium citrate, and **potassium citrate** are used for urine alkalinisation. Alkalinisers are also used to prevent urate uroliths (see section 9.4).

POTASSIUM CITRATE

UK

Indications. Urine alkalinisation for treatment of urinary tract infections; management of calcium oxalate and urate urolithiasis (see section 9.4)
Contra-indications. Renal or cardiac impairment
Dose. *Dogs, cats*: *by mouth,* 75 mg/kg twice daily *or* 2 mmol/kg twice daily

P Ⓗ **Cystopurin** (Roche Consumer Health) *UK*
Oral powder, potassium citrate 3 g/sachet; 7 g sachet

GSL Ⓗ **Potassium Citrate Mixture** (BP) *UK*
Oral solution, potassium citrate 30%, citric acid monohydrate 5%, contains about 28 mmol K+/10 mL

Australia

Indications. Urine alkalinisation; aid to muscular recovery after racing
Dose. See preparation details

A.K.M. (Action Chemical) *Austral*
Oral solution, potassium citrate 41.7 g/L, potassium acetate 41.7 g/L, for *dogs*
Dose. *Greyhounds*: *by mouth,* 10 mL twice daily for 4 days; then 10 mL on alternate days

Baladene (Inca) *Austral*
Oral solution, sodium citrate 225 g, potassium citrate 75 g, citric acid 75 g sucrose 440 g/L, for *horses, dogs*
Dose. *Horses*: *by mouth,* 50–75 mL
Greyhounds: *by mouth,* 2–4 mL

SODIUM BICARBONATE

UK

Indications. Urine alkalinisation
Dose. *Dogs, cats*: *by mouth,* 10–50 mg/kg 2–3 times daily. Adjust dose until desired urinary pH change achieved

GSL Ⓗ **Sodium Bicarbonate** (Non-proprietary) *UK*
Capsules, sodium bicarbonate 500 mg
Tablets, sodium bicarbonate 600 mg

SODIUM CITRATE

Australia

Indications. Urine alkalinisation; 'tying up' syndrome; acidosis
Dose. See preparation details

Baladene (Inca) *Austral*
Oral solution, sodium citrate 225 g, potassium citrate 75 g, citric acid 75 g sucrose 440 g/L, for *horses, dogs*
Dose. *Horses*: *by mouth,* 50–75 mL
Greyhounds: *by mouth,* 2–4 mL

Neutradex (Vetsearch) *Austral*
Oral syrup, sodium acid citrate 283.3 g/L, for *horses, greyhounds*
Withdrawal Periods. *Horses*: slaughter withdrawal period nil
Dose. *Horses*: *by mouth,* 25–50 mL
Greyhounds: *by mouth,* 4-6 mL

Neutralite (Troy) *Austral*
Oral liquid, sodium acid citrate 8 g/30 mL, for *horses, greyhounds*
Withdrawal Periods. *Horses*: slaughter withdrawal period nil
Dose. *Horses*: *by mouth,* 25 mL–50 mL
Greyhounds: *by mouth,* 5 mL

Neutra-Syrup (International Animal Health Products) *Austral*
Oral syrup, citric acid 15 g, sodium ions, 2.8 g, for *horses, greyhounds*
Withdrawal Periods. *Horses*: slaughter withdrawal period nil
Dose. *Horses*: *by mouth,* 30–60 mL daily
Greyhounds: *by mouth,* 5 mL daily

9.3 Drugs for urinary retention and incontinence

Urinary retention and incontinence may affect animals of all ages. Non-neurogenic causes include inherited lesions or acquired conditions such as cystitis, neoplasia, or urinary calculi. Neurological deficits may follow spinal trauma.
Bladder wall irritability leading to frequent micturition may be caused by cystitis and antibacterial therapy should be instigated (see section 9.2).
Rarely, idiopathic detrusor instability occurs and may respond to anticholinergic drugs. **Propantheline** is an antimuscarinic drug, which reduces urinary urgency and frequency by diminishing unstable muscle contractions but has a negligible effect on urethral spincter pressure.
Incontinence may be caused by flaccidity of the urethral sphincter. This condition commonly affects ovariohysterectomised bitches and may be responsive to oestrogen therapy (see section 8.2.1), which enhances the sensitivity of the alpha-adrenoreceptors in the smooth muscle of the bladder neck and urethra to sympathetic stimuli. drugs used for treatment include oral **estriol**, a recently introduced short acting natural oestrogen, and oral **diethylstilbestrol** at doses of up to 1.0 mg daily for 3 to 5 days, followed by weekly treatment. Alpha-adrenoreceptor stimulants may also be used to improve urethral tone, either alone or in combination with oestrogens. The dose of each drug should be reduced and titrated for each individual animal. Ephedrine has been used in the past but **phenylpropanolamine** is thought to be preferable. The dose of phenylpropanolamine should be reduced if used concurrently with oestrogen therapy. Surgery may be necessary if medical treatment alone proves unsuccessful.
Excessive urinary retention that may lead to incontinence is caused by detrusor muscle paralysis or excessive urethral sphincter contraction. Paralysis of the bladder wall may occur following spinal trauma or overdistension of the bladder due to obstruction. Parasympathomimetics, such as **bethanechol,** produce the effects of parasympathetic nerve stimulation; they possess the muscarinic rather than the nicotinic effects of acetylcholine and improve voiding by increasing the tone and contractions of the detrusor muscle. Treatment should be initiated at the lowest dose and increased after 48 hours if no improvement.

Phenoxybenzamine acts by blocking alpha-adrenoreceptors of the bladder neck and proximal urethra allowing relaxation of the urethral sphincter. Oral **diazepam** (see section 6.9.2) may assist by causing relaxation and reduction of urethral resistance; the recommended dose for dogs is 200 micrograms/kg 3 times daily and for cats is 2.5 mg 3 times daily.

Many of the above drugs take some time to have a clinically observable effect and treatment should be continued for up to 3 to 4 weeks before deciding that the condition is unresponsive to a particular drug.

BETHANECHOL CHLORIDE

UK
Indications. Urinary retention
Contra-indications. Urinary obstruction
Side-effects. Salivation, vomiting, diarrhoea
Dose. *By mouth.*
Horses: 50–100 micrograms/kg 2–3 times daily
Dogs: 5–25 mg 3 times daily
Cats: 1.25–5.0 mg 3 times daily

POM Ⓗ **Myotonine** (Glenwood) *UK*
Tablets, scored, bethanechol chloride 10 mg, 25 mg; 100

ESTRIOL

UK
Indications. Hormone-dependent urinary incontinence due to sphincter mechanism incontinence
Contra-indications. Intact bitches; animals showing polyuria-polydipsia syndrome
Side-effects. Occasionally swollen vulva, swollen mammary glands, attractiveness to males, and vomiting; rarely vaginal bleeding
Warnings. Animals should be re-examined every 6 months
Dose. *By mouth*. Dosage should be titrated according to individual response. For guidance.
Dogs: initial dose, 1 mg daily. If response, reduce to 0.5 mg daily or on alternate days. If no response to initial treatment, 2 mg once daily (maximum 2 mg/animal daily)

POM **Incurin** (Intervet)
Tablets, estriol 1 mg, for *ovariohysterectomised bitches*; 30

PHENOXYBENZAMINE HYDROCHLORIDE

UK
Indications. Urinary retention secondary to reflux dyssinergia
Contra-indications. Cardiovascular or renal disease
Side-effects. Hypotension
Dose. *By mouth.*
Dogs: 0.25–0.5 mg/kg 2–3 times daily
Cats: 0.5 mg/kg twice daily

POM Ⓗ **Dibenyline** (Goldshield) *UK*
Capsules, phenoxybenzamine hydrochloride 10 mg; 30

PHENYLPROPANOLAMINE HYDROCHLORIDE

UK, Eire
Indications. Urinary incontinence secondary to urinary sphincter incompetence
Contra-indications. Pregnant animals
Side-effects. Aggression, anorexia, hyperexcitability, lethargy, cardiac arrhythmias, hypertension
Warnings. May produce clinical signs mimicking excessive stimulation of the sympathetic nervous system, hyperexcitability may be particularly marked in cats
Dose. *By mouth.*
Dogs: 1.5 mg/kg twice daily *or* 1 mg/kg 3 times daily
Cats ♦: 1.0–1.5 mg/kg twice daily

POM **Propalin** (Vétoquinol) *UK, Eire*
Syrup, phenylpropanolamine hydrochloride 50 mg/mL, for *dogs*

NZ
Indications. Urinary incontinence secondary to urinary sphincter incompetence
Contra-indications. Pregnant animals; concurrent use of other hypertensive drugs
Side-effects. Aggression, hyperexcitability
Warnings. May produce clinical signs mimicking excessive stimulation of the sympathetic nervous system
Dose. *Dogs*: by mouth, 1.5 mg/kg twice daily

Propalin (Ethical) *NZ*
Syrup, phenylpropanolamine hydrochloride 50 mg/mL, for *dogs*

PROPANTHELINE BROMIDE

UK
Indications. Urinary incontinence due to detrusor hyperreflexia; adjunct in gastro-intestinal disorders characterised by smooth muscle spasm (see section 3.7)
Contra-indications. Glaucoma, urinary obstruction
Side-effects. Dry mouth, increased intra-ocular pressure, constipation, tachycardia
Dose. Urinary incontinence, *by mouth.*
Dogs: 400 micrograms/kg 3–4 times daily
Cats: 7.5 mg every 3 days

POM Ⓗ **Pro-Banthine** (Hansam) *UK*
Tablets, s/c, propantheline bromide 15 mg; 100, 1000

9.4 Drugs for urolithiasis

The management and treatment of urolithiasis will depend on the type of calculus present and may include surgery, dietary control, antibacterial therapy, urinary acidifiers or alkalinisers in addition to specific drug therapy.
Struvite calculi may form when urease-positive staphylococcci or *Proteus* bacteria and high concentrations of magnesium or phosphate salts are present in the bladder. Medical therapy includes appropriate antibacterials (based on urine bacteriology and antibacterial sensitivity testing) to eliminate bacteria, dietary control to reduce protein intake and induce polyuria (see section 16.8), and urinary acidifiers (see section 9.2.1). **Walpole's buffer solution** may be used to irrigate the bladder in cats with feline urological syn-

drome (FUS). It dissolves feline uroliths in the bladder but is sometimes used as a flushing solution in cats with urethral obstruction. However, the solution may worsen pre-existing urethral inflammation and is probably best confined to intravesical use.

Urate uroliths are more soluble in alkaline urine. Dietary control to reduce protein intake and urine alkalinisers (see section 9.2.2) are used as preventive treatment. **Allopurinol** reduces the formation of uric acid from purines by inhibiting xanthine oxidase.

Penicillamine reacts with cystine to form a more soluble sulphide compound that is more readily excreted. It is used as an adjunct to dietary management and urinary alkalinisation in the management of *cystinuria*.

Penicillamine is best given on an empty stomach because food interferes with its absorption. Common side-effects such as vomiting or diarrhoea can be ameliorated by dividing the daily dose or by giving the drug with food.

Thiazide diuretics (see section 4.2.1) may be used to reduce the recurrence of calcium-containing uroliths (for example, calcium oxalate calculi) in dogs. Patients undergoing chronic thiazide therapy should be monitored for adverse effects such as dehydration, hypokalaemia, and hypercalcaemia. Thiazide diuretics are not currently recommended for prophylaxis of feline calcium oxalate urolithiasis.

ALLOPURINOL

UK

Indications. Urate calculi; leishmaniosis (see section 1.4.7)

Side-effects. Erythema, hypersensitivity; predisposition to xanthine calculi

Warnings. Reduce dosage for patients with renal impairment

Dose. *Dogs*: urate calculi, *by mouth*, 10 mg/kg 3 times daily for 4 weeks then 10 mg/kg twice daily

POM Ⓗ **Allopurinol** (Non-proprietary) *UK*
Tablets, allopurinol 100 mg, 300 mg

POM Ⓗ **Zyloric** (GlaxoWellcome)
Tablets, allopurinol 100 mg, 300 mg

PENICILLAMINE

UK

Indications. Cystine calculi; copper, mercury, and lead poisoning (see Treatment of poisoning); copper hepatotoxicosis (see section 3.10)

Contra-indications. Concurrent administration of cytotoxic drugs, phenylbutazone, and gold salts in dogs

Side-effects. Anorexia, vomiting; pyrexia; nephrotic syndrome

Warnings. Penicillamine absorption decreased if concurrent administration with food, antacids, iron or zinc salts

Dose. *Dogs*: cystine calculi, *by mouth*, 15 mg/kg twice daily preferably on an empty stomach. May be mixed with food or daily dose divided if vomiting occurs (but absorption may be impaired)

POM Ⓗ **Penicillamine** (Non-proprietary) *UK*
Tablets, penicillamine 125 mg, 250 mg

POM Ⓗ **Distamine** (Dista) *UK*
Tablets, f/c, penicillamine 125 mg, 250 mg; 100

COMPOUND PREPARATIONS FOR UROLITHIASIS

UK

POM **Walpole's Buffer Solution** (Arnolds) *UK*
Glacial acetic acid, sodium acetate 1.17% (pH 4.5), for *male cats*; 25 mL
Use undiluted to irrigate bladder by bladder lavage
Indications. Acute urethral obstruction due to struvite calculi
Contra-indications. Bladder injection

Australia

Walpoles Solution (Mavlab) *Austral*
Bladder irrigation, sodium acetate 7.05 mg/mL, acetic acid 6.8 mg/mL, for *cats*
Indications. Acute urethral obstruction due to struvite calculi

New Zealand

Vetrecal (Bomac) *NZ*
Oral solution, sodium edetate 85 mg/mL, sodium tripolyphosphate 60 mg/mL, for *dogs, cats*
Indications. Urinary calculi
Dose. *Dogs, cats*: *by mouth*, treatment, 10-30 drops/5-8 kg daily for 1-4 days; prophylaxis, 5-10 drops/5-8 kg daily

10 Drugs used in the treatment of disorders of the
MUSCULOSKELETAL SYSTEM and JOINTS

Contributors:
B D X Lascelles BVSc, BSc, PhD, CertVA, DSAS (ST), DipECVS, MRCVS
T S Mair BVSc, PhD, DEIM, MRCVS

Many classes of drugs are used to suppress or abolish one or more of the cardinal signs of acute inflammation (heat, redness, swelling, pain, and loss of function) in soft tissues and joints. The principle value of these drugs is to relieve pain and reduce swelling.

Arthritis involves inflammation of certain tissues and changes in other tissues of the joint, which may result in pain. The inciting cause may be infective, immune-mediated, drug-induced, or due to trauma caused by surgery, injury, or poor conformation. Septic arthritis may occur due to a localised or systemic infection. Infective agents include *Erysipelothrix rhusiopathiae*, *Mycoplasma* spp., *Streptococcus* spp., *Staphylococcus aureus*, and *Actinomyces pyogenes*. Dependent on the causative agent, antibacterials used for treatment include lincomycin, tylosin, tiamulin, gentamicin, and oxytetracycline (see section 1.1). Vaccination against erysipelas (see sections 18.2.6 and 18.3.6) is available.

Anti-inflammatory drugs used in the management of musculoskeletal and joint disorders interfere with the synthesis, release, or action of mediators and modulators of inflammation and cartilage metabolism. These mediators and modulators include histamine, bradykinin, prostaglandins, leukotrienes, platelet-activating factor, complement components, a range of lysosomal and non-lysosomal enzymes, nitric oxide, and oxygen-derived free radicals. The many mediators that are implicated in acute and chronic inflammation may interact either synergistically or antagonistically. Anti-inflammatory drugs that antagonise the action or release of a single mediator or group of mediators often suppress, but usually do not abolish, inflammatory changes.

Not all of the drugs considered in this chapter are, strictly, anti-inflammatory. 'Chondroprotective agents', for example polysulphated glycosaminoglycan (see section 10.2), possibly retard the degradation and may promote the synthesis of cartilage matrix components in joints.

10.1 Non-steroidal anti-inflammatory drugs

Mechanism of action. Almost all non-steroidal anti-inflammatory drugs (NSAIDs) are weak carboxylic or enolic acids. They are central and peripheral analgesics, antipyretics, and have peripheral and central anti-inflammatory activity. Most act primarily by inhibiting cyclo-oxygenase leading to reduced synthesis of prostaglandins and related compounds. This mechanism probably underlies their principal therapeutic and toxic activities. However, recent studies have shown a number of additional actions at the periphery, including inhibition of superoxide radical generation, inhibition of bradykinin action, and blockade of lysosomal and non-lysosomal enzyme release, inhibition of metalloproteinases and effects on interleukin-1 activity, which may contribute to the therapeutic effects. Recent studies have also revealed actions of NSAIDs at the spinal level, in particular analgesic actions which reduce the CNS hypersensitivity which occurs as a result of peripheral inflammation or trauma. Much recent interest has focused on demonstration of the existence of two cyclo-oxygenase isoforms. COX1 is a constitutive enzyme which is thought to subserve a range of physiological roles, inhibition of which accounts for the major toxic effects of NSAIDs. COX2 is an inducible isoform, produced at inflammatory sites to generate inflammatory mediators, although COX2 is constitutively present in some tissues. Potency ratios for the inhibition of COX2:COX1 vary widely being high for aspirin, phenylbutazone, and piroxicam and lower for naproxen, carprofen, etodolac, meloxicam, and nabumetone. The development of specific COX2 antagonists is being vigorously pursued but as yet, no truly preferential COX2 inhibitors are available on the veterinary market. Selective inhibition of COX2 is claimed to improve gastrointestinal tolerance but this remains unproven in both the human and veterinary fields.

Carprofen is considered a weak cyclo-oxygenase inhibitor. Although the principal mechanism of action is unknown it is probably not attributable to cyclo-oxygenase inhibition. Weak antagonists of cyclo-oxygenase appear to have fewer side-effects than potent inhibitors of the enzyme.

Some NSAIDs, such as the 2-arylpropionic acid subgroup including carprofen, ketoprofen, and vedaprofen, contain a single chiral centre and therefore exist as two enantiomeric forms: R(-) and S(+). Such products are effectively drug combinations, since the pharmacodynamic and pharmacokinetic properties of the enantiomers may differ markedly from each other and there are also significant species differences in enantiomer pharmacokinetics. Non-chiral NSAID pharmacokinetics also differ markedly between species, and dosing intervals for one species should not be extrapolated to another.

Most NSAIDs are well absorbed following administration by mouth, although drug-induced gastric irritation in dogs and cats may lead to persistent vomiting, particularly with certain drugs such as ibuprofen, indomethacin, flunixin, and aspirin. Absorption following oral administration may be delayed in ruminants and, in horses, the formulation may profoundly affect oral bioavailablity; absorption being reduced for some oil-based products. Parenteral formulations of some drugs and compound analgesic preparations may be given by subcutaneous, intramuscular, or intravenous injection but phenylbutazone is too irritant for injection by non-vascular routes. With the exception of sodium salicylate, NSAIDs are highly bound to plasma proteins, commonly in excess of 99%, which limits extravascular penetration. However, penetration into acute inflammatory exudate is generally good and persistent partly because exudate is rich in extravasated plasma protein.

Clinical use. NSAIDs are used for their analgesic and anti-oedematous actions in acute inflammatory conditions including postoperative pain and control of joint pain in various arthritides, particularly osteoarthritis. In recent years increasing attention has been given to the perioperative use of NSAIDs to control postoperative pain. Drugs such as flunixin, carprofen, meloxicam, and ketoprofen have been shown to provide very effective postoperative analgesia comparable to and often better than some opioid analgesics. Analgesics (opioids and NSAIDs) have been shown to be more effective if administered prior to the onset of surgery. NSAIDs that are potent cyclo-oxygenase inhibitors, for example flunixin, can occasionally precipitate acute renal failure, most in notably dogs and cats. This is due to the fact that under anaesthesia, if there is a degree of relative or absolute hypovolaemia, or if there is hypotension, locally produced prostaglandins help to maintain renal afferent arteriolar dilation. The administration of a potent inhibitor of cyclo-oxygenase can remove the protective effect of these prostaglandins, and leave the kidney vulnerable to damage. In these situations, the choice of a mild inhibitor of prostaglandin production or a preferential COX2 inhibitor is preferable. Most NSAIDs therefore cannot be recommended for use until the patient has regained consciousness. In dogs, the only NSAIDs that have been shown to be safe if administered before anaesthesia are carprofen and meloxicam.

Differences in anti-inflammatory and analgesic effects between different NSAIDs are small, but there is considerable variation in individual patient tolerance and response.

NSAIDs may ameliorate symptoms of endotoxic shock, for example, in peracute mastitis and equine colic. Flunixin, ketoprofen, carprofen, meloxicam, and tolfenamic acid♦ have been used to reduce morbidity and mortality in calf pneumonia by suppressing pulmonary oedema. NSAIDs are also used to reduce pain in equine colic.

Aspirin, unlike other NSAIDs, combines with cyclo-oxygenase (COX1) covalently to produce irreversible enzyme blockade and thus prevents the production of thromboxane by platelets. Vascular endothelial cells, unlike platelets, are able to regenerate cyclo-oxygenase, and so produce prosta-

cyclin which has an anti-aggregative effect. This action has been utilised to prevent platelet aggregation in thrombo-embolic disorders.

The pharmacokinetics of NSAIDs vary between species, which leads to marked inter-species differences in dosage requirements. In general, the dosage interval should be increased in neonates and aged animals to avoid toxicity.

Side-effects. Toxicity of NSAIDs varies with the species, the individual animal within the species, and the individual drug and is therefore not readily predictable. The principle side-effects of NSAIDs are gastro-intestinal irritation and ulceration, and renal failure. Lesions may occur throughout the gastro-intestinal tract and high doses may lead to a life-threatening plasma protein-losing enteropathy in ponies. Lesions may occur after parenteral or oral administration and may be more prevalent in patients given NSAIDs in conjunction with corticosteroids. Treatment (see section 3.8.2) includes the H_2-antagonists ranitidine or cimetidine, the prostaglandin E_1 analogue misoprostol, or the 'proton pump' inhibitor omeprazole. NSAIDs can induce direct renal papillary necrosis, or renal failure if administered in dehydrated, hypovolaemic, or hypotensive animals (see above).

Other side-effects include vomiting, blood dyscrasias, delayed blood clotting, hepatotoxicity due to cholestatic and parenchymal cell damage, and occasionally skin rashes. Some NSAIDs, such as aspirin, have been shown to be teratogenic in animal studies. NSAIDs inhibit proteoglycan synthesis particularly when synthesis is greatly increased, for example, in osteoarthritis. Some manufacturers claim that different NSAIDs have different properties in this respect. It is unlikely that any of the currently available NSAIDs have a 'chondroprotective' effect, however recent work has suggested that meloxicam and carprofen may not have adverse effects on cartilage metabolism at therapeutic doses in dogs.

There is very little difference between the various NSAIDs in terms of anti-inflammatory or analgesic efficacy, the choice of NSAID should depend on the incidence of side-effects associated with use of the drug. **However, unfortunately there is insufficient information on the clinical incidence of side-effects associated with NSAID use in animals.**

ASPIRIN
(Acetylsalicylic acid)

UK
Indications. Inflammation and pain; thrombo-embolic disorders (see section 4.6)
Contra-indications. See under Carprofen, treatment before regaining consciousness after any general anaesthesia
Side-effects. Warnings. See under Carprofen
Dose. *By mouth.*
Horses: 10–100 mg/kg twice daily
Dogs: inflammation and pain, 10 mg/kg twice daily
Cats: inflammation and pain, 10 mg/kg on alternate days
Thrombo-embolic disorders: up to 75 mg every 3 days

P Ⓗ **Aspirin** (Non-proprietary) *UK*
Tablets, aspirin 75 mg, 300 mg
Tablets, dispersible, aspirin 75 mg, 300 mg
Note. GSL if pack sizes 16 or less

GSL **Rheumatine** (Sherley's)
Tablets, scored, aspirin 120 mg, for *adult dogs*; 25
Contra-indications. Cats; pregnant bitches
Dose. 1–3 tablets 3 times daily given with a milky drink or food

Australia

Indications. Inflammation, pain, pyrexia
Contra-indications. Cats; pre-existing gastro-intestinal disease
Side-effects. Vomiting, gastro-intestinal bleeding, renal calculi, anaemia; testicular atrophy and inhibition of spermatogenesis at high doses
Warnings. Care in hepatic or renal impairment; Drug Interactions – corticosteroids, digoxin, aminoglycosides; withdraw 2 weeks before major surgery
Dose. *By mouth.* Dosages vary, see manufacturers' information

Aspil 350 mg Chewable Tablets (Mavlab) *Austral*
Tablets, aspirin 350 mg, for *dogs*

Aspil Tablets (Mavlab) *Austral*
Tablets, aspirin 100 mg, for *dogs*

USA

Indications. Inflammation, pain, pyrexia
Contra-indications. Pre-existing gastro-intestinal disease
Warnings. Treatment should be discontinued if diarrhoea occurs
Dose. *By mouth.* Dosages vary, see manufacturers' information

Aspirin 60 Grain (Butler) *USA*
Tablets, aspirin 3.9 g, for *horses, cattle, sheep, pigs*
Withdrawal Periods. Should not be used in *cattle* producing milk for human consumption

Aspirin 240 Grain Boluses (Vedco) *USA*
Tablets, aspirin 15.6 g, for *horses, cattle*
Withdrawal Periods. Should not be used in *cattle* producing milk for human consumption

Aspirin 480 Grain Boluses (Vedco) *USA*
Tablets, aspirin 31.2 g, for *horses, cattle*

Aspirin Boluses 480 Grains (RXV) *USA*
Tablets, aspirin 31.2 g, for *horses, cattle*

Aspirin Bolus (AgriLabs, Aspen, DurVet, Phoenix) *USA*
Tablets, aspirin 15.6 g, for *horses, cattle*

Aspirin Boluses (AgriLabs, AgriPharm, Butler) *USA*
Tablets, aspirin 15.6 g, for *horses, cattle*

Aspirin Boluses (RXV, Wendt) *USA*
Tablets, aspirin 15.6 g, for *horses, cattle*
Withdrawal Periods. Should not be used in *cattle* producing milk for human consumption

Aspirin Powder (AgriLabs, Butler, First Priority, RXV, Vedco) *USA*
Oral powder, aspirin 2.2 kg, for *horses, cattle, sheep, pigs, dogs, cats, chickens*

Aspirin Tablets (Vedco) *USA*
Tablets, aspirin 3.9 g, for *horses, cattle, sheep, pigs*

Withdrawal Periods. Should not be used in *horses* intended for human consumption

Equi-Spirin (Vedco) *USA*
Oral granules, aspirin 2500mg/39 mL scoop, for *horses*

Palaprin 65 (VRX) *USA*
Tablets, aspirin 65 mg, for *dogs*

Palaprin 325 (VRX) *USA*
Tablets, aspirin 325 mg, for *dogs*

Vetrin Canine Aspirin (King Pharm) *USA*
Tablets, aspirin 100 mg, 325 mg, for *dogs*

CARPROFEN

UK

Indications. Inflammation and pain
Contra-indications. Patients with cardiac, renal, or hepatic disease, where there is the possibility of gastro-intestinal ulceration or bleeding, hypersensitivity to the drug; treatment with other NSAIDs concurrently or within 24 hours; racehorses prior to racing; pregnant mares
Side-effects. Prolonged use may cause gastro-intestinal lesions, inappetance, vomiting, and diarrhoea
Warnings. Caution with use in animals less than 6 weeks of age, or aged animals; avoid use in dehydrated, hypovolaemic, or hypotensive patients; avoid concurrent administration of potentially nephrotoxic drugs; safety in pregnancy may not have been established; Drug Interactions – Appendix 1 (NSAIDs); patients on long-term treatment should be monitored
Dose.
Horses, ponies: *by mouth*, 700 micrograms/kg once daily for up to 4 or 9 days
by intravenous injection, 700 micrograms/kg as a single dose. Repeat after 1 day if required
Cattle: *by subcutaneous or intravenous injection*, 1.4 mg/kg as a single dose
Dogs: *by mouth*, 2–4 mg/kg daily in divided doses for 7 days then 2 mg/kg once daily
by subcutaneous or intravenous injection, 4 mg/kg as a single dose. (May be used preoperatively)
Cats: *by subcutaneous or intravenous injection*, 4 mg/kg as a single dose. (May be used preoperatively)

POM **Rimadyl Granules** (Pfizer) *UK*
Oral granules, carprofen 210 mg/sachet, for *horses, ponies*; 2.4-g sachets
Withdrawal Periods. Should not be used in *horses* intended for human consumption
Dose. *Horses*: *by addition to a small amount of feed*, 1 sachet/300 kg

POM **Rimadyl Large Animals Solution** (Pfizer) *UK*
Injection, carprofen 50 mg/mL, for *horses, ponies, cattle less than 12 months of age*; 50 mL
Withdrawal Periods. Should not be used in *horses* intended for human consumption. *Cattle*: slaughter 21 days, should not be used in cattle producing milk for human consumption

POM **Rimadyl Small Animal Injection** (Pfizer) *UK*
Injection, carprofen 50 mg/mL, for *dogs, cats*; 20 mL

POM **Rimadyl Tablets** (Pfizer) *UK*
Tablets, scored, carprofen 20 mg, 50 mg, for *dogs*; 100, 500

Australia

Indications. Inflammation and pain

Contra-indications. Patients with cardiac, renal, or hepatic disease, hypersensitivity to the drug, blood dyscrasia; treatment with other NSAIDs concurrently or within 24 hours; pregnant animals

Warnings. Caution with use in animals less than 6 weeks of age, or aged animals or where there is the possibility of gastro-intestinal ulceration or bleeding; avoid use in dehydrated, hypovolaemic, or hypotensive patients; avoid concurrent administration of potentially nephrotoxic drugs

Dose.

Horses: *by mouth or by intravenous injection*, 700 micrograms/kg

Dogs: *by mouth*, 2–4 mg/kg daily in divided doses for 7 days then 2 mg/kg once daily

by subcutaneous or intravenous injection, 4 mg/kg

Cats: *by subcutaneous or intravenous injection*, 4 mg/kg

Zenecarp Granules (Novartis) *Austral*
Oral granules, carprofen 210 mg/ 2.4 g sachet, for *horses*
Withdrawal Periods. *Horses*: slaughter 28 days

Zenecarp Injection (Novartis) *Austral*
Injection, carprofen 50 mg/mL, for *horses, dogs, cats*
Withdrawal Periods. *Horses*: slaughter 28 days

Zenecarp Tablets (Novartis) *Austral*
Tablets, carprofen 20 mg and 50 mg, for *dogs*

Eire

Indications. Inflammation and pain

Contra-indications. Patients with cardiac, renal, or hepatic disease, where there is the possibility of gastro-intestinal ulceration or bleeding, hypersensitivity to the drug; treatment with other NSAIDs concurrently or within 24 hours; racehorses within 8 days prior to racing; pregnant animals

Warnings. Caution with use in animals less than 6 weeks of age, or aged animals; avoid use in dehydrated, hypovolaemic, or hypotensive patients; avoid concurrent administration of potentially nephrotoxic drugs

Dose.

Horses: *by mouth or by intravenous injection*, 700 micrograms/kg

Cattle: *by subcutaneous or intravenous injection*, 1.4 mg/kg

Dogs: *by mouth*, 2–4 mg/kg daily in divided doses for 7 days then 2 mg/kg once daily

by subcutaneous or intravenous injection, 4 mg/kg

Cats: *by subcutaneous or intravenous injection*, 4 mg/kg

Rimadyl Granules (Pfizer) *Eire*
Oral granules, carprofen 210 mg/sachet, for *horses*
Withdrawal Periods. *Horses*: slaughter 4 days

Rimadyl Injection (Pfizer) *Eire*
Injection, carprofen 50 mg/mL, for *horses, dogs, cats*
Withdrawal Periods. *Horses*: slaughter 4 days

Rimadyl Solution for Horses, Ponies and Young Cattle (Pfizer) *Eire*
Injection, carprofen 50 mg/mL, for *horses, cattle*
Withdrawal Periods. *Horses*: slaughter 4 days. *Cattle*: slaughter 21 days, should not be used in cattle producing milk for human consumption

Rimadyl Tablets (Pfizer) *Eire*
Tablets, carprofen 20 mg, 50 mg, for *dogs*

Zenecarp Granules (Cypharm) *Eire*
Oral granules, to mix with feed, carprofen 8.75%, for *horses*
Withdrawal Periods. Should not be used in *horses* intended for human consumption

Zenecarp Injection (Cypharm) *Eire*
Injection, carprofen 50 mg/mL, for *horses, dogs*
Withdrawal Periods. *Horses*: slaughter 4 days

Zenecarp Solution (Cypharm) *Eire*
Injection, carprofen 50 mg/mL, for *cattle*
Withdrawal Periods. Slaughter 21 days, should not be used in cattle producing milk for human consumption

Zenecarp Tablets 20 mg and 50 mg (Cypharm) *Eire*
Tablets, carprofen 20 mg, 50 mg, for *dogs*

New Zealand

Indications. Inflammation and pain

Contra-indications. Patients with cardiac, renal, or hepatic disease, hypersensitivity to the drug, blood dyscrasia; treatment with other NSAIDs concurrently or within 24 hours; pregnant animals; racehorses within 8 days prior to racing

Warnings. Caution with use in animals less than 6 weeks of age, or aged animals or where there is the possibility of gastro-intestinal ulceration or bleeding; avoid use in dehydrated, hypovolaemic, or hypotensive patients; avoid concurrent administration of potentially nephrotoxic drugs

Dose.

Horses: *by mouth or by intravenous injection*, 700 micrograms/kg

Dogs: *by mouth*, 2–4 mg/kg daily in divided doses for 7 days then 2 mg/kg once daily

by subcutaneous or intravenous injection, 4 mg/kg

Cats: *by subcutaneous or intravenous injection*, 4 mg/kg

Zenecarp Granules (Novartis) *NZ*
Oral granules, carprofen 87.5 mg/g, for *horses*
Withdrawal Periods. Slaughter 28 days

Zenecarp Injection (Novartis) *NZ*
Injection, carprofen 50 mg/mL, for *horses, dogs, cats*
Withdrawal Periods. *Horses*: slaughter 30 days

Zenecarp Solution (Novartis) *NZ*
Injection, carprofen 50 mg/mL, for *horses*
Withdrawal Periods. Slaughter 28 days

Zenecarp Tablets (Novartis) *NZ*
Tablets, carprofen 20 mg, 50 mg, for *dogs*

USA

Indications. Inflammation and pain

Contra-indications. Hypersensitivity to the drug

Warnings. Caution with use in animals less than 6 weeks of age, or aged animals; avoid use in dehydrated, hypovolaemic, or hypotensive patients; avoid use in patients with cardiac, renal, or hepatic disease, where there is the possibility of gastro-intestinal ulceration or bleeding; treatment with other NSAIDs concurrently or within 24 hours; safety in breeding, pregnant, or lactating animals has not been established; avoid concurrent administration of potentially nephrotoxic drugs

Dose. *Dogs*: *by mouth*, 2.2 mg/kg

Rimadyl (Pfizer) *USA*
Tablets, carprofen 25 mg, 75 mg, 100 mg, for *dogs*

ELTENAC

UK

Indications. Inflammation
Contra-indications. **Side-effects**. See under Carprofen
Warnings. See under Carprofen; repeated use in equine colic is not generally recommended due to pain-masking effects
Dose. *Horses*: *by intravenous injection*, 500 micrograms/kg once daily for up to 5 days

POM **Telzenac** (Schering-Plough) *UK*
Injection, eltenac 50 mg/mL, for *horses*; 20 mL, 50 mL
Withdrawal Periods. Should not be used in *horses* intended for human consumption

ETODOLAC

USA

Indications. Inflammation and pain
Contra-indications. Hypersensitivity to the drug
Warnings. Avoid use in dehydrated, hypovolaemic, or hypotensive patients; avoid use in patients with cardiac, renal, or hepatic disease, where there is the possibility of gastro-intestinal ulceration or bleeding; patients should be monitored for side-effects; treatment should be discontinued if signs of inappetance, emesis, faecal abnormalities, or anaemia seen
Dose. *Dogs*: *by mouth*, 10–15mg/kg

EtoGesic Tablets (Fort Dodge) *USA*
Tablets, etodolac 150 mg, 300 mg, for *dogs*

FLUNIXIN

See section 1.1 for combination flunixin and antibacterial preparations

UK

Indications. Inflammation and pain; endotoxic shock
Contra-indications. See under Carprofen; treatment before regaining consciousness after general anaesthesia is contra-indicated for NSAIDs which inhibit prostaglandin synthesis
Side-effects. See under Carprofen
Warnings. See under Carprofen; repeated use in equine colic is not generally recommended due to pain-masking effects
Dose.
Horses: musculoskeletal disorders, *by mouth or by intravenous injection*, 1.1 mg/kg once daily for up to 5 days
Equine colic, *by intravenous injection*, 1.1 mg/kg (**see Warnings above**)
Endotoxaemia, *by slow intravenous injection*, 250 micrograms/kg 3–4 times daily
Cattle: acute inflammatory conditions, *by intravenous injection*, 2.2 mg/kg once daily for up to 5 days
Dogs: musculoskeletal disorders, post-operative pain and inflammation, *by subcutaneous injection*, 1 mg/kg daily for up to 3 days
Endotoxic shock, *by slow intravenous injection*, 1 mg/kg up to twice daily for a maximum of 3 doses

POM **Binixin Injection 5%** (Bayer) *UK*
Injection, flunixin (as meglumine) 50 mg/mL, for *horses, cattle*
Withdrawal Periods. Should not be used in *horses* intended for human consumption. *Cattle*: slaughter 7 days, milk 12 hours

POM **Cronyxin** (Bimeda) *UK*
Injection, flunixin (as meglumine) 50 mg/mL, for *horses, cattle*
Withdrawal Periods. Should not be used in *horses* intended for human consumption. *Cattle*: slaughter 7 days, milk 12 hours

POM **Finadyne Granules** (Schering-Plough) *UK*
Oral granules, for addition to feed, flunixin (as meglumine) 25 mg/g, for *horses*; 10 g
Withdrawal Periods. *Horses*: slaughter 7 days

POM **Finadyne Injection for Dogs** (Schering-Plough) *UK*
Injection, flunixin (as meglumine) 10 mg/mL, for *dogs*; 20 mL

POM **Finadyne Paste** (Schering-Plough) *UK*
Oral paste, flunixin (as meglumine) 110 mg/division, for *horses*; 10-g metered-dose applicator
Withdrawal Periods. Should not be used in *horses* intended for human consumption

POM **Finadyne Solution** (Schering-Plough) *UK*
Injection, flunixin (as meglumine) 50 mg/mL, for *horses, cattle*
Withdrawal Periods. *Horses*: slaughter 7 days. *Cattle*: slaughter 5 days, milk 12 hours

POM **Flunixin Injection** (Norbrook) *UK*
Injection, flunixin (as meglumine) 50 mg/mL, for *horses, cattle*
Withdrawal Periods. *Horses*: slaughter 7 days. *Cattle*: slaughter 7 days, milk 36 hours

POM **Meflosyl 5% Injection** (Fort Dodge) *UK*
Injection, flunixin (as meglumine) 50 mg/mL, for *horses, cattle*
Withdrawal Periods. *Horses*: slaughter 7 days. *Cattle*: slaughter 7 days, milk 36 hours

POM **Resprixin** (Intervet) *UK*
Injection, flunixin (as meglumine) 50 mg/mL, for *horses, cattle*
Withdrawal Periods. *Horses*: slaughter 7 days. *Cattle*: slaughter 7 days, milk 36 hours

Australia

Indications. Inflammation and pain; endotoxic shock
Contra-indications. Concurrent administration of other NSAIDs, anti-inflammatory drugs, or nephrotoxic substances; cats; treatment of foals less than 72 hours of age
Side-effects. Slight irritation on intramuscular injection
Warnings. Discontinue treatment if adverse gastro-intestinal signs occur; safety in pregnant animals has not been established
Dose.
Horses: *by mouth or by intravenous injection*, 1.1 mg/kg
Cattle: *by intramuscular or intravenous injection*, 1.1–2.2 mg/kg
Pigs: *by intramuscular injection*, 1.1–2.2 mg/kg
Dogs: *by mouth*, 1 mg/kg
by intramuscular or intravenous injection, 1.1 mg/kg

Cronyxin Injection (Bimeda) *Austral*
Injection, flunixin (as meglumine) 50 mg/mL, for *horses, cattle, dogs, pigs*
Withdrawal Periods. *Cattle*: slaughter 28 days, milk 36 hours. *Horses, pigs*: slaughter 28 days

Finadyne Granules (Schering-Plough) *Austral*
Oral granules, flunixin (as meglumine) 25 mg/g, for *horses*

Finadyne Solution (Schering-Plough) *Austral*
Injection, flunixin meglumine 50 mg/mL, for *horses, cattle, sheep, goats, pigs, dogs*

Finadyne Tablets (Schering-Plough) *Austral*
Tablets, flunixin (as meglumine) 5 mg, 20 mg

Flumav (Mavlab) *Austral*
Injection, flunixin (as meglumine) 50 mg/mL, for *horses, cattle, pigs, dogs*
Withdrawal Periods. *Horses, pigs*: slaughter 28 days. *Cattle*: slaughter 28 days, milk 7 days

Flunix (Parnell) *Austral*
Injection, flunixin (as meglumine) 50 mg/mL, for *horses, cattle, pigs, dogs*
Withdrawal Periods. *Horses, pigs*: slaughter 28 days. *Cattle*: slaughter 28 days, milk 36 hours

Flunixil (Ilium) *Austral*
Injection, flunixin (as meglumine) 50 mg/mL, for *horses, dogs*
Withdrawal Periods. *Horses*: slaughter 28 days

Eire

Indications. Inflammation and pain
Contra-indications. Cardiac, hepatic, or renal disease, where ther is possibility of gastro-intestinal ulceration or bleeding; blood dyscrasia; hypersensitivity to the drug; concurrent administration of other NSAIDs or potential nephrotoxic drugs, racehorses within 8 days of racing
Warnings. Care in dehydrated, hypovolaemic, or hypotensive patients, animals less than 6 weeks of age or aged animals; Drug Interactions – highly protein-bound drugs
Dose. *Horses*: *by mouth or by intravenous injection*, 1.1 mg/kg
Cattle: *by intravenous injection*, 2.2 mg/kg

Binixin Injection (Bayer) *Eire*
Injection, flunixin meglumine 50 mg, for *horses, cattle*
Withdrawal Periods. *Horses*: slaughter 7 days. *Cattle*: slaughter 7 days, milk 36 hours

Finadyne Granules (Schering-Plough) *Eire*
Oral granules, flunixin (as meglumine) 250 mg/10 g, for *horses*
Withdrawal Periods. Slaughter 7 days

Finadyne Paste (Schering-Plough) *Eire*
Oral paste, flunixin (as meglumine) 500 mg/10 g, for *horses*
Withdrawal Periods. Should not be used in *horses* intended for human consumption

Finadyne Solution (Schering-Plough) *Eire*
Injection, flunixin (as meglumine) 50 mg/mL, for *horses, cattle*
Withdrawal Periods. *Horses*: slaughter 7 days. Cattle: slaughter 7 days, milk 36 hours

Flunixin Injection (Norbrook) *Eire*
Injection, flunixin (as meglumine) 50 mg/mL, for *horses, cattle*
Withdrawal Periods. *Horses*: slaughter 7 days. *Cattle*: slaughter 7 days, milk 36 hours

New Zealand

Indications. Inflammation and pain
Contra-indications. Concurrent administration of other NSAIDs or within 24 hours, anti-inflammatory drugs, nephrotoxic substances; cardiac, hepatic, or renal disease, where there is a possibility of gastro-intestinal ulercation or bleeding; blood dyscrasia, hypersensitivity to the drug; cats
Side-effects. Prolonged use may cause gastro-intestinal irritation and ulceration
Warnings. Use with care in pregnant animals; Drug Interactions – highly protein-bound drugs
Dose. *Horses*: *by intramuscular or intravenous injection*, 1.1 mg/kg

Cattle: *by intravenous injection*, 2.2 mg/kg
Pigs: *by intramuscular injection*,2.2 mg/kg
Dogs: *by intravenous injection*, 1.1 mg/kg

Cronyxin (Reamor) *NZ*
Injection, flunixin (as meglumine) 50 mg/mL, for *horses, cattle*
Withdrawal Periods. *Horses*: slaughter 1 day. *Cattle*: slaughter 1 day, discard milk during treatment

Finadyne (Schering-Plough) *NZ*
Injection, flunixin (as meglumine) 50 mg/mL, for *horses, cattle, pigs, dogs*
Withdrawal Periods. *Horses*: slaughter 28 days. *Cattle*: slaughter 1 day, milk withdrawal period nil. *Pigs*: slaughter 3 days

Flunix (Parnell) *NZ*
Injection, flunixin (as meglumine) 50 mg/mL, for *horses, cattle, pigs, dogs*
Withdrawal Periods. *Horses*: slaughter 28 days. *Cattle*: slaughter 1 day, milk withdrawal period nil. *Pigs*: slaughter 3 days

USA

Indications. Inflammation and pain
Warnings. Safety in pregnant animals has not been established
Dose. *Horses*: *by mouth or by intramuscular or intravenous injection*, 1.1 mg/kg

Banamine (Schering-Plough) *USA*
Oral granules, flunixin (as meglumine) 25 mg/g, for *horses*
Withdrawal Periods. Should not be used in *horses* intended for human consumption

Banamine (Schering-Plough) *USA*
Oral paste, flunixin (as meglumine) 50 mg/g, for *horses*
Withdrawal Periods. Should not be used in *horses* intended for human consumption

Banamine (Schering-Plough) *USA*
Injection, flunixin (as meglumine) 50 mg/mL, for *horses*
Withdrawal Periods. Should not be used in *horses* intended for human consumption

Equi-Phar Equigesic (Vedco) *USA*
Injection, flunixin (as meglumine) 50 mg/mL, for *horses*
Withdrawal Periods. Should not be used in *horses* intended for human consumption

Equileve (Vetus) *USA*
Injection, flunixin (as meglumine) 50 mg/mL, for *horses*
Withdrawal Periods. Should not be used in *horses* intended for human consumption

Flumeglumine (Phoenix) *USA*
Injection, flunixin (as meglumine) 50 mg/mL, for *horses*
Withdrawal Periods. Should not be used in *horses* intended for human consumption

Flu-Nix (Pro Labs) *USA*
Injection, flunixin (as meglumine) 50 mg/mL, for *horses*
Withdrawal Periods. Should not be used in *horses* intended for human consumption

Flunixamine (Fort Dodge) *USA*
Injection, flunixin (as meglumine) 50 mg/mL, for *horses*
Withdrawal Periods. Should not be used in *horses* intended for human consumption

Flunixin Meglumine (Butler, VetTek) *USA*
Injection, flunixin (as meglumine) 50 mg/mL, for *horses*
Withdrawal Periods. Should not be used in *horses* intended for human consumption

Suppressor (RXV, Western Veterinary Supplies) *USA*
Injection, flunixin (as meglumine) 50 mg/mL, for *horses*
Withdrawal Periods. Should not be used in *horses* intended for human consumption

INDOMETHACIN

Australia

Indications. Inflammation and pain

Contra-indications. Concurrent administration of other NSAIDs

Warnings. Safety in pregnant animals has not been fully evaluated; care with renal or hepatic impairment; discontinue treatment 54 hours before competition in racing horses

Dose. *By mouth*.

Horses: 10 g/450 kg

Dogs: 200 micrograms/kg once daily, then 100 micrograms/kg once daily

Cu-Algesic Granules (Biochemical Veterinary Research) *Austral*
Oral granules, copper indomethacin 10 mg/g, for *horses*
Withdrawal Periods. Slaughter 28 days

Cu-Algesic Oral Paste (Biochemical Veterinary Research) *Austral*
Oral paste, copper indomethacin 40 mg/g, for *horses*
Withdrawal Periods. Slaughter 28 days

Cu-Algesic Tablets (Biochemical Veterinary Research) *Austral*
Tablets, copper indomethacin 2 mg, for *dogs*

New Zealand

Indications. nflammation and pain

Warnings. Safety in pregnant animals has not been fully evaluated; care with renal or hepatic impairment; discontinue treatment 54 hours before competition in racing horses

Dose. *By mouth*.

Horses: 5–10 g/450 kg, then 5 g/450 kg

Dogs: 200 micrograms/kg once daily, then 100 micrograms/kg once daily

Cu-algesic Oral Paste (Parnell) *NZ*
Oral paste, copper indomethacin 20 mg/5 g, for *horses*
Withdrawal Periods. Slaughter 180 days

Cu-algesic Tablets (Parnell) *NZ*
Tablets, copper indomethacin 2 mg, for *dogs*

KETOPROFEN

UK

Indications. Inflammation and pain

Contra-indications. See under Carprofen; treatment before regaining consciousness after any general anaesthesia; racehorses 15 days prior to racing

Side-effects. See under Carprofen

Warnings. See under Carprofen; avoid intra-arterial injection

Dose.

Horses: musculoskeletal disorders, *by intravenous injection*, 2.2 mg/kg once daily for 3–5 days
Equine colic, *by intravenous injection*, 2.2 mg/kg. Repeat dose once only

Cattle: *by intramuscular or intravenous injection*, 3 mg/kg once daily for up to 3 days

Pigs: *by intramuscular injection*, 3 mg/kg as a single dose

Dogs: *by mouth*, 1 mg/kg once daily for up to 5 days

by subcutaneous, intramuscular, or intravenous injection, 2 mg/kg once daily for up to 3 days

Cats: *by mouth*, 1 mg/kg once daily for up to 5 days

by subcutaneous injection, 2 mg/kg once daily for up to 3 days

POM **Ketofen** (Merial) *UK*
Tablets, scored, ketoprofen 5 mg, for *dogs, cats*; 100
Tablets, scored, ketoprofen 20 mg, for *dogs*; 100

POM **Ketofen 1%** (Merial) *UK*
Injection, ketoprofen 10 mg/mL, for *dogs, cats*; 20 mL

POM **Ketofen 10%** (Merial) *UK*
Injection, ketoprofen 100 mg/mL, for *horses, cattle, pigs*; 10 mL, 100 mL
Withdrawal Periods. *Horses*: slaughter 1 day. *Cattle*: slaughter 1 day (by intravenous injection), 4 days (by intramuscular injection), milk withdrawal period nil. *Pigs*: 4 days

Australia

Indications. Inflammation and pain

Contra-indications. Concurrent administration of other NSAIDs, diuretics, or anticoagulants; patients with gastroduodenal ulcers, haemorrhagic syndome; hypersensitivity to ketoprofen or aspirin; severe renal or hepatic impairment; animals less than 6 weeks of age

Warnings. Safety in pregnant animals has not been established

Dose. *Horses*: *by intramuscular or intravenous injection*, 2.2 mg/kg

Dogs: *by mouth*, 1 mg/kg

by subcutaneous, intramuscular, or intravenous injection, 2 mg/kg

Cats: *by mouth*, 1 mg/kg

by subcutaneous injection, 2 mg/kg

Ketofen Injection (Merial) *Austral*
Injection, ketoprofen 10 mg/mL, for *dogs, cats*

Ketofen Tablets (Merial) *Austral*
Tablets, ketoprofen 5 mg, 20 mg, for *dogs, cats*

Ketoprofen Injection (Parnell, RWR) *Austral*
Injection, ketoprofen 100 mg/mL, for *horses*
Withdrawal Periods. Slaughter 28 days

Eire

Indications. Inflammation and pain

Contra-indications. Cardiac, hepatic, or renal disease, where there is a possibility of gastro-intestinal ulercation or bleeding; blood dyscrasia, hypersensitivity to the drug; concurrent administration of other NSAIDs or within 24 hours, nephrotoxic drugs; pregnant animals

Side-effects. Rarely vomiting and diarrhoea; transient swelling at injection site

Warnings. Care in animals less than 6 weeks of age or aged animals

Dose. *Horses*: *by intravenous injection*, 2.2 mg/kg

Cattle: *by intramuscular or intravenous injection*, 3 mg/kg

Dogs: *by mouth*, 1 mg/kg

by subcutaneous, intramuscular, or intravenous injection, 2 mg/kg

Cats: *by mouth*, 1 mg/kg

by subcutaneous injection, 2 mg/kg

Ketofen 1% (Merial) *Eire*
Injection, ketoprofen 10 mg/mL, for *dogs, cats*

Ketofen 10% (Merial) *Eire*
Injection, ketoprofen 100 mg/mL, for *cattle, horses*
Withdrawal Periods. *Horses*: slaughter 24 hours. *Cattle*: slaughter 24 hours
(iv injection), 4 days (im injection), milk withdrawal period nil

Ketofen 5 mg Tablets (Merial) *Eire*
Tablets, ketoprofen 5 mg, 20 mg, for *dogs, cats*

New Zealand

Indications. Inflammation and pain
Contra-indications. Concurrent administration of other
NSAIDs, diuretics, or anticoagulants; patients with gastroduodenal ulcers, haemorrhagic syndome; hypersensitivity to ketoprofen or aspirin; severe renal or hepatic
impairment; animals less than 6 weeks of age
Warnings. Safety in pregnant animals has not been established
Dose.
Horses: by intramuscular or intravenous injection, 2 mg/kg
or 2.2 mg/kg
Cattle: by intramuscular or intravenous injection, 3 mg/kg
Dogs: by mouth, 1 mg/kg
by subcutaneous, intramuscular, or intravenous injection, 2
mg/kg
Cats: by mouth, 1 mg/kg
by subcutaneous injection, 2 mg/kg

Ketofen (Merial) *NZ*
Tablets, ketoprofen 5 mg, 20 mg, for *dogs, cats*

Ketofen 1% (Merial) *NZ*
Injection, ketoprofen 10 mg/mL, for *dogs, cats*

Ketofen 10% (Merial) *NZ*
Injection, ketoprofen 100 mg/mL, for *horses, cattle*
Withdrawal Periods. Should not be used in *horses* intended for human con-
sumption. *Cattle*: slaughter 4 days, milk withdrawal period nil

Ketoflam (Virbac) *NZ*
Injection, ketoprofen 100 mg/mL, for *horses*
Withdrawal Periods. Slaughter 28 days

Ketoprofen Injection (Vetpharm) *NZ*
Injection, ketoprofen 100 mg/mL, for *horses*
Withdrawal Periods. Slaughter 28 days

Ketoprofen Injection for Horses & Cattle (Parnell) *NZ*
Injection, ketoprofen 100 mg/mL, for *horses, cattle*
Withdrawal Periods. *Horses*: slaughter 28 days. *Cattle*: slaughter 4 days,
milk withdrawal period nil

USA

Indications. Inflammation and pain
Contra-indications. Hypersensitivity to the drug
Dose. *Horses*: by intravenous injection, 2.2 mg/kg

Ketofen (Fort Dodge) *USA*
Injection, ketoprofen 100 mg/mL, for *horses*
Withdrawal Periods. Should not be used in *horses* intended for human con-
sumption

LYSINE ASPIRIN

Australia

Indications. Inflammation and pain; pyrexia
Contra-indications. Severe renal or hepatic disease; concurrent use with aminoglycosides or other salicylates; foals
less than 30 days of age; administration within 6 weeks of
anticoagulant therapy
Dose. *Horses*: by mouth, 20–40 mg/kg

Vetalgine (Boehringer Ingelheim) *Austral*
Injection, powder for reconstitution, lysine acetylsalicylate 10 g (= aspirin
5.5 g)/50 mL, for *horses*
Withdrawal Periods. *Horses*: slaughter 28 days

New Zealand

Indications. Inflammation, pain, pyrexia
Warnings. Care in hepatic or renal impairment
Dose.
Horses: by intravenous injection, 20 mg/kg
Cattle: by subcutaneous, intramuscular, or intravenous
injection, 26 mg/kg
Pigs: by subcutaneous, intramuscular, or intravenous injec-
tion, 10–30 mg/kg
Dogs: by subcutaneous, intramuscular, or intravenous
injection, 20–40 mg/kg

Vetalgine (Virbac) *NZ*
Injection, lysine aspirin (=aspirin 5.5 mg/mL), for *horses, cattle, pigs, dogs*
Withdrawal Periods. *Horses, pigs*: slaughter 2 days. *Cattle*: slaughter 2 days,
milk withdrawal period nil

MECLOFENAMIC ACID

UK

Indications. Inflammation and pain
Contra-indications. See under Carprofen; treatment before
regaining consciousness after any general anaesthesia; discontinue administration 5 days prior to administration of
prostaglandins for breeding purposes
Side-effects. Warnings. See under Carprofen
Dose. Horses: by mouth, 2.2 mg/kg once daily for 5–7
days, then adjust dose frequency to suit each individual
patient if further treatment is necessary

POM **Arquel V Granules** (Pharmacia & Upjohn)
Oral granules, for addition to feed, meclofenamic acid 50 mg/g, for *horses*;
10 g
Withdrawal Periods. Should not be used in *horses* intended for human consumption

Australia

Indications. Inflammation and pain
Contra-indications. Gastro-intestinal disease, renal or
hepatic impairment
Warnings. Safety in pregnant animals has not been established; may enhance the effect of oral anticoagulants; treatment should be discontinued if gastro-intestinal signs occur
Dose. Horses: by mouth, 2.2 mg/kg

Arquel (Vetrepharm) *Austral*
Oral granules, meclofenamic acid 50 mg/g granules, for *horses*
Withdrawal Periods. Slaughter 28 days

USA

Indications. Inflammation and pain

Contra-indications. Congestive heart failure, gastro-intestinal disease, renal or hepatic impairment

Warnings. Safety in pregnant animals or dogs less than 8 months of age has not been established; may enhance the effect of oral anticoagulants; treatment should be discontinued if gastro-intestinal signs occur

Dose. *Horses*: *by mouth*, 2.2 mg/kg

Dogs: *by mouth*, 1.1 mg/kg

Arquel Granules (Fort Dodge) *USA*
Oral granules, meclofenamic acid 50 mg/g, for *horses*
Withdrawal Periods. Should not be used in *horses* intended for human consumption

Arquel Tablets (Fort Dodge) *USA*
Tablets, meclofenamic acid 10 mg, 20 mg, for *dogs*

MELOXICAM

UK

Indications. Inflammation and pain

Contra-indications. See under Carprofen; treatment before regaining consciousness after any general anaesthesia; pregnant or lactating bitches

Side-effects. Warnings. See under Carprofen

Dose.

Cattle: *by subcutaneous or intravenous injection*, 500 micrograms/kg as a single dose

Dogs: *by mouth or by addition to food*, 200 micrograms/kg as a single dose for 1 day then 100 micrograms/kg once daily. Should be given soon after feeding when given by mouth.

by subcutaneous injection, 200 micrograms/kg as a single dose

POM **Metacam Oral Suspension** (Boehringer Ingelheim) *UK*
Oral suspension, meloxicam 1.5 mg/mL, for *dogs*; 32 mL, 100 mL (1 drop = 100 micrograms)

POM **Metacam 0.5% Injection** (Boehringer Ingelheim) *UK*
Injection, meloxicam 5 mg/mL, for *dogs*; 10 mL

POM **Metacam 5 mg/ml Solution for Injection for Cattle** (Boehringer Ingelheim) *UK*
Injection, meloxicam 5 mg/mL, for *cattle*; 100 mL

Australia

Indications. Inflammation and pain

Contra-indications. Last third of pregnancy or lactating bitches

Warnings. Care in animals less than 6 weeks of age or aged animals

Dose. *Dogs*: *by mouth or by addition to food*, 200 micrograms/kg as a single dose for 1 day then 100 micrograms/kg once daily

by subcutaneous injection, 200 micrograms/kg

Metacam Anti-inflammatory Injectable for Dogs (Boehringer Ingelheim) *Austral*
Injection, meloxicam 5 mg/mL, for *dogs*

Metacam Anti-inflammatory Oral Suspension for Dogs (Boehringer Ingelheim) *Austral*
Oral suspension, meloxicam 1.5 mg/mL, for *dogs*

Eire

Indications. Inflammation and pain

Contra-indications. Pregnant or lactating bitches; cardiac, hepatic or renal impairment, where gastric ulceration is suspected, haemorrhagic disorders; hypersensitivity to the drug; concurrent administration of other NSAIDs or within 24 hours

Side-effects. Occasional transient diarrhoea and vomiting; loss of appetite, faecal occult bleeding, and apathy

Warnings. Care in animals less than 6 weeks of age or aged animals; avoid use in dehydrated, hypovolaemic, or hypotensive animals; Drug Interactions – highly protein-bound drugs

Dose. *Cattle*: *by subcutaneous or intravenous injection*, 500 micrograms/kg

Dogs: *by mouth or by addition to food*, 200 micrograms/kg as a single dose for 1 day then 100 micrograms/kg once daily

by subcutaneous injection, 200 micrograms/kg

Metacam 0.5% Injection (Boehringer Ingelheim) *Eire*
Injection, meloxicam 5 mg/mL, for *dogs*

Metacam 5 mg/ml Solution for Injection for Cattle (Boehringer Ingelheim) *Eire*
Injection, meloxicam 5 mg/mL, for *cattle*
Withdrawal Periods. Slaughter 15 days, should not be used in cattle producing milk for human consumption

Metacam Oral Suspension (Boehringer Ingelheim) *Eire*
Oral suspension, meloxicam 1.5 mg/mL, for *dogs*

New Zealand

Indications. Inflammation and pain

Contra-indications. Pregnant or lactating bitches; cardiac, hepatic or renal impairment, where gastric ulceration is suspected, haemorrhagic disorders; hypersensitivity to the drug; concurrent administration of other NSAIDs, aminoglycosides, or anticoagulants

Warnings. Care in animals less than 6 weeks of age or aged animals

Dose. *Dogs*: *by mouth or by addition to food*, 200 micrograms/kg as a single dose for 1 day then 100 micrograms/kg once daily

by subcutaneous injection, 200 micrograms/kg

Metacam 0.5% (Boehringer Ingelheim) *NZ*
Injection, meloxicam 5 mg/mL, for *dogs*

Metacam Oral Suspension (Boehringer Ingelheim) *NZ*
Oral suspension, meloxicam 1.5 mg/mL, for *dogs*

METAMIZOLE SODIUM
(Dipyrone)

USA

Indications. Inflammation and pain; gastro-intestinal disorders characterised by smooth muscle spasm

Contra-indications. Concurrent administration of barbiturates, chlorpromazine, or phenylbutazone; racing animals within 5 days before a race
Dose. *By subcutaneous, intramuscular, or intravenous injection.*
Horses: 5–10 g
Dogs, cats: 27.5 mg/kg

Dipyrone 50% Injection (Vedco) *USA*
Injection, metamizole sodium (as monohydrate) 500 mg/mL, for *horses, dogs, cats*
Withdrawal Periods. Should not be used in *horses* intended for human consumption

PHENYLBUTAZONE

UK

Indications. Inflammation and pain
Contra-indications. See under Carprofen; treatment before regaining consciousness after any general anaesthesia; thyroid disease; thyroid disease
Side-effects. See under Carprofen; occasional oedema of limbs
Warnings. See under Carprofen; regular haematological monitoring required in prolonged use; Drug Interactions – see Appendix 1; coated tablets should not be broken or crushed
Dose.
Horses: by mouth, 4.4 mg/kg twice daily on day one then 2.2 mg/kg twice daily for 2–4 days, followed by 2.2 mg/kg daily or on alternate days
by slow intravenous injection, 4.4 mg/kg as a single dose
ponies: by mouth, 4.4 mg/kg on alternate days
by subcutaneous injection, 4.4 mg as a single dose
Dogs: by mouth, dosages vary, see manufacturers' information. Reduce to lowest effective dose
Cats: by mouth, 25 mg 1–2 times daily for up to 7 days. Then reduce dose to 25 mg daily or on alternate days

POM **Companazone 25** (Arnolds) *UK*
Tablets, s/c, phenylbutazone 25 mg, for *dogs, cats*; 500

POM **Equipalazone** (Arnolds) *UK*
Oral powder, for addition to feed, phenylbutazone 1 g/sachet, for *horses, ponies*
Withdrawal Periods. Should not be used in *horses* intended for human consumption

POM **Equipalazone** (Arnolds) *UK*
Injection, phenylbutazone 200 mg/mL, for *horses, ponies*; 50 mL
Withdrawal Periods. Should not be used in *horses* intended for human consumption

POM **Equipalazone E-PP** (Arnolds) *UK*
Oral paste, phenylbutazone 1 g/division, for *horses, ponies*; 35-mL metered-dose applicator
Withdrawal Periods. Should not be used in *horses* intended for human consumption

POM **Phenogel 100, 200** (Fort Dodge) *UK*
Tablets, s/c, phenylbutazone 100 mg, for *dogs 5–20 kg body-weight*; 1000
Tablets, s/c, phenylbutazone 200 mg, for *dogs more than 20 kg body-weight*; 1000

POM **Phenycare** (Animalcare) *UK*
Tablets, s/c, phenylbutazone 100 mg, 200 mg, for *dogs more than 5 kg body-weight*; 500, 1000
Contra-indications. Pregnant animals

POM **Phenylbutazone** (Loveridge) *UK*
Tablets, s/c, phenylbutazone 100 mg, for *dogs 5–20 kg body-weight*; 250, 500, 1000
Tablets, s/c, phenylbutazone 200 mg, for *dogs more than 20 kg body-weight*; 250, 500, 1000

POM **Phenylbutazone Tablets BP (Vet)** (Millpledge) *UK*
Tablets, phenylbutazone 25 mg, for *dogs, cats*

POM **Pro-Dynam Powder** (Leo) *UK*
Oral powder, for addition to feed (bran or oats), phenylbutazone 1 g/sachet, for *horses*
Withdrawal Periods. Should not be used in *horses* intended for human consumption
Contra-indications. Prior or concurrent feeding of hay

Australia

Indications. Inflammation and pain
Contra-indications. Cardiac, renal, or hepatic impairment; history of blood dyscrasias, hypersensitivity to the drug; pre-existing gastro-intestinal ulceration
Warnings. May be toxic to cats; treatment should be discontinued if gastro-intestinal signs, hepatitis, or blood dyscrasias occur; Drug Interactions – highly protein-bound drugs
Dose. Dosages vary, see manufacturers' information

Beautamav Tablets (Mavlab) *Austral*
Tablets, phenylbutazone 100 mg, for *dogs*

Butalone Granules (Apex) *Austral*
Oral granules, phenylbutazone 1 g/1.3 g granules, for *horses*
Withdrawal Periods. Slaughter 28 days

Butalone Tablets (Apex) *Austral*
Tablets, phenylbutazone 100 mg, for *horses, dogs*
Withdrawal Periods. Slaughter 28 days

Butin Antiinflammatory Oral Paste (Parnell) *Austral*
Oral paste, phenylbutazone 200 mg/mL, for *horses, dogs*
Withdrawal Periods. Slaughter 28 days

Deltazone '100' Tablets (Delvet) *Austral*
Tablets, phenylbutazone 100 mg, for *dogs*

Equibutazone (Virbac) *Austral*
Oral powder, phenylbutazone 1 g/sachet, for *horses*
Withdrawal Periods. Slaughter withdrawal period nil

Equipalazone (Delvet) *Austral*
Oral powder, phenylbutazone 1g/sachet, for *horses*

Myoton (Jurox) *Austral*
Oral granules, phenylbutazone 1 g, for *horses*
Withdrawal Periods. Slaughter 28 days

Myoton (Jurox) *Austral*
Tablets, phenylbutazone 100 mg, for *dogs*

Nabudone IM (Ilium) *Austral*
Injection, phenylbutazone sodium 200 mg/mL, cinchocaine hydrochloride 2 mg/mL, for *horses, dogs*
Withdrawal Periods. Slaughter 14 days

Nabudone P (Ilium) *Austral*
Injection, phenylbutazone sodium 200 mg/mL, for *horses, dogs*
Withdrawal Periods. Slaughter 2 weeks

P-Butazone Granules (Vetsearch) *Austral*
Oral granules, phenylbutazone 1 g/sachet, for *horses*
Withdrawal Periods. Should not be used in *horses* intended for human consumption

P-Butazone Paste (Vetsearch) *Austral*
Oral paste, phenylbutazone 1 g/5 mL paste, for *horses*
Withdrawal Periods. Should not be used in *horses* intended for human consumption

PBZ (Virbac) *Austral*
Tablets, phenylbutazone 100 mg, for *dogs, cats*

Phenylarthrite Injection (Vetoquinol) *Austral*
Injection, phenylbutazone 200 mg/mL, for *horses, dogs*
Withdrawal Periods. Should not be used in *horses* intended for human consumption

Phenylbut IV (Jurox) *Austral*
Injection, phenylbutazone sodium 200 mg/mL, for *horses*
Withdrawal Periods. Slaughter 28 days

Eire
Indications. Inflammation and pain
Contra-indications. Cardiac, renal, or hepatic impairment; history of blood dyscrasias, hypersensitivity to the drug; concurrent NSAIDs or within 24 hours
Warnings. Drug Interactions – nephrotoxic drugs; care in dehydrated, hypovolaemic, or hypotensive animals; safety in pregnant animals has not been established
Dose. *Horses*: *by mouth*, 4.4 mg/kg twice daily on day 1 then 2.2 mg/kg twice daily
by intramuscular injection, 4–6 g on day 1, then 4 g on day 2, then 2 g
by slow intravenous injection, 4 g

Phenylarthrite Injectable Solution (Vetoquinol) *Eire*
Injection, phenylbutazone 200 mg/ mL, for *horses*
Withdrawal Periods. Should not be used in *horses* intended for human consumption

Pro-Dynam (Leo) *Eire*
Oral powder, phenylbutazone 1 g/sachet, for *horses*
Withdrawal Periods. Should not be used in *horses* intended for human consumption

New Zealand
Indications. Inflammation and pain
Contra-indications. Cardiac, renal, or hepatic impairment; history of blood dyscrasias, hypersensitivity to the drug; concurrent other treatment or within 6 weeks of coumarin; gastro-intestinal disorders; cats
Warnings. Care in dehydrated, hypovolaemic, or hypotensive animals; safety in pregnant animals has not been established
Dose. Dosages vary, see manufacturers' information

Bute I.V. (Virbac) *NZ*
Injection, phenylbutazone 200 mg/mL, for *horses, dogs*

Bute Tabs (Virbac) *NZ*
Tablets, phenylbutazone 100 mg, 200 mg, for *dogs*

Equipalazone (Bomac) *NZ*
Oral powder, phenylbutazone 1 g/sachet, for *horses*

Myoton Granules (Jurox) *NZ*
Oral granules, phenylbutazone 1 g/sachet, for *horses*

Myoton Tablets (Jurox) *NZ*
Tablets, phenylbutazone 100 mg, for *dogs*

Nabudone P (Ethical) *NZ*
Injection, phenylbutazone 200 mg/mL, for *horses, dogs*

Oralject P Butazone (Bomac) *NZ*
Oral paste, phenylbutazone 200 mg/mL, for *horses*
Withdrawal Periods. Slaughter 28 days

PBZ Granules (Ethical) *NZ*
Oral granules, per sachet: phenylbutazone 1 g, for *horses*
Withdrawal Periods. Slaughter 28 days

USA
Indications. Inflammation and pain
Contra-indications. Cardiac, renal, or hepatic impairment; history of blood dyscrasias, hypersensitivity to the drugs
Warnings. Care in dehydrated, hypovolaemic, or hypotensive animals; safety in pregnant animals has not been established; treatment should be discontinued if gastro-intestinal, jaundice, or dyscrasia signs occur; monitor RBC count
Dose.
Horses: *by mouth*, 4.4–8.8 mg/kg daily
by intravenous injection, 2.2–4.4 mg/kg daily
Dogs: *by mouth*, 44 mg/kg daily (maximum 800 mg)

Bizolin-1 Gram (Boehringer Ingelheim Vetmedica) *USA*
Tablets, phenylbutazone 1 g, for *horses*
Withdrawal Periods. Should not be used in *horses* intended for human consumption

Bizolin-200 (Bio-Ceutic) *USA*
Tablets, phenylbutazone 200mg, for *dogs*

Butaject (Vetus) *USA*
Injection, phenylbutazone 200 mg/mL, for *horses*
Withdrawal Periods. Should not be used in *horses* intended for human consumption

Butatabs D (Vetus) *USA*
Tablets, phenylbutazone 100 mg, for *dogs*

Butatabs E (Vetus) *USA*
Tablets, phenylbutazone 1 g, for *horses*
Withdrawal Periods. Should not be used in *horses* intended for human consumption

Equi-Phar Phenylbutazone Injection (Vedco) *USA*
Injection, phenylbutazone 200 mg/mL, for *horses*
Withdrawal Periods. Should not be used in *horses* intended for human consumption

Equi-Phar Phenylbutazone Tablets (Vedco) *USA*
Tablets, phenylbuazone 1 g, for *horses*
Withdrawal Periods. Should not be used in *horses* intended for human consumption

Equiphen Paste (Luitpold) *USA*
Oral paste, phenylbutazone 6 g or 12 g/syringe, for *horses*
Withdrawal Periods. Should not be used in *horses* intended for human consumption

Phen-Buta-Vet Injection (Horses) (Anthony) *USA*
Injection, phenylbutazone 200 mg/mL, for *horses*
Withdrawal Periods. Should not be used in *horses* intended for human consumption

Phen-Buta-Vet Tablets (Horses) (Anthony) *USA*
Tablets, phenylbutazone 1 g, for *horse*
Withdrawal Periods. Should not be used in horses intended for human consumption

Phen-Buta-Vet Tablets (Dog) (Anthony) *USA*
Tablets, phenylbutazone 100mg, for *dogs*

Phenylbutazone (Butler) *USA*
Tablets, phenylbutazone 1 g, for *horses*
Withdrawal Periods. Should not be used in *horses* intended for human consumption

Phenylbutazone 100 mg Tablets (Vedco) *USA*
Tablets, phenylbutazone 100 mg, for *dogs*

Phenylbutazone 20% Injection (Phoenix, RXV, VetTek, Western Veterinary Supply) *USA*
Injection, phenylbutazone 200 mg/mL, for *horses*
Withdrawal Periods. Should not be used in *horses* intended for human consumption

Phenylbutazone Injection 200 mg/mL (Butler) *USA*
Injection, phenylbutazone 200 mg/mL, for *horses*
Withdrawal Periods. Should not be used in *horses* intended for human consumption

Phenylbutazone Tablets (VetTek) *USA*
Tablets, phenylbutazone 100 mg, for *dogs*

Phenylbutazone Tablets (VetTek) *USA*
Tablets, phenylbutazone 1 g, for *horses*
Withdrawal Periods. Should not be used in *horses* intended for human consumption

Phenylbutazone Injection (VetTek) *USA*
Injection, phenylbutazone 200 mg/mL, for *horses*
Withdrawal Periods. Should not be used in *horses* intended for human consumption

Pro-Bute (Pro Labs) *USA*
Injection, phenylbutazone 200 mg/mL, for *horses*
Withdrawal Periods. Should not be used in *horses* intended for human consumption

Pro-Bute (Pro Labs) *USA*
Tablets, phenylbutazone 1 g, for *horses*
Withdrawal Periods. Should not be used in *horses* intended for human consumption

---

TOLFENAMIC ACID

UK
Indications. Inflammation and pain
Contra-indications. See under Carprofen; treatment before regaining consciousness after any general anaesthesia
Side-effects. Warnings. See under Carprofen
Dose.
Cattle: *by intravenous injection,* 4 mg/kg as a single dose
Pigs: *by intramuscular injection,* 2 mg/kg as a single dose
Dogs: chronic locomotor disease, *by mouth,* 4 mg/kg once daily for 3 days given with food. May be repeated after 4 days
by subcutaneous or intramuscular injection, 4 mg/kg. May be repeated once only after 24 hours if required
Cats: febrile syndromes, *by mouth,* 4 mg/kg once daily for 3 days given with food
by subcutaneous injection, 4 mg/kg. May be repeated once only after 24 hours if required

POM **Tolfedine Tablets** (Vétoquinol) *UK*
Tablets, tolfenamic acid 6 mg, for *dogs, cats*; 100
Tablets, scored, tolfenamic acid 20 mg, 60 mg, for *dogs*; 96

POM **Tolfedine Injection 4%** (Vétoquinol) *UK*
Injection, tolfenamic acid 40 mg/mL, for *dogs, cats*; 10 mL

POM **Tolfine** (Vétoquinol) *UK*
Injection, tolfenamic acid 40 mg/mL, for *cattle, pigs*
Withdrawal Periods. *Cattle*: slaughter 7 days, first milking after treatment should not be used for human consumption. *Pigs*: slaughter 3 days

Australia
Indications. Inflammation and pain
Dose. *Dogs, cats*: *by subcutaneous or intramuscular injection,* 4 mg/kg

Tolfedine Injection (Vetoquinol) *Austral*
Injection, tolfenamic acid 40 mg/mL, for *dogs, cats*

Eire
Indications. Inflammation and pain
Contra-indications. Hepatic or renal impairment, gastroduodenal disorders, haemorrhagic disorders; hypersensitivity to the drug; concurrent administration of other NSAIDs
Side-effects. Diarrhoea and vomiting
Warnings. Safety in pregnant animals has not been established
Dose. *Dogs, cats*: *by mouth or by subcutaneous or intramuscular injection,* 4 mg/kg

Tolfedine 6 mg Tablets (Vetoquinol) *Eire*
Tablets, tolfenamic acid 6 mg, for *dogs, cats*

Tolfedine 60 mg Tablets (Vetoquinol) *Eire*
Tablets, tolfenamic acid 60 mg, for *dogs*

Tolfedine 4% Injection (Vetoquinol) *Eire*
Injection, tolfenamic acid 40 mg/mL, for *dogs, cats*

New Zealand
Indications. Inflammation and pain
Contra-indications. Cardiac, hepatic or renal impairment, where gastric ulceration is suspected, haemorrhagic disorders; hypersensitivity to the drug; concurrent administration of other NSAIDs
Warnings. Care in animals less than 6 weeks of age or aged animals; avoiduse in dehydrated, hypovolaemic, or hypotensive animals
Dose.
Cattle: *by intramuscular or intravenous injection,* 2 mg/kg
Pigs: *by intramuscular injection,* 2 mg/kg
Dogs, cats: *by mouth or by subcutaneous or intramuscular injection,* 4 mg/kg

Tolfedine (Ethical) *NZ*
Tablets, tolfenamic acid 6 mg, 20 mg, 60 mg, for *dogs, cats*

Tolfedine 4% (Ethical) *NZ*
Injection, tolfenamic acid 40 mg/mL, for *dogs, cats*

Tolfedine CS (Ethical) *NZ*
Injection, tolfenamic acid 40 mg/mL, for *cattle, pigs*
Withdrawal Periods. *Cattle*: slaughter 14 days, milk withdrawal period nil. *Pigs*: slaughter 20 days

SODIUM SALICYLATE

Australia
Indications. Inflammation and pain; thrombo-embolic disorders

Contra-indications. Renal or hepatic impairment, clotting defects, intestinal ulceration, animals less than 30 days of age, less than 7 days before surgery; concurrent aminoglycosides

Dose. *By intravenous injection.*

Horses: inflammation, 35–45 mg/kg; thrombo-embolic disorders, 5 mg/kg *or* 20 mg/kg

Dogs: inflammation, 10 mg/kg; thrombo-embolic disorders, 3 mg/kg

Salsprin (RWR) *Austral*
Injection, sodium salicylate 250 mg/mL, for *horses, dogs*
Withdrawal Periods. Slaughter 28 days

VEDAPROFEN

UK

Indications. Inflammation and pain

Contra-indications. See under Carprofen; treatment before regaining consciousness after any general anaesthesia; parturition; animals that are not eating

Side-effects. Warnings. See under Carprofen; horses should be monitored for oral lesions and treatment discontinued if necessary

Dose. *By mouth.*

Horses: initial dose, 2 mg/kg, then 1 mg/kg twice daily for up to 14 days

Dogs: 500 micrograms/kg once daily given at feeding, for up to 28 days

POM **Quadrisol for Dogs** (Intervet) *UK*
Oral gel, vedaprofen 5 mg/mL, for *dogs more than 10 kg and 12 weeks of age*; 15-mL metered dose applicator, 30-mL metered dose applicator

POM **Quadrisol for Horses** (Intervet) *UK*
Oral gel, vedaprofen 100 mg/mL, for *horses more than 6 months of age*
Withdrawal Periods. Slaughter 12 days

Australia

Indications. Inflammation and pain

Contra-indications. Cardiac, renal or hepatic impairment, gastro-intestinal disorders, hypovolaemia, dehydration; concurrent administration of other NSAIDs or corticosteroids

Side-effects. Occasional gastro-intestinal discomfort, vomiting, diarrhoea

Dose. *Dogs*: *by mouth*, 500 micrograms/kg

Quadrisol 5 (Intervet) *Austral*
Oral gel, vedaprofen 5 mg/mL, for *dogs*

10.2 Other anti-inflammatory drugs

Other classes of drugs may be used to treat inflammatory conditions such as non-infective joint disease. In addition to systemic administration, some of these drugs may be given by intra-articular injection to horses or dogs. Strict asepsis should be observed on administration by intra-articular injection; in some instances antibacterials are given concurrently.

Sodium hyaluronate is a high molecular weight mucopolysaccharide. It is the sodium salt of hyaluronic acid, which is a constituent of the high molecular weight cartilage matrix molecules, aggregated proteoglycans, and is also present in synovial fluid. This accounts for the high viscosity of synovial fluid. In some forms of joint disease depolymerisation of hyaluronic acid occurs, which affects the thixotropic properties of synovial fluid. Sodium hyaluronate is administered by intra-articular or intravenous injection for the therapy of joint diseases in the horse, especially in cases associated with synovitis. The mechanism of action is not known but may be partially attributable to restoration of normal viscosity of synovial fluid and partially due to its anti-inflammatory properties. It inhibits the production of pain-inducing mediators such as prostaglandin E$_2$, blocks superoxide anion release by macrophages, reduces polymorphonuclear neutrophil infiltration into synovial fluid, and (in septic arthritis) reduces glycosaminoglycan loss from articular cartilage.

Pentosan polysulphate sodium is a semi-synthetic glycosaminoglycan with a high molecular weight. **Polysulphated glycosaminoglycan** (PSGAG) is based on hexosamine and hexuronic acid and has a very high molecular weight. These high molecular weight polymers have been shown in some studies to improve clinical outcome in animals with osteoarthritis. Several possible modes of action have been identified. Some models have shown an enhanced production of proteoglycans from certain cells, and others a decreased rate of proteoglycan loss from degenerating articular cartilage. The ability of these compounds to inhibit a range of proteolytic enzymes including metalloproteinases such as stromelysin may be of particular importance. These compounds are 'heparin-like' in structure and high dosages may inhibit clotting mechanisms. A fibrinolytic action in subchondral bone capillaries may help alleviate pain associated with osteoarthritis.

Orgotein is a superoxide dimutase which catalyses the conversion of superoxide radicals to peroxide. It contains copper and zinc and has a molecular weight of about 33 000.

Beta-aminopropionitrile fumarate is claimed to assist in tendon repair. It inhibits the enzyme lysyl oxidase. Theoretically, initial inhibition of random crosslinking of new collagen fibres together with conservative excercise allows the subsequent formation of physiologically aligned crosslinked collagen fibres.

Preparations containing **glucosamine** and **chondroitin** sulphate are administered orally and claimed to help the repair of cartilage by providing the 'building blocks' for new proteoglycan formation. Examples of these preparations include Arthrotabs (Genitrix), Cosequin (Vétoquinol), and Synoquin (VetPlus). Various experimental models also show a potential stimulating effect on glycosaminoglycan synthesis and weak anti-inflammatory properties. A proportion of these ingested macromolecules will reach the blood stream, and some components will reach the synovial fluid. However, at present, their beneficial effect on the course of disease in dogs with osteoarthritis remains unproven. In addition, the effect of these 'neutraceuticals' when administered concurrently with other drugs such as NSAIDs is unknown.

Systemic and locally applied **corticosteroids** are extensively used for the treatment of inflammatory conditions. The general uses and side-effects of corticosteroids are described in section 7.2.1. Some corticosteroid preparations are authorised for intra-articular administration; UK products are listed below.

BETA-AMINOPROPIONITRILE FUMARATE

USA

Indications. Tendinitis
Contra-indications. Dermal irritation oropen skin lesions in injection area; intra-articular or tendon sheath injection; fractures; breeding animals; concurrent irritants or penetrating substances on affected area 10 days before until 8 weeks after treatment; concurrent corticosteroid treatment
Side-effects. Increased inflaammation and occasional lameness
Dose. *Horses*: *by intratendinous injection*, 7 mg

Bapten (Boehringer Ingelheim Vetmedica) *USA*
Injection, 0.7 mg/mL, for **horse**
Withdrawal Periods. Should not be used in **horses** intended for human consumption

CORTICOSTEROIDS (intra-articular administration)

UK

POM Ⓗ **Adcortyl Intra-articular/Intradermal** (Squibb) *UK*
Injection, triamcinolone acetonide 10 mg/mL; 1 mL, 5 mL
Dose. *Horses*: *by intra-articular injection*, 1–10 mg

POM **Depo-Medrone V** (Pharmacia & Upjohn) *UK*
See section 7.2.1 for preparation details
Dose. *Horses*: *by intrasynovial injection*, up to 120 mg
by intratendinous injection, 80-400 mg
Dogs: *by intrasynovial injection*, up to 20 mg

POM **Dexadreson** (Intervet) *UK*
See section 7.2.1 for preparation details
Dose. *Horses*: *by intra-articular injection*, 2–10 mg

ORGOTEIN

USA

Indications. Musculoskeletal inflammation
Contra-indications. Hypersensitivity to the drug or other bovine proteins
Side-effects. Rarely urticaria and pruritis in horses, anaphylaxis in dogs; occasionally paradoxical transient exacerbation of clinical signs in horses initially
Dose.
Horses: *by intramuscular injection*, 5 mg/kg
Dogs: *by subcutaneous injection*, 5 mg/kg

Palosein (OXIS) *USA*
Injection, solid for reconstitution, orgotein 5 mg, for **horses, dogs**
Withdrawal Periods. Should not be used in **horses** intended for human consumption

PENTOSAN POLYSULPHATE SODIUM

UK

Indications. Osteoarthritis and non-immune arthritides
Contra-indications. Septic arthritis, haemorrhage, hepatic or renal impairment, malignant disease; concurrent NSAIDs or other anti-inflammatory drugs or within 24 hours
Side-effects. Rarely reaction to injection within 24 hours
Warnings. Drug Interactions – see Appendix 1
Dose.
Horses ◆: *by intra-articular injection*, 250 mg/joint, repeat after 7–10 days
Dogs: *by subcutaneous injection*, 3 mg/kg, repeat 3 times at 5–7 day intervals
by intra-articular injection ◆, 10–20 mg

POM **Cartrophen Vet** (Arthropharm) *UK*
Injection, pentosan polysulphate sodium 100 mg/mL, for **dogs**; 10 mL

Australia

Indications. Osteoarthritis
Contra-indications. Septic arthritis, haemorrhage, hepatic impairment, renal impairment, clotting defects; use within 2 days of surgery
Dose.
Horses: *by subcutaneous or intramuscular injection*, 3 mg/kg
by intra-articular injection, 250 mg/joint
Dogs: *by mouth*, 10 mg/kg
by subcutaneous injection, 3 mg/kg

Cartrophen Vet Capsules (Biopharm) *Austral*
Capsules, pentosan polysulphate calcium 100 mg, for **dogs**

Cartrophen Vet injection (Biopharm) *Austral*
Injection, pentosan polysulphate sodium 100 mg/mL, for **dogs**

Pentarthron H (Nature Vet) *Austral*
Injection, pentosan polysulphate sodium 250 mg/mL, for **horses**
Withdrawal Periods. Slaughter 28 days

Pentosan Vet (Nature Vet) *Austral*
Injection, pentosan polysulphate 125 mg/mL, for **horses**
Withdrawal Periods. Slaughter 28 days

New Zealand

Indications. Osteoarthritis
Contra-indications. Septic arthritis, haemorrhage, hepatic impairment, renal impairment, clotting defects; use within 2 days of surgery
Dose.
Horses: *by intra-articular injection*, 120–240 mg/joint
Dogs: *by subcutaneous or intramuscular injection*, 3 mg/kg

Cartrophen Vet (Therapeutix) *NZ*
Injection, pentosan polysulphate 100 mg/mL, for **dogs**

Pentarthron (Virbac) *NZ*
Injection, pentosan polysulphate 120 mg/mL, for **horses, dogs**
Withdrawal Periods. Slaughter 28 days

POLYSULPHATED GLYCOSAMINOGLYCAN

UK

Indications. Non-infectious and non-immune arthritides; navicular disease♦ (see section 10.6)
Contra-indications. Advanced hepatic or renal impairment, pregnant animals, injection into infected or actively inflamed joints
Side-effects. Increased oedema at joint site
Warnings. Drug Interactions – other anticoagulant preparations
Dose. *Horses*: *by intramuscular injection*, 500 mg, repeat 6 times at 4-day intervals
by intra-articular injection, 250 mg/joint, repeat 4 times at weekly intervals

POM **Adequan** (Janssen) *UK*
Injection, polysulphated glycosaminoglycan 100 mg/mL, for **horses**; 5 mL
For intramuscular injection
Injection, polysulphated glycosaminoglycan 250 mg/mL, for **horses**; 1 mL
For intra-articular injection

Australia

Indications. Non-infectious arthritides
Contra-indications. Advanced hepatic or renal impairment, patients with increased risk of bleeding
Side-effects. Increased oedema at joint site
Dose. *Horses*: *by intramuscular injection*, 500 mg
by intra-articular injection, 250 mg/joint

Adequan IA (Boehringer Ingelheim) *Austral*
Injection, polysulphated glycosaminoglycan 250 mg/mL, for **horses**
Withdrawal Periods. Slaughter 28 days

Adequan IM (Boehringer Ingelheim) *Austral*
Injection, polysulphated glycosaminoglycan 100 mg/mL, for **horses**
Withdrawal Periods. Slaughter 28 days

Eire

Indications. Non-infectious arthritides
Contra-indications. Advanced hepatic or renal impairment; pregnant animals
Side-effects. Increased oedema at joint site
Dose. *Horses*: *by intra-articular injection*, 250 mg/joint

Adequan 250 mg/mL (Janssen) *Eire*
Injection, polysulphated glycosaminoglycan 250 mg/mL, for **horses**
Withdrawal Periods. Slaughter withdrawal period nil

New Zealand

Indications. Non-infectious arthritides
Contra-indications. Advanced hepatic or renal impairment; pregnant animals
Dose. *Horses*: *by intramuscular injection*, 500 mg

Adequan IM (Boehringer Ingelheim) *NZ*
Injection, polysulphated glycosaminoglycan 100 mg/mL, for **horses**
Withdrawal Periods. Slaughter withdrawal period nil

USA

Indications. Non-infectious arthritides
Contra-indications. Animals intended for breeding; hypersensitivity to the drug
Side-effects. Increased oedema at joint site

Dose. *Horses*: *by intramuscular injection*, 500 mg
by intra-articular injection, 250 mg/joint
Dogs: *by intramuscular injection*, 4.4 mg/kg

Adequan Canine (Luitpold) *USA*
Injection, polysulphated glycosaminoglycan 100mg/mL, for **dogs**

Adequan I.A. (Luitpold) *USA*
Injection, polysulphated glycosaminoglycan 250mg/mL, for **horses**
Withdrawal Periods. Should not be used in **horses** intended for human consumption

Adequan I.M. (Luitpold) *USA*
Injection, polysulphated glycosaminoglycan 500mg/5mL, for **horses**
Withdrawal Periods. Should not be used in **horses** intended for human consumption

SODIUM HYALURONATE
(Hyaluronate sodium)

UK

Indications. Arthritides associated with synovitis; navicular disease♦ (see section 10.6)
Contra-indications. No more than 2 joints should be treated at one time
Side-effects. Transient local reactions
Dose. *Horses*: *by intra-articular injection*, 20–40 mg/joint, repeat if required

Note. For therapeutic purposes sodium hyaluronate and hyaluronic acid may be considered equivalent in effect.

POM **Hyalovet 20** (Arnolds) *UK*
Injection, hyaluronic acid (as sodium salt) 10 mg/mL, for **horses**; 2-mL syringe
Withdrawal Periods. **Horses**: slaughter withdrawal period nil

POM **Hylartil Vet** (Pharmacia & Upjohn) *UK*
Injection, sodium hyaluronate 10 mg/mL, for **horses**; 2-mL syringe
Withdrawal Periods. **Horses**: slaughter withdrawal period nil

POM **Hyonate Injection** (Bayer) *UK*
Injection, sodium hyaluronate 10 mg/mL, for **horses**; 2 mL
Withdrawal Periods. **Horses**: slaughter withdrawal period nil

Australia

Indications. Arthritides associated with synovitis
Side-effects. Transient local swelling
Dose. *Horses*: *by intravenous injection*, 40 mg
by intra-articular injection, 20–40 mg/joint
Dogs: *by intra-articular injection*, 10–20 mg/joint

Hyonate i.v. Injection for Horses (Bayer) *Austral*
Injection, sodium hyaluronate 10 mg/mL, for **horses**

Synacid (Virbac) *Austral*
Injection, sodium hyaluronate 10 mg/mL, for **horses, dogs**
Withdrawal Periods. Slaughter 28 days

Eire

Indications. Arthritides associated with synovitis
Contra-indications. No more than 2 joints should be treated at one time
Side-effects. Transient local reactions
Dose. *Horses*: *by intra-articular injection*, 20–40 mg/joint

Hylartil Vet (Alstoe) *Eire*
Injection, sodium hyaluronate 10 mg/mL, for **horses**
Withdrawal Periods. Slaughter withdrawal period nil

Hyonate Injection (Bayer) *Eire*
Injection, sodium hyaluronate 10 mg, for *horses*
Withdrawal Periods. Should not be used in *horses* intended for human consumption

New Zealand

Indications. Arthritides associated with synovitis
Side-effects. Transient local reactions
Dose. *Horses*: *by intravenous injection*, 40 mg
by intra-articular injection, 20 mg/joint

Hyalovet (Virbac) *NZ*
Injection, hyaluronic acid (as sodium hyaluronate) 10 mg/mL, for *horses*

Hyonate (Bayer) *NZ*
Injection, sodium hyaluronate 10 mg/mL, for *horses*

USA

Indications. Arthritides associated with synovitis
Side-effects. Transient local reactions
Dose. *Horses*: *by intravenous injection*, 40 mg
by intra-articular injection, 20–40 mg/joint

Hyalovet (Fort Dodge) *USA*
Injection, sodium hyaluronate 10 mg/mL, for *horses*
Withdrawal Periods. Should not be used in *horses* intended for human consumption

Hylartin V (Luitpold) *USA*
Injection, sodium hyaluronate 10 mg/mL, for *horses*
Withdrawal Periods. Should not be used in *horses* intended for human consumption

Legend Injectable Solution (Bayer) *USA*
Injection, sodium hyaluronate 10 mg/mL, for *horses*
Withdrawal Periods. Should not be used in *horses* intended for human consumption

---

10.3 Compound preparations of anti-inflammatory and analgesic drugs

Compound preparations are available that contain combinations of NSAIDs such as phenylbutazone and ramifenazone (isopyrin), corticosteroids for example prednisolone, opioid analgesics, and non-opioid analgesics such as paracetamol. Metamizole (dipyrone) has analgesic, anti-inflammatory, and anti-pyretic properties. The drugs included in each preparation may be additive or synergistic in their toxic as well as therapeutic effects and care should be taken to ensure that the recommended dose is not exceeded. In addition, these drugs should not be administered with other NSAIDs or corticosteroids. These preparations are used for the relief of pain and inflammation in soft tissue injury and lameness due to muscular and articular pain and inflammation.

UK

P **Pardale-V Tablets** (Arnolds) *UK*
See section 6.3.3 for preparation details

POM **PLT** (Vericore VP) *UK*
Tablets, scored, cinchophen 200 mg, prednisolone 1 mg, for *dogs*; 100, 1000
Dose. *Dogs*: *by administration with food*, (8 kg body-weight) ½ tablet twice daily; (16 kg body-weight) 1 tablet twice daily; (24 kg body-weight) 1½ tablets twice daily; (>32 kg body-weight) 2 tablets twice daily. Then reduce to lowest effective dose

POM **Tomanol** (Intervet) *UK*
Injection, phenylbutazone (as sodium salt) 121.4 mg, ramifenazone 240 mg/mL, for *horses*; 100 mL
Withdrawal Periods. Should not be used in *horses* intended for human consumption
Contra-indications. Side-effects. Warnings. See under Carprofen and Phenylbutazone
Dose. *Horses*: *by slow (at least 1 minute) intravenous injection*, 3.5 mL/100 kg body-weight. Repeat daily for 2–3 days if required

Australia

Butapyrin (Jurox) *Austral*
Injection, ramifenazone 240 mg/mL, phenylbutazone sodium 130 mg/mL, for *horses*
Withdrawal Periods. Slaughter 28 days

Butasyl (Novartis) *Austral*
Injection, phenylbutazone 186 mg/mL, sodium salicylate 50 mg/mL, for *horses, dogs*

Dexa-Tomanol (Schering-Plough) *Austral*
Injection, ramifenazone 140 mg/mL, phenylbutazone sodium 70 mg/mL, dexamethasone 0.5 mg/mL, cinchocaine hydrochloride 2.2 mg/mL, for *horses, dogs*
Withdrawal Periods. Slaughter 28 days

Prisantol (Intervet) *Austral*
Injection, ramifenazone 240 mg/mL, phenylbutazone 120 mg/mL, for *horses, dogs, cats*

Tomanol (Schering-Plough) *Austral*
Injection, ramifenazole 240 mg/mL, phenylbutazone (as sodium) 120 mg/mL, for *horses, dogs*
Withdrawal Periods. Slaughter 28 days

Eire

Buscopan Compositum (Boehringer Ingelheim) *Eire*
Injection, hyoscine butylbromide 4 mg, dipyrone 500 mg, for *horses, cattle, dogs*
Withdrawal Periods. Should not be used *horses* intended for human consumption. *Cattle*: slaughter 9 days (intravenous injection), 15 days (single intramuscular injection), 18 days (by multiple intramuscular injection), milk 1 day

PLT Tablets (Cypharm) *Eire*
Tablets, cinchophen 200 mg, prednisolone 1 mg, for *dogs*

New Zealand

Dexa-Tomanol (Schering-Plough) *NZ*
Injection, cinchocaine hydrochloride 22 mg/mL, dexamethasone 0.5 mg/mL, phenylbutazone 70 mg/mL, ramifenazone 140 mg/mL, for *horses, cattle, pigs, dogs, cats*
Withdrawal Periods. *Horses*: slaughter 28 days. *Cattle*: slaughter 21 days, milk 72 hours. *Pigs*: slaughter 21 days

Tomanol (Schering-Plough) *NZ*
Injection, phenylbutazone 130 mg/mL, ramifenazone 240 mg/mL, for *horses, cattle, pigs, dogs, cats*
Withdrawal Periods. *Horses*: slaughter 28 days. *Cattle*: slaughter 21 days, milk 72 hours. *Pigs*: slaughter 21 days

USA

Cortaba (Pharmacia & Upjohn) *USA*
Tablets, methylprednisolone 0.5 mg, aspirin 300 mg, for *dogs*

10.4 Topical anti-inflammatory preparations

The topical drugs used most extensively for their anti-inflammatory properties are the corticosteroids (see section

7.2, section 14.2.1 Skin, section 12.3.1 Eye, and section 14.8 Ear). Topical drugs that may also be applied include dimethyl sulfoxide (dimethyl sulphoxide, DMSO) and particular NSAIDs such as methyl salicylate. Preparations containing copper in combination with NSAIDs and formulated in a DMSO basis have been evaluated.

DMSO is a solvent that readily dissolves both water-soluble and lipid-soluble drugs and can be used to transport drugs through skin. It also possesses some anti-inflammatory activity and causes dissolution of collagen. Its mode of action as an anti-inflammatory drug is unknown but it may act through scavenging free radicals.

Copper and copper-containing compounds may also act by the same mechanism. They possess superoxide dismutase activity. However, the therapeutic value of copper-containing compounds in joint disease remains to be established.

Combination preparations are available, which are used for tendonitis and synovitis mainly on horses.

UK
Indications. See notes above
Contra-indications. Racehorses 48 hours prior to racing
Warnings. Operators should wear impervious gloves

GSL **Lincoln Kaolin Poultice BP** (Battle Hayward & Bower) *UK*
Paste, kaolin 52%, boric acid 4.5%, glycerol 42.5%, peppermint oil 0.05%, salicylate 0.2%, thymol 0.05%, for *horses*; 1 kg, 3 kg
Withdrawal Periods. Should not be used on *horses* intended for human consumption

PML **Tensolvet** (Day Son & Hewitt) *UK*
Gel, glycol salicylate 5%, menthol 0.5%, heparin sodium 50 units/g, for *horses*; 300 g
Withdrawal Periods. Should not be used on *horses* intended for human consumption
Contra-indications. Application to broken skin; should not be massaged into skin

10.5 Cytotoxic immunosuppressants

Cytotoxic drugs with immunosuppressant properties such as cyclophosphamide and mercaptopurine have been used in the treatment of immune-based arthritides mainly in dogs. These drugs are usually given in combination with a corticosteroid such as prednisolone.

Cyclophosphamide (see section 13.1.1) is administered to dogs at a dose of 25 mg/m^2 for dogs weighing less than 10 kg, 20 mg/m^2 for dogs weighing 10 to 35 kg, and 15 mg/m^2 for dogs weighing more than 35 kg. Doses of up to 50 mg/m^2 have been used. Cyclophosphamide is given for 4 consecutive days every week *or* on alternate days for 4 doses, in combination with initial doses of **prednisolone** (see section 7.2.1) 2 to 4 mg/kg daily decreasing to 0.5 to 2 mg/kg on alternate days.

After 4 months, treatment should be changed to **mercaptopurine** (see section 13.1.2) given at a dose of 20 mg/m^2 on alternate days.

10.6 Gold

Drugs in this class include the gold salts sodium aurothiomalate and auranofin. These drugs are used in humans to suppress symptoms and retard degenerative changes in rheumatoid and other immune-based arthritides. The mechanism of action has not been fully elucidated. Some of the drugs have been used to treat immune-based arthritides in dogs but the slow onset of action, difficulty in assessing efficacy, and potential toxicity to the haematopoietic system have limited their veterinary usage.

Sodium aurothiomalate treatment regimens consist of progressively increasing doses over a period of 13 weeks although it is possible to modify dosage according to the severity of the condition and the size and breed of the animal treated.

Auranofin is administered by mouth twice daily, generally in combination with a low dose of prednisolone. Urine-protein concentration and blood cell counts should be monitored regularly in treated animals.

AURANOFIN

UK
Indications. Immune-based arthritides
Warnings. Potential haematopoietic system toxicity
Dose. *Dogs: by mouth,* initially 0.5–2.0 mg twice daily. May be increased to a maximum dose of 9 mg daily and may be used in combination with prednisolone (see section 7.2.1) 0.5 mg/kg daily. Treatment should be discontinued when the patient has been in remission for 6 months

POM Ⓗ **Ridaura** (Yamanouchi) *UK*
Tablets, f/c, auranofin 3 mg; 60

SODIUM AUROTHIOMALATE

UK
Indications. Immune-based arthritides
Warnings. Potential haematopoietic system toxicity
Dose. *By intramuscular injection.*
Horses, cattle: 10 mg, then 20 mg, then 2 injections of 50 mg, and then 9 injections of 100 mg, at weekly intervals over 13 weeks
Dogs: 10 mg, then 6 injections of 20 mg, and then 6 injections of 50 mg, at weekly intervals over 13 weeks

POM Ⓗ **Myocrisin** (JHC) *UK*
Injection, sodium aurothiomalate 20 mg/mL, 40 mg/mL, 100 mg/mL; 0.5 mL

10.7 Treatment of navicular disease

Navicular disease (navicular syndrome) is a cause of intermittent forelimb lameness in horses between 4 and 15 years of age. The hindlimbs are rarely affected. Predisposing factors include faulty conformation, foot imbalance, irregular shoeing and exercise on hard surfaces.

The exact cause of navicular disease is unknown. It is suggested that the condition arises due to interruption of blood flow to and from the navicular region. Alternatively degenerative changes in the navicular bone occur as a result of tension acting through the deep digital flexor tendon which compresses the navicular bone dorsally against the distal and middle phalanges.

The pathological changes in navicular disease include focal cartilage degeneration, cartilage erosion, subchondral bone sclerosis, focal areas of bone lysis, and oedema, congestion and fibrosis in the marrow spaces. Pain results from degenerative changes in the bone, and from strain to the surrounding soft tissue structures. Venous drainage from the marrow spaces of the navicular bones of affected horses is impaired, and the resultant venous distension and venous hypertension may be an important cause of pain.

A variety of treatments can be used in navicular disease. In many cases, effective treatment probably only arrests or delays the progression of the disease and manages the pain, rather than cures the condition. Treatment usually involves variable periods of rest, corrective trimming and shoeing, medications to improve blood flow, anti-inflammatory analgesics, and drugs to treat degenerative bone and cartilage changes.

Rest is important to allow time for soft tissue inflammation to subside and for the horse to adapt to corrective trimming and shoeing. Some horses respond favourably to corrective trimming and shoeing without the need for specific medical therapy. The aims of trimming and shoeing are to restore normal hoof balance, to correct problems such as under-run heels, shearing of the hoof wall, and heel bulb contraction, and to reduce biomechanical forces on the navicular region. A variety of different forms of trimming and shoeing can be used. Egg bar shoes are appropriate in some cases.

NSAIDs (see section 10.1), in particular phenylbutazone, are commonly used to provide pain relief. Phenylbutazone can be helpful to allow pain-free adjustment to new shoes and hoof angles following corrective farriery. The horse should also be rested during initial therapy. In some cases, phenylbutazone can be used to manage pain long term, or in association with specific athletic events.

Isoxsuprine is commonly used in the treatment of navicular disease. It is a beta-adrenergic agent with vasodilatory properties and causes direct relaxation of vascular smooth muscle. Reported success rates with this drug range from 40% to 87%, with the best results in horses affected for less than one year. However, in recent studies orally administered isoxsuprine failed to produce any demonstrable pharmacological effects. Various different dosage regimes have been recommended. The improvement in clinical signs can persist for up to 1 year after administration of isoxsuprine is discontinued, especially when foot balance has been corrected. However, in some cases continuous treatment at a low dose is required.

Propentofylline (see section 4.3.4) and pentoxifylline are xanthine derivatives, which alter the physical characteristics of the blood by increasing erythrocyte flexibility, preventing aggregation of erythrocytes and platelets, decreasing fibrinogen levels, and inhibiting the action of some inflammatory cytokines. Pentoxifylline has been shown to be erratically absorbed following oral administration in horses. Propentofylline has been shown shown to be helpful in the treatment of navicular disease.

Corticosteroids (see section 7.2) are sometimes beneficial as an adjunctive therapy in the treatment of navicular disease. These agents can be injected into the distal interphalangeal joint or navicular bursa. Many clinicians utilise this treatment only in cases where initial treatment by corrective trimming and shoeing, rest, isoxsuprine and phenylbutazone has been unsuccessful. The corticosteroid given is based on personal experience. For guidance, a dose of methylprednisolone 20 to 40 mg injected into the distal interphalangeal joint may be used.

Warfarin has been used as a treatment of navicular disease in an attempt to reduce and slow thrombosis. Serious side-effects of warfarin treatment such as the risk of haemorrhage and the interaction of warfarin with protein-bound drugs (including phenylbutazone) may occur. Warfarin is now rarely used for the treatment of navicular disease.

Sodium hyaluronate and **polysulphated glycosaminoglycan** (see section 10.2) have been used in the treatment of navicular disease. Sodium hyaluronate may be injected intrasynovially concurrently with a corticosteroid.

Surgical treatments can be used for horses with navicular disease that have not responded to more conservative treatments. Three surgical treatments are described: palmar digital neurectomy; navicular suspensory desmotomy; and desmotomy of the distal check ligament.

The treatment of laminitis is discussed in chapter 15.

ISOXSUPRINE HYDROCHLORIDE

UK

Indications. Navicular disease, and other conditions of the lower limb where vasodilatation may be beneficial; laminitis ♦

Contra-indications. Recent arterial haemorrhage; pregnant mares and mares up to 2 weeks post partum

Side-effects. Tachycardia

Dose. See preparation details

Laminitis ♦, *by mouth*, 0.6 to 4.0 mg/kg twice daily

POM **Navilox** (Vétoquinol) *UK*
Oral powder, isoxsuprine hydrochloride 30 mg/g, for *horses*; 300 g
Withdrawal Periods. Should not be used in *horses* intended for human consumption
Dose. *Horses*: 600 micrograms of isoxsuprine (20 mg of powder)/kg twice daily for 6 weeks, then once daily for 3 weeks, then on alternate days for 3 weeks. Treatment should be administered on an empty stomach 30 minutes before feeding

POM **Oralject Circulon** (Vetsearch; distributed by Millpledge) *UK*
Oral paste, isoxsuprine hydrochloride 40 mg/mL, for *horses*; 230 mL
Withdrawal Periods. Should not be used in *horses* intended for human consumption
Dose. *Horses*: 600 micrograms/kg twice daily for 3 weeks. Avoid sudden discontinuation of treatment. The dose should be reduced over a further 3-week period to 600 micrograms/kg once daily for 14 days, then on alternate days for 7 days. Treatment may be increased to 900 micrograms/kg twice daily if required and dose reduced to once daily, then on alternate days. Treatment should be administered on an empty stomach, 30 minutes before feeding

Australia

Indications. Navicular disease, and other conditions of the lower limb where vasodilatation may be beneficial
Contra-indications. Recent arterial haemorrhage; pregnant mares and mares up to 2 weeks post partum
Warnings. Avoid sudden discontinuation of treatment
Dose. *Horses*: 600 micrograms/kg twice daily for 3 weeks, then once daily for 3 weeks, then on alternate days for 7 days

Circulon Paste (Vetsearch) *Austral*
Oral paste, isoxsuprine hydrochloride 40 mg/mL, for *horses*
Withdrawal Periods. Slaughter 28 days

Eire

Indications. Navicular disease
Contra-indications. Recent arterial haemorrhage; pregnant mares and mares up to 2 weeks post partum
Warnings. Avoid sudden discontinuation of treatment
Dose. See manufacturer's information

Duviculine (Interchem) *Eire*
Capsules, isoxsuprine hydrochloride 60 , for *horses*
Withdrawal Periods. Should not be used in *horses* intended for human consumption

New Zealand

Indications. Navicular disease
Contra-indications. Recent arterial haemorrhage; pregnant mares and mares up to 2 weeks post partum
Warnings. Avoid sudden discontinuation of treatment
Dose. *Horses*: 600 micrograms/kg twice daily for 3 weeks, then daily, reducing to alternate days over 3 weeks

Oralject Circulon (Bomac) *NZ*
Oral paste, isoxsuprine hydrochloride 40 mg/mL, for *horses*
Withdrawal Periods. Slaughter 28 days

PROPENTOFYLLINE

UK

Indications. Navicular disease in horses♦; dullness, lethargy in older dogs (see section 4.3.4)
Dose. *Horses*♦: *by mouth*, 7.5 mg/kg twice daily for 6 weeks

See section 4.3.4 for preparation details

WARFARIN SODIUM

UK

Indications. Navicular disease (**but see notes above**); vascular thrombosis (see section 4.6.2)
Contra-indications. Purpura, malnutrition, haemorrhage, late pregnancy; Drug Interactions – see Appendix 1
Side-effects. Haemorrhage
Warnings. One stage prothrombin time must be measured before commencement of therapy; monitor effects of Warfarin therapy, see section 4.6.2; Drug Interactions – see Appendix 1
Dose. *Horses*: (**but see notes above**) *by mouth*, 20 micrograms/kg daily increasing gradually by 20% per week until the one stage prothrombin time is increased by 2–4 seconds (usual dose range: 16–170 micrograms/kg)

See section 4.6.2 for preparation details

11 Drugs used in the treatment of
MASTITIS

Contributor:
P W Edmondson MVB, CertCHP, FRCVS

11.1 Intramammary preparations
11.2 Preparations for the care of teats and udders

Mastitis is of economic importance in dairy cows because it causes decreased milk quality, and reduced milk yield which often leads to early culling. Peracute mastitis often results in death. Other species affected include sheep, pigs, dogs, cats, goats, and horses; male animals may also be affected. Treatment of mastitis in sheep and goats is similar to that employed for cattle.

Generally, the infecting organisms enter the udder via the teat canal during the milking process. Contamination may arise from the teats and udders of infected cows, teat abrasions, environmental sources, faulty milking equipment, and in the case of summer mastitis, the head fly *Hydrotoea irritans*.

The main mastitis pathogens are *Staphylococcus aureus*, *Streptococcus agalactiae*, *Strep. dysgalactiae*, *Strep. uberis*, *Actinomyces pyogenes* (summer mastitis); *Escherichia coli*, *Klebsiella* spp., *Enterobacter aerogenes* (coliform mastitis); some fungi; and yeasts.

These pathogens enter through the teat canal and cause infection in the mammary gland, which may be either clinical or subclinical, depending on the number and type of pathogens involved. The majority of subclinical mastitis is caused by *Staph. aureus*, *Strep. agalactiae*, and *Strep. dysgalactiae*. These are contagious mastitis organisms whose reservoir is within the udder itself and are spread from cow to cow during the milking process. Environmental organisms live outside the udder and are transferred onto the teats between milkings. A systemic reaction may also occur in some cases. Early diagnosis and treatment of clinical mastitis will increase the rate of recovery and the return to normal milk production, and lessen the damage to the mammary gland.

In **peracute clinical mastitis**, there is acute inflammation of the mammary gland with toxaemia. The causal bacteria may include coliforms, *Staph. aureus*, *A. pyogenes*, *Bacillus cereus*, or *Pseudomonas aeruginosa*. Treatment should include antibacterials and supportive therapy. Infected quarters should be stripped out frequently.

Oxytocin may be administered, by intramuscular or slow intravenous injection, to aid evacuation of the udder. Initial treatment consists of oxytocin 80 units, given by intramuscular injection before stripping out, and intramammary treatment. Then oxytocin 20 units given by intramuscular injection before each stripping out, and concurrent intramammary treatment. The build-up of endotoxin in the udder is reduced, thereby limiting the extent of toxaemia.

NSAIDs (see section 10.1) such as flunixin meglumine at a dose of 2.2 mg/kg body-weight by intravenous injection or ketoprofen at a dose of 3 mg/kg by intramuscular or intravenous injection are indicated for the treatment of toxaemia.

Fluids (see section 16.1.2) such as sodium chloride 0.9% by intravenous infusion may be administered rapidly to dehydrated cows at a dose equal to or more than 5% body-weight. Alternatively, hypertonic saline (sodium chloride 7.2%) at a dose of 2 litres may be administered by intravenous injection to aid rehydration. Intravenous administration of glucose is useful to counteract the hypoglycaemia that occurs with toxaemia.

Parenteral antibacterials (see section 1.1) such as procaine benzylpenicillin and dihydrostreptomycin in combination, potentiated sulphonamides, cephalosporins, or oxytetracycline may be given in addition to intramammary preparations.

Multivitamin preparations (see section 16.6.7) containing B vitamins may also aid recovery. Intravenous calcium may also be given.

In **acute mastitis** there is swelling and inflammation of the mammary gland with or without systemic reaction. The milk is found to be abnormal. Treatment consists of thoroughly evacuating the udder before administering intramammary preparations for lactating cows (see section 11.1.1). Oxytocin may be used to assist emptying of the udder. In cases where there is systemic involvement, parenteral antibacterials and supportive therapy are indicated.

Staph. aureus is the most common cause of **chronic mastitis** in the dairy cow. Some strains of this micro-organism are resistant to certain antibacterials (see section 11.1.1). After treatment, there is frequently a clinical improvement but infection tends to persist. Chronic mastitis can also occur with *Strep. uberis* and occasionally coliform infections. The best time to attempt to eliminate chronic mastitis infections is during the dry period (see section 11.1.2).

In cases of **subclinical mastitis** no gross abnormality of the milk is evident. The constituents of milk will be altered and the cell count will be elevated. These cases are usually treated when the animal is no longer lactating by using long-acting intramammary preparations (see section 11.1.2). Subclinical mastitis caused by *Strep. agalactiae* may be treated successfully during lactation. If the entire herd is treated with intramammary antibacterials to eliminate *Strep. agalactiae* it is essential that basic mastitis control measures have been implemented before treatment. Preparations for non-lactating animals are used to eliminate subclinical infection at the end of lactation and to prevent the establishment of new infections during the dry period, including summer mastitis due to *A. pyogenes*.

Scrupulous hygiene measures must be observed when administering any intramammary preparation to avoid introducing a more severe infection than that for which the original treatment was intended. This is especially important with treatment for the dry period. Careless administration may result in bacteria being infused into the udder leading to mastitis during the dry period or at the time of calving.

Before infusion, teat ends should be thoroughly cleaned and then disinfected using cotton wool soaked in surgical or methylated spirit until there is no sign of contamination on the cotton wool. The nozzle of the intramammary syringe should be introduced only a short distance into the teat canal and the contents administered. After infusion, the preparation should be massaged up into the udder and the teats dipped with a disinfectant solution (see section 11.2). It is important that antibacterial preparations are infused into, and not through the teat canal, because mastitis pathogens frequently colonise the canal. This also helps to protect the lining of the canal from mechanical damage caused by the end of the intramammary applicator.

Mastitis causes a significant loss of production, and prevention and control of the disease should be practised. Monitoring of herd status using bulk and individual cow somatic cell counts is important; under Directive 92/46EEC, implemented in the UK as the *Dairy Products (Hygiene) Regulations 1995* (SI 1995/1086), it is a requirement that all saleable milk has a three monthly rolling herd cell-count less than 400 000. In addition, use of pre- and post milking disinfectant preparations, attention to hygiene standards in the dairy and housing areas, and thorough plant cleaning are essential. A culling policy, together with whole herd dry cow therapy (see section 11.1.2) and a 6-monthly check on milking machine installations will help to reduce the level of mastitis in the herd. Guidance is provided in the following:

- MAFF. *A guide to clean milk production.* PB 0341. London: HMSO
- BSI. *Milking machine installations.* BS 5545. London: BSI, 1988.

A vaccine is available for control of mastitis caused by environmental pathogens (see section 18.2.11).

11.1 Intramammary preparations

11.1.1 Intramammary preparations for lactating animals

11.1.2 Intramammary preparations for non-lactating animals

11.1.1 Intramammary preparations for lactating animals

These preparations are used to treat clinical and subclinical mastitis (see notes above). Bacterial culture and sensitivity testing should be carried out on pretreatment milk samples on a regular basis so that mastitis pathogens within a herd are identified and the most suitable therapy is administered. Pretreatment samples should be refrigerated. Veterinarians should keep records, such as results of antibacterial sensi-

tivity testing and identification of bacterial isolates for individual farms. Where no information is available, initial treatment is usually empirical and chosen to provide the widest possible cover.

The most common pathogens responsible for clinical mastitis are *Strep. uberis*, coliforms, *Staph. aureus*, *Strep. dysgalactiae*, and *Strep. agalactiae*. Antibacterials included in intramammary preparations give either narrow- or broad-spectrum activity against mastitis pathogens. Details of antibacterial spectra of activity may be found in section 1.1. Some compound preparations also contain corticosteroids to help reduce inflammation within the udder. The success of treatment for *Staph. aureus* infection is very poor due to the organisms surviving within micro abscesses and macrophages, and antibacterial resistance. In addition, some strains are not killed by antibacterials if the micro-organisms are in a state of dormancy.

Antibiotic resistance to penicillins occurs with beta-lactamase producing staphylococci (70% of strains) and in these cases cephalosporins, cloxacillin, or combination preparations containing clavulanic acid should be used. Improved resolution of *Staph. aureus* infection is achieved when intramammary and systemic antibacterials are administered concurrently. A full course of treatment should be administered even if the milk returns to normal appearance before the course is completed. Partial treatment may increase the likelihood of infection recurring and may contribute to the development of bacterial resistance.

In general, milk should not be used for human consumption if the animal is in poor health or the cow has a milk yield of less than 5 litres per day. Medicinal and antibacterial residues present in milk may interfere with manufacturing processes and lead to hypersensitivity problems in humans. Withdrawal periods for meat and milk are stated by the manufacturer. If no withdrawal periods are given or a product is used outwith the data sheet recommendations, standard withdrawal periods apply. In addition, in England, Wales, and Scotland all milk should be withheld for the first 4 days after calving and, in Scotland, milk should be discarded for 2 days after the administration of any medicine. In any case of doubt, an antibacterial residue test should be carried out on a milk sample from the individual cow and a negative result obtained before milk from that cow is included in bulk milk for human consumption. The presence of antibacterials in the milk leaving the farm is likely to lead to severe financial penalties being applied by the purchasing company. See NOAH. *Antibiotic residue avoidance in milk* for further information.

Intramammary preparations should be administered after milking using the recommended procedure (see notes above).

CEFACETRILE SODIUM
(Cephacetrile)

UK

Indications. Mastitis, see notes above
Dose. See preparation details

POM **Vetimast** (Novartis)
Intramammary suspension, cefacetrile sodium 250 mg/dose, for *cattle*
Withdrawal Periods. *Cattle*: slaughter 7 days, milk 4 days
Dose. *Cattle*: *by intramammary infusion*, one dose per infected quarter.
One dose is usually sufficient for treatment

CEFOPERAZONE

UK

Indications. Mastitis, see notes above
Dose. See preparation details

POM **Pathocef** (Pfizer)
Intramammary suspension (oily), cefoperazone (as sodium salt) 250 mg/dose, for *cattle*
Withdrawal Periods. *Cattle*: slaughter 2 days, milk 3.5 days
Dose. *Cattle*: *by intramammary infusion*, one dose per infected quarter.
One dose is usually sufficient for treatment

CEFQUINOME

UK

Indications. Mastitis, see notes above
Dose. See preparation details

POM **Cephaguard LC Intramammary** (Intervet)
Intramammary suspension, cefquinome 75 mg/dose, for *cattle*
Withdrawal Periods. *Cattle*: slaughter 2 days, milk 4 days
Dose. *Cattle*: *by intramammary infusion*, one dose per infected quarter.
Repeat twice at 12-hour intervals

CLOXACILLIN

UK

Indications. Mastitis, see notes above
Dose. See preparation details

POM **Noroclox QR** (Norbrook)
Intramammary suspension, cloxacillin (as sodium salt) 200 mg/dose, for *cattle*
Withdrawal Periods. *Cattle*: slaughter 7 days, milk 2.5 days
Dose. *Cattle*: *by intramammary infusion*, one dose per infected quarter.
Repeat twice at 12-hour intervals

POM **Orbenin LA** (Pfizer)
Intramammary suspension, cloxacillin (as sodium salt) 200 mg/dose, for *cattle, sheep*
Withdrawal Periods. *Cattle*: slaughter 7 days, milk 3.5 days. *Sheep*: slaughter 7 days, should not be used in sheep producing milk for human consumption
Dose. *Cattle*: *by intramammary infusion*, one dose per infected quarter.
Repeat twice at 48-hour intervals
Sheep: *by intramammary infusion*, one dose per udder half at weaning

POM **Orbenin QR** (Pfizer)
Intramammary suspension, cloxacillin (as sodium salt) 200 mg/dose, for *cattle*
Withdrawal Periods. *Cattle*: slaughter 7 days, milk 2.5 days
Dose. *Cattle*: *by intramammary infusion*, one dose per infected quarter.
Repeat twice at 12-hour intervals

ERYTHROMYCIN

UK

Indications. Mastitis, see notes above
Dose. See preparation details

POM **Erythrocin Intramammary** (Ceva)
Intramammary solution, erythromycin 300 mg/dose, for *cattle*

Withdrawal Periods. *Cattle*: slaughter 7 days, milk 1.5 days
Dose. *Cattle*: *by intramammary infusion*, one dose per infected quarter.
Repeat twice

COMPOUND ANTIBACTERIAL PREPARATIONS FOR LACTATING ANIMALS

UK

Indications. Mastitis, see notes above

POM **Bimamast MC** (Bimeda)
Intramammary suspension, ampicillin (as trihydrate) 200 mg, cloxacillin (as sodium salt) 200 mg/dose, for *cattle*
Withdrawal Periods. *Cattle*: slaughter 7 days, milk 2.5 days
Dose. *Cattle*: *by intramammary infusion*, one dose per infected quarter.
Repeat twice at 12-hour intervals

POM **Embacillin C** (Merial)
Intramammary suspension, ampicillin (as sodium) 75 mg, cloxacillin sodium 200 mg/dose, for *cattle*
Withdrawal Periods. *Cattle*: slaughter 7 days, milk 2.5 days
Dose. *Cattle*: *by intramammary infusion*, one dose per infected quarter.
Repeat twice at 12-hour intervals

POM **Kloxerate Plus Milking Cow** (Fort Dodge)
Intramammary suspension, ampicillin (as sodium salt) 75 mg, cloxacillin (as sodium salt) 200 mg/dose, for *cattle*
Withdrawal Periods. *Cattle*: slaughter 7 days, milk 2.5 days
Dose. *Cattle*: *by intramammary infusion*, one dose per infected quarter.
Repeat twice at 12-hour intervals

POM **Lactaclox** (Norbrook)
Intramammary suspension, ampicillin (as sodium salt) 75 mg, cloxacillin (as sodium salt) 200 mg/dose, for *cattle*
Withdrawal Periods. *Cattle*: slaughter 7 days, milk 2.5 days
Dose. *Cattle*: *by intramammary infusion*, one dose per infected quarter.
Repeat twice at 12-hour intervals

POM **Lactatrim MC** (Elanco)
Intramammary suspension, sulfadiazine 200 mg, trimethoprim 40 mg/dose, for *cattle*
Withdrawal Periods. *Cattle*: slaughter 7 days, milk 2 days
Dose. *Cattle*: *by intramammary infusion*, one dose per infected quarter.
Repeat twice at 12-hour intervals

POM **Lincocin Forte S** (Pharmacia & Upjohn)
Intramammary suspension, lincomycin (as hydrochloride) 330 mg, neomycin (as sulphate) 100 mg/dose, for *cattle*
Withdrawal Periods. *Cattle*: slaughter 2 days, milk 3.5 days
Dose. *Cattle*: *by intramammary infusion*, one dose per infected quarter.
Repeat twice at 12-hour intervals

POM **Nafpenzal MC** (Intervet)
Intramammary suspension, benzylpenicillin sodium 180 mg, dihydrostreptomycin (as sulphate) 100 mg, nafcillin (as sodium salt) 100 mg/dose, for *cattle*
Withdrawal Periods. *Cattle*: slaughter 7 days, milk 3.5 days
Dose. *Cattle*: *by intramammary infusion*, one dose per infected quarter daily for 3–4 days

POM **Streptopen Milking Cow** (Schering-Plough)
Intramammary paste (oily), dihydrostreptomycin (as sulphate) 500 mg, procaine benzylpenicillin 1 g/dose, for *cattle*
Withdrawal Periods. *Cattle*: slaughter 7 days, milk 4.5 days
Dose. *Cattle*: *by intramammary infusion*, one dose per infected quarter.
Repeat twice at 12-hour intervals

POM **Streptopen QR** (Schering-Plough)
Intramammary paste (oily), dihydrostreptomycin (as sulphate) 100 mg, procaine benzylpenicillin 100 mg/dose, for *cattle*r
Withdrawal Periods. *Cattle*: slaughter 7 days, milk 3 days
Dose. *Cattle*: *by intramammary infusion*, one dose per infected quarter daily for 3 days

POM **Strypen Forte Rapid** (Merial)
Intramammary suspension, dihydrostreptomycin (as sulphate) 250 mg, procaine benzylpenicillin 300 mg/dose, for *cattle*
Withdrawal Periods. *Cattle*: slaughter 7 days, milk 3 days
Dose. *Cattle*: *by intramammary infusion*, one dose per infected quarter daily for 3 days

POM **Synermast Lactating Cow** (Virbac)
Intramammary suspension, ampicillin (as trihydrate) 200 mg, cloxacillin (as sodium salt) 200 mg/dose, for *cattle*
Withdrawal Periods. *Cattle*: slaughter 7 days, milk 2.5 days
Dose. *Cattle*: *by intramammary infusion*, one dose per infected quarter. Repeat twice at 12-hour intervals

POM **Vonapen Milking Cow** (Intervet)
Intramammary paste, neomycin (as sulphate) 300 mg, procaine benzylpenicillin 500 mg/dose, for *cattle*
Withdrawal Periods. *Cattle*: slaughter 7 days, milk 3 days
Dose. *Cattle*: *by intramammary infusion*, one dose per infected quarter daily for 3 days

Compound antibacterial and corticosteroid preparations for lactating animals

UK

POM **Aureomycin Mastitis Suspension** (Fort Dodge)
Intramammary suspension, chlortetracycline hydrochloride 426 mg, hydrocortisone 2 mg/dose, for *cattle*
Withdrawal Periods. *Cattle*: slaughter 7 days, milk 4.5 days
Dose. *Cattle*: *by intramammary infusion*, one dose per infected quarter daily as necessary

POM **Duphacerate Co** (Fort Dodge)
Intramammary paste (oily), neomycin sulphate 100 mg, prednisolone 10 mg, procaine benzylpenicillin 100 mg, streptomycin sulphate 100 mg/dose, for *cattle*
Withdrawal Periods. *Cattle*: slaughter 7 days, milk 3 days
Dose. *Cattle*: *by intramammary infusion*, one dose per infected quarter daily for 3 days

POM **Leo Yellow Milking Cow** (Leo)
Intramammary paste, dihydrostreptomycin (as sulphate) 150 mg, framycetin sulphate 50 mg, penethamate hydriodide 150 mg, prednisolone 5 mg/dose, for *cattle*
Withdrawal Periods. *Cattle*: slaughter 28 days, milk 3.5 days
Dose. *Cattle*: *by intramammary infusion*, one dose per infected quarter daily for 3 days

POM **Multiject IMM** (Norbrook)
Intramammary paste (oily), neomycin sulphate 100 mg, prednisolone 10 mg, procaine benzylpenicillin 100 mg, streptomycin sulphate 100 mg/dose, for *cattle*
Withdrawal Periods. *Cattle*: slaughter 7 days, milk 3 days
Dose. *Cattle*: *by intramammary infusion*, one dose per infected quarter daily for 3 days

POM **Synulox Lactating Cow** (Pfizer)
Intramammary suspension (oily), amoxicillin (as trihydrate) 200 mg, clavulanic acid (as potassium salt) 50 mg, prednisolone 10 mg/dose, for *cattle*
Withdrawal Periods. *Cattle*: slaughter 7 days, milk 60 hours
Dose. *Cattle*: *by intramammary infusion*, one dose per infected quarter. Repeat twice at 12-hour intervals

POM **Tetra-Delta** (Pharmacia & Upjohn)
Intramammary suspension (oily), dihydrostreptomycin (as sulphate) 100 mg, neomycin (as sulphate) 105 mg, novobiocin (as sodium salt) 100 mg, prednisolone 10 mg, procaine benzylpenicillin 100 mg/dose, for *cattle*
Withdrawal Periods. *Cattle*: slaughter 7 days, milk 3 days
Dose. *Cattle*: *by intramammary infusion*, one dose per infected quarter. Repeat after 24 or 48 hours if required

11.1.2 Intramammary preparations for non-lactating animals

Non-lactating or dry cow therapy is administered to eliminate any subclinical infection present at the end of lactation and to prevent the establishment of new infections, including summer mastitis, during the dry period. Management plays a major part in the control of mastitis during the dry period and animals should be examined frequently, preferably twice daily.

The choice of dry cow therapy depends on many factors: the mastitis pathogens present in the herd, the length of the dry period, and bacterial culture and sensitivity test results from pretreatment mastitis samples and high cell count cows. As *Staph. aureus* is the most common cause of subclinical infection, a dry cow preparation should contain an antibacterial that is effective for all strains of *Staph. aureus*. The use of parenteral antibacterials in conjunction with dry cow therapy may improve the recovery rate of quarters infected with *Staph. aureus*. Details of antibacterial spectra of activity may be found in section 1.1. Where no bacterial culture or sensitivity data are available, a broad-spectrum preparation is recommended. The main pathogens causing clinical mastitis during the dry period are *Strep. uberis*, *Strep. dysgalactiae*, and *Actinomyces pyogenes*.

Preparations are formulated with aluminium mono-stearate or in an oily basis, which may prolong effective tissue-antibacterial concentrations for up to several weeks. In herds where the expected calving date is unknown, it is unwise to use long-acting preparations. If calving does occur within the effective drug duration, milk must be discarded for the remainder of the recommended milk withdrawal period and, in addition, for a specified time such as given in the farmer-purchaser contract (the statutory period is 4 days) after calving. Some manufacturers recommend that in cows with hypocalcaemia, it may be necessary to withhold milk for a longer period than the milk withdrawal period. In any case of doubt, an antibacterial residue test should be carried out on a milk sample from the individual cow and a negative result obtained before milk from that cow is included in bulk milk for human consumption.

> Preparations for non-lactating animals should not be used in animals with a dry period of less than the milk withdrawal period of the preparation

Cows should be dried off abuptly and not milked once a day before treatment. If high yielding cows (more than 25 litres/day) are to be dried off they should be fed a reduced diet for four days before and two days after drying off to help decrease the milk yield. Immediately after the last milking, one dose of dry cow therapy is infused into the teat canal by following the recommended procedure (see notes above in the introduction to section 11.1).

The head fly, *Hydrotaea irritans*, contributes to the spread of *Actinomyces pyogenes*. Therefore during the risk period for summer mastitis, fly control measures are required (see section 2.2). Topical insecticide preparations are more effective if applied directly to the teats. Dry cows and maiden heifers should graze fields away from shaded areas, woods, and stagnant water. They should be kept away from known 'summer mastitis' pastures. Udders should be examined daily to aid early detection of infection and thus improve the likelihood of a good response to therapy. In certain instances, treatment with a preparation for non-lactating animals may be repeated after drying off in order to help reduce the risk of *A. pyogenes* infection. In these cases, particular care must be taken in selecting a suitable preparation to avoid problems with antibacterial residues in milk at calving.

CEFALONIUM

UK
Indications. Mastitis, see notes above
Contra-indications. Lactating animals, see notes above
Dose. *Cattle*: *by intramammary infusion*, one dose per quarter after the last milking before drying off

POM **Cepravin Dry Cow** (Schering-Plough)
Intramammary paste, cefalonium 250 mg/dose, for *cattle*
Withdrawal Periods. *Cattle*: slaughter 21 days, milk not less than 51 days after administration plus 4 days after calving
Contra-indications. Use within 51 days of calving

CLOXACILLIN

UK
Indications. Mastitis, see notes above
Contra-indications. Lactating animals, see notes above
Dose. *Cattle*: *by intramammary infusion*, one dose per quarter after the last milking before drying off
Summer mastitis, before the first calving, one dose per quarter

POM **Bimaclox Extra DC** (Bimeda)
Intramammary suspension (oily), cloxacillin (as benzathine salt) 1 g/dose, for *cattle*
Withdrawal Periods. *Cattle*: slaughter 30 days, milk not less than 28 days after administration plus 96 hours after calving
Contra-indications. Use within 28 days of calving

POM **Chanamast DC** (Chanelle)
Intramammary suspension (oily), cloxacillin (as benzathine salt) 500 mg/dose, for *cattle*
Withdrawal Periods. *Cattle*: slaughter 28 days, milk not less than 28 days after administration plus 120 hours after calving
Contra-indications. Use within 42 days of calving

POM **Cloxacillin 1000 Dry Cow** (Virbac)
Intramammary suspension, cloxacillin (as benzathine salt) 1 g/dose with aluminium monostearate, for *cattle*
Withdrawal Periods. *Cattle*: slaughter 30 days, milk not less 28 days after administration plus 4 days after calving
Contra-indications. Use within 28 days of calving

POM **Embaclox Dry Cow** (Merial)
Intramammary suspension, cloxacillin (as benzathine salt) 500 mg/dose with aluminium monostearate, for *cattle*
Withdrawal Periods. *Cattle*: slaughter 28 days, milk not less than 28 days after administration plus 2.5 days after calving
Contra-indications. Use within 28 days of calving

POM **Kloxerate DC (Dry Cow)** (Fort Dodge)
Intramammary suspension, cloxacillin (as benzathine salt) 500 mg/dose with aluminium monostearate, for *cattle*
Withdrawal Periods. *Cattle*: slaughter 28 days, milk not less than 28 days after administration plus 2.5 days after calving
Contra-indications. Use within 28 days of calving

POM **Noroclox DC (Dry Cow)** (Norbrook)
Intramammary suspension, cloxacillin (as benzathine salt) 500 mg/dose with aluminium monostearate, for *cattle*
Withdrawal Periods. *Cattle*: slaughter 28 days, milk not less than 28 days after administration plus 2.5 days after calving
Contra-indications. Use within 28 days of calving

POM **Orbenin Dry Cow** (Pfizer)
Intramammary suspension, cloxacillin (as benzathine salt) 500 mg/dose with aluminium monostearate, for *cattle*
Withdrawal Periods. *Cattle*: slaughter 28 days, milk not less than 28 days after administration plus 4 days after calving
Contra-indications. Use within 28 days of calving

POM **Orbenin Extra Dry Cow** (Pfizer)
Intramammary suspension (oily), cloxacillin (as benzathine salt) 600 mg/dose, for *cattle*
Withdrawal Periods. *Cattle*: slaughter 28 days, milk not less than 42 days after administration plus 4 days after calving
Contra-indications. Use within 42 days of calving

POM **Tetraclox Dry Cow Xtra** (Pharmacia & Upjohn)
Intramammary suspension (oily), cloxacillin (as benzathine salt) 600 mg/dose, for *cattle*
Withdrawal Periods. *Cattle*: slaughter 28 days, milk not less than 42 days after administration plus 4 days after calving
Contra-indications. Use within 42 days of calving

PROCAINE BENZYLPENICILLIN
(Procaine penicillin)

UK
Indications. Mastitis, see notes above
Contra-indications. Lactating animals, see notes above
Dose. *Cattle*: prophylaxis, *by intramammary infusion*, one dose per quarter after the last milking before drying off
Summer mastitis, repeat dose after 2–3 weeks

POM **Mylipen Dry Cow** (Schering-Plough)
Intramammary paste (oily), procaine benzylpenicillin 300 mg/dose, for *cattle*
Withdrawal Periods. *Cattle*: slaughter 10 days, milk not less than 28 days after administration plus 4 days after calving
Contra-indications. Use within 28 days of calving

COMPOUND ANTIBACTERIAL PREPARATIONS FOR NON-LACTATING ANIMALS

UK
Indications. Mastitis, see notes above
Contra-indications. Lactating animals, see notes above
Dose. See preparation details

POM **Bovaclox DC** (Norbrook)
Intramammary suspension, ampicillin (as trihydrate) 250 mg, cloxacillin (as benzathine salt) 500 mg/dose with aluminium monostearate, for *cattle*
Withdrawal Periods. *Cattle*: slaughter 28 days, milk not less than 30 days after administration plus 4 days after calving
Contra-indications. Use within 30 days of calving
Dose. *Cattle*: prophylaxis, *by intramammary infusion*, one dose per quarter after the last milking before drying off
Summer mastitis, repeat dose every 3 weeks during the dry period

POM **Bovaclox DC Xtra** (Norbrook)
Intramammary suspension, ampicillin (as trihydrate) 300 mg, cloxacillin (as benzathine salt) 600 mg/dose, for *cattle*
Withdrawal Periods. *Cattle*: slaughter 28 days, milk not less than 49 days after administration plus 4 days after calving
Contra-indications. Use within 49 days of calving
Dose. *Cattle*: prophylaxis, *by intramammary infusion*, one dose per quarter after the last milking before drying off
Summer mastitis, before the first calving, one dose per quarter

POM **Embacillin C Dry Cow** (Merial)
Intramammary suspension, ampicillin (as trihydrate) 250 mg, cloxacillin (as benzathine salt) 500 mg/dose with aluminium monostearate, for *cattle*
Withdrawal Periods. *Cattle*: slaughter 28 days, milk not less than 30 days after administration plus 4 days after calving
Contra-indications. Use within 30 days of calving
Dose. *Cattle*: prophylaxis, *by intramammary infusion*, one dose per quarter after the last milking before drying off
Summer mastitis, repeat dose every 3 weeks during the dry period

POM **Kloxerate Gold DC** (Fort Dodge)
Intramammary suspension, ampicillin (as trihydrate) 300 mg, cloxacillin (as benzathine salt) 600 mg/dose, for *cattle*; 5.4-g dose applicator
Withdrawal Periods. *Cattle*: slaughter 28 days, milk not less than 49 days after administration plus 4 days after calving
Contra-indications. Use within 49 days of calving
Dose. *Cattle*: prophylaxis, summer mastitis, *by intramammary infusion*, one dose per quarter after the last milking before drying off or before first calving in heifers

POM **Kloxerate Plus DC(Dry Cow)** (Fort Dodge)
Intramammary suspension, ampicillin (as trihydrate) 250 mg, cloxacillin (as benzathine salt) 500 mg/dose with aluminium monostearate, for *cattle*
Withdrawal Periods. *Cattle*: slaughter 28 days, milk not less than 30 days after administration plus 4 days after calving
Contra-indications. Use within 30 days of calving
Dose. *Cattle*: prophylaxis, *by intramammary infusion*, one dose per quarter after the last milking before drying off
Summer mastitis, repeat dose every 3 weeks during the dry period

POM **Leo Red Dry Cow** (Leo)
Intramammary paste, framycetin sulphate 100 mg, penethamate hydriodide 100 mg, procaine benzylpenicillin 300 mg/dose, for *cattle*
Withdrawal Periods. *Cattle*: slaughter 28 days, milk 3.5 days after calving or not less than 28 days after administration plus 3 days after calving if calving occurs before 28 days after last treatment
Contra-indications. Use within 28 days of calving
Dose. *Cattle*: *by intramammary infusion*, one dose per quarter after the last milking before drying off

POM **Nafpenzal DC** (Intervet)
Intramammary suspension, dihydrostreptomycin (as sulphate) 100 mg, nafcillin (as sodium salt) 100 mg, procaine benzylpenicillin 300 mg/dose, for *cattle*
Withdrawal Periods. *Cattle*: slaughter 28 days, milk not less than 28 days after administration plus 4.5 days after calving
Contra-indications. Use within 28 days of calving
Dose. *Cattle*: *by intramammary infusion*, one dose per quarter after the last milking before drying off

POM **Streptopen Dry Cow** (Schering-Plough)
Intramammary paste (oily), dihydrostreptomycin (as sulphate) 500 mg, procaine benzylpenicillin 1 g/dose, for *cattle, sheep*
Withdrawal Periods. *Cattle*: slaughter 10 days, milk not less than 32 days after administration plus 4 days after calving. *Sheep*: slaughter 10 days
Contra-indications. Use within 32 days of calving
Dose. *Cattle*: prophylaxis, *by intramammary infusion*, one dose per quarter after the last milking before drying off
Summer mastitis, repeat dose after 3–4 weeks
Sheep: *by intramammary infusion*, ½ dose per udder half not more than 2 weeks after weaning

POM **Tetra-Delta Dry Cow** (Pharmacia & Upjohn)
Intramammary suspension (oily), novobiocin (as sodium salt) 400 mg, procaine benzylpenicillin 200 mg/dose, for *cattle*

Withdrawal Periods. *Cattle*: slaughter 30 days, milk not less than 30 days after administration plus 3.5 days after calving
Contra-indications. Use within 30 days of calving
Dose. *Cattle*: *by intramammary infusion*, one dose per quarter after the last milking before drying off

POM **Vonapen Dry Cow** (Intervet)
Intramammary suspension, benzylpenicillin potassium 314 mg, neomycin 500 mg, procaine benzylpenicillin 1 g/dose, for *cattle*
Withdrawal Periods. *Cattle*: slaughter 28 days, milk not less than 35 days after administration
Contra-indications. Use within 35 days of calving
Dose. *Cattle*: *by intramammary infusion*, one dose per quarter after the last milking before drying off

11.2 Preparations for the care of teats and udders

The care and hygiene of teats and udders are important factors in mastitis control, as is proper maintenance of the milking machine to ensure blood circulation is maintained throughout milking, and to avoid excessive pressure variations on the teat ends and damage to the teats.

Teat skin can act as a reservoir for mastitis pathogens, especially *Strep. dysgalactiae*, coagulase-negative staphylococci, and *Staph. aureus*, if cut or chapped. These pathogens may originate from the environment (infection transferred onto teats between milkings) or from infected cows (infection transferred during the milking process). Teat disinfection pre- and post-milking removes these organisms and in so doing reduces the risk of mastitis. Hygiene in the milking parlour and accommodation areas in addition to the use of skin disinfectants will reduce the population of pathogenic micro-organisms on the teats.

Before milking, teats contaminated with mud or faeces should be washed with running water, to which a disinfectant such as iodine may be added. Clean teats should then be wiped dry with a single-service paper towel. The use of communal udder cloths to wash and dry teats before milking is strongly discouraged because they can spread infection from cow to cow, even if immersed in a disinfectant solution between uses. Foremilk should be examined for the presence of any clots or abnormalities.

The teats may be predipped with a disinfectant solution. Predipping reduces the number of bacteria on the teat surface before the milking unit is attached. Most of these bacteria will be environmental in origin, and therefore the risk of mastitis caused by environmental organisms will be reduced. A pre-dip solution is applied to the prepared teats before milking for the recommended contact time. It is essential that pre-dip solutions have a rapid rate of kill so as not to reduce milking speed. The teats must be wiped dry before the milking unit is attached to avoid disinfectant residues entering the bulk milk supply.

Post-milking disinfectants reduce the bacterial population on the teats after milking and assist abrasions to heal. Bacteria which may have been transferred onto the teats during the milking process will be killed thereby reducing this potential source of infection. Each teat should be coated with teat dip or spray after every milking throughout lactation. Cows should remain standing for 20 to 30 minutes after milking to allow time for the teat canal to close, avoiding bacteria entering the open teat canal, helping to reduce the risk of environmental mastitis. During this period, feed should be offered and access to the housing area prohibited. Some farmers dilute a post-dip solution and use it as both a pre and a postdip. Conventional post-dip solutions do not kill bacteria fast enough to be effective as a predip. When this diluted solution is then used as a postdip, its efficacy is likely to be compromised and its benefit will be reduced. It is only acceptable to use a solution as a pre and postdip if the solution is authorised for that use.

Cetrimide, **chlorhexidine**, and **polihexanide** are effective against Gram-positive and Gram-negative bacteria, although *Pseudomonas* spp. and *Nocardia* spp. are killed slowly. These disinfectants are inactivated by soaps and anionic substances. **Dodecylbenzenesulphonic acid** is effective against most bacteria but ineffective against bacterial spores. It has a longer duration of action compared to many dips and is quite effective in the presence of organic matter. **Glutaral** (glutaraldehyde) is effective against Gram-positive and Gram-negative bacteria; concentrated solutions may cause dermatitis. **Iodine compounds** have broad-spectrum antibacterial activity and are advantageous because they stain teats and the operator can then check for coverage. **Chlorine compounds** have broad-spectrum antibacterial activity but are rapidly neutralised in the presence of organic matter. **Chlorous acid/chlorine dioxide** are effective against Gram-positive and Gram-negative bacteria as well as viruses and fungi. COSHH regulations should be adhered to when handling disinfectants.

Pre- and post-milking disinfectants can be applied by dipping or spraying. Teat dipping tends to be more effective because the entire surface of the teat is coated in disinfectant, whereas with teat spraying, parts of the teat are frequently missed, unless applied diligently. When teat dipping, on average approximately 10 mL of solution is used per cow per milking, whereas application by spray uses 15 mL per cow. During freezing and windy weather conditions, teat dips or sprays should only be applied to cows provided solutions are allowed to dry onto the teats before the cows exit the milking parlour; alternatively creams or ointments may be used. All pre- and post-milking preparations must be stored so as to avoid contamination. Any solution remaining in the teat dip cup at the end of milking should be discarded and the cup cleaned between milkings.

Preparations for udder and teat hygiene are formulated as dips, sprays, or udderwashes, which may require dilution before use. Glycerol (glycerine), hydrous wool fat (lanolin), white and yellow soft paraffin, and sorbitol are added to preparations to promote skin hydration, to soften skin, and allow lesions to heal. Cracked teat skin harbours many more bacteria than intact skin. Emollients may be applied to dry teats immediately after milking. When the emollient concentration exceeds 10%, the killing ability of the post-dip solution is reduced. Other preparations used for skin sores and wounds may also be applied to teats and udders (see section 14.1).

BENZYL ALCOHOL

UK
Indications. Cleaning and disinfection of teats
Warnings. See under Cetrimide

GSL **Deosan Thixodip BA** (DiverseyLever)
Post-milking teat dip, benzyl alcohol 4%, for *cattle*; 20 litres. Use undiluted
Withdrawal Periods. *Cattle:* slaughter withdrawal period nil, milk withdrawal period nil

CETRIMIDE

UK
Indications. Cleaning and disinfection of teats and udders
Contra-indications. Concurrent use of soaps and anionic substances
Warnings. Do not contaminate ponds, waterways, or ditches with disinfectants. Avoid contact of product with eyes and do not use internally

GSL **Cetriad** (Fort Dodge)
Cream, cetrimide 2%, glycerol, for *cattle*; 425 g
Withdrawal Periods. *Cattle*: slaughter withdrawal period nil, milk withdrawal period nil

Vanodine Udder Cream (Evans Vanodine)
Cream, cetrimide 0.5%, glycerol, hydrous wool fat, for *cattle*; 4 kg
Withdrawal Periods. *Cattle*: slaughter withdrawal period nil, milk withdrawal period nil

CHLORHEXIDINE

UK
Indications. **Contra-indications**. **Warnings**. See under Cetrimide

GSL **Alfa Blue Plus** (Alfa Laval Agri)
Post-milking teat dip or spray, chlorhexidine gluconate 0.425%, glycerol, sorbitol; 25 litres. Use undiluted

GSL **Alfa Red +** (Alfa Laval Agri)
Post-milking teat dip or spray, chlorhexidine gluconate 0.425%, glycerol, sorbitol; 25 litres. Use undiluted

GSL **C-Dip** (Kilco)
Post-milking teat dip or spray, chlorhexidine gluconate 0.5%, glycerol, for *cattle*; 5 litres, 25 litres, 200 litres. Use undiluted
Withdrawal Periods. Slaughter withdrawal period nil, milk withdrawal period nil

GSL **Deosan Summer Teatcare Plus** (DiverseyLever)
Post-milking teat dip or spray, chlorhexidine gluconate 0.425%, glycerol, fly repellents, for *cattle*; 25 litres. Use undiluted
Withdrawal Periods. Slaughter withdrawal period nil, milk withdrawal period nil

GSL **Deosan Teatcare Plus** (DiverseyLever)
Post-milking teat dip or spray, chlorhexidine digluconate 0.425%, glycerol, for *cattle*; 25 litres, 200 litres. Use undiluted
Withdrawal Periods. Slaughter withdrawal period nil, milk withdrawal period nil

GSL **Deosan Teat-Ex** (DiverseyLever)
Post-milking teat dip or spray, chlorhexidine digluconate 0.425%, glycerol, sorbitol, for *cattle*; 25 litres. Use undiluted
Withdrawal Periods. Slaughter withdrawal period nil, milk withdrawal period nil

GSL **Deosan Uddercream** (DiverseyLever)
Cream, chlorhexidine 2%, hydrous wool fat, for *cattle*; 2 kg
Withdrawal Periods. Slaughter withdrawal period nil, milk withdrawal period nil

GSL **Star Uddercream** (DiverseyLever)
Cream, chlorhexidine gluconate 2%, hydrous wool fat, for *cattle*
Withdrawal Periods. Slaughter withdrawal period nil, milk withdrawal period nil

GSL **Summer C-Dip** (Kilco)
Post-milking teat dip or spray, chlorhexidine gluconate 0.5%, glycerol, fly repellent, for *cattle*; 5 litres, 25 litres, 200 litres. Use undiluted
Withdrawal Periods. Slaughter withdrawal period nil, milk withdrawal period nil

Summer Masodip (Evans Vanodine)
Post-milking teat dip or spray, chlorhexidine gluconate 0.425%, glycerol, fly repellents, for *cattle*; 25 litres. Use undiluted
Withdrawal Periods. Slaughter withdrawal period nil, milk withdrawal period nil

GSL **Superspray** (Novartis)
Post-milking teat dip or spray, chlorhexidine gluconate 0.425%, glycerol, for *cattle*; 25 litres, 200 litres. Use undiluted
Withdrawal Periods. Slaughter withdrawal period nil, milk withdrawal period nil

CHLORINE COMPOUNDS

UK

Indications. Cleaning and disinfection of teats and udders
Warnings. Store solutions away from direct sunlight

GSL **Agrisept** (Pharmacia & Upjohn)
Pre- and post-milking teat dip, spray, or udderwash, tablets for dissolution, available chlorine 1.4 g/litre; 40, 100
Dissolve 1 tablet in 1 litre water

DODECYLBENZENESULPHONIC ACID

UK

Indications. Cleaning and disinfection of teats and udders

GSL **Blu-Gard** (Ecolab)
Post-milking teat dip, dodecylbenzenesulphonic acid 1–2%, glycerol, sorbitol, for *cattle*; 5 litres, 20 litres. Use undiluted

GSL **Blu-Gard** (Ecolab)
Post-milking teat spray, dodecylbenzenesulphonic acid 1–2%, glycerol, sorbitol, for *cattle*; 5 litres, 20 litres, 200 litres. Use undiluted

GLUTARAL
(Glutaraldehyde)

UK

Indications. Cleaning and disinfection of teats and udders
Side-effects. Concentrated solutions may cause dermatitis
Warnings. See under Cetrimide

GSL **Leo Yellow Super Dip** (Leo)
Post-milking teat dip or spray, glutaral 1.5%, glycerox, lanolin oil, for *cattle, sheep, goats*; 5 litres
Withdrawal Periods. Slaughter withdrawal period nil, milk withdrawal period nil
Dilute 1 volume with 4 volumes water

IODINE COMPOUNDS

UK

Indications. Cleaning and disinfection of teats and udders

GSL **Coopercare 1 Concentrate** (Schering-Plough)
Post-milking teat dip, spray, or udderwash, available iodine 2%, glycerol, sorbitol, for *cattle*; 25 litres
Withdrawal Periods. **Cattle**: slaughter withdrawal period nil, milk withdrawal period nil
Teat dip or spray. Dilute 1 volume with 3 volumes water
Udderwash. Dilute 20 mL in 10 litres water

GSL **Coopercare 3 (Ready to Use)** (Schering-Plough)
Post-milking teat dip, spray, or udderwash, available iodine 0.5%, glycerol, sorbitol, for *cattle*; 25 litres
Withdrawal Periods. **Cattle**: slaughter withdrawal period nil, milk withdrawal period nil
Teat dip or spray. Use undiluted
Udderwash. Dilute 12.5 mL in 1 litre water

GSL **Deosan Iodip Concentrate** (DiverseyLever)
Post-milking teat dip or spray, available iodine 2%, glycerol, sorbitol, for *cattle*; 25 litres
Withdrawal Periods. **Cattle:** slaughter withdrawal period nil, milk withdrawal period nil
Teat dip. Dilute 1 volume with 3 volumes water
Spray. Dilute 1 volume with 4 volumes water

GSL **Deosan Super Ex-Cel** (DiverseyLever)
Post-milking teat dip or spray, available iodine 0.5%, glycerol, sorbitol, for *cattle*; 25 litres, 200 litres. Use undiluted
Withdrawal Periods. **Cattle**: slaughter withdrawal period nil, milk withdrawal period nil

GSL **Deosan Super Iodip** (Diversey Lever)
Post-milking teat dip or spray, available iodine 2%, glycerol, sorbitol, for *cattle*; 5 litres, 25 litres, 200 litres
Withdrawal Periods. **Cattle:** slaughter withdrawal period nil, milk withdrawal period nil
Teat dip. Dilute 1 volume with 3 volumes water
Teat spray. Dilute 1 volume with 4 volumes water

GSL **Dipal Concentrate** (Alfa Laval Agri)
Post-milking teat dip, spray, or udderwash, available iodine 1.5%, glycerol; 10 litres, 25 litres
Teat dip or spray. Dilute 1 volume with 2 volumes water
Udderwash. Dilute 6.25 mL in 1 litre water

GSL **Iosan CCT** (Novartis)
Post-milking teat dip, spray, or udderwash, available iodine 1.55%, for *cattle*; 25 litres
Withdrawal Periods. **Cattle**: slaughter withdrawal period nil, milk withdrawal period nil
Teat dip or spray. Dilute 1 volume with 2 volumes water
Udderwash. Dilute 25 mL in 4 litres water

GSL **Iosan Superdip** (Novartis)
Post-milking teat dip, spray, or udderwash, available iodine 0.5%, glycerol, for *cattle*; 25 litres, 200 litres
Withdrawal Periods. **Cattle**: slaughter withdrawal period nil, milk withdrawal period nil
Teat dip or spray. Use undiluted
Udderwash. Dilute 75 mL in 4 litres water

GSL **Iosan Teat Dip** (Novartis)
Post-milking teat dip, spray, or udderwash, available iodine 1.55%, glycerol, for *cattle*; 25 litres, 200 litres
Withdrawal Periods. **Cattle**: slaughter withdrawal period nil, milk withdrawal period nil
Teat dip or spray. Dilute 1 volume with 2 volumes water
Udderwash. Dilute 25 mL in 4 litres water

GSL **Lanodip 4:1** (Kilco)
Post-milking teat dip, spray, or udderwash, available iodine 2.71%, hydrous wool fat, for *cattle*; 5 litres
Withdrawal Periods. Slaughter withdrawal period nil, milk withdrawal period nil
Dilute 1 volume with 4 volumes water

GSL **Lanodip Concentrate** (Kilco)
Post-milking teat dip, spray, or udderwash, available iodine 1.5%, hydrous wool fat, for *cattle*; 5 litres, 25 litres, 200 litres
Withdrawal Periods. *Cattle*: slaughter withdrawal period nil, milk withdrawal period nil
Teat dip or spray. Dilute 1 volume with 2 volumes water
Udderwash. Dilute 3.125 mL in 1 litre water

GSL **Lanodip Gold** (Kilco)
Post-milking teat dip, spray, or udderwash, available iodine 0.53%, hydrous wool fat, for *cattle*; 5 litres, 25 litres, 200 litres
Withdrawal Periods. Slaughter withdrawal period nil, milk withdrawal period nil
Teat dip or spray. Use undiluted
Udderwash. Dilute 10 mL in 1 litre water

GSL **Lanodip Readymix** (Kilco)
Post-milking teat dip, spray, or udderwash, available iodine 0.5%, hydrous wool fat; 5 litres, 25 litres, 200 litres
Withdrawal Periods. Slaughter withdrawal period nil, milk withdrawal period nil
Teat dip or spray. Use undiluted
Udderwash. Dilute 10 mL in 1 litre water

GSL **Lanodip Super Concentrate** (Kilco)
Post-milking teat dip, spray, or udderwash, available iodine 2%, hydrous wool fat, for *cattle*; 5 litres, 25 litres, 200 litres
Withdrawal Periods. Slaughter withdrawal period nil, milk withdrawal period nil
Teat dip. Dilute 1 volume with 3 volumes water
Udderwash. Dilute 2 mL in 1 litre water

GSL **Masocare** (Evans Vanodine)
Post-milking teat dip, spray, or udderwash, available iodine 0.5%, glycerol, sorbitol, for *cattle*; 25 litres, 200 litres
Withdrawal Periods. Slaughter withdrawal period nil, milk withdrawal period nil
Teat dip or spray. Use undiluted
Udderwash. Dilute 12.5 mL in 1 litre water

GSL **Masodine 1:3** (Evans Vanodine)
Post-milking teat dip, spray, or udderwash, available iodine 2%, glycerol, sorbitol, for *cattle*; 5 litres, 25 litres, 200 litres
Withdrawal Periods. Slaughter withdrawal period nil, milk withdrawal period nil
Teat dip or spray. Dilute 1 volume with 3 volumes water
Udderwash. Dilute 2 mL in 1 litre water

GSL **Masodine 1:4** (Evans Vanodine)
Post-milking teat dip, spray, or udderwash, available iodine 2.7%, glycerol, sorbitol, for *cattle*; 5 litres, 25 litres, 200 litres
Withdrawal Periods. *Cattle*: slaughter withdrawal period nil, milk withdrawal period nil
Teat dip or spray. Dilute 1 volume with 4 volumes water
Udderwash. Dilute 2.5 mL in 1 litre water

GSL **Masodine RTU** (Evans Vanodine)
Post-milking teat dip, spray, or udderwash, iodine 0.5%, sorbitol, glycerol, for *cattle*; 25 litres, 200 litres
Withdrawal Periods. Slaughter withdrawal period nil, milk withdrawal period nil
Teat dip or spray. Use undiluted
Udderwash. Dilute 12.5 mL in 1 litre water

GSL **QuarterMate** (Alfa Laval Agri)
Pre-milking teat dip or spray, available iodine (as sodium iodide/iodine complex) 0.1%, for *cattle*; 10 litres, 25 litres, 200 litres. Use undiluted
Withdrawal Periods. Slaughter withdrawal period nil, milk withdrawal period nil

GSL **Star Ready-Dip** (DiverseyLever)
Post-milking teat dip or spray, available iodine 0.5%, glycerol, sorbitol, for *cattle*; 25 litres
Withdrawal Periods. Slaughter withdrawal period nil, milk withdrawal period nil
Teat dip or spray. Use undiluted

GSL **Star Iodocare Concentrate** (DiverseyLever)
Post-milking teat dip or spray, available iodine 2%, glycerol, sorbitol, for *cattle*
Teat dip. Dilute 1 volume with 3 volumes water
Teat spray. Dilute 1 volume with 4 volumes water

GSL **Super Concentrate Teat Dip or Spray** (Kilco)
Post-milking teat dip, spray, or udderwash, available iodine 1.5%, hydrous wool fat, for *cattle*, 5 litres, 25 litres, 200 litres
Withdrawal Periods. Slaughter withdrawal period nil, milk withdrawal period nil
Teat dip or spray. Dilute 1 volume with 2 volumes water
Udderwash. Dilute 3.125 mL in 1 litre water

GSL **Superteat** (Alfa Laval Agri)
Post-milking teat dip, spray, or udderwash, available iodine 0.5%, glycerol, for *cattle*; 25 litres, 200 litres
Teat dip or spray. Use undiluted
Udderwash. Dilute 18.75 mL in 1 litre water

Vanodine Udder Salve (Evans Vanodine)
Ointment, iodine 0.2%, hydrous wool fat; 4 kg
Withdrawal Periods. Slaughter withdrawal period nil, milk withdrawal period nil

POLIHEXANIDE
(Polyhexanide)

UK
Indications. Cleaning and disinfection of teats and udders
Contra-indications. Warnings. See under Cetrimide

GSL **Sapphire** (Evans Vanodine)
Post-milking teat dip or spray, polihexanide 0.5%, glycerol, for *cattle*; 25 litres. Use undiluted
Withdrawal Periods. *Cattle*: slaughter withdrawal period nil, milk withdrawal period nil

GSL **Sapphire Concentrate 1:9** (Evans Vanodine)
Post-milking teat dip or spray, polihexanide 5%, glycerol, for *cattle*; 2.5 litres
Dilute 1 volume with 9 volumes water

COMPOUND DISINFECTANTS FOR TEATS AND UDDERS

UK
Indications. Cleaning and disinfection of teats and udders
Warnings. See under Cetrimide

GSL **Coopercare 2 Teat Dip or Spray** (Schering-Plough)
Post-milking teat dip or spray, chlorhexidine digluconate 1.5%, cetrimide 0.25%, sorbitol, for *cattle*; 5 litres
Withdrawal Periods. *Cattle*: slaughter withdrawal period nil, milk withdrawal period nil
Dilute 1 volume with 4 volumes water

GSL **Hibitex Ready-to-Use** (Schering-Plough)
Post-milking teat dip, spray, or udderwash, benzalkonium chloride 0.1%, chlorhexidine gluconate 4.25%, glycerol, sorbitol, for *cattle*; 25 litres
Withdrawal Periods. *Cattle*: slaughter withdrawal period nil, milk withdrawal period nil
Teat dip or spray. Use undiluted
Udderwash. Dilute 150 mL in 10 litres water

GSL **Masodip** (Evans Vanodine)

Post-milking teat dip, spray, or udderwash, benzalkonium chloride 0.01%, chlorhexidine gluconate 0.425%, glycerol, sorbitol, for *cattle*; 25 litres, 200 litres

Withdrawal Periods. *Cattle*: slaughter withdrawal period nil, milk withdrawal period nil

Teat dip or spray. Use undiluted

Udderwash. Dilute 15 mL in 1 litre water

GSL **Masodip Extra** (Evans Vanodine)

Post-milking teat dip, spray, or udderwash, benzalkonium chloride 0.01%, chlorhexidine gluconate 0.425%, glycerol, sorbitol, for *cattle*

Withdrawal Periods. *Cattle*: slaughter withdrawal period nil, milk withdrawal period nil

Teat dip or spray. Use undiluted

Udderwash. Dilute 15 mL in 1 litre water

EMOLLIENTS FOR TEATS AND UDDERS

UK

There are many preparations available; this is not a comprehensive list

GSL **Antiseptic Teat Ointment** (Arnolds)

Ointment, zinc oxide 7%; 500 g, 4 kg

GSL **Golden-Udder** (Shep-Fair)

Ointment, salicylic acid 1.5%, sulphur 10%, for *cattle, sheep, goats*; 600 g

Lenimint (Nordic Star)

Ointment, Japanese peppermint oil, camphor, liquid paraffin, glycerol, for *cattle*; 2.5 litres

Lenisan (Nordic Star)

Ointment, chlorhexidine, yellow soft paraffin, for *cattle*; 5 litres

GSL **Leo Yellow Teat Ointment** (Leo)

Ointment, colophony, industrial methylated spirit, wool fat, yellow beeswax, yellow soft paraffin, zinc oleostearate, for *cattle, sheep, goats*; 400 g, 2.75 kg

Withdrawal Periods. Slaughter withdrawal period nil, milk withdrawal period nil

Vanodine Udder Ointment (Evans Vanodine)

Ointment, yellow soft paraffin, sorbitol, for *cattle*; 4 kg

Withdrawal Periods. *Cattle*: slaughter withdrawal period nil, milk withdrawal period nil

12 Drugs acting on the EYE

Contributor:
S Turner, MA, VetMB, DVOphthal, MRCVS

12.1 Administration of drugs to the eye

Many owners have difficulty in administering eye drops and eye ointments to animals and therefore the procedure should always be demonstrated to them. For example, eye drops should be applied in dogs as follows: the animal's head should be gently raised by holding the muzzle. Then with the bottle held in the other hand the upper lid should be gently pulled back and one drop applied to the bulbar conjunctiva. One drop is sufficient; more than one drop will increase lacrimation and effectively wash the drug away. It is useful to keep the head elevated for a minute after instillation or to block the ventral nasolacrimal punctum to reduce immediate drainage. Eye ointment should be applied into the conjunctival fornix inside the lower lid by everting the lid with the index finger or thumb. The softer eye ointments may be put on to the cornea but owners may be afraid of injuring the eye. Eye drops are easy to use in dogs and cats, but eye ointments are probably easier to use in larger species such as horses.

The frequency of administration of eye drops or eye ointment depends on the type and severity of the disease. The absorption and effect of a drug used topically may be dependent upon the inflamed or diseased state of the conjunctival and corneal epithelium. Eye drops generally require frequent application in order to achieve acceptable ocular and intra-ocular concentrations because rapid elimination of solutions will occur from the conjunctival sac after dilution with tears (although some newer formulations may allow once daily application). When two different eye drop formulations are to be administered, there should be an interval of at least 5 minutes between applications to avoid dilution and overflow. Drops must always be instilled before ointments if both have been prescribed. Eye ointments have a longer contact time resulting in higher ocular and intra-ocular drug concentrations and thereby necessitating less frequent application. Eye ointments may be preferred for night-time treatment.

Preparations for the eye contain suitable preservatives and provided that contamination is avoided they may be used for about one month (unless otherwise stated by the manufacturer) after which, if treatment is to be continued, a new container should be opened and the old one discarded. Some patients may develop hypersensitivity to preservatives, which may cause conjunctival hyperaemia or corneal epithelial ulceration with frequent or prolonged administration.

The potential effects of systemic absorption of drugs such as atropine, corticosteroids, or chloramphenicol should be considered.

Subconjunctival injections may be carried out in all species following the topical administration of 1 drop of a local anaesthetic. It is recommended that the drug is placed under the bulbar conjunctiva rather than the palpebral conjunctiva. The volume of injectable solution used is approximately 0.5 mL for dogs and cats, and up to 1 mL for horses and cattle.

Subpalpebral lavage systems, nasolacrimal canulation, ocular inserts, and therapeutic contact lenses have all been used with success in veterinary ophthalmology. Therapeutic contact lenses (i-protex, Veterinary Speciality Products) designed for use in horses, dogs, and cats may be useful for the management of corneal ulceration (superficial to one-third stromal thickness), injury, and in the post-operative period following corneal surgery, for example after superficial keratectomy and correction of symblepharon.

Systemic therapy may be undertaken in conjunction with topical therapy in cases of severe intra-ocular infection and inflammation. Systemic administration may be required to achieve adequate drug concentrations in the eyelid tissue and also the posterior segment of the eye, for example for the treatment of chorioretinitis. The penetration of systemically administered drugs, such as sulphonamides, depends on their ability to cross the blood:ocular barriers (blood:aqueous and blood:retinal barriers). Generally, small molecules that are not bound to plasma proteins, for example chloramphenicol, penetrate well. Inflammation may cause the breakdown of the regional blood:ocular barrier allowing improved penetration of all drugs.

12.2 Anti-infective eye preparations

12.2.1 Antibacterial preparations
12.2.2 Antifungal preparations
12.2.3 Antiviral preparations

Care should be taken to distinguish superficial ocular disease caused by infections from other conditions that may result in a red or inflamed eye. Where possible the causative organism should be identified and any initial choice of a broad-spectrum antibacterial, or combination of antibacterials, modified according to bacterial sensitivity data. The severity of an infection may determine the choice of drug and frequency of application. When prescribing antibacterials, it is considered preferable to use topical preparations of drugs that are not usually used to treat systemic infections. Primary bacterial conjunctivitis is usually acute and corticosteroids are unnecessary. The normal conjunctival flora of the dog consists of a number of species whereas the cat conjunctiva harbours relatively few micro-organisms. Hence, with the exception of conjunctivitis due to *Chlamydia* infection, primary bacterial conjunctivitis is rare in cats; viral infections are more frequently seen in this species.

Where only one eye is involved but, for prophylactic reasons, the other eye is also being treated, medication should be applied first to the unaffected eye to minimise the possibility of cross-infection.

12.2.1 Antibacterial preparations

Bacterial infections of the eye in animals may be caused by *Staphylococcus*, *Streptococcus*, *Bacillus*, *Actinobacillus*, *Chlamydia*, *Moraxella*, *Micrococcus*, or *Clostridium* spp. This list is not exhaustive and the bacteria involved vary between species. Ocular infections usually present as conjunctivitis, blepharitis, keratitis, keratoconjunctivitis, or uveitis.

The aminoglycosides **gentamicin, tobramycin** and **framycetin** have a a broad-spectrum bactericidal activity. Framycetin is active against *Proteus* spp., but its corneal penetration is poor. Tobramycin has been shown to be active against strains of *Pseudomonas aeruginosa* that have developed resistance to gentamicin and is useful for the treatment of melting ulcers in horses. **Kanamycin** is active against a range of Gram-negative organisms except *Pseudomonas* spp. and *Bacteroides* spp. It is effective against *Moraxella bovis* and can be used subconjunctivally to treat this infection in cattle.

Cefalonium has a broad-spectrum of bacteriocidal activity against Gram-negative and Gram-positive bacteria. It is effective for the treatment of infectious bovine keratoconjunctivitis (New Forest Disease, pinkeye) caused by *Moraxella bovis*.

Cloxacillin is active against a wide-range of bacteria, the main indications are infections caused by *Staphylococcus* spp. and *Bacillus* spp. This drug is effective for the treatment of infectious bovine keratoconjunctivitis and contagious ophthalmia (infectious keratoconjunctivitis) in sheep.

Chloramphenicol has a broad spectrum of activity and is lipid soluble and hence is particularly useful for intra-ocular infections.

Chlortetracycline has a bacteriostatic action against some staphylococci, streptococci, some Gram-negative bacteria, and *Mycoplasma*. Chlortetracycline is used to treat chlamydial conjunctivitis in cats. Oral **doxycycline**, at a dose of 5 mg/kg♦ once or twice daily has also been advocated for the treatment of feline chlamydial infections.

Fusidic acid has particular action against staphylococci, which are common causes of bacterial blepharitis and conjunctivitis in dogs.

The fluoroquinolones **ciprofloxacin** or **ofloxacin** have broad-spectrum bactericidal activity against Gram-negative and to a lesser extent Gram-positive organisms. They have some activity against *Mycoplasma* and *Chlamydia* spp.

Oral **clindamycin** (see section 1.1.4) has been used to treat toxoplasmosis♦ in cats, at a dose of 25 mg/kg daily in divided doses, although the resulting destruction of tachyzoites may lead to an increased inflammatory response. Sulphadiazine in combination with pyrimethamine has been used in the past but toxicity precludes treatment with this regimen.

The use of topical compound preparations containing an antibacterial and a corticosteroid requires careful judgement and the potential deleterious effects of corticosteroids (see section 12.3.1) should always be taken into account.

Subconjunctival injections may be advantageous. Chloramphenicol sodium succinate, amikacin, kanamycin, gentamicin, ampicillin, benzylpenicillin, sulphonamides, and oxytetracycline may be administered by this route.

A vaccine is available for protection against *Chlamydia psittaci* infection (see section 18.5.1) in cats.

CEFALONIUM
(Cephalonium)

UK
Indications. Bacterial eye infections, in particular infectious bovine keratoconjunctivitis

Contra-indications. Hypersensitivity to cefalonium

Dose. *Cattle*: apply as a single dose (using ½ tube ointment), repeat after 2–3 days as necessary

Dogs: apply as a single dose (using $\frac{1}{10}$ tube ointment), repeat daily as necessary

POM **Cepravin** (Schering-Plough)
Eye ointment, cefalonium (as dihydrate), for *cattle*, *dogs*; 2 g
Withdrawal Periods. Slaughter withdrawal period nil, milk withdrawal period nil

CHLORAMPHENICOL

UK
Indications. Bacterial eye infections, see notes above

Warnings. Operators should wear impermeable disposable gloves when handling the product and avoid contact with skin

Dose. *Eye drops*, apply up to 8 times daily for at least 2 days

By subconjunctival injection, 100–200 mg (0.5–1.0 mL) of chloramphenicol solution 200 mg/mL into bulbar subconjunctival tissue

POM **Chloromycetin V Redidrops** (Pharmacia & Upjohn)
Eye drops, chloramphenicol 0.5%, for *dogs, cats*; 10 mL

POM Ⓗ **Kemicetine** (Pharmacia & Upjohn)
See section 1.1.5 for preparation details

CHLORTETRACYCLINE HYDROCHLORIDE

UK

Indications. Bacterial eye infections in dogs and cats, infectious bovine keratoconjunctivitis
Dose. *Cattle*: apply ¼ tube at least once daily as necessary
Dogs, cats: apply at least 3 times daily

POM **Aureomycin Ophthalmic Ointment** (Fort Dodge)
Eye ointment, chlortetracycline hydrochloride 1%, for **cattle, dogs, cats**
Withdrawal Periods. Slaughter withdrawal period nil, milk withdrawal period nil

CIPROFLOXACIN

UK

Indications. Superficial bacterial eye infections
Warnings. Treatment recommended for a maximum of 21 days in humans
Dose. *Eye drops*, apply 4 times daily. Increase frequency of application when treating serious bacterial corneal ulceration

POM Ⓗ **Ciloxan** (Alcon)
Eye drops, ciprofloxacin (as hydrochloride) 0.3%; 5 mL

CLOXACILLIN

UK

Indications. Bacterial eye infections particularly *Staphylococcus* and *Bacillus* spp.
Contra-indications. Penicillin hypersensitivity
Dose. See preparation details

POM **Orbenin Ophthalmic Ointment** (Pfizer)
Eye ointment, cloxacillin (as benzathine salt) 16.7% with aluminium monostearate, for **horses, cattle, sheep, dogs, cats**; 3 g
Withdrawal Periods. Slaughter after last treatmeat, milk withdrawal period nil
Dose. *Horses*: apply as a single dose, repeat daily as necessary
Cattle, sheep: apply as a single dose, repeat after 2–3 days as necessary
Dogs, cats: apply as a single dose, repeat daily as necessary

POM **Opticlox Eye Ointment** (Norbrook)
Eye ointment, cloxacillin (as benzathine salt) 16.7%, for **horses, cattle, sheep, dogs, cats**; 5 g
Withdrawal Periods. Slaughter withdrawal period nil, milk withdrawal period nil
Dose. *Horses, cattle, sheep, dogs, cats*: apply as a single dose, repeat after 2–3 days if required

FRAMYCETIN SULPHATE

UK

Indications. Bacterial eye infections
Dose. *Eye drops or ointment*, apply 4 times daily

POM Ⓗ **Soframycin** (Florizel)
Eye drops, framycetin sulphate 0.5%; 10 mL
Eye ointment, framycetin sulphate 0.5%; 5 g

FUSIDIC ACID

UK

Indications. Bacterial eye infections, in particular *Staphylococcus* spp. infections
Contra-indications. Conjunctivitis due to *Pseudomonas* spp. infection
Dose. *Dogs, cats, rabbits*: apply 1–2 times daily

POM **Fucithalmic Vet** (Leo)
Eye drops (viscous), m/r, fusidic acid 1%, for **dogs, cats, rabbits**; 3 g
Withdrawal Periods. Should not be used on **rabbits** intended for human consumption

GENTAMICIN SULPHATE

UK

Indications. Bacterial eye infections, see notes above
Dose. *Dogs, cats, rabbits*: apply 3 times daily

POM **Tiacil** (Virbac)
Eye drops, gentamicin sulphate 0.3%, for **dogs, cats, rabbits**; 5 mL
Withdrawal Periods. Should not be used on **rabbits** intended for human consumption

KANAMYCIN

UK

Indications. Bacterial eye infections
Dose. *Cattle*: *by subconjunctival injection*, 30 mg

See section 1.1.3 for preparation details

OFLOXACIN

UK

Indications. Bacterial eye infections
Warnings. Treatment recommended for a maximum of 10 days in humans
Dose. *Eye drops*, apply 4 times daily

POM Ⓗ **Exocin** (Allergan)
Eye drops, ofloxacin 0.3%; 5 mL

OXYTETRACYCLINE

UK

Indications. Bacterial eye infections
Dose. *Cattle*: *by subconjunctival injection*, 25–50 mg (0.5–1.0 mL)

POM **Terramycin Q50** (Pfizer)
See section 1.1.2 for preparation details

COMPOUND ANTIBACTERIAL OPHTHALMIC PREPARATIONS

UK

POM Ⓗ **Neosporin** (Dominion)
Eye drops, gramicidin 25 units, neomycin sulphate 1700 units, polymyxin B sulphate 5000 units/mL; 5 mL
Dose. Apply 4 times daily

12.2.2 Antifungal preparations

Ocular fungal infections may be superficial, for example mycotic keratitis, or intra-ocular such as mycotic endophthalmitis; both conditions are rare in the UK.

Intra-ocular manifestations of systemic mycotic infections in dogs and cats, such as blastomycosis, cryptococcosis, geotrichosis, and histoplasmosis, usually present as a focal granulomatous posterior uveitis, often involving the retina and other tissues of the eye.

Most topical antifungal drugs have poor corneal penetration and systemic antifungals (see section 1.2) such as ketoconazole and amphotericin B are used for treatment.

12.2.3 Antiviral preparations

Feline herpesvirus (FHV) is a common cause of acute conjunctivitis and chronic keratitis and is also a potential respiratory pathogen. **Trifluridine** has been shown to be efficacious against FHV-1 *in vitro* and appears to be clinically useful. **Aciclovir** has very limited *in vitro* effect.

Some forms of equine superficial punctate keratitis may be due to equine herpesvirus infection; aciclovir may be effective in these cases.

ACICLOVIR
(Acyclovir)

UK
Indications. See notes above
Dose. *Horses, cats*: *eye ointment*, apply 5–6 times daily

POM (H) **Zovirax** (GlaxoWellcome)
Eye ointment, aciclovir 3%; 4.5 g

TRIFLURIDINE
(Trifluorothymidine)

UK
Indications. See notes above
Dose. *Cats*: *eye drops*, apply 4–5 times daily

POM (H) **Trifluridine Eye Drops 1%**
Eye drops containing trifluridine are not generally available. Readers are advised to contact their local pharmacist or Moorfields Eye Hospital, 162 City Road, London EC1V 2PD, telephone: 0275662365, facsimile: 0275662367 to obtain a supply in the UK

12.3 Corticosteroids and other anti-inflammatory preparations

12.3.1 Corticosteroids
12.2.2 Other anti-inflammatory preparations

12.3.1 Corticosteroids

The anti-inflammatory effects of **corticosteroids** are based upon their ability to suppress capillary dilatation, vascular exudation, and leucocyte migration regardless of the causative agent. In chronic conditions they inhibit neovascularisation and fibroblastic activity in the eye. This may be useful in preventing scarring and pigment deposition in the cornea but disadvantageous by retarding healing. In general, topical preparations readily penetrate the cornea. The salt of the corticosteroid used influences corneal penetration, for example, prednisolone acetate has a superior corneal penetration to prednisolone sodium phosphate.

Topical corticosteroids are particularly useful in the treatment of uveitis, various specific and non-specific inflammatory disorders of the cornea, such as chronic superficial keratitis (CSK, pannus) in the German Shepherd dog. They also assist in the reduction of post-surgical inflammation, such as that following cataract or lens extraction.

Following administration, therapeutic levels remain in the eye for only about three hours and this may necessitate frequent application to prevent treatment failure. Topical corticosteroids should not be used in the presence of corneal ulceration; systemic NSAIDs should be considered. Corticosteroids may be used in the presence of glaucoma in animals but care should obviously be taken in the differential diagnosis of a 'red eye'.

Subconjunctival injections may augment, or replace, topical instillation. Preparations of methylprednisolone acetate or triamcinolone acetonide may be effective for up to three weeks. Their use may sometimes be effective for owners experiencing difficulty in applying drops. Subconjunctival therapy may be used for the treatment of bovine iritis. Betamethasone sodium phosphate (2 mg) or dexamethasone sodium phosphate (2 mg) every 3 days or methylprednisolone (10 to 20 mg, depot injection) every 7 to 14 days may be administered by subconjunctival injection for the treatment of inflammatory ocular conditions in horses. However subconjunctival granulomas, plaques, or mineralisation can occur at the injection site. It is recommended that specialist advice be sought before using subconjunctival corticosteroid treatment in equines.

Care must be taken with the use of topical corticosteroids in horses because the alteration in ocular micro-environment can predispose to fungal infections. Similar caution must be exercised in cats with suspected herpetic keratitis because local immunosuppression caused by the corticosteroid can allow recrudescence of the herpes virus.

The use of systemic corticosteroids for ophthalmic therapy is limited because lower ocular concentrations are achieved than with topical application. However, systemic therapy may be useful for idiopathic partial serous retinal detachments, posterior uveitis, and optic neuritis. There is an association between cataractogenesis and steroid therapy in humans but this has not been described in animals. The adverse effects of prolonged administration of systemic corticosteroids may be minimised by alternate day therapy.

Periodic ophthalmia (equine recurrent uveitis) is a disease of horses resulting in recurrent photophobia, lacrimation, conjunctival injection, corneal changes (such as oedema and vascularisation), hypopyon, miosis, synechiation, and even blindness due to extensive synechiae, cataract formation, or phthisis bulbi. Some forms of the disease have been linked to *Leptospira* infection, although in many instances the aetiology remains obscure. Treatment consists of topical and possibly subconjunctival corticosteroids, NSAIDs, and if bacterial infection is suspected, systemic antibacterials. Topical atropine is used to achieve a mid-dilated pupil.

BETAMETHASONE

UK

Indications. See notes above
Contra-indications. Corneal ulceration, fungal or viral infections, see notes above
Dose. Apply every 2–3 hours

POM Ⓗ **Betnesol** (Medeva)
Drops (for eye, ear, or nose), betamethasone sodium phosphate 0.1%; 10 mL
Ointment, betamethasone sodium phosphate 0.1%; 3 g

DEXAMETHASONE

UK

Indications. See notes above
Contra-indications. Corneal ulceration, see notes above
Dose. Apply every 2–3 hours

POM Ⓗ **Maxidex** (Alcon)
Eye drops, dexamethasone 0.1%, hypromellose 0.5%; 5 mL, 10 mL

FLUOROMETHOLONE

UK

Indications. See notes above
Contra-indications. Corneal ulceration, see notes above
Dose. Apply 4 times daily

POM Ⓗ **FML** (Allergan)
Eye drops, fluorometholone 0.1%, polyvinyl alcohol 1.4%; 5 mL, 10 mL

PREDNISOLONE

UK

Indications. See notes above
Contra-indications. Corneal ulceration, see notes above
Dose. Apply 4 times daily

POM Ⓗ **Pred Forte** (Allergan)
Eye drops, prednisolone acetate 1%; 5 mL, 10 mL

POM Ⓗ **Predsol** (Medeva)
Drops (eye drops or ear drops), prednisolone sodium phosphate 0.5%; 10 mL

POM Ⓗ **Minims Prednisolone** (Chauvin)
Eye drops, prednisolone sodium phosphate 0.5%; 0.5 mL (single use)

COMPOUND CORTICOSTEROID AND ANTI-BACTERIAL OPHTHALMIC PREPARATIONS

Preparations containing antibacterial and glucocorticoid agents in combination can be useful in cases of infected inflammatory processes such as bacterial keratitis, and for prophylaxis, for example following intra-ocular surgery where control of inflammation is important but a risk of infection also exists. A specific diagnosis and rationale for combination therapy should always be established.

UK

POM **Betsolan Eye and Ear Drops** (Schering-Plough)
Drops (eye drops or ear drops), betamethasone sodium phosphate 0.1%, neomycin sulphate 0.5%, for *dogs, cats*; 5 mL
Contra-indications. Pregnant animals, corneal ulceration
Dose. Apply every 2–3 hours

POM Ⓗ **Maxitrol** (Alcon)
Eye drops, dexamethasone 0.1%, hypromellose 0.5%, neomycin (as sulphate) 0.35%, polymyxin B sulphate 6000 units/mL; 5 mL
Contra-indications. Pregnant animals, corneal ulceration
Dose. Apply 4 times daily
Eye ointment, dexamethasone 0.1%, neomycin (as sulphate) 0.35%, polymyxin B sulphate 6000 units/g; 3.5 g
Contra-indications. Pregnant animals, corneal ulceration
Dose. Apply 3 times daily

POM **Neobiotic HC Drops** (Pharmacia & Upjohn)
Drops (eye drops or ear drops), hydrocortisone acetate 1.5%, neomycin (as sulphate) 0.35%, for *dogs, cats*; 5 mL
Contra-indications. Corneal ulceration
Warnings. Safety in pregnant animals has not been established
Dose. Apply 3–6 times daily, then gradually reduce dose

12.3.2 Other anti-inflammatory preparations

Ciclosporin (see section 12.6) has an anti-inflammatory action by inhibiting T helper lymphocytes. The drug has been shown to be effective in treating canine ocular surface diseases believed to be immune-mediated. These include keratoconjunctivitis sicca, chronic superficial keratitis (pannus), and plasmacytic conjunctivitis of the third eyelid♦.

Systemic NSAIDs (see section 10.1) may be useful when corticosteroids are contra-indicated. Aspirin, by mouth, may be administered pre-operatively to reduce inflammation during intra-ocular surgery. Adequate renal perfusion should be maintained in these patients to reduce the risk of kidney damage. Carprofen is a useful analgesic anti-inflammatory for ocular conditions and is often used for surgical conditions.

Topical NSAIDs, such as **diclofenac, flurbiprofen**, and **ketorolac** have been used as pre-operative treatment of canine patients undergoing cataract extraction. They inhibit intra-operative pupillary constriction which, if it occurs, can complicate cataract extraction. Additionally, their anti-inflammatory actions are additive to those of the pre- and postoperative corticosteroids usually required in these patients. They may also prove to be useful in the management of anterior uveitis in dogs. Topical applications of NSAIDs overcome the potentially serious side-effects which may accompany systemic NSAIDs. However, NSAIDs may extend bleeding time and topical or systemic preparations should probably not be used in procedures where intra-ocular haemorrhage is a likely complication.

Antihistamines may have a limited use in reducing inflammation associated with immunoglobulin (IgE)-mediated immediate hypersensitivity reactions. Antihistamine therapy has been largely replaced by the use of corticosteroids.

DICLOFENAC SODIUM

UK

Indications. Pre-operative treatment for cataract extraction
Dose. Apply 1 drop once every 30 minutes starting 2 hours
before surgery for a total of 4 drops

POM Ⓗ **Voltarol Ophtha** (CIBA Vision)
Eye drops, diclofenac sodium 0.1%; single-dose unit

FLURBIPROFEN SODIUM

UK

Indications. Pre-operative treatment for cataract extraction
Dose. Apply 1 drop once every 30 minutes starting 2 hours
before surgery for a total of 4 drops

POM Ⓗ **Ocufen** (Allergan)
Eye drops, flurbiprofen sodium 0.03%, polyvinyl alcohol 1.4%; 0.4 mL (single use)

KETOROLAC TROMETAMOL

UK

Indications. Prophylaxis and reduction of inflammation
following ocular surgery
Contra-indications. Hypersensitivity to ketorolac
Warnings. Caution in animals with bleeding disorders
Dose. Apply 1 drop 3 times daily, starting 24 hours before
surgery

POM Ⓗ **Acular** (Allergen)
Eye drops, kerorolac trometamol 0.5%; 5 mL

12.4 Mydriatics and cycloplegics

Adrenoceptor stimulants (sympathomimetics) such as
epinephrine (adrenaline) and phenylephrine dilate the pupil
by stimulating the dilator muscle of the iris. Antimuscarinic
drugs including atropine and tropicamide paralyse the iris
sphincter muscle and the ciliary muscle (cycloplegia).
Atropine is frequently used to relieve muscle spasm, and
therefore pain, associated with anterior uveitis (iridocyclitis). It is also useful in maintaining an open pupil in the
presence of exudation and preventing the formation of anterior and posterior synechiae. Treatment is aimed at achieving a moderately dilated pupil. The duration of action,
which is several days in the normal eye, is greatly reduced
in uveitis and 3 to 4 applications daily may be necessary.
However, the duration of action in horses may be much
extended compared to other species. Atropine is contra-indicated in glaucoma and keratoconjunctivitis sicca. In
addition, the potential risk of systemic effects should be
considered in animals of low body-weight. Atropine has a
bitter taste and hypersalivation may occur following naso-lacrimal drainage. Cats, in particular, dislike the taste of
atropine and ointment may be better tolerated than drops in
this species.
Cyclopentolate is a tertiary amine antimuscarinic agent
with actions similar to atropine. It has a long duration of

action in dogs and cats but its therapeutic application in
dogs is limited due to conjunctival irritation and chemosis.
Phenylephrine is effective as a mydriatic in dogs but not in
cats. Phenylephrine is useful in the investigation of
Horner's syndrome. When Horner's syndrome is the result
of lesions in the second or third order neurones, the pupil on
the affected side will dilate more rapidly due to denervation
hypersensitivity.
Tropicamide, a non-cycloplegic, has the most rapid onset
of action, and is the mydriatic of choice for intra-ocular
examination and fundoscopy. The effect is maximal within
30 minutes and persists for several hours.

ATROPINE SULPHATE

UK

Indications. Relief of ciliary muscle spasm, maintenance
of patent pupil
Contra-indications. Keratoconjunctivitis sicca, glaucoma
Side-effects. Bitter taste, see notes above
Warnings. Systemic toxicity if applied frequently to animals of low body-weight
Dose. Apply up to 3–4 times daily

POM Ⓗ **Atropine** (Non-proprietary)
Eye ointment, atropine sulphate 1%; 3 g

POM Ⓗ **Isopto Atropine** (Alcon)
Eye drops, atropine sulphate 1%, hypomellose 0.5%; 5 mL

POM Ⓗ **Minims Atropine Sulphate** (Chauvin)
Eye drops, atropine sulphate 1%; 0.5 mL (single use)

CYCLOPENTOLATE HYDROCHLORIDE

UK

Indications. Mydriasis and cycloplegia
Contra-indications. Glaucoma
Side-effects. Conjunctival irritation
Dose. Apply 1 drop. Repeat after 15 minutes if required

POM Ⓗ **Mydrilate** (Boehringer Ingelheim)
Eye drops, cyclopentolate hydrochloride 0.5%, 1%; 5 mL

POM Ⓗ **Minims Cyclopentolate** (Chauvin)
Eye drops, cyclopentolate hydrochloride 0.5%, 1%; 0.5 mL (single use)

PHENYLEPHRINE HYDROCHLORIDE

UK

Indications. Mydriasis in dogs, investigation of Horner's
syndrome in dogs and cats
Warnings. Possible risk of systemic absorption and cardiac
effects if frequently applied to animals of low body-weight
with cardiac disease
Dose. Apply 1 drop

P Ⓗ **Phenylephrine** (Non-proprietary)
Eye drops, phenylephrine hydrochloride 10%; 10 mL

P Ⓗ **Minims Phenylephrine Hydrochloride** (Chauvin)
Eye drops, phenylephrine hydrochloride 2.5%, 10%; 0.5 mL (single use)

TROPICAMIDE

UK

Indications. Mydriasis for intra-ocular examination and fundoscopy
Conta-indications. Glaucoma, caution in breeds predisposed to primary glaucoma or goniodysgenesis. Intra-ocular pressure should be monitored
Dose. Apply one drop. Repeat after 15 minutes if required

POM Ⓗ **Mydriacyl** (Alcon)
Eye drops, tropicamide 0.5%, 1%; 5 mL

POM Ⓗ **Minims Tropicamide** (Chauvin)
Eye drops, tropicamide 0.5%, 1%; 0.5 mL (single use)

12.5 Drugs used in glaucoma

12.5.1 Miotics
12.5.2 Carbonic anhydrase inhibitors
12.5.3 Beta-adrenoceptor blocking drugs
12.5.4 Prostaglandin analogues

Glaucoma is a common condition in dogs and occurs, to a lesser extent, in other species. It almost invariably arises through impairment of aqueous drainage. The causes are many and include acquired or inherited ocular disease, uveitis, cataract, lens luxation, neoplasia, and intra-ocular haemorrhage. In some breeds of dog, glaucoma is inherited as a primary condition. Chronic open-angle glaucoma, as seen in humans, is not a significant problem in animals. Clinical signs of the early stages of glaucoma are difficult to assess and many cases present at a late stage of the disease when medical therapy alone is unlikely to succeed. In such cases, surgical intervention to facilitate aqueous drainage is the only practical alternative. The clinical history, presenting signs, intra-ocular pressure, and gonioscopic findings will influence the choice of treatment. Medical therapy will not succeed in a globe that has become enlarged, such as in hydrophthalmos or buphthalmos. Intra-ocular pressure should be measured regularly in order to monitor the effects of treatment.

Depending on the aetiology, medical therapy for glaucoma may include a combination of a miotic to increase aqueous outflow and a carbonic anhydrase inhibitor to inhibit aqueous production. Beta-adrenoceptor blocking drugs have been shown experimentally to be of use in the treatment of some forms of canine glaucoma, although the preparations found to be most efficacious were of higher concentration than commercially available preparations. Cardiac side-effects, bronchoconstriction, or both may be seen with the use of more concentrated preparations.

Emergency treatment of glaucoma. Emergency lowering of intra-ocular pressure is required when pupil block is present (such as in anterior lens luxation, extensive posterior synechiae) or in an acute rise in intra-ocular pressure due to primary angle closure glaucoma. In these cases, emergency lowering of intra-ocular pressure is used to pre-

vent continuation of retinal and optic nerve head damage and as a pre-operative measure.

Hyperosmotic agents are used in combination with a carbonic anhydrase inhibitor as follows:

- **glycerol** (see section 16.4) *by mouth*, 1–2 mL/kg
  or
  mannitol 20% solution (see section 4.2.5) by intravenous injection given over 20 to 30 minutes, 5–10 mL/kg
- **acetazolamide** (see section 12.5.2) *by intravenous injection*, 5–25 mg/kg

12.5.1 Miotics

The most useful drug is **pilocarpine**, a parasympathomimetic miotic. However, miotics alone are usually insufficient to lower intra-ocular pressure significantly. Pilocarpine penetrates the cornea, produces miosis within 15 minutes and is effective for 6 to 8 hours. Initially, frequent applications are required, thereafter it is instilled 3 to 4 times daily. Pilocarpine may produce local irritation. Cats appear to be more susceptible to the side-effects of pilocarpine. **Carbachol** has a longer duration of action than pilocarpine and can be used for open-angle glaucoma.

Miotics are contra-indicated if anterior uveitis or anterior lens luxation are present, although it has been suggested that the use of miotics immediately before surgical removal of an anteriorly luxated lens may help to prevent the lens moving posteriorly during surgery.

CARBACHOL

UK

Indications. Glaucoma, see notes above
Contra-indications. Anterior uveitis, anterior lens luxation, see notes above
Dose. *Dogs*: apply 2–3 times daily

POM Ⓗ **Isopto Carbachol** (Alcon)
Eye drops, carbachol 3%, hypromellose 1%; 10 mL

PILOCARPINE

UK

Indications. Glaucoma, see notes above; improvement of tear secretion (see section 12.6)
Contra-indications. Anterior uveitis, anterior lens luxation, see notes above
Side-effects. Local irritation
Dose. Apply 1% or 2% solution 3–4 times daily

POM Ⓗ **Pilocarpine Hydrochloride** (Non-proprietary)
Eye drops, pilocarpine hydrochloride 0.5%, 1%, 2%; 10 mL

POM Ⓗ **Minims Pilocarpine Nitrate** (Chauvin)
Eye drops, pilocarpine nitrate 1%, 2%; 0.5 mL (single use)

12.5.2 Carbonic anhydrase inhibitors

These substances act by inhibiting the carbonic anhydrase enzyme present in the ciliary epithelium, which catalyses the reversible hydration of carbon dioxide and leads to aqueous humour production. **Acetazolamide** administered orally results in a lowering of intra-ocular pressure within an hour and the effect may persist for at least 8 hours. The concentration of the available oral formulation precludes its use in animals of low body-weight; diclofenamide should be used in these cases. Acetazolamide may be administered intravenously in emergencies.

Diclofenamide (dichlorphenamide), which may only be administered orally, has a similar duration of action but has the advantage of fewer side-effects. Administering the drug in divided doses may further minimise the side-effects.

Dorzolamide is a topical carbonic anhydrase inhibitor. Although its use in animals has not been fully evaluated, if efficacious it promises to avoid the side-effects which can accompany systemic use of this class of drug.

ACETAZOLAMIDE

UK

Indications. Glaucoma, see notes above
Side-effects. Lethargy, vomiting, diarrhoea, polydipsia, polyuria, hypokalaemia
Dose. *Dogs*: *by mouth*, 5–10 mg/kg 2–4 times daily *by intravenous injection*, 5–25 mg/kg

POM Ⓗ **Diamox** (Wyeth)
Tablets, acetazolamide 250 mg
Injection, powder for reconstitution, acetazolamide (as sodium salt) 500 mg

DICLOFENAMIDE
(Dichlorphenamide)

UK

Indications. Glaucoma, see notes above
Side-effects. See under Acetazolamide
Dose. *Dogs*: *by mouth*, 5–15 mg/kg daily in 2–3 divided doses

Preparations of diclofenamide are not generally available. A supply may be obtained as a 'Special Order' from Rosemount in the UK

DORZOLAMIDE

UK

Indications. Glaucoma
Dose. *Dogs*: *eye drops*, 1 drop 3 times daily

POM Ⓗ **Trusopt** (MSD)
Eye drops, dorzolamide (as hydrochloride) 2%; 5 mL

12.5.3 Beta-adrenoceptor blocking drugs

Beta-adrenoceptor blocking drugs such as **timolol** inhibit beta adrenoceptors in the ciliary epithelium and reduce the secretion of aqueous humour; their efficacy in closed-angle glaucoma is limited.

TIMOLOL

UK

Indications. Glaucoma
Dose. *Eye drops,* apply twice daily

POM Ⓗ **Timolol** (Non-proprietary)
Eye drops, timolol (as maleate) 0.25%, 0.5%; 5 mL

12.5.4 Prostaglandin analogues

Latanoprost is a prostaglandin $F_{2\alpha}$ analogue, which exerts an ocular hypotensive effect by increasing uveoscleral outflow of aqueous humour. Intra-ocular pressure is reduced within 3 to 4 hours of instillation and lasts for 24 hours.

LATANOPROST

UK

Indications. Glaucoma
Contra-indications. Uveitis
Side-effects. Conjunctival hyperaemia, superficial punctate keratopathy, iris colour change
Dose. *Eye drops,* apply one drop once daily (preferably at night)

POM Ⓗ **Xalatan** (Pharmacia & Upjohn)
Eye drops, latanoprost 50 micrograms/mL; 2.5 mL

12.6 Drugs used in keratoconjunctivitis sicca

Keratoconjunctivitis sicca (KCS) occurs in dogs but is rare in other species. Treatment consists of the replacement of tear secretions, or the improvement of tear secretion. Management of the condition by surgical procedures may be necessary.

Ciclosporin has been shown to be effective in the treatment of some cases of KCS. Ciclosporin appears to have several beneficial actions including modulation of immune-mediated destruction of tear secreting tissue and stimulation of tear production. It also acts on the cornea to control the pigmentary keratitis that accompanies many cases of KCS. An increase in tear production is expected within 10 days, but in some dogs it may take up to 6 weeks for maximal improvement.

A number of tear replacement preparations are available. Many of the preparations contain **hypromellose** but others are available containing agents such as **carbomers** or **polyvinyl alcohol** which are designed to improve spread over the ocular surface and duration of contact of the drops. It may be necessary to try a number of different preparations to find the most satisfactory for the individual patient. The required frequency of application depends on the severity of the condition and the preparation used. For more severe cases, frequent application of up to 8 to 10 times daily may be indicated; in some patients this may prove impracticable. A mucolytic, such as **acetylcysteine**, may be beneficial where tears are particularly mucoid and viscous.

Pilocarpine (see section 12.5.1) has been used to improve tear secretion in patients that have some residual lacrimal gland function. One to two drops of a 1% solution are administered by mouth, once or twice daily, for an initial trial period of 4 to 6 weeks. Close attention to the development of systemic side-effects such as hypersalivation and nausea, should be taken particularly in animals of low body-weight.

Topical corticosteroids may be beneficial in some cases of KCS. They may be applied only when there is no corneal ulceration. They probably have an anti-inflammatory action in the tear producing tissues and also control the superficial pigmentary keratitis which results from chronicity of the condition. Owners should be warned of the potential of corticosteroids to exacerbate any corneal ulceration that may occur.

Topical antibacterials may also be indicated because secondary bacterial infections occur in some cases of KCS.

ACETYLCYSTEINE

UK
Indications. Tear deficiency; collagenase ulcers
Dose. Apply up to 8–10 times daily

POM Ⓗ **Ilube** (Alcon)
Eye drops, acetylcysteine 5%, hypromellose 0.35%; 10 mL

CARBOMERS
(Polyacrylic acid)

UK
Indications. Tear deficiency
Dose. Apply up to 8–10 times daily

P Ⓗ **GelTears** (Chauvin)
Eye drops, cabomer 940 (polyacrylic acid) 0.2%; 10 g

P Ⓗ **Viscotears** (CIBA Vision)
Eye drops, cabomer 940 (polyacrylic acid) 0.2%; 10 g

CICLOSPORIN
(Cyclosporin A, Cyclosporin)

UK
Indications. Chronic recurrent conjunctivitis due to auto-immune disease, keratoconjunctivitis sicca, chronic superficial keratitis (pannus), plasmacytic conjunctivitis of the third eyelid (plasmoma)♦; immune-mediated disease, perianal fistula, anal furunculosis, sebaceous adenitis (see section 13.2)
Contra-indications. Manufacturer advises that safety in pregnant animals has not been established. Application with suspected concurrent ocular fungal or viral infection
Side-effects. Transient mild irritation; discontinue treatment if irritation persists. Blepharitis if excess ointment has been allowed to contact the eyelids
Warnings. Operators should wear impervious gloves when applying ointment, avoid skin contact, wash hands after use
Dose. *Dogs*: apply twice daily

POM **Optimmune Ophthalmic Ointment** (Schering-Plough)
Eye ointment, ciclosporin 0.2%, for *dogs*; 3.5 g

HYPROMELLOSE

UK
Indications. Tear deficiency
Dose. Apply up to 8–10 times daily

P Ⓗ **Hypromellose** (Non-proprietary)
Eye drops, hypromellose 0.3%; 10 mL

P Ⓗ **Isopto Alkaline** (Alcon)
Eye drops, hypromellose 1%; 10 mL

P Ⓗ **Isopto Plain** (Alcon)
Eye drops, hypromellose 0.5%; 10 mL

P Ⓗ **Moisture-eyes** (Co-Pharma))
Eye drops, hypromellose 0.3%; 10 mL

P Ⓗ **Tears Naturale** (Alcon)
Eye drops, dextran '70' 0.1%, hypromellose 0.3%; 15 mL

LIQUID PARAFFIN

UK
Indications. Tear deficiency
Dose. Apply up to 4 times daily

P Ⓗ **Lacri-Lube** (Allergan)
Eye ointment, white soft paraffin 57.3%, liquid paraffin 42.5%; 3.5 g, 5 g

P Ⓗ **Lubri-Tears** (Alcon)
Eye ointment, white soft paraffin 60%, liquid paraffin 30%; 5 g

POLYVINYL ALCOHOL

UK
Indications. Tear deficiency
Dose. Apply up to 8–10 times daily

P Ⓗ **Hypotears** (CIBA Vision)
Eye drops, macrogol '8000' 2%, polyvinyl alcohol 1%; 10 mL

P Ⓗ **Liquifilm Tears** (Allergan)
Eye drops, polyvinyl alcohol 1.4%; 15 mL

P Ⓗ **Sno Tears** (Chauvin)
Eye drops, polyvinyl alcohol 1.4%; 10 mL

12.7 Local anaesthetics

Local anaesthetics should only be used for diagnostic and minor surgical procedures. They can be toxic to corneal epithelial cells and also block the afferent arm of the lacrimation reflex and corneal blink reflex. The preservatives in multidose preparations and the active drug itself may have antibacterial actions and should not be applied before taking swabs for bacterial culture. **Proxymetacaine** has a rapid onset of action and the effect persists for 15 to 20 minutes. **Tetracaine** has a more prolonged effect.

PROXYMETACAINE HYDROCHLORIDE
(Proparacaine)

UK
Indications. Topical local anaesthesia

POM Ⓗ **Minims Proxymetacaine Hydrochloride** (Chauvin)
Eye drops, proxymetacaine hydrochloride 0.5%; 5 mL (single use)

TETRACAINE HYDROCHLORIDE
(Amethocaine hydrochloride)

UK
Indications. Local anaesthesia

POM Ⓗ **Minims Amethocaine Hydrochloride** (Chauvin)
Eye drops, tetracaine hydrochloride 0.5%, 1%; 0.5 mL (single use)

12.8 Diagnostic stains

The ophthalmic stains fluorescein sodium and rose bengal are used for the diagnosis of disorders of the cornea and conjunctiva. Following instillation excess stain should be washed out of the eye with sodium chloride solution 0.9%.

The main use of **fluorescein sodium** is in the diagnosis of corneal epithelial defects, in which areas denuded of epithelium are stained bright fluorescent green. It is also used to assess the overall function of the nasolacrimal drainage system (although the results of this test should be interpreted with care because false negatives are common), and in fluorescein angiography of both anterior and posterior segments of the eye.

Rose bengal stains devitalised epithelial cells an intense dark red. It can be useful in the detection of dendritic ulcers that may result from feline herpesvirus infection in adult cats. Mucus is also stained and rose bengal is used in human ophthalmology to aid in the diagnosis of keratoconjunctivitis sicca.

FLUORESCEIN SODIUM

UK
Indications. Diagnosis of corneal epithelial defects and patency of nasolacrimal drainage system (see notes above); angiography

P Ⓗ **Fluorets** (Chauvin)
Impregnated-paper strips, fluorescein sodium 1 mg; 100

P Ⓗ **Minims Fluorescein Sodium** (Chauvin)
Eye drops, fluorescein sodium 1%, 2%; 0.5 mL (single use)

ROSE BENGAL

UK
Indications. Diagnosis of dendritic ulcers; see notes above

P Ⓗ **Minims Rose Bengal** (Chauvin)
Eye drops, rose bengal 1%; 0.5 mL (single use)

13 Drugs used in the treatment of MALIGNANT DISEASE and for IMMUNOSUPPRESSION

Contributor:
J M Dobson, MA, BVetMed, DVetMed, DipECVIM, MRCVS

13.1 Cytotoxic drugs
13.2 Immunosuppressants
13.3 Sex hormones and hormone antagonists

Conventional methods for cancer therapy in animals are surgery, radiotherapy, and chemotherapy. These techniques need not be used in isolation, indeed the combination of surgical management of a primary mass with chemotherapy directed at systemic disease is the most logical and potentially effective way of managing malignant disease.

Surgery is the the most effective form of treatment for solid tumours of skin, soft tissues, and bone. Advances in surgical technique mean that many primary tumours can be managed by surgical excision but early treatment and aggressive resection are required to maximise the success of surgery.

The use of radiotherapy in veterinary medicine is limited by the availability of and access to radiotherapy facilities. However an increasing number of specialist centres in the USA, UK, and Europe are able to offer this technique. The main role of radiotherapy is as a *local* treatment for malignant tumours, which cannot be controlled by surgery alone. Radiotherapy cannot be used to treat widespread disease because of its toxicity, although local lymph nodes may be included in treatment fields. (For further information on usage of radiotherapy see Blackwood L, Dobson J. Radiotherapy in small animal oncology. *In Practice* 1998; **20:** 566–75.)

The major indication for chemotherapy is in the treatment of systemic malignant disease such as lymphoma and other lymphoproliferative and myeloproliferative diseases. The tumour cells in these diseases are reasonably chemosensitive and the widespread nature of the disease necessitates a systemic form of therapy. Chemotherapy is not effective against large solid primary tumours of skin, soft tissues, or bone but may have a beneficial role as an adjunct to surgery in the management of some malignant solid tumours.

13.1 Cytotoxic drugs

13.1.1 Alkylating drugs
13.1.2 Antimetabolites
13.1.3 Antitumour antibiotics
13.1.4 Vinca alkaloids
13.1.5 Platinum compounds
13.1.6 Other cytotoxic drugs

Cytotoxic drugs are classified according to their characteristic sites or modes of action. Most cytotoxic drugs act upon the processes of cell growth and division.

These drugs are potent and potentially dangerous and extreme care is required in their use. Careful consideration must be given to the pharmacology and toxicity of the drug, the spectrum of drug activity, and the condition of the patient.

> In veterinary medicine, the prescribing and administration of these drugs is usually confined to specialists in the field and empirical use is to be discouraged.

The main indications for cytotoxic drugs in veterinary medicine are management of lymphoproliferative and myeloproliferative disorders including leukaemia, lymphoma (lymphosarcoma), and multiple myeloma. Cytotoxic drugs are of little value as sole agents in the management of large solid tumours such as mammary carcinoma or fibrosarcoma. They may have a palliative role as adjuncts to surgery or radiotherapy in the prevention or management of metastatic disease associated with certain tumours, for example osteosarcoma or haemangiosarcoma. In this role chemotherapy is complimentary to surgical excision of the primary tumour with the actions of the drugs directed at microscopic disease residual at the primary site or elsewhere in the body in the form of micrometastases. The efficacy of adjunctive chemotherapy in tumours such as malignant carcinomas and melanoma has not been established in veterinary medicine.

Generally, the use of cytotoxic drugs in combination protocols is favoured as the most effective approach; by combining different drug classes that have different mechanisms of action greater tumour cell kill may be achieved without increasing normal tissue toxicity. For example, combinations of cyclophosphamide (alkylating agent), vincristine (vinca alkaloid), and prednisolone (corticosteroid) are widely used in the treatment of canine and feline lymphoma. Many different protocols have been described using combinations of these and other drugs; three of the more commonly used regimens are listed in Tables 13.1, 13.2, and 13.3.

Intermittent or 'pulse' therapy is the conventionally preferred use of cytotoxic drugs because continual administration of low doses of cytotoxic agents will select for tumour cells that are resistant to those drugs. In tumour cells, drug resistance can arise through a variety of different mechanisms. Acquired drug resistance refers to the clinical situa-

Table 13.1 Combination cytotoxic therapy COP[1] (low dose)

Drug	Dose
INDUCTION	
Cyclophosphamide	50 mg/m^2 p.o. on alternate days *or* 50 mg/m^2 p.o. for the first 4 days of each week
Vincristine	500 micrograms/m^2 i.v. every 7 days
Prednisolone	40 mg/m^2 p.o. daily for 7 days then 20 mg/m^2 p.o. on alternate days and given with cyclophosphamide
MAINTENANCE AFTER A MINIMUM OF 2 MONTHS	
Cyclophosphamide	50 mg/m^2 p.o. on alternate days *or* 50 mg/m^2 p.o. for the first 4 days of each second week
Vincristine	500 micrograms/m^2 i.v. every 14 days
Prednisolone	20 mg/m^2 p.o. on alternate days of each second week
MAINTENANCE AFTER 6 MONTHS (IF DISEASE IS IN REMISSION)	
Cyclophosphamide[2]	50 mg/m^2 p.o. on alternate days *or* 50 mg/m^2 p.o. for the first 4 days of each third week
Vincristine	500 micrograms/m^2 i.v. every 21 days
Prednisolone	20 mg/m^2 p.o. on alternate days of each third week
MAINTENANCE AFTER 12 MONTHS[3]	
Cyclophosphamide[2]	50 mg/m^2 p.o. on alternate days *or* 50 mg/m^2 p.o. for the first 4 days of each fourth week
Vincristine	500 micrograms/m^2 i.v. every 28 days
Prednisolone	20 mg/m^2 p.o. on alternate days of each fourth week

[1] COP = combination cyclophosphamide, oncovin (vincristine) ,and prednisolone therapy
[2] Chlorambucil (5 mg/m^2 p.o. on alternate days) or melphalan (5 mg/m^2 p.o. on alternate days) may be used as a substitute for cyclophosphamide in animals that develop haemorrhagic cystitis. Melphalan may be used as a substitute for cyclophosphamide after 6 months to reduce the risk of haemorrhagic cystitis
[3] Doxorubicin (30 mg/m^2 i.v. every 3 weeks) or crisantaspase (10 000–20 000 units/m^2 i.m. every 7 days or as necessary) may be used for treatment of relapsing or recurrent disease

Table 13.2 Combination cytotoxic therapy COP (high dose)[1]

Drug	Dose
INDUCTION	
Cyclophosphamide	250–300 mg/m^2 p.o. every 21 days
Vincristine	750 micrograms/m^2 i.v. every 7 days for 4 weeks then 750 micrograms/m^2 i.v. every 21 days and given with cyclophosphamide
Prednisolone	1 mg/kg p.o. daily for 4 weeks then 1mg/kg p.o. on alternate days
MAINTENANCE AFTER 12 MONTHS	
Cyclophosphamide[2]	250–300 mg/m^2 p.o. every 28 days
Vincristine	750 micrograms/m^2 i.v. every 28 days and given with cyclophosphamide
Prednisolone	1 mg/kg p.o. on alternate days
Note. Treatment should be continued for a further 6 months	

[1] COP = combination cyclophosphamide, oncovin (vincristine), and prednisolone therapy
[2] The maximum recommended dose for cyclophosphamide in dogs is 250 mg/m^2

Table 13.3 Cyclic combination treatment for lymphoma

Drug		Dose
INDUCTION		
Week 1 (day 1)	Vincristine	500–750 micrograms/m^2 i.v.
	Cristantaspase	400 units/kg i.m.
	± Prednisolone	2 mg/kg p.o. daily
Week 2 (day 8)	Cyclophosphamide	200 mg/m^2 i.v. or p.o.
	± Prednisolone	1.5 mg/kg p.o. daily
Week 3 (day 15)	Vincristine	500–750 micrograms/m^2 i.v.
	± Prednisolone	1 mg/kg p.o. daily
Week 4 (day 22)	Doxorubicin	30 mg/m^2 i.v.
	± Prednisolone	500 micrograms/kg p.o. daily
Week 5 (day 29)	Vincristine	500–750 micrograms/m^2 i.v.
Week 6 (day 36)	Cyclophosphamide	200 mg/m^2 i.v. or p.o.
Week 7 (day 43)	Vincristine	500–750 micrograms/m^2 i.v.
Week 8 (day 50)	Doxorubicin	30 mg/m^2 i.v.
Week 9 (day 57)	NO TREATMENT	
MAINTENANCE		

Repeat above 8-week cycle twice with an interval of 2 weeks between between each drug administration and then for another 2 times with an interval of 3 weeks between each drug administration.
Chlorambucil (1.4 mg/kg p.o.) may be substituted for cyclophosphamide during maintenance cycles

tion in which a previously drug-responsive tumour regrows and is no longer sensitive to further treatment with the original drugs. Canine lymphoma often exhibits acquired resistance at relapse. Drugs that have similar mechanisms of action, or similar chemical structure, are likely to share resistance mechanisms. Therefore drugs used for further treatment should be selected from different drug groups. However, relapsing tumour cells can acquire resistance to drugs or drug groups to which the tumour has not been exposed previously. This phenomenon, known as multi-drug resistance (MDR), is associated with a P-glycoprotein that acts as an export pump reducing the intracellular concentration of certain drugs and thereby allowing the tumour cell to survive exposure to the drug. Drugs that are substrates for the pump include the vinca alkaloids, doxorubicin, and epirubicin.

Side-effects. Toxicity is the major treatment-limiting factor in chemotherapy. Cytotoxic drugs are not selective in their actions on growing and dividing cells, hence organs that contain populations of rapidly dividing cells, for example the bone marrow and gastro-intestinal tract, are particularly susceptible to toxic effects. Myelosuppression is the most common and potentially serious complication following administration of many cytotoxic drugs. Bone marrow suppression may lead to leucopenia, resulting in an increased risk of infection and sepsis. Infectious organisms may gain entry to the body through the respiratory, urogenital, or gastro-intestinal tracts, or through normal barriers such as skin and mucosa, which have been disrupted by the tumour, surgery, or the placement of catheters. In animal cancer patients the most frequent source of infection is the migration of enteric bacteria through damaged intestinal mucosa. *Escherichia coli* and *Klebsiella pneumoniae* are the most common pathogens. *Pseudomonas aeruginosa*, *Staphylococcus aureus*, *Bacteroides* spp., *Candida* spp., and polymicrobial infections also occur.

Thrombocytopenia may also occur following chemotherapy; anaemia is generally less common. Peripheral blood cell counts should be assessed before treatment and monitored regularly once therapy is commenced. Ideally the white blood cell count should be measured every two to three weeks depending on the protocol used. Where less aggressive chemotherapy schedules are employed, four to six weekly counts may be acceptable. Myelosuppression is usually reversible on withdrawal of the drug(s). The dosage of drugs that cause myelosuppression must be reduced or therapy withheld if critical blood cell counts are reached. It is usually recommended that the drug dosage should be reduced by 50% if the neutrophil count falls below 3 x 10^9/litre and therapy should be withheld if the neutrophil count falls below 2 x 10^9/litre. The myelosuppressed patient should also be given prophylactic, broad-spectrum antibacterials; potentiated sulphonamides (see section 1.1.6.2) or fluoroquinolone derivatives (see section 1.1.9) are preferred.

Toxic effects may also manifest in the gastro-intestinal tract and the skin. Anorexia, vomiting, and diarrhoea may occur following administration of many cytotoxic drugs. In most cases such problems are of short duration with spontaneous recovery as the gastro-intestinal epithelium regenerates. Supportive care and fluid therapy may be required. For drugs that cause vomiting that is centrally mediated, for example cisplatin, the use of anti-emetics such as metoclopramide (see section 3.4.1) is recommended.

Poor hair growth or alopecia may occur, particularly in fine or curly-coated breeds such as poodles.

Hypersensitivity reactions to cytotoxic drugs are rare but certain drugs can produce such reactions when administered to animals. Most cytotoxic drug hypersensitivities are immune-mediated reactions, for example the enzyme crisantaspase is highly immunogenic. Some drugs such as doxorubicin may directly degranulate mast cells thus releasing histamine and other vaso-active substances.

Several drugs, including vincristine, cisplatin, and doxorubicin, are extremely irritant and will cause severe local tissue necrosis if extravasation occurs; intravenous catheters should always be used for administration of such agents and these should be flushed with saline before removal.

Individual drugs may have specific toxic actions on other organs, for example cardiotoxicity of doxorubicin or nephrotoxicity of cisplatin

---

Extreme care is required in the handling, preparation, and administration of cytotoxic drugs. Many cytotoxic substances are irritant to skin and mucous membranes and are suspected of having mutagenic, teratogenic, or carcinogenic potential. Cytotoxic drugs should never be handled by pregnant women. Injectable preparations should be prepared in designated areas by specially trained staff wearing appropriate protective clothing. Animals must be adequately restrained by trained staff for administration of such drugs. Tablets must never be broken or crushed. Information on the safe use of cytotoxic drugs may be found in:

- Approved Code of practice: control of substances hazardous to health and Approved Code of practice: control of carcinogenic substances. 3rd ed. *COSHH Regulations 1988*. London: HMSO, 1992
- Precautions for the safe handling of cytotoxic drugs. *Guidance notes Medical Series 21*. London: HMSO, 1983
- Allwood M, Wright P (eds) *The Cytotoxics Handbook* 2nd ed. Radcliffe Medical Press Ltd: Oxford, 1993.

Dosage. Due to the low therapeutic index of cytotoxic drugs, in veterinary medicine the commonly used dosages and protocols are a compromise between efficacy and toxicity, being designed to cause minimal side-effects to the patient. The intensive medical support often necessary for human patients to manage the severe toxicity resulting from aggressive chemotherapy is not routinely available or feasible in veterinary practice. In this chapter, only approximate guidelines are given regarding dosages and indications.

Doses of cytotoxic drugs are calculated as a function of body surface area (m^2) rather than body-weight because the blood supply to the organs responsible for detoxification, that is the kidney and liver, is more closely related to surface area than body-weight. Tables of weight to surface area for dogs up to 50 kg body-weight and cats up to 5 kg body-weight are provided in Appendix 3.

The mode of drug metabolism and excretion should be known because drug dosage may need to be reduced in patients with hepatic or renal impairment.

13.1.1 Alkylating drugs

In veterinary medicine, alkylating drugs are the most widely used in cancer chemotherapy. They act by interfering with DNA replication.

Cyclophosphamide is widely used in the treatment of lymphoproliferative diseases in cats and dogs. Use in the treatment of multiple myeloma has been reported. Cyclophosphamide may also have a palliative role as an adjunct to surgery in the treatment of certain solid carcinomas and sarcomas.

Cyclophosphamide is converted to active alkylating metabolites by the liver and primarily excreted by the kidney. One of the metabolites, acrolein, may cause a sterile necrotising haemorrhagic cystitis. This is a serious complication which precludes further use of the drug. An increased water intake may help to avoid this complication. Prolonged therapy may also result in insidious fibrosis of the bladder.

Chlorambucil is the slowest acting and least toxic of the alkylating drugs. It is primarily used for maintenance therapy in lymphoma, in the treatment of chronic lymphocytic leukaemia and multiple myeloma. The use of chlorambucil in the treatment of polycythaemia vera has been described. Myelosuppression is reversible on discontinuation of the drug. In humans, chlorambucil is metabolised in the liver and excreted in the urine as metabolites.

Melphalan is primarily indicated in the treatment of multiple myeloma, but is also useful in lymphoproliferative disorders. It has been included in combined protocols for palliative and adjunctive treatment of osteogenic sarcoma and mammary carcinoma. Myelosuppression is the major side-effect and may be delayed in onset. Anorexia and vomiting may also occur. In humans, melphalan is excreted in the urine, about 10% as unchanged drug.

Busulfan has a selective action against granulocytes and is almost exclusively used in the treatment of chronic granulocytic leukaemia. Use in the treatment of polycythaemia vera has been described. Myelosuppression is the main side-effect although pulmonary fibrosis may occur rarely. In humans, busulfan is excreted in the urine as metabolites.

Thiotepa may be administered by instillation for topical treatment of superficial transitional cell carcinoma of the bladder. However, most canine bladder tumours are too large at the time of diagnosis for such treatment to be effective. It has been used experimentally in the management of malignant pleural and ascitic effusions.

The nitrosureas carmustine and lomustine also have an alkylating action. Unlike most other agents that do not cross the blood-brain barrier, these drugs are highly lipophilic and pass into the CSF. They have been used widely in human cancer therapy but in dogs and cats a cumulative bone marrow toxicity which is difficult to manage has been reported and therefore the drugs have not been commonly used in veterinary practice.

Carmustine is used in the treatment of malignant gliomas in humans and the use of carmustine in the treatment of canine brain tumours has been reported. With increasing use of CT scans for the diagnosis of brain tumours in animals, the use of this drug in the therapy of these tumours may be further explored. In humans, carmustine is rapidly degraded but the metabolites may be active. The drug is mainly excreted in the urine.

Lomustine has recently been shown to have some activity in the treatment of canine mast cell tumours, however further validation is required before this use can be recommended.

In general, alkylating drugs may cause myelosuppression. The gastro-intestinal system may be affected causing anorexia, vomiting, and diarrhoea. Gametogenesis may be affected. Some breeds may show thinning of the hair coat. Drug-specific side-effects are noted in the text and under monographs.

BUSULFAN
(Busulphan)

UK
Indications. Chronic granulocytic leukaemia, see notes above
Side-effects. Myelosuppression, pulmonary fibrosis
Dose. *Dogs, cats*: *by mouth*, induction dose, 3–6 mg/m^2 daily until white blood cell count approaches normal values Maintenance dose, 2 mg/m^2 daily, repeat as necessary to maintain the white blood cell count at 20–25 x 10^9/litre

POM Ⓗ **Myleran** (GlaxoWellcome) *UK*
Tablets, busulfan 500 micrograms, 2 mg; 25

CARMUSTINE
(BCNU, BiCNU)

UK
Indications. Brain tumours (e.g. malignant glioma) in dogs
Contra-indications. Severe myelosuppression
Side-effects. Cumulative and delayed bone marrow toxicity due to stem cell toxicity can lead to protracted myelosuppression, possible pulmonary fibrosis

Warnings. There is limited veterinary experience of this drug and specialist use only is recommended
Dose. *Dogs*: *by slow intravenous injection (over 20 minutes)*, 50 mg/m^2 every 6 weeks

POM Ⓗ **BiCNU** (Bristol-Myers) *UK*
Injection, powder for reconstitution, carmustine 100 mg

CHLORAMBUCIL

UK
Indications. Lymphocytic leukaemia, multiple myeloma, lymphoma, see notes above
Side-effects. Myelosuppression
Dose. *Dogs, cats*: *by mouth*, 2–5 mg/m^2 every 1–2 days

POM Ⓗ **Leukeran** (GlaxoWellcome) *UK*
Tablets, chlorambucil 2 mg, 5 mg; 25

CYCLOPHOSPHAMIDE

UK
Indications. Lymphoma, leukaemia, see notes above
Side-effects. Myelosuppression, gastro-intestinal disturbances, haemorrhagic cystitis
Dose. *Dogs, cats*: *by mouth*, 50 mg/m^2 on alternate days *or* 50 mg/m^2 for the first 4 days of each week *or* 100–300 mg/ m^2 every 3 weeks
by intravenous injection, 100–300 mg/m^2 every 3 weeks (maximum dose for *dogs*, 250 mg/m^2)

POM Ⓗ **Cyclophosphamide** (Pharmacia & Upjohn) *UK*
Tablets, s/c, cyclophosphamide (anhydrous) 50 mg; 100
Injection, powder for reconstitution, cyclophosphamide 200 mg, 500 mg, 1 g

POM Ⓗ **Endoxana** (ASTA Medica) *UK*
Tablets, s/c, cyclophosphamide 50 mg; 100
Injection, powder for reconstitution, cyclophosphamide 200 mg, 500 mg, 1 g

---

LOMUSTINE
(CCNU)

UK
Indications. Brain tumours (e.g. malignant glioma) in dogs, mast cell tumours, see notes above
Contra-indications. Severe myelosuppression
Side-effects. Cumulative bone marrow toxicity due to stem cell toxicity can lead to protracted myelosuppression, possible neurological reactions
Warnings. There is limited veterinary experience of this drug and specialist use only is recommended
Dose. *Dogs*: *by mouth*, 90 mg/m^2 as single dose every 3 weeks

POM Ⓗ **Lomustine** (Medac) *UK*
Capsules, lomustine 40 mg

MELPHALAN

UK
Indications. Multiple myeloma, lymphoma, see notes above

Side-effects. Myelosuppression (may be delayed), anorexia, vomiting

Dose. *Dogs, cats*: multiple myeloma, *by mouth*, 1–2 mg/m^2 on alternate days until plasma-protein concentrations approach normal values *or* 1–2 mg/m^2 daily for 7–14 days with repeat cycles at intervals of 2–4 weeks

Lymphoproliferative disorders, *by mouth*, up to 5 mg/m^2 on alternate days

POM (H) **Alkeran** (GlaxoWellcome) *UK*
Tablets, melphalan 2 mg, 5 mg; 25

THIOTEPA

UK

Indications. Malignant effusions, transitional cell carcinomas, see notes above

Side-effects. Myelosuppression, vomiting

Dose. *Dogs, cats*: *by instillation into the bladder*, up to 60 mg in 60–100 mL water, instilled and retained for 30 minutes every 7 days

by intravenous injection, 9 mg/m^2 as a single dose *or* 9 mg/m^2 in 2–4 divided doses on successive days. Repeat dose every 7–28 days

POM (H) **Thiotepa** (Lederle) *UK*
Injection, powder for reconstitution, thiotepa 15 mg

13.1.2 Antimetabolites

Antimetabolites interfere with DNA and RNA synthesis by interaction with enzymes.

Cytarabine acts by interfering with pyrimidine synthesis. It is primarily used to induce remission in lymphoproliferative or myeloproliferative diseases and has been used intrathecally for the treatment of CNS lymphoma in dogs. The drug is rapidly degraded after injection and is therefore more effective but also more toxic, if given by slow intravenous infusion. Cytarabine is a potent myelosuppressant leading to leucopenia, which is more severe when prolonged infusions of the drug are used. Cytarabine is metabolised in the liver and excreted in the urine as metabolites.

Fluorouracil has been used in the treatment of carcinomas of the mammary gland, gastro-intestinal tract, liver, and lung in dogs, but is at best palliative. In addition to myelosuppression, fluorouracil causes neurotoxicity, manifest as cerebellar ataxia and seizures. These effects are transitory in dogs *but fatal in cats and fluorouracil is contra-indicated in this species*. It is usually administered intravenously, but a preparation is also available for topical application, which has been used for the treatment of superficial squamous cell and basal tumours in horses. In humans, fluorouracil is catabolised in the liver and other tissues. Inactive metabolites are excreted in the urine.

Methotrexate competitively inhibits the enzyme dihydrofolate reductase, which is essential for the synthesis of purines and pyrimidines. Methotrexate may be used in the treatment of lymphoproliferative and myeloproliferative disorders. Its use has also been described in transmissible

venereal tumours, Sertoli cell tumours, osteosarcoma and other sarcomas.

The 'high-dose' regimen described for human use of methotrexate is not generally advisable in veterinary medicine because of the resultant toxic effects. Even at low doses, many dogs will show side-effects of severe diarrhoea. Methotrexate is primarily excreted unchanged by the kidney and renal tubular necrosis may occur with high-dose regimens. Myelosuppression and gastro-intestinal ulceration are common side-effects.

Mercaptopurine and **tioguanine** are natural purine analogues that act by inhibiting a number of enzymes involved in the early stages of purine synthesis particularly those involved in the formation of adenine and guanine nucleotides. These drugs have not been used extensively in veterinary oncology but there is evidence to suggest a role in the management of myeloid leukaemia in dogs and cats. In general, both drugs are well tolerated in dogs, but experience of their use in cats is limited. Myelosuppression is the major toxicity with leucopenia, thrombocytopenia, and, on occasion, anaemia. Leucopenia is not usually severe at the doses described but it can be a problem in leukaemic animals that are already neutropenic due to the disease. Nausea and vomiting have been reported although gastro-intestinal toxicity is rare. Mercaptopurine and tioguanine are metabolised in the liver.

> In general, antimetabolites may cause myelosuppression. The gastro-intestinal system may be affected causing anorexia, vomiting, and diarrhoea. Drug-specific side-effects are noted in the text and under monographs.

CYTARABINE

UK

Indications. Lymphoma, leukaemia

Side-effects. Myelosuppression

Dose. *Dogs, cats*: *by subcutaneous or intravenous injection*, 100 mg/m^2 daily for 2–4 days

by intravenous infusion, 75–100 mg/m^2 given over 24 hours

by intrathecal injection, 20 mg/m^2 every 1–5 days

POM (H) **Cytarabine** (Non-proprietary) *UK*
Injection, cytarabine 20 mg/mL
For subcutaneous, intravenous, or intrathecal use
Injection, cytarabine 100 mg/mL
Not for intrathecal injection

POM (H) **Cytosar** (Pharmacia & Upjohn) *UK*
Injection, powder for reconstitution, cytarabine 100 mg, 500 mg
For subcutaneous injection, intravenous injection or infusion; not recommended for intrathecal use

FLUOROURACIL

UK

Indications. Carcinomas but see notes above, squamous cell and basal carcinomas

Side-effects. Myelosuppression, neurotoxicity, gastro-intestinal disturbances

Contra-indications. Cats, see notes above

Dose. *Dogs*: *by intravenous injection*, 150–200 mg/m² every 7 days

POM Ⓗ **Fluorouracil** (Non-proprietary) *UK*
Injection, fluorouracil (as sodium salt) 25 mg/mL, 50 mg/mL

POM Ⓗ **Efudix** (ICN) *UK*
Cream, fluorouracil 5%; 20 g

MERCAPTOPURINE

UK

Indications. Lymphoma, leukaemia
Side-effects. Myelosuppression
Dose. *Dogs, cats*: *by mouth*, 50 mg/m² daily to effect then 50 mg/m² on alternate days or as necessary

POM Ⓗ **Puri-Nethol** (GlaxoWellcome) *UK*
Tablets, scored, mercaptopurine 50 mg; 25

METHOTREXATE

UK

Indications. Lymphoma, leukaemia, see also notes above
Contra-indications. Renal impairment
Side-effects. Renal tubular necrosis, gastro-intestinal disturbances
Dose. *Dogs, cats*: *by mouth or by intravenous injection*, 2.5 mg/m² daily. Dose frequency should be adjusted according to toxicity (see notes above)

POM Ⓗ **Methotrexate** (Non-proprietary) *UK*
Tablets, methotrexate 2.5 mg, 10 mg
Injection, methotrexate (as sodium salt) 2.5 mg/mL, 25 mg/mL, 100mg/mL (not for intrathecal use)

TIOGUANINE
(Thioguanine)

Indications. Lymphoma, leukaemia
Side-effects. Myelosuppression
Dose. *Dogs*: *by mouth*, 50 mg/m² every 1–2 days

UK
POM Ⓗ **Lanvis** (GlaxoWellcome) *UK*
Tablets, scored, tioguanine 40 mg; 25

13.1.3 Antitumour antibiotics

These drugs act by forming a stable complex with DNA and interfering with the synthesis of nucleic acids.

Doxorubicin is an anthracycline antibiotic, and is one of the most effective of the cytotoxic drugs. In veterinary medicine, doxorubicin is used to treat lymphoproliferative and myeloproliferative disorders. It is also a palliative in soft tissue and osteogenic sarcomas and in carcinomas of mammary, thyroid, and prostatic origin.

Doxorubicin is administered by slow intravenous injection and is severely irritant if injected perivascularly. Gastro-intestinal toxicity such as vomiting and diarrhoea may occur 48 to 72 hours following administration of the drug and occasionally dogs may develop haemorrhagic enterocolitis. It is myelosuppressive with the lowest leucocyte count occurring 10 to 14 days after treatment. Changes in hair coat can occur in some dog breeds. Doxorubicin also causes myocardial damage leading to a dose-dependent congestive cardiomyopathy, and cardiac monitoring is advisable. Doxorubicin is excreted in the biliary tract.

Tachyarrhythmias, cutaneous anaphylaxis, and collapse may occur during infusion; premedication with an antihistamine such as chlorphenamine (see section 14.2.2), 5 to 10 mg given by slow intravenous injection, is advisable. *Treatment with doxorubicin should be supervised by specialists familiar with its use.*

Epirubicin is a structural analogue of doxorubicin. The tumoricidal activity of both drugs is similar but epirubicin is reported to be less cardiotoxic than doxorubicin. The indications for epirubicin are essentially as for doxorubicin. Epirubicin causes myelosuppression with leucopenia 10 to 15 days post administration but the white blood cell count usually returns to normal in about 21 days. Thrombocytopenia and anaemia may follow a similar pattern but are much less common. Gastro-intestinal and dermatological toxicity are similar to doxorubicin. Epirubicin may also cause anaphylaxis and is irritant if extravasation occurs.

Mitoxantrone is an anthracenedione and is related to doxorubicin. Although mitoxantrone intercalates with DNA, its main cytotoxic effect is through stimulating strand breaks in DNA. Veterinary experience of this drug is limited although preliminary results of its use in the treatment of a variety of tumours in dogs and cats have been reported. In these species, mitoxantrone appears to have a wide spectrum of activity against lymphomas, sarcomas, and possibly carcinomas, especially in cats. Mitoxantrone may cause myelosuppression, the main sign of which is a leucopenia that is greatest at about 10 days post treatment. Mitoxantrone is cardiotoxic but its cardiac effects are reported to be significantly less severe than those of doxorubicin. Anorexia, nausea, and vomiting may also occur. Mitoxantrone is excreted mainly by the liver.

Bleomycin has not been widely used in veterinary chemotherapy. It has been used in the treatment of lymphoproliferative disorders and has shown some efficacy against squamous cell carcinoma in dogs. Bleomycin causes minimal myelosuppression but hypersensitivity reactions may occur. Lung changes including interstitial pneumonia, pleural scarring, and pulmonary fibrosis have been reported with high doses in the dog. In humans, bleomycin is degraded by tissue hydrolase but most of the drug is excreted unchanged in the urine.

Dactinomycin has not been extensively used in veterinary chemotherapy. There is limited investigational experience in the treatment of canine lymphoproliferative disorders, carcinomas, and sarcomas. Toxicities include leucopenia, anorexia, vomiting, diarrhoea, and weight loss, due to selective damage of the haemopoietic and intestinal tissues.

BLEOMYCIN

UK

Indications. Lymphoma, leukaemia
Side-effects. Hypersensitivity, pneumonitis, pulmonary fibrosis, see notes above
Dose. *Dogs*: *by intravenous injection*, 10 000–15 000 units/m^2 weekly to a maximum cumulative dose of 250 000 units/m^2

POM (H) **Bleomycin** (Non-proprietary) *UK*
Injection, powder for reconstitution, bleomycin (as sulphate) 15 000 units
Note. To conform with the European Pharmacopocia ampoules previously labelled as containing '15 units' of bleomycin are now labelled as containing 15 000 units. The amount of bleomycin in the ampoule has not changed.

DACTINOMYCIN
(Actinomycin D)

UK

Indications. Side-effects. See notes above
Dose. *Dogs*: *by intravenous injection*, 1.5 mg/m^2 every 7 days

POM (H) **Cosmegen Lyovac** (MSD) *UK*
Injection, powder for reconstitution, dactinomycin 500 micrograms

DOXORUBICIN HYDROCHLORIDE

UK

Indications. Lymphoma, leukaemia, sarcomas, carcinomas, see notes above
Contra-indications. Hepatic impairment, cardiac disease
Side-effects. Myelosuppression, gastro-intestinal toxicity, cardiac toxicity
Warnings. Drug should be handled with extreme care, severely vesicant if extravasation occurs
Dose. *Dogs*: *by slow intravenous injection*, 30 mg/m^2 every 3 weeks to a maximum cumulative dose of 240 mg/m^2
Cats: *by slow intravenous injection*, 20 mg/m^2 every 3–6 weeks

POM (H) **Doxorubicin Rapid Dissolution** (Pharmacia & Upjohn) *UK*
Injection, powder for reconstitution, doxorubicin hydrochloride 10 mg, 50 mg

POM (H) **Doxorubicin Solution for Injection** (Pharmacia & Upjohn) *UK*
Injection, doxorubicin hydrochloride 2 mg/mL; 5 mL, 25 mL

EPIRUBICIN HYDROCHLORIDE

UK

Indications. Lymphoma, leukaemia, sarcomas, carcinomas, see notes above
Contra-indications. Hepatic impairment, cardiac disease
Side-effects. Myelosuppression, gastro-intestinal toxicity, cardiac toxicity
Warnings. Drug should be handled with extreme care, severely vesicant if extravasation occurs
Dose. *Dogs*: *by slow intravenous injection*, 30 mg/m^2 every 3 weeks to a maximum cumulative dose of 240–300 mg/m^2

Cats: *by slow intravenous injection*, 20 mg/m^2 every 3–6 weeks

POM (H) **Pharmorubicin Rapid Dissolution** (Pharmacia & Upjohn) *UK*
Injection, powder for reconstitution, epirubicin hydrochloride 10 mg, 20 mg, 50 mg

POM (H) **Pharmorubicin Solution for Injection** (Pharmacia & Upjohn) *UK*
Injection, epirubicin hydrochloride 2 mg/mL; 5 mL, 25 mL

MITOXANTRONE
(Mitozantrone)

UK

Indications. Lymphoma, sarcomas, carcinomas
Contra-indications. Hepatic impairment
Side-effects. Myelosuppression, cardiac toxicity, anorexia, vomiting, diarrhoea
Warnings. Drug should be handled with extreme care
Dose. *Dogs*: *by intravenous infusion*, 5 mg/m^2 every 3 weeks
Cats: *by intravenous infusion*, 3–5 mg/m^2 every 3 weeks

POM (H) **Novantrone** (Lederle) *UK*
Intravenous infusion, mitoxantrone (as hydrochloride) 2 mg/mL; 10 mL, 12.5 mL, 15 mL

13.1.4 Vinca alkaloids

These drugs are plant alkaloids. They bind to microtubular proteins, causing metaphase arrest thus inhibiting mitosis in the metaphase. They may also cause enzyme inhibition.

Vincristine is the most widely used vinca alkaloid in veterinary medicine. The main indications are in the treatment of lymphoproliferative disorders and transmissible venereal tumour. The latter is extremely sensitive to vincristine. The experimental use of vincristine in the treatment of soft tissue sarcomas and carcinomas has also been reported. Vincristine is also of value in the management of thrombocytopenia by virtue of its stimulation of platelet release from megakaryocytes.

Vincristine causes virtually no myelosuppression but is severely vesicant if extravasation occurs. Peripheral and autonomic neuropathies rarely occur in dogs and cats. Constipation may result from long-term therapy.

Vinblastine is less frequently used than vincristine. Its uses include treatment of lymphoproliferative disorders and solid carcinomas but efficacy in the latter case is limited. Unlike vincristine, vinblastine causes myelosuppression, and will also cause severe perivascular reactions.

In humans, vincristine and vinblastine undergo hepatic metabolism and biliary excretion.

VINBLASTINE SULPHATE

UK

Indications. Lymphoma, leukaemia
Side-effects. Myelosuppression
Warnings. Severely vesicant if extravasation occurs

Dose. *Dogs, cats*: *by intravenous injection*, 2.0–2.5 mg/m² every 7 or 14 days

POM Ⓗ **Vinblastine** (Non-proprietary) *UK*
Injection, vinblastine sulphate 1 mg/mL; 10 mL

POM Ⓗ **Velbe** (Lilly) *UK*
Injection, powder for reconstitution, vinblastine sulphate 10 mg

VINCRISTINE SULPHATE

UK
Indications. Lymphoma, leukaemia, transmissible venereal tumour, see notes above
Side-effects. Neuropathies, constipation
Warnings. Severely vesicant if extravasation occurs
Dose. *Dogs, cats*: *by intravenous injection*, 500–750 micrograms/m² every 7 or 14 days

POM Ⓗ **Vincristine** (Non-proprietary) *UK*
Injection, vincristine sulphate 1 mg/mL; 1 mL, 2 mL, 5 mL

POM Ⓗ **Oncovin** (Lilly) *UK*
Injection, vincristine sulphate 1 mg/mL; 1 mL, 2 mL

13.1.5 Platinum compounds

Platinum co-ordination compounds inhibit protein synthesis by cross linking strands of DNA. These are potent drugs with a broad spectrum of activity against solid tumours. They may cause severe toxicity which limits their use in veterinary medicine.

Cisplatin has been used systemically, by intravenous infusion during saline diuresis, in the treatment of osteosarcoma, soft tissue sarcoma, and various carcinomas.
Cisplatin is nephrotoxic, causing acute proximal tubular necrosis. Vomiting and myelosuppression also occur. Pretreatment hydration and diuresis are recommended. Treatment with this drug should be supervised by specialists familiar with its use. Approximately 80% of the drug is excreted unchanged in the urine. Urine of dogs that have received cisplatin must therefore be treated as a chemical spill for at least 24 hours following treatment. Persons handling the animal during this time should wear appropriate protective clothing and any contaminated bedding should be double-wrapped and sent for chemical disposal. *Cisplatin can cause severe pulmonary reactions in cats and its use is contra-indicated in this species*.
A variety of controlled-release formulations of cisplatin are under investigation. OPLA-pt (polylactic acid impregnated with cisplatin; investigational product that is not available in the UK) has been used as an adjunct to surgical treatment of osteosarcoma in the dog. Cisplatin has also been used in gel or oil preparations for local, intralesional application in equine melanoma and equine sarcoids; a potentially hazardous procedure and not recommended.

Carboplatin is a second generation platinum analogue with a spectrum of antineoplastic activity similar to cisplatin. Carboplatin has a much shorter elimination half-life than cisplatin and is significantly less nephrotoxic and emetogenic, however, myelosuppression can be severe. Carboplatin has been used in the treatment of canine osteosarcoma and some carcinomas. It has also been used in cats. Carboplatin is excreted in urine.

CARBOPLATIN

UK
Indications. Canine osteosarcoma, some carcinomas in dogs
Contra-indications. Patients with bone marrow depression, renal impairment
Side-effects. Myelosuppression, vomiting, renal toxicity
Dose. *Dogs*: *by intravenous injection*, 300 mg/m², given over 15–30 minutes every 3–4 weeks
Cats: *by intravenous injection*, 200 mg/m², given over 15–30 minutes every 4 weeks

POM Ⓗ **Carboplatin** (Non-proprietary) *UK*
Injection, carboplatin 10 mg/mL; 15 mL, 45 mL, 60 mL

POM Ⓗ **Paraplatin** (Bristol-Myers) *UK*
Injection, carboplatin 10 mg/mL; 5 mL, 15 mL, 45 mL

CISPLATIN

UK
Indications. Sarcomas, carcinomas
Contra-indications. Renal impairment; cats, see notes above
Side-effects. Renal toxicity, myelosuppression, vomiting
Dose. *Dogs*: treatment may be repeated 4–6 times at intervals of 3–4 weeks. Treatment should be combined with prehydration, anti-emetics, and diuresis
Prehydration, *by intravenous infusion*, sodium chloride 0.9% given at a rate of 25 mL/kg per hour for 3 hours
Treatment with cisplatin, *by intravenous infusion*, 50–100 mg/m² given over 15 minutes
Anti-emetics (see section 3.4) may be given 30–60 minutes after treatment. Chlorpromazine, *by intramuscular injection*, 200–400 micrograms/kg *or* metoclopramide, *by intramuscular injection*, 0.5–1.0 mg/kg
Diuresis, *by intravenous infusion*, sodium chloride 0.9% given at a rate of 15 mL/kg per hour for 3 hours. Furosemide, *by intravenous injection*, 2.5–5.0 mg/kg may be given concurrently if urine production is reduced

POM Ⓗ **Cisplatin** (Non-proprietary) *UK*
Injection, cisplatin 1 mg/mL; 10 mL, 50 mL, 100 mL
Injection, powder for reconstitution, cisplatin 10 mg, 50 mg

13.1.6 Other cytotoxic drugs

Crisantaspase is the enzyme asparaginase produced by *Erwinia chrysanthemi*. It hydrolyses asparagine, an essential amino acid, and is used in the treatment of lymphoproliferative disorders. It has also been used in the treatment of canine melanoma and mast cell tumours. Crisantaspase may be administered by the intravenous, intramuscular, or intraperitoneal routes but anaphylaxis may follow administration and the intramuscular route appears to be the safest and most effective. Premedication with an antihistamine such as chlorphenamine (see section 14.2.2), 5 to 10 mg given by slow intravenous injection, is necessary if crisantaspase is administered by other routes. Haemorrhagic pancreatitis has been reported in dogs.

Dacarbazine has alkylating actions but also inhibits DNA and protein synthesis. It is not commonly used in veterinary medicine due to its toxic effects. However dacarbazine has been included in some combination protocols for the treatment of lymphoproliferative disorders, in particular it is used in combination with doxorubicin for rescue treatment of relapsed canine lymphoma. In addition to myelosuppression, gastro-intestinal toxicity has been reported. Dacarbazine can cause pain on injection and severe perivascular cellulitis.

Hydroxycarbamide inhibits the enzyme ribonucleotide reductase. It is administered orally and is excreted by the kidney. It is used in the treatment of polycythaemia vera and chronic granulocytic leukaemia. Myelosuppression is the main toxic effect.

Prednisolone (see section 13.2) is widely used in cancer therapy. Corticosteroids have antimitotic and cytolytic effects on lymphoid tissues and are therefore used in the treatment of lymphoproliferative disorders. They are also useful in the treatment of mast cell tumours and may be indicated in brain tumours because these drugs are able to cross the blood-brain barrier. Corticosteroids may also be used in the management of secondary complications of neoplasia and palliation of advanced disease. Although they do not directly affect a large solid mass, corticosteroids decrease the inflammation around the mass.

Toxic effects include pancreatitis and diarrhoea. Hyperadrenocorticism may result from long-term therapy. Corticosteroids cause little or no myelosuppression.

Mitotane (see section 7.6) selectively destroys the zona fasciculata and zona reticularis of the adrenal cortex and is used in the medical management of pituitary-dependent hyperadrenocorticism.

CRISANTASPASE

UK
Indications. Lymphoma, leukaemia, see notes above
Side-effects. Anaphylaxis, haemorrhagic pancreatitis
Dose. *Dogs, cats*: *by intramuscular (preferred), intravenous, or intraperitoneal injection*, 10 000–40 000 units/m² every 7 days or more

POM Ⓗ **Erwinase** (Ipsen) *UK*
Injection, powder for reconstitution, crisantaspase 10 000 units

DACARBAZINE

UK
Indications. Lymphoma, see notes above
Side-effects. Myelosuppression, anorexia, vomiting, diarrhoea, severe perivascular cellulitis
Dose. *Dogs, cats*: *by intravenous injection*, 200–250 mg/m² daily on days 1–5, repeat cycle every 21–28 days *or* 100 mg/m² every 7 days

POM Ⓗ **Dacarbazine** (Non-proprietary) *UK*
Injection, powder for reconstitution, dacarbazine (as citrate) 100 mg, 200 mg, 500 mg, 1 g

POM Ⓗ **DTIC-Dome** (Bayer) *UK*
Injection, powder for reconstitution, dacarbazine 200 mg

HYDROXYCARBAMIDE
(Hydroxyurea)

UK
Indications. Polycythaemia vera and chronic granulocytic leukaemia
Contra-indications. Renal impairment
Side-effects. Myelosuppression
Dose. *Dogs, cats*: 50 mg/kg daily *or* 80 mg/kg every 3 days

POM Ⓗ **Hydrea** (Squibb) *UK*
Capsules, hydroxycarbamide 500 mg; 100

13.2 Immunosuppressants

Immune-mediated diseases seen in veterinary practice include haemolytic anaemia, immune-mediated thrombocytopenia, systemic lupus erythematosus, myasthenia gravis, arthritides, and pemphigus variants. Many of these may be improved by glucocorticoid administration and high dose **prednisolone** is the conventional method of treatment. High doses of prednisolone should be used with extreme caution in horses because of the risk of causing laminitis. It is recommended that expert advice is sought before treating horses requiring immunosuppression.

Many cytotoxics are potent immunosuppressants and some, such as cyclophosphamide and mercaptopurine, are used in treatment of immune-mediated conditions principally in dogs (see section 10.5). **Azathioprine** is a purine analogue that contains the 6-mercaptopurine moiety. The breakdown of azathioprine causes slow liberation of mercaptopurine in the tissues. Superior immunosuppressive activity is achieved in comparison to mercaptopurine and therefore azathioprine is used clinically as an immunosuppressive agent rather than as a cytotoxic drug. In veterinary medicine the main indication for its use is in the treatment of immune-mediated diseases that cannot be adequately controlled with corticosteroids alone.

Danazol is a synthetic derivative of ethinyl testosterone, which has a synergistic action with corticosteroids in the control of immune-mediated thrombocytopenia or haemolytic anaemia. The proposed mechanism of action is mediated by a reduction in the number of immunoglobulin (Fc) receptors on the surface of macrophages and a decrease in the amount of antibody on the surface of target cells. The onset of this action may be slow and varies from 2 weeks to 2 months. Once the patient is stabilised, the dose of prednisolone may be carefully reduced and in some cases it may be possible to maintain the patient on danazol alone. Danazol is principally metabolised in the liver.

Ciclosporin is a cyclic polypeptide fungal metabolite and is a potent T cell selective, immunosuppressive drug. Developed for use in human organ transplant patients, it is now being used increasingly in the treatment of immune-mediated disease. Orally administered ciclosporin has been used successfully in the treatment of canine anal furunculosis and it is currently the subject of clinical study in a variety of immune-mediated conditions. Optimal dosages for treatment of immune-mediated disease have not been established, but these may be substantially lower than those required in organ transplant patients. The drug is orally absorbed and elimination is primarily by biliary excretion. Ciclosporin causes little myelosuppression and the main adverse effect in humans is nephrotoxicity. In human patients, hepatotoxicity, hypertension, hypertrichosis, gingival hyperplasia, and other side-effects have been reported and are mostly reversible with dose reduction. Nephrotoxicity and hepatotoxicity may be less of a problem in dogs but gastro-intestinal toxicity, gingival hypertrophy, and papillomatosis have been reported.

Topical ciclosporin (see section 12.6) is used in veterinary medicine for the treatment of keratoconjunctivitis sicca (KCS) in dogs. It modulates immune-mediated destruction of tear secreting tissue and stimulates tear production. The pigmentary keratitis that accompanies many cases of KCS is also controlled.

AZATHIOPRINE

UK

Indications. Immune-mediated disease unresponsive to corticosteroid therapy alone; severe inflammatory bowel disease (see section 3.1.3)
Side-effects. Myelosuppression
Dose. *Dogs*: *by mouth*, 1–2 mg/kg every 1–2 days

POM (H) **Azathioprine** (Non-proprietary) *UK*
Tablets, azathioprine 25 mg, 50 mg

POM (H) **Imuran** (GlaxoWellcome) *UK*
Tablets, f/c, azathioprine 25 mg, 50 mg; 100

CICLOSPORIN
(Cyclosporin)

UK

Indications. Immune-mediated disease as an immunosuppressant, perianal fistula, anal furunculosis, sebaceous adenitis; ocular disease (see section 12.6)
Contra-indications. Renal impairment and pre-existing infections (systemic administration)
Side-effects. Immunosuppression, mild gastro-intestinal signs, renal toxicity, papillomatosis
Warnings. Do not administer orally to patients with renal impairment
Dose. *Dogs*: immunosuppression, *by mouth*, 5 mg/kg 1–2 times daily

POM (H) **Neoral** (Novartis) *UK*
Capsules, ciclosporin 10 mg, 25 mg, 50 mg, 100 mg

POM (H) **Neoral** (Novartis) *UK*
Oral solution, ciclosporin 100 mg/mL
Note. Due to differences in bioavailability of ciclosporin-containing products, the brand should be specified

DANAZOL

UK

Indications. Immune-mediated thrombocytopenia and haemolytic anaemia in combination with corticosteroids
Contra-indications. Pregnant animals
Side-effects. Hepatotoxicity in dogs, androgenic effects: virilization in females, increased muscle mass, testicular atrophy, hirsuitism, alopecia
Warnings. Teratogenic; avoid use in patients with cardiac, renal, or hepatic impairment
Dose. *By mouth*.
Dogs: 4–10 mg/kg 2–3 times daily. (Suggested initial dose 5 mg/kg 3 times daily)
Cats: 5 mg/kg 3 times daily

POM (H) **Danazol** (Non-proprietary) *UK*
Capsules, danazol 100 mg, 200 mg

POM (H) **Danol** (Sanofi-Synthelabo) *UK*
Capsules, danazol 100 mg, 200 mg

PREDNISOLONE

UK

Indications. Immunosuppression, cancer therapy (see section 13.1.6 for indications); inflammatory and allergic disorders (see section 7.2.1); adrenocortical insufficiency (see section 7.2.2); myasthenia gravis (see section 6.7.4)
Side-effects. Pancreatitis, diarrhoea, see also section 7.2.1
Warnings. High doses of prednisolone should be used with extreme caution in horses because of the risk of causing laminitis
Dose.
Horses: immunosuppression, *by mouth*, 1 mg/kg on alternate days (**but see note above**)
Dogs, cats: immunosuppression, *by mouth*, induction 2–4 mg/kg daily, maintenance 0.5–2.0 mg/kg on alternate days
Cancer therapy, *by mouth*, 20–40 mg/m² daily or on alternate days

See section 7.2.1 for preparation details

13.3 Sex hormones and hormone antagonists

In male dogs, oestrogens (see section 8.2.1) and progestogens such as delmadinone (see section 8.2.2) are used for the medical treatment of benign prostatic hypertrophy and, on occasion, for the management of anal (perianal, circumanal, hepatoid gland) adenomata. If such therapy is beneficial, a hormonal dependency is demonstrated and castration is usually recommended as the long-term treatment of choice. These tumours often lose their hormonal dependency with malignant transformation. In these cases castration is rarely of benefit and the efficacy of hormonal treatment is questionable.

In bitches, mammary tumours occur commonly. The majority of these are benign and cured by surgical resection. The role of hormones in the development and progression of canine mammary tumours is controversial. Studies indicate that there is hormonal influence on the development of mammary tumours but the value of hormonal manipulation once a tumour has developed has not been established. Some canine mammary tumours do express oestrogen receptors but these tend to occur in differentiated (less aggressive) tumours rather than poorly differentiated (malignant) tumours. Therefore the use of androgens such as methyltestosterone for the treatment of canine mammary tumours is uncertain. The hormone antagonist, tamoxifen, is a complex drug having anti-oestrogenic and also oestrogenic activity depending on the target tissue and species. The drug has been found to cause pyometra in entire bitches and its efficacy in the treatment of canine mammary tumours has not been established.

14 Drugs acting on the SKIN

Contributors:
S M E Cockbill LLM, BPharm, MPharm, DAgVetPharm, MCPP, MIPharmM, FRPharmS, PhD
I S Mason BVetMed, PhD, CertSAD, MRCVS

14.1 Dermatological vehicles
14.2 Preparations for allergic, inflammatory, and other immune-mediated skin conditions
14.3 Sunscreens
14.4 Anti-infective skin preparations
14.5 Keratolytics and keratoplastic agents
14.6 Shampoos
14.7 Wound management
14.8 Preparations for the ear

The use of topical preparations acting on the skin is also described in Parasiticides (Chapter 2), under Preparations for the care of teats and udders (section 11.2), and Drugs acting on feet (Chapter 15).

Systemic disorders may also be responsible for clinical signs affecting the skin. Examples include hormonal disturbances such as hypothyroidism or hyperadrenocorticism (see chapter 7), nutritional deficiency of for example zinc (see chapter 16), or neoplasia for example exocrine pancreatic adenocarcinoma exhibited as feline paraneoplastic alopecia (FPA).

14.1 Dermatological vehicles

The skin is amenable to treatment by local application because there is immediate contact between drug and target tissue. Both vehicle and active ingredients are important in treatment. The vehicle affects the degree of hydration of the skin, may have a mild anti-inflammatory effect, and may aid the penetration of the active ingredients into the skin.

Before application of a topical preparation, it is important to prepare the area for treatment by clipping away hair or wool and removing contaminating debris with disinfectants or cleansing agents (see section 14.7.1). The importance of skin preparation and regular application of treatment to the affected area should be stressed to pet owners.

The tendency for animals to lick the affected area immediately after application can be a major problem, especially in cats, and may result in worsening of the skin condition. Licking may be reduced by applying the preparation before feeding or exercise (which distract the animal), or by using methods of restraint such as an Elizabethan collar. Licking of treated areas also makes it important to avoid using substances that are potentially toxic if ingested.

Hypersensitivity reactions to topical preparations may occur, leading to both local and systemic manifestations.

For skin disorders, formulations are available as powders, sprays, shampoos, lotions, gels, creams, and ointments. The choice of vehicle depends on the type of lesion and convenience of application.

Creams are water-miscible and readily removed by licking and washing. They are less greasy and easier to apply than ointments. Aqueous cream, which soothes and hydrates the skin, is used as an emollient in the treatment of dry, scaling lesions. Frequent application is desirable.

Aqueous Cream
emulsifying ointment 30%, phenoxyethanol 1%, in freshly boiled and cooled purified water

Ointments are greasy, normally anhydrous, insoluble in water, and more occlusive than creams. Ointments are also effective emollient preparations. Ointments are used for chronic dry lesions and should be avoided in exudative lesions. The more commonly used ointment bases consist of soft paraffin or soft paraffin and liquid paraffin with hard paraffin. Such greasy preparations may not be suitable for pets in household conditions because they may stain furniture, etc.

Emulsifying Ointment
emulsifying wax 30%, white soft paraffin 50%, liquid paraffin 20%
Hydrous Wool Fat (lanolin)
wool fat 50%, in freshly boiled and cooled purified water
White Soft Paraffin, (white petroleum jelly)
Yellow Soft Paraffin, (yellow petroleum jelly)

Dusting powders are finely divided powders that may contain one or more active ingredients. Generally, they absorb moisture, which discourages bacterial growth. Dusting powders should not be used on wet, raw surfaces because adherent crusts and caking may result; they may be used in the treatment of wound infections.

Lotions are usually aqueous solutions or suspensions, for application without friction to inflamed unbroken skin. They cool by evaporation of solvents, require frequent application, and leave a thin film of drug on the skin. Lotions are used on hairy areas and for lesions with minor exudation and ulceration. Care should be taken with nervous or excitable animals because lotions containing volatile substances can sting on application.

'Shake lotions' such as calamine lotion are used to cool dry scabbed lesions. They leave a film of dry powder.

Pastes are stiff preparations containing a high proportion of finely powdered solids. They are less occlusive than ointments and are used mainly for circumscribed, ulcerated lesions.

Zinc oxide is a mild astringent and has soothing and protective properties. Magnesium sulphate paste is used in the treatment of minor skin infections.

Compound Zinc Paste
zinc oxide 25%, starch 25%, white soft paraffin 50%
Magnesium Sulphate Paste (Morison's Paste)
dried magnesium sulphate, after drying, 45 g, phenol 500 mg, anhydrous glycerol 55 g

Gels are semisolid aqueous solutions that are easy to apply, not greasy, miscible with water, and wash off easily.

Sprays are used as pressurised aerosols or in spraying units. They may be economical to use because of the ease of application with little waste, and can be easily directed. Sealed packaging means the risk of contamination of the remaining constituents is minimised. Additionally, the cooling effect produced by the evaporation of solvents may be beneficial in certain conditions. Some animals may show signs of anxiety in response to the noise produced by the spray.

Shampoos are used as complementary therapy in association with other treatment or as sole preparations in the long-term management of certain disorders such as seborrhoea. They help to clean the skin and remove crusts and debris. Shampoos are formulated to reduce any irritant effects and are generally well tolerated. Effective rinsing is essential after the recommended contact time. Shampoos are indicated as vehicles for antipruritic and keratolytic drugs (see section 14.5) and for skin disinfecting and cleansing preparations (see section 14.7.1). Shampoos can be poor vehicles for ectoparasiticides because they are rinsed off after use and therefore afford no residual protection if the parasite is still present in the environment; this is particularly important in the treatment of flea infestation.

Collodions are painted onto the skin and allowed to dry to leave a flexible film over the site of the application. In veterinary medicine their main use is to 'seal' the teats of non-lactating cows.

Flexible Collodion

castor oil 2.5%, colophony 2.5% in a collodion basis, prepared by dissolving pyroxylin (10%) in a mixture of 3 volumes of ether and 1 volume of alcohol (90%)

Warnings. Highly flammable

Liniments are liquid preparations for external application that contain analgesics and rubefacients.

14.2 Preparations for allergic, inflammatory, and other immune-mediated skin conditions

A wide variety of causative factors may be involved in these skin conditions. The selection of the type and duration of treatment depends on the inflammatory disease present. In every case, the underlying causes should be identified and eliminated, if possible. If this can be done, long-term anti-inflammatory therapy is unnecessary.

Hypersensitivity reactions to environmental allergens, including house dust mites, forage mites, danders, moulds, pollens, insect bites particularly fleas, and foods, are common causes of chronic dermatitis in dogs and cats. Diagnosis may be possible by provocative intradermal testing. Phenothiazines may have an antihistaminic effect and their use as sedatives should be avoided before hypersensitivity testing. Contact allergy is a relatively uncommon cause of

dermatitis. Irritant contact reactions are more likely to induce inflammatory lesions on contact areas and relatively hairless parts of the skin.

Ideally, allergies should be remedied by separation of the affected animal from the source of allergens. This is usually possible in contact or food allergy but may be difficult to achieve in the other allergic skin diseases.

Allergies to dusts and pollens (atopy) can be controlled by hyposensitisation using vaccines containing the allergens to which the animal has been shown to react. Various protocols for vaccine administration are used but generally these start with vaccination at short intervals over a period of weeks during the induction phase and then at approximately monthly intervals during maintenance which continues indefinitely. Manufacturers supply appropriate protocols with the vaccines. There is a risk of adverse reactions to the vaccines, including anaphylaxis, and thus vaccination should be monitored carefully, although adverse effects are rarely seen. A good response may be obtained in about 50% of dogs.

Drug reactions may cause a very broad range of clinical signs ranging from urticaria and swelling to severe, acute, generalised and often fatal diseases such as erythema multiforme major and toxic epidermal necrolysis. Such reactions may occur in response to recently administered drugs but may also be caused by reactions to bacterial infections, tumours, and agents incorporated in the diet.

Auto-immune dermatoses such as the pemphigus complex can also be seen in drug reactions but may also arise when no causative factor can be identified. In general, hypersensitivity diseases require much less aggressive therapy than the auto-immune dermatoses.

14.2.1 Corticosteroids

14.2.2 Antihistamines

14.2.3 Topical anti-inflammatory skin preparations

14.2.4 Essential fatty acid preparations

14.2.1 Corticosteroids

Systemic corticosteroids (see section 7.2.1) are of great value in the treatment of inflammatory and immune-mediated skin conditions. Oral preparations with a short duration of action are preferred because therapy can be discontinued swiftly if adverse effects are seen. This is not possible with longer acting, injectable agents. In addition, fewer side-effects are associated with the use of short-acting oral drugs than with other formulations of corticosteroids. However, in severe, acute, life-threatening disease short-acting injectable corticosteroid formulations are favoured. In chronic diseases when corticosteroids are indicated, alternate day therapy should be used to minimise the risk of adrenal suppression. Depot corticosteroids such as methylprednisolone acetate should be reserved for cases in which the use of short acting preparations is impractical for example in dogs or cats which will not tolerate oral dosing.

The dose and type of corticosteroid used depends on the type and severity of the disease present. Typically, allergic diseases are managed with oral prednisolone at a dosage in dogs of 500 micrograms/kg daily or methylprednisolone at a dosage of 400 micrograms/kg daily until the pruritus is controlled and then the dose is tapered to achieve the minimum effective alternate day dose. The dose should be reduced once remission is achieved. Glucocorticoid therapy may lead to adverse effects (unacceptable polyuria, polydipsia, and polyphagia) in some animals and alternative forms of therapy (see below) may be needed as an adjunct or a substitute for corticosteroids. Cats typically require double the corticosteroid doses used in dogs.

Combinations of antihistamines and corticosteroids with essential fatty acids have been shown to enhance their efficacy and enable lower doses of corticosteroids to be used for allergic conditions.

In auto-immune diseases, much higher daily dosages are required (2 to 4 mg/kg prednisolone or 1.5 to 3.0 mg/kg methylprednisolone for dogs). Such high dosages may be poorly tolerated and other immunosuppressive drugs such as azathioprine, gold salts, or chlorambucil may be needed as additional therapy in order to allow a reduction in the dose of glucocorticoids. However, the management of such severe diseases with potentially toxic drugs should be undertaken with caution.

Megestrol acetate (see section 8.2.2) should not be used to control 'feline miliary dermatitis' (papular-crusting dermatitis) or eosinophilic granuloma complex. The side-effects are unacceptable and equally good effects can be obtained with corticosteroids.

14.2.2 Antihistamines

Antihistamines are antagonists of the histamine H_1 receptor and include **chlorphenamine**, **clemastine**, **diphenhydramine**, **hydroxyzine**, **promethazine**, **mepyramine**, **tripelennamine,** and **alimemazine**. Antihistamines diminish or abolish the main actions of histamine in the body by competitive, reversible blockade of histamine receptor sites. Histamine is only one of many autacoids involved in hypersensitivity reactions and so antihistamines have limited use in the treatment of allergic disorders in animals. The effects of antihistamines may not be observed for 1 to 2 weeks and they are most effective for preventing rather than for rapidly reducing pruritus. Some authorities indicate initial use of glucocorticoids in conjunction with antihistamines. Glucocorticoid therapy is stopped when pruritus is eliminated; antihistamine treatment is continued.

Systemic antihistamines may be used to control pruritus in allergic reactions such as urticaria and allergic skin problems including food allergies. It is generally accepted that about 10 to 15% of dogs are likely to respond to treatment with H_1 receptor antagonists but there is considerable individual variation between dogs and it is not possible to predict which antihistamine will be effective in any particular dog. Orally administered antihistamines reported to be effective include chlorphenamine, clemastine, diphenhydramine, hydroxyzine, and alimemazine. H_2 antagonists

have not proven effective. In cats, efficacy has been reported with chlorphenamine and clemastine.

Combination preparations of antihistamines and corticosteroids are available in some countries.

ALIMEMAZINE TARTRATE
(Trimeprazine tartrate)

UK

Indications. Pruritus in allergic skin disorders
Side-effects. CNS depression; drowsiness
Dose. *By mouth.*
Dogs: pruritus, 1–2 mg/kg 3 times daily

POM Ⓗ **Vallergan** (Castlemead)
Tablets, alimemazine tartrate 10 mg; 28
Syrup, alimemazine tartrate 1.5 mg/mL; 100 mL
Syrup forte, alimemazine tartrate 6 mg/mL; 100 mL

CHLORPHENAMINE MALEATE
(Chlorpheniramine maleate)

UK

Indications. Pruritus in allergic skin disorders, premedication for drugs that may induce an anaphylactic reaction (see section 13.1); mild sedation, compulsive scratching (see section 6.11.10)
Contra-indications. Urine retention, glaucoma, hyperthyroidism
Dose.
Dogs: pruritus in allergic skin disorders, *by mouth,* 4–8 mg 2–3 times daily (maximum dose 500 micrograms/kg twice daily)
Behaviour modification, *by mouth,* 220 micrograms/kg 3 times daily (maximum 1 mg/kg daily)
Premedication, *by slow intravenous injection over 1 minute,* 5–10 mg diluted in syringe with blood
Cats: pruritus in allergic skin disorders, *by mouth,* 2–4 mg twice daily
Behaviour modification, *by mouth,* 1–2 mg/cat 2–3 times daily (low dose), 2–4 mg/cat twice daily (high dose)
Premedication, *by slow intravenous injection over 1 minute,* 5–10 mg diluted in syringe with blood

Ⓗ **Chlorphenamine** (Non-proprietary)
P *Tablets,* chlorphenamine maleate 4 mg
POM *Injection,* chlorphenamine maleate 10 mg/mL; 1 mL

P Ⓗ **Piriton** (Stafford-Miller)
Tablets, chlorphenamine maleate 4 mg; 30, 500
Syrup, chlorphenamine maleate 400 micrograms/mL; 150 mL

CLEMASTINE

UK

Indications. Pruritus in allergic skin disorders
Dose. *By mouth.*
Dogs, cats: 100 micrograms/kg twice daily

P Ⓗ **Tavegil** (Novartis)
Tablets, scored, clemastine (as hydrogen fumarate) 1 mg; 50
Elixir, clemastine (as hydrogen fumarate) 100 micrograms/mL; 150 mL

DIPHENHYDRAMINE HYDROCHLORIDE

UK

Indications. Pruritus in allergic skin disorders; relief of coughing (see section 5.2.1); mild sedation (see section 6.11.10); motion sickness (see section 3.4.2)
Contra-indications. Urine retention, glaucoma, hyperthyroidism
Side-effects. CNS depression; drowsiness
Dose. *By mouth*.
Motion sickness. *Dogs*: 2–4 mg/kg 3 times daily
Pruritus. *Dogs*: 2 mg/kg 3 times daily
Sedation. *Dogs, cats*: 2–4 mg/kg 2–3 times daily

P (H) **Medinex** (Whitehall)
Syrup, diphenhydramine 2 mg/mL; 100 mL

P (H) **Nytol** (Stafford-Miller)
Tablets, diphenhydramine hydrochloride 25 mg, 50 mg; 20

HYDROXYZINE HYDROCHLORIDE

UK

Indications. Allergic disorders, in particular pruritus in allergic skin disorders
Dose. *By mouth*.
Horses: 1 mg/kg 3 times daily
Dogs: 2 mg/kg 3 times daily

POM (H) **Atarax** (Pfizer)
Tablets, s/c, hydroxyzine hydrochloride 10 mg, 25 mg; 10-mg tablets 84, 25-mg tablets 28

POM (H) **Ucerax** (UBC Pharma)
Tablets, f/c, scored, hydroxyzine hydrochloride 25 mg; 25
Syrup, hydroxyzine hydrochloride 2 mg/mL; 200 mL

14.2.3 Topical anti-inflammatory skin preparations

Topical corticosteroid preparations are used mainly to treat limited areas of diseased skin. They are useful for therapy of areas where the coat is thin and the animal is unable to remove the product by licking.

Repeated use for a prolonged period may cause excessive absorption of these drugs particularly if lesions are abraded or licked. This may result in localised skin atrophy, alopecia, and in some cases depigmentation. When used extensively and for prolonged periods, topical corticosteroids can induce impaired responses to exogenous ACTH administration and signs of localised hyperadrenocorticism. **See also section 7.2 for detailed text on the side-effects of corticosteroids.**

In the UK, topical corticosteroids are available as compound preparations with antimicrobials.

COMPOUND ANTI-INFLAMMATORY AND ANTI-MICROBIAL PREPARATIONS

These preparations should only be used for superficial, localised inflammatory lesions. Treatment should be for a short period, lasting days rather than weeks. They should not be used where a diagnosis of the underlying disorder has not been made.

UK

POM **Betsolan** (Schering-Plough)
Cream, betamethasone sodium phosphate 0.1%, neomycin sulphate 0.5%, for *dogs, cats*; 15 g
Contra-indications. Pregnant animals

Dermacool (Virbac)
Spray, benzalkonium chloride, hamamelis extract, menthol, parachlorometaxylenol, for *dogs*; 50 mL

POM **Dermobion Clear** (Fort Dodge)
Ointment, neomycin sulphate 0.5%, nitrofurazone 0.09%, prednisolone 0.25%, for *horses, dogs, cats*; 14 g
Withdrawal Periods. Should not be used on *horses* intended for human consumption
Contra-indications. Pregnant animals

POM **Dermobion Green** (Fort Dodge)
Ointment, neomycin sulphate 0.5%, nitrofurazone 0.09%, prednisolone 0.25% in ointment base containing chlorophyll, for *horses, dogs, cats*
Withdrawal Periods. Should not be used on *horses* intended for human consumption
Contra-indications. Pregnant animals

POM **Fuciderm** (Leo)
Gel, betamethasone (as valerate ester) 0.1%, fusidic acid 0.5%, for *dogs*; 5 g, 15 g, 30 g
Contra-indications. Pregnant bitches, fungal infections, deep pyoderma

POM **Hydrocortisone and Neomycin Cream Veterinary** (Millpledge)
Cream, hydrocortisone 0.5%, neomycin sulphate 0.5%, for *dogs, cats*; 15 g
Contra-indications. Not recommended for pregnant animals

POM **Panolog Ointment** (Novartis)
See section 14.8.1 for preparation details

POM **Surolan** (Janssen)
See section 14.8.1 for preparation details

POM **Vetodale** (Arnolds)
Cream, hydrocortisone 0.5%, neomycin sulphate 0.5%, for *dogs, cats*; 15 g
Contra-indications. Not recommended for pregnant animals

POM **Vetsovate** (Schering-Plough)
Cream, betamethasone valerate 0.122%, neomycin sulphate 0.5%, for *dogs, cats*; 15 g, 30 g
Contra-indications. Not recommended for pregnant animals.

Corticosteroids may produce irreversible effects in the skin; they can be absorbed and may have harmful effects, especially with frequent and extensive contact or in pregnancy. Operators should wear single-use disposable gloves when applying preparations containing a corticosteroid.

14.2.4 Essential fatty acid preparations

Essential fatty acids (EFAs) are polyunsaturated fatty acids that cannot be synthesised in the body. The parent EFAs are linoleic acid and alpha-linolenic acid, which are metabolised to form, respectively, the omega-6 and omega-3 series of fatty acids. The omega-6 series appears to be more important and is involved in epidermal barrier function, in cell membranes, and in the control of inflammation. The two series share enzymes and therefore compete with each other. Of particular significance is delta-6 desaturase, which converts linoleic acid to gamolenic acid (gamma-linolenic acid), an important precursor of substances involved in inflammation including prostaglandins, thromboxanes, and leukotrienes. The fatty acid, dihomo-gamma-linolenic acid (a derivative of gamolenic acid), is a precursor of the anti-inflammatory 1-series prostaglandins and thromboxanes. Eicosapentaenoic acid, an omega-3 fatty acid, is precursor of the 3-series which are also anti-inflammatory but not as potent as the 1-series.

Delta-6 desaturase is lacking in cats, which are therefore theoretically more susceptible to EFA deficiency. There is evidence that insufficiency of this enzyme also occurs in other circumstances including inhalant allergy and old age. Evening primrose oil, borage, and blackcurrant contain gamolenic acid. Cold water marine fish oils are rich in eicosapentaenoic acid while sunflower oil and corn oil contain linoleic acid. It is suggested that evening primrose oil may be the most efficient oil at promoting the synthesis of the anti-inflammatory 1-series eicosanoids. It is predicted that gamolenic acid and eicosapentaenoic acid should have additive or synergistic effects and there is clinical evidence to support this. Zinc, niacin, retinol (vitamin A), and vitamin C are cofactors favouring the conversion of dihomogammalinolenic acid to the anti-inflammatory 1-series. EFA deficiency leads to the development of a dry scurfy coat, hair loss, epidermal peeling and exudation, skin lichenification, and increased susceptibility to infection. Frank EFA deficiency is uncommon in animals fed normal diets but may occur as a result of gastro-intestinal malabsorption, and hepatic or pancreatic impairment. There is evidence that EFA supplementation can ameliorate allergic skin diseases, particularly atopy in the dog and can lead to improvements in coat condition. It may aid in the control of 'miliary dermatitis' (papular-crusting dermatitis) in cats.

Dietary supplementation with evening primrose oil, and with mixtures of evening primrose oil and marine fish oil have been shown to be effective in canine atopy. Although the effect appears to be dose related, optimum dosages and the most effective combinations of these oils have not yet been determined. Daily doses of 172 mg/kg of evening primrose oil with 44 mg/kg of marine fish oil have been used in dogs over periods of one year without ill effects. In cats, preliminary data indicate some efficacy in allergic skin disease at doses of evening primrose oil 0.5 to 1.0 g daily and fish oil up to 107 mg daily. Side-effects are rare and may include mild and transient diarrhoea and vomiting. These effects can be minimised and absorption of the oils increased if they are given with food. Evening primrose oil may lower the seizure threshold and should be used with caution in epileptics. If there is evidence of intolerance to fish then fish oil should be avoided. Recent studies have shown that high dosages of marine fish oil alone can be effective in reducing inflammation in canine atopy.

Proprietary preparations of EFAs are available; these may also contain vitamins and minerals.

ESSENTIAL FATTY ACIDS

UK

There are many preparations available. This is not a comprehensive list.

Complederm (Virbac)
Oral liquid, docosahexaenoic acid 4.45 mg, eicosapentaenoic acid 6.75 mg, gamolenic acid 2.02 mg, linoleic acid 460 mg/mL, vitamins, minerals,for *dogs, cats*; 250 mL
Dose. *Dogs, cats*: *by mouth*, 5–25 mL (depending on body-weight and condition) daily with food

GSL **EfaCoat**(Schering-Plough)
Capsules, gamolenic acid 20 mg, linoleic acid 182.5 mg, vitamin E 5 mg, for *dogs*; 100
Dose. *Dogs*: *by mouth*, 1–3 capsules daily; *puppies*: 1 capsule daily

GSL **EfaCoat Oil** (Schering-Plough)
Drops, gamolenic acid 18.4 mg, linoleic acid 145 mg/5 drops, vitamins, for *dogs, cats*; 30-mL dropper bottle
Dose. *Dogs*: *by mouth*, 8 drops
Cats: *by mouth*, 5 drops; *kittens*: 1–2 drops

GSL **EfaVet 330** (Schering-Plough)
Capsules, docosahexaenoic acid 3.4 mg, eicosapentaenoic acid 5.15 mg, gamolenic acid 15.4 mg, linoleic acid 138.6 mg, vitamins, minerals, for *dogs, cats*; 100
Dose. *Dogs, cats*: *by mouth*, 1 capsule/5 kg with food

GSL **EfaVet 660** (Schering-Plough)
Capsules, docosahexaenoic acid 6.8 mg, eicosapentaenoic acid 10.3 mg, gamolenic acid 30.8 mg, linoleic acid 277.2 mg, vitamins, minerals, for *dogs*; 100
Dose. *Dogs*: *by mouth*, 1 capsule/10 kg with food

GSL **EfaVet Regular** (Schering-Plough)
Capsules, docosahexaenoic acid 11.6 mg, eicosapentaenoic acid 17.3 mg, gamolenic acid 34.4 mg, linoleic acid 309.6 mg, vitamin E 10 mg, for *dogs, cats*; 50, 250
Dose. *Dogs, cats*: *by mouth*, 1 capsule/10 kg with food.
Note. For maintenance following EfaVet™ 330 or EfaVet™ 660 supplementation

GSL **EfaVet Regular High Strength** (Schering-Plough)
Capsules, docosahexaenoic acid 11.6 mg, eicosapentaenoic acid 17.3 mg, gamolenic acid 34.4 mg, linoleic acid 309.6 mg, vitamin E 10 mg, for *dogs*; 50, 250
Dose. *Dogs*: *by mouth*, 1 capsule/20 kg with food.
Note. For maintenance following EfaVet™ 660 supplementation

Efadose (Virbac)
Oral liquid, essential fatty acids, zinc, for *dogs, cats*; 250 mL

NorCoat (Norbrook)
Oral liquid, gamolenic acid,for *dogs, cats*

Nutriderm (Ceva)
Capsules, docosahexaenoic acid 12 mg, gamolenic acid 40 mg, linoleic acid 300 mg, eicosapentaenoic acid 18 mg, for *dogs, cats*; 60
Dose. *Dogs*: *by mouth*, (up to 12 kg body-weight) 1 capsule daily; (more than 12 kg body-weight) 2 capsules daily
Cats: *by mouth*, 1 capsule daily

GSL **Pet-Coat** (Pfizer)
Oral liquid, polyunsaturated fatty acids 780 mg/mL, vitamins, zinc, lecithin, for *dogs, cats*; 200 mL
Dose. *Dogs, cats*: *by mouth*, 1.25–7.5 mL

Viacutan (Boehringer Ingelheim)
Oral liquid, docosahexaenoic acid 6.6 mg, eicosapentaenoic acid 9.9 mg, gamolenic acid 105 mg, linoleic acid 190 mg, vitamin E 10 mg/unit dose, for *dogs, cats*; 70-mL dose applicator (1 unit dose = 0.55 mL)
Dose. *Dogs, cats*: *by mouth*, 1–2 dose units/10 kg

14.3 Sunscreens

Exposure of the skin to ultraviolet light causes damage which is related to the light intensity, duration of exposure, and skin sensitivity. Phototoxic reactions occur in skin with low levels of pigmentation which are not protected by the coat. The resulting solar dermatitis varies from a mild erythematous and scaling reaction to swelling with associated cysts, bullae, folliculitis, furunculosis, and scarring. Chronic light exposure may lead to the development of squamous cell carcinoma. Photosensitivity reactions are caused when photodynamic agents in the skin are exposed to ultraviolet light and cause tissue damage. Photodynamic agents may be generated by abnormalities of hepatic function, aberrant pigment synthesis, or may be derived from substances ingested (see Treatment of poisoning), injected, or absorbed through the skin. The increasing levels of ultraviolet light penetration, which are now being experienced are leading to an increasing amount of damage to the skin. Animals which spend a lot of time out of doors and which are sparsely coated or lacking in pigmentation are especially at risk.

Sun avoidance is the best solution but protective clothing and use of topically applied stains for example felt-tipped pen on depigmented nose are effective. Sunscreens which are water resistant and have a sun protection factor (SPF) of over 15 are useful and should be applied at least once daily but they do not eliminate damage totally and chronic effects may still occur. Extensively farmed pigs should be provided with a mud bath. Tattooing does not prevent sun exposure because the pigment is introduced into the dermis underneath the susceptible surface layers of the skin.

14.4 Anti-infective skin preparations

14.4.1 Topical antibacterial skin preparations
14.4.2 Topical antifungal skin preparations
14.4.3 Preparations for minor cuts and abrasions

An infection may be the principal cause of a skin condition or may be secondary to skin trauma or an underlying disorder such as an endocrine imbalance, hypersensitivity, immunosuppression, or nutritional deficiencies.

14.4.1 Topical antibacterial skin preparations

Bacteria commonly causing primary skin infections in animals include *Staphylococcus*, *Streptococcus*, and *Proteus* spp., *Escherichia coli*, and *Dermatophilus congolensis* ('mycotic' dermatitis, rain scald).

Dermatophilosis is seen in horses and ponies kept outdoors and is associated with wet weather. Ideally, affected animals should be housed; if lesions can be kept dry affected areas will regress spontaneously in several weeks. The organism remains viable in the environment and therefore crusts should be disposed of carefully. Topical treatment is often employed using topical antibacterials, zinc sulphate, copper sulphate, lime sulphur, and iodine-containing compounds. *Dermatophilus congolensis* is susceptible to many antibacterials; see below for systemic treatment.

Antibacterials incorporated into topical preparations include **chlortetracycline** and **oxytetracycline** (see section 15.1), which may be effective against superficial infections caused by bacteria including *Bacillus*, *Actinomyces*, *Clostridium*, streptococci, and staphylococci.

Fusidic acid is particularly effective against infections caused by staphylococci, *Actinomyces*, *Neisseria*, and some *Clostridium* spp.

Sulfanilamide is effective against common Gram-positive and Gram-negative skin pathogens.

An important aspect of topical therapy in skin infection is the removal of accumulated scales, crusts, and skin secretions, which provide a habitat for the bacteria and contain irritant bacterial metabolites. Therefore, shampoos (see section 14.6) containing keratolytic, keratoplastic, and degreasing agents may be useful as adjunctive treatment.

Topical antibacterial treatment may be used alone or in combination with systemic therapy. Systemic antibacterial treatment is necessary for all but the most superficial skin infections. Treatment for several weeks may be necessary. Recurrence will be seen unless the underlying cause is determined and treated.

In horses, cattle, sheep, and pigs, systemic therapy is based mainly on the penicillins, erythromycin, and potentiated sulphonamides (see section 1.1).

Cefalexin, clindamycin, amoxicillin with clavulanic acid, enrofloxacin, erythromycin, lincomycin, marbofloxacin, potentiated sulphonamides, and tylosin (see section 1.1) are indicated for skin infections in dogs and cats.

CHLORTETRACYCLINE HYDROCHLORIDE

UK

Indications. Skin infections, see notes above; hoof lesions (see section 15.1)

POM **Aureomycin Topical Powder** (Fort Dodge)
Dusting powder, chlortetracycline hydrochloride 2%, benzocaine 1%; 25 g
Withdrawal Periods. Slaughter withdrawal period nil, milk withdrawal period nil

POM **PEP** (Intervet)
Dusting powder, chlortetracycline hydrochloride 2%, benzocaine 1%; 25 g
Withdrawal Periods. Slaughter withdrawal period nil, milk withdrawal period nil

FUSIDIC ACID

UK

Indications. Skin infections caused by Gram-positive bacteria, see notes above; otitis externa (see section 14.8)

POM Ⓗ **Fucidin** (Leo)
Cream, fusidic acid 2%; 15 g, 30 g
Gel, fusidic acid 2%; 15 g, 30 g
Ointment, sodium fusidate 2%; 15 g, 30 g

SULFANILAMIDE
(Sulphanilamide)

UK
Indications. Skin infections, see notes above
Warnings. Safety in pregnant and lactating animals has not been established

PML **Negasunt** (Bayer)
Dusting powder, coumafos 3%, propoxur 2%, sulfanilamide 5%, for *horses*
Withdrawal Periods. Should not be used on *horses* intended for human consumption
Note. Product contains an organophosphorus compound and a carbamate; operators should wear protective clothing

14.4.2 Topical antifungal skin preparations

Most fungal infections of the skin and keratin structures of domestic animals are caused by *Trichophyton* and *Microsporum* spp. They are commonly referred to as ringworm and are zoonotic infections. *Malassezia pachydermatis* (*Pityrosporum canis*) is a cause of pruritic skin disease in dogs, particularly in seborrhoeic conditions and in otitis externa. *Candida albicans* infection causes mucocutaneous ulcerations in dogs and is rare.

Ringworm is usually a self-limiting disease. Drug therapy can often shorten the duration of the disease although in some species, notably long-haired cats and dogs, response to treatment may be poor. Paronychial infections may also be refractory to treatment.

The success of drug therapy depends on additional management aimed at reducing and limiting infection such as careful clipping around the lesions in dogs and cats, limiting grooming, isolating the animal, and using antifungal washes on the affected animal and local environment.

Griseofulvin and **ketoconazole** are used for systemic treatment of ringworm (see section 1.2). Ketoconazole is effective in *Malassezia pachydermatis* infection of the skin. **Itraconazole** (see section 1.2) is also effective against ringworm in dogs and cats and appears to be much less hepatotoxic and associated with fewer side-effects than ketoconazole. Insufficient information is available at present to provide guidance on the use of terbinafine.

Topical antifungals may be used for the treatment of ringworm, although drug toxicity due to ingestion through self-grooming, the necessity for clipping of the fur, and repeated application and limited efficacy of the preparation should be taken into account.

Topical **enilconazole** and **ketoconazole** are effective for *Malassezia pachydermatis* infection. However, the treatment of choice is a shampoo containing chlorhexidine and **miconazole** (Malaseb, Leo). Selenium sulphide containing shampoo (see section 14.5.1) may also be effective. Topical enilconazole or miconazole may be used in conjunction with systemic griseofulvin for the treatment of ringworm.

Povidone-iodine (see section 14.7.1) is also used as a fungicide.

Natamycin is a polyene antifungal antibacterial, which may be used for topical treatment and also for disinfection of the ringworm-contaminated environment and horse tackle.

A vaccine is available for immunisation against ringworm in cattle (see section 18.2.14).

ENILCONAZOLE

UK
Indications. Ringworm, *Malassezia pachydermatis*◆ infection
Dose.
Horses: *by wash*, 0.2% solution every 3 days for 4 applications
Cattle: *by wash or spray*, 0.2% solution every 3 days for 3–4 applications
Dogs: *by wash or dip*, 0.2% solution every 3 days for 4 applications

P **Imaverol** (Janssen)
Liquid concentrate, enilconazole 10%, for *horses, cattle, dogs*; 100 mL. To be diluted before use
Withdrawal Periods. Should not be used on *horses* intended for human consumption. *Cattle*: slaughter withdrawal period nil, milk withdrawal period nil
Dilute 1 volume in 50 volumes water (= enilconazole 0.2%)

KETOCONAZOLE

UK
Indications. *Malassezia pachydermatis* infection
Warnings. Use with caution in pregnant animals, hepatic impairment

P Ⓗ **Nizoral** (Johnson & Johnson MSD)
Shampoo, ketoconazole 2%; 120 mL

NorClear (Norbrook)
Shampoo, ketoconazole 1%, for *dogs, cats*

MICONAZOLE

UK
Indications. Seborrhoeic dermatitis associated with *Malassezia pachydermatis* infection and *Staphylococcus intermedius* infection in dogs; aid in control and treatment of ringworm in conjunction with systemic griseofulvin in cats
Warnings. Puppies or kittens should not come in contact with treated nursing bitches or queens until the coat has dried. Exceptionally a dog with atopy or a cat with allergic skin disease may develop a pruritic reaction after treatment; maximum treatment length in cats is 16 weeks; should only be used in conjunction with griseofulvin in cats

POM **Malaseb** (Leo)
Shampoo, chlorhexidine gluconate 2%, miconazole nitrate 2%, for *dogs, cats*; 250 mL

NATAMYCIN

UK
Indications. Ringworm
Warnings. Treated animals should not be exposed to sunlight for several hours; use galvanised or plastic containers because natamycin reacts with metals such as copper

Dose. *Horses, cattle*: *by spray*, using 1 litre per adult animal, or local application, 0.01% solution, repeat after 4–5 days and again after 14 days if required

PML **Mycophyt** (Intervet)
Suspension, powder for reconstitution and dilution, natamycin 0.01%, for *horses, cattle*; 2 g, 10 g
Reconstitute and dilute with 2 litres (for 2-g bottle) water or 10 litres (for 10-g bottle) water (= natamycin 0.01%)
Withdrawal Periods. Slaughter withdrawal period nil, milk withdrawal period nil
Note. May also be used for environmental contamination

14.4.3 Preparations for minor cuts and abrasions

These preparations are used to treat minor skin infections and abrasions, and to prevent infection following surgery or when dehorning. They are applied as necessary in the form of dusting powders, ointments, or sprays. Preparations containing benzoic acid, cresol, or phenols should not be used on cats.

UK

GSL **Aeroclens** (Battle Hayward & Bower)
Aerosol spray, benzalkonium chloride 1.61%, suitable dye; 150 g
Withdrawal Periods. Slaughter withdrawal period nil, milk withdrawal period nil

GSL **Antiseptic Ointment** (Bob Martin)
Ointment, chloroxylenol 2%, oil of camphor 4%, salicylic acid 0.5%, terebene 1%, for *dogs, cats*; 50 g

Cetrimide Cream
Cetrimide 0.5% in a suitable water-miscible basis such as cetostearyl alcohol 5%, liquid paraffin 50% in freshly boiled and cooled purified water

GSL **Cetream** (Pettifer)
Cream, cetrimide 0.5%, for *horses*; 400 g

GSL **Green Oils** (Pettifer)
Liquid, arachis oil 36.03%, chloroxylenol 0.27%, gum turpentine 31.71%, for *horses*; 250 mL, 500 mL

GSL **Green Oils Healing Gel** (Pettifer)
Gel, camphor 0.43%, chloroxylenol 0.2%, eucalyptus oil 0.87%, for *horses*; 400 g

GSL **Kitzyme Veterinary Antiseptic Ointment** (Seven Seas)
Ointment, chloroxylenol 0.7%, coal tar 0.91%, ichthammol 6.95%, zinc oxide 1.88%, for *cats*; 25 g

GSL **Kitzyme Veterinary Antiseptic Powder** (Seven Seas)
Dusting powder, chloroxylenol 1.25%, salicylic acid 2.2%, for *cats*; 25 g
Contra-indications. Cats less than 6 months of age, nursing queens

GSL **Otodex Skin Cream** (Petlife)
Cream, chlorocresol 0.5%, phenoxyethanol 0.72%, lidocaine hydrochloride 0.05%, zinc oxide 9%, for *dogs, cats*; 35 g

GSL **Hydrophane Protocon Gold** (Battle Hayward & Bower)
Gel, sulphur 10%, salicylic acid 10%, for *horses*; 250 g
Withdrawal Periods. Should not be used on *horses* intended for human consumption
Contra-indications. Application to racehorses within 12 hours of competing or white heels; bandaging of treated areas

GSL **Saniphor** (Battle Hayward & Bower)
Spray, available iodine (as povidone-iodine) 0.5%, for *horses*; 240 mL
Withdrawal Periods. Should not be used on *horses* intended for human consumption

GSL **Veterinary Antiseptic Spray** (Battle Hayward & Bower)
Aerosol spray, benzalkonium chloride 1.61%, for *sheep*; 150 g
Withdrawal Periods. Slaughter withdrawal period nil, milk withdrawal period nil

GSL **Veterinary Wound Powder** (Battle Hayward & Bower)
Dusting powder, chloramine 2%, for *horses*; 20 g, 125 g

GSL **Vetodex** (Arnolds)
Cream, chlorocresol 0.5%, lidocaine hydrochloride 0.05%, phenoxyethanol 0.72%, zinc oxide 9%, for *dogs, cats*; 35 g

GSL **Vet-Ointment** (Johnson's)
Ointment, zinc oxide 19.8%, for *dogs, cats*; 40 g

GSL **Vetzyme Veterinary Antiseptic Lotion** (Seven Seas)
Liquid, cetrimide 0.5%, fenticlor 0.1%; 100 mL. Dilute before use

GSL **Vetzyme Veterinary Antiseptic Ointment** (Seven Seas)
Ointment, chloroxylenol 0.7%, coal tar 0.91%, ichthammol 6.95%, zinc oxide 1.88%, for *dogs, cats*; 25 g

GSL **Vetzyme Veterinary Antiseptic Powder** (Seven Seas)
Dusting powder, chloroxylenol 1.25%, salicylic acid 2.2%; 25 g

GSL **Vetzyme Veterinary Skin Cream** (Seven Seas)
Cream, cetrimide 0.5%, for *dogs, cats*; 30 g

GSL **Woundcare Powder** (Animalcare)
Dusting powder, chloramine PhEur 2%, for *dogs, cats*; 20 g

14.5 Keratolytic and keratoplastic agents

14.5.1 Keratolytics
14.5.2 Retinoids
14.5.3 Caustic agents

Primary keratinisation disorders are skin diseases in which excessive scale formation occurs in epidermal structures including the hair follicle and interfollicular epidermis. They manifest as blocked follicles (comedones), superficial scale (dry, waxy, or greasy seborrhoea), and follicular casts. Secondary superficial bacterial and yeast (*Malassezia pachydermatis*) infections commonly occur. Treatment of primary keratinisation disorders may involve the use of topical or systemic substances. Topical treatments include keratolytic shampoos and antimicrobials. Systemic treatments include vitamins and minerals, in particular zinc, and essential fatty acids (see section 14.2.2). Oral and topical retinoid therapy is also used for the treatment and control of some of these conditions.

14.5.1 Keratolytics

Keratolytics promote the loosening or separation of the horny layer of the epidermis. Keratoplastic agents are substances which can modify and normalise the process of keratinisation. In order to exert this action they must be capable of penetrating into the living epidermis when applied topically; penetration is influenced by the concentration of the active agent and duration of exposure.

Coal tar, **sulphur**, and **salicylic acid** have keratoplastic actions. **Selenium sulphide** has antiseborrhoeic properties. **Benzoyl peroxide** has mild keratolytic properties. Its antimicrobial action is probably due to its oxidising effect. Irritant and allergic reactions may occur, particularly with concentrations above 3%.

Calamine has mild astringent and antipruritic actions. **Zinc oxide** acts as mild astringent and is available as compound zinc paste (see section 14.1).

In severely greasy or scaly seborrhoeic conditions, powerful keratolytic and keratoplastic preparations containing tar, sulphur, and salicylic acid are indicated. However, dermatitis caused by *Malassezia* infection must be eliminated from the differential diagnosis before keratolytic shampoos are used. In milder conditions preparations containing only salicylic acid and sulphur are appropriate. Shampoos containing tar, sulphur, or salicylic acid may have a drying effect and if not formulated to combat this may require the subsequent use of moisturisers. Often two applications of shampoo are recommended which allows degreasing and removal of superficial scale at the first application and increased penetration at the second. Prolonged exposure to the active ingredients before rinsing allows penetration and is particularly important for keratoplastic action and to permit penetration of active ingredients in the hair follicles. Manufacturer's instructions on the duration of exposure should be carefully observed except in animals with sensitive skin when the duration of treatment should be reduced.

BENZOYL PEROXIDE

UK

Indications. Canine dermatitis, pyoderma, seborrhoeic dermatitis
Side-effects. See notes above
Warnings. Operators should wear impervious gloves when applying shampoo

POM **Paxcutol** (Virbac)
Shampoo, benzoyl peroxide 2.5%, for *dogs*; 200 mL

SELENIUM SULPHIDE

UK

Indications. Skin cleansing
Warnings. Operators should wear impervious gloves when applying shampoo

GSL **Seleen** (Ceva)
Shampoo, selenium sulphide 1%, for *dogs*; 150 mL

COMPOUND ANTIPRURITIC AND KERATO-LYTIC PREPARATIONS

UK

Coal Tar Solution, BP
Coal tar 20%, polysorbate '80' 5%, in alcohol
Contra-indications. Cats

P **Dermisol Cream** (Pfizer)
See section 14.8.2 for preparation details

P **Dermisol Multicleanse Solution** (Pfizer)
See section 14.8.2 for preparation details

GSL **Golden-Coat** (Shep-Fair)
Gel, salicylic acid 1.5%, sulphur 10%, for *dogs, cats*; 60 g

GSL **Golden-Mane** (Shep-Fair)
Gel, salicylic acid 1.5%, sulphur 10%, for *horses*; 350 g

Kerect (Vericore VP)
Shampoo, salicylic acid 2%, sulphur 2%, for *dogs*; 180 mL

Sebolytic (Virbac)
Shampoo, coal tar 3%, salicylic acid 2%, sulphur 2%, for *dogs*; 200 mL
Contra-indications. Cats

Sebomild (Virbac)
Shampoo, salicylic acid 2%, sodium thiosulphate 5%, for *dogs, cats*; 200 mL

Tarlite (Vericore VP)
Shampoo, solubilised tar 3%, salicylic acid 2%, sulphur 2%, for *dogs*; 180 mL

14.5.2 Retinoids

Isotretinoin is used in Schnauzer comedo syndrome, sebaceous adenitis, and other diseases of the hair follicles and associated glands. **Tretinoin** can be used topically to control idiopathic nasal hyperkeratosis, ear margin dermatosis, and acanthosis nigrans in dogs, and severe canine and feline chin acne. **Etretinate** was used in the management of primary disorders of keratinisation but is no longer available. **Acitretin**, a metabolite of etretinate, has recently become available but has not been fully evaluated for use in dogs.

ISOTRETINOIN

Note. Isotretinoin is an isomer of tretinoin

UK

Indications. Primary keratinisation disorders; see notes above
Contra-indications. Breeding animals
Side-effects. Keratoconjunctivitis sicca; joint and leg pain; mild elevation of serum-cholesterol, triglycerides, and alanine aminotransferase concentrations; inhibition of spermatogenesis; possible extended teratogenic effect as a result of tissue storage for long periods
Warning. Monitor changes in haematology, blood biochemistry, urine and tear production, and long bones
Dose. *Dogs*: by mouth, 1–2 mg/kg daily for 8–12 weeks for control then reduce to alternate day therapy if possible

POM (H) **Roaccutane** (Roche)
Capsules, isotretinoin 5 mg, 20 mg; 56
Note. Preparations of isotretinoin are not generally available. A written order, stating case details, should be sent to the manufacturer to obtain a supply of the preparation.

TRETINOIN

UK

Indications. Primary keratinisation disorders; see notes above
Side-effects. Occasional allergic or irritant reaction, particularly in cats
Warning. Gloves should be worn when applying the preparations; should not be applied by pregnant women
Dose. *Dogs, cats*: apply daily until remission then as necessary for maintenance

POM (H) **Retin-A** (Janssen-Cilag)
Cream, tretinoin 0.025%; 60 g
Gel, tretinoin 0.01%, 0.025%; 60 g
Lotion, tretinoin 0.025%; 100 mL

14.6 Shampoos

Shampoos are used as complementary therapy in association with other treatment or as sole preparations in the long-term management of certain disorders such as seborrhoea. They help to clean the skin and remove crusts and debris. Shampoos are formulated to reduce any irritant effects and are generally well tolerated. Effective rinsing is essential after the recommended contact time.

Shampoos are available for general cleansing, conditioning, and moisturising. They are formulated to be used alone or in combination or with other treatments for skin disorders. These preparations may also have emollient, humectant, cooling, antiseptic, keratoplastic, keratolytic, astringent, or antipruritic properties. Proprietary preparations are listed in Table 14.1. Ectoparasiticide-containing shampoos are given in section 2.2. The efficacy of these is limited particularly for the control of flea infestation.

14.5.3 Caustic agents

Sodium hydroxide is a powerful caustic. Preparations are available for removal of embryo horn in calves not more than 7 days of age.

SODIUM HYDROXIDE

UK

Indications. Disbudding
Warnings. Operator must wear protective clothing; do not allow paste to become wet after application; keep cow and calf separated for 0.5 hour after application

PML **Hornex Calf Dehorning Paste** (Hornex)
Paste, sodium hydoxide 42.7%, for *calves not more than 7 days of age*

14.7 Wound management

14.7.1 Skin cleansers and disinfectants
14.7.2 Preparations for wound management

The objective of any wound management regimen is to heal the wound in the shortest time possible and with minimum pain and discomfort to the patient.

Open wounds (abrasions, lacerations, avulsions, ballistic, penetrating, hernias, and excised or surgical wounds) are most common in the domestic species and are characterised by a break in the skin. Closed wounds include contusions, bruises, ruptures, and sprains. Any wound may be classified according to the number of skin layers affected. Damage limited to the epidermis is regarded as a superficial wound which will heal rapidly by regeneration of epithelial cells. A partial thickness wound involves the deeper dermal layer and includes vessel damage. Its repair is more complex. A full thickness wound affects the subcutaneous fat layer and beyond. Its healing will require the synthesis of new connective tissue and it takes longer to heal because it contracts, whereas partial thickness wounds do not.

Wound healing follows a specific sequence of phases which result ultimately in connective tissue repair and the formation of a fibrous scar. The first phase is the inflammatory (reaction) phase which is followed by the proliferative (repair) phase, and finally by the maturation (regeneration) phase. The whole process may take from three weeks to two years with connective tissue (granulation tissue) developing about four days after the original injury. In the distal limb, particularly of horses, large tissue deficits may lead to the production of excessive, exuberant granulation tissue. The precise cause of this condition is not known but some of the factors involved are thought to be increased movement, lack of soft tissue covering, excessive contamination, and a reduction in blood supply. The use of effective pressure bandaging or cast application should be encouraged. The management of excessive granulation tissue varies and includes topical steroid/antibacterial ointments, pressure bandaging, sharp excision, or caustic astringent solutions. Many wounds of the trunk and upper limbs heal well by secondary intention with good cosmetic results but those of the distal extremities tend to heal slowly with production of excessive scar tissue and skin grafting is often useful.

Both systemic and local factors may challenge the successful continuation of each of the stages of wound repair. The systemic factors include the nutritional status of the animal, concurrent therapy such as corticosteroids, prostaglandin inhibition, oncolytic agents, and clinical conditions such as anaemia and diabetes.

The objectives of wound care are to prepare the wound for surgical closure while minimising the risk of wound infection or to control wound infection thereby promoting wound healing by secondary intention. The aim of any treatment is to return the animal to normal function and cosmetic appearance. The selection of the wound treatments for each particular case involves many interdependent factors. The duration of the injury is important because wounds have a better prognosis the sooner they are sutured or treated. The cause of the injury will influence the prognosis for healing and also the likelihood of infection. Sharp lacerations are generally less prone to infection than shearing wounds caused by barbed wire, bite wounds, or degloving. Previous treatment by the owner, for example the over-enthusiastic use of antiseptics or local antibiotics, may mean that the wound may no longer undergo primary closure by suturing. The location, depth and configuration of the wound; the degree of contamination; other systemic factors; the intended use of the animal; and the co-operation of the patient and the owner should also be considered.

14.7.1 Skin cleansers and disinfectants

The preparation of any wound before treatment is of fundamental importance. The hair should be clipped from a wide area around wound edges. Hair clippings which may enter

Table 14.1 Shampoos

Drug	Conditions	Preparations
Antibacterials		
Benzoyl peroxide[1]	Pyoderma	Paxcutol (Virbac)
Chlorhexidine	Skin cleansing	Nolvasan (Fort Dodge)
Ethyl lactate	Superficial pyoderma	Dermacleanse (Novatis), Etiderm (Virbac)
Hexetidine	Skin cleansing	Hexocil (Pharmacia & Upjohn)
Antifungal drugs		
Ketoconazole	*Malassezia pachydermatis* infection	Ⓗ Nizoral (Johnson & Johnson MSD), NorClear (Norbrook)
Miconazole/chlorhexidine	Seborrhoeic dermatitis	Malaseb (Leo)
Ectoparasiticides		
See section 2.2.2.4 for preparations containing permethrin or pyrethrins; see section 2.2.2.2 for preparations containing carbaril		
Keratolytic and keratoplastic agents		
Benzoyl peroxide[1]	Pyoderma, 'seborrhoea'	Paxcutol (Virbac)
Salicylic acid/sulphur/tar[1]	'Seborrhoea'	Sebolytic (Virbac), Tarlite (Vericore VP)
Salicylic acid/sulphur	Mild 'seborrhoea'	Kerect (Vericore VP)
Salicylic acid	Mild 'seborrhoea'	Sebomild (Virbac)
Selenium sulphide	Mild 'seborrhoea'	Seleen (Sanofi)
Skin cleansers		
	Normal to sensitive skins	Clenderm Cream or Lotion (Vétoquinol), Dermacleanse (Vericore VP), Dermasoothe (Vericore VP), Epi-Soothe (Virbac), Hylashine Shampoo (Vericore VP), Logic Dry Shampoo (Ceva), Sebocalm (Virbac)
Moisturisers		
		Humilac Spray (Virbac)

[1] May be drying and irritant to the skin

the wound are very difficult to remove and may be regarded as foreign bodies whose presence will lead to an increase in wound healing time. The wound should be protected during clipping by either the insertion of sterile moist swabs which are easily removed, or Ⓗ K-Y Jelly (Johnson & Johnson) which will be subsequently rinsed off with sterile sodium chloride 0.9% solution (Normal saline).

Alcohol 70% is commonly used for its solvent properties for the removal of superficial contamination. **Benzalkonium chloride**, **cetrimide**, and **povidone-iodine** are used for skin disinfection.

Contaminated wounds should be thoroughly lavaged with isotonic solutions such as sodium chloride 0.9% solution (Normal saline) or Ringer's solution. If the wound is less than three hours old, antibacterials in the lavage solution decrease the occurrence of wound infection. After three hours antibacterials in lavage are no more effective than lavage alone. All gross contamination should be removed if possible but lavage should not be continued excessively as this will cause tissue maceration.

Infected wounds should be treated with hypertonic solutions such as magnesium sulphate 10% solution or paste (see section 14.1), or sodium chloride 5% to 10% solution. Following removal of debris, necrotic or obviously devitalised tissue should be surgically debrided. Multiple debridements are often necessary. Antibacterial therapy and tetanus prophylaxis in horses are essential.

Non-surgical debridement involves use of agents such as Ⓗ Intrasite Gel (S & N Hlth), Ⓗ Debrisan (Pharmacia & Upjohn), or Ⓗ Aserbine (Forley) which remove debris from a wound via the establishment of an osmotic gradient within the wound without damage to new granulation tissue. Although still often used in animals, wet to dry bandaging of wounds for non-surgical debridement is contraindicated. This procedure involves the use of moistened gauze swabs packed into the wound and covered by open wove bandage or gauze and allowed to dry. When dry, removal of the packing will inevitably lead to destruction of some regenerating healthy tissue.

ALCOHOL

UK
Indications. Skin preparation before injection or surgery
Warnings. Flammable; avoid broken skin

Industrial Methylated Spirit
A mixture of 19 volumes of alcohol of an appropriate strength with 1 volume of approved wood naphtha

Surgical Spirit
Methyl salicylate 0.5 mL, diethyl phthalate 2 mL, castor oil 2.5 mL, Industrial Methylated Spirit to 100 mL

BENZALKONIUM CHLORIDE

UK
Indications. Skin disinfection
Contra-indications. Concurrent use of soaps and anionic detergents

Marinol-10% Blue (Vericore VP)
Liquid concentrate, benzalkonium chloride 10%, 5 litres. To be diluted before use
Dilute 1 volume with 100 volumes water for skin disinfection

CETRIMIDE

UK
Indications. Skin disinfection; footrot (see section 15.1)
Contra-indications. See under Benzalkonium chloride

Cetrimide Solution
Cetrimide 1% in freshly boiled and cooled purified water
Use undiluted

Cetrimide Solution Strong
A 20% to 40% aqueous solution of cetrimide, containing not more than 10% alcohol, isopropyl alcohol, or industrial methylated spirit. It may be perfumed and may contain colouring matter
Used to prepare cetrimide solution

CHLORHEXIDINE

UK
Indications. Skin disinfection and cleansing
Contra-indications. See under Benzalkonium chloride

Hibiscrub Veterinary (Schering-Plough)
Solution, Chlorhexidine Gluconate Solution BP 20% (= chlorhexidine gluconate 4%); 5litres

Nolvasan Surgical Scrub (Fort Dodge)
Solution, chlorhexidine acetate 2%; 3.75 litres

Nolvasan Shampoo (Fort Dodge)
Shampoo, chlorhexidine acetate 0.5%, for **horses, dogs, cats**; 230 mL, 5 litres

GSL Savlon Veterinary Antiseptic Concentrate (Schering-Plough)
Liquid concentrate, Chlorhexidine Gluconate Solution BP 7.5% (= chlorhexidine gluconate 1.5%), cetrimide 15%; 5 litres. To be diluted before use
Dilute 1 volume with 30 volumes alcohol 70% for skin disinfection
Dilute 1 volume with 100 volumes water for wound cleansing

Vetasept Chlorhexidine Skin Scrub Blue (Animalcare)
Solution, chlorhexidine gluconate 0.5%, industrial methylated spirits 70%; 500 mL, 4.5 litres

HEXETIDINE

UK
Indications. Skin cleansing

Hexocil (Pharmacia & Upjohn)
Shampoo, hexetidine 0.55%; 125 mL, 2.25 litres

HYDROGEN PEROXIDE

UK
Indications. Skin cleansing and disinfection of wounds

Hydrogen Peroxide Solution 3%
Hydrogen peroxide (10 volumes)
To be diluted before use, see notes above

IODINE COMPOUNDS

UK
Indications. Skin disinfection
Contra-indications. Concurrent use of other antiseptics or detergents

Pevidine Antiseptic Solution (Vericore VP)
Solution, available iodine (as povidone-iodine) 1%; 500 mL, 5 litres. May be diluted before use
Use undiluted for wound cleansing

Pevidine Surgical Scrub (Vericore VP)
Solution, available iodine (as povidone-iodine) 0.75%; 500 mL, 5 litres
Use undiluted for skin disinfection

Vetasept Povidone-Iodine Alcoholic Tincture (Animalcare)
Solution, available iodine (as povidone-iodine) 1%; 500 mL, 5 litres

Vetasept Povidone-Iodine Antiseptic Solution (Animalcare)
Solution, available iodine (as povidone-iodine) 1%; 500 mL, 5 litres

SODIUM CHLORIDE

UK
Indications. Skin and wound cleansing

Aquspray (Animalcare)
Aerosol spray, sodium chloride 0.9%; 200 mL

14.7.2 Preparations for wound management

14.7.2.1 Vapour permeable adhesive films
14.7.2.2 Foam dressings
14.7.2.3 Hydrogel dressings
14.7.2.4 Xerogel dressings
14.7.2.5 Hydrocolloid dressings

Veterinary wound management is still in its infancy. If a wound cannot be closed primarily because of a large soft tissue defect or if the wound is infected then closure must be delayed and the wound bandaged. The type of bandage applied to open wounds varies depending on whether additional debridement is necessary and to what degree movement will disrupt wound healing.

'Passive' materials, which plug and conceal, such as gauze, gamgee tissue, and absorbent cotton now have limited application in wound management. 'Interactive' materials such as the hydrocolloids, hydrogels, foams, and films are now used to enhance the healing cascade by controlling the micro-environment surrounding the wound and thus promote wound healing. 'Bioactive' materials are now being developed which will lead to improved healing by direct stimulation of one or more steps in the healing cascade.

Wounds need to be continually assessed at all stages of the healing process and an appropriate dressing regimen devised for the wound at the time. No single dressing will meet all the criteria required in all of the healing stages. Local factors which delay healing may be avoided by providing products which will produce the optimal micro-environment for healing. This micro-environment should be moist at the wound interface but remove excess exudate to avoid sloughing. The tissue temperature should be maintained and the injury protected from infective organisms, foreign particles, and toxic compounds. In addition, when the dressing is changed there should be no secondary trauma due to adherence.

The products used for wound management are categorised by the materials from which the dressings are made. They have the ability to create or maintain a moist local environment for wound healing. They have variable absorbent and adhesive properties, conformability, and ability to rehydrate necrotic tissue.

A primary dressing is one which is placed in direct contact with the surface of the wound whereas a secondary dressing is a material which covers a primary dressing and holds it in place. An island dressing comprises a central absorbent pad surrounded by an adhesive area.

Unfortunately, the current presentation, packaging, and size ranges of the available products may present difficulties for use in veterinary wound management.

14.7.2.1 Vapour-permeable films

These are polymeric, transparent films coated on one side with an adhesive. The adhesive is inactivated by contact with moisture and will not therefore stick to moist skin or the wound bed. These films are permeable to water vapour, oxygen, and carbon dioxide but occlusive to water and bacteria. The film retains a moist environment at the surface of the wound, allowing epithelium regeneration to occur more rapidly.

Vapour permeable films are used in wounds in which granulation tissue is established and wound exudate is declining. In animals, the rate of hair growth (which regrows at approximately twice the rate of human hair) can prove to be a problem both with maintenance of adhesion and removal of the dressing. Careful monitoring of the film while it is in use is essential.

UK
Bioclusive (Johnson & Johnson Medical)

Cutifilm (Beiersdorf, TSK)

Opsite Flexigrid (Hillcross Pharms)

Tegaderm (3M Health Care)

14.7.2.2 Foam dressings

These materials vary from foamed polymers that have been made into sheets to silicone foams which are formed *in situ* and used to treat large cavity wounds (Allevyn Cavity). The wound contact layer of sheet dressings is often heat-treated to give a smooth surface which absorbs fluids by capillarity. Foaming the polymer creates small, open cells which are able to hold fluids. Foam dressings have a non-adherent wound contact surface and are also available as adhesive island dressings and cavity fillers.

Foam dressings are used for wounds with moderate to heavy exudation. Their structure and softness also provide a cushion which protects and contributes to thermal insulation of the wound. They may be tailored for difficult areas. The non-adhesive foams will require a secondary dressing. Hydropolymer foam expands into the contours of the wound as it absorbs fluid. The material is used in an island configuration with an adhesive dressing (Tielle). The product can re-adhere once lifted enabling manipulation of the dressing for fit or assessment of the wound without dressing change. The hydropolymer wicks fluid into the upper layers of the dressing where it escapes through the backing. The dressing is used for dynamic fluid management for heavily exuding wounds or where extended periods between dressings changes are desirable.

UK

Allevyn (S & N Hlth)

Allevyn Cavity (S & N Hlth)

Cutinova Foam (Beiersdorf, TSK)

Lyofoam (SSL International)

Tielle (Johnson & Johnson Medical; distributed by Janssen Veterinary)

14.7.2.3 Hydrogel dressings

Sheet hydrogel dressings (Geliperm) are sheets of three dimensional networks of cross-linked hydrophilic polymers. Their formulation may incorporate up to 96% bound water but they are insoluble in water and interact by three-dimensional swelling with aqueous solutions. The polymer physically entraps water to form a solid sheet which may make them feel moist but compression of the sheet will not release any water. They have a thermal capacity which provides initial cooling to the wound surface. This plus occlusion transiently reduces pain. A secondary dressing is required.

Sheet hydrogel dressings are used on thermal or other painful wounds and inflamed skin where the avoidance of topical agents is indicated.

Amorphous hydrogel dressings are similar in composition to sheet hydrogels but the polymer has not been cross-linked. They do not have cooling properties. A secondary dressing is required. They are used for hydration of dry, sloughy, or necrotic wounds and autolytic debridement.

UK

Geliperm (Geistlich)

Intrasite Gel (S & N Hlth)

Nugel (Johnson & Johnson Medical; distributed by Janssen Veterinary)

Purilon Gel (Coloplast)

Sterigel (SSL International)

14.7.2.4 Xerogel dressings

These materials have no water in their formulation but swell to form a gel when in contact with aqueous solutions. A biodegradable gel is formed via ion exchange when the fibre is in contact with exudate and the calcium contributes to the clotting mechanism. The gel is removed with saline. Alginate dressings are flat, non-woven pads of either calcium sodium alginate fibre or pure alginate fibre. The alginate wound contact layer may be bonded to a secondary absorbent viscose pad. Alginate hanks, packing and ribbon dressings are available for deeper cavity wounds and sinuses. Alginates have been shown to be effective in the management of injuries where there has been substantial tissue loss as in degloving injuries and have reduced the number of surgical procedures which could normally have been expected in addition to accelerating healing. The non-adhesive formulations will require a secondary dressing.

Xerogel dressings are used in lacerations, post-operative wounds, donor sites, and in the management of non-bleeding wounds such as second degree burns or heavily exuding wounds where long periods are required between dressing changes.

Dextranomers (Debrisan) are xerogel polymers of polysaccharide dextran and are available as beads or paste. These are used for debridement of moist sloughy wounds whether clean or infected and small area burns.

Collagen-containing xerogels contain collagen of bovine origin which is non-antigenic due to enzyme purification. Addition of collagen to a wound bed may accelerate wound repair by the provision of a matrix for cellular migration. The dry materials absorb exudate to form a gel. The materials require a secondary dressing. They are recommended for use in any recalcitrant wound and moist sloughy wounds and ulcers whether clean or infected, and small area burns.

UK

Algosteril (Beiersdorf, TSK)

Algisite M (S & N Hlth)

Comfeel SeaSorb Filler (Coloplast)

Debrisan (Pharmacia & Upjohn)

Kaltostat (Convatec)

Sorbsan (Maersk Medical)

Tegagen (3M Healthcare)

14.7.2.5 Hydrocolloid dressings

These dressings are flexible, highly absorbent, occlusive or semi-occlusive adhesive pads formulated from hydrophilic polymers incorporated into a hydrophobic adhesive. The dressings may be backed by a polymeric film and may be contoured to fit difficult areas. However, they fail to adhere to muscular areas of greater flexion such as the neck or shoulders for a significant period. The pads do not require a secondary dressing.

When used to treat veterinary wounds, hydrocolloid dressings applied to relatively immobile muscular areas have resulted in a decrease of up to 30% in healing time from injury to hair growth. The dressings are removed by soaking with sodium chloride 0.9% (Normal saline).

Hydrocolloids dressings are used for wounds with moderate exudate such as pressure sores, minor burns, granulating wounds, and wounds exhibiting slough or necrotic tissue. Hydrocolloids pastes are used in conjunction with dressings for cavity wounds and heavily exuding wounds.

Superabsorbent hydrocolloid dressings (Combiderm) have a highly absorbent capacity and entrap exudate. These products incorporate the highly absorbent material into an island pad which is covered by a nonwoven absorbent and surrounded by an extra thin hydrocolloid as the adhesive portion. The covering acts as a transfer layer while its surface stays dry. This is used for heavily exuding ulcers.

Hydrofibre hydrocolloid dressings (Aquacel) are nonwoven pads which form a gel in contact with fluid. The resultant gel is similar to a sheet hydrogel which does not dry out or wick laterally. Therefore there is no maceration of the skin surrounding the wound but moisture is maintained in contact with the wound bed. The highly absorbent capacity reduces the frequency of dressing changes. They are used for heavily exuding wounds or wounds where an extended wear time is desired.

UK

Aquacel (Convatec)

AquaForm Hydrogel (TSK)

Combiderm (Convatec)

Comfeel (Coloplast)

Granuflex (Convatec)

Granugel (Convatec)

Tegasorb (3M Healthcare)

14.8 Preparations for the ear

14.8.1 Anti-infective ear preparations
14.8.2 Ear cleansers and sebolytics

Diseases of the pinna and external ear canal more commonly affect the smaller species of domestic animals. These structures are specialised extensions of the skin and almost any dermatological disease can affect this region.

The pinna is a site of skin disease due to various causative agents, including ectoparasitic, allergic, nutritional, and auto-immune disorders. In all species the pinna may become inflamed as a result of insect bites. Self-inflicted trauma frequently complicates any painful or pruritic disorder of the pinna.

The principal disorder of the ear canal is otitis externa. This is a multifactorial disorder with a variety of possible causes and, without proper investigation and treatment, many cases may become chronic. Chronic inflammation of the external ear canal can result in perforation of the tympanic membrane and subsequent otitis media. Otitis externa commonly affects dogs, especially those breeds with pendulous ears such as spaniels and those predisposed to allergic skin dis-

ease and keratinisation defects. The prevalence of ear disease is significantly lower in cats and farm animals.

A variety of micro-organisms may act as opportunistic pathogens. The bacteria most often isolated include *Staphylococcus* spp., *Streptococcus* spp., *Proteus* spp., *Pseudomonas* spp., and *Escherichia coli*. The yeasts *Malassezia pachydermatis* (*Pityrosporum canis*) and, less commonly, *Candida* spp. may also be encountered. The ear mite *Otodectes cynotis* is a common cause of otitis externa in dogs and cats, while *Psoroptes cuniculi* may affect rabbits.

14.8.1 Anti-infective ear preparations

Prevention of insect attacks requires the use of fly repellents, fly sprays, or flea sprays (see section 2.2.2) to minimise repeated bites. If possible the affected animal should be housed indoors away from flies while lesions heal.

For otitis externa, a variety of topical antimicrobials is used to control bacterial and yeast infection. Neomycin is the most frequently used antibacterial, but others such as polymyxin B sulphate and fusidic acid are included in available preparations. Nystatin, natamycin, and miconazole are used for fungal infections. Mites are controlled with ectoparasiticides such as pyrethrins, monosulfiram and tiabendazole. Some products have proven efficacy against ear mites although they do not contain ectoparasiticides. Selamectin (see section 2.2.1.1) may be used for the treatment of *Otodectes* in cats. Otodectic mites may also be found on other areas of the body and it may be necessary to treat the whole animal.

Many topical preparations incorporate a corticosteroid or a local anaesthetic such as tetracaine or benzocaine to aid resolution of pain and inflammation. Systemic glucocorticoids may be necessary to control severe inflammation and reduce self-trauma. Most preparations contain various combinations of the above drugs. The product selected should contain therapeutic agents likely to be efficacious against the pathogens identified by cytology, culture, or both. Solutions or lotions are preferred for exudative conditions, while oil-based preparations or ointments are useful for dry lesions. The veterinarian should ensure that the tympanum is not perforated before administering these preparations. Systemic antibacterial therapy alone may be of limited value in otitis externa because the organisms are present in the cerumen and exudate. The ear should be prepared for treatment by cleansing.

Corticosteroids may produce irreversible effects in the skin; they can be absorbed and may have harmful effects, especially with frequent and extensive contact or in pregnancy. Operators should wear single-use disposable gloves when applying preparations containing a corticosteroid.

Otitis media is usually caused by bacterial infection extending from otitis externa. Systemic antibacterial therapy should be based on culture and antibacterial and fungal sensitivity tests. Systemic glucocorticoids may also be indicated. Surgery may be necessary if the response to medical management is poor.

UK

GSL Aurotex (Arnolds)
Solution, chlorobutanol 1.1%, phenoxyethanol 1%, for *dogs, cats*; 14 mL

POM Auroto (Arnolds)
Ear drops, neomycin sulphate 0.5%, tetracaine hydrochloride 1%, tiabendazole 4%, for *dogs, cats*; 10 mL, 25 mL
Contra-indications. Animals less than 4 kg body-weight in the first half of pregnancy

POM Betsolan Eye and Ear Drops (Schering-Plough)
See section 12.3.1 for preparation details

POM Canaural (Leo)
Ear drops (oily), diethanolamine fusidate 0.5%, framycetin 0.5%, nystatin 100 000 units/g, prednisolone 0.25%, for *dogs, cats*
Contra-indications. Not recommended for use in pregnant animals

GSL Ear Drops (Johnson's)
Ear drops, piperonyl butoxide 1%, pyrethrins 0.1%, for *dogs, cats*; 15 mL
Contra-indications. Puppies or kittens less than 12 weeks of age

POM (H) Fucidin Ointment (Leo)
See section 14.4.1 for preparation details

POM GAC (Arnolds)
Ear drops, neomycin sulphate 0.5%, permethrin (*cis:trans* 25:75) 1%, tetracaine hydrochloride 1%, for *dogs, cats*; 10 mL, 25 mL

GSL Kitzyme Veterinary Ear Drops (Seven Seas)
Ear drops, dichlorophen 0.99%, for *dogs, cats*; 18 mL

POM Neobiotic HC Drops (Pharmacia & Upjohn)
See section 12.3.1 for preparation details

POM Oterna Ear Drops (Schering-Plough)
Ear drops (oily), betamethasone 0.1%, monosulfiram 5%, neomycin sulphate 0.5%, for *dogs, cats*; 20 mL
Contra-indications. Not recommended for use in pregnant animals

GSL Otodex Veterinary Ear Drops (Petlife)
Ear drops, chlorobutanol 1.1%, phenoxyethanol 1%, for *dogs, cats*; 14 mL

POM Otomax (Schering-Plough)
Ear drops , betamethasone (as valerate) 0.88 mg/mL, clotrimazole 8.8 mg/mL, gentamicin 2640 units/mL, for *dogs*
Contra-indications. Not recommended for use in pregnant or lactating animals

POM Panolog Ointment (Novartis)
Liquid (oily), neomycin (as sulphate) 0.25%, nystatin 100 000 units/mL, thiostrepton 2500 units/mL, triamcinolone acetonide 0.1%, for *dogs, cats*; 7.5 mL, 100 mL
Warnings. Avoid administration to pregnant animals

POM Pimavecort Lotion (Intervet)
Ear drops, hydrocortisone 0.5%, natamycin 1%, neomycin (as sulphate) 0.175%, for *dogs, cats*; 20 mL

GSL Ruby Veterinary Ear Drops (Spencer)
Ear drops, piperonyl butoxide 1%, pyrethrins 0.1%, for *dogs, cats*; 15 mL
Contra-indications. Puppies or kittens less than 12 weeks of age

GSL Secto Ear Drops (Sinclair)
Ear drops, piperonyl butoxide 1%, pyrethrins 0.1%, for *dogs, cats*; 15 mL
Contra-indications. Puppies or kittens less than 12 weeks of age

POM Surolan (Janssen)
Suspension (drops), miconazole nitrate 2.3%, polymyxin B sulphate 5500 units/mL, prednisolone acetate 0.5%, for *dogs, cats*; 15 mL
Warnings. Manufacturer does not recommend use in pregnant animals

POM Vetsovate Cream (Schering-Plough)
See section 14.2.1 for preparation details

POM Vetsovate Eye and Ear Drops (Schering-Plough)
See section 12.3.1 for preparation details

GSL Vetzyme Veterinary Ear Drops (Seven Seas)
Ear drops, dichlorophen 0.99%, for *dogs, cats*; 18 mL

GSL Woundcare Powder (Animalcare)
See section 14.4.3 for preparation details

14.8.2 Ear cleansers and sebolytics

A significant proportion of otic disorders in animals will improve with flushing and cleansing of the ear canal to remove wax and debris. Preparations are available using solvents such as propylene glycol, squalane, or xylene, and incorporating benzoic acid and salicylic acid.

UK

There are many preparations available. This is not a comprehensive list.

Auroclens (Arnolds)
Liquid, vegetable oil emulsion, for *dogs, cats*; 30 mL, 100 mL

Canidor (Boehringer Ingelheim)
Gel, essential oils, for *dogs, cats, rabbits*; 10 mL

Clenderm (Vétoquinol)
Solution, organic acids 2.4%, propylene glycol 40%, salicylic acid 0.037%; 100 mL, 500 mL

P Dermisol (Pfizer)
Cream, benzoic acid 0.025%, malic acid 0.375%, propylene glycol 1.75%, salicylic acid 0.006%, for *horses, cattle, dogs, cats*; 30 g, 100 g
Withdrawal Periods. *Cattle*: slaughter withdrawal period nil, milk withdrawal period nil
Contra-indications. Concurrent use of teat dips or other disinfectants

P Dermisol Multicleanse (Pfizer)
Solution, benzoic acid 0.15%, malic acid 2.25%, propylene glycol 40%, salicylic acid 0.0375%, for *horses, cattle, dogs, cats*; 100 mL, 340 mL
Withdrawal Periods. *Cattle*: slaughter withdrawal period nil, milk withdrawal period nil
Contra-indications. Concurrent use of teat dips or other disinfectants

Epi-Otic (Virbac)
Solution, lactic acid 2.5%, salicylic acid 0.1%, for *dogs, cats*; 60 mL, 125 mL

GSL Logic Ear Cleaner (Sanofi)
Solution, xylene 2%, for *dogs, cats*; 60 mL

Nolvasan Otic (Fort Dodge)
Solution, chlorhexidine acetate 0.2%, for *dogs, cats*; 60 mL

Pimaveclens (Intervet)
Solution, lactic acid, propylene glycol, salicylic acid, docusate sodium, for *dogs, cats*; 125 mL

Specicare Cat Ear Cleaner (Leo)
Solution, glycerol, propylene glycol, for *cats*; 50 mL

Specicare Dog Ear Cleaner (Leo)
Solution, borax, boric acid, isopropanol, propylene glycol, for *dogs*; 50 mL, 100 mL

15 Drugs acting on FEET

Contributors:
R W Blowey BVSc, BSc, FRCVS
Dr T S Mair BVSc, PhD, DEIM, MRCVS

15.1 Anti-infective foot preparations
15.2 Hoof care preparations

Disorders of the feet are typically characterised by lameness, although sometimes other clinical signs such as swelling, inflammation, and discharge may be seen. In farm livestock, lameness is both a major economic and welfare problem and in horses performance can be seriously impaired .

Conditions affecting horses. Thrush in horses can result from poor hoof care, unhygienic stabling, poor foot conformation, and incorrect shoeing; *Fusobacterium necrophorum* is usually found in the lesion. Thrush is characterised by areas of necrotic frog exuding black, foul smelling discharge. Treatment includes debridement of necrotic tissue and improved stable hygiene. The diseased area can be dressed with anti-infective agents such as povidone-iodine 1% solution, sulfanilamide powder, tetracycline spray, or zinc sulphate 10% solution. It may be necessary to bandage severe cases for a short time. Attention should be paid to foot balance.

Canker is a severe hypertrophic pododermatitis usually affecting the frog, but sometimes extending to the wall. Treatment consists of resection of the abnormal tissue followed by application of topical metronidazole and bandaging.

Pathogens involved in suppurative hoof lesions include *F. necrophorum*, *Actinomyces pyogenes*, *Bacteroides* spp., and *Escherichia coli*. Foot abscesses in horses should be carefully drained and poulticed. Tetanus antitoxin or a booster dose of tetanus toxoid should be administered as necessary. As the tissues heal, iodine-based spray and magnesium sulphate paste (see section 14.1) may be applied before bandaging to keep the area dry and clean. Antibacterials are generally not indicated for the treatment of subsolar abscesses. Deep penetrating wounds to the foot with sepsis involving the pedal bone, navicular bone, navicular bursa, or distal interphalangeal joint require surgical debridement, lavage, and appropriate antibiotic therapy.

Laminitis in horses can present with a spectrum of clinical signs ranging from mild lameness to severe disease with loss of the hoof capsule. Although the precise pathogenesis of the disease is uncertain, there appears to be decreased laminar perfusion, with varying degrees of inflammation and necrosis of the sensitive laminae. Causes include carbohydrate overload, endotoxaemia (such as caused by gastrointestinal disease, septic metritis and pleuritis), excessive work, and hyperadrenocorticism (Cushing's syndrome).

The management of laminitis usually involves both physical support of the distal phalanx, and treatment of laminar pain and inflammation. Initial therapy should be aimed at removing the inciting cause if possible. Heparin (see section 4.6.1) at a dose of 25 to 100 micrograms/kg three times daily by subcutaneous injection has been shown to reduce the prevalence of laminitis associated with small intestinal disease and endotoxaemia. Heparin is only effective when is administered before any clinical signs of laminitis are apparent.

NSAIDs (see section 10.1), such as flunixin, ketoprofen, meclofenamic acid, and phenylbutazone, are used to manage pain and control laminar inflammation, especially during the acute phases of the disease. Systemic administration of dimethyl sulfoxide (100 mg to 1 g/kg by intravenous injection two to three times daily) has also been used to reduce inflammation and reperfusion injury in the laminae.

Maintenance of laminar blood flow is important to reduce some of the deleterious effects of acute laminitis. Peripheral vasodilation has been attempted by use of the alpha-adrenergic blockers acepromazine. These drugs may help to reduce the hypertension associated with acute laminitis, although the efficacy of these treatments is unproven.

Isoxsuprine (see section 10.6) has also been used as a peripheral vasodilator in laminitis ♦ at a dose of 0.6 to 4 mg/kg orally twice daily.

Heparin and aspirin have been used to reduce inappropriate intravascular coagulation and to maintain perfusion in the laminar capillary network. Aspirin (see section 10.1), given at a dose of 20 mg/kg orally daily, blocks thromboxane-mediated platelet aggregation. Heparin (see section 4.6.1) has an anticoagulant effect by enhancing the activity of antithrombin III and prolonging blood clotting times and also a potential beneficial effect on the laminar basement membrane. It is given at a dose of 40 to 100 units/kg by subcutaneous injection three times daily.

Nitric oxide donors have been used in an attempt to increase laminar blood flow. Glyceryl trinitrate (see section 4.3.3) ointment applied locally to the coronary band or the digital arteries have been shown to increase the laminar blood flow and to reduce the bounding digital pulse in acute laminitis. A dose of 2.5 cm of 2% ointment applied to each digital vessel of affected feet is applied topically.

Corrective trimming and shoeing are essential components of the treatment of acute laminitis. Frog pads or styrofoam pads apply support to the frog and deeper structures of the foot. The use of special shoes, such as heart bar shoes, and dorsal wall resection may be helpful in some cases. In advanced cases and unresponsive cases, deep digital flexor tenotomy may be performed to reduce the rotational forces on the distal phalanx.

Conditions affecting cattle. Sole ulcers and white line disorders (haemorrhage, separation, and abscessation), are associated with inflammatory changes within the foot, namely laminitis or more correctly coriosis. In some animals clinical signs of acute coriosis may be seen and include pain, altered gait, and heat in the hooves. However it is the sequellae of chronic coriosis (ulcers, white line disease, and hoof abnormalities) which cause most of the lameness. The cow seems to have an inherent phase of coriosis at parturition, although it is only when other factors predisposing to coriosis, for example nutritional imbalance, excessive standing, poor cow comfort, and inadequate management occur during the periparturient period that severe disease occurs. The sole of the hoof is 5 to 10 mm thick and as horn grows at approximately 5 mm per month, it takes at least 4 to 8 weeks for the damaged horn, produced at the time of parturition and immediately afterwards, to grow to the surface. Therefore peak incidence of lameness is seen 6 to 14 weeks after calving. Many hoof lesions are essentially of a physical nature and treatment of uncomplicated cases involves paring away under-run horn, draining abscesses, and allowing the corium to regenerate new horn.

Other lesions of the bovine hoof include foreign body penetration, vertical and horizontal fissures ('sandcracks'), 'false soles', and growth abnormalities, the most common of which is overgrowth. Coriosis, leading to increased pressure within the foot, can produce growth distortions such as 'hardship grooves' (concentric horizontal grooves encircling the anterior hoof wall) and a dorsal rotation of the toe, producing a concave anterior wall. Severe coriosis resulting from, for example a toxic mastitis or metritis, can produce a total, but temporary, cessation of horn formation and may result in a complete horizontal fissure. This can cause lameness 6 to 8 months later when the distal fragment of hoof moves over the corium at the toe. Dietary supplementation with biotin (20 mg/cow daily) has been shown to decrease the incidence of white line disease and vertical fissures.

The main lesions affecting the skin of the bovine claw are interdigital necrobacillosis ('foul'), digital dermatitis, interdigital skin hyperplasia ('corns', 'growths'), and mud fever. 'Foul' is a necrotising bacterial infection of the dermis caused by *Fusobacterium necrophorum*, *Porphyromonas* spp., and *Prevotella* spp. (*Bacteroides melaninogenicus*). The possible presence of an interdigital foreign body should be eliminated before treatment of 'foul' with parenteral antibacterials is instigated. Concurrent topical treatment reduces the spread of infection. The peracute condition of 'super foul' appears to involve the same organisms, although more prompt, prolonged, and aggressive antibacterial therapy is required. The local application of antibacterials such as clindamycin, has also been suggested. 'Super foul' is most commonly seen in herds infected with digital dermatitis.

Digital dermatitis is a superficial erosive epidermitis caused by a spirochaete of the *Treponeme* spp., the full identity of which has yet to be determined. A reservoir of infection persists in the interdigital pouch (at the rear of the interdigital cleft) and the typical lesion radiates circumferentially from this pouch. Other common sites for dermatitis include the interdigital cleft, the anterior aspect of the hoof (where infection may involve the coronary band and produce a vertical fissure), and the bulbs of the heels. Lesions in the inter-

digital cleft may be specifically referred to as 'interdigital dermatitis'; *Dichelobacter nodosus* may be involved in these lesions. Chronic neglected lesions of the heel develop a proliferative epidermitis known as 'hairy warts'. Treatment of individual animals is by topical antibacterial aerosol spray, usually oxytetracycline. Herd treatments involve the use of an antibacterial foot bath; oxytetracycline♦ (200 g to 600 g/100 litres), lincomycin♦ (100 g/100 litres), lincomycin and spectinomycin♦ Linco-Spectin 100, Pharmacia & Upjohn (150 g of powder/150 litres), and erythromycin♦ (46 g/100 litres) have all been used. Lincomycin is rapidly degraded in the environment and may be preferred. Maximum benefit is obtained if the heels are washed with a pressure hose before entering the foot bath, or if two foot baths are used in series, the first containing water to wash the feet, remove superficial debris, and allow better penetration of the antibacterial. Control of digital dermatitis is achieved by attention to environmental hygiene and regular footbaths with formaldehyde 10% (daily for one week, repeated on alternate weeks).

Interdigital skin hyperplasia may be a sequel to chronic inflammatory conditions such as low-grade 'foul' or digital dermatitis, although there is also a hereditary predisposition. Early lesions may resolve spontaneously after dishing the axial hoof wall to minimise compression of the lesion during locomotion; more advanced lesions required amputation.

Mud fever is uncommon in cattle. Extremely muddy and damp conditions are required. Treatment involves washing affected limbs with antiseptic and spraying with iodine teat disinfectants containing an emollient. Parenteral antibacterials may also be used.

Lesions within the foot mainly affect the pedal bone for example fractures and necrosis, or are infections secondary to ulcers, white line abscesses , or 'foul'.

Conditions affecting sheep and goats. Footrot, a bacterial infection caused by *Dichelobacter nodosus* (*Bacteroides nodosus*), is the main cause of lameness in sheep and goats. Recent outbreaks of peracute disease, in some cases leading to total shedding of the hoof, have also implicated a organism similar to the spirochaete causing digital dermatitis. A dermatitis affecting the interdigital cleft ('scald', 'strip') is thought to be caused by the same organisms and can be treated with topical antibacterial aerosol spray (usually oxytetracycline). Typical lesions lead to separation of the horn wall from the underlying corium. For treatment, all under-run wall must be removed and the area sprayed with antibacterial or disinfectant. Parenteral antibacterials, such as oxytetracycline, are also used in advanced cases and promote healing. *D. nodosus* is a strict anaerobe and exposing the lesion to air facilitates healing. Neglected lesions, leading to secondary joint infections with organisms such as *A. pyogenes*, require more protracted parenteral antibacterials. A proliferative dermatitis extending dorsally from the skin of the heel bulbs is often referred to as 'strawberry footrot' because of the nature of the lesion. A combination of the orf virus and *Dermatophilus congolensis* may be involved and is exacerbated by wet muddy conditions under foot. Cleaning the lesion, in addition to topical and parenteral antibacterials facilitates healing.

Conditions affecting pigs. In the first week of life the feet of piglets are highly susceptible to bruising, especially when concrete floors are rough, damp or poorly bedded. The junction of the abaxial wall with the bulb of the heel is a particularly common site of injury and often leads to a secondary bacterial infection of the foot, requiring parenteral antibacterial therapy. Similar lesions occur in sows and are again associated with rough floors, wet conditions under foot (leading to soft horn), and sudden foot movements (for example from aggression) leading to physical separation of the wall from the heel bulb. The ideal treatment is to lift the foot and remove all under-run horn. Unfortunately few farmers do this and a large number of cases develop secondary infections, leading to a swollen foot with a chronic discharge. These cases are known as 'bush foot'.

Haemorrhages and fissures in the anterior hoof wall have been attributed to biotin deficiency and biotin is often added to pig rations in an attempt to prevent lameness and to reverse hoof problems. Joint infections caused by *Mycoplasma hyosynoviae* or *Erysipelothrix rhusiopathiae* may occur. *M. hyosynoviae* is common and responds well to treatment with lincomycin or tiamulin.

The other major causes of lameness and leg weakness in sows are conditions affecting the bones and joints of the upper leg and spine.

Conditions affecting dogs and cats. See chapter 14 for information on dogs and cats

Conditions affecting chickens. In poultry, the majority of causes of lameness are associated with bone and joint abnormalities of the limb and do not involve the feet. The most common foot lesion is erosion of the foot pad caused by wet litter. Dietary changes resulting in scouring are often implicated. The high fat content of partially digested faeces seems to be particularly erosive. Insufficient litter in high humidity, poorly insulated, and poorly ventilated buildings in the winter can also be contributory factors. Under such conditions, long-standing erosions and other causes of skin damage predispose to a deeper infection of the footpads, often known as 'bumble foot' and commonly involving staphylococcal species.

In domestically-housed chickens, mange caused by *Cnemidocoptes mutans* can be a problem, leading to 'scaly leg'. Occasionally osteopetrosis (leucosis virus infection) may occur and is characterised by foot and leg swelling; there is no treatment.

General treatment of foot conditions.

Lesions of the hoof should be treated by removing all under-run horn, thereby exposing the underlying healthy corium. In most cases the corium will be covered by a layer of germinative tissue and growth of new horn is rapid. Sole ulcers are the exception to this, because the corium itself will have been damaged. Opinions vary concerning the value of dressings. In cattle there is a risk that they will be left on for too long, impede drainage, and therefore retard rather than improve healing. In addition, the presence of a dressing may make the affected claw the major weight-bearing area. As a consequence, many practitioners no longer use a dressing and the general opinion is that undressed feet heal equally as well as dressed feet. Fixing a block to the sole of the sound claw, thereby removing weight bearing from the affected claw, is excellent practice and promotes both healing and comfort. Blocks may be nailed on or glued on. A glue-on PVC shoe (Cowslip Plus, Giltspur) gives excellent support. With such support there is often no longer a need to house lame cows separately, although this is good practice while lameness persists because lame cows may find cubicles especially difficult to use.

Topical antibacterials are commonly applied to sheep lesions such as scald and footrot, and lesions involving the digital skin of cattle such as digital dermatitis and 'foul'. Disinfectants and antiseptics may also be used, although single applications are of limited value against digital dermatitis because the causative organism is sited below the surface of the epidermis: disinfectants (and particularly formaldehyde) 'seal' the surface of the skin and although surface contamination may be eliminated, the infection persists deeper within the epidermis. Prolonged footbathing with disinfectants may be beneficial.

Parenteral antibacterials help to resolve sheep footrot lesions and long-acting oxytetracycline preparations (see section 1.1.3) are frequently used. They are becoming increasingly common as part of the standard treatment, even where no secondary infection exists. A wide range of antibacterials is effective against 'foul' in cattle, with long-acting penicillin (see section 1.1.1.1) or oxytetracycline (see section 1.1.3) usually used in younger stock. Tilmicosin (see section 1.1.4) is widely used for footrot and 'foul' in many countries but is not authorised for this indication in the UK. Ceftiofur (see section 1.1.1.5) is often used in lactating dairy cows because of its nil milk withholding period; cefalexin, cefquinome, or tylosin may also be used. Mycoplasmal arthritis in pigs generally responds well to lincomycin or tiamulin.

Ideally, deep-seated lesions in all species which involve the tendon sheaths, navicular bursa or even the pedal joint require drainage in addition to prolonged and aggressive antibacterial therapy such as high doses for 7 to 14 days. Again a wide range of antibacterials is used including oxytetracycline, tylosin, and lincomycin. High concentrations of tylosin and lincomycin are achieved in joints following parenteral administration.

A vaccine is available for footrot in sheep (see section 18.2.7)

15.1 Anti-infective foot preparations

These products can be applied by aerosol spray, hand spray, or by foot bath and are commonly used for both the treatment and prevention of foot lesions, particularly for scald and footrot in sheep and goats, slurry heel, 'foul' and digital dermatitis in cattle, and general foot problems in pigs.

Paring away under-run horn and cleaning the lesions before application improves response to therapy. Individual cow, or even whole herd, treatments against digital dermatitis may be carried out using a hand-held garden sprayer, especially if a jet rather than spray application is used. Aqueous solutions of oxytetracycline♦ (10 g/litre) and lincomycin♦ (1 to 5 g/litre) are commonly used at a dosage of approximately 5 mL per foot. Lincomycin is very stable in an aqueous solution.

Foot baths are more commonly used for group treatments. Ideally they should be under cover to avoid dilution with rain water, and sited so that animals can be dispersed into a clean dry area, thus allowing time for the chemical to work. The bath should allow a fluid depth of approximately 7 to 10 cm for cattle and 4 to 6 cm for sheep. Baths which are too deep may cause scalding of the skin on the legs, contamination and damage to teats, or both. Baths should be 2.5 m long for cattle and 3.0 m for sheep, that is long enough to prevent the animal from jumping over it. The floor should be non-slip and ridged to spread the claws, allowing fluid to come into contact with interdigital space. Placing straw in the footbath makes it more acceptable to the animals.

The chemicals used in foot baths should kill the pathogenic organisms rapidly without causing damage to the skin and other sensitive structures of the foot. Solutions commonly used include antibacterials (for digital dermatitis) and formaldehyde, copper sulphate, and zinc sulphate. Zinc sulphate is less toxic and less irritant than formaldehyde or copper sulphate, the latter two having been banned from use in some countries because of their potential human health, environmental effects, or both. All three products are claimed to harden the hoof as well as disinfect it. Lincomycin is highly toxic to cattle if ingested and it is important to ensure that cows do not drink the footbath solution. Care must be taken to ensure that cows do not drink from the solution as they walk through the bath and animals should not be allowed to linger beside freshly made up foot baths. It is probably a wise precaution to soil the bath slightly before the first cow approaches. In general the foot bath should be emptied after each herd or flock treatment. Spent footbath solution should be disposed of correctly.

CETRIMIDE

UK
Indications. Footrot in sheep; wound cleansing and dressing

Cetrimide Solution
See section 14.6 for preparation details

Cetrimide Solution Strong
See section 14.6 for preparation details

GSL **Deosan Footrot Aerosol** (Diversey Lever)
Spray, cetrimide 10%, for *sheep*; 150 g
Withdrawal Periods. Slaughter withdrawal period nil, milk withdrawal period nil

GSL **Foot Rot Aerosol** (Battle Hayward & Bower)
Spray, cetrimide 10%, for *sheep*; 150 g
Withdrawal Periods. Slaughter withdrawal period nil, milk withdrawal period nil

COPPER SULPHATE

UK
Indications. Footrot in sheep; foot lesions in cattle
Side-effects. Stains wool
Warnings. Toxic, particularly to sheep. Ineffective when solution is dirty. Corrodes metal foot baths
Dose.
Cattle: *foot bath*, copper sulphate 5–10% solution *or* copper sulphate 5%-formaldehyde 10% solution twice daily
Sheep: *foot bath*, copper sulphate 5–10% solution
Local application, ointment, powder, or 5% solution

Copper Sulphate
Powder, copper sulphate. To be prepared as a solution for use

GSL **Lame-Less Copper Plus** (Net-Tex)
Foot bath, powder for reconstitution, copper sulphate, zinc sulphate, for *cattle*; 10 kg
Dilute 1 kg in 20 litres water

FORMALDEHYDE SOLUTION

Formaldehyde is available as formaldehyde solution (formalin) which is diluted before use, the percentage strength being expressed in terms of formaldehyde solution rather than formaldehyde (CH_2O). For example, in the UK, formaldehyde solution 3% consists of 3 volumes of Formaldehyde Solution BP diluted to 100 volumes with water and thus contains 1.02 to 1.14% w/w of formaldehyde (CH_2O).

UK
Indications. Hardening of hooves; footrot in cattle, sheep, and pigs♦
Side-effects. Skin irritation may occur with excessive strength of solution or frequency of use
Warnings. Toxic and irritant. Use in well-ventilated areas. Wear protective clothing in preparation and use of foot bath. Do not use at a concentration of more than 10% solution
Dose. *Cattle♦, sheep, pigs♦*:
Foot bath, 10% solution daily for treatment
Local application, 5–10% solution

GSL **Formaldehyde Foot Rot Liquid** (Alfa Laval Agri)
Foot bath, formaldehyde 38%, for *sheep*; 25 litres. To be diluted before use
Dilute 1 volume with 19 volumes water

Zal Formalin-S (DiverseyLever)
Foot bath, formaldehyde 35%, for *sheep*; 25 litres. To be diluted before use
Dilute 1 volume with 19 volumes water

OXYTETRACYCLINE HYDROCHLORIDE

UK
Indications. Footrot and topical infections in horses♦, cattle, sheep, and pigs

POM **Alamycin Aerosol** (Norbrook)
Spray, oxytetracycline hydrochloride 3.6%, suitable dye, for *cattle, sheep, pigs*; 140 g
Withdrawal Periods. Slaughter withdrawal period nil, milk withdrawal period nil

POM Duphacycline Aerosol (Fort Dodge)
Spray, oxytetracycline hydrochloride 3.6%, suitable dye, for *cattle, sheep, pigs*; 140 g
Withdrawal Periods. Slaughter withdrawal period nil, milk withdrawal period nil

POM Embacycline Aerosol (Merial)
Spray, oxytetracycline hydrochloride 3.6%, suitable dye, for *cattle, sheep, pigs*; 140 g
Withdrawal Periods. Slaughter withdrawal period nil, milk withdrawal period

POM Engemycin Aerosol (Intervet)
Spray, oxytetracycline hydrochloride 3.58%, suitable dye, for *cattle, sheep, pigs*; 140 g
Withdrawal Periods. Slaughter withdrawal period nil, milk withdrawal period nil

POM Oxycare Aerosol (Animalcare)
Spray, oxytetracycline hydrochloride 3.6%, suitable dye, for *cattle, sheep, pigs*; 140 g
Withdrawal Periods. Slaughter withdrawal period nil, milk withdrawal period

POM Terramycin Aerosol (Pfizer)
Spray, oxytetracycline hydrochloride 3.92%, suitable dye, for *sheep, cattle*; 150 mL
Withdrawal Periods. Slaughter withdrawal period nil, milk withdrawal period nil

POM Tetcin Aerosol (Vétoquinol)
Spray, oxytetracycline hydrochloride 3.6%, for *sheep, pigs*; 140 g
Withdrawal Periods. Slaughter withdrawal period nil, milk withdrawal period nil

ZINC SULPHATE

UK

Indications. Footrot in sheep; foot infections in cattle
Dose. *Foot bath*.
Cattle: zinc sulphate solution daily
Sheep: zinc sulphate solution after each trimming

GSL Deosan Hoof-care (Diversey Lever)
Foot bath, powder for reconstitution, zinc sulphate (as heptahydrate) 98%, for *cattle, sheep*; 20 kg
Withdrawal Periods. *Cattle, sheep*: slaughter withdrawal period nil, milk withdrawal period nil
Dissolve 1 kg in 10 litres water

GSL Golden-Hoof (Shep-Fair)
Foot bath, powder for reconstitution, zinc sulphate heptahydrate 98%, for *cattle, sheep*; 10 kg, 20 kg
Dissolve 1 kg in 10 litres water

GSL Golden-Hoof Plus (Shep-Fair)
Foot bath, powder for reconstitution, zinc sulphate heptahydrate 98%, wetting agents, for *cattle, sheep*; 10 kg, 20 kg

Zal Surefoot (DiverseyLever)
Foot bath, powder for reconstitution, zinc sulphate heptahydrate 100%, for *cattle, sheep*; 15 kg
Withdrawal Periods. *Cattle, sheep*: slaughter withdrawal period nil

GSL Zincoped (Battle Hayward & Bower)
Foot bath, powder for reconstitution, zinc sulphate heptahydrate 95%, for *sheep*; 12.5 kg, 20 kg
Withdrawal Periods. Slaughter withdrawal period nil, milk withdrawal period nil
Dissolve 1 kg in 10 litres water

15.2 Hoof care preparations

Many preparations are said to assist in maintaining the integrity of hoof horn, although the efficacy of some is difficult to assess.

Beneficial effects on hoof structure have been demonstrated when supplementary **biotin** is added to the diet. A daily dose of 20 mg biotin per cow has been shown to reduce the incidence of white line lameness in the UK, and vertical fissures (sand cracks) in beef cattle in North America. In pigs, biotin at a dose of 500 to 1500 mg/tonne is often added to the feed in an attempt to prevent lameness due to poor hoof horn quality. In extreme cases up to 3000 mg/tonne has been used to reverse hoof problems. Biotin has been shown to be beneficial in horses which are not biotin deficient. Long-term biotin supplementation in horses may improve hoof quality and certain hoof deficits when given either alone or in combination with additional calcium and good quality protein.

Zinc is often promoted as reducing lameness, and while it is known to improve the rate of healing of skin lesions, its effect on the feet of livestock has yet to be proven. Chelated or organic mineral complexes may give better absorption and improve the effectiveness of mineral supplementation.

Methionine also appears to assist in improving horse hoof horn integrity but its efficacy is better when given in combination with biotin. Compound preparations containing vitamins and minerals are available.

Application of vegetable oil-based products to the horse hoof will improve appearance of the hoof but the efficacy of these preparations is unproven and may even cause deterioration of the horn.

PREPARATIONS FOR HOOF CARE

UK

There are many preparations available. This is not a comprehensive list.

Biometh-Z (Vétoquinol)
Oral powder, for addition to feed, biotin, methionine, zinc gluconate, for *horses*; 750 g, 1.5 kg
Dose. *Horses*: 15 g of powder daily

Biotin + Zinc & Methionine (Day Son & Hewitt)
Oral powder, for addition to feed, biotin, methionine, zinc (as zinc methionine), for *horses*; 270 g, 810 g
Dose. *Horses*: 6–15 g of powder daily

Bio-Trition (Equine Products)
Oral powder, for addition to feed, biotin, lysine, zinc methionine, for *horses, donkeys*; 500 g, 1.5 kg, 4 kg
Dose. *Horses*: (adults) 25 g of powder daily in feed; (ponies, foals, donkeys) 15 g of powder daily in feed

Farrier's Formula (Equi Life)
Oral powder, for addition to feed, ascorbic acid, biotin, choline, copper, hydroxyproline, glycine, inositol, iodine, methionine, proline, tyrosine, zinc, for *horses*; 5 kg, 10 kg, 20 kg
Dose. *Horses*: 170 g of powder (1 measure)/450 kg body-weight daily

Keracare (Crown)
Cubes, biotin 7.5 mg, for *horses*
Dose. *Horses*: 7.5–22.5 mg daily

Kera-fac (Vericore LP)
Oral powder, for addition to feed, biotin 600 micrograms/g, calcium 100 mg/
g, iron (as sulphate) 2 mg/g, methionine 200 micrograms/g, zinc (as sulphate) 4 mg/g, for **horses**; 2.5 kg
Dose. *Horses*: 12.5–37.5 g of powder daily

TAR
(Stockholm Tar)

Tar or Stockholm tar, which has antiseptic properties, may
be used following treatment of an infected frog in horses or
footrot in cattle and sheep. It is used alone or with a packing
material to fill defects in the wall, sole, or frog and helps to
prevent entry of gravel and reinfection.

UK

Indications. Hoof and horn disorders

Stockholm Tar (Battle Hayward & Bower)
Tar (wood tar), for **horses, cattle, sheep**; 450 g, 1 kg, other sizes available

16 Drugs affecting
NUTRITION and BODY FLUIDS

Contributors:
S J Browne BVSc, MRCVS
P A Harris MA, VetMB, PhD, MRCVS
C B Johnson BVSc, DVA, DipECVA, MRCVS
P R Scott DVM&S, CertCHP, DSHP, FRCVS

16.1 Electrolyte and water replacement
16.2 Plasma substitutes
16.3 Parenteral nutrition
16.4 Drugs for ketosis
16.5 Minerals
16.6 Vitamins
16.7 Compound multivitamin and mineral preparations
16.8 Complete dietetic foods

16.1 Electrolyte and water replacement

16.1.1 Oral administration
16.1.2 Parenteral administration

The objectives of fluid therapy, whether oral or parenteral, include the correction of extracellular fluid (ECF) volume, plasma pH, blood-glucose concentration, and plasma concentrations of K^+ and Na^+; restoration of cellular K^+; and the provision of nutrients.

Any severely dehydrated, shocked, or collapsed animal almost certainly requires parenteral, preferably intravenous, fluid therapy before oral rehydration therapy.

16.1.1 Oral administration

Oral fluid therapy is the primary treatment in most cases of diarrhoea irrespective of the causal agent. The basic mechanism underlying the use of oral rehydration solutions is the intestinal co-transport of sodium and glucose leading to increased water uptake and reversal of dehydration. Therefore sodium and glucose are present in most oral rehydration solutions in approximately equimolar amounts and the solution is isotonic with plasma. Sodium concentrations vary from 50 mmol/L to 120 mmol/L. As a rule the higher the sodium concentration, the more efficacious the solution will be in terms of water uptake by the animal. Potassium is usually present to assist in repairing likely deficits. Fatty acid anions such as citrate, acetate, and propionate may be included to assist in correction of acidosis; they are metabolised to bicarbonate by the animal. Normal plasma contains bicarbonate 25 mmol/L and any oral rehydration solution should yield at least 25 mmol/L in order to avoid the possible development of dilutional acidosis. To effectively correct acidosis, higher bicarbonate yields of up to 100 mmol/L are desirable.

Some solutions (for example Energaid Elanco) contain higher glucose and sodium concentrations. Fears that such hypertonic solutions may worsen diarrhoea due to osmosis or produce hypernatraemia are unfounded in calves. The risk is probably greater in puppies and kittens.

While the main indication for oral fluid therapy is diarrhoea, it is of value in any situation where fluid loss and acidosis is present or anticipated, for example post operative rehydration, as an adjunct to parenteral fluid therapy, to minimise risk of diarrhoea due to stress of transport or weaning, and prevention and treatment of exertional fluid loss. Concentrated solutions are used in the treatment of pregnancy toxaemia in sheep.

In general, milk feeding in calves should not be restricted for longer than 24 to 48 hours because an energy deficit may be produced in the animal and may result in villous atrophy of the intestinal mucosa. If possible, animals should be maintained on milk or food during therapy, even though it may appear to worsen the diarrhoea as judged by the volume and consistency of the faeces.

Table 16.1 shows the approximate composition (after reconstitution) of oral rehydration solutions available in the UK. Most proprietary solutions are for use in calves but appear equally efficacious in all species. The volume of fluid required and the frequency of administration generally depend on the severity of the condition. Solutions should be prepared according to the manufacturer's instructions. Further dilution may be required for use in exotic species (see Prescribing for exotic birds and Prescribing for reptiles).

16.1.2 Parenteral administration

Parenteral solutions are used with the aim of restoring the normal concentrations of natural constituents of ECF.

In evaluating an animal for possible fluid therapy, the state of hydration, electrolyte balance, acid-base balance, renal function, and calorific balance should be considered. Evaluation should be based on history, physical examination, ECG, and laboratory testing.

The choice of parenteral fluid will depend on losses incurred. Table 16.2 lists some typical clinical conditions and parenteral solutions that may be appropriate.

The potential effects of parenteral solutions are best judged by comparing the composition with that of normal plasma. Parenteral solutions may be classified according to their clinical use: restoration of ECF volume, specific restoration of plasma volume (see section 16.2), acidifiers, alkalinisers, ECF diluents, 'maintenance solutions', nutrient solutions (see section 16.3), and concentrated additives. Parenteral solutions are preferably administered intravenously or intraosseously. Non-irritant isotonic solutions may be given by intraperitoneal or subcutaneous injection. Subcutaneous injection is associated with poor absorption when peripheral perfusion is reduced.

Table 16.1 Oral rehydration solutions available in the UK

| | Millimoles per litre | | | | | | | | | | |
Product	Na$^+$	K$^+$	Cl$^-$	HCO$_3^-$	Precursor[1]	Glucose %	Ca/Mg	Other components	Species	Reconstitution/dilution details	Pack size
Canine/Feline Electrolyte (Pedigree)	40	20	40	20		5	–/–	tea extract	dogs, cats	Reconstitute 1 sachet in 500 mL water	27.3-g sachets
Effydral (Fort Dodge)	120	15	55	80	citrate	3.2	–/–		calves, pigs	Dissolve 1 tablet in 1 litre water	48
Electydral (Novartis)	80	25	54	50	acetate, propionate	1.4	–/+		calves	Reconstitute 1 sachet in 1.5 litres water	35-g sachets
Energaid (Elanco)	133	20	60	93	acetate, citrate, propionate	6.76	–/–		calves	Reconstitute 1 sachet in 2 litres	165-g sachets
Ion-Aid (Merial)	74	24	74			2.3	+/+	glycine, phosphate	calves, lambs, pigs	Reconstitute 2-compartment sachet in 2.27 litres water	89.7-g sachets
Ionalyte (Intervet)	145	11	108	57	acetate	0	+/+		foals, cattle, pigs, dogs, cats	Dilute 1 volume with 15 volumes water	1 litre
Lactolyte (Bimeda)	77	32	55	40	acetate, propionate	0	+/+	dehydrated whey, phosphate	calves	Reconstitute 1 sachet in 2 litres water	90-g sachets
Lectade (Pfizer)	73	16	73	4	citrate	2.2	–/–	phosphate	horses, calves, lambs, pigs, dogs, cats	Reconstitute small animal paired sachets in 500 mL water, large animal paired sachets in 2–4 litres water	paired sachets
Lectade Plus (Pfizer)	50	20	39	29	citrate	3.1	–/–	glycine, phosphate	calves	Reconstitute paired sachets in 2 litres water	paired sachets
Liquid Lectade (Pfizer)	74	16	73	13	citrate	2.2	–/–	phosphate	horses, calves, sheep	Dilute 1 volume with 11.5 volumes water; use undiluted for pregnancy toxaemia in sheep	960 mL
Life-Aid P (Norbrook)	76	15	74	2	propionate	2.5	–/–	glycine, phosphate	calves, pigs	Reconstitute paired sachets in 2 litres water	Paired sachets
Life-Aid Xtra (Norbrook)	90	25	60	50	acetate, citrate, propionate	3.2	–/–	phosphate	calves	Reconstitute 1 sachet in 2 litres water	83.7-g sachet

Table 16.1 Oral rehydration solutions available in the UK

Product	Millimoles per litre					Glucose %	Ca/ Mg	Other components	Species	Reconstitution/ dilution details	Pack size
	Na⁺	K⁺	Cl⁻	HCO₃⁻	Precursor¹						
Liquid Life-Aid (Norbrook)	79	15	74	2	propionate	2.5	–/–	glycine, phosphate	calves, sheep, pigs	Dilute 1 volume with 11.5 volumes water; use undiluted for pregnancy toxaemia in sheep (see section 16.4)	960 mL
Pectilec (Arnolds)	90	10	73	25	citrate	1.9	–/+	fibrous pulp, phosphate	calves, lambs, piglets	Reconstitute 1 sachet in 1 litre water *or* 1 sachet in 2 litres milk or milk replacer	50-g sachets
Scourproof (Forum)	84	15	48	52	acetate	1.6	–/+	ispagula husk, wheat bran	calves	Reconstitute 1 sachet in 1.5 litres water	67-g sachets

¹ 1 mmol acetate = 1 mmol bicarbonate
  1 mmol citrate = 3 mmol bicarbonate
  1 mmol propionate = 1 mmol bicarbonate
Precursor converted to bicarbonate in the body

Some solutions may be incompatible with particular drugs or with other solutions, for example, calcium with bicarbonate-containing solutions (see Drug Incompatibilities – Appendix 2).

Fluid replacement

The *restoration of ECF volume* can be achieved only by solutions of plasma-like sodium concentration (130–160 mmol/litre), preferably administered intravenously. Intravenous infusions used include sodium chloride 0.9%, Hartmann's solution (lactated Ringer's solution, compound sodium lactate infusion), and Darrow's solution. Darrow's solution contains a high potassium concentration and low sodium concentration. It is not suitable for initial restoration of ECF volume in cases of neonatal diarrhoea when, despite potassium depletion, hyperkalaemia is likely as a result of acidosis and poor perfusion of tissues generally and the kidneys in particular. Darrow's solution is rarely used in veterinary medicine.

ECF diluents provide a parenteral source of water that is made temporarily isotonic, such as contained in glucose 5% intravenous infusion. Calorie content is trivial compared with daily requirements although there is temporary relief of hypoglycaemia.

'Maintenance solutions' substitute for normal oral intake of water and dietary electrolytes and are provided after initial fluid balance is restored. They contain approximately 20% of the plasma-sodium concentration plus other electrolytes, notably potassium, and sufficient glucose (usually about 4%) for isotonicity. Intravenous glucose solution may be used in lambs to provide energy for a short period.

Table 16.2 Parenteral fluid therapy for various disorders

Condition	Disturbances	Fluid	Suggested additives
Anorexia	short-term	sodium chloride 0.18% + glucose 4% *or* glucose 5%	potassium chloride (20–30 mmol/L)
	long-term: depletion of calories and protein	parenteral nutrition (see section 16.3)	
Drought, unable to drink/swallow, diabetes insipidus, polyuric renal failure, pyrexia	primary water loss	sodium chloride 0.18% + glucose 4%	potassium chloride (10–20 mmol/L) if therapy longer than 3 days
Vomiting	loss of water, H^+, Na^+, Cl^-, K^+, metabolic alkalosis	Ringer's solution *or* sodium chloride 0.9%	potassium chloride (10–20 mmol/L) if therapy longer than 3 days
Vomiting (bile-stained)	loss of water, H^+, HCO_3^-, Cl^-, Na^+, metabolic acidosis	Hartmann's solution	
Diarrhoea	loss of water, Na^+, HCO_3^-, Cl^-, (K^+ if long term), metabolic acidosis	Hartmann's solution	potassium chloride (10–20 mmol/L) if therapy is prolonged bicarbonate (1–3 mmol/kg) if condition is severe and therapy is prolonged
Bowel obstruction	loss of water, Na^+, HCO_3^-, Cl^-, metabolic acidosis	plasma expander + Hartmann's solution	bicarbonate (1–3 mmol/kg)
Urethral obstruction, ruptured urinary bladder	accumulation of K^+, H^+, metabolic acidosis	sodium chloride 0.9% + glucose 5% *or* sodium chloride 0.18% + glucose 4% *or* sodium chloride 0.9%	bicarbonate (1–3 mmol/kg) if in hypovolaemic shock
Haemorrhage	blood loss, hypovolaemic shock	plasma expander *or* Hartmann's solution, whole blood if PCV is low	
Burns, peritonitis, pancreatitis	loss of plasma and ECF, hypovolaemic shock	plasma expander + Hartmann's solution	bicarbonate (1–3 mmol/kg)

The calculation of fluid required is based on:

- Replacement of fluid deficits existing at time of presentation

  Depends on degree of dehydration on presentation plus accumulated daily maintenance losses plus accumulated losses through diarrhoea, vomiting, etc.

- Replacement of daily maintenance losses

  Daily fluid requirements including loss through skin, respiratory tract, and urine are usually 44 to 66 mL/kg daily (average 50 mL/kg) for an adult animal and 130 mL/kg daily for a neonate. Such replacement is required until the patient is able to take sustainable oral fluids

- Replacement of continuing abnormal losses

  Abnormal fluid losses such as through vomiting or diarrhoea depend on the individual clinical case. As an estimate, fluid loss through vomiting is 2 mL/kg body-weight per vomit and through diarrhoea may be up to 200 mL/kg body-weight daily.

Examples of fluid loss calculation.

A 20 kg dog vomiting 4 times daily for 3 days, having been ill for 5 days will, at a conservative estimate, accumulate a deficit of at least 3.5 litres. This is calculated as follows:

- Irreversible losses at 25 mL/kg/day for 5 days

  $25 \times 20 \times 5 = 2500$ mL
- Urinary losses at 25 mL/kg/day for first day of illness only

  $25 \times 20 \times 1 = 500$ mL
- Vomiting losses at 2 mL/kg/vomit for 3 days

  $2 \times 20 \times 4 \times 3 = 480$ mL.

A horse with acute diarrhoea, such as occurs with salmonellosis, rapidly develops a large fluid deficit of 100 litres or more.

The **rate of administration** will depend on the severity of the clinical condition. Initially, fluids may be given rapidly (up to 50 mL/kg/hour) and subsequently reduced to 5 to 15 mL/kg/hour. Some manufacturers recommend that half the initial fluid deficit should be corrected in 1 to 2 hours. The *maximum* satisfactory rate (in the absence of cardiovascular or pulmonary disease) of infusion may be calculated by:

$$\text{mLs of fluid/hour} = BW \times 90$$

BW = body-weight of patient in kg

Authorities recommend that these high infusion rates should only be used for resuscitation of animals in shock, only for short periods of time (20 to 30 minutes), and in the absence of pulmonary or cardiac dysfunction. Cardiopulmonary function should be monitored during infusion at high rates and restoration of urine output must be confirmed. Clinical signs of excessively rapid administration include restlessness, moist lung sounds, tachycardia, tachypnoea, nasal discharge, coughing, vomiting, and diarrhoea.

To convert the flow rate in mL/kg/hour to drops/minute the following formula can be used:

$$\text{Drops/minute} = \frac{\text{Drops/mL} \times \text{FR} \times \text{BW}}{60}$$

Drops/mL = number of drops delivered by the infusion set per mL

FR = flow rate in mL/kg/hour

BW = body-weight of patient in kg

Electrolyte replacement

Concentrated additives are added to existing solutions to increase the content of one particular electrolyte, for example, bicarbonate or potassium, with minimal change in volume. They must be adequately mixed before administration to the animal.

Disturbances of plasma-sodium concentration reflect water rather than sodium imbalance. Therefore, hyponatraemia is generally corrected by repair of ECF volume and hypernatraemia by controlled access to water given orally or gradual use of glucose 5% intravenous infusion or sodium chloride 0.45% intravenous infusion, to avoid sudden changes in plasma-sodium concentration. Sodium chloride 0.45% is also used for neonates.

Herbivores may become hypokalaemic when anorexic because their normal diet contains high concentrations of potassium. Treatment of mild hypokalaemia in dogs and cats includes dietary supplementation with foods having a high potassium content such as vegetables, fruit, and meat. If the plasma-potassium concentration falls below 2.5 mmol/litre, parenteral solutions are required. Plasma-potassium concentrations and heart rate should be monitored throughout the intravenous infusion because intravenous potassium administration is potentially life threatening.

Initial clinical signs of hyperkalaemia include listlessness, weakness, and hypotension and may lead to cardiac arrhythmias. Plasma-potassium concentration may not be a true reflection of total potassium concentration in the body and cell-potassium deficits can exist in the presence of hyperkalaemia. By providing intravenous fluid therapy to correct metabolic acidosis and dehydration and restore renal function, correction of hyperkalaemia is facilitated in the majority of patients. In the short term, glucose solution 5% or 10% given at a dose of 1 mL/kg with insulin 0.5 unit/kg promotes movement of potassium ions back into cells.

Acid-base balance

Acidifiers such as potassium chloride contain no bicarbonate precursors and are used to repair metabolic alkalosis. They may improve a mild acidosis despite their composition, by increasing ECF volume and thereby improving renal perfusion and function. *Alkalinisers* are required for the repair of metabolic acidosis. These solutions contain bicarbonate or one of its precursors such as lactate or acetate. Lactate is converted to bicarbonate within 1 to 2 hours solely in the liver and is not suitable for use in patients with hepatic impairment. Hartmann's solution contains lactate at a concentration similar to normal plasma; higher concentrations of bicarbonate or its precursor may be needed for severe acidosis. To calculate the amount of bicarbonate required to correct acidosis use the following formula:

$$HCO_3^- (mmol) = (0.3–0.5) BW \times base\ deficit\ (mmol/L)$$

Base deficit = normal plasma-bicarbonate concentration minus the actual plasma-bicarbonate concentration
BW = body-weight of patient in kg

In the absence of measured plasma-bicarbonate deficit, but with a history suggesting metabolic acidosis, an initial bicarbonate dose of 1–2 mmol/kg may be given and repeated if required after some hours.
Table 16.3 shows the approximate composition of parenteral fluids used in veterinary medicine.

GLUCOSE
(Dextrose monohydrate)

UK
Indications. See Table 16.2 and notes above
Warnings. Use with care in diabetic patients
Dose. See Table 16.2 and notes above

See Table 16.3 for preparation details

POTASSIUM CHLORIDE
UK
Indications. See Table 16.2 and notes above
Contra-indications. Renal failure, hyperkalaemia; atrioventricular block
Warnings. Rapid injection may be cardiotoxic, ECG should be monitored; must be diluted with not less than 50 times its volume of sodium chloride 0.9% or other suitable diluent and mixed well
Dose. Should not exceed 3–5 mmol K+/kg daily, given at maximum infusion rate of 0.5 mmol/kg per hour

See Table 16.3 for preparation details

SODIUM BICARBONATE
UK
Indications. See Table 16.2 and notes above
Warnings. Incompatible with calcium-containing solutions (see Drug Incompatibilities – Appendix 2)
Dose. See notes above

See Table 16.3 for preparation details

SODIUM CHLORIDE
UK
Indications. See Table 16.2 and notes above
Warnings. Not suitable for protracted use unless there is heavy and continued loss of electrolytes. Oral potassium supplements may be necessary
Dose. See notes above

See Table 16.3 for preparation details

SODIUM LACTATE

UK
Indications. See Table 16.2 and notes above
Contra-indications. Hepatic impairment, patients with cardiac arrhythmias
Dose. See notes above

See Table 16.3 for preparation details

16.2 Plasma substitutes

Haemorrhage occurs most commonly as a result of trauma but may also occur internally following surgery; rupture of tumours, abdominal ulceration in cattle, or guttural pouch mycosis in horses; or post partum. Haemorrhage may be associated with coagulopathies or platelet abnormalities due to poisoning with warfarin or bracken, or acquired or congenital bleeding disorders.
Shock is the failure of adequate perfusion of cells, tissues, and organs. Causes of shock are numerous and include hypovolaemia resulting from haemorrhage, fluid and electrolyte loss due to vomiting and diarrhoea, heat stroke, and burns; toxic shock due to sepsis or endotoxaemia; and vasogenic shock due to traumatic injury, anaphylaxis, or electrocution.
Hypertonic saline may be used in the initial treatment of severe hypovolaemia in horses, cattle, dogs, and cats. Sodium chloride 7.2% solution is administered by intravenous infusion at a dose of 4 mL/kg. Hypertonic saline has a positive iontropic action and also draws water from intracellular space into the extracellular space leading to a rapid increase in extracellular and therefore plasma volume. It is important that treatment with hypertonic saline is followed by full replacement of fluid deficits using isotonic solutions because long-term depletion of intracellular fluid may have detrimental effects on cellular function. Hypertonic saline is contra-indicated if there is impaired renal function or in horses suffering from exhaustion or water deprivation.
Plasma substitutes such as **gelatin** and **dextrans** are artificial colloids that restore circulating volume by mimicking the action of plasma proteins such as albumin. Plasma substitutes are retained in the circulation longer than electrolyte solutions due to their higher molecular weight. The use of colloids and electrolyte solutions in preference to whole blood in the early stages of shock ensures that the 'sludging phenomenon', which occurs in the peripheral microcirculation, is minimised.
Dextran 40 produces a greater expansion of plasma volume than the higher molecular weight Dextran 70, although the expansion has a shorter duration because of more rapid renal excretion. Dextran 40 also inhibits sludging of red blood cells and is used to improve blood flow and reduce intravascular aggregation and thrombus formation in conditions associated with impaired circulation.
Solutions of hydroxyethyl starch, **hexastarch,** may also be used as plasma expanders in a similar manner to dextrans.

Table 16.3 Composition of parenteral fluids in the UK (*see* monographs for contra-indications and warnings)

| | Millimoles per litre | | | | | Glucose | | Other | |
	Na^+	K^+	Cl^-	HCO_3^-	Precursor	%	Ca/Mg	components	Species
GLUCOSE									
Vetivex 6 (Ivex)						5	–/–		horses, cattle, dogs, cats
SODIUM CHLORIDE									
Aqupharm No 1 (Animalcare)[1]	150		150				–/–		dogs, cats
Aqupharm No 9 (Animalcare) *Ringer's solution*	147	4	155				+/–		dogs, cats
Vetivex 1 (Ivex)[1]	150		150				–/–		horses, cattle, dogs, cats
Vetivex 9 (Ivex) *Ringer's solution*	147	4	155.5				+/–		horses, cattle, dogs, cats
Vetivex 20 (Ivex)[2]	1232		1232						horses, cattle, dogs, cats
SODIUM CHLORIDE and GLUCOSE									
Aqupharm No 3 (Animalcare)	154		154			5	–/–		dogs, cats
Aqupharm No 18[3] (Animalcare)	30		30			4	–/–		dogs, cats
Duphalyte (Fort Dodge)	18	3	5	18	acetate	5	+/+	vitamins, amino acids	horses, cattle, pigs, dogs, cats
Vetivex 3 (Ivex)	150		150			5	–/–		horses, cattle, dogs, cats
Vetivex 18 (Ivex)[3]	30		30			4			horses, cattle, dogs, cats
SODIUM LACTATE									
Aqupharm No 11 (Animalcare) *Hartmann's solution, Lactated Ringer's solution*	131	5	111	29	lactate		+/–		dogs, cats
Isolec (Ivex) *Hartmann's solution, Lactated Ringer's solution*	131	5	111	29	lactate		+/–		horses, cattle, dogs, cats
ADDITIVES Ⓗ									
Potassium chloride solution, strong		2000	2000				–/–		
Sodium bicarbonate 1.26%	150			150			–/–		
Min-I-Jet Sodium Bicarbonate (Medeva) 4.2%	500			500			–/–		
Min-I-Jet Sodium Bicarbonate (Medeva) 8.4%	1000			1000			–/–		

All entries:
POM or PML
Withdrawal Periods. Slaughter withdrawal period nil, milk withdrawal period nil

[1] Sodium chloride 0.9% (Normal saline) contains Na^+ 150 mmol/L and Cl^- 150 mmol/L
[2] Sodium chloride 7.2% (hypertonic saline) contains Na^+ 1232 mmol/L and Cl^- 1232 mmol/L
[3] Sodium chloride 0.18% + glucose 4% contains Na^+ 30 mmol/L, Cl^- 30 mmol/L, and glucose 4%

Severe haemorrhage may lead to hypovolaemia and is life-threatening. Restoration of circulating blood volume with plasma-replacement solutions is a priority before replacing ECF loss. If packed-cell volume (PCV) falls below 150 mL/litre in cattle or 210 mL/litre in horses, dogs, or cats, whole blood transfusion should be considered. These figures are variable because hypovolaemia will affect PCV and are given for guidance only. PCV of less than 200 mL/litre is often tolerated in patients with chronic anaemia.

Crossmatching of donor and recipient blood is not always possible but, fortunately, reactions are rarely seen on first transfusion in animals. However, it is advisable, where possible, that blood should be typed and cross-matched before infusion. A healthy adult animal of the same species as the patient must be used as a donor. Donor animals should be regularly tested for infectious diseases, for example cats should be tested for feline leukaemia virus, feline immuno-deficiency virus, and *Haemobartonella felis*. **One percent of the donor's body-weight (or 10 mL/kg) is the amount of blood that may be safely taken at one time**.

Before transfusion, corticosteroids (see section 7.2) such as dexamethasone may be administered to reduce transfusion reactions such as dyspnoea, pyrexia, urticaria, and haemoglobinuria. Intravenous administration of blood into the patient should be performed slowly, administering 10 to 20 mL/kg depending on the severity of the condition. More rapid transfusion may be given depending on rate of ongoing haemorrhage. Intraperitoneal transfusion may be of value, especially in neonates.

The amount of blood to be transfused may be calculated from the following formulae:

$$\text{Blood volume} = \frac{K \times BW \text{ (required PCV - recipient PCV)}}{\text{donor PCV}}$$
required

BW = body-weight of patient in kg
K = 90 for dogs and cats
PCV = packed cell volume

However, the clinician is reminded that the above equation should be used for guidance and close attention should be paid to the response of the patient to therapy.

If blood is given at the same time as gelatin-containing products, it can be given through the same giving set since these products do not clot blood. They can also be used to reconstitute packed red cells.

DEXTRANS

UK
Indications. Plasma expansion in shock
Dose. *By intravenous infusion*, volume equal to estimated plasma volume deficit

POM Ⓗ **Gentran 40** (Baxter) *UK*
Intravenous infusion, dextran 40 intravenous infusion in glucose intravenous infusion 5% or sodium chloride intravenous infusion 0.9%; 500 mL

POM Ⓗ **Gentran 70** (Baxter) *UK*
Intravenous infusion, dextran 70 intravenous infusion in glucose intravenous infusion 5% or sodium chloride intravenous infusion 0.9%; 500 mL

POM Ⓗ **Rheomacrodex** (Cambridge) *UK*
Intravenous infusion, dextran 40 intravenous infusion in glucose intravenous infusion 5% or sodium chloride intravenous infusion 0.9%; 500 mL

GELATIN

UK
Indications. Plasma expansion in shock
Side-effects. Mild urticarial reactions
Warnings. Care with administration to animals susceptible to circulatory overloading
Dose. *Horses, dogs, cats*: *by intravenous infusion*, volume equal to estimated fluid loss; see also manufacturer's data sheet

POM **Gelofusine Veterinary** (Braun) *UK*
Intravenous infusion, succinylated gelatin (modified fluid gelatin, average molecular-weight 30 000) 40 g/litre, containing Na⁺ 154 mmol, Cl⁻ 125 mmol/litre, for *horses, dogs, cats*; 500 mL
Withdrawal Periods. Should not be used in *horses* intended for human consumption

POM **Haemaccel** (Intervet) *UK*
Intravenous infusion, polygeline (degraded gelatin, average molecular-weight 35 000) 35 g/litre, containing Na⁺ 145 mmol, K⁺ 5 mmol, Ca²⁺ 5 mmol, Cl⁻ 160 mmol/litre, for *horses, dogs, cats*; 500 mL
Withdrawal Periods. Slaughter withdrawal period nil

HEXASTARCH

UK
Indications. Plasma expansion in shock
Dose. *By intravenous infusion*, volume equal to estimated plasma volume deficit

POM Ⓗ **eloHAES** (Fresenius) *UK*
Intravenous infusion, hexastarch (average molecularweight 200 000) 6% in sodium chloride 0.9% intravenous infusion

16.3 Parenteral nutrition

Parenteral nutrition is intended to provide calories and protein precursors to animals as a substitute for a normal diet. It should only be used as a short term measure or where any method of enteral nutrition is contra-indicated. Parenteral nutrition can be provided as a solution containing glucose and protein hydrolysates or amino acids or a lipid emulsion. Daily calorific requirements should ideally be provided as 40 to 60% lipid with the remainder as carbohydrate. This is less important in short-term therapy, but in prolonged treatment an imbalance in nutrition can lead to hyperlipaemia or other metabolic problems.

Lipid emulsions may be given via peripheral veins, but glucose and amino acid solutions are hypertonic and should only be given via central veins. Nutrient solutions increase the risk of systemic infection and thrombophlebitis. Catheters and equipment used for parenteral nutrition should be placed and maintained using scrupulous asepsis.

UK

Indications. Provision of nutrients where enteral nutrition is contra-indicated

Warnings. Increased risk of thrombophlebitis and systemic infections

Dose. *Daily calorie requirements.*

Dogs, cats:

BER $= 30 \times$ BW $+ 70$

BER = basal energy requirement in kcal/day
BW = body-weight of patient in kg
Note. Actual energy requirements may be 2 times BER in post operative patients and those with systemic sepsis.

Daily protein requirements.
Dogs: 2–4 g of amino acids/kg
Cats: 4–6 g of amino acids/kg

POM Ⓗ **FreAmine III 8.5%** (Fresenius Kabi) *UK*
Solution, amino acids 79.1 g (nitrogen 13 g), Na⁺ 10, acetate 72 mmol, phosphate 10 mmol, Cl⁻ <3 mmol/litre; 500 mL, 1 litre

POM Ⓗ **FreAmine III 10%** (Fresenius Kabi) *UK*
Solution, amino acids 93 g (nitrogen 15.3 g), Na⁺ 10, acetate 89 mmol, phosphate 10 mmol, Cl⁻ <3 mmol/litre; 500 mL, 1 litre

POM Ⓗ **Intralipid 10%** (Fresenius Kabi) *UK*
Emulsion, total energy 1098 kcal, fractionated soya oil 100 g, glycerol 22.5 g, phosphate 15 mmol/litre; 100 mL, 500 mL

POM Ⓗ **Intralipid 20%** (Fresenius Kabi) *UK*
Emulsion, total energy 2006 kcal, fractionated soya oil 200 g, glycerol 22.5 g, phosphate 15 mmol/litre; 100 mL, 250 mL, 500 mL

POM Ⓗ **Intralipid 30%** (Fresenius Kabi) *UK*
Emulsion, total energy 3001 kcal, fractionated soya oil 300 g, glycerol 16.7 g, phosphate 15 mmol/litre; 333 mL

POM Ⓗ **Plasma-Lyte 148 (Dextrose 5%)** (Baxter) *UK*
Solution, total energy 200 kcal, K⁺ 16 mmol, Mg²⁺ 1.5 mmol, Na⁺ 40 mmol, Cl⁻ 40 mmol, Ca²⁺ 2.5 mmol/litre; 1 litre

POM Ⓗ **Plasma-Lyte M (Dextrose 5%)** (Baxter) *UK*
Solution, total energy 200 kcal, K⁺ 16 mmol, Mg²⁺ 1.5 mmol, Na⁺ 40 mmol, Cl⁻ 40 mmol, Ca²⁺ 2.5 mmol/litre; 1 litre

POM Ⓗ **Synthamin 17 without electrolytes** (Baxter) *UK*
Solution, amino acids 104.5 g (nitrogen 16.5 g), Cl⁻ 40 mmol/litre; 500 mL

POM Ⓗ **Vamin 9 Glucose** (Fresenius Kabi) *UK*
Solution, amino acids 70.2 g (nitrogen 9.4 g), total energy 399 kcal, K⁺ 20 mmol, Mg²⁺ 1.5 mmol, Na⁺ 50 mmol, Cl⁻ 50 mmol, Ca²⁺ 2.5 mmol/litre; 500 mL, 1 litre

POM Ⓗ **Vamin 18 (Electrolyte-Free)** (Fresenius Kabi) *UK*
Solution, amino acids 114 g (nitrogen 18 g)/litre; 500 mL, 1 litre

16.4 Drugs for ketosis

(bovine acetonaemia; ovine pregnancy toxaemia, twin lamb disease)

Several disorders may occur in ruminants, particularly cattle, when the animal experiences an inadequate energy supply.

In dairy cattle, primary ketosis results from high glucose demand of the mammary gland for lactose synthesis. This increased requirement for glucose causes a decreased amount of available oxaloacetate for the oxidative metabolism of acetate via the tricarboxylic acid (TCA, Kreb's cycle) and results in the accumulation of the ketone bodies acetoacetate, betahydroxybutrate, and acetone in blood, milk, and urine. Primary ketosis is generally self limiting with a precipitous drop in milk yield and considerable weight loss followed by gradual improvement in appetite and milk yield. In the early post partum period a reduced appetite secondary to mastitis, metritis, or left abomasal displacement may cause secondary ketosis resulting from poor appetite.

Starvation ketosis can occur during late gestation in range beef cattle carrying twin fetuses when maintained on either very poor grazing or fed low energy value roughages with no concentrate feeding. In sheep, energy requirements increase rapidly during the last 6 weeks of gestation, particularly in those ewes with 3 or 4 fetuses *in utero*, leading to ovine pregnancy toxaemia (twin lamb disease). Prognosis for these conditions with symptomatic treatments in either species is guarded unless the fetuses can be aborted. Ovine pregnancy toxaemia is fatal in all but the earliest cases due to the rapid accumulation of fat in the parenchymatous organs, especially the liver.

Rapid mobilisation of body fat in highly conditioned cows, that is body condition score greater than 4.0 on a scale 1.0 (very thin) to 5.0 (obese), in the immediate post partum period can result in fatty liver disease (fat cow syndrome). This syndrome is associated with an increased incidence of periparturient metabolic disease such as parturient paresis (milk fever) and infectious diseases such as mastitis and metritis due to environmental pathogens.

Treatment of dairy cattle with ketosis is aimed at providing replacement glucose, generally by intravenous injection of glucose 50% solution in addition to administration of glucose precursors such as propionate, lactate, glycerol, or propylene glycol given by mouth; overdosage may lead to diarrhoea. A glucocorticoid by injection is given concurrently. This further reduces milk yield thereby bringing the cow into positive energy status, promotes gluconeogenesis, and stimulates appetite. Dexamethasone♦ may induce parturition during the last 10 days of gestation in ewes with pregnancy toxaemia thereby improving prognosis. Many ewes with pregnancy toxaemia develop metabolic acidosis and additional treatment with intravenous solutions containing sodium bicarbonate may be necessary.

Ovine pregnancy toxaemia and starvation ketosis in cattle can be controlled by feeding an appropriate diet to supply sufficient dietary energy during late gestation. For prevention of ketosis during lactation, cows should be in condition score 2.5 to 3.0 at calving and be provided with well balanced, energy rich feed.

AMMONIUM LACTATE

UK
Indications. Ketosis
Dose. *Cattle*: *by mouth*, 200 g daily for 5 days

GLUCOSE
(Dextrose monohydrate)

UK
Indications. Ketosis
Dose.
Cattle: *by subcutaneous or slow intravenous injection*, 400–800 mL of glucose 40–50%
Sheep: *by subcutaneous or slow intravenous injection*, 100–200 mL of glucose 40–50%

PML **Glucose 40%** (Arnolds) *UK*
Injection, glucose 40% (400 mg/mL), for *cattle, sheep*; 400 mL
Withdrawal Periods. Slaughter withdrawal period nil, milk withdrawal period nil

GLYCEROL
(Glycerin)

UK
Indications. Ketosis; glaucoma (see section 12.5)
Dose. Ketosis, *by mouth*.
Cattle: 180 mL twice daily for 2 days then 90 mL twice daily for 2 days
Sheep: 90 mL daily

GSL **Glycerol** (Non-proprietary)

PROPYLENE GLYCOL

UK
Indications. Ketosis in cattle and sheep; pregnancy toxaemia in sheep
Dose. See preparation details

GSL **Forketos** (Arnolds) *UK*
Oral solution, propylene glycol 800 mg, cobalt (as sulphate) 210 micrograms/mL, for *cattle, sheep*; 1 litre, 25 litres
Withdrawal Periods. Slaughter withdrawal period nil, milk withdrawal period nil
Dose. *Cattle*: *by mouth*, 150–200 mL daily
Sheep: 2 mL/kg (maximum 120 ml). May be repeated after 7–8 hours if required

GSL **Ketol** (Intervet) *UK*
Oral liquid, for addition to drinking water or feed or to prepare an oral solution, propylene glycol 0.8 mL/mL, for *cattle, sheep*; 1 litre, 20 litres
Withdrawal Periods. Slaughter withdrawal period nil, milk withdrawal period nil
Dose. *By mouth*.
Cattle: 225 mL twice daily for 1 day then 115 mL twice daily for 3 days
Sheep: 115 mL daily

GSL **Ketosaid** (Norbrook) *UK*
Oral liquid, propylene glycol 0.99 mL/mL, for *cattle, sheep*
Withdrawal Periods. *Cattle, sheep*: slaughter withdrawal period nil, milk withdrawal period nil
Dose. *By mouth*.
Cattle: 200 mL twice daily for 1 day then 100 mL twice daily for 3 days
Sheep: 100 mL daily for 4 days

PML **Ketosis Drench** (Bttle Hayward & Bower) *UK*
Oral liquid, propylene glycol 0.8 mL/mL, cobalt (as sulphate heptahydrate) 210 micrograms/mL, for *cattle, sheep*
Withdrawal Periods. Slaughter withdrawal period nil, milk withdrawal period nil
Dose. *By mouth*.
Cattle: 150–200 mL daily
Sheep: 2 mL/kg (maximum 120 ml). May be repeated after 7–8 hours if required

GSL **Liquid Lectade** (Pfizer) *UK*
See Table 16.1 for preparation details
Dose. *Sheep*: pregnancy toxaemia, *by mouth*, 160 mL, repeat every 4–8 hours as necessary

GSL **Liquid Life-Aid** (Norbrook) *UK*
See Table 16.1 for preparation details
Dose. *Sheep*: pregnancy toxaemia, *by mouth*, 160 mL, repeat 3–6 times daily as necessary

PML **Twin Lamb** (Trilanco) *UK*
Oral liquid, propylene glycol containing cobalt sulphate 990 micrograms, potassium iodide 1.76 mg/mL, for *sheep*; 1 litre
Dose. *Sheep*: *by mouth*, 100 mL daily

SODIUM PROPIONATE

UK
Indications. Ketosis
Dose. *Cattle*: *by mouth*, 100–250 g daily

16.5 Minerals

16.5.1 Calcium
16.5.2 Magnesium
16.5.3 Phosphorus
16.5.4 Compound calcium, magnesium, and phosphorus preparations
16.5.5 Cobalt
16.5.6 Copper
16.5.7 Iodine
16.5.8 Iron
16.5.9 Manganese
16.5.10 Potassium
16.5.11 Selenium
16.5.12 Sodium
16.5.13 Zinc
16.5.14 Compound trace elements

Deficiencies of the major minerals can occur for one or more reasons. There may be increased demand associated with certain metabolic states, for example higher calcium requirements at the start of lactation. There may be inadequate supply in the feed or reduced availability in the feed, caused by the interference from other minerals such as occurs between magnesium and potassium after the use of fertilisers on pasture.

The need for treatment with the major minerals in ruminants is restricted almost entirely to calcium, magnesium, and phosphorus. Severe sodium deficiency in cattle may occur on maize silage diets but deficiencies of the other major mineral elements such as potassium and sulphur are rare in ruminants. Additional sodium, chloride, and occasionally potassium plus calcium may be required by competition horses especially those that sweat copiously, compete under adverse climatic conditions, or both.

Ruminant diets which rely upon conserved forages and cereal byproducts with inappropriate mineral supplementation can contain insufficient concentrations of trace elements and primary deficiencies of cobalt, copper, and selenium may occur. Secondary deficiency states may result from interference with the absorption of these trace elements by sulphate, molybdenum, or iron. A primary iron deficiency is almost entirely restricted to the rapidly growing piglet.

The causes of many excessive plasma-mineral concentrations include disorders of the endocrine system, neoplasia, accidental overdosage, and renal impairment.

Nutrient requirements of domestic species including horses, cattle, sheep, pigs, dogs, and cats are published by National Academy of Sciences Press, Washington DC.

16.5.1 Calcium

Calcium is an important electrolyte, a major component of bones and teeth, and is required for maintenance of a normal cardiac rhythm, blood clotting, and initiation of neuromuscular and metabolic activities.

Homoeostasis of calcium is mainly regulated by parathyroid hormone, calcitonin, and vitamin D.

In dairy cows, short-term hypocalcaemia almost always occurs at, or soon after, parturition when mammary gland secretions more than doubles the cow's requirement for calcium. This increased demand is not always balanced by an increase in the intestinal absorption of calcium or by the mobilisation of calcium from bone, and the concentration of ionised calcium in the plasma may fall. In ewes, hypocalaemia may occur in late pregnancy associated with a sudden dietary change or stressful event such as gathering or movement to other pastures. In beef cattle and sheep, hypocalcaemia may occur when animals are fed a diet high in oxalate-containing plants such as *Oxalis* species. Hypocalcaemic tetany has occasionally been described in heavily lactating mares especially those which have been recently stressed, for example by transportation. Mild hypocalcaemia has often been reported in horses with abdominal crises and may contribute to post operative ileus and weakness. In bitches eclampsia may occur in late pregnancy or early lactation.

Signs of hypocalcaemia in cattle are characterised by an initial short period of excitement, muscle tremors, and a stiff gait. The animal becomes ataxic followed by muscular weakness leading to sternal recumbency with a characteristic S bend of the neck or the head may be held averted against the flank. In sheep the clinical signs of hypocalcaemia are most commonly seen during the last month of pregnancy and include weakness leading to sternal recumbency, depression progressing to stupor, and ruminal bloat. In mares signs of lactation tetany may include profuse sweating, muscle tremor, weakness, ileus, stiffness and incoordination, staggering high-stepping gait, synchronous

diaphragmatic flutter, and may lead to tetanic seizures. In dogs hypocalcaemia is characterised by behavioural aberrations, muscle twitches, ataxia, paresis, and ultimately tetany and grand mal seizures.

In hypocalcaemia, the amount of calcium provided therapeutically is usually insufficient to counteract the increased demand from the mammary gland, but the objective of therapy is to correct the immediate imbalance to allow time for the homoeostatic mechanisms to adapt. An almost immediate and dramatic response follows intravenous infusion of calcium in all species. In ruminants, either calcium borogluconate 20% (calcium 15.2 mg/mL) or calcium borogluconate 40% (calcium 30.4 mg/mL) is administered by slow intravenous infusion while monitoring the heart rate and rhythm. A similar volume of calcium borogluconate 40% is administered by subcutaneous injection behind the shoulder in two divided sites. In dogs, calcium gluconate 10% (calcium 8.9 mg/mL) is administered intravenously. Subcutaneous injection of calcium salts in dogs and cats may cause necrosis at the site of injection and in cattle subcutaneous swelling may persist for several days. The amount of calcium provided therapeutically is small in comparison with the animal's daily requirement and it is essential to ensure that appetite is maintained. If eclampsia occurs in bitches, ideally puppies should not be allowed to feed from the dam but should be hand-reared.

The absorption of calcium from the gastro-intestinal tract and mobilisation of calcium from bone may be accelerated by the administration of vitamin D or related compounds (see section 16.6.4). If they are to be administered before calving it is necessary to accurately predict the date of calving or induce parturition with glucocorticoids or prostaglandin preparations. Alfacalcidol or colecalciferol may be used for the prevention of hypocalcaemia in dairy cattle. In cattle, feeding an acidifying diet during the last 2 to 3 weeks of gestation dramatically reduces the prevalence of hypocalcaemia. Growing cattle fed high cereal rations with inappropriate mineral content are prone to pathological fractures.

In dogs and cats, oral calcium supplementation during the latter stages of pregnancy may help to prevent hypocalcaemia. Growing animals, in particular dogs, may develop skeletal undermineralisation if the diet is deficient in calcium or contains a low calcium:phosphorus ratio. Adequate minerals are obtained from a balanced commercial food and additional mineral supplementation may lead to bone deformation in giant breeds.

Synchronous diaphragmatic flutter is most commonly found in exhausted dehydrated horses. Hypocalcaemia, in particular, as well as hypokalaemia, and alkalosis may all contribute to increased phrenic nerve irritability so that it becomes stimulated in response to atrial depolarisation. As hypocalcaemia is the most likely deficit, treatment includes the administration of calcium by *slow* intravenous infusion (500 mL calcium borogluconate 20% diluted 1:4 in sodium chloride 0.9%) and given according to the patient's response. During administration, the heart should be auscultated or the pulse palpated so that on detection of any cardiac irregularity, the infusion can be immediately stopped. In some cases restoration of the ECF and circulating blood volume may be sufficient to correct the abnormality. Calcium administration has been suggested for its cardioprotective properties in hyperkalaemic horses such as patients with hyperkalaemic periodic paralysis or anuric renal failure; care should be taken with intravenous administration of calcium in such patients as described above.

Hypercalcaemia is occasionally seen and tends to result from chronic renal failure or neoplasia. It may occasionally occur in conjunction with other conditions such as paraneoplastic syndromes and vitamin D toxicosis.

CALCIUM SALTS

UK

Indications. Prevention and treatment of hypocalcaemia
Side-effects. Persistent swelling or necrosis at subcutaneous injection site, see notes above
Warnings. Administer calcium 40% to cows only by subcutaneous injection if toxaemia or cardiac insufficiency suspected
Dose. Expressed as calcium; see also notes above
Treatment.
Horses, cattle: *by subcutaneous or slow intravenous injection*, 3–12 g according to the patient's response, dependent on clinical signs and blood analysis
Sheep: *by subcutaneous or slow intravenous injection*, 0.5–1.5 g according to the patient's response, dependent on clinical signs and blood analysis
Dogs, cats: *by slow intravenous injection*, 75–500 mg according to the patient's response, dependent on clinical signs and blood analysis

Prophylaxis.
Dogs, cats: see oral preparation details

Notes. 1 mg calcium = 11.2 mg calcium gluconate = 13.2 mg calcium borogluconate

Calcium gluconate 10% = calcium (as gluconate) 8.9 mg/mL
Calcium borogluconate 20% = calcium (as borogluconate) 15.2 mg/mL
Calcium borogluconate 40% = calcium (as borogluconate) 30.4 mg/mL

POM Ⓗ **Calcium Gluconate** (Non-proprietary) *UK*
Injection, calcium (as gluconate) 8.9 mg/mL; 10 mL

PML **Calcibor CBG 20** (Arnolds) *UK*
Injection, calcium (as borogluconate) 15 mg/mL, for *cattle*; 400 mL
Withdrawal Periods. *Cattle*: slaughter withdrawal period nil, milk withdrawal period nil

PML **Calcibor CBG 40** (Arnolds) *UK*
Injection, calcium (as borogluconate) 30 mg/mL, for *cattle*; 400 mL
Withdrawal Periods. *Cattle*: slaughter withdrawal period nil, milk withdrawal period nil

PML **Calciject 40** (Norbrook) *UK*
Injection, calcium borogluconate 400 mg/mL, for *cattle*; 400 mL
Withdrawal Periods. *Cattle*: slaughter withdrawal period nil, milk withdrawal period nil

Canovel Calcium Tablets (Pfizer) *UK*
Tablets, calcium, for *dogs, cats*; 30, 150
Dose. *By mouth.*
Dogs: (<9 kg body-weight) ½ tablet daily; (>9 kg body-weight) 1 tablet/9 kg daily
Cats: ½ tablet daily

Hi-Cal (Bimeda) *UK*
Oral paste, calcium (as propionate) 40g/dose applicator, for *cattle*

16.5.2 Magnesium

Magnesium is an essential electrolyte, a cofactor in numerous enzyme systems, and involved in phosphate transfer, muscle contractility, and neuronal transmission.

Magnesium deficiency may occur in ruminants on lush pasture ('grass staggers') associated with heavy fertiliser application containing nitrogen and potash. Grazing on such pastures that may lead to hypomagnesaemia in ruminants does not appear to affect horses in a similar manner. Hypomagnesaemia may also occur in outwintered cows exposed to adverse weather conditions.

Hypomagnesaemia may be a cause of sudden death in young suckled beef calves. Acute magnesium deficiency is more commonly seen in beef cows during early lactation. Affected cattle become ataxic and excitable and collapse with tetanic convulsions of the limbs and neck. Tetany, seizures, and death have been described in critically ill foals with profound hypomagnesaemia.

Chronic magnesium deficiency may be associated with a decreased appetite and a reduction in milk yield. Hypomagnesaemia is often encountered in dry cows in herds with a high prevalence of milk fever (hypocalcaemia). In horses, clinical hypomagnesaemia has been occasionally found in association with other electrolyte disturbances in conditions such as transit tetany and synchronous diaphragmatic flutter.

Intravenous administration of magnesium sulphate may precipitate fatal effects on the cardiovascular and respiratory systems in cattle. Clinical experience suggests that slow intravenous administration of 50 mL of magnesium sulphate 25% solution added to 400 mL calcium borogluconate 40% solution reduces the possibility of seizures. Afterwhich 400 mL of magnesium sulphate 25% solution is administered subcutaneously. Hypomagnesaemic tetany is almost invariably due to a long-term dietary magnesium deficiency. It is essential to ensure adequate daily magnesium supplementation, particularly to lactating cattle. This metabolic disease is more commonly encountered in extensively managed beef cows with inadequate dietary supplementation. Long-term supplementation with magnesium may be achieved by compound feedstuffs containing high concentration of calcined magnesite, provision of adequate fibre in the ration, direct supplementation using slow-release magnesium alloy ruminal boluses or addition of magnesium compounds to the drinking water.

MAGNESIUM SALTS

UK

Indications. Prevention and treatment of magnesium deficiency

Warnings. Intravenous administration of magnesium salts may precipitate seizures

Dose.

Cattle: *by mouth*, see preparation details

by subcutaneous injection, 200–400 mL of magnesium sulphate 25% according to the patient's response

Sheep: *by mouth*, see preparation details

by subcutaneous injection, 50–100 mL of magnesium sulphate 25% according to the patient's response

PML **Magnesium Sulphate Injection BP(Vet) 25%** (Arnolds) *UK*
Injection, magnesium sulphate 250 mg/mL, for *cattle*; 400 mL
Withdrawal Periods. *Cattle*: slaughter withdrawal period nil, milk withdrawal period nil

PML **Magniject** (Norbrook) *UK*
Injection, magnesium sulphate 250 mg/mL, for *cattle*, *sheep*; 400 mL
Withdrawal Periods. *Cattle*, *sheep*: slaughter withdrawal period nil, milk withdrawal period nil

Rumag Aqua (Rumenco) *UK*
Oral solution, for addition to drinking water, magnesium 50 mg/mL, for *cattle*
Dose. *Cattle*: *by addition to drinking water*, 0.33 litre/animal daily

Rumag Sugalic (Rumenco) *UK*
Oral liquid, for addition to feed, magnesium 38 mg/mL in molasses base, for *cattle*
Dose. *Cattle*: *by addition to feed*, 0.5 litre/animal daily

PML **Rumbul** (Agrimin) *UK*
Ruminal bolus, m/r, magnesium (as magnesium/aluminium/copper alloy) 15 g, for *calves more than 50 kg body-weight, sheep more than 30 kg body-weight*; 20
Withdrawal Periods. Slaughter withdrawal period nil, milk withdrawal period nil
Dose. *Calves*: (>50 kg body-weight) two 15-g boluses. Repeat after 3 weeks if calf predominantly on milk diet
Sheep: (>30 kg body-weight) one 15-g bolus given 2 days before period of risk. Repeat after 3 weeks if required
Ruminal bolus, m/r, magnesium (as magnesium/aluminium/copper alloy) 40 g, for *dairy cattle more than 300 kg body-weight*; 10
Withdrawal Periods. Slaughter withdrawal period nil, milk withdrawal period nil
Dose. *Cattle*: (>300 kg body-weight) two 40-g boluses given 2–3 days before period of risk. Repeat after 4 weeks if required

---

16.5.3 Phosphorus

Phosphorus is a key component in energy and protein metabolism and also as a structural part of bone. Homoeostasis is controlled by vitamin D and calcium.

Acute phosphorus deficiency is uncommon in farm animals but may be encountered in older beef suckler cows during the first 6 weeks of lactation. Hypophosphataemia may occur in association with parturient paresis in dairy cows but specific supplementation is not usually required. Phosphorus deficiency in the lactating cow has been associated with the development of post-parturient haemoglobinuria after the onset of acute haemolysis. More commonly, phosphorus deficiency causes chronic hypophosphataemia, which may result in skeletal defects, lameness, and low milk production.

Phosphorus containing compounds may be used if animals fail to respond to calcium therapy for parturient paresis. Chronic hypophosphataemia may occur in ruminants. However, high phosphorus concentration in cereals suggest that this may only occur when certain byproducts are fed and clinical signs should be alleviated by correct mineral supplementation.

Foals fed excessive amounts of phosphorus may show lesions of osteochondrosis although clinical signs of nutritional secondary parathyroidism do not tend to be seen providing adequate calcium is fed. Nutritional secondary parathyroidism in horses due to an excessive dietary intake of phosphorus or oxalates coupled with an inadequate supply of calcium may result, especially in younger horses, in a shifting lameness or a condition referred to as 'big head'. The latter is less commonly seen today.

PHOSPHORUS SALTS

UK

Indications. Treatment and prevention of hypophosphataemia

Warnings. Avoid perivascular injection

POM **Foston** (Intervet) *UK*
Injection, toldimfos sodium 200 mg/mL, for *cattle*, *dogs*; 50 mL
Withdrawal Periods. *Cattle*: slaughter withdrawal period nil, milk withdrawal period nil
Dose. Acute hypophosphataemia. *By subcutaneous, intramuscular, or intravenous injection*.
Cattle: 10–25 mL
Dogs: 1–3 mL
Chronic hypophosphataemia. *By subcutaneous or intramuscular injection*.
Cattle: 2.5–5.0 mL every 2 days for 5–10 doses
Dogs: 1–2 mL every 2 days for 5–10 doses

POM **Phosphorus Supplement Injection** (Arnolds) *UK*
Injection, phosphorus (as calcium hypophosphite) 18 mg/mL, for *cattle*; 400 mL
Withdrawal Periods. *Cattle*: slaughter withdrawal period nil, milk withdrawal period nil
Dose. *Cattle*: *by intravenous or subcutaneous injection*, up to 400 mL

16.5.4 Compound calcium, magnesium, and phosphorus preparations

Compound mineral preparations containing calcium with magnesium and phosphorus have been used in ruminants in certain geographical areas with reported clinical efficacy. Some cases of milk fever in cows may be associated with subclinical hypomagnesaemia before calving, and cows that relapse repeatedly after treatment with calcium solutions may be hypophosphataemic. The precise biochemistry of the disorder should be determined by blood analysis before treatment, if practicable. Sheep may exhibit similarly complicated biochemical abnormalities for which compound mineral preparations may be beneficial.

Compound mineral preparations are often given by subcutaneous administration shortly before calving for the prevention of milk fever.

UK

PML Calcibor CM20 (Arnolds) *UK*
Injection, calcium (as borogluconate) 15 mg, magnesium hypophosphite 50 mg/mL, for *sheep*; 400 mL
Withdrawal Periods. Slaughter withdrawal period nil, milk withdrawal period nil
Dose. *Sheep*: *by subcutaneous injection*, 50–100 mL

PML Calcibor CM40 (Arnolds) *UK*
Injection, calcium (as borogluconate) 30 mg, magnesium hypophosphite 50 mg/mL, for *cattle*; 400 mL
Withdrawal Periods. Slaughter withdrawal period nil, milk withdrawal period nil
Dose. *Cattle*: *by subcutaneous or slow intravenous injection*, 400 mL

PML Calcibor CM+D Injection (Arnolds) *UK*
Injection, calcium (as calcium gluconate and calcium borogluconate) 6g/400 mL, magnesium (as magnesium hypophosphite) 1.84 g/400 mL, glucose 80 g/400 mL, for *cattle*
Withdrawal Periods. Slaughter withdrawal period nil, milk withdrawal period nil
Dose. *Cattle*: *by slow intravenous injection*, 400 mL and *by subcutaneous injection*, 400 mL

PML Calciject 20 CM (Norbrook) *UK*
Injection, calcium borogluconate 14.8 mg, magnesium 4.6 mg/mL, for *cattle, sheep*; 400 mL
Withdrawal Periods. Slaughter withdrawal period nil, milk withdrawal period nil
Dose. *Cattle*: *by subcutaneous or slow intravenous injection*, 400–800 mL
Sheep, pigs: *by subcutaneous or slow intravenous injection*, 50–80 mL

PML Calciject 40 CM (Norbrook) *UK*
Injection, calcium borogluconate 40%, magnesium hypophosphite hexahydrate 50 mg/mL, for *cattle*; 400 mL
Withdrawal Periods. Slaughter withdrawal period nil, milk withdrawal period nil
Dose. *Cattle*: *by subcutaneous or slow intravenous injection*, 200–400 mL

PML Calciject LV (Norbrook) *UK*
Injection, calcium 42 mg, magnesium 7.8 mg/mL, for *cattle*; 100 mL
Withdrawal Periods. Slaughter withdrawal period nil, milk withdrawal period nil
Dose. *Cattle*: *by subcutaneous or slow intravenous injection*, 100–200 mL

PML Calciject PMD (Norbrook) *UK*
Injection, calcium borogluconate 200 mg/mL, glucose 200 mg, magnesium hypophosphite 50 mg/mL, for *horses, cattle, sheep, goats, pigs*; 400 mL
Dose. *By subcutaneous or slow intravenous injection. Horses*: 150–300 mL
Cattle: 200–400 mL
Sheep, goats, pigs: 15–50 mL

PML Ewecal (Young's) *UK*
Injection, calcium (as calcium borogluconate, calcium gluconate, calcium hydroxide) 41.66 mg, magnesium (as magnesium chloride) 7.8 mg/mL, for *sheep*; 100 mL
Withdrawal Periods. Slaughter withdrawal period nil, milk withdrawal period nil
Dose. *Sheep*: *by subcutaneous injection*, 10–20 mL

PML Maxacal (Crown) *UK*
Injection, calcium (as calcium borogluconate, calcium gluconate, calcium hydroxide) 41.66 mg, magnesium (as magnesium chloride) 7.8 mg/mL, for *cattle*; 100 mL
Withdrawal Periods. Slaughter withdrawal period nil, milk withdrawal period nil
Dose. *Cattle*: (500 kg body-weight) *by subcutaneous or slow intravenous injection*, 100 mL

PML Maxacal S (Crown) *UK*
Injection, calcium (as calcium borogluconate, calcium gluconate, calcium hydroxide) 41.66 mg, magnesium (as magnesium chloride) 7.8 mg/mL, for *sheep*; 100 mL
Withdrawal Periods. Slaughter withdrawal period nil, milk withdrawal period nil
Dose. *Sheep*: *by subcutaneous injection*, 10–20 mL

16.5.5 Cobalt

Cobalt is an essential trace element and deficiency may occur in animals on pasture providing inadequate cobalt. Cobalt is a component of cyanocobalamin and hydroxocobalamin, which are forms of vitamin B_{12} (see section 16.6.2). Vitamin B_{12} is synthesised by the rumen microflora and therefore cobalt supplements should be given by mouth.

Cobalt deficiency predominantly affects young growing ruminants, however the signs of cobalt deficiency in ruminants are not specific. There is decreased appetite, loss of body-weight, and failure to thrive. Pica often develops and wool growth is poor. There is non-specific reduction in immunity in sheep and an associated increased prevalence of helminthiasis, and bacterial infections such as pasteurellosis and clostridial disease. Growing cattle are less prone to cobalt deficiency. Injection of cyanocobalamin (see section 16.6.2) is useful for the treatment of the effects of cobalt deficiency in ruminants.

Oral supplements are available to prevent cobalt deficiency.

COBALT OXIDE

UK

Indications. Prevention and treatment of cobalt deficiency
Contra-indications. Administration of ruminal boluses to animals under 8 weeks of age
Dose. See preparation details

Aquatrace Cobalt (Brinicombe) *UK*
Tablets, dispersible, cobalt 3 g/sachet, for *cattle*
Withdrawal Periods. *Cattle*: slaughter withdrawal period nil, milk withdrawal period nil
Dose. *Cattle*: *by addition to drinking water in dispenser*, 1 sachet is sufficient for 25 animals for 7 days

GSL SI-RO-CO Cobalt Pellets (Cox) *UK*
Ruminal bolus, m/r, cobalt oxide 3 g, for *sheep*; 100
Dose. *Sheep*: one 3-g ruminal bolus
Ruminal bolus, m/r, cobalt oxide 9 g, for *cattle*; 30
Dose. *Cattle*: one 9-g ruminal bolus

16.5.6 Copper

Copper is an integral component of several important enzymes and essential for the production of bone, haemoglobin, melanin, and keratin. Copper deficiency is common in young growing ruminants in certain geographical areas. Primary deficiency may occur as a result of inadequate dietary intake and secondary deficiency because of high levels of molybdenum, iron, or sulphur in the diet. Increased concentrations of molybdenum and sulphur favour the formation of complexes, which reduce copper absorption. Horses do not seem to be as sensitive to molybdenum interference with copper utilisation as ruminants and excessive molybdenum is not normally considered to be a significant factor in copper deficiency in equines.

In growing cattle, primary and secondary copper deficiency can cause unthriftiness, loss of coat colour, and diarrhoea. 'Pine' is sometimes used to describe unthriftiness due to copper or cobalt deficiency in calves. If copper deficiency is prolonged, the structure of the collagen is altered resulting in deformity of long bones.

Copper deficiency during mid gestation can result in the birth of lambs with enzootic ataxia ('swayback') due to demyelination. It has been recommended that when a case of swayback is confirmed in a flock, each lamb should be given copper (0.2 mL of copper (as copper heptonate) 12.5 mg/mL for a lamb 5 kg body-weight). Delayed swayback may be encountered in 2 to 4 month-old lambs. In growing lambs copper deficiency is associated with failure to thrive and a poor open fleece.

Copper deficiency in young horses has been suggested to be a contributory cause to certain forms of developmental orthopaedic disease (DOD). Anecdotal reports of oral copper supplementation being of benefit in certain cases of poor performance have not been scientifically verified.

In ruminants, treatment of copper deficiency is by parenteral injection of copper salts or oral administration of copper oxide needles. There is great variation in the susceptibility of different sheep breeds to copper toxicity and a diagnosis of copper deficiency must be established before supplementation commences. Serum-copper concentration and assays for copper containing enzymes are helpful but liver copper content remains the most useful indicator of true deficiency.

Copper salts such as calcium copper edetate and cuproxoline are rapidly mobilised from the site of intramuscular or subcutaneous administration and may be toxic in sheep. The recommended doses for sheep provide only a small amount of copper. Preparations based on methionine or heptonate complexes are not so readily mobilised from the site of injection and are therefore more commonly used in sheep.

The oral administration of copper can also correct copper deficiencies but more slowly than parenteral treatment because of the time taken for intestinal absorption and possible inhibition by dietary sulphates, iron, and molybdenum. In horses, oral administration of copper, where required, is recommended.

Absorbed excess copper provided by either oral or parenteral preparations is stored in body tissues predominantly in the liver. In sheep, once the concentration of copper in the liver has exceeded a critical value, sudden release of copper into the blood may cause intravascular haemolysis leading to a haemolytic crisis and death. Some sheep breeds are especially susceptible, notably the Suffolk, Texel, Welsh, and rare breeds such as the Soay and North Ronaldsay.

Excessive liver-copper storage, an inherited disease, may occur in Bedlington terriers and rarely in other breeds. Treatment for copper hepatotoxicosis includes penicillamine or trientine (see section 3.10). Control includes restriction of copper intake and provision of a high fat diet to stimulate biliary secretion and copper excretion.

COPPER SALTS

UK

Indications. Prevention and treatment of copper deficiency; to improve growth rate and feed conversion efficiency in pigs (see section 17.2)

Contra-indications. Concurrent administration of other copper-containing preparations; hepatic or renal impairment

Warnings. Administer only to animals at risk or suffering from copper deficiency, sheep are particularly susceptible to copper toxicity

Dose. Dependent on copper-serum concentrations and liver analyses before and after treatment

Aquatrace Copper (Brinicombe) *UK*
Tablets, dispersible, copper 30 g/sachet, for *cattle*; 200-g sachets
Withdrawal Periods. *Cattle*: slaughter withdrawal period nil, milk withdrawal period nil
Contra-indications. Concurrent administration of iodine
Dose. *Cattle*: *by addition to drinking water in dispenser*, 1 sachet is sufficient for 25 animals for 7 days

PML **Copacaps Cattle** (Merial) *UK*
Ruminal bolus, m/r, copper (as oxide) 8.8 g, for *cattle more than 100 kg body-weight*; 50
Withdrawal Periods. *Cattle*: slaughter withdrawal period nil, milk withdrawal period nil
Dose. *Cattle*: (100–200 kg body-weight) one 8.8-g ruminal bolus; (>200 kg body-weight) two 8.8-g ruminal boluses

PML **Copacaps Ewe/Calf** (Merial) *UK*
Ruminal bolus, m/r, copper (as oxide) 2.1 g, for *calves, sheep*; 200
Withdrawal Periods. *Cattle, sheep*: slaughter withdrawal period nil, milk withdrawal period nil
Dose. *Calves*: one 2.1-g ruminal bolus per 25 kg body-weight (maximum dose 8 ruminal boluses)
Sheep: (approximately 50 kg body-weight) two 2.1-g ruminal boluses; *lambs*: (20–40 kg body-weight) one 2.1-g ruminal bolus

GSL **Copinox Cattle** (Bayer) *UK*
Ruminal bolus, for *cattle more than 100 kg body-weight*
Dose. *Cattle*: one 27-g ruminal bolus

GSL **Copinox Ewe/Calf** (Bayer) *UK*
Ruminal bolus, for *calves and sheep less than 100 kg body-weight*
Dose. *Calves, sheep*: one 4-g ruminal bolus

GSL **Copinox Lamb** (Bayer) *UK*
Ruminal bolus, for *lambs more than 10 kg body-weight*
Dose. *Lambs*: one 2-g bolus

PML **Copper Sulphate** (UKASTA) *UK*
Oral powder, for addition to feed copper (as copper sulphate) 254 g/kg, for *dairy cattle, dairy goats, pigs* (see section 17.2)
Withdrawal Periods. *Cattle, goats*: slaughter withdrawal period nil, milk withdrawal period nil. *Pigs*: slaughter withdrawal period nil
Dose. *Cattle, goats*: up to 2 g/head

PML **Copprite** (Pfizer) *UK*
Ruminal bolus, m/r, copper (as oxide) 1.7 g, 3.4 g, 20.4 g, for *cattle, sheep*; 1.7-g ruminal bolus 100, 3.4-g ruminal bolus 50, 20.4-g ruminal bolus 24
Dose. *Cattle*: (<100 kg body-weight) two 3.4-g ruminal boluses; (100–300 kg body-weight) one 20.4-g ruminal bolus; (>300 kg body-weight) one or two 20.4-g ruminal boluses
Sheep: one 3.4-g ruminal bolus; *lambs*: one 1.7-g ruminal bolus

PML **Coppaclear** (Crown) *UK*
Injection, copper (as heptonate) 12.5 mg/mL, for *sheep*
Withdrawal Periods. *Sheep*: slaughter 7 days
Dose. *Sheep*: *by intramuscular injection*, 25 mg given 10 weeks before lambing

POM **Coprin** (Schering-Plough) *UK*
Injection, copper (as calcium copper edetate) 100 mg/unit dose, for *cattle*; dose applicator
Withdrawal Periods. *Cattle*: slaughter 7 days, milk withdrawal period nil
Dose. *Cattle*: *by subcutaneous injection*, (<100 kg body-weight) ½ unit dose; (>100 kg body-weight) 1–2 unit doses every 4 months as necessary

PML **Cuvine** (Vericore VP) *UK*
Injection, copper (as heptonate) 12.5 mg/mL, for *sheep*; 100 mL
Withdrawal Periods. *Sheep*: slaughter 7 days
Dose. *Sheep*: *by intramuscular injection*, 25 mg given 10 weeks before lambing

PML **Swaycop** (Young's) *UK*
Injection, copper (as heptonate) 12.5 mg/mL, for *sheep*
Withdrawal Periods. *Sheep*: slaughter 7 days
Dose. *Sheep*: *by intramuscular injection*, 25 mg given 10 weeks before lambing

PML **Veticop** (Virbac) *UK*
Injection, copper (as copper methionate complex) 20 mg/mL, for sheep
Withdrawal Periods. Slaughter 28 days
Dose. *Sheep*: *by subcutaneous injection*, 40 mg given 10 weeks before lambing

16.5.7 Iodine

Dietary iodine is required for the synthesis of tri-iodothyronine and thyroxine by the thyroid gland.

Primary iodine deficiency occurs as a result of low dietary intake. Secondary deficiency may result from feeding plants such as *Brassica* spp. containing thiocyanates, which inhibit iodine uptake by the thyroid gland.

Deficiency may result in compensatory hyperplasia of the thyroid gland (goitre), alopecia, prolonged gestation, and an increased incidence of stillbirths and weak offspring. The association between weak calf syndrome and iodine deficiency is not well established.

Many concentrated foods and mineral supplements (see section 16.7) contain sufficient iodine to ensure that the overall dietary concentration exceeds 1 mg/kg feed. However, reliance on home-grown silage and lack of supplementation to pregnant cattle may result in iodine deficiency. Greater concentrations may be needed if the diet also contains kale, rape-seed, linseed, groundnut, or soya bean.

Toxic dietary intakes in horses can result from excessive iodine or from feeding certain feedingstuffs high in iodine such as kelp and may result in toxic goitre in foals. The most vulnerable animals are foals from mares who are supplemented with high levels of iodine. The iodine is concentrated across the placenta and milk, and foals receive relatively higher intakes than the mare.

IODINE

UK
Indications. Iodine deficiency

Aquatrace Iodine (Brinicombe) *UK*
Tablets, dispersible, iodine 11.37 g/sachet, for *cattle*; 300-g sachets
Withdrawal Periods. *Cattle*: slaughter withdrawal period nil, milk withdrawal period nil
Contra-indications. Concurrent administration of copper
Dose. *Cattle*: *by addition to drinking water in dispenser*, 1 sachet is sufficient for 25 animals for 7 days

16.5.8 Iron

Iron is an essential constituent of haemoglobin and is involved in many oxidative processes.

Acute iron deficiency affects piglets that are maintained under conditions of intensive husbandry and rely on an all milk diet. The piglet's requirement for approximately 7 mg of iron daily is not provided by the milk diet alone. Acute hypochromic anaemia develops within the first three weeks of life and clinical signs appear at 3 to 6 weeks of age. The piglets appear pale and hairy. Their food intake and growth rate decline and diarrhoea is common.

In piglets, iron is always administered in the form of a complex such as iron dextran or gleptoferron, in order to avoid the toxic effects caused by ions of free iron. Iron supplements are usually given in the first week of life. The iron is stored in body tissues until required for haematopoiesis. Occasionally, there may be residual staining of the tissues at, or near, the site of injection. Anaphylactic reactions have been reported occasionally.

Iron deficiency resulting in iron-deficiency anaemia may occur in any species. Iron deficiency in dogs and cats may occur as a result of chronic blood loss, haemolysis, and secondary to a number of clinical conditions such as feline leukaemia or chronic renal failure. Dietary deficiency is rarely seen in dogs and cats. Chronic blood loss may be associated in some species with gastro-intestinal parasites (for example haemonchosis) or ectoparasites (such as sucking lice). In horses, haemorrhagic gastric ulceration and exercise induced pulmonary haemorrhage are other possible causes of blood loss, although it is rare that any apparent anaemia in athletic horses is associated with iron deficiency. Nutritional iron deficiency is not considered to be a practical problem in foals or mature horses. Treatment should not be instituted without prior confirmation of iron deficiency. Excessive supplementation can result in toxicity. Diagnosis of the cause and correction of chronic blood loss is essential. Oral treatment should be used in dogs and cats unless continuing severe blood loss or malabsorption of iron due to gastro-intestinal damage is present.

IRON COMPLEXES

UK
Indications. Prevention and treatment of iron-deficiency anaemia
Contra-indications. Parenteral administration in dogs and cats with hepatic or renal impairment, cardiac disease
Side-effects. Occasionally residual staining at site of injection; oral treatment may cause vomiting, constipation and diarrhoea in dogs and cats; parenteral iron may cause arrhythmias, anaphylaxis, shunting of iron to reticuloendothelial stores in dogs and cats.
Dose. *Dogs ♦: by mouth,* 100–300 mg daily
by intramuscular injection, 25 mg/kg weekly (**but see notes above**)
Cats ♦: by mouth, 50–100 mg daily
by intramuscular injection, 25 mg/kg weekly (**but see notes above**)

Piglets: *by intramuscular injection*, 200 mg

PML **Ferrofax 20%** (Vericore LP) *UK*
Injection, iron (as iron dextran) 200 mg/mL, for *piglets*; 100 mL
Withdrawal Periods. *Pigs*: slaughter withdrawal period nil

PML **Gleptosil** (Alstoe) *UK*
Injection, iron (as gleptoferran) 200 mg/mL, for *piglets*; 100 mL
Withdrawal Periods. *Pigs*: slaughter withdrawal period nil

PML **Leodex 20%** (Leo) *UK*
Injection, iron (as iron dextran) 200 mg/mL, for *piglets*; 100 mL
Withdrawal Periods. *Pigs*: slaughter withdrawal period nil

PML **Scordex** (Crown) *UK*
Injection, iron (as iron dextran) 200 mg/mL, for *piglets*; 100 mL
Withdrawal Periods. *Pigs*: slaughter withdrawal period nil

PML **Tri-Dex** (Trilanco) *UK*
Injection, iron (as iron dextran) 100 mg/mL, for *piglets*; 100 mL

16.5.9 Manganese

A deficiency of manganese is uncommon, but may occur in ruminants if the diet contains less than 20 mg manganese per kg feed or high concentrations of calcium and phosphorus. The clinical signs of deficiency include poor growth, weakness, infertility, birth of stillborn or weak offspring, and an increase in the proportion of male offspring. Most concentrated foods and dietary supplements contain manganese. Deficiency is most likely to occur in herbivores consuming only herbage grown in regions where the soil is deficient in manganese and high in calcium.

The manganese requirements of horses are not well understood. Suggested effects of deficiency on bone development are currently unproven.

MANGANESE

UK

Indications. Manganese deficiency
Dose. See preparation details

Aquatrace Manganese (Brinicombe) *UK*
Tablets, dispersible, manganese 35 g/sachet, for *cattle*; 300-g sachets
Withdrawal Periods. Slaughter withdrawal period nil, milk withdrawal period nil
Dose. *Cattle*: *by addition to drinking water in dispenser*, 1 sachet is sufficient for 25 animals for 7 days

16.5.10 Potassium

Potassium is an essential electrolyte that is important for the maintenance of intracellular osmotic pressure. In association with sodium, potassium helps maintain membrane potential and can influence nerve transmission and muscle function. Dietary sources of potassium include molasses and vegetable matter.

Potassium deficiency is uncommon in dogs and cats. However it has been seen in healthy adult cats on a low potassium vegetarian diet or an acidifying diet, and chronic diarrhoea may result in increased faecal potassium losses. Potassium deficiency is most commonly reported in cats with polyuric renal failure. Hypokalaemic polymyopathy has been reported in certain cat breeds, in particular Bur-

mese have an inherited predisposition to this condition. Clinical signs of deficiency are episodic muscular weakness, ventroflexion of the head and a stiff gait with no symptoms between episodes and relapses within days or weeks. A diagnosis should be made from the plasma-potassium concentration before supplementation is instituted.

Potassium supplementation (with Slow-K) may be required when administering some diuretics (see section 4.2), although in patients with mild hypokalaemia withdrawal of the diuretic and normal feeding may be sufficient.

Care should be taken when giving potassium salts or potassium rich feeds to horses prone to hyperkalaemic periodic paralysis.

POTASSIUM SALTS

UK

Indications. Potassium deficiency
Contra-indications. Renal impairment, adrenal impairment
Side-effects. Gastro-intestinal irritation, vomiting, diarrhoea, melaena
Warnings. Caution in patients with cardiac disease, renal impairment
Dose. See preparation details

P Ⓗ **Slow-K** (Alliance) *UK*
Tablets, m/r, s/c, potassium chloride 600 mg (8 mmol each of K^+ and Cl^-)
Dose. *Dogs, cats*: *by mouth*, 74.5–223.5 mg/kg (1–3 mmol/kg) once daily

Tumil-K (Arnolds) *UK*
Tablets, potassium gluconate 468 mg, for *cats*; 100
Oral powder, for addition to feed, potassium gluconate 468 mg/650 mg of powder, for *cats*; 116 g (650 mg of powder = ¼ 5-mL spoonful)
Dose. *Cats*: *by mouth*, 468 mg/4.5 kg body-weight twice daily with food

16.5.11 Selenium

The essential role of selenium is as part of the enzyme glutathione peroxidase, whose function is to prevent free radical damage to tissues.

Deficiency is seen in young or rapidly growing calves and lambs causing muscular degeneration in cardiac, respiratory, or skeletal muscles; vitamin E/selenium responsive myopathy may also affect skeletal and cardiac muscles especially in young foals. It is reported that moderate selenium deficiency may result in illthrift, reduced growth rate, and compromised immunocompetence.

Selenium status can be assessed by measuring the activity of glutathione peroxidase in red blood cells. Plasma-selenium concentration tends to be a better indicator of very recent selenium status and toxicity than glutathione peroxidase.

There is a complex interaction between the requirements for selenium and vitamin E whereby either nutrient may substitute, in part, for the other.

Confirmed deficiencies may be treated by the parenteral administration of selenium salts, but amounts greater than 400 micrograms of readily available selenium per kg body-weight may cause acute toxicity in sheep. There have been anecdotal reports of anaphylactoid responses in horses to vitamin E/selenium preparations given by injection. The administration of selenium containing anthelmintic preparations may prevent the development of deficiency states in ruminants.

Acute and chronic selenium toxicity can occur in horses, can be fatal, and is usually due to excessive supplementation. Clinical signs of acute toxicity include respiratory distress, diarrhoea, recumbancy, and death. Chronic toxicity is characterised by emaciation, lameness, hoof horn sloughing, or loss of mane and tail hair.

SELENIUM SALTS

UK
Indications. Selenium deficiency
Dose. See preparation details

Aquatrace Selenium (Brinicombe) *UK*
Tablets, dispersible, selenium 875 mg/sachet, for *cattle*; 200-g sachets
Withdrawal Periods. *Cattle*: slaughter withdrawal period nil, milk withdrawal period nil
Dose. *Cattle*: *by addition to drinking water in dispenser*, 1 sachet is sufficient for 25 animals for 7 days

POM **Deposel Injection** (Vericore VP) *UK*
Depot injection (oily), selenium (as barium selenate) 50 mg/mL, for *cattle, sheep*; 5 mL
Withdrawal Periods. Slaughter withdrawal period nil, milk withdrawal period nil
Dose. *Cattle, sheep*: *by subcutaneous injection*, 1 mg/kg
See also section 16.6.5 for Compound Selenium and Vitamin E preparations

16.5.12 Sodium

Sodium is an essential electrolyte. The concentration of sodium in extracellular fluid is controlled by hormonal mechanisms. Concentrated feed contains added salt for palatability and ruminants receiving this diet are unlikely to become sodium deficient.

Sodium deficiency is unusual in species other than grazing herbivores not receiving concentrated feed supplements. Additional sodium, chloride, and occasionally potassium may be required by competition horses. Many pastures in the UK provide less than the required 1.5 g per kg feed to avoid deficiency in ruminants. The requirement is higher for lactating animals and animals with mastitis owing to the loss of sodium in the milk, although milk yield is often reduced.

Sodium deficiency occurs in high yielding cattle subsisting solely on a grass-based diet or receiving a high intake of maize silage. The body's initial response to sodium deficiency, beyond that which can be countered by sodium conservation, is to reduce the extracellular fluid volume. This results in polycythaemia and an increase in packed-cell volume and haemoglobin concentration, which is commonly observed in grazing cattle in the UK during summer. Greater deprivation results in pica for salt including drinking stagnant water and urine and ultimately polyuria and polydipsia due to renal failure. Prevention and treatment are achieved by providing salt blocks or compound mineral feed blocks.

Salt poisoning can occur, particularly in pigs due to excessive salt concentration either in the diet or water supply and is more usually associated with swill feeding. Temporary loss of water supply may cause hypernatraemia followed by sudden death due to brain oedema once the water supply is restored.

16.5.13 Zinc

Zinc has been shown experimentally to be important in the hepatic synthesis of protein, and severe zinc deficiency may lead to growth cessation. Pigs and certain breeds of cattle may exhibit clinical signs of zinc deficiency when their diet contains less than 50 mg per kg of feed of zinc and over 5 g per kg of feed of calcium. Parakeratosis develops with the skin becoming crusty and cracked, and growth rate is decreased. This condition is occasionally seen in young calves after protracted diarrhoea. Supplementation of the diet with at least 100 mg of zinc per kg feed is usually effective in treating and preventing deficiency. In Friesian cattle, a genetic deficiency associated with malabsorption of zinc has been recorded.

Skin disease in dogs responding to zinc supplementation (zinc-responsive dermatosis) occurs as two clinical syndromes. Certain breeds, notably Alaskan Malamutes and Siberian Huskies have a genetic defect impairing absorption of zinc from the intestine. In such dogs, the disease can occur despite feeding a well-balanced diet; it usually appears in young animals. The coat is often dry and dull. Erythema, scaling, crusting, and alopecia develop particularly around the mouth, eyes, ears, scrotum, prepuce, and vulva; crusting and hyperkeratosis may be marked at pressure points including the elbows and footpads. A second syndrome is seen in puppies from a variety of breeds fed diets deficient in zinc or containing substances that reduce its availability for absorption, such as calcium. Malaise and secondary infections are also seen.

In the first syndrome, lifelong supplementation with zinc is usually necessary. Zinc may be administered as zinc sulphate or zinc methionine and given with food. If vomiting occurs, the dose should be reduced. In the second syndrome, supplementation with zinc may be required while a balanced diet is introduced and may be necessary until the dog reaches maturity.

Zinc deficiency and excess have been suggested, but not proven, to be implicated in developmental orthopaedic disease (DOD) in young horses. Zinc has ben suggested to improve hoof quality in horses (see section 15.2). Adequate copper and zinc should be provided and fed in the appropriate ratio (Zn:Cu 3–4:1)

ZINC SALTS

UK
Indications. Zinc deficiency; improvement of hoof quality (see section 15.2)

Aquatrace Zinc (Brinicombe) *UK*
Tablets, dispersible, manganese 43.75 g/sachet, for *cattle*; 300-g sachets

Withdrawal Periods. Slaughter withdrawal period nil, milk withdrawal period nil
Dose. *Cattle*: *by addition to drinking water in dispenser*, 1 sachet is sufficient for 25 animals for 7 days

P (H) **Solvazinc** (Thames) *UK*
Tablets, zinc sulphate monohydrate 125 mg; 30
Dose. *Dogs*: *by mouth*, 10 mg/kg daily

Zincaderm (Virbac) *UK*
Tablets, methionine 35 mg, vitamin A 1250 units, zinc (as zinc methionine) 15 mg, for *dogs, cats*; 48
Dose. *Dogs, cats*: *by mouth*, 1 tablet/10 kg body-weight for at least 2–3 weeks

(H) **Zincomed** (Medo Pharmaceuticals) *UK*
Capsules, zinc sulphate 220 mg; 30, 250
Dose. *Dogs*: *by mouth*, 10 mg/kg daily

P (H) **Zincosol** (Bioceuticals) *UK*
Tablets, zinc sulphate monohydrate 220 mg; 50
Dose. *Dogs*: *by mouth*, 10 mg/kg daily

16.5.14 Compound trace element preparations

Trace elements are essential dietary constituents, which are required in relatively small amounts. The main function is to act as cofactors in various enzyme systems. Deficiencies of copper, cobalt, and/or selenium may occur in young, rapidly growing calves and lambs in certain well defined geographical areas. Prevention by oral supplementation with preparations containing combinations of all three elements may be advisable, however the possibility of chronic copper toxicity in sheep must always be considered.

UK

All-Trace (Agrimin) *UK*
See section 16.7 for preparation details

Aquatrace Trio Cattle (Brinicombe) *UK*
Tablets, dispersible, copper 35 g, iodine 11.37, selenium 875 mg/sachet, for *cattle*; 300-g sachets
Withdrawal Periods. *Cattle*: slaughter withdrawal period nil, milk withdrawal period nil
Dose. *Cattle*: *by addition to drinking water in dispenser*, 1 sachet is sufficient for 25 animals for 7 days

Aquatrace Trio Plus (Brinicombe) *UK*
Tablets, dispersible, cobalt 3.5 g, copper 35 g, selenium 875 mg/sachet, for *cattle*; 300-g sachets
Withdrawal Periods. *Cattle*: slaughter withdrawal period nil, milk withdrawal period nil
Dose. *Cattle*: *by addition to drinking water in dispenser*, 1 sachet is sufficient for 25 animals for 7 days

Cosecure for Cattle (Telsol) *UK*
Ruminal bolus, s/r, cobalt 500 mg and copper 13.4 g in sodium phosphate glass matrix, selenium (as sodium selenate) 300 mg, for *cattle more than 100 kg body-weight and 2 months of age*; 100-g bolus 20
Dose. *Cattle*: two 100-g ruminal boluses

Cosecure for Deer (Telsol) *UK*
Ruminal bolus, s/r, cobalt 330 mg and copper 8.84 g in sodium phosphate glass matrix, selenium (as sodium selenate) 99 mg, for *adult deer*; 66-g bolus
Dose. *Deer*: one 66-g ruminal bolus

Cosecure for Lambs (Telsol) *UK*
Ruminal bolus, s/r, cobalt 80 mg and copper 2.1 g in sodium phosphate glass matrix, selenium (as sodium selenate) 24 mg, for *lambs up to 25 kg body-weight and more than 5 weeks of age*; 16-g bolus 50
Dose. *Lambs*: one 16-g ruminal bolus

Cosecure for Sheep (Telsol) *UK*
Ruminal bolus, s/r, cobalt 165 mg and copper 4.4 g in sodium phosphate glass matrix, selenium (as sodium selenate) 50 mg, for *sheep more than 25 kg body-weight*; 33-g bolus 50
Dose. *Sheep*: one 33-g ruminal bolus

Zincosel/Densecure for Lambs (Telsol) *UK*
Ruminal bolus, s/r, cobalt 80 mg and zinc 2.5 g in sodium phosphate glass matrix, selenium (as sodium selenate) 24 mg, for *lambs up to 20 kg body-weight and more than 5 weeks of age*; 16-g bolus
Dose. *Sheep*: one 16-g ruminal bolus

Zincosel/Densecure for Sheep (Telsol) *UK*
Ruminal bolus, s/r, cobalt 165 mg and zinc 5 g in sodium phosphate glass matrix, selenium (as sodium selenate) 50 mg, for *sheep more than 25 kg body-weight*; 33-g bolus
Dose. *Sheep*: one 33-g ruminal bolus

Ionox (Bayer) *UK*
Ruminal bolus, s/r, cobalt 500 mg, iodine 3.4 g, selenium 500 mg, for *cattle*; 55-g bolus
Dose. *Cattle*: (200–399 kg body-weight) one 55-g bolus; (>400 kg body-weight) one 55-g bolus but may be increased to two 55-g boluses at certain times such as mid-late pregnancy, 2 months before service

Zincosel for Cattle (Telsol) *UK*
Ruminal bolus, s/r, cobalt 500 mg and zinc 15.4 g in sodium phosphate glass matrix, selenium (as sodium selenate) 150 mg, for *cattle more than 100 kg body-weight and 2 months of age*; 100-g bolus
Dose. *Cattle*: two 100-g ruminal boluses

16.6 Vitamins

16.6.1 Vitamin A substances
16.6.2 Vitamin B substances
16.6.3 Vitamin C substances
16.6.4 Vitamin D substances
16.6.5 Vitamin E substances
16.6.6 Vitamin K substances
16.6.7 Multivitamin preparations

Traditionally, vitamins have been classified into water-soluble, such as the vitamin B group and vitamin C, and fat-soluble including vitamins A, D, E, and K. Nutrient requirements for domestic animals are published by National Academy of Sciences Press, Washington DC.

Vitamins are used for the prevention and treatment of specific deficiency diseases and when the diet is known to be vitamin deficient. They are also often used for general supportive therapy and during recovery from debilitating diseases such as chronic neonatal diarrhoea and helminthiasis in ruminant species. The administration of excessive amounts of fat-soluble vitamins, especially vitamin A or vitamin D, can be harmful because they accumulate in the body and may cause pathological changes.

16.6.1 Vitamin A substances

Vitamin A and its precursor beta-carotene are present in growing plants, which form the primary source of the vitamin. Synthetic water soluble beta-carotene sources may not be well utilised in horses. Vitamin A is also derived from animal fat products, in particular fish oils and liver. Cats, unlike other species, are unable to convert beta-carotene to vitamin A and therefore require a dietary supply of vitamin A such as is found in fish oils, liver, or synthetic vitamin A. Deficiency is commonest in growing cattle fed poor quality hay where much of the vitamin content of the forage has been lost due to bleaching and during storage. Deficiency is also seen in young growing ruminants fed an intensive cereal-based diet without appropriate supplementation. The rate of absorption of vitamin A and other fat-soluble vitamins is dependent on other fat constituents in the diet, bile salts, and pancreatic enzymes. The liver can store large quantities of vitamin A and provides a reserve, particularly for carnivores. Diets deficient in vitamin A produce no ill effect until the liver stores are depleted and the plasma concentration falls below 220 units/litre. The daily requirement of vitamin A is 20 to 100 units/kg body-weight. Liquid paraffin can prevent the absorption of vitamin A from the intestine; animals given prolonged liquid paraffin therapy may show signs of vitamin A deficiency.

A deficiency of vitamin A interferes with bone growth, with the maintenance of tissues, particularly secretory epithelial tissue, and with the growth of the embryo. In young animals, deficiency arrests the growth of the skull causing neurological effects such as blindness due to pressure on the growing brain and cranial nerve roots. Older animals may develop a rough coat with scaly, cracked skin, and dry mucous membranes. They may fail to grow and reproduce and may exhibit neurological dysfunction. Animals of all ages may develop night blindness due to a deficiency of retinal rhodopsin. Vitamin A deficiency has not been reported in horses to cause abnormal bone remodelling as seen in other species.

Dietary supplementation is a convenient way to prevent, and to some extent reverse, the effects of the deficiency, although the neurological deficits due to cranial growth inhibition may not be completely reversible.

Overdosage from excessive dietary intake of liver or vitamin A-containing supplements most commonly occurs in cats and dogs and may result in vertebral fusion. Excessive vitamin A intakes in young foals may result in a decreased growth rate and have been suggested to increase the risk of developmental orthopaedic disease (DOD). Mild vitamin A toxicity in horses may result in slowed growth, dull hair, and poor muscle tone. Severe toxicity may be characterised by depression, alopecia, ataxia, severe bone deformation, and death.

VITAMIN A
(Retinol)

UK

Indications. Dose. See Prescribing for reptiles and Prescribing for exotic birds

POM Ⓗ **Vitamin A Palmitate** (Cambridge) *UK*
Injection, vitamin A (as palmitate) 50 000 units/mL; 2 mL

16.6.2 Vitamin B substances

The complex of B vitamins includes thiamine (B_1), nicotinic acid (niacin), riboflavin (B_2, riboflavine), choline, pantothenic acid, pyridoxine (B_6), biotin (see also section 15.2), folic acid, and vitamin B_{12}. All of these can be synthesised by the microflora in the gastro-intestinal tract of ruminants and hind gut of horses and deficiencies are, therefore, uncommon in these species. However, absorption of the microbiologically synthesised thiamine may not meet the total needs in horses under some circumstances. B vitamins, required by non-ruminants, are derived from a variety of plant and animal sources. Dried yeast provides a rich supply of these vitamins. B vitamins are not stored in the body to any great extent and prolonged inappetance or chronic diarrhoea may lead to a deficiency. Deficiencies affect the nervous and gastro-intestinal systems and skin.

Vitamin B_{12} is a collective term for the cobalamins of which **cyanocobalamin** and **hydroxocobalamin** are the principal compounds. They are cobalt-containing vitamins. Ruminants are able to use cobalt to synthesise vitamin B_{12} in the rumen and deficiency occurs when inadequate cobalt is present in the diet. In carnivores, vitamin B_{12} deficiency may occur as a result of inadequate absorption of the vitamin from the gastro-intestinal tract or increased body requirements.

In all species, vitamin B_{12} is required for maintenance of tissues, protein synthesis, and haematopoiesis. Clinical signs of deficiency include anorexia, unthriftiness, anaemia, and incoordination.

It has been suggested that daily oral administration of folic acid may be of benefit in stable fed, competition horses. Certain orally administered synthetic folic acid supplements may interfere with the absorption or utilisation of natural forms of folate causing folate deficiency and therefore inducing clinical problems when co-administered with certain therapeutic agents.

It has been reported that additional long-term **biotin** supplementation may improve hoof quality and certain hoof deficits particularly when given in combination with an adequate and well balanced diet (see section 15.2).

Thiamine deficiency may occur as a result of inadequate dietary intake or destruction of the vitamin by excessive heating during processing of diets for carnivores. Secondary thiamine deficiency may occur in carnivores, because of the thiaminase present in raw fish, and in horses because of the thiaminase present in bracken and horsetails (*Equisetum* spp.). Bracken poisoning in horses is characterised by progressive ataxia followed by convulsions or paresis and terminal coma. Treatment includes thiamine or dried brewers yeast.

In ruminant species, particularly growing sheep aged 4 to 6 months, thiamine deficiency may result following increased thiaminase activity in the rumen. Changes in diet, recent anthelmintic treatment, or other factors may disturb the rumen microflora with proliferation of thiaminase-producing bacteria. Outbreaks of cerebrocortical necrosis (polioencephalomalacia) have been associated with diets containing a high concentration of sulphur.

Secondary thiamine deficiency can be successfully treated with intravenous thiamine provided therapy is started shortly after the onset of neurological signs.

BIOTIN

UK

Indications. Treatment of biotin deficiency; treatment in horses (see section 15.2)

Biotin (Animalcare) *UK*
Tablets, biotin 50 micrograms, for *dogs, cats*; 500
Dose. *Dogs, cats*: *by mouth*, 2 tablets twice daily for 3 days then 1 tablet twice weekly

CYANOCOBALAMIN

UK

Indications. Treatment of vitamin B_{12} deficiency
Dose. *By subcutaneous or intramuscular injection*.
Horses, cattle: 1–3 mg 1–2 times weekly
foals, calves: 0.5–1.5 mg 1–2 times weekly
Sheep, pigs: 250–750 micrograms 1–2 times weekly
Dogs, cats: 250–500 micrograms 1–2 times weekly

PML **Anivit B_{12}** (Animalcare) *UK*
Injection, cyanocobalamin 250 micrograms/mL, for *horses, cattle, sheep, pigs, dogs, cats*; 50 mL
Withdrawal Periods. Slaughter withdrawal period nil, milk withdrawal period nil
Injection, cyanocobalamin 1 mg/mL, for *horses, cattle*; 50 mL
Withdrawal Periods. Slaughter withdrawal period nil, milk withdrawal period nil

PML **Intravit 12** (Norbrook) *UK*
Injection, cyanocobalamin 500 micrograms/mL, for *horses, cattle, sheep, pigs*; 100 mL
Withdrawal Periods. Slaughter withdrawal period nil, milk withdrawal period nil

PML **Vitamin B_{12}** (Battle Hayward & Bower) *UK*
Injection, cyanocobalamin 250 micrograms/mL, for *horses, cattle, sheep, pigs*; 100 mL
Withdrawal Periods. Slaughter withdrawal period nil, milk withdrawal period nil

PML **Vitbee** (Arnolds) *UK*
Injection, cyanocobalamin 250 micrograms/mL, for *foals, calves, sheep*; 50 mL
Withdrawal Periods. Slaughter withdrawal period nil, milk withdrawal period nil
Injection, 1 mg/mL, for *horses, cattle*; 50 mL
Withdrawal Periods. Slaughter withdrawal period nil, milk withdrawal period nil

THIAMINE
(Vitamin B_1)

UK

Indications. Treatment of thiamine deficiency
Dose. *Horses* ♦: *by intramuscular or slow intravenous injection*, 0.25–1.25 mg/kg twice daily for up to 7 days
Cattle, sheep: *by intramuscular or slow intravenous injection*, 5–10 mg/kg, repeat every 3 hours as necessary

Pigs ♦: *by intramuscular or slow intravenous injection*, 0.25–1.25 mg/kg twice daily for up to 7 days
Cats ♦: *by intramuscular injection*, 50 mg 1–2 times daily

POM **Vitamin B1** (Bimeda) *UK*
Injection, thiamine hydrochloride 100 mg/mL, for *cattle, sheep*; 50 mL
Withdrawal Periods. Slaughter withdrawal period nil, milk withdrawal period nil

16.6.3 Vitamin C substances
(Ascorbic acid)

Ascorbic acid is synthesised by all animals except primates and guinea pigs. Deficiency may occur in these species when the diet contains inadequate supplies of fresh fruit and vegetables or food is stored incorrectly.

It is believed that the requirements for vitamin C in healthy horses are met by tissue synthesis. It has, however, been suggested that horses that have been severely stressed may require additional sources although no dietary requirement has been conclusively identified. The efficiency of intestinal absorption is thought to be very poor in horses.

ASCORBIC ACID

UK

Indications. See notes above; adjunct in the treatment of paracetamol poisoning (see Treatment of poisoning); urinary acidification (see section 9.2.1)

POM Ⓗ **Ascorbic acid** (Non-proprietary) *UK*
Tablets, ascorbic acid 50 mg, 100 mg, 500 mg
Injection, ascorbic acid 100 mg/mL; 5 mL

16.6.4 Vitamin D substances

The term vitamin D is used for a range of compounds including ergocalciferol (calciferol, vitamin D_2), colecalciferol (vitamin D_3), alfacalcidol (1α-hydroxycholecalciferol), and calcitriol (1,25-dihydroxycholecalciferol).

D vitamins are found in plants and animals as sterols, which are converted to vitamins by ultraviolet light. Ergocalciferol is derived from plants. Colecalciferol is synthesised from the sterols present in skin on exposure to sunlight. It may be converted to calcitriol in the liver and kidney. Calcitriol is now believed to be the active form of the vitamin and is 10 times more potent than colecalciferol.

Vitamin D is absorbed and stored in tissues, in particular the liver and fat. Low plasma-calcium concentration initiates the conversion of stored vitamin D to functional vitamin D by enzyme systems principally regulated by parathyroid hormone and plasma-calcium concentrations. Vitamin D enhances the absorption of calcium from the intestine and the reabsorption of calcium from the renal tubules and acts, together with parathyroid hormone and calcitonin, to regulate the processes of bone resorption and formation during remodelling of the skeleton.

The increased absorption of calcium after administration of vitamin D can be used in dairy cows to prevent clinical hypocalcaemia, which may occur at parturition due to the increased calcium demand at the onset of lactation. The timing of the injection of vitamin D is important and for optimum effectiveness should fall between 8 and 2 days before calving. Induced parturition can be used to facilitate accurate timing of vitamin D treatment. The efficacy of vitamin D is influenced by blood pH which can be manipulated by feeding acidifying diets during late gestation, thereby reducing clinical hypocalcaemia.

A deficiency of vitamin D results in the failure of bone to calcify correctly and may lead to rickets in young animals and osteomalacia in adults. These conditions may be treated and prevented by the administration of vitamin D preparations either parenterally or in the diet.

Excessive administration of vitamin D preparations may result in metastatic calcification of the major blood vessels, the kidney, and other organs. Sodium clodronate (see section 7.7.2) has been used in dogs as a palliative treatment for hypercalcaemia of hypervitaminosis D.

ALFACALCIDOL
(1α-Hydroxycholecalciferol)

UK
Indications. Prevention of hypocalcaemia (milk fever)
Contra-indications. Concurrent use of other vitamin D₃ preparations
Side-effects. Excessive dosage may result in calcification of blood vessels and organs, see notes above
Warnings. May induce hypomagnesaemia, ensure magnesium intake is adequate
Dose. *Cattle*: *by subcutaneous injection*, 350 micrograms 24–48 hours before calving. Repeat once only after 72–96 hours if calving has not occurred

POM **Vetalpha** (Schering-Plough) *UK*
Injection, alfacalcidol 35 micrograms/mL, for *dairy cattle*; 10 mL
Withdrawal Periods. *Cattle*: slaughter 3 days, milk 3 days

COLECALCIFEROL
(Cholecalciferol, Vitamin D₃)

UK
Indications. Prevention of hypocalcaemia (milk fever)
Side-effects. See under Alfacalcidol
Dose. See preparation details

PML **Duphafral D₃ 1000** (Fort Dodge) *UK*
Injection, colecalciferol 25 mg/mL, for *cattle*; 10 mL
Withdrawal Periods. *Cattle*: slaughter 28 days, milk 28 days
Dose. *Cattle*: by intramuscular injection, 250 mg 2–8 days before calving

COMPOUND CALCIUM and VITAMIN D PREPARATIONS

UK
Calcivet (Vetafarm) *UK*
Oral liquid, calcium borogluconate 400 mg, colecalciferol 625 micrograms, magnesium sulphate 10 mg/mL, for *birds*; 100 mL, 250 mL, other sizes available
Dose. *Birds*: prophylaxis, 20 mL/litre drinking water
Egg binding, *by mouth*, 0.2 mL/100 g body-weight hourly

Pet-Cal (Pfizer) *UK*
Tablets, calcium hydrogen phosphate 2.04 g, colecalciferol 5 micrograms, for *dogs, cats*; 30, 150
Dose. *By mouth*.
Dogs: (< 9 kg body-weight) ½ tablet daily; (>9 kg body-weight) 1 tablet/9 kg body-weight daily
Cats: ½ tablet daily

16.6.5 Vitamin E substances

Vitamin E or tocopherols is the group name for substances with vitamin E activity. The main naturally-occurring substance is *d*-alpha tocopherol and the principal compounds used in preparations are *d*-alpha tocopheryl acid succinate and *dl*-alpha tocopheryl acetate. Vitamin E is present in growing plants and in cereals. Vitamin E is an antioxidant and is necessary for the stability of muscular tissue. It has a similar role to selenium (see section 16.5.11) and each can to some extent replace the other.

Vitamin E deficiency occurs most commonly in young, rapidly growing calves and lambs aged 3 to 6 weeks. In growing ruminants, vitamin E deficiency may occur in animals receiving a diet of poor quality straw and root crops. Muscles that are deficient in vitamin E become stiff, swollen, and painful, and degenerative changes are visible microscopically. The disease is called 'white muscle disease'. Both skeletal and heart muscle are susceptible causing a stiff gait leading to inability to stand and sudden death respectively. 'White muscle disease' has also been reported in foals. Feeding propionic acid treated cereals or some fishmeals to pregnant sheep and cattle may increase the likelihood of white muscle disease in the offspring. Parenteral therapy with vitamin E and selenium often produces a complete restoration of health when skeletal muscle is involved but recovery will depend on the extent of muscular damage and which muscles are affected.

Equine degenerative myeloencephalopathy (EDM) or equine motor neurone disease (EMND) is believed to be associated with a vitamin E deficiency. Cases tend to occur in stabled horses, horses with access to dirt paddocks only, or horses fed mature grass hay usually with a high grain ration. Lack of antioxidant action of vitamin E in the CNS is believed to predispose the type 1 oxidative neurones to oxidative injury and death with subsequent degeneration of axons in the peripheral nerves and denervation atrophy of skeletal muscle, in particular type 1 muscles needed for maintenance of posture. Decreased serum-vitamin E concentration is not always present. Treatment includes dietary vitamin E supplementation plus the feeding of fresh, green forage. Affected animals may improve or stabilise but many do not fully recover.

The role of vitamin E supplementation in reducing free radical induced damage during and following intensive exercise in horses is under evaluation.

Prevention of vitamin E deficiency requires a daily intake of approximately 1 g of vitamin E for cows, 150 mg for calves, 75 mg for ewes, and 25 mg for lambs.

VITAMIN E
(Tocopherols)

UK

Indications. See notes above
Dose. See preparation details

Note. Vitamin E activity per 1 mg = *dl*-alpha tocopheryl acetate 1 unit = *d*-alpha tocopheryl acid succinate 1.21 units = *d*-alpha tocopheryl acetate 1.36 units = *d*-alpha tocopherol 1.49 units

Tocovite 50, 100, 200 (Arnolds) *UK*
Tablets, *d*-alpha tocopheryl acid succinate 41 mg, 83 mg, 165 mg, for *horses, calves, lambs, dogs*; 100
Dose. *By mouth*.
Horses: 0.83–2.48 g daily
Calves: 165–248 mg daily
Lambs, dogs: 41–83 mg daily

COMPOUND SELENIUM and VITAMIN E PREPARATIONS

UK

Indications. Prevention and treatment of selenium/vitamin E deficiency

POM **Dystosel** (Intervet) *UK*
Injection, *dl*-alpha tocopheryl acetate 68 mg, selenium (as potassium selenate) 1.5 mg/mL, for *cattle, sheep, pigs*; 50 mL
Withdrawal Periods. *Cattle*: slaughter 28 days, milk withdrawal period nil. *Sheep*: slaughter 28 days, should not be used in sheep producing milk for human consumption. *Pigs*: slaughter 28 days
Dose. *By subcutaneous or intramuscular injection*.
Cattle: 1–2 mL/45 kg, repeat after 2–4 weeks if required
Ewes: 2 mL/45 kg; *lambs*: 0.5–1.0 mL, repeat after 2–4 weeks if required
Pigs: 1 mL/25 kg, repeat after 2–4 weeks if required

POM **Vitenium** (Vericore VP) *UK*
Injection, *dl*-alpha tocopheryl acetate 150 mg, selenium 500 micrograms/mL, for *horses, cattle, sheep, pigs*; 100 mL
Withdrawal Periods. Should not be used in *horses* intended for human consumption. *Cattle*: slaughter 28 days, milk withdrawal period nil. *Sheep, pigs*: slaughter 28 days
Dose. *Horses: by intramuscular injection*, up to 20 mL; *foals*: 2–5 mL
Cattle: by subcutaneous or intramuscular injection, up to 15 mL; *calves*: 2–5 mL
Sheep: by subcutaneous or intramuscular injection, up to 5 mL; *lambs*: 0.5–3.0 mL
Pigs: by subcutaneous or intramuscular injection, up to 5 mL; *piglets*: 0.5–2.0 mL

POM **Vitesel** (Norbrook) *UK*
Injection, *dl*-alpha tocopheryl acetate 68 mg, selenium (as potassium selenate) 1.5 mg/mL, for *calves, sheep, pigs*; 50 mL
Withdrawal Periods. *Calves, sheep, pigs*: slaughter 8 weeks
Dose. *By subcutaneous or intramuscular injection*.
Calves: 1–2 mL/45 kg, repeat after 2–4 weeks if required
Ewes: 2 mL/45 kg; *lambs*: 0.5–1.0 mL, repeat after 2–4 weeks if required
Pigs: 1 mL/25 kg, repeat after 2–4 weeks if required
See also section 16.5.11 for preparations containing selenium

16.6.6 Vitamin K substances

Sources of vitamin K include green leafy plants, fish meal, and liver. Phylloquinone in pasture or in good quality hay together with the menaquinones synthesised by intestinal bacteria are believed to meet the needs of horses. Sufficient amounts of vitamin K are synthesised and absorbed from the gastro-intestinal tract in most species, but not poultry. Vitamin K is necessary for the synthesis of blood clotting factors in the liver.

Oral coumarin anticoagulants, used in many rodenticides, act by interfering with vitamin K metabolism in the hepatic cells and their effects can be antagonised by giving vitamin K. **Phytomenadione** (vitamin K_1) is usually administered for 7 days but treatment may need to be continued for several weeks in some cases (see Treatment of poisoning). In severe cases, blood transfusion may be required. One stage prothrombin time should be monitored. **Menadione** (vitamin K_3) is ineffective and should not be used.

16.6.7 Multivitamin preparations

Multivitamin preparations may be used for the prevention and treatment of vitamin deficiencies, particularly during periods of illness, convalescence, stress, and unthriftiness. Cod-liver oil is a rich source of vitamin D and also a good source of vitamin A and several unsaturated fatty acids.

UK

There are many preparations available. This is not a comprehensive list.

Indications. See notes above
Side-effects. Occasional anaphylactic reaction especially in horses following intravenous injection; intravenous injections should be administered slowly
Dose. See manufacturer's data sheet

POM **Anivit 4BC** (Animalcare) *UK*
Injection, ascorbic acid 70 mg, nicotinamide 23 mg, pyridoxine (as hydrochloride) 7 mg, riboflavin (as sodium phosphate) 500 micrograms, thiamine (as hydrochloride) 35 mg/mL, for *horses, cattle, sheep, pigs*; 50 mL, 100 mL
Withdrawal Periods. Slaughter withdrawal period nil, milk withdrawal period nil

POM **Bimavite Plus** (Bimeda) *UK*
Injection, ascorbic acid 70 mg, nicotinamide 22.5 mg, pyridoxine hydrochloride 7 mg, riboflavin (as phosphate) 800 micrograms, thiamine hydrochloride 35 mg/mL, for *cattle, sheep*; 50 mL, 100 mL
Withdrawal Periods. Slaughter withdrawal period nil, milk withdrawal period nil

BSP (Vetark) *UK*
Oral liquid, ascorbic acid, biotin, colecalciferol, folic acid, nicotinic acid, pantothenic acid, pyridoxine hydrochloride, riboflavin, thiamine hydrochloride, vitamin A, for *birds, reptiles*; 50 mL

PML **Combivit** (Norbrook) *UK*
Injection, ascorbic acid 70 mg, nicotinamide 23 mg, pyridoxine hydrochloride 7 mg, riboflavin sodium phosphate 500 micrograms, thiamine hydrochloride 35 mg/mL, for *horses, cattle, sheep*; 50 mL, 100 mL
Withdrawal Periods. Slaughter withdrawal period nil, milk withdrawal period nil

PML **Duphafral ADE Forte** (Fort Dodge) *UK*
Injection, *dl*-alpha tocopheryl acetate 50 mg, colecalciferol 1.25 mg, vitamin A 500 000 units/mL, for *cattle, sheep, pigs*; 50 mL
Withdrawal Periods. Slaughter 28 days

PML Duphafral Extravite (Fort Dodge) *UK*
Injection, ascorbic acid 70 mg, nicotinamide 23 mg, pyridoxine hydrochloride 7 mg, riboflavin sodium phosphate 500 micrograms, thiamine hydrochloride 35 mg/mL, for *horses, cattle, sheep*; 50 mL, 100 mL
Withdrawal Periods. Slaughter withdrawal period nil, milk withdrawal period nil

PML Duphafral Multivitamin 9 (Fort Dodge) *UK*
Injection, dl-alpha tocopheryl acetate 20 mg, colecalciferol 25 micrograms, cyanocobalamin 20 micrograms, dexpanthenol 25 mg, nicotinamide 35 mg, pyridoxine hydrochloride 3 mg, riboflavin 5 mg, thiamine hydrochloride 10 mg, vitamin A 15 000 units/mL, for *horses, cattle, sheep, pigs*; 100 mL
Withdrawal Periods. Slaughter 28 days, milk withdrawal period nil

PML Multivitamin (Arnolds) *UK*
Injection, dl-alpha tocopheryl acetate 20 mg, colecalciferol 25 micrograms, cyanocobalamin 50 micrograms, dexpanthenol 25 mg, nicotinamide 35 mg, pyridoxine hydrochloride 3 mg, riboflavin sodium phosphate 5 mg, thiamine hydrochloride 10 mg, vitamin A 15 000 units/mL, for *horses, cattle, sheep, pigs*; 100 mL
Withdrawal Periods. Slaughter 28 days, milk withdrawal period nil

PML Multivitamin (Norbrook) *UK*
Injection, dl-alpha tocopheryl acetate 20 mg, colecalciferol 25 micrograms, cyanocobalamin 25 micrograms, dexpanthenol 25 mg, nicotinamide 35 mg, pyridoxine hydrochloride 3 mg, riboflavin sodium phosphate 5 mg, thiamine hydrochloride 10 mg, vitamin A 15 000 units/mL, for *horses, cattle, sheep, pigs*; 100 mL
Withdrawal Periods. Slaughter 28 days, milk withdrawal period nil

PML Multivitamin (Trilanco) *UK*
Injection, colecalciferol 25 micrograms, cyanocobalamin 50 micrograms, dexpanthenol 25 mg, nicotinamide 35 mg, pyridoxine 3 mg, riboflavin sodium phosphate 5 mg, thiamine 10 mg, vitamin A 15 000 units, vitamin E 20 mg/mL, for *horses, cattle, sheep, goats, pigs*; 100 mL

SA Vits (Vetark) *UK*
Oral liquid, ascorbic acid, biotin, colecalciferol, folic acid, nicotinic acid, pantothenic acid, pyridoxine hydrochloride, riboflavin, thiamine hydrochloride, vitamin A, for *rabbits, small pets*; 50 mL

16.7 Compound multivitamin and mineral preparations

Compound multivitamin and mineral preparations are used as general tonics or supplements, although their therapeutic efficacy has not been established.
These preparations are useful in all species for the treatment of specific deficiencies and supportive therapy during convalescence, for example following septicaemia or toxaemia, parasitic infections, malabsorption syndrome, hepatitis, and post-operative stress. Continuous or excessive administration should be avoided because interactions with other minerals and vitamins in the normal diet can have adverse effects. Most proprietary diets contain adequate concentrations of minerals and vitamins.
Some oral liquid preparations may contain caffeine and care should be taken if administering them to animals used in competitions.

UK
There are many preparations available. This is not a comprehensive list.

Indications. Side-effects. See notes above
Dose. See manufacturer's data sheet

ACE-High (Vetark) *UK*
Oral powder, ascorbic acid, biotin, calcium, colecalciferol, choline chloride, cobalt, copper, folic acid, iodine, iron, manganese, nicotinic acid, pantothenic acid, phosphorus, pyridoxine hydrochloride, riboflavin, selenium, sodium chloride, thiamine hydrochloride, vitamin A, zinc, for *fish, birds, reptiles*; 50 g

Activol (Arnolds) *UK*
Oral emulsion, calcium pantothenate, nicotinamide, riboflavin, thiamine, vitamin A, vitamin B$_{12}$, vitamin E, fatty acids, for *dogs*; 125 mL

Activol Multi-Tabs (Arnolds) *UK*
Tablets, calcium, colecalciferol, cobalt, copper, iodine, magnesium, manganese, phosphorus, pyridoxine, riboflavin, nicotinic acid, sodium, thiamine, vitamin A, vitamin B$_{12}$, vitamin E, zinc, for *dogs*; 50, 150

Activol Multi-Tabs (Arnolds) *UK*
Tablets, calcium, colecalciferol, choline, cobalt, copper, iodine, inositol, magnesium, manganese, pantothenic acid, phosphorus, pyridoxine, riboflavin, nicotinic acid, sodium, thiamine, vitamin A, zinc, for *cats*; 50, 150

All-Trace (Agrimin) *UK*
Ruminal bolus, dl-alpha tocopheryl acetate, colecalciferol, cobalt, copper, iodine, manganese, selenium, sulphur, vitamin A, zinc, for *cattle*; 20

Aquatrace Ex-Sel Cattle (Brinicombe) *UK*
Oral liquid, cobalt, colecalciferol, copper, iodine, manganese, niacin, pantothenic acid, pyridoxine, selenium, thiamine, vitamin A, vitamin B12, vitamin E, zinc, for *cattle*
Withdrawal Periods. Slaughter withdrawal period nil, milk withdrawal period nil

Aquatrace Ex-Sel Sheep (Brinicombe) *UK*
Oral liquid, cobalt, colecalciferol, copper, iodine, manganese, niacin, pantothenic acid, pyridoxine, selenium, thiamine, vitamin A, vitamin B12, vitamin E, zinc, for *sheep*
Withdrawal Periods. Slaughter withdrawal period nil, milk withdrawal period nil

Arkvits (Vetark) *UK*
Oral powder, ascorbic acid, biotin, calcium, colecalciferol, choline chloride, cobalt, copper, folic acid, iodine, iron, manganese, nicotinic acid, pantothenic acid, phosphorus, pyridoxine hydrochloride, riboflavin, selenium, sodium chloride, thiamine hydrochloride, vitamin A, zinc, for *rabbits, reptiles*; 50 g, 250 g

Avimix (Vetark) *UK*
Oral powder, ascorbic acid, biotin, calcium, colecalciferol, choline chloride, cobalt, copper, folic acid, iodine, iron, manganese, nicotinic acid, pantothenic acid, phosphorus, pyridoxine hydrochloride, riboflavin, selenium, sodium chloride, thiamine hydrochloride, vitamin A, zinc, for *birds*; 50 g, 250 g

GSL Canovel Vitamin Mineral (Pfizer) *UK*
Tablets, dl-alpha tocopheryl acetate, calcium, calcium pantothenate, cobalt, copper, ergocalciferol, iodine, iron, manganese, nicotinic acid, phosphorus, pyridoxine hydrochloride, riboflavin, selenium, sodium chloride, sugars, thiamine hydrochloride, vitamin A, yeast, zinc, for *dogs*; 50
Oral powder, dl-alpha tocopheryl acetate, biotin, calcium, calcium pantothenate, colecalciferol, cobalt, copper, cyanocobalamin, folic acid, iodine, iron, manganese, nicotinic acid, phosphorus, pyridoxine, riboflavin, selenium, thiamine, vitamin A, vitamin K, zinc, for *dogs*; 200 g, 2.5 kg

Collotone (Harkers) *UK*
Oral solution, for addition to drinking water, caffeine citrate, green ferric ammonium citrate, iron and magnesium citrate, sodium glycerophosphate, thiamine hydrochloride, for *pigeons*; 200 mL

Equisup 23 (Vétoquinol) *UK*
Oral powder, ascorbic acid, biotin, colecalciferol, choline, cobalt, copper, cyanocobalamin, dexpanthenol, folic acid, iodine, iron, lysine, manganese, menadione, methionine, nicotinic acid, pyridoxine, riboflavin, selenium, thiamine, vitamin A, vitamin E, zinc, for *horses*; 1.5 kg

Equi-ton (Intervet) *UK*
Oral liquid, dl-alpha tocopheryl acetate, colecalciferol, choline bitartrate, cyanocobalamin, dexpanthenol, ferric ammonium citrate, inositol, nicotinamide, pyridoxine hydrochloride, riboflavin, thiamine hydrochloride, vitamin A, for *horses*; 1 litre

POM **Haemo 15** (Arnolds) *UK*
Injection, biotin, choline chloride, cobalt gluconate, copper gluconate, cyanocobalamin, dexpanthenol, ferric ammonium citrate, glycine, inositol, lysine hydrochloride, nicotinamide, pyridoxine hydrochloride, methionine, riboflavin sodium phosphate, for *horses*; 100 mL
Withdrawal Periods. Should not be used in *horses* intended for human consumption

Leo Cud (Leo) *UK*
Oral powder, dl-alpha tocopheryl acetate, aneurine mononitrate, casein, colecalciferol, cobalt sulphate, copper sulphate, disodium hydrogen phosphate, glucose, maize starch, manganese dioxide, methionine, nicotinamide, riboflavin, sodium bicarbonate, sodium propionate, thiamine hydrochloride, vitamin A, dried yeast, skimmed milk powder, for *cattle, sheep, goats*; 80 g, 160 g

Minivit (Vétoquinol) *UK*
Oral solution, dl-alpha tocopheryl acetate, ascorbic acid, colecalciferol, dexpanthenol, menadione, nicotinamide, pyridoxine hydrochloride, riboflavin, thiamine hydrochloride, vitamin A, for *puppies, kittens, rodents, birds, tortoises*; 7 mL

Nutri-Plus (Virbac) *UK*
Oral gel, dl-alpha tocopheryl acetate, calcium pantothenate, colecalciferol, cyanocobalamin, folic acid, iodine, iron, magnesium, manganese, nicotinamide, pyridoxine hydrochloride, riboflavin, thiamine hydrochloride, vitamin A, for *dogs, cats*; 120.5 g

Nutrobal (Vetark) *UK*
Oral powder, ascorbic acid, biotin, calcium, colecalciferol, choline chloride, cobalt, copper, folic acid, iodine, iron, manganese, nicotinic acid, pantothenic acid, phosphorus, pyridoxine hydrochloride, riboflavin, selenium, sodium chloride, thiamine hydrochloride, vitamin A, zinc, for *birds, reptiles*; 100 g, 250 g

Pardevit (Bayer) *UK*
Oral liquid, dl-alpha tocopheryl acetate, colecalciferol, cobalt, selenium, vitamin A, for *cattle, sheep*; 500 mL, 1 litre, 2.5 litres

Pet-Tabs (Pfizer) *UK*
Tablets, dl-alpha tocopheryl acetate, calcium, cobalt, copper, cyanocobalamin, ergocalciferol, iodine, iron, linoleic acid, magnesium, manganese, nicotinic acid, phosphorus, pyridoxine hydrochloride, riboflavin, thiamine mononitrate, vitamin A, zinc, for *dogs*; 50, 150

GSL **Pet-Tabs Feline** (Pfizer) *UK*
Tablets, dl-alpha tocopheryl acetate, calcium pantothenate, choline, cobalt, copper, ergocalciferol, inositol, iodine, iron, linoleic acid, magnesium, manganese, nicotinic acid, phosphorus, pyridoxine hydrochloride, riboflavin, thiamine mononitrate, vitamin A, zinc, for *cats*; 100

Poly-Aid (Vetafarm) *UK*
Oral powder, dl-alpha tocopheryl acetate, ascorbic acid, colecalciferol, vitamin A, mineral salts, glucose plymers, vitamins, for *birds*; 20 g, 40 g, other sizes available

SA-37 (Intervet) *UK*
Tablets, d-alpha tocopheryl acetate, arachidonic acid, ascorbic acid, biotin, calcium, colecalciferol, choline, cobalt, copper, cyanocobalamin, dexpanthenol, folic acid, iodine, iron, lecithin, linoleic acid, linolenic acid, manganese, nicotinic acid, phosphorus, potassium, pyridoxine hydrochloride, riboflavin, thiamine hydrochloride, vitamin A, vitamin K, zinc, for *dogs, cats*; 100, 500

SA-37 (Intervet) *UK*
Oral powder, d-alpha tocopheryl acetate, arachidonic acid, ascorbic acid, biotin, calcium, colecalciferol, choline, cobalt, copper, cyanocobalamin, dexpanthenol, folic acid, iodine, iron, lecithin, linoleic acid, linolenic acid, manganese, nicotinic acid, phosphorus, potassium, pyridoxine hydrochloride, riboflavin, thiamine hydrochloride, vitamin A, vitamin K, zinc, for *dogs, cats, pet birds*; 100 g, 200 g, 2 kg

Tasvite (Schering-Plough) *UK*
Oral liquid, alpha tocopherol acetate, colecalciferol, cobalt (as cobalt sulphate heptahydrate), selenium, thiamine, vitamin A, for *horses, cattle, sheep*; 1 litre

Trans-fer (Net-Tex) *UK*
Oral liquid, iron, copper, folic acid, vitamin B complex, for *piglets*; 110 mL, 500 mL

POM **Vitatrace** (Vétoquinol) *UK*
Injection, cobalt gluconate, copper gluconate, cyanocobalamin, dexpanthenol, ferric ammonium citrate, nicotinamide, pyridoxine hydrochloride, riboflavin, thiamine hydrochloride, for *horses, cattle, sheep, pigs*; 100 mL

16.8 Complete dietetic foods

The modification of energy and nutrient intake is of value in the management of many conditions, and in some it is essential for a successful outcome. In addition to regulating the intake of specific nutrients, a dietetic food must continue to meet the animal's requirements for energy, essential amino acids, vitamins, and minerals. Special diets are frequently required for long-term maintenance and therefore only complete diets have been included in this section. Diets should be selected on the basis of their nutritional characteristics, and an accurate diagnosis of a disorder is essential in order to choose the correct diet.

In the UK, dietetic pet foods are regulated under the *Feeding Stuffs Regulations 1995* (SI 1995/1412), which state the requirements for labelling of diets for the nutritional management of clinical cases (termed dietetic pet foods or feeding stuffs for particular nutritional purposes). However this legislation does not apply to any leaflet or other literature.

Table 16.4 lists complete dietetic pet foods for feeding to dogs and cats classified under their appropriate nutritional purpose(s); some diets have more than one purpose. These purposes are often expressed in official language, although the meaning is sufficiently understandable. An important point to appreciate is that the legislature considered that most indications for dietary management would be temporary. Consequently manufacturers are obliged to state a recommended maximum length of treatment, even in situations where indefinite feeding of the diet would be both justified and desirable.

There are many dietary products available in the UK; Table 16.4 lists those for medical conditions (as stated by the legislation) and those that are labelled in accordance with the Regulations. Some diets are available in different flavours.

Primary objectives in the dietary management of **renal insufficiency** (see section 1 of Table 16.4) are firstly to minimise the intake of phosphorus, reducing its accumulation which is associated with disease progression. Secondly the diet should restrict protein intake reducing the accumulation of nitrogenous toxins that are responsible for most of the clinical signs of uraemia. Adequate non-protein calories should be provided, sodium intake should be reduced to control systemic hypertension, and the intake of water soluble B vitamins increased to compensate for increased losses due to polyuria. There should also be an increase in the intake of buffering agents to control metabolic acidosis and, in cats, of potassium to avoid hypokalaemia.

In **liver disease** (see section 12 of Table 16.4), protein intake should be controlled to reduce ammonia production and thereby help to prevent encephalopathy, yet ensure a sufficient amount for liver cell regeneration and the maintenance of plasma-protein concentration. An increase in non-protein calories will support liver cell regeneration and a low sodium intake will discourage ascites. With liver failure it is recommended that dogs should receive 10 to 14% of calories from protein and 30 to 50% from each of carbohydrate and fat. Cats should receive at least 20% of their calories from protein.

Experts on canine and feline liver disease now believe the legislators' requirement for a low level of fat in the diet for patients with liver disease is unnecessary or even contra-indicated, with the provision of an adequate amount of energy taking precedence.

The management of liver disease is helped by the provision of digestible complex carbohydrates rather than simple sugars. This reduces insulin requirements and the glucose load presented to the liver. Carbohydrates also promote an insulin to glucagon ratio that favours an anabolic state in which amino acids absorbed from the small intestine are converted to protein rather than glucose. This reduces the production of ammonia that accompanies the utilisation of amino acids for gluconeogenesis. The inclusion of both soluble and insoluble dietary fibre plays an important role in the management of hepatic encephalopathy by modifying the production, absorption, and elimination of ammonia and other neurotoxic microbial byproducts from the large intestine.

Dietary supplementation with zinc and restriction of copper will provide protection from further liver injury associated with hepatocellular copper accumulation.

The requirement for B vitamins increases with energy intake and doubling of maintenance dietary requirements has been recommended. A deficiency of vitamin E is thought to contribute to ongoing hepatic injury due to production of superoxide radicals and peroxides; vitamin E supplementation is also considered to be of benefit.

In **exocrine pancreatic insufficiency** (see section 9 of Table 16.4), the diet should be highly digestible, containing only a small amount of fibre, and have a reduced concentration of fat to avoid steatorrhoea.

In cases of severe **diarrhoea,** or when vomiting accompanies diarrhoea, parenteral electrolyte and water replacement (see section 16.1) should be considered. In acute diarrhoea it is conventional to withhold all food for 24 hours and then to feed small quantities 4 to 6 times daily. An easily digestible diet with a reduced concentration of fat should be provided. A similar dietary regimen may be effective in some cases of inflammatory bowel disease. Alternatively, a hypoallergenic diet is more appropriate to manage the hypersensitivity reaction which causes, or is caused by,

inflammatory bowel disease. Highly digestible diets or hypoallergenic diets will control many cases of colitis but some individuals respond better to a diet containing increased fibre which increases the water binding capacity and normalises colonic motility. See sections 8 and 9 of Table 16.4. Dogs and cats prone to constipation may benefit from a diet containing 10% or more fibre on a dry matter basis which promotes water retention and stimulates normal peristalsis.

The main manifestations of **food allergy** in the dog and cat are skin lesions and, less often, gastro-intestinal disturbances. The most common allergens in the dog are beef, milk and dairy products, and wheat; in the cat, allergens include beef, milk and dairy products, and fish. Dietary management (see section 7 of Table 16.4) involves elimination of the protein source(s) responsible for the hypersensitivity reaction. This is best achieved by feeding a diet containing a limited number of novel proteins in restricted amounts. To establish whether a particular trial diet (elimination diet) will result in an improvement may require feeding the diet for up to 10 weeks. Such a 'hypoallergenic' diet is valuable for both diagnosis and management. Subsequent provocative exposure to different protein sources is required to determine which is/are responsible for the allergic response.

Diets for the management of **congestive heart failure** (see section 10 of Table 16.4) should contain a restricted concentration of sodium to control cardiovascular preload and circulatory congestion together with hypertension and fluid retention due to an increase in venous pressure. An increased intake of potassium and vitamin B substances is desirable to replace losses due to diuresis and a moderately low protein concentration reduces the retention of nitrogenous wastes resulting from concurrent renal insufficiency. Diets for cats with dilated cardiomyopathy should contain extra taurine.

Clinical diets have an important role in the management of canine and feline crystalluria and **urolithiasis** (often associated with feline lower urinary tract disease), involving not only a reduction in the availability of their constituents and an adjustment of the urinary pH to discourage precipitation of the relevant mineral type but also a product that will encourage an increased water turnover. Management of struvite (magnesium ammonium phosphate) crystals and uroliths requires the use of diets which produce adequate urinary acidification and are low in magnesium and phosphorus, and (in the dog) protein (see sections 2 and 3 of Table 16.4). It is imperative to eliminate urinary tract infections due to urease-producing organisms, which will convert urea to ammonia and consequently elevate the urinary pH.

Calcium oxalate calculi are best managed by alkalinisation of the urine and a reduction in the dietary intake of calcium and oxalate (see section 5 of Table 16.4). Urate calculi are controlled with diets that have a low purine and protein content and produce urinary alkalinisation (see section 4 of Table 16.4). Low protein diets are also advocated for cystine calculi (see section 6 of Table 16.4).

To achieve weight reduction in **obesity** (see section 15 of Table 16.4), the energy intake should be reduced to 40% of the metabolisable energy requirement (at the ideal weight) for dogs, and 60% for cats. The energy density of the diet is reduced primarily by minimising its fat content. Decreasing the density of the diet, or increasing the volume, will help promote a satisfying feeling of 'fullness' (satiety) without providing calories. This can be achieved by kibble extrusion (dry diets), enhanced moisture content (canned diets), or by inclusion of higher concentration of indigestible fibre. Ideally a number of small meals and several short periods of exercise should be provided throughout the day.

Nutritional support is vital to the survival of **critically ill patients** (for example those suffering from trauma, burns, sepsis, and pyrexia) as well as speeding the recovery of convalescent patients (for example after surgery) and those suffering from debilitation, cachexia, and anorexia. Primary calorie sources should be proteins and lipids, with reduced concentration of carbohydrates (see section 16 of Table 16.4). There should be a high content of essential and branched chain amino acids, glutamine, essential fatty acids, and zinc. Palatability and digestibility of the diet should be high. If an animal cannot be persuaded for example, by hand feeding or 'force feeding', to maintain an adequate intake of nutrients then tube feeding may be necessary. Information on parenteral nutrition is given in section 16.3.

In dogs and cats suffering from **diabetes mellitus** (see section 11 of Table 16.4) an increased dietary fibre content promotes slower and more consistant absorption of glucose (reducing postprandial blood glucose fluctuations). A high concentration of digestible complex carbohydrates accentuates the benefit of fibre, and the restriction of fat to 7 to 17% of dry matter minimises hyperlipidaemia and hepatic lipidosis. Glycaemic control can be improved by feeding frequent small meals throughout the period of insulin activity. Changing the type and amount of a diet will affect insulin requirements and may result in destabilisation.

Table 16.4 Complete dietetic pet foods for dogs and cats

Preparations for dogs	*Preparations for cats*

1 Support of renal function in chronic renal insufficiency (and temporary renal insufficiency)

Characteristics: low concentration of phosphorus and restricted concentration of protein but of high quality used for initially up to 6 months (temporary renal insufficiency: 2–4 weeks)

Canine Low Phosphorus Low Protein, canned (Pedigree)	Feline Low Phosphorus Low Protein, canned (Whiskas)
Canine Low Phosphorus Low Protein, dry (Pedigree)	Feline Low Phosphorus Low Protein, dry (Whiskas)
Canine Low Phosphorus Medium Protein, canned (Pedigree)	Prescription Diet Feline g/d, dry (Hill's)
Canine Low Phosphorus Medium Protein, canned (Pedigree)	Prescription Diet Feline k/d, canned (Hill's)
Eukanuba Renal Phase 1 Formula, dry (Iams)	Prescription Diet Feline k/d, dry (Hill's)
Eukanuba Renal Phase 2 Formula, dry (Iams)	Purina Feline CNM NF, dry (Ralston)
Prescription Diet Canine g/d, dry (Hill's)	
Prescription Diet Canine k/d, canned (Hill's)	
Prescription Diet Canine k/d, dry (Hill's)	
Prescription Diet Canine u/d, canned (Hill's)	
Prescription Diet Canine u/d, dry (Hill's)	
Purina Canine CNM NF, dry (Ralston)	

2 Dissolution of struvite stones (and feline lower urinary tract disease)

Characteristics: urine acidifying properties, low concentration of magnesium in dogs and cats; and restricted concentration of protein but of high quality in dogs; used for 5–12 weeks

Prescription Diet Canine s/d, canned (Hill's)	Feline Low pH Control, canned (Whiskas)
Canine Low pH Control, canned (Pedigree)	Feline Low pH Control, dry (Whiskas)
Canine Low pH Control, dry (Pedigree)	Prescription Diet Feline s/d, canned (Hill's)
	Prescription Diet Feline s/d, dry (Hill's)
	Purina Feline CNM UR, dry (Ralston)

3 Reduction of struvite stone recurrence (and feline lower urinary tract disease)

Characteristics: urine acidifying properties and moderate concentration of magnesium used for up to 6 months

Prescription Diet Canine c/d, canned (Hill's)	Eukanuba Struvite Urinary Formula, canned (Iams)
Prescription Diet Canine c/d, dry (Hill's)	Eukanuba Struvite Urinary Formula, dry (Iams)
Canine Low pH Control, canned (Pedigree)	Feline Low pH Control, canned (Whiskas)
Canine Low pH Control, dry (Pedigree)	Feline Low pH Control, dry (Whiskas)
	Prescription Diet Feline c/d, canned (Hill's)
	Prescription Diet Feline c/d, dry (Hill's)
	Purina Feline CNM UR, dry (Ralston)

4 Reduction of urate stone formation

Characteristics: low concentration of purines, low concentration of protein but of high quality used for up to 6 months but lifetime in cases of irreversible disturbance of uric acid metabolism

Prescription Diet Canine u/d, canned (Hill's)
Prescription Diet Canine u/d, dry (Hill's)
Canine Low Phosphorus Low Protein, canned (Pedigree)

5 Reduction of oxalate stone formation

Characteristics: low concentration of calcium, low concentration of vitamin D and urine alkalising properties used for up to 6 months

Prescription Diet Canine u/d, canned (Hill's)	Eukanuba Oxalate Urinary Formula, canned (Iams)
Prescription Diet Canine u/d, dry (Hill's)	Eukanuba Oxalate Urinary Formula, dry (Iams)
Canine Low pH Control, canned (Pedigree)	Feline Low pH Control, canned (Whiskas)
	Prescription Diet Feline x/d, canned (Hill's)

Table 16.4 Complete dietetic pet foods for dogs and cats

Preparations for dogs	Preparations for cats

6 Reduction of cystine stone formation

Characteristics: low concentration of protein, moderate concentration of sulphur amino acids, and urine alkalising properties used for initially up to 1 year

Prescription Diet Canine u/d, canned (Hill's) Prescription Diet Canine u/d, dry (Hill's) Canine Low Phosphorus Low Protein, canned (Pedigree)	

7 Reduction of ingredient and nutrient intolerances

Characteristics: selected protein source(s) and/or selected carbohydrate source(s) used for 3–8 weeks; if signs of intolerance disappear this feed can be used indefinitely

Canine Selected Protein, canned (Pedigree) Canine Selected Protein, dry (Pedigree) Eukanuba Response Formula FP, canned (Iams) Eukanuba Response Formula FP, dry (Iams) Prescription Diet Canine d/d, canned (Hill's) Prescription Diet Canine d/d, dry (Hill's)	Eukanuba Response Formula LB, canned (Iams) Feline Selected Protein, dry (Whiskas) Feline Selected Protein, canned (Whiskas) Prescription Diet Feline d/d, canned (Hill's)

8 Reduction of acute intestinal absorptive disorders

Characteristics: increased concentration of electrolytes and highly digestible ingredients used for 1–2 weeks

Canine Selected Protein, canned (Pedigree) Canine Selected Protein, dry (Pedigree) Eukanuba Intestinal Formula (Iams) Prescription Diet Canine i/d, canned (Hill's) Prescription Diet Canine i/d, dry (Hill's)	Eukanuba Intestinal Formula (Iams) Feline Selected Protein, canned (Whiskas) Feline Selected Protein, dry (Whiskas) Prescription Diet Feline i/d, canned (Hill's) Prescription Diet Feline i/d, dry (Hill's)

9 Compensation for maldigestion (and exocrine pancreatic insufficiency)

Characteristics: highly digestible ingredients and low concentration of fat used for 3–12 weeks, but lifetime in chronic pancreatic insufficiency

Canine Low Fat, canned (Pedigree) Canine Low Fat, dry (Pedigree) Eukanuba Intestinal Formula (Iams) Prescription Diet Canine i/d, canned (Hill's) Prescription Diet Canine i/d, dry (Hill's) Purina Canine CNM EN, dry (Ralston)	Eukanuba Intestinal Formula (Iams) Feline Selected Protein, dry (Whiskas) Purina Feline CNM EN, dry (Ralston) Prescription Diet Feline i/d, canned (Hill's) Prescription Diet Feline i/d, dry (Hill's)

10 Support of heart function in chronic cardiac insufficiency

Characteristics: low concentration of sodium and increased potassium:sodium ratio used for initially up to 6 months

Canine Low Sodium, canned (Pedigree) Prescription Diet Canine h/d, canned (Hill's) Purina Canine CNM CV, dry (Ralston)	Feline Low Phosphorus Low Protein, canned (Whiskas) Feline Low Phosphorus Low Protein, dry (Whiskas) Prescription Diet Feline h/d, canned (Hill's) Purina Feline CNM CV, dry (Ralston)

11 Reduction of glucose supply (diabetes mellitus)

Characteristics: low concentration of rapid glucose-releasing carbohydrates used for initially up to 6 months

Canine High Fibre, canned (Pedigree) Canine High Fibre, dry (Pedigree) Prescription Diet Canine w/d, canned (Hill's) Prescription Diet Canine w/d, dry (Hill's) Purina Canine CNM DCO, dry (Ralston)	Feline Concentration, canned (Whiskas) Feline Low Caloric, canned (Whiskas) Prescription Diet Feline w/d, canned (Hill's) Prescription Diet Feline w/d, dry (Hill's) Purina Feline CNM OM, dry (Ralston)

Table 16.4 Complete dietetic pet foods for dogs and cats

Preparations for dogs	*Preparations for cats*

12 Support of liver function in case of chronic liver insufficiency

Characteristics: high quality protein, moderate concentration of protein, low concentration of fat in dogs, moderate concentration of fat in cats, high concentration of EFAs and highly digestible carbohydrate used for initially up to 6 months

Canine Hepatic Support, canned (Pedigree) Canine Hepatic Support, dry (Pedigree) Prescription Diet Canine l/d, canned (Hill's) Prescription Diet Canine l/d, dry (Hill's) Purina Canine CNM NF, dry (Ralston)	Feline Selected Protein, dry (Whiskas) Prescription Diet Feline l/d, canned (Hill's) Prescription Diet Feline l/d, canned (Hill's) Purina Feline CNM NF, dry (Ralston)

13 Regulation of lipid metabolism in hyperlipidaemia

Characteristics: low concentration of fat and high concentration of EFAs used for initially up to 2 months

Canine Low Fat Diet, canned(Pedigree) Canine Low Fat Diet, dry (Pedigree) Eukanuba Intestinal Formula (Iams) Prescription Diet Canine w/d, canned (Hill's) Prescription Diet Canine w/d, dry (Hill's) Purina Canine CNM EN, dry (Ralston) Purina Canine CNM OM, dry (Ralston)	Feline Selected Protein, dry (Whiskas) Prescription Diet Feline w/d, canned (Hill's) Prescription Diet Feline w/d, dry (Hill's) Purina Feline CNM OM, dry (Ralston)

14 Reduction of copper in the liver

Characteristics: low concentration of copper for initially used for up to 6 months

Canine Hepatic Support Diet, canned (Pedigree)
Canine Hepatic Support Diet, dry (Pedigree)
Prescription Diet Canine l/d, canned (Hill's)
Prescription Diet Canine l/d, dry (Hill's)

15 Reduction of excessive body-weight

Characteristics: low energy density used until target body-weight is achieved

Canine Calorie Control Diet, dry (Pedigree) Canine Low Calorie Diet, canned (Pedigree) Eukanuba Restricted-Calorie Formula, dry (Iams) Prescription Diet Canine r/d, canned (Hill's) Prescription Diet Canine r/d, dry (Hill's) Prescription Diet Canine w/d, canned (Hill's) Prescription Diet Canine w/d, dry (Hill's) Purina Canine CNM GL, dry (Ralston) Purina Canine CNM OM, dry (Ralston)	Eukanuba Restricted-Calorie Formula, dry (Iams) Feline Calorie Control Diet, dry (Whiskas) Feline Low Calorie Diet, canned (Whiskas) Prescription Diet Feline r/d, canned (Hill's) Prescription Diet Feline r/d, dry (Hill's) Prescription Diet Feline w/d, canned (Hill's) Prescription Diet Feline w/d, dry (Hill's) Purina Feline CNM OM, dry (Ralston)

16 Nutritional restoration, convalescence (and hepatic lipidosis in cats)

Characteristics: high energy density, high concentration of essential nutrients and highly digestible ingredients used until restoration is achieved

Canine Concentration Diet, canned (Pedigree) Canine Concentration Instant Diet, dry (Pedigree) Eukanuba High Caloric Formula, canned (Iams) Eukanuba High Caloric Formula, dry (Iams) Fortol Complete Liquid Feed (Arnolds) Prescription Diet Canine/Feline a/d, canned (Hill's) Prescription Diet Canine n/d, canned (Hill's) Prescription Diet Canine p/d, canned (Hill's) Purina Critical Care Nutrition for Dogs and Cats (Ralston)	Eukanuba High Caloric Formula, canned (Iams) Eukanuba High Caloric Formula, dry (Iams) Feline Concentration Diet, canned (Whiskas) Feline Concentration Instant Diet, dry (Whiskas) Prescription Diet Canine/Feline a/d, canned (Hill's) Purina Critical Care Nutrition for Dogs and Cats (Ralston)

Table 16.4 Complete dietetic pet foods for dogs and cats

Preparations for dogs	*Preparations for cats*

17 Support of skin function in dermatosis and excessive loss of hair
Characteristics: high concentration of EFAs used for up to 2 months

Canine Concentration Diet, canned (Pedigree)	Eukanuba Response Formula LB, canned (Iams)
Canine Concentration Instant Diet, dry (Pedigree)	Feline Concentration Diet, canned (Whiskas)
Eukanuba Response Formula FP, canned (Iams)	Feline Concentration Instant Diet, dry (Whiskas)
Eukanuba Response Formula FP, dry (Iams)	Prescription Diet Feline d/d, canned (Hill's)
Prescription Diet Canine d/d, canned (Hill's)	Prescription Diet Feline p/d, canned (Hill's)
Prescription Diet Canine d/d, dry (Hill's)	
Prescription Diet Canine p/d, canned (Hill's)	

18 Support of patient with neoplasia
Characteristics: high fat (in particular omega3 fatty acids), high protein (in particular arginine), low carbohydrate

Canine Concentration Diet, canned (Pedigree)	Feline Concentration Diet, canned (Whiskas)
Canine Concentration Instant Diet, dry (Pedigree)	Feline Concentration Instant Diet, dry (Whiskas)
Prescription Diet Canine n/d, canned (Hill's)	

17 PRODUCTION ENHANCERS

Contributor:
Professor D M Pugh BVSc, MA, MSc, DrMedVet, MRCVS

17.1 Antibacterial production enhancers
17.2 Probiotics
17.3 Enzymes
17.4 Other production enhancers

Many preparations have been evaluated and used to enhance the efficiency of animal production. There is both variation and similarity between EU member states and other countries as to which products may legally be used for production enhancement. Illicit uses have led to an array of control measures while policy divergences have lead to the threat of trade disputes at the international level.

Within the EU, substances or preparations which are approved for use for specified purposes for inclusion in animal diets are listed in the classified Annexes of EC Directive 70/524/EEC. The Directive includes antibiotics (class A), growth promoters (class J), coccidiostats (class D), mineral, and vitamins in addition to additives such as colourants, preservatives, and antioxidants. The authorisation of feed additives is separate from the authorisation of medicinal products, including those administered in feed and it is anomalous that coccidiosats are included under Directive 70/524/EEC. The similarity between additives is that they are all routinely included in finished feeds at the point of manufacturer.

The permitted production enhancers are marketed as feed additives for inclusion by approved compounders in premixtures or in bulk feedingstuffs at the time of their manufacture. Production enhancers, that were previously authorised as PML products in the UK, are now zootechnical feed additives (*The Feedingstuffs (Zootechnical Products) Regulations 1999*). Zootechnical feed additives may be incorporated in the feed at specified concentrations for particular species as indicated in the relevant Annex entry of Directive 70/524/EEC; there is no provision for incorporation in any way not in accordance with the Annex entry, for example at higher concentrations or for different species. Manufacturers may choose to market a production enhancer differently in various countries which is permitted as long as within the Annex entry; product information provided below is for preparations marketed in the UK.

The purpose of production enhancers is to improve liveweight gain, improve feed conversion efficiency, or both in order to increase the scale of production, efficiency of production, or both. Production enhancers are most widely used in pig and poultry diets and increasingly in rations for intensively-reared cattle and animals bred for fur, notably rabbits, mink, and chinchilla. Use in rabbits kept for meat production is also possible.

The use of antibiotic production enhancers has raised concerns over the potential impact on human medicine of microbial resistance of animal origin and for worker safety; these considerations do not appear to be founded on direct scientific evidence of harm. In addition, fears over animal welfare and a preference for 'natural' production systems have lead to an EU precautionary banning of the additive antibiotics avoparcin, bacitracin zinc, tylosin, spiramycin, and virginiamycin and the growth promoters under Annex J are also no longer available.

Preparations containing micro-organisms (probiotics) or enzymes are now included under EC Directive 70/524/EEC, implemented in the UK under the *Feeding Stuffs Regulations 1995*. Under this legislation, the identity and contents of permitted organisms or enzymes are listed in the Schedules; product-specific approval may lead to listing of individual products.

Both micro-organism and enzyme-containing products will be used in efforts to offset the production consequences of the loss of the banned antibiotics and growth promoters and veterinarians should be able to offer advice on this matter.

17.1 Antibacterial production enhancers

Most production enhancers available in the EU are antibiotics that are not used for therapeutic or prophylactic purposes in animals or humans, and with activity against Gram-positive bacteria only. This strategy aims to conserve the utility of antibiotics used for treatment in human medicine, veterinary practice, or both. However, there is evidence that some antibiotics that have been used as production enhancers but never for animal or human therapy, for example avoparcin, may select in favour of enterococci that are simultaneously resistant to glycopeptides which are used in human but not veterinary medicine. Similarly other feed additives, such as virginiamycin, which are related to agents used to treat enterococcal infections in humans, or which belong to an antibacterial group, other members of which are used in human or veterinary therapeutics, for example tylosin, have been reconsidered for use as production enhancers. Avoparcin, bacitracin zinc, spiramycin, tylosin, and virginiamycin are banned for use as production enhancers in the EU. These agents, where appropriate, may be used for therapeutic purposes.

Not all antibiotics possess production-promoting activity and production promoting potential does not appear to be dependent on a common molecular structure.

It is a requirement of Directive 70/524/EEC that antibiotic feed additives should not be used in combination. In addition, they may be mixed into animal feed only at appropriately registered and inspected feed mills and only within the final concentration ranges in finished feed specified in the legislation.

Antibacterial production enhancers may increase live-weight gain by up to 10% in poultry, pigs, and calves and up to 16% in adult cattle. This, together with increased feed conversion efficiency, reduces the time and the quantity of feed required to raise the animal. Important environmental benefits such as reducing the amount of nitrogen excreted and making available for human consumption cereals previously put into animal feed are also claimed.

Most antibacterial production enhancers are not absorbed from the gastro-intestinal tract to any great extent. This and their consequent absence from animal produce or presence in trace amounts of no toxicological concern explains the prevalence of zero withdrawal periods for these preparations.

In ruminants, the primary site of action is on the microflora of the rumen, enhancing the microbial production of the gluconeogenic fatty acid propionate, and to some extent acetate, at the expense of butyrate. Beyond the rumen in the small intestine, the production enhancer will have actions similar to those suggested for monogastric species. Production enhancers may act by suppressing harmful bacterial metabolites, potentially pathogenic organisms, or by biasing competition between organisms. Alternatively, they may act by altering metabolic activity or enhancing the intestinal absorption of nutrients.

The antibiotics may be administered to calves, lambs, and pigs up to 6 months of age. In poultry, these agents are usually given up to 6 to 9 weeks of age, excluding those authorised for use in laying hens, which may be given for a longer period. Some production enhancers are also authorised for use in turkeys and recommended age ranges may vary between preparations. Growing (older than 6 months) and finishing (in the 3 months before slaughter) cattle can also be treated with certain preparations. The term fattening cattle is a more general term sometimes used; it can be regarded as referring to older cattle destined for beef production.

Avilamycin is an oligosaccharide antibiotic used as a production enhancer in pigs and broiler chickens. Everninomycin (everninomicin), a related antibacterial agent, is now under evaluation in humans. If this agent is authorised for use in humans, it is likely that avilamycin will cease to be available for production enhancement.

Flavophospholipol (bambermycin) is a phosphorus-containing glycolipid antibacterial. It is used as a production enhancer in cattle, pigs, poultry, rabbits, and fur producers. Flavophospholipol is structurally distinct from antibiotic classes either under evaluation or used in human therapy. It is therefore unlikely to create resistance which will pose a danger for humans and should, logically, remain available as a production enhancer.

Monensin is an ionophore antibiotic used as an anticoccidial (see section 1.4.1), and as a production enhancer in beef cattle and dairy heifers up to the time of first service. Ingestion of feed containing monensin has been fatal in horses. **Salinomycin**, an ionophore, is also used for prevention of coccidiosis (see section 1.4.1), and for production promotion in pigs. Ionophores are not used in human medicine.

Therefore there can be no resistance-based argument to ban these agents from production enhancement use. It is probable that further members of this class may be authorised. However, when ionophores are used as production enhancers or coccidiostats their narrow margin of safety should be considered and caution exercised when using concurrent ionophores for therapy.

Large feed-compounding companies routinely add a specific production enhancer to their proprietary diets and this practice often governs the animal producer's choice of agent. Often the production enhancer is changed regularly every 6 to 12 months.

AVILAMYCIN

UK
Indications. To improve growth-rate and feed conversion efficiency
Contra-indications. Do not use simultaneously with other feed antibiotic or growth promoter
Dose.
Pigs: (up to 16 weeks of age) 20–40 g/tonne feed; (16–26 weeks of age) 10–20 g/tonne feed
Broiler chickens, turkeys: 5 *or* 10 g/tonne feed

ZFA **Maxus G200** (Elanco) *UK*
Premix, avilamycin 200 g/kg, for *pigs, broiler chickens, turkeys*
Withdrawal Periods. *Pigs, poultry*: slaughter withdrawal period nil

FLAVOPHOSPHOLIPOL
(Bambermycin)

UK
Indications. To improve growth-rate and feed conversion efficiency
Contra-indications. See under Avilamycin
Dose.
Cattle. Calves: (up to 26 weeks of age) 6–16 g/tonne feed *or* 8–16 g/tonne milk replacer
Fattening cattle: *by addition to complete feed*, 2–10 g/tonne
by addition to supplementary feed or free-access minerals, (100 kg body-weight) maximum daily dose 40 mg, (>100 kg body-weight) 40 mg plus 1.5 mg for each additional 10 kg body-weight
by addition to feed blocks, 80 mg/kg feed block
Pigs: (up to 6 months of age) 1–20 g/tonne feed; (up to 3 months of age) 10–20 g/tonne milk replacer or piglet creep feed
Broiler chickens: (up to 16 weeks of age) 1–20 g/tonne feed
Laying hens: 2–5 g/tonne feed
Turkeys: (up to 26 weeks of age) 1–20 g/tonne feed
Rabbits: 2–4 g/tonne feed

PML **Flaveco 40** (ECO)
Premix, flavophospholipol 80 g/kg, for *cattle, pigs, laying hens, broiler chickens, turkeys, rabbits*; 25 kg
Withdrawal Periods. *Cattle, pigs, poultry, rabbits*: slaughter withdrawal period nil

ZFA **Flavomycin 80** (Intervet) *UK*
Premix, flavophospholipol 80 g/kg, for *cattle, pigs, laying hens, broiler chickens, turkeys, rabbits*; 25 kg
Withdrawal Periods. *Cattle, pigs, poultry, rabbits*: slaughter withdrawal period nil

MONENSIN

UK

Indications. To improve growth-rate and feed conversion efficiency in cattle; prophylaxis of coccidiosis in poultry (see section 1.4.1)
Contra-indications. See under Avilamycin
Warnings. Should not be given within 7 days before or after the administration of tiamulin (Drug Interactions – see Appendix 1). Toxic to horses and other Equidae
Dose.

Cattle: *by addition to complete feed*, 10–40 g/tonne
by addition to supplementary feed, (100 kg body-weight) maximum daily dose 140 mg, (>100 kg body-weight) 140 mg plus up to 6 mg for each additional 10 kg body-weight
by addition to feed block, 400 g/tonne feed block

PML **Ecox 200** (ECO) UK
Premix, monensin (as monensin sodium) 100 g/kg, for *beef cattle, poultry* (see section 1.4.1)
Withdrawal Periods. *Cattle*: slaughter withdrawal period nil. *Poultry*: slaughter 3 days

ZFA **Romensin G100** (Elanco) *UK*
Premix, monensin (as monensin sodium) 100 g/kg, for *cattle, except lactating dairy cattle*; 25 kg
Withdrawal Periods. *Cattle*: slaughter withdrawal period nil, should not be used in lactating dairy cattle
Note. See manufacturer's data sheet for further dosages

SALINOMYCIN SODIUM

UK

Indications. To improve growth-rate and feed conversion efficiency in pigs; prophylaxis of coccidiosis in poultry (see section 1.4.1)
Contra-indications. **Side-effects**. **Warnings**. Not to be given within 4 days before or 7 days after the administration of tiamulin (Drug Interactions – see Appendix 1). Toxic to horses and other Equidae
Dose. *Pigs*: (up to 16 weeks of age and 35–40 kg body-weight) 30–60 g/tonne feed; (up to 26 weeks of age) 15–30 g/tonne feed

ZFA **Bio-Cox 120G** (Alpharma) *UK*
Premix, salinomycin sodium 120 g/kg, for *chickens* (see section 1.4.1), *pigs*
Withdrawal Periods. *Pigs*: slaughter withdrawal period nil

PML **Sal-Eco 120** (ECO)
Premix, salinomycin sodium 120 g/kg, for *chickens* (see section 1.4.1), *pigs*
Withdrawal Periods. *Pigs*: slaughter withdrawal period nil. *Poultry*: slaughter 5 days

ZFA **Salocin 120** (Intervet) *UK*
Premix, salinomycin sodium 120 g/kg, for *pigs*; 25 kg
Withdrawal Periods. *Pigs*: slaughter withdrawal period nil

17.2 Probiotics

Probiotics are products whose favourable effect on health and production indices is usually attributed to an effect on the environment of the gut. They contain micro-organisms in vegetative or arrested states, but capable of colony formation in the gut. There is evidence that probiotics reduce the adverse effects of other organisms and even inhibit the colonization of the gut by pathogens. This may be due to competition for space and nutrients (competitive exclusion), production of inhibiting substances (bacteriocins), or both. Lactobacilli can reduce the concentrations of microbial metabolites such as ammonia and amines that are harmful to the host.

Many approved probiotics are lised under UK and EU legislation. Micro-organisms used in probiotics are specific strains of either brewers yeast, or bacteria which can be found within the normal gut flora. The various strains available in products are *Bacillus cereus* var *toyoi* (CNCM 1-1012/NCIB 40112), *Bacillus licheniformis* (DSM 5749), *Bacillus subtilis* (DSM 5750), *Saccharomyces cerevisiae* (NCYC Sc47) and *Bacillus cereus* (ATCC 14893/CIP 5832). Under Directive 70/524/EEC, minimum and maximum inclusion levels in finished feed are given and expressed as CFU (Colony-Forming Units) per g, mL, or kg.

Many probiotic preparations are based on organisms normally resident in the gastro-intestinal tract, for example enterococci. A major safety concern is that probiotics should not introduce or aid in the dissemination of resistance determinants. For similar reasons, neither should they produce an antibiotic of relevance to therapy. Other probiotic micro-organisms belong to families, some members of which are toxin producing, for example *Bacillus cereus*. Therefore approved products are strain specific and producers have to show strain stability.

UK

There are many preparations available. Authorised products are listed below.

Indications. To prevent diarrhoea and improve growth-rate
Contra-indications. Concurrent use of antibacterials

PML **Provita Protech** (Provita Eurotech) *UK*
Oral liquid, containing *Lactobacillus acidophilus* strains LA-101, LA-107, *Enterococcus faecium* strain SF-10, for *calves up to 12 weeks of age*; 100-mL dose applicator (1 unit dose = 2.5 mL)
Withdrawal Periods. *Calves*: slaughter withdrawal period nil
Dose. *Calves*: *by mouth*, initial dose 5 mL, followed by 2.5 mL daily for 2 days given in the morning before feed

17.3 Enzymes

Enzymes enhance the digestibility of low quality and other carbohydrates, principally of cereal origin, in the diet of production animals. The enzymes such as glucanases, xylanases, and amylases are usually produced as single activities by specialist biotechnology companies. They are then assembled into feed additive products, sometimes containing more than one enzyme activity. As for micro-organisms, the information requirement for marketing authorisations is very much less demanding than that for new antibiotic feed additves. For enzymes, the most important toxicological concerns relate to exposure of workers and potential hypersensitisation and irritant properties.

Many enymes are listed under the UK and EU legislation including phytases, galactosidases, glucanases, xylanases, amylases, bacillolysin, aspergillopepsin, triacylglycerol lipase, polygalacturonase, xylosidase, and subtilisin. All the enzymes are fermentation products of either bacterial or fungal origin. The available products are described as liquids, slurries, solids, powders, coated preparations, granulates, or microgranulates. Potency is expressed as units of lytic activity against a stated substrate per g or mL.

17.4 Other production enhancers

Certain **copper** salts may be incorporated into the diet of pigs in excess of nutritional requirements and have a production-enhancing effect. The efficacy of copper salts as production enhancers is probably related to their antimicrobial activity. Some reports have shown that copper salts and antibacterial production enhancers have an additive effect and they may be combined in pig feeds.

Arsenical compounds have been used in the past as production enhancers in pig and poultry diets but are now superseded by the use of antibiotics.

Steroid hormone growth promoters, the somatotrophins, and beta-adrenoceptor stimulants (beta-agonists) are used for production enhancement in some countries. Under EC Directive 96/22/EEC, implemented as the *Animals and Animal Products (Examinaton for Residues and Maximum Residue Limits) Regulations 1997* in the UK, hormonal growth promoters and beta-adrenoceptor stimulants (under certain circumstances) are banned for use in food-producing animals within the EU.

COPPER SALTS

UK

Indications. To improve growth-rate and feed conversion efficiency in pigs; correction of copper deficiency in dairy cattle and dairy goats (see section 16.5.6)

Warnings. Care should be taken that sheep do not have access to effluent from treated animals

Dose. *Pigs*: (up to 16 weeks of age) 175 g/tonne feed; (16–26 weeks of age) 100 g/tonne feed

ZFA **Copper Carbonate** (UKASTA) *UK*
Oral powder, for addition to feed, copper (as copper carbonate) 551 g/kg, for *pigs*
Withdrawal Periods. *Pigs*: slaughter withdrawal period nil

ZFA **Copper Sulphate** (UKASTA) *UK*
Oral powder, for addition to feed, copper (as copper sulphate) 254 g/kg, for *pigs*
Withdrawal Periods. *Cattle, goats*: slaughter withdrawal period nil, milk withdrawal period nil. *Pigs*: slaughter withdrawal period nil

ZFA **Cupric Oxide** (UKASTA) *UK*
Oral powder, for addition to feed, copper (as cupric oxide) 785 g/kg, for *pigs*
Withdrawal Periods. *Pigs*: slaughter withdrawal period nil

18 VACCINES and IMMUNOLOGICAL PREPARATIONS

Contributors:
M Bennett BVSc, PHD, MRCVS
P A Flecknell MA, VetMB, PhD, DLAS, MRCVS
S A Lister BVetMed, BSc, CertPMP, MRCVS
L M Sommerville BVMS, MRCVS
A E Wall BVM&S, MSc, CertVOphthal, MRCVS

18.1 Immunological preparations for horses
18.2 Immunological preparations for cattle, sheep, and goats
18.3 Immunological preparations for pigs
18.4 Immunological preparations for dogs
18.5 Immunological preparations for cats
18.6 Immunological preparations for birds
18.7 Immunological preparations for rabbits
18.8 Immunological preparations for fish

Immunity in animals may be acquired by either passive or active means. **Passive immunity** results from the transfer of maternal antibodies to offspring or by the injection of antiserum to an animal of any age. *Antiserum* is serum usually obtained from immunised animals and contains antibodies to specific antigens. An *antitoxin* is antiserum containing antibodies to a specific bacterial toxin.

Domestic mammals acquire passive immunity by intestinal absorption of antibodies from colostrum ingested within the first few hours of life. In birds, maternal antibody is transferred to the yolk, from where the developing chick absorbs it. There is no maternally-derived passive immunity in fish. The degree of protection conferred depends upon the amount and specificity of the antibodies transferred. Passive immunity lasts only as long as antibodies remain reactive in the blood after which the animal loses any resistance to that specific infection. Generally, passive immunity persists from 3 to to 12 weeks in mammals and for up to 3 weeks in poultry. If vaccines are given by parenteral administration during this period, they may be ineffective or induce only a short duration of immunity. Subsequent administration of vaccines may be indicated if long-term immunisation is required.

Commercially available preparations of antisera are usually produced by immunising horses or cattle to obtain sera containing the appropriate antibodies or antitoxins. Such preparations are frequently used to provide temporary protection, for example, against tetanus. The intravenous injection of antiserum, especially if repeated a number of times, may produce hypersensitivity reactions. The potency of an antitoxic serum is expressed in terms of the International Unit (IU) defined by the World Health Organization and abbreviated to 'unit' in *The Veterinary Formulary*.

Active immunity develops as a result of infection with a micro-organism, or by administration of a vaccine prepared from live or inactivated organisms, antigenic fractions, or from detoxified exotoxins produced by organisms. Vaccines are preparations of antigenic material, which are administered to induce active immunity in the recipient animal against specific bacterial, parasitic, or viral infections. Vaccines may be single component or mixed, combined preparations. Although the immune response is usually specific for each agent, cross-protection can occur, for example between canine distemper and measles viruses. The measles virus belongs to the same genus as the distemper virus but can be distinguished antigenically; the measles vaccine, when used to prevent distemper, is an example of a heterotypic (heterologous) vaccine.

Live vaccines are usually produced with live micro-organisms that have lost their pathogenicity by treatment with gentle heating, sublethal chemicals, or passage through another host cell and are called modified live or attenuated vaccines. Live vaccines may also be nonpathogenic forms of the infecting organism such as in toxoplasmosis vaccines, or related less pathogenic organisms for example Shope fibroma virus used to vaccinate rabbits against myxomatosis. Live vaccines retain many of the surface antigens of the organism from which they are derived. They replicate and disseminate throughout the host's body but do not normally cause disease. They stimulate production of antibodies locally, systemically, or both.

Local antibodies may be stimulated by vaccines that promote immunity at mucosal surfaces, such as the nasal or intestinal mucosa. Living bacteria or viruses in these vaccines colonise and replicate on the surface of the appropriate mucosa. Temperature-sensitive strains of virus may be used in intranasal vaccines. These viruses undergo replication in the cooler nasal mucosa and upper respiratory tract; core body temperature inhibits replication at other sites in the body. Immunity derived from such vaccines develops rapidly and they may be used to protect noninfected animals during a herd outbreak of a disease such as infectious bovine rhinotracheitis.

The degree of protection afforded by live vaccines varies, depending upon the antigen and the animal, but is usually high and of long duration, although it is generally less than that following natural infection.

Antibodies, especially maternally-derived, may inhibit the replication of the live micro-organism in the vaccine and thus interfere with the process of immunisation for several weeks. Therefore, further doses of vaccine may be recommended, given at suitable intervals to allow time for interfering antibodies to decline.

Inactivated (killed) vaccines contain sufficient antigen to stimulate antibody production but generally require two doses, with an appropriate interval between (or initial stimulation with a live vaccine), in order to produce a satisfactory immune response and protection. As a consequence of the process necessary to inactivate many micro-organisms, the surface antigens may be modified. The organisms in these vaccines do not replicate. Other vaccines contain genetically engineered subunits of the pathogen, for example feline leukaemia vaccine.

These inactivated vaccines may contain adjuvants that enhance the immune reaction. Adjuvants commonly used are aluminium hydroxide, aluminium phosphate, alum, and carbomer, or an appropriate mineral oil such as liquid paraffin. Therefore, inactivated vaccines may cause local irritation and swelling at the site of injection. Asepsis on administration is very important. These vaccines must always be administered by injection as recommended by the manufacturer. Booster doses of inactivated vaccines are usually employed to maintain an enduring immunity. These are often administered annually and manufacturer's recommendations should be followed.

Toxoids are toxins obtained from micro-organisms and treated by heat or chemical means to destroy their deleterious properties without destroying their ability to stimulate the formation of antibodies, for example tetanus toxoid. Toxoid vaccines usually contain adjuvants.

Autogenous vaccines are prepared from cultures of material derived from a lesion of the animal to be vaccinated, for example wart vaccines. Unauthorised immunological products may be used only if they are autogenous vaccines prepared from material taken from one animal for use solely in that same animal. A UK emergency vaccine authorisation will be needed before an autogenous vaccine may be used in poultry.

Emergency vaccines are produced using micro-organisms from an animal, and are intended solely for administration to the herd or flock to which the animal belongs. They are used when commercial vaccines are not available. A UK emergency vaccine authorisation is required before a vaccine prepared from material taken from one animal is used in animals on the same premises. Applications should be made to the VMD.

Contra-indications and side-effects of vaccines.   The possibility of undesirable side-effects should be considered when vaccines are used and the manufacturer's data sheet or pack insert should be consulted. Unhealthy or febrile animals should not be vaccinated. Animals should not be vaccinated within several weeks of receiving immunosuppressive drugs or corticosteroids. When administering live vaccines derived from bacteria, care must be taken in the use of antibacterials. When herds or flocks are being vaccinated with live vaccines, the transmission of infection due to the organism in the vaccine should be borne in mind, for example the introduction of orf virus into a susceptible flock or infection of younger more susceptible stock in a multi-age flock or herd. With vaccines containing live herpesviruses the probability of latent infections and their effects on future export of animals from the herd may require consideration. The full vaccination course as recommended by the manufacturer should always be administered.

Some live vaccines, such as feline panleucopenia virus, may be able to cross the placenta and cause abortion or fetal abnormalities. In general, inactivated vaccines are safer than live vaccines in pregnant animals but handling and vaccinating animals in late pregnancy is associated with some risk. Stressing animals to be vaccinated should be avoided. Some inactivated vaccines may cause a transient swelling at the injection site. Some side-effects such as coat colour change at the site of injection in certain cat breeds may be permanent.

Temporary clinical signs such as coughing may be seen after administration of some vaccines, for example canine tracheobronchitis vaccine administered by intranasal instillation. Occasionally, animals exhibit a hypersensitivity reaction post-vaccination. Clinical signs of hypersensitivity reactions are species-dependent and subject to individual variation. Signs tend to occur rapidly after injection and may include respiratory distress, vomiting, diarrhoea, salivation, and urticaria. The risk of anaphylactic reaction is particularly increased following repeated doses of heterologous antiserum, such as tetanus antitoxin. Epinephrine (see section 4.5) or corticosteroids (see section 7.2.1) should be administered promptly in the event of a reaction.

In any animal population there may be a small number of individuals which fail to respond fully to vaccination. However, non-effectiveness of vaccines, that is failure to prevent clinical disease in a group vaccinated with a specific vaccine, is regarded as an adverse effect and should be reported to the VMD (see *British Veterinary Association Code of Practice on Medicines*).

Accidental self-injection with oil-based vaccines can cause severe pain and intense swelling, which may result in ischaemic necrosis and loss of a digit. Prompt medical attention is essential. A copy of the warning given in the product leaflet or data sheet should be shown to the doctor (or nurse) on duty.

Storage and handling of vaccines. Care must be taken to store and transport all vaccines and other immunological preparations under the conditions recommended by the manufacturer, otherwise the preparation may become denatured and totally ineffective. Vaccines should be stored according to the manufacturer's recommendations. Refrigerated storage at 2°C to 8°C is usually necessary. Some poultry vaccines are stored in liquid nitrogen. Unless otherwise specified, vaccines should not be frozen and should be protected from light. Live antigens may be inactivated by disinfectants or alcohol and become ineffective.

Only sterile needles and syringes should be used for vaccination and injections should be given with aseptic precautions to avoid the possibility of abscess formation or the transmission of incidental infections. Animals should not be vaccinated through dirty, wet skin. The repeated use of single needles and syringes within herds and flocks is not recommended. Containers that have held live vaccines can be potentially hazardous and should be made safe in accordance with HSE and COSHH recommendations and regulations.

Injectable vaccines should be stored and reconstituted as recommended by the manufacturer and liquid preparations should always be adequately shaken before use to ensure uniformity of the material to be injected. It is important that vaccines are administered correctly. For example live vaccines (such as feline viral respiratory disease complex vaccines) injected subcutaneously may cause disease if accidently administered orally or intranasally. This may occur if an aerosol is made during reconstitution of the vaccine or if a drop of vaccine is left on the skin and subsequently licked off. Manufacturers recommend that the skin is wiped with spirit after vaccination to reduce the potential risk of ingestion.

18.1 Immunological preparations for horses

18.1.1 Enteritis
18.1.2 Equine herpesvirus
18.1.3 Equine influenza
18.1.4 Equine viral arteritis
18.1.5 Rabies
18.1.6 Tetanus
18.1.7 Combination vaccines for horses
18.1.8 Immunoglobulins for horses

The immunisation programme employed for individual horses depends on their use and amount of contact with other horses. It is advisable that horses are always vaccinated against tetanus and equine influenza. The Jockey Club and Fédération Equestre Internationale (FEI) require horses to be vaccinated regularly against equine influenza. Vaccination against the equine herpesvirus, which causes rhinopneumonitis and abortion, is sometimes recommended.

Generally, vaccines are injected intramuscularly or occasionally subcutaneously, into the neck, pectoral, or gluteal regions dependent on the antigen present in the vaccine.

With some vaccines there is a recommendation to avoid strenuous exercise particularly following primary vaccination. Inactivated vaccines may rarely cause a post-vaccination reaction characterised by limb stiffness. Local and systemic adverse reactions have been reported with influenza vaccines and with equine herpesvirus 1 vaccine following a recent respiratory infection with the herpesvirus.

18.1.1 Enteritis

Rotavirus is the most common cause of diarrhoea in young foals. Other causative agents include bacteria, protozoa, other viruses and environmental and management factors.

An inactivated vaccine, which is used as an aid in the prevention of disease caused by equine rotavirus in foals, is available under a provisional marketing authorisation. Efficacy in use data is collected. Pregnant mares are vaccinated to provide passive transfer of rotavirus antibodies to foals. Mares are vaccinated at the 8th, 9th, and 10th of pregnancy.

UK
Indications. Vaccination against equine rotavirus
Contra-indications. Side-effects. Warnings. See notes at beginning of chapter
Dose. See notes above and preparation details

POM **Duvaxyn R** (Fort Dodge) *UK*
Injection, rotavirus vaccine, inactivated, prepared from equine rotavirus strain H2, containing a suitable oil as adjuvant, for *horses*
Withdrawal Periods. Should not be used in *horses* intended for human consumption
Dose. *Horses*: *by intramuscular injection*, 1 mL

18.1.2 Equine herpesvirus

Infection with equine herpesvirus 1 and equine herpesvirus 4 may cause respiratory disease, abortion, neonatal death, and paresis. The respiratory form, known as equine viral rhinopneumonitis, is characterised by fever, coughing, and nasal and ocular discharge.

Inactivated vaccines are available which may be used in horses of all ages except foals. The vaccination programme depends on the vaccine used. The primary course consists of 2 vaccines given at an interval of 3 to 6 weeks, depending on the vaccine used. Booster vaccinations should be given every 6 to 12 months, depending on the vaccine used. The Horserace Betting Levy Board publishes a *Code of Practice on Equid Herpesvirus 1 (EHV-1)*.

UK
Indications. Vaccination against equine herpesvirus
Contra-indications. Side-effects. Warnings. See notes at beginning of chapter
Dose. See preparation details

POM **Duvaxyn EHV** (Fort Dodge) *UK*
Injection, equine herpesvirus vaccine, inactivated, prepared from equine herpesvirus 1 and equine herpesvirus 4 grown on continuous cell lines, containing carbomer as adjuvant, for *horses and ponies more than 5 months of age*; 1-dose vial
Dose. *Horses*: *by intramuscular injection*, 1 dose. Repeat after 4–6 weeks. Thereafter a booster vaccination should be given every 6 months. (Immuno-compromised foals may receive a vaccination from 3 months of age which should be followed by the primary course.)

POM **Pneumabort-K** (Fort Dodge) *UK*
Injection, equine herpesvirus vaccine, inactivated, prepared from equine herpesvirus 1, containing a suitable oil as adjuvant, for *horses*; 2-mL syringe
Dose. *Pregnant mares*: (previously vaccinated) *by intramuscular injection*, 2 mL during the fifth, seventh, and ninth months of pregnancy; (previously unvaccinated, more than 5 months pregnant), *by intramuscular injection*, 2 mL. Repeat every 2 months until foaling
Maiden or barren mares in stable or pasture contact with pregnant mares should be vaccinated as for pregnant mares
In-contact horses: *by intramuscular injection*, 2 mL at time of contact. Repeat after 3–4 weeks. Booster vaccination given after 6 months, then every 12 months.

18.1.3 Equine influenza

Equine influenza is a respiratory disease caused by Orthomyxoviridae type A influenza viruses. The disease is characterised by a mild fever and a persistent cough. Vaccination against equine influenza is required for horses entering a property or competing under the rules of the Jockey Club or the FEI. To comply with the rules of the Jockey

Club and FEI (see Prescribing for animals used in competitions), vaccination should follow the manufacturer's guidelines and revaccination must be completed annually. (If a combination equine influenza and tetanus vaccine (see section 18.1.7) is administered, it is necessary to allow a minimum 4-week interval between first and second primary vaccines to allow the tetanus component to be effective.) Certification by a veterinarian that the horse is correctly vaccinated and pictorially identified is necessary. FEI and the Jockey Club require the certification to be stamped with the veterinary practice stamp.

The initial vaccination course consists of 2 injections given 4 to 6 weeks apart. Further doses are usually given 5 to 7 months and 12 to 18 months after the primary course. It is usually recommended that booster doses be given every 12 months but 6 monthly vaccination may be used in the presence of viral challenge (see manufacturer's recommendations). Mares may be vaccinated 8 to 4 weeks before foaling. Foals born to vaccinated mares should not be vaccinated before 4 months of age for equine influenza but earlier vaccination is recommended for tetanus.

Combined equine influenza virus and tetanus vaccines (see section 18.1.7) may be used for the initial vaccination course and every alternate annual booster vaccination.

UK

Indications. Vaccination against equine influenza
Contra-indications. Side-effects. Warnings. See notes at beginning of chapter; temporary swelling at injection site, occasional increase in body temperature on the day following vaccination
Dose. See preparation details, see notes above for vaccination programmes

POM **Duvaxyn IE Plus** (Fort Dodge) *UK*
Injection, equine influenza vaccine, inactivated, prepared from influenza A virus strains Equi/1 Prague 56, Equi/2 Miami 63, Equi/2 Suffolk 89, containing carbomer as adjuvant, for *horses and ponies more than 5 months of age*; 1-dose vial or syringe
Withdrawal Periods. *Horses*: slaughter withdrawal period nil
Dose. *Horses, ponies*: by intramuscular injection, 1 dose

POM **Equip F** (Schering-Plough) *UK*
Injection, equine influenza ISCOM vaccine, inactivated, prepared from influenza A virus strains Equi/1 Newmarket, Equi/2 Brentwood, Equi/2 Borlange 91, for *horses*; 2 mL
Dose. *Horses*: by intramuscular injection, 2 mL

POM **Prevac Pro** (Intervet) *UK*
Injection, equine influenza vaccine, inactivated, prepared from influenza A virus strains Equi/1 Prague 56, Equi/2 Newmarket 1/93 (American type strain), Equi/2 Newmarket 2/93 (European type strain), containing aluminium hydroxide as adjuvant, for *horses and ponies more than 4 months of age*; 1 mL
Withdrawal Periods. Slaughter withdrawal period nil
Dose. *Horses, ponies*: by intramuscular injection, 2 mL

18.1.4 Equine viral arteritis

Equine viral arteritis (EVA) is a contagious disease of worldwide distribution, which is particularly prevalent in non-thoroughbred horses. Most horses develop sub-clinical infection but some may exhibit clinical signs of fever, depression, and peripheral oedema. Mares may abort and

stallions frequently become long-term carriers of the virus. Transmission by the respiratory route occurs during acute infection and by the venereal route through semen from chronically infected stallions.

Artervac (Fort Dodge) is available and approved for use in horses in Britain under an Animal Test Certificate. The manufacturer should be contacted for further information.

Some countries prohibit the importation of animals seropositive to EVA without veterinary certification of vaccination. Therefore veterinarians should always take a blood sample before vaccination and ensure that animal is tested for antibody to EVA; available at the Animal Health Trust.

Under the *Equine Viral Arteritis Order 1995* (SI 1995/ 1755) and *Equine Viral Arteritis Order (Northern Ireland) 1996* (SI 1996/34), the disease is notifiable in shedding stallions and in mares that have been served 14 days before the suspected presence of the disease. The legislation indicates the procedures to follow concerning transport and use of a restricted stallion.

Prevention and control of the disease in the UK is based on the Horserace Betting Levy Board *Code of Practice on Equine Viral Arteritis (EVA)*. Horses imported from a country where EVA is known to occur or suspected should be isolated on arrival for 21 days. Blood samples taken on arrival and 14 days later should be tested for antibodies. It is also recommended that mares and stallions are tested for antibodies before mating. BEVA and the HBLB have jointly published a leaflet (*Equine Viral Arteritis*. April, 1999) explaining how breeders can help reduce the risk of EVA spreading.

18.1.5 Rabies

See section 18.4.6

18.1.6 Tetanus

Tetanus is caused by the toxin of *Clostridium tetani* and may affect all species. Horses are particularly susceptible to the neurotoxin. Although animals are affected when wounds become infected with clostridial spores, the disease is not always associated with visible lesions in horses. Clinical signs include hyperaesthesia, tetany, and tonic convulsions.

Immunity to tetanus is generated by a primary course consisting of 2 doses of toxoid given 4 to 6 weeks apart. A further dose should be given 12 months after the primary course, followed by booster doses every 1 to 2 years for horses and annually for other species. Previously immunised pregnant mares should be given a booster dose about one month before foaling. Foals from immunised mares will generally not require vaccination until 4 months of age. However, foals whose immune status is doubtful should be given tetanus antitoxin shortly after birth and again at 6 weeks of age, when a primary vaccination course may be commenced.

Animals that have not been vaccinated or whose immune status is doubtful should be given antitoxin prophylactically when exposed to risk of infection, for example, following injury. If desired, toxoid may be given simultaneously at a separate injection site using a different syringe. The antitoxin may be given at the site of injury or point of entry of the infection, if known. When used for treatment, antitoxin should initially be given intravenously. Treatment may be repeated daily as necessary.

UK

Indications. Prevention and treatment of tetanus
Contra-indications. Side-effects. Warnings. See notes at beginning of chapter
Dose. See preparation details and notes above

Antitoxins

POM **Tetanus Antitoxin Behring** (Intervet) *UK*
Injection, Cl. tetani antitoxin, derived from horses, containing 1000 units/mL, for *horses, cattle, sheep, pigs, dogs*; 50 mL
Dose. Treatment. *Horses, cattle*: *by epidural or intravenous injection*, 30 000 units, with concurrent administration of 15 000 units given *by subcutaneous or intramuscular injection*. Repeat daily as necessary
Prophylaxis. *By subcutaneous or intramuscular injection.Horses, cattle*: 7500 units; *foals, calves*: 3000 units
Sheep: 3000 units
Pigs: 1500–3000 units
Dogs: 500–1000 units

Vaccines

POM **Duvaxyn T** (Fort Dodge) *UK*
Injection, tetanus vaccine, inactivated, *Cl. tetani* toxoid, containing aluminium phosphate as adjuvant, for *horses and ponies more than 3 months of age*; 1 mL
Dose. *Horses, ponies: by intramuscular injection*, 1 mL

POM **Equip T** (Schering-Plough) *UK*
Injection, tetanus vaccine, inactivated, *Cl. tetani* toxoid, containing aluminium phosphate as adjuvant, for *horses*; 2-mL syringe
Dose. *Horses: by intramuscular injection*, 2 mL

POM **Tetanus Toxoid Concentrated** (Intervet) *UK*
Injection, tetanus vaccine, inactivated, *Cl. tetani* toxoid, containing aluminium hydroxide as adjuvant, for *horses, other mammalian species*; 1 mL
Dose. *Horses, other mammalian species: by subcutaneous or intramuscular injection*, 1 mL

18.1.7 Combination vaccines for horses

UK

POM **Duvaxyn IE-T Plus** (Fort Dodge) *UK*
Injection, combined equine influenza and tetanus vaccine, inactivated, prepared from influenza A virus strains Equi/1 Prague 56, Equi/2 Miami 63, Equi/2 Suffolk 89, *Cl. tetani* toxoid, containing aluminium hydroxide and carbomer as adjuvants, for *horses and ponies more than 5 months of age*
Withdrawal Periods. Slaughter withdrawal period nil
Dose. *Horses: by intramuscular injection*, 1 dose

POM **Equip FT** (Schering-Plough) *UK*
Injection, combined equine influenza ISCOM and tetanus vaccine, inactivated, prepared from influenza A virus strains Equi/1 Newmarket, Equi/2 Brentwood, Equi/2 Borlange 91, *Cl. tetani* toxoid, containing aluminium phosphate as adjuvant, for *horses*; 2-mL syringe
Dose. *Horses: by intramuscular injection*, 2 mL

POM **Prevac T Pro** (Intervet) *UK*
Injection, combined equine influenza and tetanus vaccine, inactivated, prepared from influenza A virus strains Equi/1 Prague 56, Equi/2 Newmarket 1/93 (American type strain), Equi/2 Newmarket 2/93 (European type strain), *Cl. tetani* toxoid, containing aluminium hydroxide as adjuvant, for *horses and ponies more than 4 months of age*; 2 mL
Withdrawal Periods. Slaughter withdrawal period nil
Dose. *Horses, ponies: by intramuscular injection*, 2 mL

18.1.8 Immunoglobulins for horses

Immunoglobulins (or antibodies) combine with specific antigens. Endotoxin-specific immunoglobulins act by neutralising endotoxin produced by a wide variety of Gram-negative bacteria including *Salmonella* spp., *E. coli* serotypes, *Serratia marcescens, Shigella flexneri, Klebsiella pneumoniae*, and *Pseudomonas aeruginosa*. These bacteria may be a component of a number of diseases such as gastroenteritis, septic metritis, septicaemia, or shock. Other appropriate treatment such as antibacterials, NSAIDs, and fluid therapy should also be instigated.

Antitoxins for tetanus are available (see section 18.1.6).

UK

Indications. Treatment and prophylaxis of endotoxaemia
Contra-indications. Side-effects. Warnings. Safety   in pregnant animals has not been established
Dose. See preparation details

POM **Stegantox 60** (Schering-Plough) *UK*
Injection, powder for reconstitution, 3 mg endotoxin-specific immunoglobulin G/mL, for *horses*; 20 mL
Dose. *Horses: by slow intravenous injection*, 300 micrograms/kg. May be repeated twice at 24-hour intervals

18.2 Immunological preparations for cattle, sheep, and goats

The immunisation programme used for ruminants depends on the management system, location, and the history of the herd or flock.

Cattle are often vaccinated against blackleg and tetanus but, in some herds, immunisation against other conditions, such as 'husk' (lungworm disease), rotavirus, and infectious bovine rhinotracheitis (IBR) is also necessary.

Sheep flocks are generally vaccinated to prevent clostridial diseases and pasteurellosis but vaccination against other diseases, such as ovine abortion and louping ill, is sometimes necessary depending on the flock and its history. Collapse and death have been reported following vaccination of pregnant ewes; it is important that any stress is avoided. Vaccination in goats is similar to that employed for sheep.

In cattle, the site for vaccination by subcutaneous injection is usually the neck, while for intramuscular injection, the gluteal muscle, neck, or shoulder region is recommended. For sheep and goats, the anterior third of the neck is usually recommended. Aseptic precautions should be observed especially with preparations in multidose containers.

18.2.1 Anthrax

Anthrax is caused by *Bacillus anthracis* and characterised by sudden death. Anthrax is a zoonotic infection. No commercial vaccine is available for routine vaccination of horses, ruminants, and pigs in the UK. MAFF should be contacted for information regarding emergency supplies of vaccine.

18.2.2 Bovine pneumonia

Enzootic pneumonia in calves is usually caused primarily by viruses, with secondary bacterial invasion, exacerbated by inadequate housing and ventilation. Causative viruses include adenovirus, herpesvirus, parainfluenza virus 3 (PI3), respiratory syncytial virus (RSV), reovirus, and rhinovirus. Vaccination with live virus vaccines is generally a very effective means of preventing disease caused by the specific virus.

18.2.2.1 Bovine parainfluenza virus
18.2.2.2 Bovine herpesvirus
18.2.2.3 Respiratory syncytial virus
18.2.2.4 Pasteurellosis
18.2.2.5 Combination vaccines for bovine pneumonia

18.2.2.1 Bovine parainfluenza virus

Depending on the age of the calf and therefore the concentration of maternally-derived antibody, the vaccine is administered intranasally either as a single dose at 12 weeks of age or more, or as a vaccination course with one dose being given at 3 to 4 weeks of age followed by a second dose at 10 to 12 weeks of age.

UK

Indications. Vaccination against bovine parainfluenza virus

Contra-indications. Side-effects. Warnings. See notes at beginning of chapter

Dose. See preparation details, see notes above for vaccination programmes

POM **Imuresp** (Pfizer) *UK*
Intranasal solution, powder for reconstitution, PI3 vaccine, living, prepared from virus strain RLB 103ts, temperature-specific, for *calves, growing cattle*; 5-dose vial
Dose. *Calves, growing cattle: by intranasal application*, 2 mL into one nostril

18.2.2.2 Bovine herpesvirus

Bovine herpesvirus 1 is the causative agent of infectious bovine rhinotracheitis (IBR) characterised by an upper respiratory-tract infection, which may lead to pneumonia. The virus may also cause other syndromes such as infectious pustular vulvovaginitis. Vaccination provides immunity against both the respiratory and genital forms of the disease. Calves over 3 to 4 weeks of age may be vaccinated but if under 3 months of age, revaccination at 10 to 12 weeks is recommended. Annual revaccination is advised.

Vaccination will not prevent the disease in cattle that are already infected but it may reduce disease in a developing outbreak. Intranasal vaccination will provide protection within 40 to 72 hours coinciding with the presence of interferon in nasal secretions. Antibodies are detectable in serum by day 7 to 10 post-vaccination whether the vaccine is given by the intranasal or intramuscular route. Maternally-derived antibody does not prevent development of active immunity following intranasal vaccination in calves. Cattle that have been vaccinated become seropositive and thus may be unacceptable for export. Following vaccination, some cattle develop pyrexia and clinical signs of respiratory disease, which may last for 3 to 5 days.

UK

Indications. Vaccination against infectious bovine rhinotracheitis

Contra-indications. Side-effects. Warnings. See notes at beginning of chapter and notes above

Dose. See preparation details, see notes above for vaccination programmes

POM **Bovilis IBR** (Intervet) *UK*
Injection or intranasal solution, powder for reconstitution, IBR vaccine, living, prepared from virus, grown on cell-line tissue culture, for *cattle more than 4 weeks of age*; 5-dose vial, 25-dose vial
Note. Reconstitute with Unisolve
Withdrawal Periods. Slaughter withdrawal period nil, milk withdrawal period nil
Dose. *Cattle: by intramuscular injection*, 2 mL; *by intranasal application (preferred)*, 1 mL into each nostril

POM **Tracherine** (Pfizer) *UK*
Intranasal solution, powder for reconstitution, IBR vaccine, living, prepared from virus strain RLB 106 ts, temperature-sensitive, for *cattle*; 5-dose vial
Dose. *Cattle: by intranasal application*, 2 mL into one nostril

18.2.2.3 Respiratory syncytial virus

Live and inactivated vaccines are available for the immunisation of calves against disease caused by the respiratory syncytial virus (RSV). The live vaccine may be used simultaneously with bovine parainfluenza virus vaccine and infectious bovine rhinotracheitis vaccine.

For protection with either vaccine, calves are vaccinated 2 or 3 times with an interval of 3 weeks between doses. When using the live vaccine, calves under 4 months of age should be vaccinated similarly with an additional vaccination at 4 months of age.

UK

Indications. Vaccination against respiratory syncytial virus

Contra-indications. Side-effects. Warnings. See notes at beginning of chapter

Dose. See preparation details, see notes above for vaccination programmes

Live vaccines

POM **Rispoval RS** (Pfizer) *UK*
Injection, powder for reconstitution, RSV vaccine, living, prepared from bovine virus, for *calves more than 1 week of age*; 5-dose vial
Dose. *Calves*: *by intramuscular injection*, 2 mL

Inactivated vaccines

POM **Torvac** (Vericore VP) *UK*
Injection, RSV vaccine, inactivated, prepared from bovine virus, containing Quil-A as adjuvant, for *calves*; 20 mL
Withdrawal Periods. Slaughter withdrawal period nil, milk withdrawal period nil
Dose. *Calves*: *by subcutaneous injection*, 2 mL

18.2.2.4 Pasteurellosis

Vaccination is available to reduce the clinical signs and lesions resulting from respiratory disease caused by *Mannheimia haemolytica* (*Pasteurella haemolytica*) infection. Cattle are vaccinated at a minimum age of 4 weeks and again 21 to 28 days later. Thereafter annual booster vaccinations may be given at intervals of not more than 12 months.

UK

Indications. Vaccination against pasteurellosis
Contra-indications. Side-effects. Warnings. See notes at beginning of chapter and notes above; transient oedema or granulomas at vaccination site in cattle; transient increased body temperature
Dose. See preparation details, see notes above for vaccination programmes

POM **Pastobov** (Merial) *UK*
Injection, pasteurellosis vaccine, inactivated, prepared from *P. haemolytica* type A1 antigens, for *cattle more than 4 weeks of age*
Withdrawal Periods. *Cattle*: nil withdrawal periods
Dose. *Cattle*: by subcutaneous or intramuscular injection, 2 mL, repeat after 3-4 weeks. Revaccinate before each risk period and no later than one year after the first vaccination

POM **Tecvax Pasteurella 1/6** (Vétoquinol)
Injection, pasteurellosis vaccine, inactivated, prepared from *P. haemolytica* biotype A serotypes 1 and 6, containing Quil A as adjuvant, for *cattle more than 4 weeks of age*
Withdrawal Periods. *Cattle*: nil withdrawal periods
Dose. *Cattle*: by intramuscular injection, 2 mL, repeat after 3 weeks. Revaccinate at least 2 weeks before each risk period

18.2.2.5 Combination vaccines for bovine pneumonia

UK

Indications. See individual vaccines
Contra-indications. Side-effects. Warnings. See notes at beginning of chapter
Dose. See preparation details

POM **Bovilis IBR + PI3** (Intervet) *UK*
Intranasal solution, powder for reconstitution, combined IBR and PI3 vaccine, living, prepared from IBR virus strain INT 1, PI3 virus strain INT 2 grown in cell tissue culture, for *cattle more than 1 week of age*; 5-dose vial, 25-dose vial
Note. Reconstitute with Unisolve
Withdrawal Periods. Slaughter withdrawal period nil, milk withdrawal period nil
Dose. *Cattle*: *by intranasal application*, 1 mL into each nostril at any age more than 1 week, repeat at 12 weeks of age. Animals more than 12 weeks of age require 1 vaccination. Annual revaccination is recommended

POM **Bovipast RSP** (Intervet) *UK*
Injection, combined RSV, PI3, and pasteurellosis vaccine, inactivated, prepared from RSV virus strain EV 908, PI3 virus strain SF-4, *Pasteuralla haemolytica* serotype A1, containing aluminium hydroxide and Quil A as adjuvantsfor *cattle*
Withdrawal Periods. Slaughter withdrawal period nil, milk withdrawal period nil
Dose. *Cattle*: *by subcutaneous injection*, 5 mL at 2 weeks of age or more. Repeat after 4 weeks. Booster revaccination should be given 2 weeks before each risk period

POM **Imuresp RP** (Pfizer) *UK*
Intranasal solution, powder for reconstitution, combined IBR and PI3 vaccine, living, prepared from IBR virus strain RLB 106 ts, PI3 virus strain RLB 103 ts, temperature-specific, for *calves, growing cattle*; 5-dose vial
Dose. *Calves, growing cattle*: *by intranasal application*, 2 mL into one nostril at 3 weeks of age, repeat at 10 weeks of age. Animals more than 12 weeks of age require 1 vaccination. Annual revaccination is recommended

18.2.3 Clostridial infections

Sheep are routinely vaccinated against clostridial infections; vaccination is also recommended for cattle, goats, and pigs.

The exotoxins produced by clostridial species exhibit a variety of pathogenic effects. *Cl. chauvoei* (*Cl. feseri*) causes blackleg disease and post-parturient gangrene in sheep. *Cl. haemolyticum* (*Cl. novyi* type D) is the causative agent of bacillary haemoglobinuria and *Cl. novyi* (*Cl. oedematiens*) causes black disease. The various serotypes of *Cl. perfringens* (*Cl. welchii*) cause different diseases; type B causes lamb dysentery, type C causes struck, and type D causes pulpy kidney disease. *Cl. chauvoei* or *Cl. septicum*, either alone or in combination, cause clostridial metritis. Exotoxins of *Cl. septicum* are responsible for braxy and *Cl. tetani* exotoxins cause tetanus (see section 18.1.6).

Single and multicomponent vaccines are available. Several clostridial infections may commonly occur in a particular geographical area. Therefore, it is usual practice to vaccinate routinely with combination vaccines capable of producing immunity to 4 to 8 clostridial infections. The vaccination programmes may vary with manufacturer's recommendations and provided these are followed vaccination against clostridial disease gives very effective protection.

Antitoxins are available for passive immunisation of sheep and lambs and for use in cattle, goats, and piglets where these species are at risk. The preparations may be expected to confer passive immunity for 3 to 4 weeks.

The available *Cl. perfringens* antitoxins contain either individual antitoxins or a combination of antitoxins. They are able to neutralise either the beta toxin or the beta and epsilon toxins produced by *Cl. perfringens* type B, the beta toxin produced by type C, or the epsilon toxin produced by type D.

Vaccination programmes for multicomponent **vaccines** may vary with the degree of risk in an area. Generally, **sheep** are given 2 doses with an interval of 4 to 6 weeks between doses and this primary course is completed 3 to 4 weeks before a period of risk such as lambing. For subsequent pregnancies, ewes are usually given a single injection 2 to 4 weeks before lambing. Lambs born to vaccinated ewes are protected by maternally-derived antibodies for up to 12 to 16 weeks of age, when they should receive 2 doses of vaccine with an interval of 4 to 6 weeks between doses. Lambs, if born to unvaccinated ewes, should generally be vaccinated in the first 2 weeks of life, and again 4 to 6 weeks later. A booster dose each autumn is recommended but in areas of higher risk, a booster dose every 6 months may be appropriate.

For **cattle** and **goats**, 2 doses are given at an interval of 3 to 6 weeks and administered 2 to 4 weeks before a period of risk. Annual booster doses are recommended. For **pigs**, initially 2 doses are administered at an interval of at least 3 weeks. Thereafter sows are vaccinated once at approximately 6 to 3 weeks before each farrowing.

UK

Indications. Prevention and treatment of clostridial infections

Contra-indications. Side-effects. Warnings. See notes at beginning of chapter

Dose. See preparation details, see notes above for vaccination programmes

See Table 18.1 for an alphabetical listing of the available antitoxins and vaccines, and the diseases against which they induce immunity.

Antitoxins

PML **Lambisan** (Intervet) *UK*
Injection, combined lamb dysentery, pulpy kidney, and struck antiserum, derived from horses, *Cl. perfringens* type B and D antitoxins, beta antitoxin not less than 1200 units, epsilon antitoxin not less than 120 units/mL, for *calves, sheep, piglets*; 100 mL
Dose. *By subcutaneous or intramuscular injection.*
Calves: 25 mL
Sheep: 12.5 mL; *lambs*: 5 mL
Piglets: 5 mL

Vaccines

PML **Blackleg Vaccine** (Intervet) *UK*
Injection, inactivated, *Cl. chauvoei* cells and toxoid, containing aluminium hydroxide as adjuvant, for *cattle, sheep*; 50 mL
Dose. *Cattle, sheep*: *by subcutaneous or intramuscular injection*, 2 mL

PML **Blackleg Vaccine** (Schering-Plough) *UK*
Injection, inactivated, *Cl. chauvoei* cells and toxoid, containing alum as adjuvant, for *cattle, sheep*; 50 mL
Dose. *Cattle*: *by subcutaneous injection*,.2 mL
Sheep: *by subcutaneous injection*,.1 mL

PML **Covexin 8** (Schering-Plough) *UK*
Injection, combined bacillary haemoglobinuria, black disease, blackleg, braxy, lamb dysentery, pulpy kidney, struck, and tetanus vaccine, inactivated, *Cl. chauvoei* toxoid, *Cl. haemolyticum* toxoid, *Cl. novyi* toxoid, *Cl.*

perfringens type B, C, and D toxoids, *Cl. septicum* toxoid, *Cl. tetani* toxoid, containing alum as adjuvant, for *cattle, sheep*; 100 mL, 250 mL, 500 mL
Dose. *Cattle*: *by subcutaneous injection*,.5 mL
Sheep: *by subcutaneous injection*,.(2–8 weeks of age) 2 mL; (>8 weeks of age) initial dose 5 mL then 2 mL

PML **Heptavac** (Intervet) *UK*
Injection, combined black disease, blackleg, braxy, clostrial metritis, lamb dysentery, pulpy kidney, struck, and tetanus vaccine, inactivated, *Cl. chauvoei* cells and toxoid, *Cl. novyi* type B toxoid, *Cl. perfringens* type B, C, and D toxoids, *Cl. septicum* toxoid, *Cl. tetani* toxoid, containing aluminium hydroxide as adjuvant, for *sheep, pigs*; 50 mL, 100 mL, other sizes available
Dose. *Sheep*: *by subcutaneous injection*,.2 mL
Pigs: *by subcutaneous injection*,.5 mL

PML **Heptavac-P Plus** (Intervet) *UK*
Injection, combined black disease, blackleg, braxy, clostrial metritis, lamb dysentery, pasteurellosis, pulpy kidney, struck, and tetanus vaccine, inactivated, *Cl. chauvoei* cells and toxoid, *Cl. novyi* type B toxoid, *Cl. perfringens* type B, C, and D toxoids, *Cl. septicum* toxoid, *Cl. tetani* toxoid, antigens of *P. haemolytica* serotypes A, T, containing aluminium hydroxide as adjuvant, for *sheep*; 50 mL, 100 mL, other sizes available
Dose. *Sheep*: *by subcutaneous injection*, 2 mL

PML **Lambivac** (Intervet) *UK*
Injection, combined lamb dysentery, pulpy kidney, struck, and tetanus vaccine, inactivated, *Cl. perfringens* type B, C, and D toxoids, *Cl. tetani* toxoid, containing aluminium hydroxide as adjuvant, for *cattle, sheep, goats, pigs*; 50 mL, 100 mL
Dose. *Cattle, sheep, goats*: *by subcutaneous injection*, 2 mL
Pigs: *by subcutaneous injection*, 5 mL

PML **Ovivac** (Intervet) *UK*
Injection, combined blackleg, braxy, pulpy kidney, and tetanus vaccine, inactivated, *Cl. chauvoei* cells and toxoid, *Cl. perfringens* type D toxoid, *Cl. septicum* toxoid, *Cl. tetani* toxoid, containing aluminium hydroxide as adjuvant, for *sheep*; 50 mL, 100 mL
Dose. *Sheep*: *by subcutaneous injection*, 2 mL

PML **Ovivac-P Plus** (Intervet) *UK*
Injection, combined blackleg, braxy, pasteurellosis, pulpy kidney, and tetanus vaccine, inactivated, *Cl. chauvoei* cells and toxoid, *Cl. perfringens* type D toxoid, *Cl. septicum* toxoid, *Cl. tetani* toxoid, antigens of *P. haemolytica* serotypes A, T, containing aluminium hydroxide as adjuvant, for *sheep*; 100 mL, 500 mL
Dose. *Sheep*: *by subcutaneous injection*, 2 mL

PML **Tribovax -T Combined Cattle Vaccine** (Schering-Plough) *UK*
Injection, combined bacillary haemoglobinuria, black disease, blackleg, braxy, and tetanus vaccine, inactivated, *Cl. chauvoei* toxoid, *Cl. haemolyticum* toxoid, *Cl. novyi* toxoid, *Cl. septicum* toxoid, *Cl. tetani* toxoid, containing alum as adjuvant, for *cattle*; 100 mL
Dose. *Cattle*: *by subcutaneous injection*, 4 mL

18.2.4 Contagious pustular dermatitis

Contagious pustular dermatitis, commonly known as orf or scabby mouth, is caused by a parapoxvirus and characterised by scabby, pustular lesions mainly on the muzzle and lips of sheep and goats.

Sheep and lambs should be vaccinated 3 to 4 weeks before the expected period of disease risk. Lambs can be vaccinated from 1 to 2 days of age. Duration of immunity is about 6 months therefore revaccination should be given every 5 to 12 months depending on the degree of challenge in the area. The vaccine should not be used on farms or in flocks where orf is not a problem, nor used to vaccinate ewes less than 6 to 8 weeks before lambing.

The vaccines are administered by scarification of the skin. Vaccinated sheep develop mild lesions of orf at the site of vaccination, which is usually the inside of the thigh or

Table 18.1 Immunological preparations for clostridial infections available in the UK

	Bacillary haemo- globinuria	Black disease	Black -leg	Braxy	Lamb dysen -tery	Pulpy kidney	Struck	Tetanus	Other infections
Antitoxins									
Lambisan (Intervet)					●	●	●		
Tetanus Antitoxin Behring (Intervet)								●	
Vaccines									
Blackleg Vaccine (Intervet)			●						
Blackleg Vaccine (Schering-Plough)			●						
Covexin 8 (Schering-Plough)	●	●	●	●	●	●	●	●	
Duvaxyn T (Fort Dodge)								●	
Equip T (Schering-Plough)								●	
Heptavac (Intervet)		●	●	●	●	●	●	●	clostridial metritis
Heptavac-P Plus (Intervet)		●	●	●	●	●	●	●	clostridial metritis, pasteurellosis
Lambivac (Intervet)					●		●	●	
Ovivac (Intervet)		●	●			●		●	
Ovivac-P Plus (Intervet)		●	●			●		●	pasteurellosis
Tetanus Toxoid Concentrated (Intervet)								●	
Tribovax-T (Schering-Plough)	●	●	●	●				●	

axilla. Sheep will shed highly infective live field virus and virus-infected scabs for 3 to 8 weeks after vaccination. Therefore during this period vaccinated animals should not come in contact with unvaccinated sheep and should not be allowed access to the lambing pens or pasture where ewes and their lambs will subsequently be grazed.

Contagious pustular dermatitis is a zoonotic disease. Therefore care should be taken when handling infected sheep or the vaccine.

UK

Indications. Vaccination against contagious pustular dermatitis

Contra-indications. Use on farms where the disease is not endemic. Vaccination of ewes less than 6–8 weeks before lambing or during lactation; see also notes at beginning of chapter

Side-effects. Warnings. See notes above and at beginning of chapter

Dose. See preparation details, see notes above for vaccination programmes

POM **Scabivax** (Schering-Plough) *UK*
Liquid for scarification, contagious pustular dermatitis vaccine, living, prepared from scab material from sheep infected with a selected strain of virus, for *sheep*; 50-dose vial
Dose. *Sheep: by scarification*, 1 application

POM **Vaxall Orf** (Fort Dodge) *UK*
Liquid for scarification, powder for reconstitution, contagious pustular dermatitis vaccine, living, prepared from virus strain 1880, for *sheep*; 50-dose vial
Withdrawal Periods. *Sheep*: slaughter 28 days
Dose. *Sheep: by scarification*, 1 application

18.2.5 Enteritis

Enteritis in ruminants may be caused by many organisms including bacteria, viruses, and parasites. Antisera and vaccines are available for the prevention and treatment of enteritis caused by *Escherichia coli*, *Salmonella*, *Pasteurella*, coronavirus, rotavirus, and by clostridial organisms (see section 18.2.3). Vaccines may contain either serotypes of a single bacterium or a combination of bacterial serotypes.

18.2.5.1 Escherichia coli infections
18.2.5.2 Bovine viral diarrhoea
18.2.5.3 Salmonella infection
18.2.5.4 Combination immunological preparations for enteritis in cattle and sheep

18.2.5.1 Escherichia coli infections

Two doses of vaccine are given at an interval of at least 2 weeks. The second dose should be given 4 weeks before lambing. Annual revaccination 4 weeks before lambing is recommended.

UK

Indications. Vaccination against *E. coli*
Contra-indications. Side-effects. Warnings. See notes at beginning of chapter

Dose. See preparation details, see notes above for vaccination programmes

PML **Coliovac** (Intervet) *UK*
Injection, E. coli vaccine, inactivated, prepared from *E. coli* O antigens 8, 9, 11, 15, 20, 26, 35, 78, 86, 101, 115, 137; K antigens 30, 32, 35, B41, 60, 61, V79, 80, 85, 99, V165 antigens, soluble F41 and K99 antigens, containing aluminium hydroxide as adjuvant, for *sheep*; 100 mL, 250 mL
Dose. *Sheep: by subcutaneous injection*, 2 mL

18.2.5.2 Bovine viral diarrhoea

Calves born to cows, that have become infected with bovine virus diarrhoea virus (BVDV) when pregnant, may have congenital defects or tolerance to the virus. Immunotolerant calves are persistently infected, continually excrete the virus, and are therefore a source of infection, particularly to pregnant cows.

Breeding cows are vaccinated 28 days before insemination and the dose is repeated after 3 to 4 weeks. The vaccination course of 2 doses should be repeated at each subsequent breeding.

UK

Indications. Vaccination against bovine viral diarrhoea
Contra-indications. See notes at beginning of chapter
Side-effects. Transient pyrexia, transient reaction at injection site for 2–3 weeks
Warnings. See notes at beginning of chapter
Dose. See preparation details, see notes above for vaccination programmes

POM **Bovidec** (Vericore VP) *UK*
Injection, bovine viral diarrhoea virus, inactivated, prepared from non-cytopathogenic strain of virus, containing Quil-A as adjuvant, for *female breeding cattle*; 20 mL
Withdrawal Periods. *Cattle*: slaughter withdrawal period nil, milk withdrawal period nil
Dose. *Cattle: by subcutaneous injection*, 4 mL

POM Bovilis BVD (Intervet)
Injection, bovine viral diarrhoea virus, inactivated, prepared from cytopathogenic BVD virus strain C86, containing aluminium salts as adjuvant, for *cows and heifers from 8 months of age*; 20 mL
Withdrawal Periods. *Cattle*: slaughter withdrawal period nil, milk withdrawal period nil
Dose. *Cattle: by subcutaneous injection*, 4 mL

18.2.5.3 Salmonella infection

Salmonella vaccine may be used in the face of a disease outbreak and may contribute to reduction of *Salmonella* contamination of the environment. Where diagnosis has been confirmed, all at risk adult cattle that are not showing overt clinical signs of salmonellosis are vaccinated and the vaccination repeated after 21 days. Pregnant cows may be vaccinated; if not calved within 8 weeks of the second dose of vaccine, a third dose should be administered at 3 to 4 weeks before calving. Healthy calves may be vaccinated from 3 weeks of age; two vaccinations are given at an interval of 14 to 21 days.

All cattle should receive a booster vaccination at least 2 weeks prior to a period of risk or at intervals of not more than 12 months. Pregnant cattle should be vaccinated 3 to 4 weeks before calving.

All stock showing overt clinical signs of salmonellosis should receive appropriate treatment and be fully vaccinated once they have recovered. Any unvaccinated stock must be managed separately to vaccinated stock, with no contact between the groups. Hygiene precautions must be instituted, where possible, to prevent transfer of infection from one group to another.

UK

Indications. Vaccination against salmonella infection
Contra-indications. See notes at beginning of chapter
Warnings. See notes at beginning of chapter
Dose. See preparation details, see notes above for vaccination programmes

POM **Bovivac S** (Intervet) *UK*
Injection, *Salmonella* vaccine, inactivated, prepared from *S. dublin* and *S. typhimurium*, containing aluminium hydroxide as adjuvant, for *cattle*
Dose. *By subcutaneous injection.*
Adult cattle: 5 mL; *calves*: 2 mL

18.2.5.4 Combination immunological preparations for enteritis in cattle and sheep

Antisera are used prophylactically and therapeutically especially in young ruminants for enteric infections caused by certain serotypes of *E. coli* and *Salmonella* spp. Repeated daily administration of antiserum may be necessary for treatment. Antisera are given soon after birth or before periods of challenge and may be administered at intervals of 10 to 14 days during periods of risk.

Vaccines contain important antigens of *E. coli*, such as K99 or selected, inactivated serotypes. Vaccines also contain *Salmonella* spp., *P. multocida* serotypes, coronavirus, or rotavirus. Initial vaccination of cattle and sheep may involve a course of 2 vaccine doses given at an interval of 14 to 21 days. Previously unvaccinated cows and ewes should be vaccinated, with the second dose administered about 3 weeks before calving or the lambing season so that the colostrum will contain protective antibodies. Thereafter, pregnant animals may be given an annual booster approximately 3 weeks before the expected date of parturition or earlier for rotavirus infection.

UK

Indications. Prevention and treatment of enteritis
Contra-indications. **Side-effects**. **Warnings**. See notes at beginning of chapter
Dose. See preparation details, see notes above for vaccination programmes

Antisera

PML **Bovisan DPS** (Intervet) *UK*
Injection, combined *E. coli*, *Pasteurella*, and *Salmonella* antiserum, derived from horses, prepared from *E. coli* serotypes, *P. multocida* Roberts types 1, 2, 3, 4, *S. dublin*, *S. typhimurium*, for *calves, sheep*; 100 mL
Dose. *By subcutaneous or intramuscular injection.*
Treatment. Repeat after 24 hours if required
Calves: 40 mL

Sheep: 10 mL
Prophylaxis. Repeat at intervals of 10–14 days during the period of risk
Calves: 20 mL
Sheep: 5 mL

PML **Ecosan** (Intervet) *UK*
Injection, combined *E. coli* and *Salmonella* antiserum, derived from cattle, prepared from *E. coli* serotypes, *S. dublin*, *S. typhimurium*, for *calves, sheep*; 100 mL
Dose. *By subcutaneous, intramuscular, or intravenous injection.*
Treatment. Repeat after 24 hours if required
Calves: 20 mL
Sheep: 10 mL
Prophylaxis. May be repeated at intervals of 10–14
Calves: 10 mL
Sheep: 5 mL

Antisera-vaccine combinations

PML **Grovax** (Intervet) *UK*
Injection, combined *E. coli*, *Pasteurella*, and *Salmonella* antiserum/vaccine, prepared from selected *E. coli* serotypes, *P. multocida* Roberts types 1, 2, 3, 4, *S. dublin* strains, *S. typhimurium* strains, in combination with antisera derived from cattle to the same organisms, for *cattle*; 100 mL
Dose. *By subcutaneous injection.*
Treatment.
Calves: 40 mL, repeat if required
Prophylaxis.
Cattle: 40 mL, repeat dose at least 2 weeks before calving in pregnant animals; *calves*: 20–30 mL

Vaccines

POM **Lactovac** (Intervet) *UK*
Injection, combined coronavirus, bovine rotavirus and *E. coli* vaccine, inactivated, prepared from coronavirus strain 800, rotavirus strains 1005/78 and Holland, *E. coli* K99 and F41 antigens, containing aluminium hydroxide and Quil A as adjuvants, for *cattle*; 5 mL, 20 mL
Withdrawal Periods. Nil withdrawal periods
Dose. *Cattle: by intramuscular injection,* 5 mL given during the later stages of pregnancy, repeat after 4–5 weeks, the second dose being given 2–3 weeks before calving. Annual vaccination 2–6 weeks before calving

POM **Rotavec Corona** (Schering-Plough) *UK*
Injection, combined bovine rotavirus, coronavirus, and *E. coli* vaccine, inactivated, prepared from virus antigens, *E. coli* K99 antigens, containing aluminium hydroxide and a light mineral oil as adjuvants, for *cattle*
Dose. *Cattle: by intramuscular injection,* 2 mL as a single dose between 12 and 3 weeks before calving

POM **Rotavec K99** (Schering-Plough) *UK*
Injection, combined bovine rotavirus and *E. coli* vaccine, inactivated, prepared from virus antigens, *E. coli* K99 antigens, containing aluminium hydroxide and a light mineral oil as adjuvants, for *cattle*; 5 mL, 20 mL
Dose. *Cattle: by intramuscular injection,* 1 mL as a single dose between 12 and 4 weeks before calving

---

18.2.6 Erysipelas

Infection with *Erysipelothrix rhusiopathiae* (*Ery. insidiosa*) occurs in lambs and in older sheep as a joint infection and bacteraemia and arises, for example, after dipping in contaminated baths. Sheep may be vaccinated to increase their immunity. Two doses are given at an interval of 2 to 6 weeks, with the second dose administered 2 weeks before the expected period of risk. In pregnant ewes, the second dose is given 3 weeks before lambing.

See section 18.3.6 for erysipelas in pigs and section 18.6.11 for erysipelas in turkeys.

UK
Indications. Vaccination against erysipelas
Contra-indications. **Side-effects**. **Warnings**. See notes at beginning of chapter
Dose. See preparation details, see notes above for vaccination programmes

PML **Erysorb ST** (Intervet) *UK*
Injection, erysipelas vaccine, inactivated, prepared from *Ery. rhusiopathiae*, containing aluminium hydroxide as adjuvant, for *sheep, turkeys* (see section 18.6.11); 100 mL
Dose. *Sheep: by subcutaneous injection*, 2 mL

18.2.7 Footrot

Vaccination against footrot in sheep should be part of an overall foot care programme (see Chapter 15). Vaccines may be used to aid prevention or treatment of footrot. Sheep do not mount an immune response to footrot; the vaccine elicits a high level of circulating antibody that lasts for about 4 months before waning. For prophylactic use, the timing of vaccination is important and should be carried out before the expected period of disease risk.

Available vaccines are prepared from *Dichelobacter nodosus (Bacteroides nodosus, Fusiformis nodosus)*. Two doses may be given at an interval of 4 to 8 weeks. Lambs may be vaccinated at 4 weeks of age. Pregnant ewes should not be vaccinated 4 weeks before or after lambing. Booster doses can be given at 4 to 6 monthly intervals if required.

A persistent reaction, lasting for several weeks, may occur at the site of injection and may produce local pigment changes in the wool. Therefore vaccination should be avoided within 6 to 8 weeks of shearing or 6 months before sale or showing. In pedigree flocks, vaccination of the resident flock will reduce the incidence of disease and show and sale animals can be treated by conventional methods.

UK
Indications. Vaccination against footrot
Contra-indications. Vaccination of lambs under 2 to 4 weeks of age, pregnant ewes within 4 weeks of lambing
Side-effects. **Warnings**. See notes above, see notes at beginning of chapter
Dose. See preparation details, see notes above for vaccination programmes

PML **Footvax** (Schering-Plough) *UK*
Injection, footrot vaccine, inactivated, prepared from 10 strains of *Dichelobacter nodosus*, containing a suitable oil as adjuvant, for *sheep*; 50 mL
Contra-indications. Lactating dairy sheep
Dose. *Sheep: by subcutaneous injection*, 1 mL

PML **Vaxall Norot** (Fort Dodge) *UK*
Injection, footrot vaccine, inactivated, prepared from 9 serotypes of *Dichelobacter nodosus*, containing a suitable adjuvant, for *sheep*; 50 mL
Dose. *Sheep: by subcutaneous injection*, 1 mL

18.2.8 Leptospirosis

Leptospirosis in cattle can be caused by *Leptospira interrogans* serovar *hardjo* and *Leptospira borgpetersenii* serovar *hardjo*. The latter appears to be the predominant strain in cattle. Infertility, abortion, and agalactia can result from

infection. Infected cattle excrete leptospirae in urine which spread to other cattle through the mouth, eye, and nose. Vaccination of the entire herd may be necessary to control the disease.

Leptospirosis is a zoonotic disease generally acquired from cattle urine or placentas. Vaccination does not decrease the need for precautions to reduce the risk of transmission of leptospirosis from animals to humans.

A primary vaccination course of 2 doses is given at an interval of 4 to 6 weeks administered after 5 months of age. If calves are vaccinated before 5 months of age, a further course should be given starting at that age. The course should be completed before the main season of transmission. A single annual booster injection is recommended at turnout to spring pasture.

Vaccinated cattle may be seropositive and therefore may be unacceptable for export to some countries.

UK
Indications. Vaccination against leptospirosis
Contra-indications. **Side-effects**. **Warnings**. See notes at beginning of chapter and notes above
Dose. See preparation details, see notes above for vaccination programmes

POM **Leptavoid -H** (Schering-Plough) *UK*
Injection, leptospirosis vaccine, inactivated, prepared from *L. interrogans* serovar *hardjo*, containing alum as adjuvant, for *cattle*; 20 mL, 50 mL
Withdrawal Periods. Slaughter withdrawal period nil
Dose. *Cattle: by subcutaneous injection*, 2 mL

POM **Spirovac** (Pfizer) *UK*
Injection, leptospirosis vaccine, inactivated, prepared from *L. interrogans* serovar *hardjo*, containing aluminium hydroxide as adjuvant, for *cattle*; 50 mL, 100 mL
Withdrawal Periods. Slaughter withdrawal period nil, milk withdrawal period nil
Dose. *Cattle: by subcutaneous injection*, 2 mL

18.2.9 Louping ill

Louping ill is caused by a flavivirus transmitted by the tick, *Ixodes ricinus*. The disease is characterised by fever, incoordination, paralysis, and convulsions.

Initial vaccinations for cattle should be completed 2 weeks, and for sheep and goats 4 weeks, before exposure to tick-infested pastures. In cattle, 2 vaccinations are given at an interval of 3 weeks to 6 months. In sheep and goats, a single dose, administered by subcutaneous injection on the chest, suffices. The vaccination course should be completed before the last month of pregnancy for cows, ewes, and does being immunised for the first time. Colostral immunity transferred to lambs will give protection for 2 to 3 months. Vaccination gives good protection and therefore a booster dose need only be given to cattle every 12 months and to sheep and goats every 2 years.

UK
Indications. Vaccination against louping ill
Contra-indications. **Side-effects**. **Warnings**. See notes at beginning of chapter

Dose. See preparation details, see notes above for vaccination programmes

PML **Louping-Ill Vaccine** (Schering-Plough) *UK*
Injection, inactivated, prepared from virus grown on tissue culture, containing a suitable mineral oil as adjuvant, for *cattle, sheep, goats*; 20 mL
Dose. *Cattle*: *by subcutaneous injection*, 2 mL
Sheep, goats: *by subcutaneous injection*, 1 mL

> Accidental self-injection with oil-based vaccines can cause severe pain and intense swelling, which may result in ischaemic necrosis and loss of a digit. Prompt medical attention is essential

18.2.10 Lungworm

Lungworm ('husk', bovine verminous pneumonia) infection may lead to pneumonia with secondary bacterial invasion. Vaccines contain a suspension of live, attenuated, larvae of *Dictyocaulus viviparus*. The larvae induce immunity while migrating from the gastro-intestinal tract to the lung where they are destroyed. The vaccination course, given to cattle over 8 weeks of age, consists of 2 doses given at an interval of approximately 4 weeks. Following the second dose, full immunity will not develop until 2 weeks after vaccination and cattle should be kept away from contaminated pasture for this period.

Where the risk of infection is present, calfhood vaccination is advisable. However to enhance the immunity induced by the vaccine, subsequent exposure to a contaminated pasture is essential. Immunity may be interfered with by the use of certain anthelmintic programmes, such as modified-release ruminal boluses or simultaneous vaccination with live vaccines which may prevent infection of pasture. Vaccinated stock should not be placed with unvaccinated animals on the same pasture.

Transient bouts of coughing may occur 7 to 10 days after vaccination. Occasionally, respiratory disease may be precipitated in animals with subclinical infectious pneumonia.

UK

Indications. Vaccination against lungworm
Contra-indications. Vaccination with other live vaccines 14 days before or after vaccination against lungworm; use of anthelmintics 8 weeks before first dose and for 14 days after second dose of lungworm vaccine; see also notes at beginning of chapter
Side-effects. Transient coughing
Warnings. The shelf life of vaccine is short; storage, if required should be at 2–6°C
Dose. See preparation details, see notes above for vaccination programmes

POM **Bovilis Huskvac** (Intervet) *UK*
Oral suspension, lungworm vaccine, living, prepared from third-stage *D. viviparus* larvae, for *calves 8 weeks of age or older*; 25 mL
Withdrawal Periods. Slaughter withdrawal period nil
Dose. *Calves*: *by mouth*, 25 mL

18.2.11 Mastitis

Coliform mastitis is caused by *Escherichia coli*, *Klebsiella* spp., and *Enterobacter aerogenes*. These pathogens are found in the environment. A vaccine is available to control clinical coliform mastitis by induction of antibodies to *E. coli*. Good management practices are essential for control of mastitis in the herd (see chapter 11). Coliform mastitis is responsible for the majority of post-calving toxic mastitis cases in dairy cows. This vaccine uses a core antigen and provides immunity against all coliforms. It does not reduce the new infection rate, but decreases the severity of infection and in so doing increases the proportion of cows who self cure. Consequently the incidence of clinical cliform mastitis is reduced.

Heifers and cows are vaccinated 3 times: at drying-off, 28 days after drying-off, and 2 weeks post partum. Animals must be vaccinated at the end of each lactation.

UK

Indications. Vaccination against coliform mastitis
Contra-indications. **Side-effects**. **Warnings**. See notes at beginning of chapter
Dose. See preparation details, see notes above for vaccination programmes

POM **Enviracor** (Pharmacia & Upjohn) *UK*
Injection, mastitis vaccine, inactivated, prepared from E. coli strain J-5, containing aluminium hydroxide and mineral oil as adjuvants, for *cattle*
Withdrawal Periods. *Cattle*: slaughter withdrawal period nil, milk withdrawal period nil
Dose. *Cattle*: *by subcutaneous injection*, 2 mL

18.2.12 Ovine abortion

Abortions, embryonic deaths, stillbirths, and the birth of weak, non-viable lambs can be caused by many factors. Most serious problems are usually the result of infection by the protozoan *Toxoplasma gondii*, a *Pestivirus* (causing border disease) and micro-organisms such as *Chlamydia* spp., *Salmonella* spp., *Listeria*, or *Campylobacter* spp. Vaccines are available for chlamydiosis (enzootic ovine abortion) and toxoplasmosis, which are the most common infectious causes of reproductive loss in sheep.

Vaccines should be administered well in advance of mating so that a satisfactory immunity can develop before the ewes become pregnant or encounter the infectious agent.

18.2.12.1 Chlamydiosis
18.2.12.2 Toxoplasmosis

18.2.12.1 Chlamydiosis

Chlamydia psittaci infection is an important cause of abortion in the last 2 to 3 weeks of gestation and of lambs born dead or weak. Irrespective of the time of infection the bacterium remains quiescent until after mid-pregnancy, when it multiplies in the uterus causing abortion. Massive numbers of chlamydiae are shed which can infect in-contact ewes and lambs. Carrier ewes may introduce infection to a flock with serious consequences.

Ewe lambs that are intended for breeding may be vaccinated from 5 months of age. Shearlings and older ewes should be vaccinated during the 4-month period before mating with a live vaccine or one month before tupping with an inactivated vaccine. Vaccination of ewes already infected with *Chlamydia* will not prevent abortion although vaccination of ewes incubating the disease may reduce the incidence of abortion.

Enzootic ovine abortion is zoonotic. Pregnant women are advised to avoid helping to lamb or milk ewes and avoid contact with aborted or new born lambs or the placenta. They should seek medical advice if fever or flu-like symptoms are experienced after coming in contact with sheep.

UK

Indications. Vaccination against chlamydiosis
Contra-indications. Pregnant animals, animals less than 4 weeks before mating (live vaccine), animals currently being treated with antibacterials, in particular tetracyclines
Side-effects. See notes at beginning of chapter
Warnings. Chlamydiosis vaccine should not be handled by pregnant women, women of child-bearing age, and immunocompromised people. Operators should wear gloves when handling the vaccine
Dose. See preparation details, see notes above for vaccination programmes

Live vaccines

POM **Enzovax** (Intervet) *UK*
Injection, powder for reconstitution, chlamydiosis vaccine, living, prepared from *Chlamydia psittaci* strain 1B, for *sheep*; 10-dose vial, 20-dose vial, other sizes available
Withdrawal Periods. *Sheep*: slaughter 7 days
Note. Reconstitute with Unisolve
Dose. *Sheep*: *by subcutaneous or intramuscular injection*, 2 mL

POM **Tecvax Chlamydia** (Vétoquinol) *UK*
Injection, powder for reconstitution, chlamydiosis vaccine, living, prepared from *Chlamydia psittaci* strain ts1B, for *sheep*
Withdrawal Periods. *Sheep*: slaughter 7 days
Dose. *Sheep*: *by subcutaneous or intramuscular injection*, 2 mL

Inactivated vaccines

POM **Mydiavac** (Vericore VP) *UK*
Injection (oily), chlamydiosis vaccine, inactivated, prepared from *Chlamydia psittaci*, for *sheep*; 20 mL, 100 mL
Withdrawal Periods. *Sheep*: slaughter withdrawal period nil
Dose. *Sheep*: *by intramuscular injection*, 1 mL

18.2.12.2 Toxoplasmosis

Toxoplasmosis is a protozoal infection caused by *Toxoplasma gondii* (see section 1.4). In sheep, toxoplasmosis can cause heavy losses as a result of early embryonic death, abortion, or the birth of weak, infected lambs. A vaccine containing living tachyzoites of *Toxoplasma gondii* is used in breeding sheep. Ewe lambs intended for breeding may be vaccinated from 5 months of age, and shearlings and older ewes during the 4-month period before mating. Animals should not be vaccinated less than 3 weeks before mating. Vaccination may be repeated every 2 years.

Toxoplasmosis is a zoonotic disease and living tachyzoites in the toxoplasmosis vaccine are capable of causing disease in humans. Therefore, appropriate precautions must be taken, including measures against self-injection and prevention of exposure to the vaccine through the eyes or mouth. The vaccine should be administered under the direct supervision of a veterinarian.

UK

Indications. Vaccination against toxoplasmosis
Contra-indications. Pregnant animals; vaccination less than 3 weeks before mating; vaccination with other live vaccines within 4 weeks of vaccination against toxoplasmosis
Side-effects. See notes above and at beginning of chapter
Warnings. Toxoplasmosis vaccine should not be handled by pregnant women, women of child-bearing age, and immunocompromised people
Dose. See preparation details, see notes above for vaccination programmes

POM **Toxovax** (Intervet) *UK*
Injection, toxoplasmosis vaccine, living, prepared from *Toxoplasma gondii* strain S48, containing living tachyzoites, for *sheep*; 10-dose vial, 20-dose vial, other sizes available
Withdrawal Periods. *Sheep*: slaughter at least 6 weeks
Note. Reconstitute with Unisolve
Dose. *Sheep*: *by intramuscular injection*, 2 mL of diluted vaccine

> Accidental self-injection, ingestion, intranasal or intraocular administration of living tachyzoites may cause disease in humans and prompt medical attention is essential

18.2.13 Ovine pasteurellosis

Pasteurella haemolytica and *P.trehalosi* may cause either a septicaemic or pneumonic form of pasteurellosis.

Sheep that have not been previously vaccinated should be given a course of 2 doses at an interval of 4 to 6 weeks. Thereafter annual booster vaccinations may be given at intervals of not more than 12 months. In adult breeding ewes, the annual vaccination is given 4 to 6 weeks before lambing. In areas of high pasteurellosis incidence, an additional vaccination may be given 2 to 3 weeks before the period of risk.

UK

Indications. Vaccination against pasteurellosis
Contra-indications. **Side-effects**. **Warnings**. See notes at beginning of chapter and notes above
Dose. See preparation details, see notes above for vaccination programmes

PML **Ovipast Plus** (Intervet) *UK*
Injection, pasteurellosis vaccine, inactivated, prepared from *P. haemolytica* and *P. trehalosis* serotypes, containing aluminium hydroxide as adjuvant, for *sheep*; 100 mL, 500 mL
Dose. *Sheep*: *by subcutaneous injection*, 2 mL

18.2.14 Rabies

See section 18.4.6

18.2.15 Ringworm

Ringworm in cattle is caused by *Trichophyton verrucosum*. Initially the whole herd should be given 2 vaccinations at an interval of 10 to 14 days. Thereafter, in a closed herd, young calves are vaccinated at 2 weeks of age and again 10 to 14 days later. Any newly introduced animals should receive a full vaccination course.

Ringworm is a highly contagious skin disease. Treatment is discussed under sections 1.2 and 14.4.2. It is important to ensure that infective spores are eliminated from buildings and equipment. Ringworm is a zoonotic disease.

UK

Indications. Vaccination against ringworm
Contra-indications. Vaccination during the last 2 months of pregnancy
Side-effects. **Warnings**. Occasional small crust formation at the site of injection. See notes at beginning of chapter and notes above
Dose. See preparation details, see notes above for vaccination programmes

POM **Ringvac Bovis LTF-130** (Intervet) *UK*
Injection, powder for reconstitution, ringworm vaccine, living, prepared from *Trichophyton verrucosum* strain LTF-130, for *cattle*; 5-calf dose vial
Dose. *By intramuscular injection.*
Cattle: 4 mL; *calves 2–16 weeks of age*: 2 mL

18.2.16 Tetanus

See section 18.1.6

18.2.17 Immunoglobulins for ruminants

Immunoglobulins (or antibodies) combine with specific antigens. A preparation containing specific immunoglobulin G against E. coli f5 (K99) is available. If given within the first 12 hours of life will protect calves against enterotoxicosis caused by E. coli. Normal colostrum should also be given. The preparation is produced from colostrum collected from cows kept under field conditions. Consequently it may also contain antibodies to other organisms, including BVD virus. This should be borne in mind when planning subsequent vaccination protocols.

Antitoxins for tetanus are available (see section 18.1.6).

UK

Indications. Prophylaxis of enterotoxicosis
Dose. See preparation details

POM **Locatim Oral Solution** (Vétoquinol)
Oral solution, E.coli f5 (K99) specific immunoglobulin G, *for calves up to 12 hours old*
Withdrawal Periods. Withdrawal periods nil
Dose. *Calves: by mouth or by addition to milk or milk replacer*, 60 mL within 12 hours (preferably 4 hours) of birth

18.3 Immunological preparations for pigs

18.3.1   Anthrax
18.3.2   Atrophic rhinitis
18.3.3   Aujeszky's disease
18.3.4   Clostridial infections
18.3.5   Enteritis
18.3.6   Erysipelas
18.3.7   Porcine parvovirus
18.3.8   Porcine pneumonia
18.3.9   Tetanus
18.3.10 Combination vaccines for pigs

Immunisation programmes used for pigs depend upon which diseases are liable to be encountered. Breeding pigs are generally vaccinated against erysipelas. Fattening pigs are vaccinated against erysipelas when necessary. Vaccination against parvovirus, Aujeszky's disease, colibacillosis, and clostridial disease may be required in some herds, the latter especially in pigs reared extensively. Subcutaneous and intramuscular injections are usually given behind the ear in adult pigs, and in the flank or axillary region in piglets.

18.3.1 Anthrax

No proprietary vaccine is available against anthrax (see section 18.2.1)

18.3.2 Atrophic rhinitis

The aetiology of atrophic rhinitis is complex. Immunisation against the bacterial components of atrophic rhinitis syndrome is possible with inactivated vaccines prepared from cultures of *Bordetella bronchiseptica* and *Pasteurella multocida* toxoid.

Sows or gilts are given a primary course of 2 doses at an interval of 6 weeks. A single booster injection during each subsequent pregnancy will provide passive protection for the piglets. The interval between booster vaccination and farrowing should not be greater than 150 days. The optimum time for revaccination is 6 to 2 weeks before farrowing, although pigs may be vaccinated at service, pregnancy testing, or weaning to reduce handling, especially in outdoor units.

UK

Indications. Vaccination against atrophic rhinitis
Contra-indications. **Side-effects**. **Warnings**. See notes at beginning of chapter; occasional temporary swelling at site of injection
Dose. See preparation details, see notes above for vaccination programmes

PML **Porcilis AR-T** (Intervet) *UK*
Injection, atrophic rhinitis vaccine, inactivated, prepared from *B. bronchiseptica*, *P. multocida* toxoid, containing a suitable oil as adjuvant, for *pigs*; 20 mL, 50 mL
Withdrawal Periods. **Pigs**: slaughter withdrawal period nil
Dose. *Pigs: by intramuscular injection*, 2 mL

18.3.3 Aujeszky's disease

Aujeszky's disease is caused by a herpesvirus, porcine herpesvirus 1, and is characterised by respiratory, reproductive, and CNS signs. In Britain, a slaughter and eradication policy is in operation for the control of Aujeszky's disease. Live vaccines are available in Northern Ireland for administration to healthy piglets. The first dose is given from 8 weeks of age and the second vaccination 3 to 4 weeks later. In gilts, sows, and boars, a third dose is given 2 weeks before service or at 6 months of age for boars. A single booster dose should be given not less frequently than every 6 months.

A scheme to eradicate Aujeszky's disease in pigs in Northern Ireland is in operation. Depending on the current disease status of the individual herd, farmers may decide whether to control the disease by vaccination or to employ blood testing of breeding stock and demonstrate the herd free from the disease.

UK

Indications. Vaccination against Aujeszky's disease
Contra-indications. Side-effects. Warnings. Not for use in Britain (see above). See also notes at beginning of chapter
Dose. See preparation details, see notes above for vaccination programmes

POM **Nobi-Porvac Aujeszky Live** (Intervet) *UK*
Injection, powder for reconstitution, Aujeszky's disease vaccine, living, prepared from virus strain Begonia, for *pigs*; 10-dose vial, 25-dose vial, other sizes available
Withdrawal Periods. *Pigs*: slaughter withdrawal period nil
Dose. *Pigs*: *by intramuscular injection*, 2 mL
Note. Available only in Northern Ireland

POM **Suvaxyn Aujeszky** (Fort Dodge) *UK*
Injection, powder for reconstitution, Aujeszky's disease vaccine, living, prepared from virus strain Bartha K61, for *pigs*; 10-dose vial, 50-dose vial
Dose. *Pigs*: *by intramuscular injection*, 2 mL
Note. Available only in Northern Ireland

18.3.4 Clostridial infections

Clostridial infections can cause enteritis, hepatitis, or tetanus in pigs. Antiserum is available for the passive protection of piglets. Active immunity can be achieved by the injection of toxoid. Two doses are recommended at an interval of about 3 weeks. Vaccination of sows 6 weeks and 3 weeks before farrowing provides passive protection to piglets through the colostrum. In subsequent pregnancies a single booster dose should be given to sows 6 to 3 weeks before farrowing.

UK

Antitoxins

PML **Lambisan** (Intervet) *UK*
See section 18.2.3 for preparation details

Vaccines

PML **Gletvax 6** (Schering-Plough) *UK*
See section 18.3.5.2 for preparation details

PML **Heptavac** (Intervet) *UK*
See section 18.2.3 for preparation details

PML **Lambivac** (Intervet) *UK*
See section 18.2.3 for preparation details

18.3.5 Enteritis

18.3.5.1 Escherichia coli infections
18.3.5.2 Combination preparations for enteritis

Enteritis in neonatal and young pigs may be caused by bacteria including *E. coli*, *Salmonella* spp., *Cl. perfringens* enterotoxin, viruses, parasites, and influenced by inadequate housing or management procedures.

18.3.5.1 Escherichia coli infections

Vaccines are available for the protection of piglets against *E. coli* infections, which contain selected serotypes or strains of the organism or important antigens. Vaccines contain toxoids, cellular antigens, or both. Parenteral administration is not recommended during the last 2 to 3 weeks of gestation. Combination preparations are also available.

Sows and gilts are vaccinated to provide passive immunity for piglets via the colostrum.

UK

Indications. Vaccination against *E. coli* infection
Contra-indications. Side-effects. Warnings. See notes at beginning of chapter and notes above
Dose. See preparation details

Oral vaccines

MFS **Intagen** (Alpharma) *UK*
Premix, *E. coli* vaccine, inactivated, prepared from residues and extracts of *E. coli* serotypes, for *pigs*; 25 kg
Dose. *Pigs*: *by addition to feed*, (up to 5 kg body-weight) 10 kg/tonne feed; (5–15 kg body-weight) 5 kg/tonne feed; (>15 kg body-weight) 2.5 kg/tonne feed; (sows) 1.5 kg/tonne feed for at least the last 8 weeks before farrowing

Parenteral vaccines

> Accidental self-injection with oil-based vaccines can cause severe pain and intense swelling, which may result in ischaemic necrosis and loss of a digit.. Prompt medical attention is essential

POM **Neocolipor** (Merial) *UK*
Injection, *E. coli* vaccine, inactivated, prepared from *E. coli* strains expressing F4ab (K88ab), F4ac (K88ac), F4ad (K88ad), F5 (K99), F6 (987P), and F41 adhesions, containing aluminium hydroxide as adjuvant, for *pigs*
Withdrawal Periods. *Pigs*: slaughter withdrawal period nil
Dose. *Pigs*: *by intramuscular injection*, 2 mL 5–7 weeks before farrowing, repeat 2 weeks before farrowing. Revaccinate 2 weeks before each farrowing

PML **Porcilis Porcol 5** (Intervet) *UK*
Injection, *E. coli* vaccine, inactivated, *E. coli* LT toxoid and antigens K88ab, K88ac, K99, 987P, containing a suitable oil as adjuvant, for *pigs*
Dose. *Pigs*: *by intramuscular injection*, 2 mL, repeat after 5–6 weeks. Revaccinate every 6 months

PML **Suvaxyn E. Coli P4** (Fort Dodge) *UK*
Injection, E. coli vaccine, inactivated, prepared from *E. coli* antigens F41, K88, K99, 987P, containing a suitable adjuvant, for *pigs*; 20 mL
Dose. *Pigs: by intramuscular injection,* 2 mL at 4 weeks and 2 weeks before farrowing. Revaccinate 2 weeks before each farrowing

18.3.5.2 Combination preparations for enteritis

UK

PML **Gletvax 6** (Schering-Plough) *UK*
Injection, combined *E. coli* and *Cl. perfringens* vaccine, inactivated, E. coli antigens K88ab, K88ac, K99, 987P, *Cl. perfringens* types B, C, and D toxoid, containing aluminium hydroxide as adjuvant, for *pigs*; 50 mL
Dose. *Pigs: by subcutaneous or intramuscular injection,* 5 mL at service *or* up to 6 weeks before farrowing, repeat dose 2 weeks before farrowing. Revaccinate 2 weeks before each farrowing

PML **Colisorb** (Intervet) *UK*
See section 18.3.10 for preparation details

18.3.6 Erysipelas

In pigs, erysipelas is characterised by acute septicaemia, endocarditis, or chronic arthritis. The disease is caused by *Erysipelothrix rhusiopathiae* (*Ery. insidiosa*). Vaccination consists of a course of 2 doses given at an interval of 2 to 4 weeks. Revaccination is usually necessary every 6 to 12 months.

Piglets from non-immune sows may be vaccinated at approximately 7 days of age and the dose repeated 2 to 3 weeks later. Piglets from immune sows may be vaccinated at 8 or 6 weeks of age with the dose repeated after 2 weeks. Depending on the vaccine used, pregnant sows and gilts are vaccinated 6 and 2 or 3 weeks before farrowing and boosters administered 3 weeks before each farrowing. For vaccines that are contra-indicated for use in pregnant animals, sows are revaccinated each lactation.

UK

Indications. Vaccination against erysipelas
Contra-indications. Side-effects. Warnings. See notes at beginning of chapter and notes above
Dose. See preparation details, see notes above for vaccination programmes

PML **Erysorb Plus** (Intervet) *UK*
Injection, erysipelas vaccine, inactivated, prepared from *Ery. rhusiopathiae* serotype 1 strain P15/10 and serotype 2 strain CN3342 and CN3461, containing aluminium hydroxide as adjuvant, for *pigs*; 50 mL, 100 mL
Dose. *Pigs: by subcutaneous injection,* 2 mL

PML **Porcilis Ery** (Intervet) *UK*
Injection, erysipelas vaccine, inactivated, prepared from *Ery. rhusiopathiae* strain M2 serotype 2, containing *dl*-alpha tocopherol as adjuvant, for *pigs more than 10 weeks of age*; 50 mL, 100 mL
Withdrawal Periods. *Pigs:* slaughter withdrawal period nil
Contra-indications. Pregnant animals
Side-effects. Transient increased body temperature, swelling at injection site, reluctance to move
Dose. *Pigs: by intramuscular injection,* 2 mL

PML **Suvaxyn Erysipelas** (Fort Dodge) *UK*
Injection, erysipelas vaccine, inactivated, prepared from selected *Ery. rhusiopathiae* strains, containing a suitable adjuvant, for *pigs more than 7 days of age, turkeys* (see section 18.6.11); 100 mL
Dose. *Pigs: by subcutaneous injection,* 2 mL

18.3.7 Porcine parvovirus

Porcine parvovirus (PPV) infection is characterised by stillbirths, mummified fetuses, embryonic death, and infertility (SMEDI syndrome). Vaccines are used in breeding pigs to protect embryos and fetuses against the disease. Vaccination is usually delayed until about 6 months of age because maternally-derived antibodies interfere with the immune response. For most vaccines, 2 doses are required and gilts are given a primary vaccination at least 2 weeks before the first service. A subsequent dose is generally administered after farrowing and before the next service. Sows are also vaccinated 2 or more weeks before service. Boars are vaccinated at about 6 months of age and revaccinated 6 months later. Booster doses are given at least annually thereafter.
The recommendations for individual vaccines vary and manufacturer's details should be consulted regarding vaccine programmes.

UK

Indications. Vaccination against porcine parvovirus infection
Contra-indications. Side-effects. Warnings. See notes at beginning of chapter
Dose. See preparation details, see manufacturer's details for vaccination programmes

POM **Suvaxyn Parvo** (Fort Dodge) *UK*
Injection, porcine parvovirus vaccine, inactivated, prepared from virus grown on porcine tissue culture, containing a suitable adjuvant, for *pigs from 6 months of age*; 20 mL
Dose. *Pigs: by intramuscular injection,* 2 mL

POM **Suvaxyn Parvo 2** (Fort Dodge) *UK*
Injection, porcine parvovirus vaccine, inactivated, prepared from virus grown on porcine tissue culture, containing a suitable oil as adjuvant, for *pigs from 5 months of age*; 20 mL
Contra-indications. Pregnant animals
Dose. *Pigs: by intramuscular injection,* 2 mL

> Accidental self-injection with oil-based vaccines can cause severe pain and intense swelling, which may result in ischaemic necrosis and loss of a digit. Prompt medical attention is essential

18.3.8 Porcine pneumonia

Many large pig herds encounter the problem of pneumonia. Primary viral infections can be complicated by secondary bacterial or mycoplasmal infections resulting in severe pneumonia. Vaccines against mycoplasma and respiratory bacteria are available which, combined with therapeutic and management procedures, can be used to combat disease.

18.3.8.1 Enzootic pneumonia
18.3.8.2 Pasteurellosis
18.3.8.3 Pleuropneumonia
18.3.8.4 PRRS

18.3.8.1 Enzootic pneumonia

Piglets may be vaccinated from 5 days to 10 weeks of age, depending on the vaccine used. In general, vaccination consists of a course of 2 doses given at an interval of 2 to 4 weeks. Animals of more than one week of age at the time of first vaccination may already have pulmonary lesions due to *Mycoplasma* infection.

UK

Indications. Vaccination against enzootic pneumonia
Contra-indications. Side-effects. Warnings. See notes at beginning of chapter
Dose. See preparation details, see notes above for vaccination programmes

POM **Hyoresp** (Merial) *UK*
Injection, enzootic pneumonia vaccine, inactivated, prepared from *Mycoplasma hyopneumoniae*, containing aluminium hydroxide as adjuvant, for *pigs more than 5 days of age*
Withdrawal Periods. *Pigs*: slaughter withdrawal period nil
Dose. *Pigs*: *by intramuscular injection*, 2 mL, repeat after 3-4 weeks for animals less than 10 weeks of age.

POM **Stellamune Mycoplasma** (Pfizer) *UK*
Injection, enzootic pneumonia vaccine, inactivated, prepared from *Mycoplasma hyopneumoniae*, containing a suitable adjuvant, for *pigs*; 100 mL
Dose. *Pigs*: *by intramuscular injection*, 2 mL

POM **Suvaxyn M.hyo** (Fort Dodge) *UK*
Injection, enzootic pneumonia vaccine, inactivated, prepared from *Mycoplasma hyopneumoniae*, containing a suitable adjuvant, for *growing pigs from 1 week of age*; 100 mL
Contra-indications. Pregnant animals
Dose. *Pigs*: *by intramuscular injection*, 2 mL

18.3.8.2 Pasteurellosis

Pneumonia with pleurisy caused by *Pasteurella* spp. can occur as a complication of chronic mycoplasmal pneumonia in intensively reared herds or as a primary sporadic pneumonia in younger pigs. Affected pigs have great difficulty in breathing, exhibit a frothy tracheal exudate and fever, and may die.

Vaccines should be administered as 2 doses given at an interval of 3 to 4 weeks. Booster vaccinations are given after 6 to 12 months.

UK

Indications. Vaccination against pasteurellosis
Contra-indications. Side-effects. Warnings. See notes at beginning of chapter
Dose. See preparation details, see notes above for vaccination programmes

PML **Pastacidin** (Intervet) *UK*
See section 18.2.12.1 for preparation details
Dose. *Pigs*: *by subcutaneous injection*, 1 mL

18.3.8.3 Pleuropneumonia

Porcine pleuropneumonia is caused by *Actinobacillus pleuropneumoniae (Haemophilus pleuropneumoniae)*. The acute disease is characterised by severe dyspnoea and fever; sporadic coughing is seen in animals with chronic pleurop-

neumonia. Poor ventilation and overcrowding may exacerbate the condition.

A course of 2 vaccinations, given at an interval of 2 weeks, is administered to growing pigs. Pigs may be vaccinated from 6 weeks of age. The second vaccination should be administered at least 3 weeks before the expected challenge.

UK

Indications. Vaccination against pleuropneumonia
Contra-indications. Side-effects. Warnings. See notes at beginning of chapter and notes above, pregnant animals; transient hyperthermia and malaise
Dose. See preparation details, see notes above for vaccination programmes

POM **Suvaxyn APP** (Fort Dodge) *UK*
Injection, pleuropneumonia vaccine, inactivated, prepared from *Actinobacillus pleuropneumoniae* serotypes 3, 6, and 8, containing a suitable adjuvant, for *growing pigs from 6 weeks of age*
Dose. *Pigs*: *by intramuscular injection*, 2 mL

18.3.8.4 PRRS

Porcine reproductive and respiratory syndome (PRRS) virus causes abortions, stillbirths, and weak newborn piglets followed by a period of severe respiratory disease.

Weaners and fattening pigs are vaccinated once. The vaccine should not be used in in-contact breeding animals including boars, or pregnant or lactating sows. Vaccination is not recommended on PRRS virus-free sites that also have reproductive pigs. Vaccine virus may incidentally spread to in-contact pigs. Strict hygiene precautions should be maintained to ensure the virus is not transferred to breeding boars and sows.

POM **Porcilis PRRS** (Intervet)
Injection, PRRS virus vaccine, living, prepared from PRRS virus strain DV, containing a suitable adjuvant, for pigs from 6 weeks of age
Withdrawal Periods. Slaughter withdrawal period nil
Dose. *Pigs*: *by intramuscular injection*, 2 mL

18.3.9 Tetanus

See section 18.1.6

18.3.10 Combination vaccines for pigs

UK

Indications. See preparation details
Contra-indications. Side-effects. Warnings. See notes at beginning of chapter
Dose. See preparation details

PML **Colisorb** (Intervet) *UK*
Injection, combined *E. coli* and erysipelas vaccine, inactivated, cells of *E. coli* serotypes of porcine origin, *E. coli* soluble antigens K88, K99, 987P, and labile toxin B fragment, and cells of *Ery. rhusiopathiae* serotypes 1 and 2, containing aluminium hydroxide as adjuvant, for *pigs*; 20 mL, 50 mL
Dose. *Pigs*: *by subcutaneous injection*, 2 mL at 6 and 3 weeks before farrowing. Revaccinate 3 weeks before each farrowing
POM **Erysorb Parvo** (Intervet) *UK*

Injection, combined erysipelas and porcine parvovirus vaccine, inactivated, prepared from *Erysipelothrix rhusiopathiae* strains, porcine parvovirus, containing aluminium hydroxide as adjuvant, for *pigs more than 6 months of age*

Withdrawal Periods. *Pigs*: slaughter withdrawal period nil

Dose. *Pigs*: *by subcutaneous injection*, 2 mL, repeat after 2-3 weeks. Both injection s should be administered before mating with the second given not earlier than 12 weeks before mating. Revaccinate every 6 months

POM Porcilis Ery + Parvo (Intervet) *UK*

Injection, combined erysipelas and porcine parvovirus vaccine, inactivated, prepared from *Erysipelothrix rhusiopathiae* strain M2 serotype 2, porcine parvovirus strain 014, containing a suitable adjuvant, for *pigs*; 10-dose vial, 25-dose vial, 50-dose vial

Withdrawal Periods. *Pigs*: slaughter withdrawal period nil

Contra-indications. Pregnant animals

Dose. *Pigs*: *by intramuscular injection*, 2 mL at 2 weeks before first mating

POM Suvaxyn M hyo - Parasuis (Fort Dodge) *UK*

Injection, combined enzootic pneumonia and Glässers disease vaccine, inactivated, prepared from *Mycoplasma hyopneumoniae, Haemophilus parasuis* serotypes 4 and 5, for *growing pigs from one week of age*

Withdrawal Periods. *Pigs*: slaughter withdrawal period nil

Side-effects. Mild transient erythema at the injection site, transient hyperthermia, lethargy, and malaise may follow vaccination

Contra-indications. Pregnant animals

Dose. *Pigs*: *by intramuscular injection*, 2 mL at 1-10 weeks of age, repeat after 2-3 weeks and at least 3 weeks before expected risk period

18.4 Immunological preparations for dogs

18.4.1 Canine distemper
18.4.2 Canine parvovirus
18.4.3 Infectious canine hepatitis
18.4.4 Infectious tracheobronchitis
18.4.5 Leptospirosis
18.4.6 Rabies
18.4.7 Tetanus
18.4.8 Combination vaccines for dogs
18.4.9 Immunoglobulins for dogs

Many factors may affect fixed canine vaccination programmes such as the animal's age, health, and maturity, the presence of maternally-derived antibodies, the antigenic mass of the vaccine used, and the presence of infection in the environment. It is now considered better to devise schedules appropriate to individual circumstances. This should be taken into account when interpreting the guidelines in the text below, and the manufacturer's recommendations.

Debate continues about possible side-effects of canine vaccines. A link between vaccination and prevalence of auto-immune haemolytic anaemia and immune-mediated thrombocytopenia has been suggested but is unproven. **The current recommendations are that booster vaccinations should be given in accordance with manufacturer's instructions.**

The National Greyhound Racing Club require that racing greyhounds are vaccinated against distemper, infectious canine hepatitis, leptospirosis, and parvovirus (see Prescribing for animals used in competitions).

18.4.1 Canine distemper

Canine distemper virus (CDV) causes a highly contagious disease of dogs and other carnivores, which is characterised by respiratory, gastro-intestinal, and occasionally, nervous signs. Respiratory signs alone may occur and distemper virus can be involved in infectious tracheobronchitis (see section 18.4.4).

The presence of maternally-derived antibody in puppies will interfere with successful immunisation. Generally, maternally-derived antibody will have declined to non-interfering levels by 12 weeks of age, although some individuals will have lost this immunity by 8 to 9 weeks of age. Therefore, when there is low risk of exposure, with puppies in isolation, one vaccination at 10 to 12 weeks of age should provide sufficient protection. An additional later vaccination may be necessary for puppies born to bitches that experienced an active infection or had been vaccinated just before pregnancy. If young puppies are at risk, earlier vaccination schedules should be used. Accordingly, an initial dose may be given at 6 to 8 weeks of age, and repeated at 10 to 12 weeks, depending on the vaccine. Some authorities advise routine vaccination at 8 and 10 or 12 weeks in all cases in order to reduce the immunity gap.

Where high and unavoidable levels of challenge virus are likely, such as in a pet shop or stray dogs' home, active immunity should be induced in puppies as early as possible. Some canine distemper vaccines can overcome low to moderate levels of maternally-derived antibody. Canine distemper vaccine may be used from 6 weeks, but puppies should be vaccinated again at 10 to 12 weeks of age, depending on the vaccine.

An initial booster vaccination should be given at one year of age and theoretically distemper titres should last for several years. Recommendations for revaccination for complete protection vary from one to two years.

Non-domestic carnivore species that are susceptible to canine distemper include foxes, mink, ferrets, and exotic zoo species. In general, clinical signs resemble those of distemper in domestic dogs. Information from manufacturers should be sought before using vaccines in these species because vaccination may cause disease. Quarantine measures, good hygiene, and good management are also important in a control programme.

Vaccines for canine distemper are available in combination with other canine vaccines (see section 18.4.7). A combination antisera preparation is available (see section 18.4.9).

18.4.2 Canine parvovirus

Canine parvovirus (CPV) infection is an enteric disease that first appeared in the canine population in 1978. The main target sites for multiplication of virus are the lymphatic tissues and intestinal epithelium, and, in neonatal puppies, the myocardium. Myocarditis is rare because most bitches are now immune, puppies being protected by maternally-derived antibody. In older dogs, disease signs may vary from subclinical infection to severe haemorrhagic gastro-enteritis.

CPV is closely related to feline panleucopenia virus (FPV) and, initially, FPV vaccines were used to protect dogs. However, these have now been superseded by homologous CPV vaccines, which generally induce a longer-lasting and more consistent response.

Most problems with CPV vaccination have arisen because of the high level of challenge virus in the environment, and because low levels of maternally-derived antibody may interfere with vaccination but not protect against infection. Puppies may become susceptible before they can respond to vaccination. In addition, the duration of maternally-derived antibodies to CPV may be quite variable and sometimes long-lasting, ranging from 4 to 20 weeks, depending on the level of immunity in the dam.

The duration of maternally-derived antibody in puppies may be predicted from the bitch's titre and a known antibody half-life of approximately 9 days. However, where practicable, each puppy's antibody level should be assessed individually to determine the optimum age for vaccination because there may be great variability in colostral intake between puppies within a litter. Alternatively, puppies may be vaccinated at 2 to 4 week intervals from 6 to 12 or 18 weeks of age, the precise timing depending on when the puppy is presented, the exposure risk, and the vaccine used. Although immunity following modified live vaccine administration may be of longer duration, annual booster vaccination is recommended.

CPV is extremely resistant in the environment. Adequate disinfection procedures, in addition to vaccination, are essential if a clinical case occurs.

A combination antisera preparation is available (see section 18.4.9).

UK

Indications. Vaccination against canine parvovirus (CPV) infection

Contra-indications. Live vaccines should not be used in pregnant animals, see notes at beginning of chapter

Side-effects. **Warnings**. See notes at beginning of chapter

Dose. See preparation details, see notes above for vaccination programmes

POM **Eurican P** (Merial) *UK*
Injection, powder for reconstitution, CPV vaccine, living, prepared from virus strain CPU C780916, for *dogs*; 1-dose vial
Note. May be reconstituted with Eurican L
Dose. *Dogs*: *by subcutaneous or intramuscular injection*, 1 dose

POM **Kavak P69** (Fort Dodge) *UK*
Injection, CPV vaccine, living, prepared from virus grown on tissue culture, for *dogs*; 1-dose vial
Note. May be reconstituted with Kavak L
Dose. *Dogs*: *by subcutaneous injection*, 1 dose

POM **Nobivac Parvo-C** (Intervet) *UK*
Injection, powder for reconstitution, CPV vaccine, living, prepared from virus grown on cell-line tissue culture, for *dogs*; 1-dose vial
Note. May be reconstituted with Nobivac Lepto
Dose. *Dogs*: *by subcutaneous injection*, 1 dose

POM **Quantum Dog CPV** (Schering-Plough) *UK*
Injection, CPV vaccine, living, prepared from virus, for *dogs*; 1-dose vial
Dose. *Dogs*: *by subcutaneous injection*, 1 dose

POM **Vanguard CPV** (Pfizer) *UK*
Injection, CPV vaccine, living, prepared from virus grown on NL-DK-1 established canine cell line, for *dogs*; 1 mL
Dose. *Dogs*: *by subcutaneous injection*, 1 mL

18.4.3 Infectious canine hepatitis

Infectious canine hepatitis (ICH) is caused by canine adenovirus type 1 (CAV 1). The virus has a predilection for hepatic cells, vascular endothelium, and lymphoid tissue. Disease signs may vary from inapparent to a severe form characterised by depression, anorexia, thirst, abdominal pain, and vomiting. In some cases, sudden death may occur, especially in young puppies, and the virus may be involved in the 'fading puppy' syndrome.

Transient corneal opacity or 'blue eye' may occur in some dogs 1 to 3 weeks after acute ICH infection and may be the only clinical sign observed if acute infection is asymptomatic. This is due to virus-antibody complexes and generally heals spontaneously, although complications and, occasionally, blindness may result in some cases. In many recovered animals, the virus persists in the kidney and may be shed in the urine for at least 6 months.

In the UK, CAV 1 is also regarded as a possible cause of infectious tracheobronchitis (see section 18.4.4). The closely related CAV 2, which does not cause ICH, is also involved in the aetiology of infectious tracheobronchitis. Originally, modified live CAV 1 vaccines were used to control ICH, but in a small percentage of dogs the vaccines induced ocular lesions similar to those seen in the natural disease. Since dogs vaccinated with CAV 2 become immune to both CAV 1 and CAV 2 infection, and CAV 2 vaccines have the advantages that they do not induce 'blue eye', or give rise to possible viral persistence with lesions in the kidney, and viral excretion in the urine, CAV 2 has replaced CAV 1 in canine adenovirus vaccines.

Vaccination may be carried out from 6 to 8 weeks of age, but a second dose should always be given at 10 or 12 weeks of age, depending on the vaccine. In general, maternally-derived antibody appears to be less of a problem with ICH vaccination in comparison with other major canine viral infections. Since the disease has been well controlled by vaccination, there is little challenge virus in the environment, and the virus-host immunity balance is generally stable.

Immunity following live virus vaccination probably lasts several years, but booster vaccination every 1 to 2 years is recommended. Inactivated vaccines are also available, which may be given to pregnant animals. The immunity induced is not so long-lasting and annual boosters are required. Vaccines for infectious canine hepatitis are available in combination with other canine vaccines (see section 18.4.8).

A combination antisera preparation is available (see section 18.4.9).

18.4.4 Infectious tracheobronchitis

A number of agents are involved in canine infectious tracheobronchitis, also known as the kennel cough syndrome. Although several viruses are implicated in the aetiology, the major cause appears to be *Bordetella bronchiseptica,* hence the alternative name of bordetellosis. The bacteria appear to attach specifically to cilia of the trachea and bronchi, and persist in the dog several months after infection. However, coughing occurs predominantly only in the first week or two after infection, when bacterial growth is greatest.

Viruses such as CDV (see section 18.4.1), canine adenovirus types 1 and 2 (CAV 1 and CAV 2), canine parainfluenza (PI) virus, and canine herpesvirus may also be involved in the aetiology of the disease. Some of these agents only cause very mild disease and the characteristic syndrome seen is often a result of combined viral and bacterial infection. CAV 1 is also involved in infectious canine hepatitis (see section 18.4.3). Combination (see section 18.4.8) and individual vaccines are available against several of these viruses.

18.4.4.1 Bordetella bronchiseptica
18.4.4.2 Parainfluenza
18.4.4.3 Combination preparations

18.4.4.1 Bordetella bronchiseptica

Originally, systemic vaccination by injection against *B. bronchiseptica* was found not to be consistently satisfactory, and adverse reactions at the injection site were common. Intranasal vaccines are reasonably effective, with few side-effects, although transient coughing may occur a few days after vaccination. The vaccine appears to induce good local immunity, which is not interfered with by maternally-derived antibody. Therefore, puppies over 2 weeks of age may be vaccinated. Immunity takes 5 days to develop and thus dogs should be isolated during this period. Revaccination every 6 to 10 months is recommended, depending on potential exposure. Pregnant animals and dogs under treatment with antibacterials active against *B. bronchiseptica* should not be vaccinated.

UK

Indications. Vaccination against infectious tracheobronchitis
Contra-indications. Pregnant animals, concurrent treatment with antibacterials active against *B. bronchiseptica*, see notes at beginning of chapter
Side-effects. **Warnings**. See notes at beginning of chapter; transient coughing after vaccination
Dose. *Dogs*: (2 weeks of age or more) *by intranasal instillation*, 1 mL into 1 nostril or 0.5 mL into each nostril; see notes above for vaccination programmes

POM **Intrac** (Schering-Plough) *UK*
Intranasal solution, powder for reconstitution, infectious tracheobronchitis vaccine, living, prepared from *B. bronchiseptica* strain S 55, for **dogs more than 2 weeks of age**; 1 mL

18.4.4.2 Parainfluenza

Canine parainfluenza (PI) virus is a major cause of infectious tracheobronchitis in North America and elsewhere and is considered to play some part in the aetiology of the disease in the UK.

Vaccination against PI virus infection involves 2 vaccinations, given at an interval of 3 to 4 weeks, with the second dose administered at 12 weeks of age or over. If required, vaccination may be provided from 6 weeks of age. Annual booster vaccination is recommended.

UK

Indications. Vaccination against parainfluenza
Contra-indications. Pregnant animals, see notes at beginning of chapter
Side-effects. **Warnings**. See notes at beginning of chapter
Dose. See preparation details, see notes above for vaccination programmes

POM **Kavak Parainfluenza** (Fort Dodge) *UK*
Injection, powder for reconstitution, PI vaccine, living, prepared from PI virus type 2 grown on an established cell line, for *dogs*; 1-dose vial
Note. May be reconstitited with Kavak L
Dose. *Dogs*: *by subcutaneous injection*, 1 dose

18.4.4.3 Combination preparations for infectious tracheobronchitis

A combined vaccine is available that affords protection about 72 hours after vaccination. Puppies may be vaccinated from 2 weeks of age. Clinical signs of upper respiratory tract disease may sometimes be seen post vaccination. If signs persist, the animal should be treated with appropriate antibacterials.

UK

Indications. Vaccination against infectious tracheobronchitis
Contra-indications. Concurrent treatment with antibacterials, see notes at beginning of chapter
Side-effects. **Warnings**. See notes at beginning of chapter; transient coughing after vaccination
Dose. *Dogs*: (2 weeks of age or more) *by intranasal instillation*, 0.4 mL into 1 nostril; see notes above for vaccination programmes

POM **Nobivac KC** (Intervet) *UK*
Intranasal solution, powder for reconstitution, combined living infectious tracheobronchitis vaccine, prepared from *B. bronchiseptica* strain B-C2, PI strain Cornell, for *dogs more than 2 weeks of age*; 0.4 mL

18.4.5 Leptospirosis

Leptospirosis in dogs is predominantly caused by the 2 serotypes of *Leptospira interrogans*: *L. interrogans* serovar *canicola* (primary host, the dog) or *L. interrogans* serovar *icterohaemorrhagiae* (primary host, the rat). The disease is characterised by acute haemorrhage, hepatitis and jaundice usually caused by *L. interrogans* serovar *icterohaemorrhagiae* infection, or acute interstitial nephritis (mainly *L. interrogans* serovar *canicola* infection). Often infection is subclinical. Leptospirosis is a zoonotic disease.

Maternally-derived immunity to *Leptospira interrogans* is not a problem in puppies with respect to vaccination, because it is absent by 8 weeks of age. For primary vaccination, 2 doses are given at an interval of 2 to 6 weeks, starting at about 8 weeks of age. Annual booster vaccination is recommended.

Although the organism may be spread by direct contact with an infected animal, the main infection source is from urine or urine-contaminated water or soil. Recovered animals may shed leptospirae into the urine for some time. Thus, while vaccination is generally effective in controlling the disease, if a clinical case occurs, antibacterial therapy should be administered. Antibacterials recommended for treatment of clinical leptospirosis include benzylpenicillin♦ (see section 1.1.1.1) given by intramuscular or intravenous injection 24 mg/kg twice daily, or oral ampicillin or amoxicillin (see section 1.1.1.3) 10 mg/kg twice daily. Once renal function is restored, dogs should be treated for a further 2 weeks to eliminate infection from the kidneys; streptomycin (see section 1.1.3) 15 mg/kg administered by intramuscular injection twice daily is used. In addition to therapy, contaminated premises should be disinfected.

A combination antisera preparation is available (see section 18.4.9).

UK

Indications. Vaccination against leptospirosis
Contra-indications. Side-effects. Warnings. See notes at beginning of chapter
Dose. See preparation details, see notes above for vaccination programmes

POM **Canigen L** (Virbac) *UK*
Injection, leptospirosis vaccine, inactivated, prepared from *L. interrogans* serotypes, for *dogs*; 1 mL
Dose. *Dogs*: *by subcutaneous injection*, 1 mL

POM **Eurican L** (Merial) *UK*
Injection, leptospirosis vaccine, inactivated, prepared from *L. interrogans* serotypes, for *dogs*; 1-dose vial
Dose. *Dogs*: *by subcutaneous or intramuscular injection*, 1 dose

POM **Kavak L** (Fort Dodge) *UK*
Injection, leptospirosis vaccine, inactivated, prepared from *L. interrogans* serotypes, for *dogs more than 6 weeks of age*; 1-dose vial
Dose. *Dogs*: *by subcutaneous or intramuscular injection*, 1 dose

POM **Nobivac Lepto** (Intervet) *UK*
Injection, leptospirosis vaccine, inactivated, prepared from *L. interrogans* serotypes, for *dogs more than 8 weeks of age*; 1 mL
Dose. *Dogs*: *by subcutaneous injection*, 1 mL

POM **Vanguard Lepto ci** (Pfizer) *UK*
Injection, leptospirosis vaccine, inactivated, prepared from *L. interrogans* serotypes, for *dogs*; 1 mL
Dose. *Dogs*: *by subcutaneous or intramuscular injection*, 1 mL

18.4.6 Rabies

Rabies is a neurotropic disease capable of affecting virtually all mammals. It exists worldwide, except in places such as the UK and Australasia where it has been excluded by rigorous quarantine. In countries where the disease is enzootic, a number of species including dogs, jackals, racoons, and bats are possible reservoir hosts. In Europe, the red fox is the most important species involved, and may serve as a source of infection for other animals, including dogs and cats, and thence to humans.

The incubation period for rabies in dogs and cats varies from about 9 days to more than a year, but clinical signs usually develop within 2 to 4 weeks of exposure. The clinical signs of classical rabies develop in 3 phases. The prodromal phase lasts 2 to 3 days and is characterised by subtle changes in temperament, mild pyrexia, slow corneal and palpebral reflexes, and signs of irritation at the site of virus entry. During the furious phase the animal becomes increasingly irritable and aggressive, develops progressive disorientation and muscular incoordination, and may have seizures. This phase usually lasts for a day or so, but may continue for up to one week, after which the animal enters the dumb or paralytic phase and develops progressive and terminal paralysis. Laryngeal and pharyngeal paralysis lead to drooling and frothing at the mouth and respiratory paralysis causes coma and death after 2 to 4 days. Atypical or chronic rabies is believed to be rare, although more common than previously thought. In atypical rabies the prodromal or furious phases can last for several months during which virus may be shed in saliva; some dogs and cats are believed to have clinically recovered.

If rabies is suspected, the animal must be held in isolation on the premises where seen and the local DVO notified immediately. Anyone coming in contact with the animal should change contaminated clothing and undertake immediate personal disinfection. No other animals should enter the premises and the names and addresses of any possible contacts (for example, in the surgery waiting room) should be recorded.

Most wild animals entering the UK (other than from the Republic of Ireland) can do so only under licence and should, in general, undergo 6 months quarantine. Quarantine will only apply to domestic animals such as horses, cattle, sheep, pigs, if there is suspicion of contact with infected animals (but note that other disease-based restrictions may apply to these species). Under the *Pets Travel Scheme (PETS)* implemented in the UK, pet dogs and cats may be brought into the UK through certain routes without being placed under quarantine if certain requirements are met. The animal must be identified by microchip and then vaccinated against rabies. Supplies of rabies vaccine in the UK are now freely available to veterinarians. About 30 days after vaccination, a blood sample should be taken from the animal and tested for rabies antibodies at an authorised laboratory. If a protective antibody titre of at least 0.5 units/mL is demonstrated, the owner should then obtain a Pet Health Certificate from a LVI in the UK. Manufacturers have indicated that some animals, in particular young animals, may not show this level of antibody titre after one vaccination; veterinarians may consider giving two vaccinations to such animals.

Further information on requirements for PETS may be obtained from:
• PETS Helpline
telephone: (0)870 2411710

facsimile: (0)20 79046834

e-mail: pets@ahvg.maff.gsi.gov.uk

• MAFF: www.maff.gov.uk/animalh/quarantine

In addition to vaccination, 24 to 48 hours before returning to the UK, the animal must be treated for ticks using an approved acaricide, and the tapeworm *Echinococcus multilocularis* using praziquantel.

Dogs and cats may be vaccinated from 4 weeks of age, in which case a further dose should be given at 11 or 12 weeks of age (vaccination from 3 months of age is required for PETS). Dogs and cats more than 11 or 12 weeks of age need only be given one dose of vaccine. Booster vaccinations should be administered every 2 years in dogs and cats. However health regulations and requirements in certain countries specifiy that dogs must be revaccinated annually. Horses and cattle are usually vaccinated at 6 months of age. They may be vaccinated from 2 months of age and then revaccinated at 6 months of age. An annual booster vaccination is required to maintain immunity in horses and cattle.

UK

Indications. Vaccination against rabies

Contra-indications. Pregnant animals, see notes at beginning of chapter

Side-effects. Warnings. See notes at beginning of chapter

Dose. See preparation details, see notes above for vaccination programmes

POM **Nobivac Rabies** (Intervet) *UK*

Injection, rabies vaccine, inactivated, prepared from virus grown on cell-line tissue culture, containing aluminium phosphate as adjuvant, for *horses, cattle, dogs, cats*; 1 mL

Dose. *Horses, cattle*: *by intramuscular injection*, 1 mL

Dogs, cats: *by subcutaneous or intramuscular injection*, 1 mL

POM **Rabisin** (Merial) *UK*

Injection, rabies vaccine, inactivated, prepared from virus strain GS 57 Wistar, containing aluminium hydroxide as adjuvant, for *dogs, cats*; 1 mL

Dose. *Dogs*: *by subcutaneous or intramuscular injection*, 1 mL

Cats: *by subcutaneous injection*, 1 mL

18.4.7 Tetanus

See section 18.1.6

18.4.8 Combination vaccines for dogs

An alphabetical list of combination vaccines for dogs and the infections to which they confer immunity is given in Table 18.2.

UK

Indications. See individual vaccines

Contra-indications. Live vaccines should not be used in pregnant animals, see notes at beginning of chapter

Side-effects. Warnings. See notes at beginning of chapter

Dose. See preparation details, see manufacturer's details for vaccination programmes

POM **Canigen PPi** (Virbac) *UK*

Injection, powder for reconstitution, combined CPV and PI vaccine, living, prepared from viruses grown on cell-line tissue culture, for *dogs*; 1-dose vial

Note. May be reconstituted with Canigen L

Dose. *Dogs*: *by subcutaneous injection*, 1 dose

POM **Canigen DHPPi** (Virbac) *UK*

Injection, powder for reconstitution, combined CDV, CPV, ICH, and PI vaccine, living, prepared from CDV, CPV, CAV 2, and PI virus type 2, all grown on cell-line tissue culture, for *dogs*; 1-dose vial

Note. May be reconstituted with Canigen L

Dose. *Dogs*: *by subcutaneous injection*, 1 dose

POM **Eurican DHPPi** (Merial) *UK*

Injection, powder for reconstitution, combined CDV, CPV, and ICH vaccine, living, prepared from CDV, CPV, CAV 2, and PI virus type 2, for *dogs*; 1-dose vial

Note. May be reconstituted with Eurican L

Dose. *Dogs*: *by subcutaneous injection*, 1 dose

POM **Kavak DA₂PiP69** (Fort Dodge) *UK*

Injection, powder for reconstitution, combined CDV, CPV, ICH, and PI vaccine, living, prepared from CDV, CPV, CAV 2, and PI virus type 2, for *dogs*; 1-dose vial

Note. May be reconstituted with Kavak L

Dose. *Dogs*: *by subcutaneous injection*, 1 dose

POM **Kavak Galaxy** (Fort Dodge) *UK*

Injection, 2 fractions for reconstitution, Kavak DA₂PiP69 and Kavak L, for *dogs*; two 1-dose vials

Dose. *Dogs*: *by subcutaneous injection*, 1 combined dose

POM **Nobivac DH** (Intervet) *UK*

Injection, powder for reconstitution, combined CDV and ICH vaccine, living, prepared from CDV strain grown on cell-line tissue culture, CAV 2 strain grown on cell-line tissue culture, for *dogs*; 1-dose vial

Note. May be reconstituted with Nobivac Lepto

Dose. *Dogs*: *by subcutaneous injection*, 1 dose

POM **Nobivac DHPPi** (Intervet) *UK*

Injection, powder for reconstitution, combined CDV, CPV, ICH, and PI vaccine, living, prepared from CDV, CPV, CAV 2, and PI virus, all grown on cell-line tissue culture, for *dogs*; 1-dose vial

Note. May be reconstituted with Nobivac Lepto

Dose. *Dogs*: *by subcutaneous injection*, 1 dose

POM **Nobivac PPi** (Intervet) *UK*

Injection, powder for reconstitution, combined CPV and PI vaccine, living, prepared from viruses grown on cell-line tissue culture, for *dogs*; 1-dose vial

Note. May be reconstituted with Nobivac Lepto

Dose. *Dogs*: *by subcutaneous injection*, 1 dose

POM **Nobivac Puppy DP** (Intervet) *UK*

Injection, powder for reconstitution, combined CDV and CPV vaccine, living, prepared from viruses grown on cell-line tissue culture, for *puppies 6 to 7 weeks of age*; 1-dose vial

Dose. *Puppies*: *by subcutaneous injection*, 1 dose

POM **Quantum Dog 7** (Schering-Plough) *UK*

Injection, 2 fractions for reconstitution, combined living CDV, CPV, ICH, and PI and inactivated leptospirosis vaccine, prepared from CDV, CPV, CAV 2, PI virus type 2, and *L. interrogans* serotypes, for *dogs*; two 1-dose vials

Dose. *Dogs*: *by subcutaneous injection*, 1 combined dose

POM **Quantum Dog CPV-L** (Schering-Plough) *UK*

Injection, combined living CPV and inactivated leptospirosis vaccine, prepared from CPV and *L. interrogans* serotypes, for *dogs*; 1-dose vial

Dose. *Dogs*: *by subcutaneous injection*, 1 dose

POM **Vanguard 7** (Pfizer) *UK*

Injection, 2 fractions for reconstitution, living CDV, CPV, ICH, and PI, and inactivated leptospirosis vaccine, prepared from CDV strain Snyder-Hill, CPV strain NL-35-D, CAV 2 strain CAV-2 Manhattan, PI virus NL-CPI-5 strain, grown on an established canine cell line, *L. interrogans* serotypes, for *dogs*; two 1-dose vials

Dose. *Dogs*: *by subcutaneous injection*, 1 combined dose

Table 18.2 Combination vaccines for dogs available in the UK

	Canine distemper virus	Canine parvovirus	Infectious canine hepatitis	Leptospirosis	Parainflenza
Canigen PPi (Virbac)		•			•
Canigen DHPPi (Virbac)	•	•	•		•
Eurican DHPPi (Merial)	•	•	•		
Kavak DA$_2$ PiP69 (Fort Dodge)	•	•	•		•
Kavak Galaxy (Fort Dodge)	•	•	•	•	•
Nobivac DH (Intervet)	•		•		
Nobivac DHPPi (Intervet)	•	•	•		•
Nobivac PPi (Intervet)		•			•
Nobivac Puppy DP (Intervet)	•	•			
Quantum Dog 7 (Schering-Plough)	•	•	•	•	•
Quantum Dog CPV-L (Schering-Plough)		•		•	
Vanguard 7 (Pfizer)	•	•	•	•	•
Vanguard CPV-L (Pfizer)		•		•	

POM **Vanguard CPV-L** (Pfizer) *UK*
Injection, combined living CPV and inactivated leptospirosis vaccine, prepared from CPV strain NL-35-D, *L. interrogans* serotypes, for *dogs*; 1 mL
Dose. *Dogs*: *by subcutaneous injection*, 1 mL

> Accidental self-injection with oil-based vaccines can cause severe pain and intense swelling, which may result in ischaemic necrosis and loss of a digit. Prompt medical attention is essential

18.4.9 Immunoglobulins for dogs

Endotoxin-specific immunoglobulins act by neutralising endotoxin produced by a wide variety of Gram-negative bacteria including *Salmonella* spp., *E. coli* serotypes, *Serratia marcescens*, *Shigella flexneri*, *Klebsiella pneumoniae*, and *Pseudomonas aeruginosa*. These bacteria may contribute to a number of diseases such as gastro-enteritis, septic metritis, septicaemia, or shock. Other appropriate treatment such as antibacterials, NSAIDs, and fluid therapy may be necessary to counteract the clinical signs of toxaemia.

UK

Indications. Treatment and prophylaxis of endotoxaemia
Contra-indications. Side-effects. Warnings. Safety in pregnant animals has not been established
Dose. See preparation details

POM **Stegantox 10** (Schering-Plough) *UK*
Injection, powder for reconstitution, 2 mg endotoxin-specific immunoglobulin G/mL, for *dogs*
Dose. *Dogs*: *by slow intravenous injection*, 500 micrograms/kg. May be repeated after 24 hours

A preparation of combined antisera is available to provide passive immunity to dogs against parvovirus infection (see section 18.4.2), canine distemper (see section 18.4.1), and infectious canine hepatitis (see section 18.4.3).

The antisera preparation may be used in animals exposed to infection. Antiserum will provide passive immunity to parvovirus, distemper, and hepatitis for up to 14 days but to ensure antibody titres above protective levels, it is recommended that repeat doses are given at 10 day intervals. The serological status of animals should be determined prior to active immunisation against parvovirus.

POM **Maxagloban P** (Intervet) *UK*
Injection, combined CDV, CPV, and ICH antiserum, prepared from canine serum containing antibodies to CDV, CPV, and ICH virus, for *dogs*; 5 mL
Dose. *By subcutaneous or intramuscular injection*. *Dogs*: treatment, 0.4 mL/kg
Prophylaxis, 0.2 mL/kg (increase to 1 mL/kg for parvovirus if risk of infection is high)

18.5 Immunological preparations for cats

18.5.1 Chlamydiosis
18.5.2 Feline leukaemia
18.5.3 Feline panleucopenia
18.5.4 Feline viral respiratory disease complex
18.5.5 Rabies
18.5.6 Combination vaccines for cats

Immunisation programmes for cats may depend on whether the animal is kept in a multi-cat household or cattery. Post vaccination reactions have been reported in cats vaccinated with inactivated vaccines. Clinical signs are notably marked lethargy of short duration. Vaccine induced fibrosarcomata at the site of injection have been reported in North America and their incidence in the UK is increasing.

18.5.1 Chlamydiosis

Feline chlamydial infection (feline pneumonitis) is a bacterial infection caused by *Chlamydophila felis* (*Chlamydia psittaci*), which results in severe and sometimes persistent conjunctivitis, and marked ocular discharge. Other effects may include mild sneezing and nasal discharge.

The vaccine (available in combination vaccines, see section 18.5.6) protects reasonably well against clinical disease, but not infection. Specific antibacterials may also be used to control both disease and infection. Therapy should include both topical and systemic treatment. Antibacterial eye ointment (see section 12.2.1) containing chlortetracycline should be applied frequently. Systemic therapy includes oral doxycycline (see section 1.1.2) 5 mg/kg♦ one to two times daily. Treatment should be continued for 4 weeks or until 2 weeks after cessation of clinical signs. All cats in the group, whether or not clinically affected, should be treated.

18.5.2 Feline leukaemia

Infection with feline leukaemia virus (FeLV) may lead to several outcomes, depending mainly on the age of the cat when it is infected and the dose of infecting virus. Following exposure, some cats undergo transient infection and recover; some cats appear to recover but remain latently infected, although most of these eventually eliminate the infection; and some cats develop persistent viraemia. Young kittens are most susceptible to the virus, and over 16 weeks of age, only a minority of exposed cats will develop persistent infection. Most persistently viraemic cats die within 2 to 3 years of exposure as a result of FeLV-related diseases such as lymphosarcoma, myeloid leukaemia, anaemia, and immunosuppression.

Cats may be vaccinated from 9 weeks of age with a second dose 2 to 4 weeks later, depending on the vaccine. Pregnant queens may or may not be vaccinated, depending on the vaccine. Annual booster vaccination is recommended where cats are exposed to infection; if not exposed or when exposure is predicted in previously unexposed cats, earlier revaccination may be required, although there are no guide-lines for this situation.

Vaccination will not induce protection in cats that are already viraemic. Therefore, it is sometimes recommended that all cats should be tested for the presence of viraemia before vaccination. This may be done using the widely available FeLV ELISA test, by virus isolation, or both. The vaccines do not interfere with methods for detecting the presence of p27 circulating viral antigen.

There has been considerable debate concerning the relative efficacy of the FeLV vaccines available in the UK. The published evidence is largely contradictory with vaccines which appear very efficacious in one trial showing less effi-cacy in other trials.

Traditionally, control of FeLV infection in colonies has been successfully achieved by the testing and removal of persistently infected cats. Vaccination can be a useful adjunct to control, but it is unwise to discontinue testing and rely on vaccination alone, because a small proportion of vaccinated animals may not be protected against persistent infection. Such cats may develop FeLV-related disease and will also be infectious to others.

UK

Indications. Vaccination against feline leukaemia
Contra-indications. Side-effects. Warnings. Occasional transient malaise post vaccination. See notes above, see notes at beginning of chapter
Dose. See preparation details, see notes above for vaccina-tion programmes

POM **Fevaxyn FeLV** (Fort Dodge) *UK*
Injection, feline leukaemia vaccine, inactivated, prepared from whole virus subgroups A and B, containing a suitable adjuvant, for *cats*; 1 mL
Contra-indications. Pregnant cats
Dose. *Cats*: *by subcutaneous injection*, 1 mL

POM **Leucogen** (Virbac) *UK*
Injection, feline leukaemia vaccine, inactivated, p45 FeLV envelope antigen, containing aluminium hydroxide and a saponin derivative as adjuvants, for *cats*; 1 mL
Contra-indications. Vaccination of pregnant queens not recommended
Dose. *Cats*: *by subcutaneous or intramuscular injection*, 1 mL

POM **Leukocell 2** (Pfizer) *UK*
Injection, feline leukaemia vaccine, inactivated, glycoprotein gp 70 envelope antigen, viral antigens subtypes A, B, C, and FOCMA, containing a suitable adjuvant, for *cats*; 1 mL
Dose. *Cats*: *by subcutaneous injection*, 1 mL

POM **Nobivac FeLV** (Intervet) *UK*
Injection, feline leukaemia vaccine, inactivated, p45 FeLV envelope antigen, containing aluminium hydroxide and a saponin derivative as adjuvants, for *cats*; 1 mL
Contra-indications. Vaccination of pregnant queens not recommended
Dose. *Cats*: *by subcutaneous or intramuscular injection*, 1 mL

POM **Quantum Cat FeLV** (Schering-Plough) *UK*
Injection, feline leukaemia vaccine, inactivated, viral antigens subtypes A, B, C, and FOCMA, containing a suitable adjuvant, for *cats*; 1-dose vial
Dose. *Cats*: *by subcutaneous injection*, 1 dose

18.5.3 Feline panleucopenia

Feline panleucopenia (FPL), or feline infectious enteritis, is a highly infectious disease of domestic cats, other Felidae,

and certain other species such as mink. There is only one serotype of the virus and it is highly immunogenic. When vaccination has been carried out, it has been extremely suc-cessful in controlling the disease.

Live vaccines are available. Live vaccines probably induce a more rapid onset of protection than inactivated vaccines, and are more likely to be able to overcome low levels of maternally-derived antibody. Live vaccines are contra-indi-cated during pregnancy because FPL virus may cross the placenta and induce cerebellar hypoplasia in kittens.

Vaccination (especially with live vaccines) should not be performed in unhealthy animals because wild-type FPL virus is immunosuppressive.

In most kittens, maternally-derived antibody has declined to non-interfering levels by 12 weeks of age. Therefore, from this age onwards, for most vaccines, one dose is usually suf-ficient. An additional dose should be given at 16 weeks of age when maternally-derived antibody is likely to be unusu-ally high, for example if the queen has been exposed to nat-ural infection or disease. Young kittens from 6 to 8 weeks of age onwards may be vaccinated, but require additional doses at 2 to 4 week intervals, ensuring the last dose is at 12 weeks or later.

Antibody titres, following vaccination with live vaccine, have been shown to persist for at least 4 years, and for over one year following administration of inactivated vaccines. An initial booster vaccination at one year of age is, how-ever, advisable, with revaccination every 1 to 2 years there-after, particularly in high risk situations or where natural boosting is unlikely.

Following an outbreak of FPL, vaccination should be accompanied by thorough cleansing of premises with an appropriate disinfectant because the virus is extremely sta-ble and high levels of virus may accumulate in the environ-ment.

UK

Indications. Vaccination against feline panleucopenia (FPL)
Contra-indications. Live vaccines should not be used in pregnant animals, see notes at beginning of chapter
Side-effects. Warnings. See notes above, see notes at beginning of chapter
Dose. See preparation details, see notes above for vaccina-tion programmes

POM **Feliniffa P** (Merial) *UK*
Injection, powder for reconstitution, FPL vaccine, living, prepared from virus, for *cats*; 1-dose vial
Note. May be reconstituted with Feliniffa RC
Contra-indications. Kittens of Burmese, Siamese, and similar breeds; avoid anthelmintic treatment within 7 days
Dose. *Cats*: *by subcutaneous injection*, 1 dose

18.5.4 Feline viral respiratory disease complex

Feline herpesvirus 1 (Feline viral rhinotracheitis, FVR) and feline calicivirus are the two main causes of upper respira-tory-tract disease in cats and account for the majority of cases. Bacteria, particularly *Bordetella bronchiseptica*, may also be implicated in feline respiratory disease complex. Feline calicivirus infection is generally milder than feline herpesvirus and is often associated with mouth ulceration and also a febrile lameness syndrome. There is only one strain of feline herpesvirus, but there are a number of strains of feline calicivirus. Most are closely related antigenically, and strains selected for vaccine use have broad antigenicity. Nevertheless, current vaccines do not protect against some strains and widespread use of particular vaccines may encourage selection for these.

In previously healthy, unexposed cats, vaccines induce reasonable protection against clinical disease, although not necessarily against infection. Both respiratory viruses are extremely widespread and clinically healthy carriers are common. Therefore, management measures, such as early weaning and isolation, are often necessary to ensure that kittens are not already incubating the disease, or are perhaps already carriers at the time of vaccination.

Live virus vaccines (see section 18.5.6 for combination vaccines) are normally quite safe but apparent vaccine reactions do sometimes occur. These may take the form of mild respiratory and oral signs, or sometimes lameness, some 6 to 7 days after vaccination. Most cases are probably caused by co-incidental infection with field virus, but some may be due to vaccine virus itself. There are occasional reports that if a vaccine is inadvertently given via the oral or respiratory route, for example, if a cat licks the injection site or an aerosol is made with the syringe, then clinical signs may develop. Also, under some circumstances, live vaccines may occasionally generalise. Therefore, in completely virus-free colonies of cats an inactivated vaccine might be preferable. It is inadvisable to vaccinate pregnant queens with live vaccines.

In general, kittens should be vaccinated initially at 9 weeks of age, when in most cases maternally-derived antibody has declined to non-interfering levels. A second dose is given 2 to 4 weeks later. However, the duration of maternally-derived antibody can be quite variable; for feline herpesvirus, antibody may last for 2 to 10 weeks and for feline calicivirus, antibody may persist for up to 10 to 14 weeks. Little work has been done in relating maternally-derived antibody levels to either protection or interference with vaccination.

Annual revaccination is usually recommended, but in some high-risk situations, vaccination every 6 months may be advisable.

UK

Indications. Vaccination against feline calicivirus infection and feline herpesvirus infection

Contra-indications. Live vaccines should not be used in pregnant animals, see notes at beginning of chapter

Side-effects. **Warnings**. See notes above, see notes at beginning of chapter

Dose. See preparation details, see notes above for vaccination programmes

POM **Feliniffa RC** (Merial) *UK*
Injection, combined feline calicivirus and feline herpesvirus vaccine, inactivated, containing a suitable oil as adjuvant, for *cats*; 1-dose vial
Note. May be reconstituted with Feliniffa P
Dose. *Cats: by subcutaneous injection*, 1 dose

Accidental self-injection with oil-based vaccines can cause severe pain and intense swelling, which may result in ischaemic necrosis and loss of a digit. Prompt medical attention is essential

---

18.5.5 Rabies

See section 18.4.6

18.5.6 Combination vaccines for cats

An alphabetical list of combination vaccines for cats and the infections to which they confer immunity is given in Table 18.3.

UK

Indications. See individual preparations
Contra-indications. Pregnant animals, see notes at beginning of chapter
Side-effects. **Warnings**. See notes at beginning of chapter
Dose. See preparation details, see manufacturer's details for vaccination programmes

POM **Feligen RCP** (Virbac) *UK*
Injection, powder for reconstitution, combined feline calicivirus, FPL, and feline herpesvirus vaccine, living, prepared from FPL virus DSV strain LR72, feline herpesvirus strain F2, feline calicivirus strain F9, for *cats*; 1-dose vial
Dose. *Cats: by subcutaneous injection*, 1 dose

POM **Felocell CVR** (Pfizer) *UK*
Injection, powder for reconstitution, combined feline calicivirus, FPL, and feline herpesvirus vaccine, living, prepared from FPL virus strain 'Snow Leopard', feline herpesvirus strain FVRm, feline calicivirus strain F9, grown on NLFK-1 feline kidney cell line, for *cats*; 1 mL
Dose. *Cats: by subcutaneous or intramuscular injection*, 1 mL

POM **Fel-O-Vax 4** (Fort Dodge) *UK*
Injection, powder for reconstitution, combined feline calicivirus, FPL, feline herpesvirus, and feline chlamydiosis vaccine, inactivated, prepared from viruses and *Chlamydophila felis*, for *cats*; 1-dose vial
Dose. *Cats: by subcutaneous injection*, 1 dose

POM **Fevaxyn Pentofel** (Fort Dodge) *UK*
Injection, powder for reconstitution, combined feline calicivirus, FPL, feline herpesvirus, FeLV, and feline chlamydiosis vaccine, inactivated, prepared from viruses and *Chlamydophila felis*, for *cats*; 1-dose syringe
Dose. *Cats: by subcutaneous injection*, 1 dose

POM **Katavac CHP** (Fort Dodge) *UK*
Injection, powder for reconstitution, combined feline calicivirus, FPL, and feline herpesvirus vaccine, living, prepared from viruses grown on an established feline cell line, for *cats*; 1-dose vial
Dose. *Cats: by subcutaneous injection*, 1 dose

POM **Katavac Eclipse** (Fort Dodge) *UK*
Injection, 2 fractions for reconstitution, Katavac CHP and Fevaxyn FeLV, for *cats*; two 1-dose vials
Dose. *Cats: by subcutaneous injection*, 1 combined dose

POM **Nobivac Tricat** (Intervet) *UK*
Injection, powder for reconstitution, combined feline calicivirus, FPL, and feline herpesvirus vaccine, living, prepared from viruses grown on cell-line tissue culture, for *cats*; 1-dose vial
Dose. *Cats*: *by subcutaneous or intramuscular injection*, 1 dose

POM **Quantum Cat CVRP** (Schering-Plough) *UK*
Injection, powder for reconstitution, combined feline calicivirus, FPL, and feline herpesvirus vaccine, living, prepared from viruses grown on a continuous cell line, for *cats*; 1-dose vial
Dose. *Cats*: *by subcutaneous or intramuscular injection*, 1 dose

Table 18.3 Combination vaccines for cats available in the UK

	Chlamydiosis	*Feline leukaemia*	*Feline panleucopenia*	*Feline calicivirus and feline herpesvirus*
Feligen RCP (Virbac)			●	●
Felocell CVR (Pfizer)			●	●
Fel-O-Vax 4 (Fort Dodge)	●		●	●
Fevaxyn Pentofel (Fort Dodge)	●	●	●	●
Katavac CHP (Fort Dodge)			●	●
Katavac Eclipse (Fort Dodge)		●	●	●
Nobivac Tricat (Intervet)			●	●
Quantum Cat CVRP (Schering-Plough)			●	●

18.6 Immunological preparations for birds

18.6.1   Avian coccidiosis
18.6.2   Avian encephalomyelitis
18.6.3   Avian infectious bronchitis
18.6.4   Avian infectious bursal disease
18.6.5   Avian reovirus
18.6.6   Chicken anaemia virus
18.6.7   Duck virus enteritis
18.6.8   Duck virus hepatitis
18.6.9   Duck septicaemia
18.6.10 Egg drop syndrome 1976
18.6.11 Erysipelas
18.6.12 Fowl pox
18.6.13 Infectious laryngotracheitis
18.6.14 Marek's disease
18.6.15 Newcastle disease
18.6.16 Paramyxovirus 3 disease
18.6.17 Pasteurellosis
18.6.18 Pigeon paramyxovirus
18.6.19 Pigeon pox
18.6.20 Post-natal colibacillosis
18.6.21 Salmonellosis
18.6.22 Swollen head syndrome
18.6.23 Turkey haemorrhagic enteritis
18.6.24 Turkey rhinotracheitis
18.6.25 Combination vaccines for birds

Vaccine administration. Vaccines may be administered to birds in the drinking water, by spraying, by beak dipping, by intranasal or intra-ocular instillation, by injection of birds, by injection of eggs during incubation, or by wing-stab or footstab techniques. To avoid any adverse interactions vaccines should not be administered within 7 days of a previous vaccination, unless administered simultaneously as a recognised combination vaccine, and in any case only in accordance with the manufacturer's recommendations.

When administering live virus vaccines in the **drinking water** it is often advisable to add skimmed milk powder, at the rate of 2 to 4 g/litre, to the water that is to be used to dilute the vaccine. This prolongs the life of the virus. Whole milk should not be used for this purpose because the fat content may block automatic drinking systems and lead to separation and hence poor distribution of the vaccine.

Before vaccination, water can be withheld for up to two hours. Withholding water for longer than this, especially in hot weather, can lead to excessive competition when water is reconnected, overcompensation of water intake, wet droppings, and deterioration in litter conditions. Drinking water dispensers ('drinkers') should be checked to ensure that there are sufficient available to allow birds to drink the water containing the vaccine over 1 to 2 hours without undue competition. Vaccine can be administered in the water via in-line dose medicators, the header tank, or by filling of individual drinking water dispensers. This should be done with the least disturbance to the birds, although birds should remain active and be encouraged to drink usu-

ally by simultaneously offering food as a stimulus to drink. The amount of water required varies with the age of bird, the type of bird, and the vaccine used. The manufacturer's directions should be followed.

Live virus vaccines may be administered by **spraying**. The vaccine is diluted using freshly boiled and cooled purified water, and sprayed over the birds using machinery adjusted to suit the particular environment and requirements. Spray volumes and equipment should be regularly checked and monitored. Operators should wear suitable face masks.

Specialist advice should be sought from the vaccine manufacturer as to the most appropriate equipment to deliver consistent and appropriate droplet size for the vaccine being administered.

Coarse spraying in the hatchery is suitable for day-old chicks. For use on chicks, the amount of vaccine sufficient for 1000 birds is diluted in 300 to 400 mL of water at 25°C. Larger volumes may be appropriate for some vaccines. When spraying, it is important that all the birds are wetted and then allowed to stand in their boxes to dry, avoiding draughts. Older birds are penned together in groups in dim light. The vaccine is diluted in water at a rate of 1 to 1.5 litres per 1000 doses. The birds are sprayed from a distance of approximately 45 centimetres from above ensuring that droplets fall on them. The light intensity should be returned to normal to allow birds to 'drink' droplets from the bodies of other birds. Thereafter the birds are allowed to dry for 10 to 15 minutes, avoiding direct heat because this may affect the efficacy of the vaccine.

Aerosol spraying is used on birds that are 10 days of age or over. The vaccine is diluted in 30 to 40 mL of water per 1000 doses. After preparing the vaccine and machines, the lighting is dimmed and the ventilation reduced. Spray is directed over the heads of the birds for about 2 minutes for 5000 birds, keeping the ventilation and lights off for a total time of 10 minutes. Longer periods without ventilation may stress the birds. Advice on the most appropriate droplet size and volume, together with equipment, may vary for different vaccines and such advice should always be sought from the manufacturer of a particular vaccine.

Other methods of vaccination include **intranasal** or **intra-ocular instillation**. Sufficient vaccine for 1000 doses is diluted in 40 to 50 mL of sterile water at 25°C such that one drop contains the required dose. The vaccine is then instilled into one eye or one nostril. In the latter case, the other nostril is held closed until the bird has inhaled the vaccine.

Vaccines may also be administered by **injection**. Intramuscular injection of an inactivated oil-based vaccine is usually given into the breast or thigh muscles. Other vaccine solutions may be given by subcutaneous or intramuscular injection into the fold of the skin at the back of the neck in poultry or the base of the neck in pigeons. Pigeons should not be fed for 12 hours before vaccination because a distended crop may distort the anatomy of the injection site. Duck virus hepatitis vaccine is given by the **footstab** technique, which is described in section 18.6.8. Some living vaccines may be authorised for vaccination of eggs during incubation.

> Before vaccinating a flock, it is important that a veterinary surgeon with experience in dealing with poultry should be consulted because vaccination programmes vary from site to site.

18.6.1 Avian coccidiosis

To avoid problems of drug resistance and the continuous use of medication to control *Eimeria* spp. in domestic poultry, a live attenuated oral vaccine is available for the control of coccidiosis in chickens. The vaccine consists of recognised selected precocious strains of each of the pathogenic species of coccidia that affect chickens. The precocious strains are those with a short pre-patent period, which means that they have short developmental stages and hence cause minimal damage to the intestines of birds but are capable of stimulating immunity.

The vaccine is given as a single dose at one day of age or between 5 and 9 days of age, depending on the vaccine. A single dose is sufficient to protect broilers, broiler breeders in rear, and replacement layer pullets.

UK

Indications. Vaccination against avian coccidiosis
Contra-indications. Side-effects. Warnings. See notes at beginning of chapter
Dose. See notes at beginning of section 18.6 for methods of administration, see notes above for vaccination programmes

POM **Paracox** (Schering-Plough) *UK*
By addition to drinking water or feed, avian coccidiosis vaccine, living, prepared from *Eimeria* spp., for *chickens 5 to 9 days of age*; 100 mL, 500 mL
Withdrawal Periods. *Poultry*: slaughter withdrawal period nil

POM **Paracox 5** (Schering-Plough) *UK*
By addition to feed, avian coccidiosis vaccine, living, prepared from *Eimeria* spp., for *chickens at one day of age*; 100 mL, 500 mL
Withdrawal Periods. *Poultry*: slaughter withdrawal period nil

18.6.2 Avian encephalomyelitis

Viral encephalomyelitis or epidemic tremor is caused by a picornavirus. The disease is manifested by CNS signs such as ataxia and tremors in young chicks. Infection in laying birds may result in reduced egg production and hatchability.

Vaccination of layers and breeders with a live vaccine will protect both laying birds and their progeny. Live vaccines are administered in drinking water. All breeders and layer hens should be vaccinated between 10 and 16 weeks of age. Chicks under 3 weeks of age should not be exposed to vaccine or vaccinated stock.

UK

Indications. Vaccination against avian encephalomyelitis
Contra-indications. Eggs for hatching should not be taken for the first 4–5 weeks after vaccination; see also notes at beginning of chapter
Side-effects. Warnings. May cause a clinical reaction in chicks; decreased egg production in older birds; see also notes at beginning of chapter
Dose. See notes at beginning of section 18.6 for methods of administration, see notes above for vaccination programmes

PML **AE–Vac** (Fort Dodge) *UK*
By addition to drinking water, powder for reconstitution, avian encephalomyelitis vaccine, living, prepared from virus, for *chickens between 10 weeks of age and 4 weeks before laying*; 1000-dose vial

PML **Nobilis AE 1143** (Intervet) *UK*
By addition to drinking water, powder for reconstitution, avian encephalomyelitis vaccine, living, prepared from virus strain Calnek 1143, for *chickens 8 weeks of age and over*; 1000-dose vial
Withdrawal Periods. *Poultry*: slaughter withdrawal period nil, should not be used in layers and at least 1 month before commencement of laying

18.6.3 Avian infectious bronchitis

Avian infectious bronchitis is caused by a coronavirus and infection can result in lesions in the respiratory tract, oviduct, and kidneys. Egg production may fall and egg quality problems are common in infected layers.

Live virus vaccines are available; the organisms are either highly attenuated (H120) or less attenuated (H52). The figures indicate the number of egg passages through which the strains are passed to produce the desired degree of attenuation. A cloned live vaccine, which is reported to be more immunogenic and causes fewer vaccine reactions, is also available (Nobilis IB Ma5, Intervet).

All vaccination programmes for parent stock should commence with a mild live vaccine (H120 or cloned) at 3 weeks of age, followed by a booster dose at 7 weeks of age with a mild live vacccine or H52. Broilers are usually afforded protection by using a mild live vaccine administered by spray to day-old chicks in the hatchery, and also sometimes live vaccine given in the drinking water or by spray at 2 to 4 weeks of age.

Infectious bronchitis variant infections have been identified in poultry in the UK and other European countries. One specific variant denoted variously as 793/B, 4-91, or CR88 has been associated with respiratory disease in broilers and egg production problems in layers. Live vaccines specifically developed against this serotype are available (Nobilis IB 4-91, Intervet and Gallivac IB 88, Merial). Vaccination programme recommendations are specific for the different vaccines. Other variants continue to emerge and specific new variant vaccines will be sought.

UK

Indications. Vaccination against avian infectious bronchitis
Contra-indications. Use of H52 or inactivated vaccine for primary vaccination, or on premises where primary vaccination has not been carried out

Side-effects. **Warnings**. See notes at beginning of chapter, vaccination during the laying period may be accompanied by a transient drop in egg production

Dose. See preparation details, see notes at beginning of section 18.6 for methods of administration, see notes above for vaccination programmes

POM **Gallivac IB88** (Merial) *UK*
By spraying, powder for reconstitution, avian infectious bronchitis vaccine, living, prepared from virus strain CR88121 (793B), for *chickens at 14 days of age*
Withdrawal Periods. *Poultry*: slaughter withdrawal period nil
Note. Should not be used in future layers or breeders, or chickens in lay

POM **Nobilis IB 4-91** (Intervet) *UK*
By addition to drinking water, by coarse spraying, by intranasal or intra-ocular instillation, powder for reconstitution, avian infectious bronchitis vaccine, living, prepared from virus strain 4-91, for *chickens more than 8 days of age*; 1000-dose vial, 2500-dose vial, other sizes available
Withdrawal Periods. *Poultry*: slaughter withdrawal period nil
Note. Should not be used in layers or broiler breeders

PML **Nobilis IB H-52** (Intervet) *UK*
By addition to drinking water, powder for reconstitution, avian infectious bronchitis vaccine, living, prepared from virus Mass. type strain H52, for *chickens*; 1000-dose vial
Withdrawal Periods. *Poultry*: slaughter withdrawal period nil, egg withdrawal period nil

PML **Nobilis IB H-120** (Intervet) *UK*
By addition to drinking water, powder for reconstitution, avian infectious bronchitis vaccine, living, prepared from virus Mass. type strain H120, for *chickens*; 1000-dose vial, 2500-dose vial, other sizes available
Withdrawal Periods. *Poultry*: slaughter withdrawal period nil, egg withdrawal period nil

PML **Nobilis IB Ma5** (Intervet) *UK*
By addition to drinking water, by spraying, by intranasal or intra-ocular instillation, powder for reconstitution, avian infectious bronchitis vaccine, living, prepared from virus Mass. type strain Ma5, for *chickens*; 1000-dose vial, 2500-dose vial, other sizes available
Withdrawal Periods. *Poultry*: slaughter withdrawal period nil, egg withdrawal period nil

PML **Poulvac H120** (Fort Dodge) *UK*
By addition to drinking water, coarse or aerosol spraying, powder for reconstitution, avian infectious bronchitis vaccine, living, prepared from virus Mass. type strain H120, for *chickens from 1 day of age*; 1000-dose vial, 2500-dose vial, 5000-dose vial
Withdrawal Periods. *Poultry*: slaughter withdrawal period nil

PML **Poulvac IBMM** (Fort Dodge) *UK*
By addition to drinking water (birds more than 4 days of age)*, by spraying, by intranasal or intra-ocular instillation*, powder for reconstitution, avian infectious bronchitis vaccine, living, prepared from virus modified Mass. strain, for *chickens from 1 day of age*; 1000-dose vial, 5000-dose vial

18.6.4 Avian infectious bursal disease

In the UK, infections occur with serotype 1 avian infectious bursal disease virus, which may show varying pathogenicity. Since 1988, an acute highly virulent strain has been active in broilers and replacement layers. Early infection of susceptible birds can result in immunosuppression, while later infection can result in very high mortality.

Live vaccines may be classified as mild, intermediate, or hot depending on their inherent effect on the bursa of Fabricius. Mild vaccines, for example Nobilis Gumboro PBG 98 (Intervet), do not afford protection against virulent challenge but may be used as a primer for replacement breeders. Intermediate strength vaccines such as Poulvac Bursine 2

(Fort Dodge), Gallivac IBD (Merial), or Nobilis Gumboro D78 (Intervet), and hot strain vaccines including Nobilis Gumboro 228E (Intervet) and Poulvac Bursa Plus (Fort Dodge) are effective in broilers.

Broilers with no maternally-derived antibodies may be vaccinated from one day of age with live virus vaccine. Birds with maternally-derived antibodies are vaccinated at 2 to 5 weeks of age, depending on the level and spread of the maternally-derived antibody. Breeding stock receive live virus vaccine at 4 to 5 weeks and, in some cases at 8 weeks, followed by inactivated vaccine at 14 to 18 weeks of age. Replacement layer pullets are vaccinated similarly to broilers; live vaccine is administered via the drinking water from 14 days of age.

Accidental self-injection with oil-based vaccines can cause severe pain and intense swelling, which may result in ischaemic necrosis and loss of a digit. Prompt medical attention is essential

---

UK

Indications. Vaccination against avian infectious bursal disease

Contra-indications. **Side-effects**. **Warnings**. See notes at beginning of chapter

Dose. See preparation details, see notes at beginning of section 18.6 for methods of administration, see notes above for vaccination programme

Live vaccines, mild

PML **Nobilis Gumboro PBG 98** (Intervet) *UK*
By addition to drinking water or spraying, powder for reconstitution, infectious bursal disease vaccine, living (mild), prepared from virus strain PBG 98, for *chickens from 1 day of age*; 1000-dose vial, 2500-dose vial, 5000-dose vial
Withdrawal Periods. *Poultry*: slaughter withdrawal period nil, egg withdrawal period nil

Live vaccines, intermediate

POM **Gallivac IBD** (Merial) *UK*
By addition to drinking water, or by coarse spraying (day-old chicks only), powder for reconstitution, infectious bursal disease vaccine, living (potentiated intermediate), prepared from virus strain S706, for *chickens from 1 day of age*; 1000-dose vial, 2000-dose vial, 2500-dose vial, 5000-dose vial
Withdrawal Periods. *Poultry*: slaughter withdrawal period nil, egg withdrawal period nil

POM **Poulvac Bursine 2** (Fort Dodge) *UK*
By addition to drinking water, or by coarse spraying (day-old chicks only), powder for reconstitution, infectious bursal disease vaccine, living (intermediate), prepared from virus, for *broiler chickens from 1 day of age, layer hens from 14 days of age*; 1000-dose vial, 5000-dose vial, 10 000-dose vial
Withdrawal Periods. *Poultry*: slaughter withdrawal period nil, egg withdrawal period nil

POM **Nobilis Gumboro D78** (Intervet) *UK*
By addition to drinking water, powder for reconstitution, infectious bursal disease vaccine, living (intermediate), prepared from virus strain D78, for *chickens more than 14 days of age*; 1000-dose vial, 2500-dose vial, 5000-dose vial
Withdrawal Periods. *Poultry*: slaughter withdrawal period nil, egg withdrawal period nil

Live vaccines, hot

POM **Nobilis Gumboro 228E** (Intervet) *UK*
By addition to drinking water, powder for reconstitution, infectious bursal disease vaccine, living (hot), prepared from virus strain 228E, for *chickens more than 10 days of age*; 500-dose vial, 1000-dose vial, other sizes available
Withdrawal Periods. *Poultry*: slaughter withdrawal period nil, should not be used in birds in lay

POM **Poulvac Bursa Plus** (Fort Dodge) *UK*
By addition to drinking water, powder for reconstitution, infectious bursal disease vaccine, living (hot), prepared from low attenuation virus, for *chickens from 14 days of age*; 500-dose vial, 1000-dose vial, 5000-dose vial
Withdrawal Periods. *Poultry*: slaughter withdrawal period nil

Combination antisera and live vaccines

POM **Bursamune in Ovo** (Fort Dodge)
Injection, combination infectious bursal disease antiserum and live vaccine, prepared from virus and antiserum, for *embryonated broiler chicken eggs*
Withdrawal Periods. Slaughter withdrawal period nil
Dose. *Eggs*: by intra-ovo injection, 0.05 mL at 18 days of incubation

18.6.5 Avian reovirus

Reoviruses have been isolated from a variety of tissues in chickens affected by assorted disease conditions including viral arthritis, tenosynovitis, malabsorption syndrome, respiratory disease, and enteric disease. Clinical disease depends on the virus pathotype involved.

Breeding stock are vaccinated at 16 to 20 weeks of age in order to afford protection against reovirus in offspring. Birds should not be vaccinated less than 4 weeks before commencement of lay. The optimal effect will be seen in birds primed by live reovirus challenge.

UK

Indications. Vaccination against avian reovirus
Contra-indications. **Side-effects**. **Warnings**. See notes at beginning of chapter
Dose. See preparation details, see notes above for vaccination programmes

POM **Nobilis Reo** (Intervet) *UK*
Injection, avian reovirus vaccine, inactivated, prepared from 2 immunogenic strains of virus grown in cell-line tissue culture, containing a suitable oil as adjuvant, for *chicken breeding stock*; 500 mL
Withdrawal Periods. *Poultry*: slaughter withdrawal period nil
Dose. *Poultry*: by subcutaneous or intramuscular injection, 0.5 mL

18.6.6 Chicken anaemia virus

Chicken anaemia virus or chicken anaemia agent (CAA), a circoviridae virus, is a very resistant virus, and the cause of avian infectious anaemia, first described in Japan in 1979. Disease is usually seen in broilers up to 3 weeks of age and results from vertical transmission from infected breeders, with no circulating antibody. Affected birds show signs associated with immunosuppression, classically gangrenous dermatitis due to secondary bacterial skin infection, and anaemia. Effective vaccination of breeders prevents viraemia and congenital infection in broiler progeny.

The vaccination programme will depend on the site. Poultry should be vaccinated at least 6 weeks before the commencement of lay and should be at least 6 weeks of age.

UK

Indications. Vaccination against chicken anaemia virus
Contra-indications. **Side-effects**. **Warnings**. See notes at beginning of chapter
Dose. See preparation details, see manufacturer's information for vaccination programmes

POM **Nobilis CAV P4** (Intervet) *UK*
Injection, powder for reconstitution, chicken anaemia virus vaccine, living, prepared from virus, for *broiler breeder chickens more than 6 weeks of age*; 500-dose vial, 1000-dose vial, other sizes available
Note. Reconstitute with specific diluent
Withdrawal Periods. *Poultry*: slaughter withdrawal period nil, should not be used in birds in lay or at least 6 weeks before commencement of laying
Dose. *Poultry*: by subcutaneous or intramuscular injection, 0.2 mL

18.6.7 Duck virus enteritis

Duck virus enteritis (duck plague) is an acute highly contagious disease caused by a herpesvirus.

A live virus vaccine is available for vaccinaton of healthy flocks. It can also be used in case of emergency for the vaccination of healthy birds where the disease is present in order to limit the spread of the disease. Before vaccination of diseased flocks, clinically affected birds should be culled.

Birds are vaccinated at 4 weeks of age when disease challenge is mild or absent. When expected risk of infection is high, birds may be vaccinated from one day of age; these birds should be revaccinated at 4 weeks of age or later when maternal antibody levels have declined.

UK

Indications. Vaccination against duck virus enteritis
Contra-indications. **Side-effects**. **Warnings**. See notes at beginning of chapter
Dose. See preparation details, see notes above for vaccination programmes

PML **Nobilis Duck Plague** (Intervet) *UK*
Injection, powder for reconstitution, duck virus enteritis vaccine, living, prepared from virus strain Utrecht, for *ducks, geese*; 500-dose vial, 100-dose vial
Withdrawal Periods. *Ducks, geese*: slaughter withdrawal period nil
Dose. *Ducks, geese*: by subcutaneous or intramuscular injection, 0.25 mL

18.6.8 Duck virus hepatitis

Duck virus hepatitis is an acute highly contagious disease of young ducklings during the first 3 weeks of life.

A live virus vaccine is administered to susceptible day-old ducklings by footstab technique. The vaccine is administered by using a needle, which is gently stabbed through the footweb and slowly withdrawn.

UK

Indications. Vaccination against duck virus hepatitis
Contra-indications. **Side-effects**. **Warnings**. See notes at beginning of chapter
Dose. See preparation details, see notes above for vaccination application and programmes

PML **Duck Virus Hepatitis** (Animal Health Trust) *UK*
Injection, duck virus hepatitis vaccine, living, prepared from virus Rispen H53 passage strain grown in chicken eggs, for **day-old ducklings**; 2 mL, 4 mL
Dose. *Ducks*: *by footstab*, 0.004 mL

18.6.9 Duck septicaemia

Duck septicaemia is caused by *Riemerella anatipestifer* (*Pasteurella anatipestifer*, *Moraxella anatipestifer*). Emergency inactivated vaccines may be made by laboratories (licensed by the VMD) for use on individual farms where this condition is a problem. The following are manufacturers of emergency vaccines in the UK:

* Axiom Veterinary Laboratories
* Leeds Veterinary Laboratories
* Ridgeway Biologicals.
*

18.6.10 Egg drop syndrome 1976

Egg drop syndrome 1976 is caused by an avian adenovirus. The disease is characterised by a fall in egg number with loss of shell strength and pigmentation. Replacement breeding and layer flocks are vaccinated before commencement of lay at 14 to 18 weeks of age. One vaccination is usually sufficient to provide immunity, although in some circumstances a second vaccination may be necessary.

UK

Indications. Vaccination against egg drop syndrome 1976
Contra-indications. Side-effects. Warnings. See notes at beginning of chapter
Dose. See preparation details, see notes above for vaccination programmes

PML **Nobilis EDS** (Intervet) *UK*
Injection, egg drop syndrome 1976 vaccine, inactivated, prepared from virus BC14, containing a suitable oil as adjuvant, for **chickens 14–18 weeks of age**; 500 mL
Withdrawal Periods. *Poultry*: slaughter withdrawal period nil
Dose. *Poultry*: *by subcutaneous injection*, 0.5 mL

> Accidental self-injection with oil-based vaccines can cause severe pain and intense swelling, which may result in ischaemic necrosis and loss of a digit. Prompt medical attention is essential

18.6.11 Erysipelas

Erysipelothrix rhusiopathiae (*Ery. insidiosa*) causes infection in turkeys resulting in sudden mortality. Birds are vaccinated before they reach 14 weeks of age.

UK

Indications. Vaccination against erysipelas
Contra-indications. Side-effects. Warnings. See notes at beginning of chapter
Dose. See preparation details

PML **Suvaxyn Erysipelas** (Fort Dodge) *UK*
Injection, erysipelas vaccine, inactivated, prepared from selected *Ery. rhusiopathiae* strains, containing a suitable adjuvant, for **pigs** (see section 18.3.6), **turkeys more than 8 weeks of age**
Dose. *Turkeys*: *by subcutaneous injection*, (up to 4.5 kg body-weight) 0.5 mL, (>4.5 kg body-weight) 1 mL. Repeat dose every 3 months

18.6.12 Fowl pox

Fowl pox causes cutaneous lesions and diphtheritic lesions of the mouth and upper respiratory tract. No vaccines are currently available in the UK.

18.6.13 Infectious laryngotracheitis

Infectious laryngotracheitis is caused by a herpesvirus capable of causing variable disease, loosely termed acute, mild, or asymptomatic. The virus exhibits typical herpesvirus latency where persistent infection and intermittent excretion are significant in the spread of the disease. Lesions are restricted to the trachea and range from frank blood clots with exudate to more chronic caseous diphtheritic changes. Chickens are vaccinated at more than 4 weeks of age. The vaccine is usually given by intra-ocular instillation. Incorporation into the drinking water is less effective, while use of the spraying method may result in severe losses.

If rearing and laying sites are contaminated, the first vaccination at 4 to 5 weeks of age will need boosting with a further vaccination at 16 to 20 weeks of age. If there are no problems on the rearing site, birds are vaccinated by intra-ocular instillation when they are moved to the laying farms. All birds on the site should be vaccinated.

Advice should be taken from a veterinary surgeon with experience of dealing with poultry before a vaccination programme is started against this infection. Vaccination of layer hens in presence of disease may result in reduced egg production.

Vaccinated birds should not be taken to a site where there are any non-vaccinated birds because the virus is shed from vaccinated birds during the laying period.

UK

Indications. Vaccination against infectious laryngotracheitis
Contra-indications. Side-effects. Warnings. See notes at beginning of chapter and notes above
Dose. See notes at beginning of section 18.6 for methods of administration, see notes above for vaccination programmes

PML **I L T Vaccine** (Fort Dodge) *UK*
By intra-ocular instillation, infectious laryngotracheitis vaccine, living, for **chickens from 4 weeks of age**; 1000-dose vial
Withdrawal Periods. *Poultry*: slaughter withdrawal period nil, egg withdrawal period nil

18.6.14 Marek's disease

Marek's disease is a lymphoproliferative disease of chickens caused by a lymphotropic herpesvirus. Mortality and clinical signs are variable and peripheral nerve involvement may lead to leg and wing paralysis.

Freeze dried vaccines prepared from turkey herpes-virus (THV) and 'wet' cell-associated live vaccines prepared from turkey herpesvirus, attenuated Marek's virus, or non-pathogenic Marek's viruses, are available. The 'wet' vaccines are stored in ampoules in liquid nitrogen and under these conditions (-196.5°C) may be expected to retain their potency for 2 years. The diluent supplied by the manufacturer is stored at 2°C to 8°C. When required for use, the vaccine is rapidly thawed in water at 37°C and then mixed gently with the diluent using a wide bore needle to avoid damage to the vaccine. Reconstituted vaccine should be used within one hour. Because of the nature of the storage conditions, ampoules may shatter, and operators handling these vaccines should be suitably protected, especially from the possibility of glass particles penetrating the eyes. As an alternative to storage in liquid nitrogen, the 'wet' vaccines may be stored in solid carbon dioxide in which case it may be expected to retain its potency for one month from date of purchase. Freeze-dried lyophilised 'dry' live vaccines are also available, which are easier to handle; vaccines are stored at 2°C to 8°C, and the diluent in a cool place below 18°C.

Chicks are ideally vaccinated at day-old in the hatchery, although chickens up to 3 weeks of age may be vaccinated. Vaccination is occasionally repeated at 2 to 4 weeks of age. In conditions of severe challenge, the 'wet' vaccines are more effective than the 'dry' vaccines. In some circumstances, day-old chicks may need to be given a dose of each.

To address more recent problems of virulent Marek's disease in poultry breeding and commercial laying stock in the UK, vaccines incorporating the Rispens strain of Marek's disease virus such as Cryomarex Rispens (Merial), Poulvac Marek CVI (Fort Dodge), or Nobilis Rismavac (Intervet) have been successful, often in combination with THV vaccines.

UK

Indications. Vaccination against Marek's disease
Contra-indications. **Side-effects**. **Warnings**. See notes at beginning of chapter. Liquid nitrogen causes serious freeze burns and thawing ampoules may occasionally explode after removal from liquid nitrogen. Operators should wear appropriate protective clothing
Dose. See preparation details, see notes above for vaccination programmes

PML **Cryomarex Rispens** (Merial) *UK*
Injection, powder for reconstitution, Marek's disease vaccine, living, deep-frozen, cell-associated, prepared from virus strain Rispens CVI988, for *day-old chicks*; 1000-dose vial
Note. Reconstitute with specific diluent
Withdrawal Periods. *Poultry*: slaughter withdrawal period nil
Dose. *Poultry*: *by subcutaneous or intramuscular injection*, 0.2 mL

PML **Nobilis Marek THV lyo** (Intervet) *UK*
Injection, powder for reconstitution, Marek's disease vaccine, living, freeze-dried, cell-free, prepared from turkey herpesvirus strain PB-THV 1, for *day-old chicks, chickens up to 3 weeks of age*; 250-dose vial, 1000-dose vial, 2000-dose vial
Note. Reconstitute with specific diluent
Withdrawal Periods. *Poultry*: slaughter withdrawal period nil
Dose. *Poultry*: *by subcutaneous or intramuscular injection*, 0.2 mL

PML **Nobilis Marexine CA 126** (Intervet) *UK*
Injection, powder for reconstitution, Marek's disease vaccine, living, deep-frozen, cell-associated, prepared from turkey herpesvirus strain FC 126, for *day-old chicks, chickens up to 3 weeks of age*; 1000-dose vial, 2000-dose vial
Note. Reconstitute with specific diluent
Withdrawal Periods. *Poultry*: slaughter withdrawal period nil
Dose. *Poultry*: *by subcutaneous or intramuscular injection*, 0.2 mL

PML **Nobilis Rismavac** (Intervet) *UK*
Injection, powder for reconstitution, Marek's disease vaccine, living, deep-frozen, cell-associated, prepared from virus strain CVI 998, for *chickens*; 1000-dose vial, 2000-dose vial
Note. Reconstitute with specific diluent
Withdrawal Periods. *Poultry*: slaughter withdrawal period nil
Dose. *Poultry*: *by subcutaneous or intramuscular injection*, 0.2 mL

PML **Nobilis Rismavac + CA126** (Intervet) *UK*
Injection, powder for reconstitution, Marek's disease vaccine, living, deep-frozen, cell-associated, prepared from Marek's disease virus CVI 998, turkey herpesvirus strain FC 126, for *chickens*; 1000-dose vial, 2000-dose vial
Note. Reconstitute with specific diluent
Withdrawal Periods. *Poultry*: slaughter withdrawal period nil
Dose. *Poultry*: *by subcutaneous or intramuscular injection*, 0.2 mL

PML **Poulvac Marek CVI** (Fort Dodge) *UK*
Injection, powder for reconstitution, Marek's disease vaccine, living, deep-frozen, cell-associated, prepared from Marek's disease virus strain Rispens CVI 988 grown on tissue culture, for *day-old chicks*; 1000-dose vial
Note. Reconstitute with specific diluent
Withdrawal Periods. *Poultry*: slaughter withdrawal period nil
Dose. *Poultry*: *by intramuscular injection*, 1 dose

PML **Poulvac Marek CVI + HVT** (Fort Dodge)
Injection, powder for reconstitution, Marek's disease vaccine, living, deep-frozen, cell-associated, prepared from Marek's disease virus strain Rispens CVI 988 grown on tissue culture, turkey herpesvirus, for *day-old chicks*
Withdrawal Periods. *Poultry*: slaughter withdrawal period nil
Dose. *Poultry*: *by subcutaneous injection 0.5 mL intramuscular injection*, 0.2 mL

PML **Poulvac MD-Vac** (Fort Dodge) *UK*
Injection, powder for reconstitution, Marek's disease vaccine, living, freeze-dried, prepared from turkey herpesvirus grown on chicken tissue culture, for *day-old chicks*; 1000-dose vial
Note. Reconstitute with specific diluent
Dose. *Poultry*: *by intramuscular injection*, 0.1 mL

PML **Poulvac MD-Vac (Frozen-Wet)** (Fort Dodge) *UK*
Injection, powder for reconstitution, Marek's disease vaccine, living, deep-frozen, prepared from turkey herpesvirus Witter strain, for *day-old chicks*; 1000-dose vial
Note. Reconstitute with specific diluent
Withdrawal Periods. *Poultry*: slaughter withdrawal period nil
Dose. *Poultry*: *by intramuscular injection*, 0.2 mL

18.6.15 Newcastle disease

Newcastle disease ('fowl pest') is a notifiable disease of poultry. The disease is caused by a group of closely related viruses which form the avian paramyxovirus type 1 (PMV-1) serotype. Viruses vary in their virulence from lentogenic (mild) to velogenic (highly virulent). Strains may show a tendency to cause nervous, visceral, or respiratory disease. Live freeze-dried vaccines and oil-based inactivated vaccines are available for vaccination against Newcastle disease in chickens, turkeys, and game birds. PMV-1 vaccines are also available for use in pigeons (see section 18.6.18). Vaccination programmes depend upon the degree of challenge in any geographical area. In areas of little challenge or no challenge, chicken and turkey broilers are not vaccinated. Replacement pullets receive a live virus vaccine at 3 weeks and 10 weeks of age, followed by an inactivated vaccine between 16 and 18 weeks of age. In areas of high challenge, broilers are vaccinated with live vaccines at one day of age, 3 weeks, and 5 weeks of age. Replacement pullets receive the same regimen followed by a further course of live vaccine at 10 weeks and inactivated vaccine at 16 weeks. Revaccination with live vaccine during lay may be necessary in exceptional circumstances. Similar programmes may be recommended for game birds where challenge from wild birds is considered a risk.

The live vaccine can be more effective when administered by the aerosol spraying method than via the drinking water. More birds are covered and a more rapid immune response is produced in individual birds. The response depends on droplet size, previous priming, and the strain of live vaccine used. It is important to follow the manufacturer's directions on these aspects.

The Diseases of Poultry Order 1994 (SI 1994/3141) gives procedures to be followed regarding movement of birds, disinfection of premises, and vaccination to ensure continued protection from Newcastle disease.

UK

Indications. Vaccination against Newcastle disease
Contra-indications. **Side-effects**. **Warnings**. See notes at beginning of chapter. Live Newcastle disease vaccines may cause conjunctivitis in humans and operators should wear appropriate protective clothing
Dose. See preparation details, see notes at beginning of section 18.6 for methods of administration, see notes above for vaccination programmes

Live vaccines

PML **Nobilis ND Clone 30** (Intervet) *UK*
By addition to drinking water, or by spraying, powder for reconstitution, Newcastle disease vaccine, living, prepared from virus strain Clone 30, for *chickens*; 1000-dose vial, 2500-dose vial
Withdrawal Periods. *Poultry*: slaughter withdrawal period nil

PML **Nobilis ND Hitchner** (Intervet) *UK*
By addition to drinking water, powder for reconstitution, Newcastle disease vaccine, living, prepared from virus strain Hitchner B1, for *chickens*; 1000-dose vial, 2500-dose vial, 5000-dose vial
Withdrawal Periods. *Poultry*: slaughter withdrawal period nil, egg withdrawal period nil
Note. May be administered by spraying or beak dipping in emergency after prior consultation with the manufacturer

PML **Poulvac Hitchner B1** (Fort Dodge) *UK*
By addition to drinking water, by spraying, by intranasal or intra-ocular instillation, powder for reconstitution, Newcastle disease vaccine, living, prepared from virus strain Hitchner B1, for *chickens, turkeys, game birds*; 1000-dose vial, 5000-dose vial
Withdrawal Periods. *Poultry*: slaughter withdrawal period nil, egg withdrawal period nil

PML **Poulvac NDW** (Fort Dodge) *UK*
By spraying, by intranasal or intra-ocular instillation, powder for reconstitution, Newcastle disease vaccine, living, prepared from attenuated strain of virus, for *chickens*; 5000-dose vial
Withdrawal Periods. *Poultry*: slaughter withdrawal period nil, egg withdrawal period nil

Inactivated vaccines

> Accidental self-injection with oil-based vaccines can cause severe pain and intense swelling, which may result in ischaemic necrosis and loss of a digit. Prompt medical attention is essential

PML **Nobilis Newcavac** (Intervet) *UK*
Injection, Newcastle disease vaccine, inactivated, prepared from virus strain Clone 30, containing a suitable oil as adjuvant, for *chickens, turkeys, guinea fowl, pheasants, ducks*; 1000-dose vial
Withdrawal Periods. *Poultry*: slaughter withdrawal period nil
Dose. *Poultry, game birds*: *by subcutaneous or intramuscular injection*, 0.5 mL

18.6.16 Paramyxovirus 3 disease

In turkeys, avian paramyxovirus type 3 (PMV-3) infection has been associated with reduced egg production and mild respiratory disease in breeding hens. Protection of birds in lay can be achieved using the combination inactivated vaccine TUR3, Merial (see section 18.6.25).

18.6.17 Pasteurellosis

Pasteurellosis covers a variety of conditions associated with *Pasteurella* spp. infections. The predominant condition is fowl cholera due to *P. multocida* infection.

Inactivated vaccines for fowl cholera alone and combination vaccines against erysipelas and *Pasteurella* are available. The latter (see section 18.6.25) appears to give better protection against fowl cholera than the former. They are mainly used in turkeys, although they are occasionally necessary for broiler breeder flocks and pheasants.

Turkey breeding flocks may be vaccinated at 12, 16, and 28 weeks of age. Occasionally vaccination has to be brought forward, if challenge occurs at an earlier age. There is very little protection from the first dose of vaccine. It is inadvisable to give the oil-based vaccine to birds in lay.

Fattening turkeys and breeding chickens are given 2 vaccines at an interval of 4 to 5 weeks, with the initial vaccine administered at 8 to 12 weeks of age.

Outbreaks of disease may still occur following this type of vaccination programme if challenge is with a serotype not covered by the available vaccines.

Emergency vaccines (see section 18.6.9) may be prepared by licensed laboratories where the *Pasteurella* serotype is not covered by those in the commercial vaccines.

UK

Indications. Vaccination against pasteurellosis
Contra-indications. Birds in lay
Side-effects. **Warnings**. See notes at beginning of chapter
Dose. See preparation details, see notes above for vaccination programmes

PML **Pabac** (Fort Dodge) *UK*
Injection, pasteurellosis vaccine, inactivated, prepared from polyvalent types of *Pasteurella multocida*, containing a suitable oil as adjuvant, for *chickens, turkeys, geese, ducks*; 500 mL
Withdrawal Periods. *Poultry*: slaughter 6 weeks; should not be used in layer hens
Dose. *Poultry*: *by subcutaneous injection*, 0.5 mL

18.6.18 Pigeon paramyxovirus

Paramyxovirus type 1 (PMV-1) infection can cause profuse green diarrhoea, marked nervous signs, and mortality, especially in young birds. The virus can potentially spread to commercial poultry.

Birds may be vaccinated at any time over 3 to 6 weeks of age by subcutaneous injection at the base of the neck with an aqueous inactivated vaccine. All pigeons in the loft should be vaccinated. Vaccination should be carried out at least 2 weeks before the beginning of the racing season or show season. A booster vaccination should be given every 12 months.

Live Newcastle disease vaccine♦ (see section 18.6.15) Hitchner B1 strain may be administered by intra-ocular instillation to pigeons to stimulate a rapid immune response against paramyxovirus. Live vaccine gives protection for a short period only and revaccination should be carried out every 3 months. This vaccine should not be given in the drinking water to pigeons because they may receive an inadequate dose by this method.

During an acute outbreak of paramyxovirus disease the live Hitchner B1 strain vaccine may be given by intra-ocular instillation simultaneously with an injection of the inactivated vaccine.

Under *The Diseases of Poultry Order 1994* (SI 1994/3141), all racing pigeons entered in races or shows, which take place wholly or partly in Great Britain, must be vaccinated against avian paramyxovirus type 1. The legislation gives procedures to be followed regarding movement of birds, disinfection of premises, and vaccination to ensure continued protection of poultry from Newcastle disease.

UK

Indications. Vaccination against pigeon paramyxovirus infection
Contra-indications. Side-effects. Warnings. See notes at beginning of chapter
Dose. See preparation details, see notes above for vaccination programmes

P **Colombovac PMV** (Fort Dodge) *UK*
Injection, pigeon paramyxovirus vaccine, inactivated, prepared from avian paramyxovirus (PMV-1), containing a suitable adjuvant, for *pigeons*; 10 mL, 20 mL
Withdrawal Periods. *Pigeons*: slaughter withdrawal period nil
Dose. *Pigeons*: *by subcutaneous injection*, 0.2 mL
Note. POM in Northern Ireland

P **Nobivac Paramyxo** (Intervet) *UK*
Injection, pigeon paramyxovirus vaccine, inactivated, prepared from avian paramyxovirus (PMV-1), containing a suitable oil as adjuvant, for *pigeons*; 20 mL, 50 mL
Withdrawal Periods. *Pigeons*: slaughter withdrawal period nil
Dose. *Pigeons*: *by subcutaneous injection*, 0.25 mL

18.6.19 Pigeon pox

Pigeon pox is caused by a poxvirus and is characterised by lesions of the mouth and eyes.

Birds are vaccinated from 5 weeks of age and all birds in the loft should be vaccinated at the same age. Annual vacci-nation is given outside the racing season between 30 September and 31 December.

Birds are vaccinated on the lower leg or breast. A few feathers are removed and the vaccine is brushed into the plucked follicles; the vaccine should be applied in one direction only. A reaction should be observed in about 4 days. In birds that produce little or no reaction, the vaccination may be repeated in 5 to 7 days; birds that are already immune from previous vaccination are unlikely to show any reaction.

During the period between vaccination and healing of the vaccination site, birds are infectious and should be isolated from other stock until the reaction has subsided.

UK

Indications. Vaccination against pigeon pox
Contra-indications. Side-effects. Warnings. See notes at beginning of chapter
Dose. See notes above for application and vaccination programme

PML **Nobivac Pigeon Pox** (Intervet) *UK*
By topical application, powder for reconstitution, pigeon pox vaccine, living, prepared from virus, for *pigeons more than 5 weeks of age*; 50-dose vial
Withdrawal Periods. *Pigeons*: slaughter withdrawal period nil
Note. Vaccine should not be exposed to sunlight

18.6.20 Post-natal colibacillosis

E. coli infection with recognised avian serotypes can lead to significant mortality in local and generalised infection of broilers, and contributes to peritonitis and septicaemia in commercial layers and broiler breeders. Vaccination of breeding stock will help reduce challenge to young chicks and may afford protection in laying birds.

Breeder birds are vaccinated at 6 to 12 weeks of age and again at 14 to 18 weeks of age. There should be an interval of at least 6 weeks between vaccinations. Vaccination of broiler breeders provides partial immunisation of broiler chickens up to one month of age.

UK

Indications. Vaccination against post-natal colibacillosis
Contra-indications. Side-effects. Warnings. See notes at beginning of chapter
Dose. See preparation details, notes above for vaccination programmes

POM **Nobilis E. coli inac** (Intervet) *UK*
Injection, post-natal colibacillosis vaccine, inactivated, prepared from F-11 and FT *E. coli* antigens, for *broiler breeder chickens*; 250 mL, 500 mL
Withdrawal Periods. *Poultry*: slaughter withdrawal period nil
Dose. *Poultry*: *by subcutaneous or intramuscular injection*, 0.5 mL

18.6.21 Salmonellosis

Salmonellosis as a specific disease of poultry is rare, except in broilers where there is heavy site contamination and early challenge or through vertical transmission from a breeder flock. Such disease is usually the result of infection with one of the so called 'invasive' strains.

Salmonella infection of poultry flocks has been associated with human infection through consumption of eggs and poultry meat. For the past 10 years, numerically, the most significant has been due to *Salmonella enteritidis*. Efficient vaccination of layer breeders, broiler breeders, and commercial layers is considered one of a number of useful control strategies in limiting spread of infection when used in combination with other measures. A specific inactivated *S. enteritidis* vaccine is available for breeding stock to eliminate spread via vertical transmission and commercial egg layers to reduce contamination rate in eggs for human consumption. The usual dosage regimen for breeders and commercial layers is two doses given at an interval of 6 weeks and between 10 and 18 weeks of age.

UK

Indications. Vaccination against salmonellosis
Contra-indications. Side-effects. Warnings. See notes at beginning of chapter
Dose. See preparation details

POM **Salenvac** (Intervet) *UK*
Injection, salmonellosis vaccine, inactivated, prepared from *Salmonella enteritidis* phage type 4, containing aluminium hydroxide as adjuvant, for *poultry*; 250 mL, 500 mL
Withdrawal Periods. *Poultry*: slaughter withdrawal period nil
Dose. *Poultry*: *by intramuscular injection*, 0.1 mL at 1 day of age, 0.5 mL at 10 weeks of age, and 0.5 mL at 18 weeks of age

18.6.22 Swollen head syndrome

The avian pneumovirus originally associated with turkey rhinotracheitis (TRT) in turkeys has been demonstrated as a contributory factor in acute respiratory syndromes of broilers. Egg production problems and nervous signs have been reported in commercial layers, layer breeders, and broiler breeders following infection with the same virus. Vaccines based on the original turkey isolate (Nobilis TRT, Intervet, or Poulvac TRT, Fort Dodge) and one based on a specific chicken isolate (Nemovac, Merial) are available to vaccinate broilers.

Live vaccines may also be used as live primers for breeding stock and commercial layers, followed with an injectable inactivated vaccine.

UK

Indications. Vaccination against swollen head syndrome
Contra-indications. Side-effects. Warnings. See notes at beginning of chapter
Dose. See notes at beginning of section 18.6 for methods of administration. Vaccination programmes will depend on the site and advice should be sought from the site veterinarian, the manufacturer, or both

POM **Nemovac** (Merial) *UK*
By addition to drinking water, swollen head syndrome vaccine, living, for *broiler chickens*; 1000-dose vial
Withdrawal Periods. *Poultry*: slaughter withdrawal period nil, should not be used in layer hens

POM **Nobilis TRT** (Intervet) *UK*
By spraying, intranasal, or intraocular instillation, turkey rhinotracheitis vaccine, living, prepared from virus, for *turkeys* (see section 18.6.24), *broiler chickens*; 500-dose vial, 1000-dose vial, other sizes available
Withdrawal Periods. *Poultry*: slaughter withdrawal period nil

POM **Poulvac TRT** (Fort Dodge) *UK*
By spraying or intraocular instillation, powder for reconstitution, turkey rhinotracheitis vaccine, living, prepared from virus strain Clone K, for *turkeys from 1 day of age* (see section 18.6.24), *broiler chickens from 1 day of age*; 1000-dose vial, 2000-dose vial, 5000-dose vial
Withdrawal Periods. *Poultry*: slaughter withdrawal period nil, should not be used in birds in lay

18.6.23 Turkey haemorrhagic enteritis

Haemorrhagic enteritis in turkeys is caused by an adenovirus and is characterised by acute diarrhoea and high mortality.

A live vaccine is available in the UK under an exceptional marketing authorisation. The vaccine is available only on specific order from Merial. Use of the vaccine must be monitored by the company and reported to the VMD. Broiler turkey poults are vaccinated at 4 weeks of age.

UK

Indications. Vaccination against turkey haemorrhagic enteritis
Contra-indications. Side-effects. Warnings. See notes at beginning of chapter; not for vaccination of breeders and future layers; avoid other vaccination within 14 days; avoid stress prior to vaccination

POM **Dindoral** (Merial)
By addition to drinking water, turkey haemorrhagic enteritis vaccine, living, prepared from virus strain Domermuth, for *broiler turkey poults*
Withdrawal Periods. Slaughter withdrawal period nil

18.6.24 Turkey rhinotracheitis

Turkey rhinotracheitis (TRT) is caused by pneumovirus infection. Live and inactivated vaccines are available. The live vaccine is available for protection of turkeys against rhinotracheitis and broilers against the adverse effects of TRT virus infection.

The live vaccination programme will depend on the site and advice should be sought. The vaccine should not be used on sites where TRT has not been diagnosed unless challenge is anticipated. Use of the vaccine may not be appropriate on some multi-age sites.

The inactivated vaccine is used in birds of 28 weeks of age. The birds should receive the live TRT vaccine, followed 4 to 6 weeks later by vaccination with the inactivated vaccine.

UK

Indications. Vaccination against turkey rhinotracheitis
Contra-indications. Side-effects. Warnings. See notes at beginning of chapter
Dose. See notes at beginning of section 18.6 for methods of administration

Live vaccines

POM **Nobilis TRT** (Intervet) *UK*

By spraying, intranasal, or eyedrop instillation, powder for reconstitution, turkey rhinotracheitis vaccine, living, prepared from virus, for *turkeys, broiler chickens* (see section 18.6.22); 500-dose vial, 1000-dose vial, other sizes available

Withdrawal Periods. *Poultry:* slaughter withdrawal period nil

Dose. *Turkeys:* vaccination programme will depend on the site and advice should be sought

POM **Poulvac TRT** (Fort Dodge) *UK*

By spraying or eyedrop instillation, powder for reconstitution, turkey rhinotracheitis vaccine, living, prepared from virus strain Clone K, for *turkeys from 1 day of age, broiler chickens from 1 day of age* (see section 18.6.22); 1000-dose vial, 2000-dose vial, 5000-dose vial

Withdrawal Periods. *Poultry:* slaughter withdrawal period nil, should not be used in birds in lay

Inactivated vaccines

POM **Nobilis TRT inac** (Intervet) *UK*

Injection, turkey rhinotracheitis vaccine, inactivated, prepared from virus, containing a suitable oil as adjuvant, for *turkeys*; 500 mL

Withdrawal Periods. *Turkeys:* slaughter withdrawal period nil, should not be used in laying birds or at least 4 weeks before commencement of lay

Dose. *Turkeys: by subcutanous or intramuscular injection,* 0.5 mL

18.6.25 Combination vaccines for birds

An alphabetical list of combination vaccines for poultry and the infections to which they confer immunity is given in Table 18.4.

UK

Indications. See preparation details

Contra-indications. Side-effects. Warnings. See notes at beginning of chapter

Dose. See notes at beginning of section 18.6 for methods of administration, see manufacturer's details for vaccination programme

P **Colombovac PMV/Pox** (Fort Dodge)

Injection, combined paramyxovirus and pigeon pox vaccine, prepared from inactivated avian paramyxovirus (PMV-1), live pigeon pox virus strain DD, for *pigeons*

Withdrawal Periods. Slaughter withdrawal period nil

Dose. *Pigeons: by subcutaneous injection,* 0.2 mL

PML **Nobilis IB + G + ND** (Intervet) *UK*

Injection, combined avian infectious bronchitis, avian infectious bursal disease, and Newcastle disease vaccine, inactivated, prepared from avian infectious bronchitis virus strain M41, avian infectious bursal disease virus strain D78, Newcastle disease virus strain Clone 30, containing a suitable oil as adjuvant, for *chickens 14–20 weeks of age*; 500 mL

Withdrawal Periods. *Poultry:* slaughter withdrawal period nil

Dose. *Poultry: by subcutaneous or intramuscular injection,* 0.5 mL

PML **Nobilis IB + ND + EDS** (Intervet) *UK*

Injection, combined avian infectious bronchitis, egg drop syndrome 1976, and Newcastle disease vaccine, inactivated, prepared from avian infectious bronchitis virus Mass. strain M41, egg drop syndrome virus strain BC14, Newcastle disease virus strain Clone 30, containing a suitable oil as adjuvant, for *chickens 14–20 weeks of age*; 1000-dose vial

Withdrawal Periods. *Poultry:* slaughter withdrawal period nil

Dose. *Poultry: by subcutaneous or intramuscular injection,* 0.5 mL

PML **Nobilis Ma5 + Clone 30** (Intervet) *UK*

By spraying, intranasal or eyedrop instillation, or addition to drinking water, powder for reconstitution, combined avian infectious bronchitis and Newcastle disease vaccine, living, prepared from infectious bronchitis strain Ma5, Newcastle disease virus strain Clone 30, for *chickens more than 1 day of age*; 500-dose vial, 1000-dose vial, 2500-dose vial

Withdrawal Periods. Slaughter withdrawal period nil, egg withdrawal period nil

Side-effects. Vaccination during laying period may cause transient drop in egg production

PML **Nobilis REO + IB + G + ND** (Intervet) *UK*

Injection, combined avian infectious bronchitis, avian infectious bursal disease, Newcastle disease, and reovirus vaccine, inactivated, prepared from avian infectious bronchitis virus Mass. strain M41, immunogenic strains of avian infectious bursal disease virus, Newcastle disease virus strain Clone 30, two immunogenic strains of reovirus, containing a suitable oil as adjuvant, for *chickens 16–20 weeks of age*; 500 mL

Withdrawal Periods. *Poultry:* slaughter withdrawal period nil

Dose. *Poultry: by subcutaneous or intramuscular injection,* 0.5 mL

PML **Nobilis TRT+ IBm + G + ND** (Intervet) *UK*

Injection, combined avian infectious bronchitis, avian infectious bursal disease, Newcastle disease, and turkey rhinotracheitis vaccine, inactivated, prepared from avian infectious bronchitis virus strains Mass. and a variant to D207/D274 serotype, immunogenic strain of avian infectious bursal disease virus, immunogenic strain of Newcastle disease virus, immunogenic strain of turkey rhinotracheitis virus, containing a suitable oil as adjuvant, for *chickens 14–20 weeks of age*; 500 mL

Withdrawal Periods. *Poultry:* slaughter withdrawal period nil

Dose. *Poultry: by subcutaneous or intramuscular injection,* 0.5 mL

PML **Pasteurella-Erysipelas Vaccine** (Intervet) *UK*

Injection, inactivated, prepared from *Ery. rhusiopathiae* strains, *P. multocida* Roberts types 2, 4 of avian origin, containing aluminium hydroxide as adjuvant, for *turkeys, other avian species*; 250 mL, 500 mL

Dose. *Poults more than 6 weeks of age: by subcutaneous or intramuscular injection,* 0.5 mL

Adults: by subcutaneous or intramuscular injection, 1 mL

POM **TUR 3** (Merial)

Injection, combined Newcastle disease, paramyxovirus 3, and turkey rhinotracheitis vaccine, inactivated, prepared from viruses, containing a suitable oil as adjuvant, for *future breeder turkeys*; 150 mL

Withdrawal Periods. Slaughter withdrawal period nil, should not be used in laying birds

Dose. *Turkeys: by intramuscular injection,* 0.3 mL at 8–10 weeks before onset of laying. Repeat at 2–4 weeks before onset of laying

Table 18.4 Combination vaccines for poultry available in the UK

	Avian infectious bronchitis	Avian infectious bursal disease	Egg drop syndrome 1976	Ery-sipelas	Newcastle disease	Para-myxo virus 3	Pasteur-ellosis	Reo-virus	Turkey rhino-tracheitis
Nobilis IB + G + ND (Intervet)	●	●			●				
Nobilis IB + ND + EDS (Intervet)	●		●		●				
Nobilis Ma5 + Clone 30 (Intervet	●				●				
Nobilis REO + IB + G + ND (Intervet)	●	●			●			●	
Nobilis TRT + IBm + G + ND (Intervet)	●	●			●				●
Pasteurella-Erysipelas Vaccine (Intervet)				●			●		
TUR 3 (Merial)					●	●			●

18.7 Immunological preparations for rabbits

18.7.1 Myxomatosis
18.7.2 Viral haemorrhagic disease

Vaccines are usually given for the prevention of disease in exhibition rabbits and those kept for meat or fur production. With the increase in popularity of pet rabbits, vaccination is becoming increasingly important particularly for those kept in rural or semirural locations.

18.7.1 Myxomatosis

Myxomatosis infection affects rabbits and hares, although the English hare is not susceptible to the disease. The disease is caused by myxoma virus, which resembles fibroma virus contained in the vaccine. The virus is transmitted from wild rabbits by mosquitoes and rabbit fleas to domestic animals. The incubation period is 2 to 8 days, and affected animals usually develop swelling of the eyelids and periorbital tissue, and purulent conjunctivitis. Subcutaneous swelling then extends to the face, ears, and anogenital area. Death usually occurs 11 to 18 days after development of clinical signs. Occasionally an animal will survive and lesions regress over a 1 to 3 month period.

Vaccination will protect rabbits from infection. Control during an outbreak also includes use of ectoparasiticides (see section 2.2.1).

UK

Indications. Vaccination against myxomatosis
Contra-indications. Pregnant animals
Side-effects. Occasional transient swelling at injection site
Dose. *Rabbits*: *by intradermal injection,* **0.1 mL and** *by subcutaneous injection,* **0.9 mL**. Revaccinate every 6–12 months

POM **Nobivac Myxo** (Intervet) *UK*
Injection, powder for reconstitution, myxomatosis vaccine, living, prepared from Shope fibroma virus grown on cell-line tissue culture, for *rabbits more than 6 weeks of age*; 1-dose vial
Withdrawal Periods. *Rabbits*: slaughter withdrawal period nil

18.7.2 Viral haemorrhagic disease

Viral haemorrhagic disease (VHD) is a disease of rabbits, which has recently been introduced into the UK.

VHD is caused by a calicivirus and characterised by an acute, often fatal infection. The incubation period is 1 to 3 days and rabbits may die suddenly without development of clinical signs. In other animals clinical signs include anorexia, pyrexia, apathy, prostration, severe signs of CNS disturbance such as convulsions or opisthotonus, dyspnoea, and a mucoid foaming or haemorrhagic nasal discharge. Animals which survive the acute phase of the disease develop jaundice and die a few weeks later. Pathological findings include hepatic necrosis and haemorrhages in various organs.

Domestic rabbits may be vaccinated against the disease. The vaccination programme varies depending on the risk of infection. Revaccination every 12 months is recommended.

UK

Indications. Vaccination against viral haemorrhagic disease (VHD)
Contra-indications. See notes at beginning of chapter
Side-effects. Occasional local reaction at injection site, transient general malaise
Dose. *Rabbits*: (at least 10–12 weeks of age) *by subcutaneous injection,* 1 mL
Risk of infection high, (less than 10 weeks of age), *by subcutaneous injection,* 1 mL. Repeat after 1 month

POM **Cylap** (Fort Dodge) *UK*
Injection, VHD vaccine, inactivated, prepared from virus, containing a suitable oil as adjuvant, for *rabbits*; 1-dose vial
Note. May be used in pregnant animals if animals handled with care

> Accidental self-injection with oil-based vaccines can cause severe pain and intense swelling, which may result in ischaemic necrosis and loss of a digit. Prompt medical attention is essential

18.8 Immunological preparations for fish

18.8.1 Enteric redmouth disease
18.8.2 Erythrodermatitis
18.8.3 Furunculosis
18.8.4 Vibriosis
18.8.5 Combination vaccines for fish

Although effective vaccines have been developed for fish, little is known of the immune response in these animals and its relationship to the protection afforded by vaccination. Cellular protection appears to be more important than humoral immune response.

Vaccines are administered to fish by intraperitoneal injection, by dipping in a vaccine solution (immersion), by passing under a spray of vaccine solution, or by addition to feed. Fish should be anaesthetised before vaccination by injection (see Prescribing for fish).

The dip method is less stressful and less time-consuming than intraperitoneal injection. Dipping allows mass vaccination of small fish (less than 15 g body-weight) and is cost-effective. However, the protection afforded by dipping is not as great as that by intraperitoneal injection. Spraying is not a commonly used method of vaccination.

In general, the higher the water temperature, the quicker the development of immunity. At water temperatures of 10°C immunity will develop within 14 to 21 days. Temperatures below 5°C may result in an inadequate immune response. For effective vaccination of fish and to minimise failure, water temperature should be above 3.5°C and preferably above 5°C. Time should be allowed for immunity to develop.

Fish should be large enough for vaccination. The minimum body-weight is 1 g for dipping and 15 g for intraperitoneal injection. Fish over 5 g body-weight will develop immunity that will last longer than those of 1 to 5 g. For this reason, it may be necessary to give fish weighing 1 to 2 g a booster vaccination when their body-weight is approximately 5 g.

Fish should be handled carefully, avoiding stress, which could result in a disease outbreak. In particular, vaccination by injection can often lead to secondary fungal infection. Care must be taken to control this infection in recently vaccinated fish. Clean water should be used and fish should be healthy. Bacterial gill disease and excess mucus in the gills will prevent vaccine uptake and result in inadequate immune response. In general, protection lasts for one year. Salmon in the sea for longer than one year may have waning immunity. Revaccination should be considered after one year. This will also apply to rainbow trout broodstock and some carp.

In salmon, vaccination in the spring before transfer to seawater may not be possible if the fresh-water temperature is too low. It may, therefore, be necessary to vaccinate fish in the previous autumn and if possible give a booster dose in the following spring. Development of immunity may be reduced because of osmotic changes in salmon undergoing smoltification.

Accidental self-injection with oil-based vaccines can cause severe pain and intense swelling, which may result in ischaemic necrosis and loss of a digit. Prompt medical attention is essential

18.8.1 Enteric redmouth disease

Enteric redmouth disease (yersiniosis) caused by the bacteria *Yersinia ruckeri* is mainly a disease of rainbow trout and exhibits the usual clinical signs associated with Gram-negative septicaemia such as extensive haemorrhages of the skin, fins, and internal organs. Chronic forms of the disease are characterised by skin darkening, exophthalmia, and blindness.

Vaccination provides good protection and dipping is the commonly used method. Dip vaccines are effective but are usually repeated when the fish are over 5 g body-weight. Annual revaccination is recommended. However rainbow trout harvested at 300 to 400 g (table size) will be adequately protected during their short lifetime by one vaccination. Atlantic salmon fry at 1 to 2 grams body-weight are occasionally vaccinated where the disease is endemic.

UK

Indications. Vaccination against enteric redmouth
Contra-indications. Side-effects. See notes at beginning of chapter
Dose. See preparation details

PML **AquaVac ERM** (AVL) *UK*
Dip, enteric redmouth vaccine, inactivated, prepared from *Y. ruckeri* strain Hagerman 1, for ***rainbow trout***; 1 litre
Dose. *Fish*: dilute 1 volume with 9 volumes water.
By dip (fish 1 g body-weight or more), for 30 seconds

PML **AquaVac ERM Oral** (AVL) *UK*
Oral liquid, for addition to feed, enteric redmouth vaccine, inactivated, prepared from *Y. ruckeri* strain Hagerman 1, for ***rainbow trout***; 1 litre
Dose. *Fish*: *by addition to feed,* daily for 15 days

PML **Ermogen** (Vericore AP) *UK*
Dip, enteric redmouth vaccine, inactivated, prepared from *Y. ruckeri* strain Hagerman, for ***rainbow trout***; 1 litre
Dose. *Fish*: dilute 1 volume with 9 volumes water.
By dip (fish 5 g body-weight or more), for 30 seconds

The water temperature of the vaccine solution should not vary more than 2°C to 5°C from the water temperature in the original holding facility

18.8.2 Erythrodermatitis

Erythrodermatitis (ulcer disease) is caused by *Aeromonas salmonicida* and affects cyprinids such as carp; it may also affect goldfish. The organism is a variant of the one that causes furunculosis in salmonids (see section 18.8.3).

18.8.3 Furunculosis

Furunculosis caused by the Gram-negative organism *Aeromonas salmonicida* affects all salmonid species such as rainbow trout and salmon. Atlantic salmon are most susceptible whereas rainbow trout are comparatively resistant to infection. The disease often presents as an acute condition in young fish and a chronic condition in older stock. Clinical signs include skin darkening, haemorrhages throughout the internal organs, and characteristic skin furuncles or 'boils'.

Improved husbandry techniques and the use of more efficient oil-based vaccines have helped to reduce the effect of this serious economic disease. However protection against furunculosis is difficult to achieve. Dip vaccination results in the development of a very low level of immunity, has not been effective in the field, and is largely superseded by vaccination by injection. Injectable vaccines containing an oil adjuvant together with improved husbandry and management have dramatically reduced the incidence of furunculosis on salmon farms. Oral vaccination provides at best temporary protection against furunculosis. It should be used for booster vaccination or temporary protection before effective long-term protection provided by injectable vaccines. Second or repeat vaccination is not required with oil-adjuvated injectable vaccines.

Diseased fish should not be vaccinated because the organism can produce a number of cellular products that may be immunosuppressive.

UK

Indications. Vaccination against furunculosis
Contra-indications. See notes at beginning of chapter
Side-effects. Intraperitoneal injection with oil-adjuvanted vaccine will cause peritoneal reaction which may result in visceral adhesions

POM **Alphaject 1200** (Vetrepharm) *UK*
Injection (oily), furunculosis vaccine, inactivated, prepared from *A. salmonicida*, containing suitable oil as adjuvant, for *Atlantic salmon 16 g or more body-weight*
Withdrawal Periods. *Fish*: slaughter withdrawal period nil
Dose. *Fish: by intraperitoneal injection*, 0.2 mL to anaesthetised fish

PML **AquaVac FNM Plus** (AVL) *UK*
Injection, furunculosis vaccine, inactivated, prepared from *A. salmonicida*, containing Alhydrgel as adjuvant for *Atlantic salmon more than 20 g body-weight*; 500 mL
Dose. *Fish: by intraperitoneal injection*, 0.1 mL to anaesthetised fish

PML **AquaVac Furovac 5** (AVL) *UK*
Dip, furunculosis vaccine, inactivated, prepared from *A. salmonicida*, for *Atlantic salmon, cyrinids, and trout more than 5 g body-weight*; 1 litre
Dose. *Fish*: dilute 1 volume with 9 volumes water.
By dip, for 60 seconds
Injection, furunculosis vaccine, inactivated, prepared from *A. salmonicida*, for *Atlantic salmon, cyrinids, and trout more than 20 g body-weight*; 1 litre
Dose. *Fish: by intraperitoneal injection*, 0.1 mL to anaesthetised fish

PML **AquaVac Furovac 5 Oral** (AVL) *UK*
Oral liquid, for addition to feed, furunculosis vaccine, inactivated, prepared from *A. salmonicida*, for *salmon, trout*; 1 litre
Dose. *Fish: by addition to feed,* daily for 10 days

POM **Furogen 2** (Vericore AP) *UK*
Injection (oily), furunculosis vaccine, inactivated, prepared from *A. salmonicida*, containing a suitable oil as adjuvant, for *Atlantic salmon*; 1 litre
Dose. *Fish: by intraperitoneal injection*, 0.1 mL to anaesthetised fish

PML **Furogen b Immersion** (Vericore AP) *UK*
Dip, furunculosis vaccine, inactivated, prepared from *A. salmonicida*, for *Atlantic salmon, rainbow trout*; 1 litre
Dose. *Fish*: dilute 1 volume with 9 volumes water.
By dip, (fish 5 g body-weight or more) for 60 seconds

18.8.4 Vibriosis

Vibriosis is caused by *Vibrio anguillarum* and affects many species of marine fish. Rainbow trout farmed in the sea are particularly susceptible. Other *Vibrio* spp. can be involved in secondary infection. *V. salmonicida* causes cold water vibriosis (HITRA disease) in Atlantic salmon. Usually seen at colder temperatures, this disease has been observed in fish in Norway and the Shetland Isles. Affected fish are dark and anorexic with distinct haemorrhages on the viscera and also have ascites and anaemia.

Vaccination against *V. anguillarum* is more commonly undertaken in marine-grown rainbow trout than Atlantic salmon. The immersion (dip) vaccine used in rainbow trout destined for the sea is effective. However these fish are usually transferred to the sea at one year of age and over 100 g body-weight when their immunity will be waning. A booster vaccination at this time may be necessary.

The bacteria *Vibrio viscosus* has been implicated in the 'wintersore disease' lesions seen in Atlantic salmon smoults recently introduced to seawater. This disease mainly occurs in colder winter months, and is characterised by large eroded areas of skin over the flanks leading to deeper muscle lesions and death.

UK

Indications. Vaccination against vibriosis
Contra-indications. Side-effects. See notes at beginning of chapter

PML **AquaVac Vibrio 1** (AVL) *UK*
Dip, vibriosis vaccine, inactivated, prepared from *V. anguillarum* biotype I, *V. anguillarum* (*V. ordalii*) biotype II, for *rainbow trout*; 1 litre
Dose. *Fish*: dilute 1 volume with 9 volumes water.
By dip, (fish 2 g body-weight or more) for 30 seconds

18.8.5 Combination vaccines for fish

UK

POM **AquaVac FHV** (AVL) *UK*
Injection (oily), combined furunculosis and vibriosis vaccine, inactivated, prepared from *A. salmonicida*, *V. anguillarum* biotypes I, II, *V. salmonicida*, containing a Montanide ISA 711 as adjuvant, for *Atlantic salmon more than 20 g body-weight*; 500 mL
Contra-indications. Breeding fish
Dose. *Fish: by intraperitoneal injection*, 0.2 mL to anaesthetised fish

POM **Alphaject 4000** (Vetrepharm) *UK*
Injection (oily), combined furunculosis, vibriosis, and cold water vibriosis vaccine, inactivated, prepared from *A. salmonicida* var *salmonicida*, *V. anguillarum* serotypes 01, 02, containing a suitable adjuvant, for *Atlantic salmon 45 g body-weight or more*
Withdrawal Periods. *Fish*: slaughter withdrawal period nil
Dose. *Fish: by intraperitoneal injection*, 0.2 mL to anaesthetised fish

POM **Alphaject 5200** (Vetrepharm) *UK*
Injection (oily), combined furunculosis, vibriosis, cold water vibriosis, and 'wintersore disease' vaccine, inactivated, prepared from *A. salmonicida* var *salmonicida*, *V. anguillarum* serotypes 01, 02, *V. salmonicida*, *V. viscosus*, containing a suitable adjuvant, for *Atlantic salmon 42 g body-weight or more*
Withdrawal Periods. *Fish*: slaughter withdrawal period nil
Dose. *Fish: by intraperitoneal injection*, 0.2 mL to anaesthetised fi

19 HERBAL MEDICINES

Contributor:
C E I Day MA, VetMB, MRCVS

So-called alternative or complementary therapies are becoming widely used particularly in Europe and the USA. The main forms of therapy included under this title are: acupuncture (not discussed here), herbal medicine (phytotherapy), homoeopathy, and aromatherapy.

Traditional *herbal medicine* diverges in philosophy and practical use from modern conventional medicine. It involves the use of plants in therapeutic doses, often using a number of different herbs in combination, to treat a patient's clinical signs. The herbs are selected according to the individual animal's perceived needs on the basis of their direct pharmacological actions, but are used in a more holistic fashion than modern conventional medicines (see below).

Homoeopathy is often confused with herbal medicine. Homoeopathy is based on the principle of 'like should be treated by like' and involves the administration, usually in extreme dilutions, of those remedies that, in larger doses, are able to produce symptoms in a healthy individual most closely mimicking those expressed by the diseased patient. The mechanism of action is unclear but research based on energy realms continues. Specific postgraduate study in veterinary homoeopathy is available and should be undertaken prior to using this exacting form of therapy.

Aromatherapy or the use of essential oils is also frequently confused with herbal medicine. Aromatic oils used in aromatherapy are extracted from plants but those oils are pharmacologically very powerful and have specific effects which are different from the whole plant. The potential side-effects or toxicity of plants may be enhanced by the method of extraction in some cases. The use of and the principles of action of essential oils also requires specific prior study becasue toxicity is a potential risk.

Administration of herbal medicines. Herbal medicines are available in several different forms. The most common form is whole plant or the active portion of the plant, dried and chopped or powdered. This may be administered via the food, made into tablets, or incorporated in a sugar coating for ease of administration. The herb may alternatively be made into a liquid in several ways. It can be made into a tea or tisane by infusion. Plants containing those active ingredients which are more difficult to extract can be decoted (prepared slowly over a low heat in a pan). Those containing a significant proportion of volatile oils may best be prepared by maceration (soaked in cold water for about twelve hours), the resultant mixture is warmed gently, strained to remove residual plant debris, and may be sweetened with honey or syrup for palatability. Alternatively, an alcoholic extract (tincture) of a plant may be made and stored in glass dropper bottles for simplicity of dosing.

This form is not widely acceptable to animals unless diluted or added to food.

Herbal medicines may also be employed for external use, being made into compresses, ointments, or creams for direct application to lesions. Poultices of various herbs are a traditional form of treatment for injuries and ulcers.

In a more modern approach, the pharmacologically-active ingredients from plant material may be identified, extracted, purified, and used as the medicine, discarding the remainder of the plant. This is not the traditional and empirically developed method and the resultant medicine is clearly different in nature from the original plant substance. Arguments surround this method. Proponents believe it is a safer, more effective, more easily controlled means of applying herbal medicine. Opponents maintain that the method removes a plant 'drug' from its holistic whole-plant context, thus changing its mode of action, removing synergists, and rendering the resultant medicine more likely to produce side-effects.

Traditional herbal medicines are selected to help the body to regain balance and restore homoeostasis. Modern drugs modify specific biochemical and physiological processes of the body. This is the fundamental difference between traditional herbal medicine and modern science. It is in this more complex and esoteric field that the concurrent use of either modern drugs or chemically extracted active ingredients of plants, alongside herbal medicines, may disturb the delicate intended purpose of the traditional herbalist. **Concurrently administered modern medicines have the potential to delay or to destroy the balancing action of herbal medicines and, as a general rule, should not be used at the same time.** It is recommended to allow at least one week to elapse between the use of modern drugs and herbal medicines, unless there has been an intended depot or residual effect of the modern drug, in which case the period should be extended accordingly.

Herbs are classified in modern herbal medicine according to their spheres of action. Many herbs contain ingredients which provide the whole plant with several such actions combined in the one medicine. Recognised actions include alterative, anodyne, anthelmintic, anticatarrhal, antiemetic, anti-inflammatory, antilithic, antibacterial, antifungal, antispasmodic, aperient/laxative, aromatic, astringent, bitter, cardiac, carminative, cathartic/purgative, cholagogue and anticholagogue, demulcent, diaphoretic, diuretic, ecbolic, emetic, emollient, expectorant, febrifuge, galactagogue, hepatic, hypnotic, nervine, rubefacient, sedative, sialogogue, soporific, stimulant, styptic, tonic, vesicant, and vulnerary.

Alternatively, herbal medicines may be classified according to the category of constituents in the composition. Constituents include acids, alcohols, alkaloids, anthraquinones, bitters, carbohydrates, cardiac glycosides, coumarins, flavones, flavonoid glycosides, phenols, saponins, tannins, and volatile oils.

Herbal medicines are traditionally selected according to the perceived needs of the patient and based upon the individual herb's constituents in relation to the above mentioned actions. Whether single herbs are used or a combination of herbs is selected depends upon the spread of activity of each herb and whether or not it supplies the necessary spectrum of action in the body.

It is of fundamental importance in herbal medicine that plants are identified correctly. They should be harvested from unpolluted areas (where possible) and should, if cultured, be grown without the use of modern agrochemicals. It is advisable that where possible, indigenous species should be used because they may prove more suited to the patient's constitution than exotic herbs.

Use of herbal medicines. The types of conditions for which herbal medicines are commonly used in veterinary practice include anxieties and mental conditions, locomotor disorders, digestive or cardiovascular disturbances, parasitism, pregnancy and parturition, and skin conditions. A full list for an experienced herbalist could cover the entire spectrum of disease.

Proprietary preparations of herbal medicines are available (see below). These preparations contain ingredients that conform to the identification and specifications given in the British Herbal Pharmacopoeia. Single herbs and combinations of herbs are tested in the context of certain disease situations or in general health applications and may then receive a marketing authorisation for use in that application. The formulae are based on traditional practice and the wisdom behind the selection is based upon years of human experience and practice. However, the use of these medicines does not recognise the importance of the individual patient in the same way as does traditional herbalism nor does it select combinations of plants according to the perceived unique needs of the individual patient. Nevertheless, the products have been used for many years with success in their stated fields and serve as a useful bridge to herbal medicine for the practitioner not experienced or trained in the folklore wisdom of traditional herbal medicine.

Side-effects of herbal medicines. The safety of herbal medicines is of paramount importance. For proprietary preparations the manufacturer's guidelines on dosage should be strictly observed. If concurrent conventional medication is being administered for the same purpose, the *combined* dosage may become an important factor and must be taken into account if the modern drug is likely to have a similar action or is related to the herbal medicine.

The administration of more toxic agents such as Aristolochia, Bryony, Deadly Nightshade, Foxglove, Hemlock, Horsetail, Lobelia, Monkshood, Mugwort, and St John's Wort should be avoided because dosage and application are of critical importance and because experience, skill, and close monitoring of the patient are required for their safe usage.

Plants may contain toxic substances and care must be employed in their use. They should only be used in combination if their effects are known to be synergistic, since their actions have the potential not only to counteract each other but also to combine in a more toxic whole. Similar warnings apply to the concurrent use of conventional drugs, in that the properties of the two can combine, the sum of the whole being different in quality from the parts or even potentially toxic. It is therefore also strongly recommended to avoid the simultaneous use of conventional medicines and herbal medicines unless the combined activity is quite clear and is not potentially harmful.

Drug residues must be taken into consideration when treating animals used in competitions or food-producing animals. Herbal medicines should not be used before slaughter of food-producing animals or before competition unless they are known to be potentially available as part of that animal's *natural diet* in a grazing context.

Herbal 'substitutes' for modern drugs are currently being marketed. These should only be used if the claims can be supported by data of quality, safety, and efficacy and if they are not likely to suppress signs of disease such that proper medical attention may be delayed.

As with the use of all medicines, warnings should always be given to observe the animal carefully during the administration of herbal medicines in order to identify any allergy or idiosyncratic reaction. In additon, herbal medicines should be used with caution during pregnancy. Many nervines, stimulants, or tonics may affect the fetus. If there is doubt, herbal medicines should not be administered to pregnant animals.

Storage of herbal medicines. In general, herbs should be collected fresh each year and stocks not accumulated such that supplies overrun the year's requirements. Dried herbs should be stored in glass containers in a warm, dry, dust-free atmosphere, protected from light. They should not be tightly packed and should be dated for ease of stock control. Proprietary preparations should be stored in accordance with manufacturer's guidelines and not kept beyond the expiry date specified.

UK

Indications. See preparation details
Contra-indications. Allergy to any of the raw ingredients
Side-effects. See preparation details
Warnings. Consult a veterinarian if condition fails to improve
Dose. See manufacturer's information

GSL **Damiana and Kola Tablets** (Dorwest Herbs)
Tablets, s/c, extract damiana 4:1 57.5 mg, extract saw palmetto 6:1 7.5 mg, kola nuts 45 mg, for *dogs*, *cats*; 100, 200
Indications. Manufacturer recommends for relief of lack of alertness and stamina

GSL **Denex** (Denes)
Tablets, aqueous extract of barberry 32.4 mg, aqueous extract of dandelion root 32.4 mg, aqueous extract of kava kava 32.4 mg, eucalyptus oil PhEur 10.8 mg, for *dogs*, *cats*; 50
Indications. Manufacturer recommends for liver disorders, some kidney problems, cystitis and other similar diseases

GSL **Garlic Tablets** (Denes)
Tablets, garlic 194.4 mg, garlic oil 0.56 mg, for *dogs, cats*; 50, 100, 400
Indications. Manufacturer recommends for prophylaxis for infection, worms, and fleas
Side-effects. Occasionally stomach irritation, constipation with overdosage

GSL **Garlic Tablets** (Dorwest Herbs)
Tablets, s/c, garlic 30 mg, garlic oil 0.001 mL, for *dogs, cats*; 100, 200, 500
Indications. Manufacturer recommends for prophylaxis for general health, external and internal parasites; symptomatic relief of cough and other upper respiratory conditions

GSL **Garlic and Fenugreek Tablets** (Dorwest Herbs)
Tablets, s/c, fenugreek 16 mg, garlic oil 220 micrograms, for *dogs, cats*; 100, 200, 500
Indications. Manufacturer recommends for symptomatic relief of rheumatism, arthritis, skin conditions, coughs, and minor infections

GSL **Gastric Tablets** (Denes)
Tablets, light kaolin 160 mg, liquorice 10 mg, peppermint oil PhEur 0.001 mL, sodium bicarbonate 40 mg, for *dogs, cats*; 50
Indications. Manufacturer recommends for diarrhoea, appetite and digestive disorders, travel sickness

GSL **Greenleaf Tablets** (Denes)
Tablets, chlorophyll 32.8 mg, ferrous sulphate 32 mg, nettles 41 mg, for *dogs, cats*; 50, 100, 400
Indications. Manufacturer recommends for prophylaxis against disease; inflammatory conditions, particularly dermatitis and arthritis
Side-effects. Diarrhoea with overdosage

GSL **Kelp Seaweed Tablets** (Dorwest Herbs)
Tablets, s/c, extract Fucus 5:1 20 mg, Fucus 150 mg, for *dogs, cats*; 100, 200, 500
Indications. Manufacturer recommends for symptomatic relief of rheumatic pain, poor hair growth and pigmentation; aid in treatment of obesity

GSL **Kidney Tablets** (Denes)
Tablets, aqueous extract of buchu 45 mg, aqueous extract of cascara BP 30 mg, aqueous extract of parsley piert 45 mg, aqueous extract of Uva ursi 45 mg, cayenne 15 mg, colophony BP 7.5 mg, juniper oil 0.001 mL, for *dogs, cats*; 50

Indications. Manufacturer recommends for kidney problems, cystitis, bladder stones, and other urinary problems

GSL **Malted Kelp Tablets** (Dorwest Herbs)
Tablets, extract malt 90 mg, Fucus 360 mg, for *dogs, cats*; 100, 200, 500
Indications. Manufacturer recommends for symptomatic relief of poor hair growth and pigmentation; loss of appetite

GSL **Mixed Vegetable Tablets** (Dorwest Herbs)
Tablets, celery plant 30 mg, celery seed 30 mg, horseradish 30 mg, parsley 20 mg, watercress 70 mg, for *dogs, cats*; 100, 200, 500
Indications. Manufacturer recommends for symptomatic relief of rheumatism, arthritis, skin, and kidney disorders; diuretic to aid normal urinary elimination

GSL **Natural Herb Tablets** (Dorwest Herbs)
Tablets, aloes 45 mg, cascara 30 mg, dandelion root 30 mg, senna leaf 90 mg, valerian root 30 mg, for *dogs, cats*; 100, 200
Indications. Manufacturer recommends for symptomatic relief of constipation; aid in treatment of furballing in cats

GSL **Nerve Tablets** (Denes)
Tablets, Asafetida tincture BP 21.6 mg, gentian 64.8 mg, hops 8.1 mg, scullcap 48.6 mg, valerian 64.8 mg, for *dogs, cats*; 100, 400
Indications. Manufacturer recommends for excitability, nervousness, hysteria, and other nervous disorders

GSL **Raspberry Leaf Tablets** (Denes)
Tablets, raspberry leaf 129.6 mg, for *dogs, cats*; 100
Indications. Manufacturer recommends for pregnancy and pseudopregnancy

GSL **Raspberry Leaf Tablets** (Dorwest Herbs)
Tablets, extracted raspberry leaf 3:1 150 mg, for *dogs, cats*; 100, 200, 500
Indications. Manufacturer recommends for symptomatic relief of problems associated with parturition; aid in prevention of pseudopregnancy

GSL **Scullcap and Valerian Tablets** (Dorwest Herbs)
Tablets, s/c, extract gentian 2:1 24 mg, extract mistletoe 3:1 50 mg, extract valerian 5:1 50 mg, scullcap 30 mg, for *dogs, cats*; 100, 200, 500
Indications. Manufacturer recommends for symptomatic relief of anxiety, nervousness, excitability, and travel sickness; adjunct in the treatment of epilepsy

Appendix 1: Drug Interactions

Contributor:
RG Cooke BSc, PhD

In veterinary practice, multiple drug therapy is frequently used. It is important to realise that particular combinations of drugs may interact rather than exert their independent effects. The interaction may result either in a loss of therapeutic activity or an increase in the therapeutic, toxic, or side-effects of one or both of the drugs.

Drug interactions *in vivo* may be either pharmacodynamic or pharmacokinetic. A **pharmacodynamic** interaction occurs when one drug has an agonistic or antagonistic action on an effect of the other drug. An interaction may occur when two drugs act at the same receptor site or when they act at different receptor sites that both produce similar effects on a tissue. This type of interaction is normally predictable on the basis of the mechanism of drug action and may be expected in all cases of concurrent administration of the two drugs. Furthermore, it can be expected to occur with all similar drugs within a particular group. An example of this type of interaction is that between aminoglycoside antibacterials and non-depolarising muscle relaxants at the neuromuscular junction, leading to an enhanced neuromuscular blockade.

A **pharmacokinetic** interaction occurs when one drug modifies the absorption, distribution, metabolism, or excretion of another drug. This type of interaction may not be seen in every case of co-administration and may depend on variables such as the state of health or age of the patient and the time interval between administration of the two drugs. There may also be differences in susceptibility to such interactions between various species.

Drug interaction at the site of subcutaneous, intramuscular, or intravenous injection is rare and the majority of interactions affecting absorption are seen following oral administration. Absorption of drugs from the gastro-intestinal tract will depend on their solubility and degree of ionisation. Factors that affect these parameters may modify the extent of drug absorption. For example, the absorption of tetracyclines from the gastro-intestinal tract can be reduced in the presence of various metal ions, with which they form insoluble chelates.

The absorption of a drug may be dependent on its gastro-intestinal transit time. A drug that increases gastro-intestinal motility may adversely affect the absorption of another drug. This usually leads to lower plasma-drug concentrations being achieved resulting in apparent therapeutic failure. Less frequently, an interaction may occur in which a reduction in gastro-intestinal motility may lead to higher plasma-drug concentrations resulting in toxicity.

Interactions affecting drug distribution are often associated with the action of one drug on the plasma-protein binding of another. Plasma-protein binding sites are non-specific and any drug that binds to plasma proteins is capable of displacing another, thereby increasing the proportion of free drug able to diffuse from plasma to its site of action. However, it is only drugs that exhibit a high degree of protein binding that demonstrate an increase in effect when displaced. This becomes particularly significant if the drug displaced has a low therapeutic index. An example of this type of drug is warfarin, which may be displaced by compounds such as sulphonamides or NSAIDs, leading to an enhanced anticoagulant effect and a risk of haemorrhage.

Interactions affecting drug metabolism may occur in the liver. The presence of some drugs in the liver can result in an increase in the liver enzyme concentration after only a few days. Induction of the hepatic microsomal enzyme system by one drug can gradually increase the rate of metabolism of another, resulting in lower plasma-drug concentrations and reduced effect. For example, administration of phenobarbital may lead to the increased metabolism of drugs including griseofulvin, phenytoin, and hydrocortisone and consequently a reduction in their therapeutic activity.

More rarely, inhibition of liver enzymes may occur. For example, chloramphenicol may increase the effects of barbiturates by inhibiting their breakdown by liver enzymes. This may continue for several weeks after treatment with chloramphenicol has ceased.

Interactions affecting drug excretion may be seen when a drug or an active metabolite is excreted in the urine. Drugs that cause alkalinisation of the urine will facilitate the ionisation of weak acids and increase their excretion and conversely reduce the excretion of weak bases. Drugs that acidify urine will have the opposite effects. Drugs that render the urine more alkaline include sodium bicarbonate and sodium citrate, while ammonium chloride or ascorbic acid will make the urine more acidic. Examples of drugs that are weak bases include quinine, pethidine, and amfetamine, and weak acids include sulphonamides, salicylates, and phenylbutazone.

Considering the frequent use of multiple drug therapy in veterinary medicine, it is surprising how infrequently drug interactions are reported. This may be because non-fatal interactions are not considered noteworthy, that therapeutic failure is accepted, or that interactions are not considered as a cause of adverse effects. However, if practitioners consider the general pharmacology of the drugs involved when they are using multiple drug therapy then it should be possible to reduce the incidence of drug interactions. Undoubtedly, many interactions remain to be discovered and any suspected interaction should be reported to the manufacturer and the VMD.

List of drug interactions

The following is an alphabetical list of drugs and their interactions. Each drug or group is listed in the alphabetical list and also against the drug or group with which it interacts. The interaction may only be listed once. Therefore, when checking for a potential interaction, it may be necessary to refer to the entries for each of the drugs involved. These drug interactions are *potential* hazards and may not have been proven in particular species or breeds; the symbol • denotes interactions listed in UK veterinary data sheets. This list is not comprehensive; absence from the list does not imply safety.

ACE inhibitors
•Diuretics: increased risk of hyperkalaemia with potassium sparing diuretics; increased risk of hypotension
•General anaesthetics: increased risk of hypotension
Insulins: possible hypoglycaemic activity with reduced insulin requirement

Acepromazine *see* Phenothiazine derivatives

Acetazolamide
Aspirin: reduced excretion of acetazolamide
Corticosteroids, corticotropin: increased risk of hypokalaemia
Diuretics: increased risk of hypokalaemia with loop and thiazide diuretics
Quinidine: increased plasma-quinidine concentration reported rarely

Adrenoceptor stimulants
Beta-adrenoceptor blocking drugs: enhanced hypertensive effect especially with non-selective beta-adrenoceptor blocking drugs
•Clomipramine: enhanced effect of adrenoceptor stimulants
Cyclopropane, enflurane, •halothane, isoflurane, methoxyflurane: arrhythmias with •epinephrine or isoprenaline
Insulins: possible increase in insulin requirement
•Selegiline: risk of either reduced or enhanced effect of adrenoceptor stimulants
•Theophylline: synergistic effects leading to increased side-effects such as cardiac arrhythmias
•Tilmicosin: increased potential lethality in pigs with epinephrine; reduced efficacy with dobutamine

Alfacalcidol
•Vitamin D containing preparations: enhanced effect

Alimemazine *see* Phenothiazine derivatives

Allopurinol
Cyclophosphamide: enhanced bone-marrow toxicity
Mercaptopurine: enhanced effect of mercaptopurine

Alpha$_2$-adrenoceptor stimulants
• Sympathomimetic amines

Altrenogest *see* Progestogens

Aluminium hydroxide *see* Antacids

Aluminium salts
• Fluoroquinolones: reduced bioavailability of fluoroquinolones

Ambutonium *see* Antimuscarinic drugs

Amiloride *see* Diuretics

Aminoglycosides
Amphotericin B: increased risk of nephrotoxicity
•Cephalosporins: increased risk of nephrotoxicity
Cisplatin: increased risk of nephrotoxicity and possibly ototoxicity
•Diuretics: increased risk of ototoxicity with loop diuretics
Enflurane, ether: enhanced neuromuscular blockade

Methoxyflurane: enhanced neuromuscular blockade; increased risk of nephrotoxicity
Muscle relaxants: enhanced neuromuscular blockade with non-depolarising muscle relaxants
Neostigmine: antagonism of interacting drug
•Potentially nephrotoxic or ototoxic drugs: increased risk of toxicity
•Thiopental: enhanced effect of thiopental with kanamycin or streptomycin

Amphotericin B
Aminoglycosides: increased risk of nephrotoxicity

Anabolic steroids
Insulins: possible hypoglycaemic activity with reduced insulin requirement
Warfarin: enhanced anticoagulant effect

Antacids
Aspirin: large doses of antacids increase aspirin excretion
Barbiturates, chlorpromazine, •fluoroquinolones, ketoconazole, penicillamine, phenylbutazone, •tetracyclines: antacids cause reduced absorption of interacting drug
Quinidine: increased plasma-quinidine concentration reported rarely

Anti-arrhythmic drugs
Combinations of 2 or more anti-arrhythmic drugs: enhanced myocardial depression
See also under individual drugs

Anticholinergics *see* Antimuscarinic drugs

Anticholinesterase compounds *see* Organophosphorus compounds; s*ee also under* individual drugs

Antidiabetic drugs
Beta-adrenoceptor blocking drugs: enhanced hypoglycaemic effect
•Corticosteroids, corticotropin, levothyroxine, progestogens: antagonism of hypoglycaemic effect
Diuretics: antagonism of hypoglycaemic effect with loop and thiazide diuretics

Antiepileptic drugs
•Phenothiazine derivatives: antagonism of anticonvulsant effect; *see also under* individual drugs

Antihistamines
Combination with any other CNS depressant drug: enhanced depressant effects

Antimuscarinic drugs
•Clenbuterol: tachycardia with atropine
•Clomipramine: enhanced effect of antimuscarinics
Ketoconazole: reduced ketoconazole absorption
•Metoclopramide: antagonism because interacting drugs have opposing effects on gastro-intestinal motility
•Phenothiazine derivatives: reduced plasma-phenothiazine concentration

Apramycin *see* Aminoglycosides

Aspirin

Acetazolamide: reduced excretion of acetazolamide

Antacids: large doses of antacids increase aspirin excretion

Diuretics: antagonism of diuretic effect with spironolactone

Heparin: enhanced anticoagulant effect

Insulins: possible hypoglycaemic activity with reduced insulin requirement

Methotrexate: reduced methotrexate excretion

Metoclopramide: increased aspirin absorption

Phenytoin: transient potentiation

Warfarin: increased risk of bleeding due to antiplatelet effect

Atenolol *see* Beta-adrenoceptor blocking drugs

Atropine *see* Antimuscarinic drugs

Barbiturates

Antacids: reduced barbituate absorption

•Clomipramine: enhanced effect of barbiturates

•Corticosteroids, corticotropin: increased risk of potassium loss; increased corticosteroid metabolism

•Chloramphenicol,   •metronidazole,   progestogens, •theophylline: barbiturates cause reduced plasma concentration of interacting drug

•Doxycycline: reduced half-life and effect of doxycycline

•Phenylbutazone: reduced metabolism of barbiturates

Warfarin: reduced anticoagulant effect

See also under individual drugs *and* Antiepileptic drugs

Benazepril *see* ACE inhibitors

Bendroflumethiazide *see* Diuretics

Benzodiazepines

•Clomipramine: enhanced effect of benzodiazepines

•Isoflurane: reduced isoflurane requirement for induction and maintenance

Beta-adrenoceptor blocking drugs

Antidiabetic drugs: enhanced hypoglycaemic effect

Adrenoceptor stimulants: enhanced hypertensive effect, especially with non-selective beta-adrenoceptor blocking drugs

Chlorpromazine: increased plasma-chlorpromazine concentration

Cimetidine: increased plasma concentration of beta-adrenoceptor drugs

•Clenbuterol: antagonism of effect

Diuretics: increased risk of ventricular arrhythmias in the presence of hypokalaemia

General anaesthetics: enhanced hypotensive effects

Lidocaine and similar anti-arrhythmic drugs: increased risk of myocardial depression and bradycardia

Neostigmine: antagonism of interacting drug

•Tilmicosin: increased effect of tilmicosin

Verapamil: atrioventricular block

Beta-blockers *see* Beta-adrenoceptor blocking drugs

Betamethasone *see* Corticosteroids

Bromocriptine

Metoclopramide: antagonism of hypoprolactinaemic effect

Bromophos *see* Organophosphorus compounds

Buprenorphine *see* Opioid analgesics

Butorphanol *see* Opioid analgesics

Butyrophenones

•Cabergoline: reduced effect of cabergoline

•Metoclopramide: increased risk of extrapyramidal effects

Cabergoline

•Butyrophenones,   metoclopramide,   •phenothiazines: reduced effect of cabergoline

•Hypotensive drugs (e.g. alpha-adrenoceptor blocking drugs, calcium-channel blockers): enhanced effect of interacting drug

Calcium salts

Cardiac glycosides: large doses of intravenous calcium can precipitate arrhythmias

Diuretics: increased risk of hypercalcaemia with thiazide diuretics

•Fluoroquinolones, •tetracyclines: reduced absorption of interacting drugs

Captopril *see* ACE inhibitors

Carbamazepine

•Clomipramine: increased plasma-carbamazepine concentration

Phenytoin: reduced plasma-phenytoin concentration

Carbaril

Combinations of 2 or more compounds with anticholinesterase activity such as organophosphorus compounds: enhanced toxicity

Cardiac glycosides

Calcium salts, •Haemaccel: large doses of intravenous calcium can precipitate arrhythmias

•Diuretics: increased toxicity if hypokalaemia occurs; enhanced effect of digoxin with furosemide or spironolactone

Muscle relaxants: arrhythmias with depolarising muscle relaxants

Phenobarbital, •phenylbutazone, phenytoin: reduced effect of digitoxin

Quinidine: enhanced effect of digoxin

Cephalosporins

•Aminoglycosides: increased risk of nephrotoxicity

•Diuretics: enhanced nephrotoxicity with loop diuretics

Chloramphenicol

•Barbiturates: reduced   plasma-chloramphenicol concentration; •reduced barbiturate metabolism and prolonged duration of pentobarbital anaesthesia

•Clindamycin: antagonism of effect

•Phenylbutazone, •phenytoin: reduced metabolism of interacting drug

Sulphonylureas: enhanced hypoglycaemic effect

Warfarin: enhanced anticoagulant effect

Chlorpromazine

Antacids: reduced absorption of chlorpromazine

Beta-adrenoceptor blocking drugs: increased plasma-chlorpromazine concentration

General anaesthetics: enhanced hypotensive effect

Depolarising muscle relaxants: enhanced neuromuscular blockade

Chlorpropamide *see* Sulphonylureas *and* Antidiabetic drugs

Chlorpyrifos *see* Organophosphorus compounds

Cimetidine

Beta-adrenoceptor blocking drugs, •clomipramine, diazepam, fluorouracil, metronidazole, pethidine, propranolol, quinidine, or theophylline: cimetidine causes increased plasma concentration of interacting drug

Erythromycin, phenytoin: reduced metabolism of interacting drug

Ketoconazole: reduced ketoconazole absorption

Lidocaine: increased risk of lidocaine toxicity

Warfarin: enhanced anticoagulant effect

Cisplatin

Aminoglycosides: increased risk of nephrotoxicity and possibly ototoxicity

Clenbuterol

•Atropine: tachycardia

•Beta-adrenoceptor blocking drugs: antagonism of effect

•General anaesthetics, •other adrenoceptor stimulants, •vasodilators: enhanced hypotensive effect

•Dinoprost (PGF$_{2\alpha}$), •oxytocin: reduced uterine relaxant effect of clenbuterol

Clindamycin

•Chloramphenicol, •macrolides: antagonism of effect

•Muscle relaxants: enhanced neuromuscular blockade with non-depolarising muscle relaxants

Clofenvinfos *see* Organophosphorus compounds

Clomipramine

•Adrenoceptor stimulants, •antimuscarinics, •barbiturates, •benzodiazepines, •coumarin anticoagulants, •general anaesthetics, •neuroleptics, •quinidine: enhanced effect of interacting drug

•Carbamazepine, •phenytoin: increased plasma concentration of interacting drug

•Cimetidine: increased plasma-clomipramine concentration

•Monamine oxidase inhibitors: enhanced effect of clomipramine

CNS depressants

Antihistamines, •opioid analgesics, •phenothiazine derivatives: enhanced depressant effects

Corticosteroids

Acetazolamide: increased risk of hypokalaemia

•Anticoagulants: reduced effect of anticoagulants

•Antidiabetic drugs (e.g. insulin): antagonism of hypoglycaemic effect

•Barbiturates, •phenylbutazone, •phenytoin, •rifampicin: increased risk of potassium loss; •increased corticosteroid metabolism

•Diuretics: antagonism of diuretic effect; increased risk of hypokalaemia with loop and thiazide diuretics

Metoclopramide: aggression

•NSAIDs: increased risk of gastro-intestinal ulceration

•Pentosan polysulphate sodium: antagonism of effect

Corticotropin

Acetazolamide, barbiturates, diuretics, phenytoin: increased risk of hypokalaemia

Antidiabetic drugs: antagonism of hypoglycaemic effect

Metoclopramide: aggression

Coumafos *see* Organophosphorus compounds

Cyclophosphamide

Allopurinol: enhanced bone-marrow toxicity

Cyclopropane

Adrenoceptor stimulants: arrhythmias with epinephrine or isoprenaline

•Doxapram: increased risk of cardiac arrhythmias

Cythioate *see* Organophosphorus compounds

Danofloxacin *see* Fluoroquinolones

Detomidine

•Potentiated sulphonamides: increased risk of cardiac arrhythmias

•Pethidine: generalised excitement

Dexamethasone *see* Corticosteroids

Diazepam

Cimetidine: increased plasma-diazepam concentration

Phenytoin: reduced phenytoin metabolism

Dichlorvos *see* Organophosphorus compounds

Diethylcarbamazine

•Levamisole, •organophosphorus compounds: enhanced toxicity

Diethylstilbestrol *see* Oestrogens

Difloxacin *see* Fluoroquinolones

Digitoxin *see* Cardiac glycosides

Digoxin *see* Cardiac glycosides

Dihydrostreptomycin *see* Aminoglycosides

Diltiazem

Insulins: possible increase in insulin requirement

Dimpylate *see* Organophosphorus compounds

Dinoprost

•Clenbuterol: reduced uterine relaxant effect of clenbuterol

Diphenhydramine

Muscle relaxants: enhanced neuromuscular blockade

Diuretics

•ACE inhibitors, potassium supplements: increased risk of hyperkalaemia with potassium-sparing diuretics

Acetazolamide: increased risk of hypokalaemia with loop and thiazide diuretics

•Aminoglycosides: enhanced ototoxicity with loop diuretics

Antidiabetic drugs: antagonism of hypoglycaemic effect with loop and thiazide diuretics

Aspirin: antagonism of diuretic effect of spironolactone

Beta-adrenoceptor blocking drugs: increased risk of ventricular arrhythmias in the presence of hypokalaemia

Calcium salts: increased risk of hypercalcaemia with thiazide diuretics

•Cardiac glycosides: •increased toxicity if hypokalaemia occurs; enhanced effect of digoxin with furosemide or spironolactone

•Cephalosporins: increased risk of nephrotoxicity with loop diuretics

•Corticosteroids, corticotropin: antagonism of diuretic effect; •increased risk of hypokalaemia with loop and thiazide diuretics

Insulins: possible increase in insulin requirement with thiazide diuretics

Lidocaine: lidocaine effect antagonised by hypokalaemia with loop and thiazide diuretics

Diuretics (*continued*)

NSAIDs: antagonism of diuretic effect; increased risk of hyperkalaemia with potassium-sparing diuretics

Oestrogens: antagonism of diuretic effect

Quinidine: toxicity of quinidine increased by hypokalaemia with loop and thiazide diuretics

•Sulphonamides: increased risk of sulphonamide allergy

Dobutamine *see* Adrenoceptor stimulants

Doxapram

•Cyclopropane, •enflurane, •halothane, •isoflurane, •methoxyflurane: increased risk of cardiac arrhythmias

•Morphine: may induce convulsions

Doxycycline

•Barbiturates, •phenytoin: reduced half-life and effect of doxycycline

Ecothiopate

Muscle relaxants: enhanced neuromuscular blockade with depolarising muscle relaxants

Eltenac *see* NSAIDs

Enalapril *see* ACE inhibitors

Enflurane

Adrenoceptor stimulants: arrhythmias with epinephrine or isoprenaline

Aminoglycosides: enhanced neuromuscular blockade

•Doxapram: increased risk of cardiac arrhythmias

Enrofloxacin *see* Fluoroquinolones

Epinephrine *see* Adrenoceptor stimulants

Erythromycin

•Lincomycin: antagonism of effect

Ciclosporin, digoxin, midazolam, phenytoin, quinidine, terfenadine, •theophylline, warfarin: enhanced effects of interacting drug

Estradiol *see* Oestrogens

Ether

Aminoglycosides: enhanced neuromuscular blockade

Ethinylestradiol *see* Oestrogens

Ethylestrenol *see* Anabolic steroids

Etiproston

•Oxytocin: enhanced ecbolic effect

Etorphine *see* Opioid analgesics

Fentanyl *see* Opioid analgesics

Fenthion *see* Organophosphorus compounds

Flumetasone *see* Corticosteroids

Fluorogestone *see* Progestogens

Fluoroquinolones

•Aluminium salts, •calcium salts, •iron salts, •magnesium salts: reduced bioavailability of fluorquinolones

•Nitrofurantoin: impaired efficacy of fluoroquinolones when used for urinary tract infection

•NSAIDs: increased risk of seizures

•Theophylline: reduced clearance of theophylline

Fluorouracil

Cimetidine: increased plasma-fluorouracil concentration

Fluoxetine

•Selegiline: enhanced toxicity of fluoxetine

Folic acid

Phenytoin: reduced plasma-phenytoin concentration

Framycetin *see* Aminoglycosides

Furosemide *see* Diuretics

General anaesthetics

Beta-adrenoceptor blocking drugs, chlorpromazine, •clenbuterol: enhanced hypotensive effect

•Clomipramine: enhanced effect of general anaesthetics

•Selegiline: risk of reduced or enhanced effect of general anaesthetics

Gentamicin *see* Aminoglycosides

Glibenclamide *see* Sulphonylureas *and* Antidiabetic drugs

Glipizide *see* Sulphonylureas *and* Antidiabetic drugs

Glycopyrronium *see* Antimuscarinic drugs

Griseofulvin

•Phenobarbital, •phenylbutazone: increased griseofulvin metabolism

Progestogens: reduced plasma-progestogen concentration

Warfarin: reduced anticoagulant effect

Halothane

•Adrenoceptor stimulants: arrhythmias with •epinephrine or isoprenaline

•Doxapram: increased risk of cardiac arrhythmias

•Ketamine: half-life of ketamine prolonged

•Muscle relaxants: increased effect of non-depolarising muscle relaxants

•Theophylline: arrhythmogenic effects

Haloxon *see* Organophosphorus compounds

Heparin

Aspirin: enhanced anticoagulant effect

Hydrochlorothiazide *see* Diuretics

Hydrocortisone *see* Corticosteroids

Hyoscine *see* Antimuscarinic drugs

Insulins

ACE inhibitors, anabolic steroids, aspirin, beta-adrenoceptor blocking drugs, mebendazole, oxytetracycline: possible hypoglycaemic activity with reduced insulin requirement

Beta-adrenoceptor blocking drugs (less common interaction), diltiazem, dobutamine, epinephrine, levothyroxine, thiazides, thyroid hormones: possible increase in insulin requirement

Iodofenphos *see* Organophosphorus compounds

Iron salts

Penicillamine: reduced penicillamine absorption

•Fluoroquinolones, tetracyclines, zinc salts: reduced absorption of interacting drugs

Isoflurane

•Acepromazine, •alpha$_2$-adrenoceptor stimulants, •benzodiazepines, •opioids: reduced isoflurane required for induction and maintenance

Adrenoceptor stimulants: arrhythmias with epinephrine or isoprenaline

•Doxapram: increased risk of cardiac arrhythmias

•Muscle relaxants: increased effect of non-depolarising muscle relaxants

Isoprenaline *see* Adrenoceptor stimulants

Kanamycin *see* Aminoglycosides

Kaolin mixtures

Lincomycin, tetracyclines: reduced absorption of interacting drugs

Ketamine

•Halothane: half-life of ketamine prolonged

•Theophylline: reduced seizure theshold

Ketoconazole

Antacids, antimuscarinic drugs, cimetidine, ranitidine: reduced ketoconazole absorption

Phenytoin: increased plasma-phenytoin concentration; reduced plasma-ketoconazole concentration

Warfarin: enhanced anticoagulant effect

Ketoprofen *see* NSAIDs

Levamisole

•Organophosphorus   compounds,   •diethylcarbamazine: enhanced toxicity

Levothyroxine

Insulins: increased requirement for insulin

•Phenylbutazone: falsely low total plasma-levothyroxine concentration

Phenytoin: increased levothyroxine metabolism

Warfarin: enhanced anticoagulant effect

Lidocaine

Beta-adrenoceptor blocking drugs: increased risk of myocardial depression and bradycardia

Cimetidine: increased risk of lidocaine toxicity

Diuretics: lidocaine effect antagonised by hypokalaemia with loop and thiazide diuretics

Lincomycin

Kaolin mixtures: reduced lincomycin absorption

•Erythromycin: antagonism of effect

Muscle relaxants: enhanced neuromuscular blockade with non-depolarising muscle relaxants

Neostigmine: antagonism of interacting drug

Macrolides

•Clindamycin: antagonism of effect

Magnesium salts

Muscle relaxants: enhanced neuromuscular blockade with non-depolarising muscle relaxants

•Fluoroquinolones, •tetracyclines: reduced absorption of interacting drugs

Malathion *see* Organophosphorus compounds

Marbofloxacin

•Theophylline: increased plasma-theophylline concentration

See also under Fluoroquinolones

Meclofenamic acid *see* NSAIDs

Mebendazole

Insulins: possible hypoglycaemic activity with reduced insulin requirement

Medroxyprogesterone *see* Progestogens

Megestrol *see* Progestogens

Meloxicam *see* NSAIDs

Mercaptopurine

Allopurinol: enhanced effect of mercaptopurine

Methadone *see* Opioid analgesics

Methohexital *see* Barbiturates

Methotrexate

Aspirin, •phenylbutazone: reduced methotrexate excretion

Phenytoin: enhanced anti-folate effect

Methoxyflurane

Adrenoceptor stimulants: arrhythmias with epinephrine or isoprenaline

Aminoglycosides: enhanced   neuromuscular   blockade; nephrotoxicity

•Doxapram: increased risk of cardiac arrhythmias

Methylprednisolone *see* Corticosteroids

Metoclopramide

•Antimuscarinic drugs, opioid analgesics: antagonism as interacting drugs have opposing effects on gastrointestinal motility

Aspirin: increased aspirin absorption

Bromocriptine: antagonism of hypoprolactinaemic effect

•Butyrophenones, •phenothiazines: increased risk of extrapyramidal effects

Cabergoline: reduced effect of cabergoline

Corticosteroids, corticotropin: aggression

Paracetamol: increased paracetamol absorption

Metoprolol *see* Beta-adrenoceptor blocking drugs

Metronidazole

•Barbiturates: increased metabolism of metronidazole

Cimetidine: increased plasma-metronidazole concentration

Phenytoin: reduced phenytoin metabolism

•Warfarin: enhanced anticoagulant effect

Miconazole

Phenytoin: reduced phenytoin metabolism

Sulphonylureas: enhanced hypoglycaemic effect

Warfarin: enhanced anticoagulant effect

Monamine oxidase inhibitors

•Clomipramine: enhanced effect of clomipramine

Monensin

•Tiamulin: reduced monensin metabolism; severe growth retardation

•Valnemulin: severe growth retardation

Morphine *see* Opioid analgesics

Muscle relaxants

Aminoglycosides, •clindamycin, •halothane, isoflurane, lincomycin, magnesium salts, polymyxin B sulphate: enhanced neuromuscular blockade with non-depolarising muscle relaxants

Cardiac glycosides: arrhythmias with depolarising muscle relaxants

Chlorpromazine,   diphenhydramine,   ecothiopate, neostigmine,   •organophosphorus   compounds, promethazine: enhanced neuromuscular blockade with depolarising muscle relaxants

Quinidine: enhanced neuromuscular blockade

Nadolol *see* Beta-adrenoceptor blocking drugs

Nalidixic acid

Warfarin: enhanced anticoagulant effect

Nandrolone *see* Anabolic steroids

Narasin

•Tiamulin, •valnemulin: severe growth retardation

Neomycin

Phenoxymethylpenicillin: reduced penicillin absorption

Warfarin: enhanced anticoagulant effect

Neostigmine

Aminoglycosides, beta-adrenoceptor blocking drugs, lincomycin, quinidine: antagonism of neostigmine

Neostigmine (*continued*)

Muscle relaxants: enhanced neuromuscular blockade with depolarising muscle relaxants

Nicergoline

•Alpha$_2$-adrenoceptor stimulants: antagonism of effect

•Vasodilators: enhancement of effect

NSAIDs

•Aminoglycosides, •corticosteroids, •other NSAIDs, •pentosan polysulphate sodium, •potentially nephrotoxic drugs, •warfarin and other anticoagulants: enhanced effects of interacting drug

Diuretics: antagonism of diuretic effect; increased risk of hyperkalaemia with potassium-sparing diuretics

•Fluoroquinolones: increased risk of seizures

•Methoxyflurane: possible toxic effect on kidneys

Oestrogens

Diuretics: antagonism of diuretic effect

Phenytoin: reduced plasma-oestrogen concentration

Warfarin: impaired action

Opioid analgesics

•Combination with any other CNS depressant drug: enhanced depressant effects

Metoclopramide: antagonism as interacting drugs have opposing effects on gastro-intestinal motility

•Doxapram: convulsions may be induced with morphine

•Selegiline: enhanced depressant effect of morphine

Organophosphorus compounds

•Combinations of 2 or more organophosphorus compounds or compounds with anticholinesterase activity, •levamisole, •diethylcarbamazine, phenothiazine derivatives: enhanced toxicity

•Muscle relaxants: enhanced neuromuscular blockade with depolarising muscle relaxants

See also under individual drugs

Oxymetholone *see* Anabolic steroids

Oxytocin

•Clenbuterol: reduced uterine relaxant effect of clenbuterol

Paracetamol

Metoclopramide: increased paracetamol absorption

Warfarin: enhanced anticoagulant effect with regular high doses of paracetamol

Penicillamine

Antacids, iron salts, zinc salts: reduced penicillamine absorption

Penicillins

•Phenylbutazone: alteration in half-life and tissue penetration

Pentazocine *see* Opioid analgesics

Pentosan polysulphate sodium

•NSAIDs: enhanced effects of interacting drug

•Corticosteroids: antagonism of effect

Pethidine

Cimetidine: increased plasma-pethidine concentration

•Detomidine: generalised excitement

•Selegiline: enhanced toxicity of pethidine

See also under Opioid analgesics

Phenobarbital, primidone

Cardiac glycosides: reduced effect of digitoxin

•Chloramphenicol, •metronidazole, progestogens: phenobarbital (or primidone) causes reduced plasma concentration of interacting drug

•Griseofulvin: increased griseofulvin metabolism

Phenytoin, sodium valproate: increased sedation

Warfarin: reduced anticoagulant effect

See also under Barbiturates

Phenothiazine derivatives

•Antiepileptic drugs: antagonism of anticonvulsant effect

Antimuscarinic drugs: reduced plasma-phenothiazine concentration

•Cabergoline: reduced effect of cabergoline

•Metoclopramide: increased risk of extrapyramidal effects

•Isoflurane: reduced isoflurane requirement for induction and maintenance with acepromazine

•Organophosphorus compounds: inhibition of acetylcholinesterase and enhanced toxicity

•Procaine hydrochloride: enhanced hypotension, enhanced prolonged-acting activity

•Combination with any other CNS depressant drug: enhanced depressant effects

Phenoxymethylpenicillin

Neomycin: reduced penicillin absorption

Phenylbutazone

•Barbiturates: reduced metabolism of interacting drug

•Cardiac glycosides, •griseofulvin: increased metabolism and reduced effect of interacting drug

•Chloramphenicol: reduced phenylbutazone metabolism

Antacids, •colestyramine: reduced enteral absorption of phenylbutazone

•Corticosteroids, •other NSAIDs, •sulphonamides: displacement from plasma proteins and enhanced effect of interacting drug

•Levothyroxine: falsely low total plasma-levothyroxine concentration

•Methotrexate: reduced methotrexate excretion

•Penicillins: alteration in half-life and tissue penetration

•Phenytoin: reduced phenytoin metabolism

•Sulphonylureas: enhanced hypoglycaemic effect

•Warfarin: enhanced anticoagulant effect

See also under NSAIDs

Phenylephrine *see* Adrenoceptor stimulants

Phenytoin

Aspirin, sodium valproate: transient potentiation

Carbamazepine, folic acid, •theophylline: reduced plasma-phenytoin concentration

Cardiac glycosides: reduced effect of digitoxin

•Chloramphenicol, cimetidine, diazepam, ketoconazole, metronidazole, miconazole, •phenylbutazone, sulphonamides (some): reduced phenytoin metabolism

•Clomipramine: increased plasma-phenytoin concentration

•Corticosteroids, corticotropin: increased potassium loss; increased corticosteroid metabolism

•Doxycycline: reduced half-life and effect of doxycycline

Ketoconazole: increased plasma-phenytoin concentration; reduced plasma-ketoconazole concentration

Levothyroxine: increased levothyroxine metabolism

Methotrexate: increased anti-folate effect

Phenytoin (*continued*)

Phenobarbital, primidone, sodium valproate: increased sedation

Oestrogen, progestogens, •theophylline, vitamin D: phenytoin causes reduced plasma concentration of interacting drug

Warfarin: both enhanced and reduced anticoagulant effects reported

See also under Antiepileptic drugs

Phosmet *see* Organophosphorus compounds

Pimobendan**NEW*****

•Propranolol, •verapamil: reduced action of pimobendan

Pindolol *see* Beta-adrenoceptor blocking drugs

Polymyxin B sulphate

Muscle relaxants: enhanced neuromuscular blockade with non-depolarising muscle relaxants

Polysulphated glycosaminoglycan

•Other anticoagulants: enhanced anticoagulant effect

Potassium

Diuretics: increased risk of hyperkalaemia with potassium-sparing diuretics

Potentiated sulphonamides *see* Sulphonamides, potentiated

Prednisolone *see* Corticosteroids

Primidone *see* Phenobarbital

Procaine benzylpenicillin

•Sulphonamides: antagonism of effect

Procaine hydrochloride

•Phenothiazines: enhanced hypotension, and prolonged-acting activity

•Sulphonamides: antagonism of effect

Prochlorperazine *see* Phenothiazine derivatives

Progesterone *see* Progestogens

Progestogens

Antidiabetic drugs: antagonism of hypoglycaemic effect

Barbiturates, griseofulvin, phenytoin: reduced plasma-progestogen concentration

Theophylline: increased plasma-theophylline concentration

Warfarin: reduced anticoagulant effect

Proligestone *see* Progestogens

Promethazine

Depolarising muscle relaxants: enhanced neuromuscular blockade

Propantheline *see* Antimuscarinic drugs

Propoxur

Combinations of 2 or more compounds with anticholinesterase activity such as organophosphorus compounds: enhanced toxicity

Propranolol

Cimetidine: increased plasma-propranolol concentration

Pyrantel

•Piperazine: mutual antagonism

Quinidine

Acetazolamide, antacids: increased plasma-quinidine concentration reported rarely

Cardiac glycosides: enhanced effect of digoxin

Cimetidine: increased plasma-quinidine concentration

•Clomipramine: enhanced effect of quinidine

Diuretics: toxicity increased by hypokalaemia with loop and thiazide diuretics

Muscle relaxants: enhanced neuromuscular blockade

Neostigmine: antagonism of neostigmine

Warfarin: enhanced anticoagulant effect

Ranitidine

Ketoconazole: reduced ketoconazole absorption

Rifampicin

Anti-arrhythmics, anticoagulants, antiepileptics, beta-adrenoceptor blocking drugs, •corticosteroids: increased metabolism of interacting drug

Salinomycin

•Tiamulin, •valnemulin: severe growth retardation

Selegiline

•CNS active drugs (e.g. alpha$_2$-adrenoceptor stimulants, tranquillisers, general anaesthetics): risk of either reduced or enhanced effects of interacting drug

•Fluoxetine, pethidine: enhanced toxicity of interacting drug

•Morphine: enhanced depressant effect of interacting drug

Selenium

•Ionophore antibacterials: increased risk of selenium toxicity

Sodium valproate

Phenobarbital, phenytoin, primidone: increased sedation

See also under Antiepileptic drugs

Spectinomycin *see* Aminoglycosides

Spironolactone *see* Diuretics

Streptomycin *see* Aminoglycosides

Sucralfate

Warfarin: impaired absorption

Sulphonamides

•Diuretics: increased risk of sulphonamide allergy

•Phenylbutazone: displacement from plasma proteins and enhanced effect of sulphonamides

Phenytoin: reduced phenytoin metabolism with some sulphonamides

•Procaine group local anaesthetics, •procaine benzylpenicillin, •vitamin B complex: antagonism of effect

Thiopental: enhanced effect of thiopental

Warfarin: enhanced anticoagulant effect

Sulphonamides, potentiated

•Detomidine, halothane, •romifidine, •xylazine: increased risk of cardiac arrhythmias

Sulphonylureas

Chloramphenicol, miconazole, •phenylbutazone: enhanced hypoglycaemic effect

See also under Antidiabetic drugs

Suxamethonium *see* Muscle relaxants

Sympathomimetics *see* Adrenoceptor stimulants

Tamoxifen

Warfarin: enhanced anticoagulant effect

Tetracyclines

•Antacids, •dairy products (not doxycycline), kaolin mixtures: reduced tetracycline absorption

•Aluminium salts, •calcium salts, •citric acid, iron salts, •magnesium salts, zinc salts: reduced absorption of interacting drugs

Tetracyclines (*continued*)

•Corticosteroids: increased risk of gastro-intestinal toxicity (especially in horses)

Insulins: possible reduced insulin requirement with oxytetracycline

Warfarin: enhanced anticoagulant effect

Theophylline

•Adrenoceptor stimulants: synergistic effects leading to increased side-effects such as cardiac arrhythmias

•Barbiturates, •phenytoin: reduced plasma-theophylline concentration

Cimetidine, •erythromycin, •marbofloxacin, progestogens: increased plasma-theophylline concentration

•Halothane: arrhythmogenic effects

•Ketamine: reduced seizure theshold

Thiopental

•Chloramphenicol, •kanamycin, •streptomycin, sulphonamides: enhanced effect of thiopental

See also under Barbiturates

Thyroid hormones

Insulins: possible increase in insulin requirement

Tiamulin

•Narasin, •salinomycin: severe growth retardation

•Monensin: reduced monensin metabolism; severe growth retardation

Tilmicosin

•Beta-adrenoceptor blocking drugs: increased effect of tilmicosin

•Dobutamine: reduced effect of tilmicosin

•Epinephrine: increased potential lethality of tilmicosin in pigs

Timolol *see* Beta blockers

Tolbutamide *see* Sulphonylureas *and* Antidiabetic drugs

Tolfenamic acid *see* NSAIDs

Triamcinolone *see* Corticosteroids

Triamterene *see* Diuretics

Trihexyphenidyl *see* Antimuscarinic drugs

Trimethoprim *see* Sulphonamides, potentiated

Tubocurarine *see* Muscle relaxants

Valnemulin

•Monensin, •narasin, •salinomycin: severe growth retardation

Vedaprofen *see* NSAIDs

Verapamil

Beta-adrenoceptor blocking drugs: atrioventricular block

Vitamin B

•Sulphonamides: antagonism of effect

Vitamin D

•Alfacalcidol: enhanced effect

Phenytoin: reduced plasma-vitamin D concentration

Vitamin K

Warfarin: reduced anticoagulant effect

Warfarin

Aspirin: increased risk of bleeding due to antiplatelet effect

Barbiturates, griseofulvin, oestrogens, progestogens, phenobarbital, primidone, vitamin K: reduced anticoagulant effect

Anabolic steroids, aspirin, chloramphenicol, cimetidine, erythromycin, ketoconazole, levothyroxine, metronidazole, miconazole, nalidixic acid, neomycin, paracetamol (regular treatment with high doses), quinidine, sulphonamides, tamoxifen, tetracyclines, •phenylbutazone, and possibly other NSAIDs: enhanced anticoagulant effect

Phenytoin: both enhanced and reduced anticoagulant effects reported

Sucralfate: impaired absorption

Xylazine

•Potentiated sulphonamides: cardiac arrhythmias

Zinc salts

Iron salts, tetracyclines: reduced absorption of interacting drugs

Penicillamine: reduced penicillamine absorption

Appendix 2: Drug Compatibilities and Incompatibilities

Contributor:
RG Cooke BSc, PhD

Drugs intended for parenteral administration may interact *in vitro* due to physical or chemical incompatibility. This may result in loss of potency, increase in toxicity, or other adverse effects. The solution may become opalescent or precipitation may occur, but in many instances there may be no visual indication of incompatibility. Precipitation reactions are numerous and varied and may occur as a result of pH changes, concentration changes, 'salting-out' of insoluble anion-cation salts, complexation, or other chemical changes.

In general, drugs should only be added to infusion containers when constant plasma concentrations are needed or when the administration of a more concentrated drug solution would be harmful.

In general, drugs should not be added to blood, mannitol, lipid emulsions, or sodium bicarbonate solutions. Information on drug incompatibilities is given below. The suitability of additions may also be checked by reference to manufacturer's literature.

> Drugs should not be mixed in infusion containers or syringes unless the components are of known compatibility.

Where drug solutions are added together they should be thoroughly mixed by shaking and checked for absence of particulate matter before use. A strict aseptic procedure should be adopted in order to prevent accidental entry and subsequent growth of micro-organisms in the infusion container or syringe. Ready prepared solutions should be used whenever possible.

In veterinary practice, due to the size and weight of the variety of species treated, it often necessary to further dilute ready prepared solutions in order to administer the correct drug dosage. Therefore, the list below also includes some information on compatible drugs and intravenous infusions.

List of drug compatibilities and incompatibilities

The following is an alphabetical list of drugs and their incompatibilities with other drugs and intravenous infusions. Some compatibilities are also listed, in particular appropriate intravenous solutions to make up intravenous infusions indicated in the chapters. To avoid excessive cross-referencing, those drugs that should not be mixed with any other drugs are only listed once. Therefore, when checking a potential incompatibility, it may be necessary to refer to the entries for each of the drugs or fluids involved. This list is not comprehensive; absence from the list does not imply safety.

Drug	*Compatibilities*	*Incompatibilities*
Acepromazine		phenylbutazone
Aminoglycosides		heparin sodium, hydrocortisone sodium succinate, norepinephrine acid tartrate
Amphotericin B	reconstitute in water for injections then infuse in glucose 5% intravenous infusion	sodium chloride intravenous infusion
Ampicillin (and other semi-synthetic penicillins)	sodium chloride 0.9%, compound sodium lactate, water for injections	dextran solutions, glucose intravenous infusion
Apramycin		should not be mixed with other solutions
Atropine sulphate		acepromazine maleate, chlorpromazine hydrochloride, heparin sodium, methohexital sodium

List of drug compatibilities and incompatibilities *(continued)*

Drug	Compatibilities	Incompatibilities
Barbiturates		all other drugs
Benzylpenicillin sodium	sodium chloride 0.9%, water for injections	glucose intravenous infusion[1], other drugs
Bretylium	glucose 5% intravenous infusion	
Calcium borogluconate (and possibly other calcium-containing solutions)		menbutone, methylprednisolone sodium succinate, prednisolone sodium phosphate, promethazine hydrochloride, sodium bicarbonate intravenous infusion, streptomycin sulphate, tetracyclines all drugs in the form of carbonate, phosphate, or sulphate salts
Carbenicillin		aminoglycosides, gentamicin sulphate, hydrocortisone sodium succinate, vitamins B and C
Ceftiofur	water for injections	
Cephalosporins		gentamicin sulphate, tetracyclines
Chloramphenicol sodium succinate		aminophylline, chlorpromazine hydrochloride, erythromycin, gentamicin sulphate, heparin sodium, hydrocortisone sodium succinate, penicillins, suxamethonium, tetracyclines, vitamins B and C
Cisplatin	sodium chloride 0.9% + glucose 5%	
Cloxacillin sodium	sodium chloride 0.9%, Ringer's solution	glucose intravenous infusion >5%, sodium lactate intravenous infusion
Compound sodium lacate intravenous infusion		methylprednisolone sodium succinate, sodium bicarbonate intravenous infusion
Cytarabine	water for injections (protect from light)	
Dextran solutions		ampicillin, oxytocin
Diazepam	glucose 5% or sodium chloride 0.9% intravenous infusions at concentrations not exceeding 40 mg diazepam in 500 mL (use within 6 hours)	should not normally be mixed with other intravenous infusions or drugs
Dobutamine	sodium chloride 0.9%, glucose 5%	
Doxapram hydrochloride		alkaline solutions such as aminophylline, furosemide, thiopental
Electrolyte solutions		sulphadiazine sodium, sulphisoxazole diolamine

List of drug compatibilities and incompatibilities *(continued)*

Drug	Compatibilities	Incompatibilities
Epinephrine	sodium chloride 0.9%	potassium chloride, sodium bicarbonate intravenous infusion, other solutions with pH > 5.5
Erythromycin		chloramphenicol sodium succinate, tetracyclines
Esmolol	sodium chloride 0.9%, glucose 5%	
Furosemide		should not be mixed with other solutions
Gelatin	sodium chloride 0.9%, glucose, Ringer's solution, heparinsed blood	citrated blood
Gentamicin sulphate		carbenicillin and other penicillins, cephalosporins, chloramphenicol sodium succinate, heparin sodium, any solution in the concentration of gentamicin which exceeds 1 g/litre
Glucose intravenous infusion		ampicillin, benzylpenicillin sodium, cloxacillin sodium, heparin sodium, sulphadiazine sodium, tetracyclines
Heparin sodium		aminoglycosides, atropine sulphate, benzylpenicillin sodium, chloramphenicol sodium succinate, gentamicin sulphate, glucose intravenous infusions[1], hydrocortisone sodium succinate, pethidine hydrochloride, promethazine hydrochloride, streptomycin sulphate, tetracyclines, tylosin
Hydrocortisone sodium succinate		aminoglycosides, chloramphenicol sodium succinate, chlorpromazine hydrochloride, heparin sodium, norepinephrine acid tartrate, promethazine hydrochloride, tetracyclines, tylosin
Insulin (soluble)	sodium chloride 0.9%	
Isoprenaline	water for injections (protect from light)	
Ivermectin	propylene glycol, water for injections (use immediately, do not store)	
Ketamine	medetomidine	should not be mixed with other drugs, excluding medetomidine
Lincomycin		penicillins
Magnesium sulphate		sodium bicarbonate intravenous infusion, tetracyclines

List of drug compatibilities and incompatibilities (continued)

Drug	Compatibilities	Incompatibilities
Medetomidine	ketamine	should not be mixed with other drugs, excluding ketamine
Menbutone		calcium salts, procaine benzylpenicillin, vitamin B complex
Methylprednisolone sodium	water for injections For intravenous infusion, reconstitute in water for injections, then infuse in glucose 5%, glucose 5% + sodium chloride 0.9%, sodium chloride 0.9%	benzylpenicillin sodium, calcium-containing solutions, compound sodium lactate intravenous infusion, pethidine hydrochloride, tetracycline, thiopental sodium, vitamins B and C
Metoclopramide	water for injections (protect from light)	
Mitoxanthrone	sodium chloride 0.9%, glucose 5%	
Norepinephrine acid tartrate	glucose 5% intravenous infusion	aminoglycosides, hydrocortisone sodium succinate, sodium bicarbonate intravenous infusion, sodium chloride 0.9%, sulphadiazine sodium
Oxytocin	sodium chloride 0.9%, sodium chloride 0.18% + glucose 4%	dextran solutions
Penicillins		chloramphenicol sodium succinate, gentamicin sulphate, lincomycin, tetracyclines
Pethidine hydrochloride		heparin sodium, methylprednisolone sodium succinate, sodium bicarbonate intravenous infusion, thiopental sodium
Phenylbutazone sodium		acepromazine maleate, chlorpromazine hydrochloride
Polysulphated glycosaminoglycan		should not be mixed with other drugs
Potassium chloride		epinephrine, sulphadiazine sodium
Prednisolone sodium phosphate		calcium gluconate, promethazine hydrochloride
Procaine benzylpenicillin		menbutone
Promethazine hydrochloride		should not be mixed with other drugs
Ringer's solution		sodium bicarbonate intravenous infusion
Sodium bicarbonate intravenous infusion		calcium-containing solutions, compound sodium lactate intravenous infusion, epinephrine, magnesium sulphate, norepinephrine acid tartrate, pethidine hydrochloride, Ringer's solution, streptomycin sulphate, tetracyclines, vitamins B and C

List of drug compatibilities and incompatibilities (continued)

Drug	Compatibilities	Incompatibilities
Sodium chloride intravenous infusion 0.9%		norepinephrine acid tartrate
Sodium clodronate	sodium chloride 0.9%	
Sodium nitroprusside	glucose 5% (use immediately, protect from light)	
Streptomycin sulphate		calcium gluconate, heparin sodium, penicillins, sulphadiazine sodium, sodium bicarbonate intravenous infusion, tylosin
Sulfadiazine sodium		electrolyte solutions, glucose 10% intravenous infusion, potassium chloride
Sulfafurazole diolamine		electrolyte solutions
Sulfamethoxazole with trimethoprim	sodium chloride 0.9%, glucose 5%	
Sulfonamides		should not be mixed with other drugs
Suxamethonium chloride		thiopental or other alkaline solutions
Tetracyclines		calcium gluconate, cephalosporins, chloramphenicol sodium succinate, chlorpromazine hydrochloride, glucose intravenous infusion[1], heparin sodium, hydrocortisone sodium succinate, penicillins, sodium bicarbonate intravenous infusion, tylosin any solution with high calcium, magnesium, or sodium content
Thiopental sodium	sodium chloride 0.9%, water for injections	methylprednisolone sodium succinate, suxamethonium chloride, acids, acid salts, oxidising agents, dextrose-saline solution
Tylosin		heparin sodium, hydrocortisone sodium succinate, streptomycin sulphate, tetracyclines
Vitamin B complex		should not be mixed with other drugs
Vitamins B and C		chloramphenicol sodium succinate, chlorpromazine hydrochloride, methylprednisolone sodium succinate, sodium bicarbonate intravenous infusion
Zidovudine	water for injections	

[1]caution: conflicting literature

Appendix 3: Conversions and Units

Mass

g	oz
28.3	1.0
454.0	16.0 (1 lb)

kg	lb
1.0	2.2
2.0	4.4
3.0	6.6
4.0	8.8
5.0	11.0
6.0	13.2
6.35	14.0 (1 stone)
10.0	22.05
20.0	44.1
50.0	110.23
50.8	112.0 (1 hundredweight, 1 cwt)
100.0	220.46
200.0	440.9
500.0	1102.3
1000.0	2204.6
1016.0	2240.0 (1 ton)

1 tonne	=	1000 kilograms (kg)
1 kilogram (kg)	=	1000 grams (g)
1 gram (g)	=	1000 milligrams (mg)
1 milligram (mg)	=	1000 micrograms (µg)
1 microgram (µg)	=	1000 nanograms (ng)
1 nanogram (ng)	=	1000 picograms (pg)

Conversion figures for imperial to metric

ounces	×	28.349	=	g
pounds	×	0.453	=	kg
stones	×	6.350	=	kg
hundredweights	×	50.802	=	kg
tons	×	1016.050	=	kg
tons	×	1.016	=	tonnes

Volume

mL	fl oz
50	1.8
100	3.5
150	5.3
200	7.0
500	17.6
568	20.0 (1 pint)
1000	35.2

litres	gallons
1.0	0.22
4.55	1.0
10.0	2.2
100.0	22.0
1000.0	220.0

1 litre	=	1000 millilitres (mL)
1 millilitre	=	1000 microlitres (µL)

Conversion figures for imperial to metric

fluid ounces	×	28.413	=	mL
fluid ounces	×	0.028	=	litres
pints	×	0.568	=	litres
gallons	×	4.546	=	litres

Other conversions and units

1 kilocalorie (kcal)	=	4186.8 joules (J)
1 gallon of water	=	10.0 pounds
	=	4.55 kg
1 gallon	=	0.16 cu. feet
1 inch (in)	=	25.4 mm
1 foot (ft)	=	0.305 metre (305.0 mm)
1 yard (yd)	=	0.914 metre (914.0 mm)
1 metre (m)	=	39.37 in
	=	3.28 ft
	=	1.09 yd

Temperature

°C	°F	°C	°F
0	32	39	102.2
10	50	40	104.0
25	77	41	105.8
35	95	42	107.6
36	96.8	43	109.4
37	98.6	44	111.2
38	100.4	45	113.0

Parts per million (ppm)

1 ppm		
	=	1 mg/litre
	=	1 mL/1000 litres
	=	1 g/1000 litres
	=	1 mg/kg

Parts per billion (ppb)

1 ppb		
	=	1 microgram/litre
	=	1 microgram/kg

Conversion tables from body-weight to surface area

Weight (kg) to surface area (m^2) for dogs

kg	m^2	kg	m^2	kg	m^2
0.5	0.06	17.0	0.66	34.0	1.05
1.0	0.10	18.0	0.69	35.0	1.07
2.0	0.15	19.0	0.71	36.0	1.09
3.0	0.20	20.0	0.74	37.0	1.11
4.0	0.25	21.0	0.76	38.0	1.13
5.0	0.29	22.0	0.78	39.0	1.15
6.0	0.33	23.0	0.81	40.0	1.17
7.0	0.36	24.0	0.83	41.0	1.19
8.0	0.40	25.0	0.85	42.0	1.21
9.0	0.43	26.0	0.88	43.0	1.23
10.0	0.46	27.0	0.90	44.0	1.25
11.0	0.49	28.0	0.92	45.0	1.26
12.0	0.52	29.0	0.94	46.0	1.28
13.0	0.55	30.0	0.96	47.0	1.30
14.0	0.58	31.0	0.99	48.0	1.32
15.0	0.60	32.0	1.01	49.0	1.34
16.0	0.63	33.0	1.03	50.0	1.36

Weight (kg) to surface area (m^2) for cats

kg	m^2	kg	m^2	kg	m^2
2.0	0.159	3.0	0.208	4.0	0.252
2.2	0.169	3.2	0.217	4.2	0.260
2.4	0.179	3.4	0.226	4.4	0.269
2.6	0.189	3.6	0.235	4.6	0.277
2.8	0.199	3.8	0.244	4.8	0.285
				5.0	0.292

Moles, millimoles, and millequivalents

A **mole** (mol) is the amount of substance that contains as many entities (atoms, molecules, ions, electrons, or other particles or specified groups of particles) as there are atoms in 0.012 kg of carbon-12. A **millimole** (mmol) is one thousandth of this amount and for ions is the ionic mass (the sum of the relative atomic masses of the elements of an ion) expressed in milligrams. A **milliequivalent** is this quantity divided by the valency of the ion. Non-ionic compounds such as dextrose cannot be expressed in terms of milliequivalents. Thus one mole of NaCl (molecular weight 58.45) weighs 58.45 g, and 58.45 mg of NaCl contains one millimole. This amount of NaCl contains 23.0 mg of Na^+ (1 mmol of Na^+) and 35.45 mg of Cl^- (1 mmol of Cl^-) and therefore 1 milliequivalent each of sodium and chloride ions.

Tonicity

When two solutions, each containing the same number of solute particles are separated by a *perfect* semipermeable membrane, they are stated to be **iso-osmotic**, that is they are in osmotic equilibrium. There is no net movement across the membrane. However, in biological systems semipermeable membranes permit the passage of some solute particles. When two solutions, separated by such a membrane, are in osmotic equilibrium they are said to be **isotonic** with respect to that membrane. Solutions administered parenterally or applied to mucous surfaces should be isotonic if used in large volume. For small volumes, such as eye drops, nasal drops, or subcutaneous injections, isotonicity is desirable but not essential.

Appendix 4: Weights of Animals

The weight of an individual within a species or breed varies greatly, and ideally **each animal should be accurately weighed** before an appropriate drug dosage is administered. The following weight ranges are for guidance only and refer to adult animals.

Species	Body-weight	Species	Body-weight
Horses	400–1000 kg	African grey parrot	310–530 g
Cattle	600–700 kg	Amazon parrot	250–500 g
Sheep	45–100 kg	Budgerigar	30–85 g
Goats	45–100 kg	Canary	12–29 g
Deer	200–300 kg	Cockatiel	70–108 g
Pigs	60–200 kg	Lesser sulphur crested cockatoo	228–315 g
Dogs	50–80 kg Saint Bernard 25–32 kg (Labrador Retriever) 7–10 kg (Fox Terrier) 2–4 kg 'toy' breeds (e.g. Maltese Terrier, Yorkshire Terrier, Dachsund)	Lovebird	42–55 g
		Macaw	850–1500 g
		Mynah bird	180–260 g
Cats	3–5 kg	Zebra finch	10–16 g
Pigeons	350–500 g		
Ostriches	120–170 kg (male) 90–130 kg (female)	Ferret	500–1500 g
		Chinchilla	400–800 g
		Gerbil	50–130 g

Body-weight estimation for horses

$$W \text{ (kg)} = \frac{\text{Length (cm)}^{0.97} \times \text{Girth (cm)}^{1.78}}{3011}$$

length = point of elbow to point of buttock
girth = umbilical girth

Species	Body-weight
Guinea Pig	750–1500 g
Hamster	100–150 g
Golden Chinese Hamster	40–60 g
Mouse	20–40 g
Rabbit	
Dwarf	1–2 kg
Others	3–6 kg
Rat	300–800 g

Appendix 5: Dosage Estimation from Body-weight

Contributor:

J K Kirkwood, BVSc, PhD, CBiol, FIBiol, MRCVS

This section addresses the problem of estimating drug dosage for species of animals for which there are no measurements of disposition kinetics available and limited availability of species-specific authorised preparations.

There are approximately 4000 species of mammals, 9000 species of birds, and 7000 species of reptiles and amphibians. Therapy of many species has to be based upon extrapolation from treatment regimens that have been studied and found effective in other species. While species may be similar enough to justify attempts to extrapolate from one to another, differences between them make the task difficult and at times hazardous. In addition to the difficulty of dose estimation, the nature of the non-domestic species and the systems of management under which they are kept often set constraints on administration regimens. Readers are reminded that if the animal is a food-producing species, only products authorised for use in food-producing animals may be administered.

In the absence of known contra-indications to drug treatment, the simplest approach to estimating an appropriate dosage regimen is to extrapolate from recommendations for closely related species of a comparable body size. For example, doses for the horse may be a basis for extrapolating to other Equidae or more broadly to other Perissodactyla. If a drug has been found to be safe and effective in a range of domestic species and man, it is likely to be safe in other species although there may be exceptions. For example, ivermectin is safe in many species of birds and mammals but is toxic in collie dogs and also Chelonia.

When prescribing a drug for a species in which it has not been evaluated, it is important to consider the taxonomic position of the animal. Rates of drug absorption, metabolism, and excretion tend to increase with body temperature and decrease with increasing body-size between species.

Metabolic pathways of major importance in one species may be unimportant or non-existent in another. Such variation can influence the kinetics of some drugs. For example, the elimination of salicylates, such as aspirin, is much slower in the cat than in other domestic species. Closely related species are more likely to have similar metabolic pathways.

Rates of drug metabolism are likely to be associated with body temperature. The metabolic rate of reptiles is at least 10 times lower than that of mammals of comparable body-size, even when reptiles are kept at high ambient temperatures. This may cause a difference in drug-clearance rate. Therefore it may be appropriate, in the absence of specific information, to reduce the frequency of drug administration in reptiles compared to that used in mammals (see also Prescribing for reptiles).

The rates of many physiological processes are also dependent on body-size. For example, between species the rate of energy expenditure is proportional to approximately the three-quarter power of body-weight ($W^{0.75}$). In general, volume per time functions, such as glomerular filtration rate and volume of urine produced per hour, increase with $W^{0.75}$. The duration of physiological events, such as blood circulation time or the time taken for the clearance of substances from the circulation, tend to increase with approximately $W^{0.25}$. Therefore, it could be predicted that, if all else is equal, the half-life of a drug would be 10 times shorter in an animal of 5 g than one of 50 kg (that is 10 000 times heavier).

Estimation of dosage regimen. The dangers of extrapolating dosage from one species to another have been well documented, but until there has been more research into drug kinetics in all species of terrestrial vertebrates, there is often no alternative but to extrapolate.

The **dose** required, in mg/kg, to produce a given peak plasma-drug concentration may vary in proportion with body-size. For example, there are indications that smaller doses in mg/kg of drugs such as ketamine may be required in larger-sized animals than in smaller individuals but this has not been fully substantiated. For several other drugs, however, initial plasma concentration, following administration of a given dose in mg/kg, does not appear to vary in relation to body-size in different species.

The **dose frequency** may be more readily predicted. Suppose it is well established that for one species the dose of a drug needed to sustain therapeutic levels is 10 mg/kg once daily. Assuming that drug clearance is related to $W^{0.25}$ and that all else is equal, it would be appropriate to adjust the frequency of administration of a 10 mg/kg dose to an animal of a different species using the following equation:

$$F_2 = F_1 \frac{W_1^{0.25}}{W_2^{0.25}}$$

where W_1 and F_1 are the body-weight (kg) and recommended dose frequency for the species for which dosage is known, and W_2 and F_2 are body-weight and estimated dose frequency for the animal for which the information is required. Therefore, if W_2 is 10 000 times less than W_1, the dose frequency, if all else is assumed to be equal, should be 10 times greater.

The information given in the table indicates how the predicted dose frequency alters with the weight ratio W_1/W_2.

In estimating the dose frequency for ectothermic animals, the lower metabolic rate should be borne in mind and information on dosage adjustment is given in Prescibing for reptiles.

Estimation of dose frequency

W_1/W_2	F_2/F_1
10 000	10.0
1000	5.6
100	3.2
10	1.8
1.0	1.0
0.1	0.56
0.01	0.32
0.001	0.18
0.0001	0.10

Animal$_1$ = dose frequency known
Animal$_2$ = dose frequency required
W = body-weight (kg)
F = dose frequency

Index of Manufacturers and Organisations

This index comprises a list of manufacturers of preparations listed in *The Veterinary Formulary* and organisations associated with veterinary practice.

Abbott, UK.
Abbott Laboratories Ltd, Abbott House, Norden Road, Maidenhead, Berkshire, SL6 4XE, UK.
Telephone: +44 (0)1628 773355
Facsimile: +44 (0)1628 644185

Abbott, USA.
Abbott Laboratories, 1400 Sheridan Rd, North Chicago, IL 60064, USA.
Telephone: +1 847 938 7662
Facsimile: +1 847 938 0659

Action, Austral.
Action Chemical Co Pty Ltd, 224 High Street, Cranbourne, Vic. 3977, Australia.
Telephone: +61 (0)3 5996 1818
Facsimile: +61 (0)3 5996 7943

AEVA, Austral.
Australian Equine Veterinary Association, PO Box 1570, Artarmon, NSW 2064, Australia.
Telephone: +61 (0)2 9411 5342

Agri Labs, USA.
Agri Labs Ltd, 20927 State Route K, St Joseph, MO 64505, USA.
Telephone: +1 816 233 9533
Facsimile: +1 816 233 9546

Agricultural and Veterinary Pharmacists Group, UK.
RPSGB, 1 Lambeth High Street, London, SE1 7JN, UK.
Telephone: +44 (0)20 7735 9141
Facsimile: +44 (0)20 7735 7629

Agriculture and Agrifoods Canada, Canad.
Race Track Division, 930 Carling Avenue, Ottawa, Ontario, K1A 0C5, Canada.
Telephone: +1 613 759 1000

Agrimin, UK.
Agrimin Ltd, 11c The Flarepath Elsham Wold Industrial Estate, Brigg, Lincolnshire, DN20 0SP, UK
Telephone: +44 (0)1652 688046
Facsimile: +44 (0)1652 688049

AgriPharm, USA.
AgriPharm, c/o RXV Products, 6301 Deramus, Kansas City, MO 64120, USA.
Telephone: +1 816 483 9220
Facsimile: +1 816 483 9455

Agrotech, Austral.
Agrotech Australia Pty Ltd, 30 Talofa Place, Castle Hill, NSW 2154, Australia.
Telephone: +61 (0)2 9899 4360
Facsimile: +61 (0)2 9899 4361

Agvet, NZ.
Agvet Consultants Ltd, 702-709 Hopetoun Street, Auckland 1, New Zealand.
Telephone: +64 (0)9 366 6218
Facsimile: +64 (0)9 366 6217

Alcon, UK.
Alcon Laboratories (UK) Ltd, Pentagon Park, Boundary Way, Hemel Hempstead, Hertfordshire, HP2 7UD, UK.
Telephone: +44 (0)1442 341234
Facsimile: +44 (0)1442 341200

Alfa Laval Agri, UK.
Alfa Laval Agri Ltd, Oakfield, Cwmbran, Gwent, NP44 7XE, UK.
Telephone: +44 (0)1633 838071
Facsimile: +44 (0)1633 873460

Allerderm/Virbac, USA.
Allerderm/Virbac Inc, 3200 Meacham Boulevard, Fort Worth, TX 76137, USA.
Telephone: +1 800 338 3659

Allergan, UK.
Allergan Ltd, Coronation Road, High Wycombe, Buckinghamshire, HP12 3SH, UK.
Telephone: +44 (0)1494 444722
Facsimile: +44 (0)1494 473593

Alliance, UK.
Alliance Pharmaceuticals Ltd, Avonbridge House, Bath Road, Chippenham, Wiltshire, SN15 2BB, UK.
Telephone: +44 (0)1249 466966
Facsimile: +44 (0)1249 466977
E-mail:
info@alliancepharm.co.uk

Alpharma, UK.
Alpharma, Portland House, 1 Bishop Street, Mansfield, Nottinghamshire, NG18 1HL, UK
Telephone: +44 (0)976 294026

Alpharma, USA.
Alpharma Animal Health Division, One Executive Drive, Fort Lee, NJ 07024, USA.
Telephone: +1 201 947 7774
Facsimile: +1 201 947 3879

Alstoe, Eire.
Alstoe Animal Health, Alstoe Ltd, 37-39 Burton Street, Melton Mowbray, Leicestershire, LE13 1AF, UK.
Telephone: +353 (0)1 830 9446
Facsimile: +353 (0)1 830 3276

Alstoe, UK.
Alstoe Ltd Animal Health, Granary Chambers, 37–39 Burton Street, Melton Mowbray, Leicestershire, UK.
Telephone: +44 (0)1664 411663
Facsimile: +44 (0)1664 481527

Ancare, NZ.
Ancare New Zealand Ltd, 48 Diana Drive, Glenfield, Auckland 10, New Zealand.
Telephone: +64 (0)9 444 1693
Facsimile: +64 (0)9 444 9948

Anchor, USA.
Anchor Division, Boehringer Ingelheim Vetmedica, Health Inc, 2621 N Belt Highway, St Joseph, MO 64506, USA.
Telephone: +1 800 821 7467
Facsimile: +1 816 236 2789

Animal Health, NZ.
Animal Health Advisory, 702-709 Hopetoun Street, Auckland 1, New Zealand.
Telephone: +64 (0)9 366 6218
Facsimile: +64 (0)9 366 6217

Animal Health Trust, UK.
Animal Health Trust, PO Box 5, Newmarket, Suffolk, CB8 8JH, UK.
Telephone: +44 (0)1638 750659
Facsimile: +44 (0)1638 750794
E-mail:
100546.3721@compuserve.com

Animalcare, UK.
Animalcare Ltd, Common Road, Dunnington, York, YO19 5RU, UK.
Telephone: +44 (0)1904 488661
Facsimile: +44 (0)1904 488184

Anpharm, UK.
Antigen Pharmaceuticals (UK), Antigen House, 82 Waterloo Road, Hillside, Southport, PR8 4QW, UK.
Telephone: +44 (0)1704 562777
Facsimile: +44 (0)1704 562888

Anthony, USA.
Anthony Products Co, 5539 Ayon Avenue, Irwindale, CA 91706, USA.
Telephone: +1 626 301 1453
Facsimile: +1 626 812 0524

APBC, UK.
Association of Pet Behaviour Counsellors, PO Box 46, Worcester, WR8 9YS, UK.
Telephone: +44 (0)1386 751151
Facsimile: +44 (0)1386 751151
E-mail:
apbc@petbcent.demon.co.uk

APDT, UK.
Association of Pet Dog Trainers, Peacock's Farm, Northchapel, Petworth, West Sussex, GU28 9JB, UK.

Apex, Austral.
Apex Laboratories Pty Ltd, 61 Chivers Road, Somersby, NSW 2250, Australia.
Telephone: +61 (0)2 4340 0555
Facsimile: +61 (0)2 4340 0888

APS, NZ.
APS Chemicals, 119 Carbine Road, Mount Wellington, Auckland, New Zealand.
Telephone: +64 (0)9 276 4019
Facsimile: +64 (0)9 276 7231

Argent, USA.
Argent Chemical Laboratories, 8702 152nd Avenue, NE Redmond, WA 98052, USA.
Telephone: +1 425 885 3777 or +1 800 426 6258
Facsimile: +1 425 885 2112

Armitage, UK.
Armitage Bros Ltd, Armitage House, Colwick, Nottingham, Nottinghamshire, NG4 3BA, UK.
Telephone: +44 (0)1159 614984
Facsimile: +44 (0)1159 617496

Arnolds, UK.
Arnolds Veterinary Products Ltd, Cartmel Drive, Harlescott, Shrewsbury, SY1 3TB, UK.
Telephone: +44 (0)1743 441632
Facsimile: +44 (0)1743 462111
E-mail: technical@arnolds.co.uk

Arthropharm, UK.
Arthropharm (Europe) Ltd, 42 Upper Ramone Park, Portadown, Co. Armagh, BT63 5TD, UK.
Telephone: +44 (0)1762 331078
Facsimile: +44 (0)1762 331078

Aspen, USA.
Aspen Veterinary Resources Ltd, 1812 Jasper, N Kansas City, MO 64116, USA.
Telephone: +1 816 283 0550
Facsimile: +1 816 283 0770

Aspiring Animal Services, NZ.
Aspiring Animal Services Ltd, Ballantyne Road, RD 2, Wanaka, New Zealand.
Telephone: +64 (0)3 443 7951
Facsimile: +64 (0)3 443 7951

ASTA Medica, UK.
ASTA Medica Ltd, 168 Cowley Road, Cambridge, CB4 0DL, UK.
Telephone: +44 (0)1223 423434
Facsimile: +44 (0)1223 420943

Astra, UK.
AstraZeneca, Home Park, Kings Langley, Hertfordshire, WD4 8DH, UK.
Telephone: +44 (0)800 7830033
Facsimile: +44 (0)1923 260431

Ausrichter, Austral.
Ausrichter Pty Ltd, 2/21 Chester Street, Camperdown, NSW 2050, Australia.
Telephone: +61 (0)2 9517 1166
Facsimile: +61 (0)2 9516 5810

Australian Petroleum, Austral.
Australian Petroleum Pty Ltd, MCL Centre, 19-29 Martin Place, Sydney, NSW 2000, Australia.
Telephone: +61 (0)2 9250 5169
Facsimile: +61 (0)2 9250 5758

AVA, Austral.
Australian Veterinary Association, 134 Hampden Road, Artarmon, 2064, NSW, Australia.

AVL, UK.
Aquaculture Vaccines Ltd, Aquaculture Centre, 24-26 Gold Street, Saffron Walden, Essex, CB10 1EJ, UK.
Telephone: +44 (0)1799 528167
Facsimile: +44 (0)1799 525546
E-mail: vaccines@avl.co.uk

Axiom, UK.
Axiom Veterinary Laboratories, 5 George Street, Teignmouth, Devon, TQ14 8AH, UK.
Telephone: +44 (0)1626 778844
Facsimile: +44 (0)1626 779570

Baker Norton, UK.
Division of Norton Healthcare Ltd, Albert Basin, Royal Docks, London, E16 2QJ, UK.
Telephone: +44 (0)8705 020304
Facsimile: +44 (0)8705 323334

Battle Hayward & Bower, UK.
Battle Hayward & Bower Ltd, Crofton Drive, Lincoln, LN3 4NP, UK.
Telephone: +44 (0)1522 529206
Facsimile: +44 (0)1522 538960

Baxter, UK.
Baxter Healthcare Ltd, Caxton Way, Thetford, Norfolk, IP24 3SE, UK.
Telephone: +44 (0)1842 767189
Facsimile: +44 (0)1842 767134

Bayer, Austral.
Bayer Australia Ltd, 875 Pacific Highway, Pymble, NSW 2073, Australia.
Telephone: +61 (0)2 9391 6000
Facsimile: +61 (0)2 9391 6225

Bayer, Eire.
Bayer Limited, Chapel Lane, Swords, Co. Dublin, Eire.
Telephone: +353 (0)1 813 2222
Facsimile: +353 (0)1 813 2288

Bayer, NZ.
Bayer (NZ) Ltd, Argus Place, Glenfield, Auckland, New Zealand.
Telephone: +64 (0)9 443 3093
Facsimile: +64 (0)9 443 3094

Bayer, UK.
Bayer plc, Animal Health Business Group, Eastern Way, Bury St Edmunds, Suffolk, IP32 7AH, UK.
Telephone: +44 (0)1284 763200
Facsimile: +44 (0)1284 702810

For information on authorised human medicines:
Bayer plc, Pharmaceutical Division, Bayer House, Strawberry Hill, Newbury, Berkshire, RG14 1JA, UK.
Telephone: +44 (0)1635 563000
Facsimile: +44 (0)1635 563393
E-mail: medical.affairs@bayer.co.uk

Bayer, USA.
Bayer Corporation, PO Box 390, Shawnee Mission, KS 66201, USA.
Telephone: +1 800 422 9874
Facsimile: +1 913 962 2878

BCVA, UK.
British Cattle Veterinary Association, The Green, Frampton-on-Severn, Gloucestershire, GL2 7EP, UK.
Telephone: +44 (0)1452 740816
Facsimile: +44 (0)1452 741117
E-mail: 106534.2075@compuserve.com

Beesy, UK.
Beesy Ltd, 11 St James Park, Chelmsford, Essex, CM1 2JG, UK.

Beiersdorf, UK.
Beiersdorf UK Ltd, Yeomans Drive, Blakelands, Milton Keynes, Buckinghamshire, MK14 5LS, UK.
Telephone: +44 (0)1908 211444
Facsimile: +44 (0)1908 211555

Bell and Croyden, UK.
John Bell and Croyden, 54 Wigmore Street, London, W1H 0AU, UK.
Telephone: +44 (0)20 7935 5555
Facsimile: +44 (0)20 7935 9605

BEVA, UK.
British Equine Veterinary Association, 5 Finlay Street, London, SW6 6HE, UK.
Telephone: +44 (0)20 7610 6080
Facsimile: +44 (0)20 7610 6823

Bimeda, Austral.
Bimeda Australia, 45 Clarence Street, Sydney, NSW 2113, Australia.
Telephone: +61 (0)2 9956 7105
Facsimile: +61 (0)2 9956 7105

Bimeda, UK.
A division of Cross Vetpharm Group (UK) Ltd, Bryn Cefni Business Park, Llangefni, Anglesey, LL77 7XA, UK.
Telephone: +44 (0)1248 725400
Facsimile: +44 (0)1248 724232
E-mail: sales@bimeda.co.uk

Bio-Ceutic, USA.
Bio-Ceutic Division, Boehringer Ingelheim Vetmedica Inc, 2621 N Belt Highway, St Joseph, MO 64506, USA.
Telephone: +1 800 821 7467
Facsimile: +1 816 236 2789

Bioceuticals, UK.
Bioceuticals Ltd, 26 Zennor Road, London, SW12 0PS, UK.
Telephone: +44 (0)20 8675 5664

Bioceutics, Austral.
Bioceutics Pty Ltd, 52 Carrington Road, Randwick, NSW 2031, Australia.
Telephone: +61 (0)2 9314 5100
Facsimile: +61 (0)2 9314 5166

Biochemical Veterinary Research, Austral.
Biochemical Veterinary Reseach Pty Ltd, Lot 6 Gantry Place, Braemar, NSW 2575, Australia.
Telephone: +61 (0)2 4871 3155
Facsimile: +61 (0)2 4871 3161

Biopharm, Austral.
Biopharm Australia Pty Ltd, 111 Bronte Road, Bondi Junction, NSW 2022, Australia.
Telephone: +61 (0)2 9389 0000
Facsimile: +61 (0)2 9387 5473

Blue Cross, Austral.
Blue Cross Veterinary Products Pty Ltd, 9 Old Beecroft Road, Cheltenham, NSW 2119, Australia.
Telephone: +61 (0)2 9876 3941
Facsimile: +61 (0)2 9876 3825

Bob Martin, UK.
The Bob Martin Company, Wemberham Lane, Yatton, Somerset, BS19 4BS, UK.
Telephone: +44 (0)1934 838061
Facsimile: +44 (0)1934 876184

Boehringer Ingelheim Vetmedica, USA.
Boehringer Ingelheim Vetmedica Inc, 2621 N Belt Highway, St Joseph, MO 64506, USA.
Telephone: +1 800 821 7467
Facsimile: +1 816 236 2789

Boehringer Ingelheim, Austral.
Boehringer Ingelheim Pty Ltd, Animal Health Division, 50 Broughton Road, Artarmon, NSW 2064, Australia.
Telephone: +61 (0)2 9428 4011
Facsimile: +61 (0)2 9427 4654

Boehringer Ingelheim, Eire.
Boehringer Ingelheim Vetmedica, Ellesfield Road, Bracknell, Berkshire, RG12 8YS, UK.
Telephone: +44 (0)1344 746959
Facsimile: +44 (0)1344 741349

Boehringer Ingelheim, NZ.
Boehringer Ingelheim Vetmedica (NZ) Ltd, 47 Druces Road, Manukau City, New Zealand.
Telephone: +64 (0)9 262 1356
Facsimile: +64 (0)9 262 1462

Boehringer Ingelheim, UK.
Boehringer Ingelheim Ltd, Ellesfield Avenue, Bracknell, Berkshire, RG12 8YS,UK.
Telephone: +44 (0)1344 424600
Facsimile: +44 (0)1344 741444

For information on authorised human medicines:
Boehringer Ingelheim Ltd, Ellesfield Avenue, Bracknell, Berkshire, RG12 4YS, UK.
Telephone: +44 (0)1344 424600
Facsimile: +44 (0)1344 741444

Boehringer Ingelheim/NOBL, USA.
Boehringer Ingelheim/NOBL, 1568 N Main Avenue, Sioux Center, IA 51250, USA.
Telephone: +1 800 323 7527
Facsimile: +1 712 722 0883

Bomac, NZ.
Bomac Laboratories Ltd, Cnr Wiri Station Road and Hobill Avenue, Manukau City, New Zealand.
Telephone: +64 (0)9 262 3169
Facsimile: +64 (0)9 262 3008

BP(Vet), UK.
British Pharmacopoeia Commission, Market Towers, 1 Nine Elms Lane, London, SW8 5NQ, UK.
Telephone: +44 (0)20 7273 0561
Facsimile: +44 (0)20 7273 0566

Braun, UK.
B Braun Medical Ltd, Thorncliffe Park, Sheffield, S35 2PW, UK.
Telephone: +44 (0)114 2259000
Facsimile: +44 (0)114 2259111

BresaGen, Austral.
BresaGen Ltd, 38-39 Winwood Street, Thebarton, SA 5031, Australia.
Telephone: +61 (0)8 8234 2660
Facsimile: +61 (0)8 8234 6268

Brinicombe, UK.
Denis Brinicombe, Fordton Industrial Estate, Crediton, Devon, EX17 3BZ, UK.
Telephone: +44 (0)1363 775115
Facsimile: +44 (0)1363 772114
E-mail: sales@brinicombe.co.uk

Bristol-Myers, UK.
Bristol-Myers Squibb Pharmaceuticals Ltd, 141-149 Staines Road, Hounslow, Middlesex, TW3 3JA, UK.
Telephone: +44 (0)20 8572 7422
Facsimile: +44 (0)20 8754 3789

Britannia, UK.
Britannia Pharmaceuticals Ltd, 41-51 Brighton Road, Redhill, Surrey, RH1 6YS, UK.
Telephone: +44 (0)1737 773741
Facsimile: +44 (0)1737 762672
E-mail:
medicalservices@forum-group.co.uk

The British Horseracing Board
42 Portman Square, London, W1H 9FH, UK.
Telephone: +44 (0)20 7396 0011

British Horse Society, UK.
British Horse Society, British Equestrian Centre, 16-17 Stoneleigh Deer Park, Kenilworth, Warwickshire, CV8 2XZ, UK.
Telephone: +44 (0)1926 707707

British Rabbit Council, UK.
Purefoy House, 7 Kirkgate, Newark, Nottingham, NG24 1AD, UK.
Telephone: +44 (0)1636 676042
Facsimile: +44 (0)1636 611683

BSAVA, UK.
British Small Animal Veterinary Association, Woodrow House, 1 Telford Way, Waterwells Business Park, Quedgeley, Gloucestershire, GL2 4AB, UK.
Telephone: +44 (0)1452 726700
Facsimile: +44 (0)1452 726701

BSI, UK.
British Standards Institute, 389 Chiswick High Road, London, W4 4AL, UK.
Telephone: +44 (0)20 8996 9000
Facsimile: +44 (0)20 8996 7400

Butler, USA.
The Butler Company, 5000 Bradenton Avenue, Dublin, OH 43017-7153, USA.
Telephone: +1 614 761 9095
Facsimile: +1 614 761 9096

BVA, UK.
British Veterinary Association, 7 Mansfield Street, London, W1G 9NQ, UK.
Telephone: +44 (0)20 7636 6541
Facsimile: +44 (0)20 7436 2970

BVA Publications, UK.
T G Scott, 6 Bourne Enterprise Centre, Wrotham Road, Borough Green, Kent, TN15 8DG, UK.
Telephone: +44 (0)1732 884023
Facsimile: +44 (0)1732 884034

Cambridge, UK.
Cambridge Laboratories, Richmond House, Old Brewery Court, Sandyford Road, Newcastle upon Tyne, NE2 1XG, UK.
Telephone: +44 (0)191 261 5950
Facsimile: +44 (0)191 222 1006

Carr & Day & Martin, UK.
Carr & Day & Martin Ltd, Lloyds House, Alderley Road, Wilmslow, Cheshire, SK9 1QT, UK.
Telephone: +44 (0)1625 545200
Facsimile: +44 (0)1625 548488

Castlemead, UK.
Castlemead Healthcare Ltd, PO Box 57, Ware, SG10 6LL, UK.
Telephone: +44 (0)7071 224986
Facsimile: +44 (0)7070 728892

CCD, Austral.
C.C.D. Animal Health, Division of Ridley Agriproducts, 351 Wentworth Avenue, Pendle Hill, NSW 2145, Australia.
Telephone: +61 (0)2 9631 0888
Facsimile: +61 (0)2 9896 1881

Ceva, UK.
Ceva Animal Health Ltd, 7 Awberry Court, Hatters Lane, Watford, Hertfordshire, WD1 8YJ, UK.
Telephone: +44 (0)1923 212212
Facsimile: +44 (0)1923 243001

Chanelle, Eire.
Chanelle Pharmaceuticals Manufacturing Ltd, Loughrea, Co. Galway, Eire.
Telephone: +353 (0)91 841788/ 841565
Facsimile: +353 (0)91 841303/ 842937

Chanelle, UK.
Chanelle Animal Health Ltd, 7 Rodney Street, Liverpool, L1 9HZ, UK.
Telephone: +44 (0)568 750432
Facsimile: +44 (0)568 750432

Chauvin, UK.
Chauvin Pharmaceuticals Ltd, Ashton Road, Harold Hill, Romford, Essex, RM3 8SL, UK.
Telephone: +44 (0)1708 383838
Facsimile: +44 (0)1708 371316

Chemavet, NZ.
Chemavet, Division of Pharmaco (NZ) Ltd, 49 George Street, Newmarket, Auckland, New Zealand.
Telephone: +64 (0)9 377 3336
Facsimile: +64 (0)9 307 1307

Chugai, UK.
Chugai Pharma UK Ltd, Mulliner House, Flanders Road, Turnham Green, London, W4 1NN, UK.
Telephone: +44 (0)20 8987 5680
Facsimile: +44 (0)20 8987 5661

CIBA Vision, UK.
CIBA Vision (UK) Ltd, Flanders Road, Hedge End, Southampton, SO30 2LG, UK.
Telephone: +44 (0)1489 775580
Facsimile: +44 (0)1489 798074

Coloplast, UK.
Coloplast Ltd, Peterborough Business Park, Peterborough, PE2 6FX, UK.
Telephone: +44 (0)1733 392000
Facsimile: +44 (0)1733 233348

Concord, UK.
Concord Pharmaceuticals Ltd, Melville House, High Street, Dunmow, Essex, CM6 1AF, UK.
Telephone: +44 (0)845 602 0137
Facsimile: +44 (0)1371 874883
E-mail:
enquiries@concord-pharma.com

Controlled Medications, Austral.
Controlled Medications Pty Ltd, (trading as All Farm Animal Health), 4 Handley Crescent, Dandenong, Victoria 3175, Australia.
Telephone: +61 (0)3 9792 2201
Facsimile: +61 (0)3 9791 8349

ConvaTec, UK.
ConvaTec Ltd, Harrington House, Milton Road, Ickenham, Uxbridge, Middlesex, UB10 8PU, UK.
Telephone: +44 (0)1895 628400
Facsimile: +44 (0)1895 628456

Co-Operative Animal Health, Eire.
Co-Operative Animal Health Limited, Tullow, Co. Carlow, Eire.
Telephone: +353 (0)503 51251
Facsimile: +353 (0)503 51856

Coopers, Austral.
Coopers Animal Health, Austral.
Contact: Schering-Plough, Austral.

Co-Pharma, UK.
Co-Pharma Ltd, Talbot House, Church Street, Rickmansworth, Hertfordshire, WD3 1DE, UK.
Telephone: +44 (0)1923 710934
Facsimile: +44 (0)1923 770199

Cortecs, UK.
Cortecs Healthcare Ltd, Abbey Road, Wrexham Industrial Estate, Wrexham, Clwyd, LL13 9PW, UK.
Telephone: +44 (0)1978 661351
Facsimile: +44 (0)1978 661673

Country Life Animal Health, Austral.
Country Life Animal Health, Division of Parnell Laboratories (Aust) Pty Ltd, Austral.
Contact: Parnell, Austral.

Cox, UK.
Cox, Unit 1, Greencroft Industrial Park, Stanley, Co Durham, DH9 7YA, UK.
Telephone: +44 (0)1207 529000
Facsimile: +44 (0)1207 529966
E-mail:
enquiries@coxsurgical.co.uk

CP, UK.
CP Pharmaceuticals Ltd, Ash Road North, Wrexham Industrial Estate, Wrexham, Clwyd, LL13 9UF, UK.
Telephone: +44 (0)1978 661261
Facsimile: +44 (0)1978 661702
E-mail:
mail@cppharma.co.uk

Crawford, UK.
Crawford Pharmaceuticals, Furtho House, 20 Towcester Road, Milton Keynes, MK19 6AQ, UK.
Telephone: +44 (0)1908 262346
Facsimile: +44 (0)1908 567730

Creosote Council, UK.
The Creosote Council, Tar Industries Services, C/- 9 Deerlands Road, Wingerworth, Chesterfield, Derbyshire, S42 6UL, UK.
Telephone: +44 (0)1246 200306
Facsimile: +44 (0)1246 200306

Crown, UK.
Crown Veterinary Pharmaceuticals, Novartis Animal Health UK Ltd, New Cambridge House, Litlington, Hertfordshire, UK.
Telephone: +44 (0)1763 850500
Facsimile:+44 (0)1763 850600

Cypharm, Eire.
Cypharm Limited, 11a Parkmore Estate, Longmile Road, Dublin 12, Eire.
Telephone: +353 (0)1 450 2664
Facsimile: +353 (0)1 456 9075

Daniels, USA.
Daniels Pharmaceuticals, 1945 Craig Road, St Louis, MO 63146, USA.
Telephone: +1 800 525 8466
Facsimile: +1 314 469 5749

DARD, UK.
Department of Agriculture and Rural Development, Veterinary Service, Dundonald House, Upper Newtownards Road, Belfast, BT4 3SB, UK.
Telephone: +44 (0)1232 524580
Facsimile: +44 (0)1232 525012

David, Austral.
David Veterinary Laboratories, Austral.
Contact: Pharmachem, Austral.

Davis, USA.
Davis Manufacturing & Packaging Inc, 541 Proctor Avenue, Scottdale, GA 30079, USA.
Telephone: +1 404 292 2424
Facsimile: +1 404 292 3049

Day Son & Hewitt, UK.
Day Son & Hewitt Ltd, St George's Quay, Lancaster, LA1 5QJ, UK.
Telephone: +44 (0)1524 381821
Facsimile: +44 (0)1524 32080
E-mail: info@day-son-hewitt.co.uk

Delmarva, USA.
Delmarva Laboratories Inc, 1500 Huguenot Road, Ste 106 Midlothian, VA 23113, USA.
Telephone: +1 804 794 7064
Facsimile: +1 804 794 7835

Delvet, Austral.
Delvet Pty Ltd, 7 Kelray Place, Asquith, NSW 2077, Australia.
Telephone: +61 (0)2 9476 6022
Facsimile: +61 (0)2 9476 6123

Denes, UK.
Denes Natural Pet Care Ltd, 2 Osmond Road, Hove, East Sussex, BN3 1TE, UK.
Telephone: +44 (0)1273 325364
Facsimile: +44 (0)1273 325704

Dermacare, Austral.
Dermacare-Vet Pty Ltd, 3331 Pacific Highway, Springwood, Qld 4127, Australia.
Telephone: +61 (0)7 3808 4761
Facsimile: +61 (0)7 3808 7967

Dexcel, UK.
Dexcel Pharma Ltd, Bishop Crewe House, North Street, Daventry, Northamptonshire, NN11 5PN, UK.
Telephone: +44 (0)1327 312266
Facsimile: +44 (0)1327 312262
E-mail: DexcelPharma@compuserve.com

Dista, UK.
Dista Products Ltd, UK.
Contact: Lilly, UK.

DiverseyLever, UK.
DiverseyLever Ltd, Weston Favell Centre, Northampton, NN3 8PD, UK.
Telephone: +44 (0)1604 783505
Facsimile: +44 (0)1604 783506

Dominion, UK.
Dominion Pharma Ltd, Dominion House, Lion Lane, Haslemere, Surrey, GU27 1JL, UK.
Telephone: +44 (0)1428 661078
Facsimile: +44 (0)1428 661075
E-mail: dominion@dompharm.com

Donkey Sanctuary, UK.
The Donkey Sanctuary, Sidmouth, Devon, EX10 0NU, UK.
Telephone: +44 (0)1395 578222

Dorwest Herbs, UK.
Dorwest Herbs, Shipton Gorge, Bridport, Dorset, DT6 4LP, UK.
Telephone: +44(0)1308 897272
Facsimile: +44 (0)1308 897929
E-mail: dorwest@cix.co.uk

Dover, Austral.
Dover Laboratories Pty Ltd, Austral.
Contact: Jurox, Austral.

Du Pont, UK.
Du Pont Pharmaceuticals Ltd, Wedgewood Way, Stevenage, Hertfordshire, SG1 4QN, UK.
Telephone: +44 (0)800 7313339
Facsimile: +44 (0)1438 842533

Duck Producers Association, UK.
Duck Producers Association Ltd, Imperial House, 15-19 Kingsway, London, WC2B 6UA, UK.
Telephone: +44 (0)20 7240 9889
Facsimile: +44 (0)20 7240 7757

DurVet, USA.
DurVet Inc, 100 SE Magellan Drive, Blue Springs, MO 64014, USA.
Telephone: +1 816 229 9101
Facsimile: +1 816 224 3080

DVM, USA.
DVM Pharmaceuticals Inc, 4400 Biscayne Boulevard, Miami, FL 33137, USA.
Telephone: +1 800 367 4902
Facsimile: +1 305 575 6200

ECO, UK.
Eco Animal Health Ltd, 78 Coombe Road, New Malden, Surrey, KT3 4QS, UK.
Telephone: +44 (0)20 84478899
Facsimile: +44 (0)20 84479292
E-mail: sales@ecoanimalhealth.com

Ecolab, UK.
Henkel-Ecolab Ltd, 830 Yeovil Road, Slough, Berkshire, SL1 4JL, UK.
Telephone: +44 (0)1753 534211
Facsimile: +44 (0)1753 693495

Elanco, Austral.
Elanco Animal Health, Division of Eli Lilly Australia Pty Ltd, 112 Wharf Road, West Ryde, NSW 2114, Australia.
Telephone: +61 (0)2 9325 4555
Facsimile: +61 (0)2 9325 4420

Elanco, Eire.
Elanco Animal Health, Dunderrow, Kinsale, Co. Cork, Eire.
Telephone: +353 (0)21 775 858
Facsimile: +353 (0)21 775 152

Elanco, NZ.
Elanco Animal Health, Division of Eli Lilly & Co (NZ) Ltd, 9 Gladding Place, Manukau City, New Zealand.
Telephone: +64 (0)9 262 1370
Facsimile: +64 (0)9 262 1408

Elanco, UK.
Elanco Animal Health, Eli Lilly and Company Limited, Kingsclere

Road, Basingstoke, Hampshire, RG21 6XA, UK.
Telephone: +44 (0)1256 353131
Facsimile: +44 (0)1256 315081
E-mail: elanco_uk_info@lilly.com

Elanco, USA.
Elanco Animal Health, Lilly Corporate Center, Indianapolis, IN 46285, USA.
Telephone: +1 800 428 4441
Facsimile: +1 919 967 8353

EMEA, UK.
European Agency for the Evaluation of Medicinal Products, 7 Westferry Circus, Canary Wharf, London, E14 4HB, UK.
Telephone: +44 (0)20 7418 8400
Facsimile: +44 (0)20 7418 8416

Equi Life, UK.
Equi Life Ltd, Mead House Farm, Dauntsey, Chippenham, Wiltshire, SN15 4JA, UK.
Telephone: +44 (0)870 4440676
Facsimile: +44 (0)870 4440677
E-mail: rae@equilife.co.uk

Equine Products, UK.
Equine Products UK Ltd, 22 Riversdale Court, Newburn Haugh Industrial Estate, Newcastle upon Tyne, NE15 8SG, UK.
Telephone: +44 (0)191 264 5536
Facsimile: +44(0)191 264 0487
E-mail: info@equine-camel.co.uk

ESAVS, Ger.
European School for Advanced Veterinary Studies, Am Kirchplatz 2, D-55765 Birkenfeld, Germany.
Telephone: +49 (0)67 82 2329
Facsimile: +49 (0)67 82 4314
E-mail: ESAVS.BIR@t-online.de

Ethical, NZ.
Ethical Agents Ltd, 54 Hobill Avenue, Wiri, Auckland, New Zealand.
Telephone: +64 (0)9 262 1388
Facsimile: +64 (0)9 262 1411

Eudaemonic, USA.
Eudaemonic Corporation, 7031 N 16th Street, Omaha, NE 68112, USA.
Telephone: +1 800 553 4550
Facsimile: +1 402 453 1052

Evans Vanodine, UK.
Evans Vanodine International plc, Brierley Road, Walton Summit, Preston, PR5 8AH, UK.
Telephone: +44 (0)1772 322200
Facsimile: +44 (0)1772 626000
E-mail:sales@evansvanodine.co.uk

Evsco, USA.
Evsco Pharmaceuticals Affiliate of IGI Inc, PO Box 685 (Harding Highway), Buena, NJ 08310, USA.
Telephone: +1 609 691 2411
Facsimile: +1 609 697 9711

Exelpet, Austral.
Exelpet Products, Effem Foods Ltd, Kelly Street, Wodonga, Vic. 3690, Australia.
Telephone: +61 (0)2 6055 5200
Facsimile: +61 (0)2 6055 5347

Exeter Bee Supplies, UK.
Merrivale Road, Exeter Road Industrial Estate, Okehampton, Devon, EX20 1UD, UK.
Telephone: +44 (0)1837 54084
Facsimile: +44 (0)1837 54085

Farnam, USA.
Farnam Companies Inc, 301 W Osborn Road, Phoenix, AZ 85013, USA.
Telephone: +1 800 720 0032
Facsimile: +1 602 285 1803

Farriers Registration Council, UK.
Sefton House, Adam Court, Newark Road, Peterborough, PE1 5PP, UK.
Telephone: +44 (0)1733 319911
Facsimile: +44 (0)1733 319910

FAWC, UK.
Farm Animal Welfare Council, Ministry of Agriculture, Fisheries & Food, 1A Page Street, London SW1P 4PQ, UK.
Telephone: +44 (0)20 7904 6000

FCI, Belg.
Fédération Cynologique Internationale, Rue Leopold II, 14b-6530, Thuin, Belgium.

FEI, Switz.
Fédération Équestre Internationale, Avenue Mon-Repos 24, PO Box 157, CH-1000 Lausanne 5, Switzerland.
Telephone: +41 21 312 56 56
Facsimile: +41 21 312 86 77

Ferring, UK.
Ferring Pharmaceuticals UK, The Courtyard, Waterside Drive, Langley, Berkshire, SL3 6EZ, UK.
Telephone: +44 (0)1753 214800
Facsimile: +44 (0)1753 214801

FIL, NZ.
FIL Industries Ltd, 142-144 Newton Street, Mount Maunganui South, New Zealand.
Telephone: +64 (0)7 575 2162
Facsimile: +64 (0)7 575 2161

First Priority, USA.
First Priority Inc, 1585 Todd Farm Drive, Elgin, IL 60123, USA.
Telephone: +1 847 289 1600
Facsimile: +1 847 289 1223

Fleabusters, USA.
Fleabusters/RX For Fleas Inc, 6555 NW 9th Avenue, Suite 412, Fort Lauderdale, FL 33309, USA.
Telephone: +1 954 351 9244
Facsimile: +1 954 351 9266

Florizel, UK.
Florizel Ltd, PO Box 138, Stevenage, SG2 8YN, UK.
Telephone: +44 (0)1462 436156
Facsimile: +44 (0)1462 457402

Foran, Eire.
Foran Animal Health (A division of Foran Chemicals Ltd), 2 Cherry Orchard Industrial Estate, Dublin 10, Eire.
Telephone: +353 (0)1 626 8058
Facsimile: +353 (0)1 626 8059

Forley, UK.
Telephone: +44 (0)
Facsimile: +44 (0)

Fort Dodge, Austral.
Fort Dodge Australia Pty Ltd, 23 Victoria Avenue, Castle Hill, NSW 2154, Australia.
Telephone: +61 (0)2 9899 2111
Facsimile: +61 (0)2 9899 2151

Fort Dodge, Eire.
Fort Dodge Laboratories Ireland, Finisklin Industrial Estate, Sligo, Eire.
Telephone: +353 (0)71 70005
Facsimile: +353 (0)71 70009

Fort Dodge, NZ.
Fort Dodge Animal Health Ltd, 4 Fisher Crescent, Mount Wellington, Auckland, New Zealand.
Telephone: +64 (0)9 276 9393
Facsimile: +64 (0)9 276 9292

Fort Dodge, UK.
Fort Dodge Animal Health, Flanders Road, Hedge End, Southampton, SO30 4QH, UK.
Telephone: +44 (0)1489 781711
Facsimile: +44 (0)1489 788306

Fort Dodge, USA.
Fort Dodge Animal Health, 9401 Indian Creek Parkway, Suite 1500, Overland Park, KS 66210, USA.
Telephone: +1 913 664 7000/7122
Facsimile: +1 800 441 0885

Forum, UK.
Forum (Holdings) Ltd, 41-51 Brighton Road, Redhill, Surrey, RH1 6YS, UK.
Telephone: +44 (0)1737 773711
Facsimile: +44 (0)1737 773116

Fresenius Kabi, UK.
Fresenius Kabi Ltd, Parenteral Nutrition Division, Hampton Court, Tudor Road, Manor Park, Runcorn, Cheshire, WA7 1UF, UK.
Telephone: +44 (0)1928 594313
Facsimile: +44 (0)1928 594314

Fresenius, UK.
Fresenius Ltd, Melbury Park, Birchwood, Warrington, WA3 6FF, UK.
Telephone: +44 (0)1925 898000
Facsimile: +44 (0)1925 898002

Galen, UK.
Galen Ltd, Seagoe Industrial Estate, Craigavon, Northern Ireland, BT63 5UA.
Telephone: +44 (0)28 3833 4974
Facsimile: +44 (0)28 3835 0206

GC Hanford, USA.
GC Hanford MFG Company, 304 Oneida Street, PO Box 1017, Syracuse, NY 13201, USA.
Telephone: +1 315 476 7418
Facsimile: +1 315 478 1124

GCCF, UK.
Governing Council of the Cat Fancy, 4-6 Penel Orlieu, Brigwater, Somerset, TA6 3PG, UK.
Telephone: +44 (0)1278 427575

Geistlich, UK.
Geistlich Pharma, Newton Bank, Long Lane, Chester, CH2 2PF, UK.
Telephone: +44 (0)1244 347534
Facsimile: +44 (0)1244 319327

Genitrix, UK.
Genitrix Ltd, The Stables Business Centre, Forest Road, Horsham, West Sussex, RH12 4HL, UK.
Telephone: +44 (0)1403 253528
Facsimile: +44 (0)1403 253571
E-mail: mail@genitrix.co.uk

Giltspur, UK.
Giltspur Scientific Ltd, 6-8 Avondale Industrial Estate, Ballyclare, Co Antrim, Northern Ireland, BT39 9AU, UK.
Telephone: +44 (0)1960 322040
Facsimile: +44 (0)1960 354885

Glaxo Wellcome, UK.
GlaxoWellcome UK, Stockley Park West, Uxbridge, Middlesex, UB11 1BT, UK.
Telephone: +44 (0)20 8990 9000
Facsimile: +44 (0)20 8990 4321

Glenwood, UK.
Glenwood Laboratories Ltd, Jenkins Dale, Chatham, Kent, ME4 5RD, UK.
Telephone: +44 (0)1634 830535
Facsimile: +44 (0)1634 831345
E-mail: g.wooduk@virgin.net

Global Genetics, UK.
Unit 1, Morton Farm, Eye, Leominster, HR6 0DP, UK.
Telephone: +44 (0)1568 612402
Facsimile: +44 (0)1568 616088

Global, USA.
Global Pharmaceutical Corporation, Castor & Kensington Avenue, Philadelphia, PA 19124-5014, USA.
Telephone: +1 215 289 2220 ext 311/308
Facsimile: +1 215 289 2223

Goldshield, UK.
Goldshield Pharmaceuticals Ltd,

NLA Tower, 12-16 Addiscombe Road, Croydon, CR0 0XT, UK.
Telephone: +44 (0)20 8649 8500
Facsimile: +44 (0)20 8686 0807

Goodwinol, USA.
Goodwinol Products Corporation, PO Box 407, Pierce, CO 80650, USA.
Telephone: +1 970 834 1229
Facsimile: +1 970 834 0180

Hansam, UK.
Hansam Healthcare Ltd, 60 Ondine Road, London, SE15 4EB, UK.
Telephone: +44 (0)845 6020137
Facsimile: +44 (0)20 7207 6850

Happy Jack, USA.
Happy Jack Inc, PO Box 475, Highway 258 S, USA.
Telephone: +1 252 747 2911
Facsimile: +1 252 747 4111

Hawgreen, UK.
Hawgreen Ltd, PO Box 157, Hatfield, AL10 8ZP, UK.
Telephone: +44 (0)7071 220777
Facsimile: +44 (0)7070 600678

HBLB, UK.
Horserace Betting Levy Board, 52 Gosvenor Gardens, London, SW1W 0AU, UK.
Telephone: +44 (0)20 73330043
Facsimile: +44 (0)20 73330041
E-mail: hblb@hblb.org.uk

Heska, USA.
Heska Corporation, 1825 Sharp Point Drive, Fort Collins, CO 80525, USA.
Telephone: +1 888 437 5287
Facsimile: +1 970 221 2393

Hill's, UK.
Hill's Pet Nutrition Ltd, The Beacons, Beaconsfield Road, Hatfield, Hertfordshire, AL10 8EQ, UK.
Telephone: +44 (0)1707 276660
Facsimile: +44 (0)1707 271859

Hillcross PharmS, UK.
AAH Pharmaceuticals Ltd, Sapphire Court, Walsgrave Triangle, Coventry, CV2 2TX, UK.
Telephone: +44 (0)24 7643 2000
Facsimile: +44 (0)24 7643 2001

Hi-Perfom, Austral.
Hi-Perform Veterinary Products, Division of Equisci International Pty Ltd, 45 Campbell Drive, Wahroonga, NSW 2076, Australia.
Telephone: +61 (0)2 9489 7051
Facsimile: +61 (0)2 9489 8127

Hoechst Marion Roussel, UK.
Hoechst Marion Roussel Ltd, Aventis Pharma Ltd, Aventis House, 50 Kings Hill Avenue, Kings Hill, West Malling, Kent, ME19 4AH, UK.

Telephone: +44 (0)1732 584000
Facsimile: +44 (0)870 5239605

Hoechst Roussel Vet, Eire.
Hoechst Roussel Vet, Cookstown Industrial Estate, Tallaght, Dublin 24, Eire.
Telephone: +353 (0)1 451 1544
Facsimile: +353 (0)1 459 6068

Hoechst-Roussel, Austral.
Hoechst Roussel Vet Pty Ltd, 381 Woolcock Street, Garbutt, Qld 4814, Australia.
Telephone: +61 (0)7 4779 2401

Hoechst-Roussel, USA.
Hoechst-Roussel Vet, PO Box 4915, Independence Boulevard, Warren, NJ 07059, USA.
Telephone: +1 800 247 4838
Facsimile: +1 908 231 4569

Hornex, UK.
Hornex (Europe) Ltd, R S H Watherston, 5 Lennox Street Lane, Edinburgh, Scotland, EH4 1PZ, UK
Telephone: +44 (0)131 332 4763
Facsimile: +44 (0)131 315 3492

HPA, UK.
The Hurlingham Polo Association, Winterlake, Kirtlington, Kidlington, Oxford, OX5 3HG, UK.
Telephone: +44 (0)1869 350277
Facsimile: +44 (0)1869 350625

HSE, UK.
Health & Safety Executive, National Agricultural Centre, Stoneleigh, Kenilworth, Warwickshire,CV8 2LZ, UK.
Telephone: +44 (0)2476 696518
Facsimile: +44 (0)2476 696542

HSE Books, UK.
PO Box 1999, Sudbury, Suffolk, CO10 2WA, UK.
Telephone: +44 (0)1787 881165
Facsimile: +44 (0)1787 313995

Hymed, USA.
The Hymed Group Corporation, 1890 Bucknell Drive, Bethlehem, PA 18015, USA.
Telephone: +1 610 865 9876
Facsimile: +1 610 691 5930

Iams, UK.
Unit 2, Meadow Brook Industrial Estate, Maxwell Way, Crawley, West Sussex, RH10 2SA, UK.
Telephone: +44 (0)1293 572100
Facsimile: +44 (0)1293 572130

ICN, UK.
ICN Pharmaceuticals Ltd, 1 Elmwood, Chineham Business Park, Crockford Lane, Basingstoke, Hampshire, RG24 8WG, UK.
Telephone: +44 (0)1256 707744
Facsimile: +44 (0)1256 707334

ID Russell, USA.
ID Russell Co Laboratories, 1301 Iowa Avenue, Longmont, CO 80501, USA.
Telephone: +1 303 678 7112
Facsimile: +1 303 678 8953

IDIS, UK.
IDIS Ltd World Medicines, Millbank House, 171 Ewell Road, Surbiton, Surrey, KT6 6AX, UK.
Telephone: +44 (0)20 8410 0700
Facsimile: +44 (0)20 8410 0800
E-mail: idis@idis.co.uk

Ilium, Austral.
Ilium Veterinary Products, Austral.
Contact: Troy, Austral.

Immuno-Chemical, NZ.
Immuno-Chemical Products, 31 Morningside Drive, Mount Albert, Auckland, New Zealand.
Telephone: +64 (0)9 815 0624
Facsimile: +64 (0)9 815 0623

Inca, Austral.
Inca (Flight) Company Pty Ltd, 22-23 Forthorn Place, St Marys, NSW 2760, Australia.
Telephone: +61 (0)2 9833 1728
Facsimile: +61 (0)2 9833 2136

Intagra, USA.
Intagra Inc, 8500 Pilsbury Avenue, South Minneapolis, MN 55420, USA.
Telephone: +1 612 881 5535
Facsimile: +1 612 881 7002

Interchem, Eire.
Interchem Limited, Animal Health Division, 29 Cherry Orchard Industrial Estate, Dublin 10, Eire.
Telephone: +353 (0)1 626 7211
Facsimile: +353 (0)1 626 5818

International Animal Health Products, Austral.
International Animal Health Products Pty Ltd, 18 Healy Circuit, Huntingwood, NSW 2148, Australia.
Telephone: +61 (0)2 9672 7944
Facsimile: +61 (0)2 9672 7988

International Donkey Protection Trust, UK.
Contact: The Donkey Sanctuary, UK.

Interpharm, Eire.
Interpharm Animal Health, Interpharm Limited, 112 Ashbourne Industrial Estate, Ashbourne, Co. Meath, Eire.
Telephone: +353 (0)1 835 1888
Facsimile: +353 (0)1 835 1917

Intervet, Austral.
Intervet (Australia) Pty Ltd, Unit 3, 4 Gladstone Road, Castle Hill, NSW 2154, Australia.
Telephone: +61 (0)2 9680 6999
Facsimile: +61 (0)2 9680 6900

Intervet, Eire.
Intervet Ireland Limited, Farnham Drive, Finglas, Dublin 11, Eire.
Telephone: +353 (0)1 864 2433
Facsimile: +353 (0)1 864 2434

Intervet, UK.
Intervet UK Ltd, Walton Manor, Walton, Milton Keynes, Buckinghamshire, MK7 7AJ, UK.
Telephone: +44 (0)1908 665050
Facsimile: +44 (0)1908 672680
E-mail: ukvet.support@intervet.com

Intervet, USA.
Intervet Inc, PO Box 318, 405 State Street, Millsboro, DE 19966, USA.
Telephone: +1 800 992 8051
Facsimile: +1 302 934 4281

Ipsen, UK.
Ipsen Ltd, 1 Bath Road, Maidenhead, Berkshire, SL6 4UH, UK.
Telephone: +44 (0)1628 771417
Facsimile: +44 (0)1628 770199

Irish Homing Union
'N' rings, 34 Adelaide Avenue, Belfast, BT9 7FY, UK.
Telephone: +44 (0)28 90 644 231
'S' rings, 69 Lorcan Crescent, Santry, Dublin 9, Eire.
Telephone: + 353 (0)1 842 1016

James A Mackie (Agricultural), UK.
James A Mackie (Agricultural), PO Box 14771, Alloa, Clackmannanshire, FK10 2EW, UK.
Telephone: +44 (0)1259 215136
Facsimile: +44 (0)1259 211053
E-mail: mackieaquacultur@tory.org.uk

Janssen, Eire.
Janssen Animal Health, Division of Janssen-Cilag Ltd, PO Box 79, Saunderton, High Wycombe, Buckinghamshire, HP14 4HJ, UK.
Telephone: +44 (0)1494 567555
Facsimile: +44 (0)1494 567556

Janssen, UK.
Janssen Animal Health, Division of Janssen-Cilag Ltd, PO Box 79, Saunderton, HighWycombe, Buckinghamshire, HP14 4HJ, UK.
Telephone: +44 (0)1494 567555
Facsimile: +44 (0)1494 567556

Janssen-Cilag, UK.
Janssen-Cilag Ltd, PO Box 79, Saunderton, High Wycombe, Buckinghamshire, HP14 4HJ, UK.
Telephone: +44 (0)1494 567567
Facsimile: +44 (0)1494 567568

JHC, UK.
JHC Healthcare Ltd, The Maltings, Bridge Street, Hitchin, Hertfordshire, SG5 2DE, UK.

Jockey Club, UK.
The Jockey Club, 42 Portman Square, London, W1H 0EN, UK.
Telephone: +44 (0)20 7486 4921

Johnson & Johnson Medical, UK.
Johnson & Johnson Medical, Coronation Road, Ascot, Berkshire, SL5 9EY, UK.
Telephone: +44 (0)1344 871000
Facsimile: +44 (0)1344 872599

Johnson & Johnson MSD, UK.
Johnson & Johnson MSD, Enterprise House, Station Road, Loudwater, High Wycombe, Buckinghamshire, HP10 9UF, UK.
Telephone: +44 (0)1494 450778
Facsimile: +44 (0)1494 450487

Johnson & Johnson, UK.
Johnson & Johnson Ltd, Foundation Park, Roxborough Way, Maidenhead, Berkshire, SL6 3UG, UK.
Telephone: +44 (0)1628 822222
Facsimile: +44 (0)1628 821222

Joseph Lyddy, Austral.
Joseph Lyddy, 315 Canterbury Road, Canterbury, Vic. 3126, Australia.
Telephone: +61 (0)3 9836 0277
Facsimile: +61 (0)3 9830 1432

Jurox, Austral.
Jurox Pty Ltd, 85 Gardiners Road, Rutherford, NSW 2320, Australia.
Telephone: +61 (0)2 4931 8200
Facsimile: +61 (0)2 4931 8222

Jurox, NZ.
Jurox New Zealand Ltd, PO Box 16, Patumahoe, South Auckland, New Zealand.
Telephone: +64 (0)9 236 3915
Facsimile: +64 (0)9 236 3915

KC Pharmacal, USA.
KC Pharmacal Inc, 8345 Melrose Drive, Lenexa, KS 66214, USA.
Telephone: +1 913 888 0945
Facsimile: +1 913 888 4940

KelatoCORP, Austral.
KelatoCORP Animal Health, Division of Chelated Laboratories Pty Ltd, 1 Manton Road, Oakleigh South, Vic. 3167, Australia.
Telephone: +61 (0)3 9540 0222
Facsimile: +61 (0)3 9540 0244

Kemlea Bee Supplies, UK.
Starcroft Apiaries, Catsfield, Battle, East Sussex, TN33 9DT, UK.
Telephone: +44 (0)1424 774830
Facsimile: +44 (0)1424 774026

The Kennel Club, UK.
1 Clarges Street, London, W1Y

8AB, UK.
Telephone: +44 (0)870 6066750
Facsimile: +44 (0)20 7518 1058

Kilco, UK.
Kilco Hygiene, 1A Trench Road, Mallusk, Newtownabbey, Co Antrim, Northern Ireland, UK.
Telephone: +44 (0)2890 342928
Facsimile: +44 (0)2890 342494

King, USA.
King Pharmaceuticals Animal Health, 501 Fifth Street, Bristol, TN 37620, USA.
Telephone: +1 800 336 7783
Facsimile: +1 423 989 8006

Knoll, UK.
Knoll Ltd, 9 Castle Quay, Castle Boulevard, Nottingham, NG7 1FW, UK.
Telephone: +44 (0)115 912 5000
Facsimile: +44 (0)115 912 5069

LAB, UK.
Laboratories for Applied Biology, 91 Amhurst Park, London, N16 5DR, UK.
Telephone: +44 (0)20 8800 2252
Facsimile: +44 (0)20 8809 6884

Land O'Lakes, USA.
Land O'Lakes Inc, 2827 8th Avenue S, Fort Dodge, IA 50501, USA.
Telephone: +1 515 576 7311
Facsimile: +1 515 574 2820

Landco, USA.
Landco Corporation, PO Box 1878, Post Falls, ID 83877, USA.
Telephone: +1 800 356 4029
Facsimile: +1 208 667 8360

Lederle, UK.
Contact: Wyeth, UK.

Leeds Veterinary Laboratories, UK.
Leeds Veterinary Laboratories Ltd, Millcroft, Gate Way Drive, Yeadon, Leeds, LS19 7XY, UK.
Telephone: +44 (0)113 2507556
Facsimile: +44 (0)113 2500198
E-mail: lvl@lvlabs.demon.co.uk

Legear, USA.
Legear, Division of Goodwinol Products Corporation, PO Box 407, Pierce, CO 80650, USA.
Telephone: +1 970 834 1229
Facsimile: +1 970 834 0180

Leo, Eire.
Leo Laboratories Limited, 285 Cashel Road, Dublin 12, Eire.
Telephone: +353 (0)1 490 8924
Facsimile: +353 (0)1 708 2052

Leo, UK.
Leo Laboratories Ltd, Longwick Road, Princes Risborough, Buckinghamshire, HP27 9RR, UK.
Telephone: +44 (0)1844 347333

Facsimile: +44 (0)1844 342278
E-mail:
AH.enquiries@leopharma.co.uk

For information on authorised human medicines:
Leo Pharmaceuticals, Longwick Road, Princes Risborough, Buckinghamshire, HP27 9RR, UK.
Telephone: +44 (0)1844 347333
Facsimile: +44 (0)1844 342278

Life Science, USA.
Life Science Products, PO Box 8111, St Joseph, MO 64508, USA.
Telephone: +1 816 279 3449
Facsimile: +1 816 279 4725

Lilly, UK.
Eli Lilly & Co Ltd, Dextra Court, Chapel Hill, Basingstoke, Hampshire, RG21 5SY, UK.
Telephone: +44 (0)1256 315000
Facsimile: +44 (0)1256 315858

Livestock Improvement, NZ.
Livestock Improvement Corporation Ltd, Private Bag 3016, Hamilton, New Zealand.
Telephone: +64 (0)7 856 0631
Facsimile: +64 (0)7 856 2428

Lloyd, NZ.
Lloyd Laboratories NZ Ltd, 233 Porchester Road, PO Box 167, Takanini, New Zealand.
Telephone: +64 (0)9 296 5147
Facsimile: +64 (0)9 298 6343

Lloyd, USA.
Lloyd Laboratories Division, Lloyd Inc, PO Box 86, Shenandoah, IA 51601, USA.
Telephone: +1 712 246 4006
Facsimile: +1 712 246 5245

Loveland, USA.
Loveland Industries Inc, PO Box 1289, Greeley, CO 80632-1289, USA.
Telephone: +1 970 346 8920
Facsimile: +1 970 356 8926

Loveridge, UK.
J M Loveridge plc, Southbrook Road, Southampton, SO15 1BH, UK.
Telephone: +44 (0)23 80222008
Facsimile: +44 (0)23 80639836
E-mail:
JMLpharmco@btinternet.com

Luitpold, USA.
Luitpold Pharmaceuticals Inc, One Luitpold Drive, Shirley, NY 11967, USA.
Telephone: +1 516 924 4000
Facsimile: +1 516 924 1731

3M HealthCare, UK.
3M Health Care Ltd, 3M House, Morley Street, Loughborough, Leicestershire, LE11 1EP, UK.
Telephone: +44 (0)1509 611611
Facsimile: +44 (0)1509 237288

Macleod, USA.
Macleod Pharmaceuticals Inc, 2600 Canton Court, Suite C, Fort Collins, CO 80525, USA.
Telephone: +1 970 482 7254
Facsimile: +1 970 482 7454

Maersk Medical, UK.
Maersk Medical Ltd, Thornhill Road, North Moons Moat, Redditch, Worcestershire, B98 9NL, UK.
Telephone: +44 (0)1527 64222
Facsimile: +44 (0)1527 592111

MAFF, UK.
Ministry of Agriculture, Fisheries and Food, 1A Page Street, London, SW1P 4PQ, UK.
Telephone: +44 (0)20 7904 6000

MAFF Publications, UK.
Admail 6000, London, SW1A 2XX, UK.
Telephone: +44 (0)845 955 6000
Facsimile: +44 (0)20 8694 8776

Maisemore Apiaries, UK.
Old Road, Maisemore, Gloucester, GL2 8HT, UK.
Telephone: +44 (0)1452 700289
Facsimile: +44 (0)1452 700196

Martindale, UK.
Martindale Pharmaceuticals Ltd, Bampton Road, Harold Hill, Romford, Essex, RM3 8UG, UK.
Telephone: +44 (0)1708 386660
Facsimile: +44 (0)1708 384032

Mavlab, Austral.
Mavlab Pty Ltd, 33 Rowland Street, Slacks Creek, Qld 4127, Australia.
Telephone: +61 (0)7 3808 1399
Facsimile: +61 (0)7 3808 4328

Meat and Livestock Commission, UK.
PO Box 44, Winterhill House, Snowdon Drive, Winterhill, Milton Keynes, MK6 1AX, UK.
Telephone: +44 (0)1908 677577

Medac, UK.
Medac (UK), 13 Lynedoch Crescent, Glasgow, G3 6EQ, UK.
Telephone: +44 (0)141 332 8464
Facsimile: +44 (0)141 332 8619

Medeva, UK.
Medeva Pharma Ltd, Medeva House, Regent Park, Kingston Road, Leatherhead, Surrey, KT22 7PQ, UK.
Telephone: +44 (0)1372 364132
Facsimile: +44 (0)1372 364018

Medo Pharmaceuticals, UK.
Medo Pharmaceuticals, Schwarz House, East Street, Chesham, Buckinghamshire, HP5 1DG, UK.
Telephone: +44 (0)1494 772071
Facsimile: +44 (0)1494 773934

Med-Pharmex, USA.
Med-Pharmex Inc, 2727 Thompson Creek Road, Pomona, CA 91767, USA.
Telephone: +1 909 593 7875
Facsimile: +1 909 593 7862

Merial, Austral.
Merial Australia Pty Ltd, 6/79 George Street, Parramatta, NSW 2150, Australia.
Telephone: +61 (0)2 9893 0000
Facsimile: +61 (0)2 9893 0099

Merial, Eire.
Merial Animal Health Ltd, 4 Adelaide Court, Adelaide Road, Dublin 2, Eire.
Telephone: +353 (0)1 478 0244
Facsimile: +353 (0)1 478 0944

Merial, NZ.
Merial New Zealand Ltd, Level 3, Merial Building, Osterley Way, Manukau City, New Zealand.
Telephone: +64 (0)9 980 1600
Facsimile: +64 (0)9 980 1601

Merial, UK.
Merial, Sandringham House, 110 Sandringham Avenue, Harlow Business Park, Harlow, Essex, CM19 5TG, UK.
Telephone: +44 (0)1279 775858
Facsimile: +44 (0)1279 775888

Merial, USA.
Merial, 2100 Ronson Road, Iselin, NJ 08830-3077, USA.
Telephone: +1 888 637 4251

Millpledge, UK.
Millpledge Pharmaceuticals, Whinleys Estate, Clarborough, Retford, Nottinghamshire, DN22 9NA, UK.
Telephone: +44 (0)1777 708440
Facsimile: +44 (0)1777 860020
E-mail: sales@millpledge.com

Mobil Oil, Austral.
Mobil Oil Australia Ltd, 417 St Kilda Road, Melbourne, Vic. 3004, Australia.
Telephone: +61 (0)3 9252 3111
Facsimile: +61 (0)3 9252 3014

Monmouth, UK.
Monmouth Pharmaceuticals, 20 Nugent Road, The Surrey Research Park, Guildford, Surrey, GU2 5AF, UK.
Telephone: +44 (0)1483 565299
Facsimile: +44 (0)1483 563658

Monsanto, USA.
Monsanto Company, 800 N Lindbergh Boulevard, St Louis, MO 63167, USA.
Telephone: +1 314 694 2123
Facsimile: +1 314 694 2791

Moorfields Eye Hospital, UK.
162 City Road, London, EC1V

2PD, UK.
Telephone: +44 (0)20 7253 3411
Facsimile: +44 (0)20 7253 4696

MSD, UK.
Merck Sharp & Dohme Ltd, Hertford Road, Hoddesdon, Hertfordshire, EN11 9BU, UK.
Telephone: +44 (0)1992 467272
Facsimile: +44 (0)1992 451066

NACAM, Neth.
Netherlands Association for Companion Animal Medicine, Bilstraat 455-457, NL-3572 AX, Utrecht, The Netherlands.
Telephone: +31 30 2 31 09 86
Facsimile: +31 30 2 32 89 27

National Academy of Sciences Press, USA.
2101 Constitution Avenue, NW Washington, DC 20418, USA.
Telephone: +1 202 334 3313

National Bee Unit, UK.
Central Science Laboratory, Room 10GA01/2, Sand Hutton, York, YO4 1LZ, UK.
Telephone: +44 (0)1904 462510
Facsimile: +44 (0)1904 462240
E-mail: m.bew@CSL.gov.uk

National Coursing Club, UK.
National Coursing Club, 16 Clock Tower Mews, Newmarket, Suffolk, CB8 8LL, UK.
Telephone: +44 (0)1638 667381
Facsimile: +44 (0)1638 669224

National Farmers Union, UK.
Agriculture House, 164 Shaftesbury Avenue, London, WC2, UK.
Telephone: +44 (0)20 7331 7200
Facsimile: +44 (0)20 7331 7313

National Trainers Federation, UK.
9 High Street, Lambourn, Hungerford, Berkshire, RG17 8XN, UK.
Telephone: +44 (0)1488 71719

Nature Vet, Austral.
Nature Vet Pty Ltd, 299 Castlereagh Road, Agnes Banks, NSW 2753, Australia.
Telephone: +61 (0)2 4578 1022
Facsimile: +61 (0)2 4578 2913

NCDL, UK.
National Canine Defence League, 17 Wakley Street, London, EC1V 7RQ, UK.
Telephone: +44 (0)20 7837 0006
Facsimile: +44 (0)20 7833 2701

Net-Tex, UK.
Net-Tex Agricultural Ltd, Priestwood, Harvel, Nr Meopham, Kent, DA13 0DA, UK.
Telephone: +44 (0)1474 813999
Facsimile: +44 (0)1474 812112
E-mail: info@net-tex.co.uk

NGRC, UK.
National Greyhound Racing Club, Twyman House, 16 Bonny Street, London, NW1 9QD, UK.
Telephone: +44 (0)20 7267 9256
Facsimile: +44 (0)20 7482 1023

Nightshade, UK.
Scientific Publishing Sales, Sir Joseph Banks Building, Royal Botanic Gardens, Kew, Richmond, Surrey, TW9 3AE, UK.
Telephone: +44 (0)20 83325219
Facsimile: +44 (0)20 83325646
E-mail: books@rbgkew.org.uk

Nishikoi, UK.
Nishikoi Aquaculture Ltd, White Hall, Wethersfield, Essex, CM7 4EP, UK.
Telephone: +44 (0)1371 851424
Facsimile: +44 (0)1371 851429

NOAH, UK.
National Office of Animal Health Ltd, 3 Crossfield Chambers, Gladbeck Way, Enfield, Middlesex, EN2 7HF, UK.
Telephone: +44 (0)20 8367 3131
Facsimile: +44 (0)20 8363 1155

Norbrook, Eire.
Norbrook Laboratories (Ireland) Limited, Rossmore Industrial Estate, Monaghan, Co. Monaghan, Eire.
Telephone: +353 (0)47 81180
Facsimile: +353 (0)47 81187

Norbrook, UK.
Norbrook Laboratories Ltd, 105 Armagh Road, Newry, Co. Down, BT35 6PU, UK.
Telephone: +44 (0)28 30260200
Facsimile: +44 (0)28 30260201
E-mail: enquiries@norbrook.co.uk

Nordic Star, UK.
Nordic Star Ltd, 11 Greenway Lane, Bath, BA2 4LJ, UK.
Telephone: +44 (0)1225 481477
Facsimile: +44 (0)1225 316137

Norgine, UK.
Norgine Ltd, Chaplin House, Moorhall Road, Harefield, Middlesex, UB9 6NS, UK.
Telephone: +44 (0)1895 826600
Facsimile: +44 (0)1895 825865

North of England Homing Union
58 Ennerdale Road, Walkerdene, Newcastle-upon-Tyne, NE6 4DG, UK.
Telephone: +44 (0)191 262 5440
Facsimile: +44 (0)191 262 5388

North West Homing Union
10 Ward Street, Lostock Hall, Preston, Lancashire, PR5 5HR, UK.
Telephone: +44 (0)1772 468 748

Norton Consumer, UK.
Norton Consumer (Division of Norton Healthcare Ltd), Albert Basin, Royal Docks, London, E16 2QJ, UK.
Telephone: +44 (0)8705 202304
Facsimile: +44 (0)8705 323334

Novartis, Austral.
Novartis Animal Health Australasia Pty Ltd, 140-150 Bungaree Road, Pendle Hill, NSW 2145, Australia.
Telephone: +61 (0)2 9688 0444
Facsimile: +61 (0)2 9896 8260

Novartis, Eire.
Novartis Agribusiness Ireland Limited, Industrial Estate, Cork Road, Waterford, Eire.
Telephone: +353 (0)51 377 201
Facsimile: +353 (0)51 377 209

Novartis, NZ.
Novartis New Zealand Ltd, Animal Health Sector, 43-45 Patiki Road, Avondale, Auckland, New Zealand.
Telephone: +64 (0)9 828 3149
Facsimile: +64 (0)9 820 3773

Novartis, UK.
Novartis Animal Health UK Ltd, New Cambridge House, Litlington, Nr Royston, Hertfordshire, SG8 0SS, UK.
Telephone: +44 (0)1763 850500
Facsimile: +44 (0)1763 850600

For information on authorised human medicines:
Novartis Pharmaceuticals UK, Frimley Business Park, Frimley, Camberley, Surrey, GU16 5SG, UK.
Telephone: +44 (0)1276 692255
Facsimile: +44 (0)1276 698449

Novartis, USA.
Novartis Animal Health US Inc, 1500 Pinecroft Road, Suite 400, Greensboro, NC 27407, USA.
Telephone: +1 800 637 0281
Facsimile: +1 336 547 1030

Novo Nordisk, UK.
Novo Nordisk Pharmaceutical Ltd, Novo Nordisk House, Broadfield Park, Brighton Road, Pease Pottage, Crawley, West Sussex, RH11 9RT, UK.
Telephone: +44 (0)1293 613555
Facsimile: +44 (0)1293 613535

NPTC, UK.
National Proficiency Tests Council, National Agriculture Centre, Stoneleigh, Kenilworth, Warwickshire, CV8 2LG, UK.
Telephone: +44 (0)2476 696553
Facsimile: +44 (0)2476 696128

Nufarm, Austral.
Nufarm Ltd (trading as Nufarm Animal Health), 103-105 Pipe Road, Laverton North, Vic. 3026, Australia.

Telephone: +61 (0)3 9282 1000
Facsimile: +61 (0)3 9282 1022

Nufarm, NZ.
Nufarm Ltd, 2 Sterling Avenue, Manurewa, Auckland, New Zealand.
Telephone: +64 (0)9 268 2920
Facsimile: +64 (0)9 267 8444

Nutra Vet, Austral.
Contact: Apex, Austral.

Nutrimol, Austral.
Nutrimol Pty Ltd, 926 Mountain Highway, Bayswater, Vic. 3153, Australia.
Telephone: +61 (0)3 9720 2266
Facsimile: +61 (0)3 9720 2288

Nutritech, NZ.
Nutritech International Ltd, 12 Fisher Crescent, Mount Wellington, Auckland, New Zealand.
Telephone: +64 (0)800 736 339
Facsimile: +64 (0)9 276 6357

Nylos, USA.
Nylos Trading Co Inc, Veterinary Pharmaceuticals Division, PO Box D 3700, Pomona, NY 10970, USA.
Telephone: +1 914 354 8787
Facsimile: +1 914 354 8703

NZVet, NZ.
NZVet Ltd, 33 Birmingham Drive, Middleton, Christchurch, New Zealand.
Telephone: +64 (0)3 338 7400
Facsimile: +64 (0)3 338 3088

OATA, UK.
Ornamental Aquatic Trade Association, Unit 5, Narrow Wine Street, Trowbridge, Wiltshire, BA14 8YY, UK.
Telephone: +44 (0)1225 777177
Facsimile: +44 (0)1225 775523
E-mail: info@oata.demon.co.uk

Oldcastle, Eire.
Oldcastle Laboratories Limited, Cogan Street, Oldcastle, Co. Meath, Eire.
Telephone: +353 (0)49 41160

Organon-Teknika, UK.
Organon-Teknika, Organon Laboratories Ltd, Cambridge Science Park, Milton Road, Cambridge, CB4 0FL, UK.
Telephone: +44 (0)1223 423650

Orphan, USA.
Orphan Medical Inc, 13911 Ridgedale Drive, Minnetonka, MN 55305, USA.
Telephone: +1 888 867 7426
Facsimile: +1 612 541 9209

Osborn, USA.
Osborn, Division of Merial Ltd, 4545 Oleatha Avenue, St Louis, MO 63116, USA.

Telephone: +1 888 637 4251
Facsimile: +1 314 752 8084

Oxis, USA.
Oxis International Inc, 6040 N Cutter Circle, Suite 317, Portland, OR 97217, USA.
Telephone: +1 800 547 3686 or +1 503 283 3911
Facsimile: +1 503 283 4058

P & D Pharmaceuticals, UK.
P & D Pharmaceuticals, 38 Woolmer Way, Bordon, Hampshire, GU35 9QF, UK.
Telephone: +44 (0)1420 487501
Facsimile: +44 (0)1420 478315
E-mail: pd.pharm@which.net

Pacific Vet, Austral.
Pacific Vet Pty Ltd, 1/151 Herald Street, Cheltenham, Vic. 3192, Australia.
Telephone: +61 (0)3 9532 1162
Facsimile: +61 (0)3 9532 1163

Pacificvet, NZ.
Pacificvet Ltd, 3 Hickory Place, Hornby, Christchurch, New Zealand.
Telephone: +64 (0)3 349 8438
Facsimile: +64 (0)3 349 8863

Parke-Davis, UK.
Parke-Davis & Co Ltd, Lambert Court, Chestnut Avenue, Eastleigh, Hampshire, SO53 3ZQ, UK.
Telephone: +44 (0)23 8062 0500
Facsimile: +44 (0)23 8062 9818

Parnell, Austral.
Parnell Laboratories (Aust) Pty Ltd, 6 Century Estate, 476 Gardeners Road, Alexandria, NSW 2015, Australia.
Telephone: +61 (0)2 9667 4411
Facsimile: +61 (0)2 9667 4139

Parnell, NZ.
Parnell Laboratories NZ Ltd, Unit 3, 179 Harris Road, East Tamaki, Auckland, New Zealand.
Telephone: +64 (0)9 273 7270
Facsimile: +64 (0)9 273 7260

Pastoral, NZ.
Pastoral Consultants (NZ) Ltd, C/- H Quinlivan, PO Box 479, Fielding, New Zealand.
Telephone: +64 (0)6 322 1323
Facsimile: +64 (0)6 322 1044

PCL, NZ.
PCL Industries Ltd (Feed, Nutrition & Health Division), 3 Red Hills Road, Massey, Auckland, New Zealand.
Telephone: +64 (0)9 833 9069
Facsimile: +64 (0)9 832 4929

Pedigree, UK.
Pedigree Masterfoods, A division of Mars UK Ltd, Waltham-on-the-Wolds, Melton Mowbray,

Leicestershire, LE14 4RS, UK.
Telephone: +44 (0)800 717800
Facsimile: +44 (0)1664 415232
E-mail:
wal.customer.care@eu.effem.com

Penn, UK.
Penn Pharmaceuticals Ltd, Tafarnaubach Industrial Estate, Tredegar, Gwent, NP2 3AA, UK.
Telephone: +44 (0)1495 711222
Facsimile: +44 (0)1495 711225

Peptech, Austral.
Peptech Animal Health Pty Ltd, 1/35-41 Waterloo Road, North Ryde, NSW 2113, Australia.
Telephone: +61 (0)2 9870 8788
Facsimile: +61 (0)2 9870 8787

Peptech, NZ.
Peptech Animal Health, Prebbleton Farm Clinic, 56 Blakes Road, Prebbleton, Christchurch, New Zealand.
Telephone: +64 (0)3 349 9946
Facsimile: +64 (0)3 349 3000

Performer, USA.
Performer Brand, Agri Laboratories Inc, 20927 State Route K, St Joseph, MO 64505, USA.
Telephone: +1 800 542 8916
Facsimile: +1 816 233 9546

Pet Food Manufacturers' Association, UK.
Pet Food Manufacturers' Association, Suite 1-2, 12-13 Henrietta Street, London, WC2E 8LH, UK.
Telephone: +44 (0)20 7379 9009
Facsimile: +44 (0)20 7379 8008

Pet Health Council, UK.
Pet Health Council, 4 Bedford Square, London, WC1B 3RA, UK.
Telephone: +44 (0)20 7631 3795
Facsimile: +44 (0)20 7631 0602

Petlife, UK.
Petlife International Ltd, Minster House, Western Way, Bury St Edmunds, Suffolk, IP33 3SP, UK.
Telephone: +44 (0)1284 761131
Facsimile: +44 (0)1284 769943
E-mail:
petlife@vetbed-uk.demon.co.uk

Pettifer, UK.
Thomas Pettifer & Company Ltd, Newchurch, Romney Marsh, Kent, TN29 0DZ, UK.
Telephone: +44 (0)1303 874455
Facsimile: +44 (0)1303 874801

Pfizer Consumer Care, UK.
Pfizer Consumer Healthcare, Wilsom Road, Alton, Hampshire, GU34 2TJ, UK.
Telephone: +44 (0)1420 84801
Facsimile: +44 (0)1420 89376

Pfizer, Austral.
Pfizer Animal Health, Division of Pfizer Pty Ltd, 38-42 Wharf Road, West Ryde, NSW 2114, Australia.
Telephone: +61 (0)2 9850 3333
Facsimile: +61 (0)2 9850 3399

Pfizer, Eire.
Pfizer Animal Health, Parkway House, Ballymount Road Lower, Dublin 12, Eire.
Telephone: +353 (0)1 408 9700
Facsimile: +343 (0)1 408 9750

Pfizer, NZ.
Pfizer Laboratories Ltd, Level 4, Corner Osterley Way & Ronwood Drive, Manukau City, New Zealand.
Telephone: +64 (0)9 262 3568
Facsimile: +64 (0)9 262 3582

Pfizer, UK.
Pfizer Ltd, Ramsgate Road, Sandwich, Kent, CT13 9NJ, UK.
Telephone: +44 (0)1304 616161
Facsimile: +44 (0)1304 616221
E-mail: Tony.Simon@pfizer.com

For information on authorised human medicines:
Pfizer Ltd, Ramsgate Road, Sandwich, Kent, CT13 9NJ, UK.
Telephone: +44 (0)1304 616161
Facsimile: +44 (0)1304 656221

Pfizer, USA.
Pfizer Animal Health, 812 Springdale Drive, Exton, PA 19341, USA.
Telephone: +1 800 366 5210
Facsimile: +1 610 363 3783

Pharmachem, Austral.
Pharmachem, Unit 3/70 Raynham Street, Salisbury, Qld 4107, Australia.
Telephone: +61 (0)7 3277 2311
Facsimile: +61 (0)7 3275 3095

Pharmacia & Upjohn, Austral.
Pharmacia & Upjohn Pty Ltd, Animal Health Business, Suite 1A, Level 5, The Spruson & Ferguson Centre, 460 Church Street, Paramatte, NSW 2150, Australia.
Telephone: +61 (0)2 9890 7177
Facsimile: +61 (0)2 9890 5391

Pharmacia & Upjohn, Eire.
Pharmacia & Upjohn Ltd, Animal Health Division, Hatton House, Hunters Road, Weldon North Estate, Corby, Northamptonshire, NN17 5JE, UK.
Telephone: +44 (0)1536 276400
Facsimile: +44 (0)1536 263365

Pharmacia & Upjohn, NZ.
Pharmacia & Upjohn (NZ) Ltd, 3 Fisher Crescent, Mount Wellington, Auckland, New Zealand.
Telephone: +64 (0)9 270 0328
Facsimile: +64 (0)9 276 5209

Pharmacia & Upjohn, UK.
Pharmacia & Upjohn Animal Health Limited, Hatton House, Hunters Road, Weldon North Estate, Corby, Northamptonshire, NN17 5JE, UK.
Telephone: +44 (0)1536 276400
Facsimile: +44 (0)1536 263365

For information on authorised human medicines:
Pharmacia & Upjohn Ltd, Davy Avenue, Knowlhill, Milton Keynes, MK5 8PH, UK.
Telephone: +44 (0)1908 661101
Facsimile: +44 (0)1908 690091

Pharmacia & Upjohn, USA.
Pharmacia & Upjohn Inc, 7000 Portage Road, Kalamazoo, MI 49001, USA.
Telephone: +1 800 253 8600
Facsimile: +1 616 833 3305

Pharmaderm, USA.
Pharmaderm, Veterinary Division of Atlanta Inc, 60 Baylis Road, Melville, NY 11747, USA.
Telephone: +1 800 432 6673
Facsimile: +1 516 454 1572

Pharmax, UK.
Pharmax Ltd, Bourne Road, Bexley, Kent, DA5 1NX, UK.
Telephone: +44 (0)1322 550550
Facsimile: +44 (0)1322 558776

Pharmtech, Austral.
Pharmtech Pty Ltd, Suite 7, 61-63 MacAlister Street, Sale, Vic. 3850, Australia.
Telephone: +61 (0)3 5144 3883
Facsimile: +61 (0)3 5144 4736

Phoenix, NZ.
Phoenix Pharm Distributors Ltd, Unit 7, 84-90 Hillside Road, Glenfield, Auckland, New Zealand.
Telephone: +64 (0)9 410 5566
Facsimile: +64 (0)9 410 6305

Phoenix, USA.
Phoenix Pharmaceutical Inc, 4621 Easton Road, PO Box 6457, St Joseph, MO 64503, USA.
Telephone: +1 816 364 5777
Facsimile: +1 816 364 4969

Pro Labs, USA.
Pro Labs Ltd, Agri Laboratories Inc, 20927 State Route K, St Joseph, MO 64505, USA.
Telephone: +1 800 542 8916
Facsimile: +1 816 233 9546

Procter & Gamble Pharm., UK.
Procter & Gamble Pharmaceuticals UK Ltd, Lovett House, Lovett Road, Staines, Middlesex, TW18 3AZ, UK.
Telephone: +44 (0)1784 495000
Facsimile: +44 (0)1784 495253

Procter & Gamble, UK.
Procter & Gamble UK, The Heights, Brooklands, Weybridge, Surrey, KT13 0XP, UK.
Telephone: +44 (0)1932 896000
Facsimile: +44 (0)1932 896200

Provita Eurotech, UK.
Provita Eurotech Ltd, 21 Bankmore Road, Omagh, County Tyrone, Northern Ireland, BT79 0EU, UK.
Telephone: +44 (0)28 8225 2352
Facsimile: +44 (0)28 8224 1734

Purina Mills, USA.
Purina Mills Inc, 1401 S Hanley Road, Brentwood, MO 63144, USA.
Telephone: +1 314 768 4380
Facsimile: +1 314 768 4143

R McKay, NZ.
R McKay Ltd, 11 Royd Avenue, Fendelton, Christchurch, New Zealand.
Telephone: +64 (0)3 351 6379

Ralston, UK.
Ralston Purina International (UK) Ltd, 79 High Street, Chobham, Surrey, GU24 8AF, UK.
Telephone: +44 (0)1276 855135
Facsimile: +44 (0)1276 855102

Ranvet, Austral.
Ranvet Pty Ltd, 65 Queen Street, Beaconsfield, NSW 2015, Australia.
Telephone: +61 (0)2 9319 6631
Facsimile: +61 (0)2 9319 0970

RCVS, UK.
Royal College of Veterinary Surgeons, Belgravia House, 62/64 Horseferry Road, London, SW1P 2AF, UK.
Telephone: +44 (0)20 7222 2001
Facsimile: +44 (0)20 7222 2004
E-mail: admin@rcvs.org.uk
extaffairs@rcvs.org.uk

Reamor, NZ.
Reamor (NZ) Ltd, 306 Titirangi Road, Titirangi, Auckland, New Zealand.
Telephone: +64 (0)9 817 6525
Facsimile: +64 (0)9 817 2595

Rhône Poulenc, Austral.
Rhône-Poulenc Animal Nutrition Pty Ltd, 66 Antimony Street, Carole Park, Qld 4300, Australia.
Telephone: +61 (0)7 3271 1244
Facsimile: +61 (0)7 3271 3335

Rhône-Poulenc Rorer, UK.
Rhône-Poulenc Rorer Ltd, Aventis Pharma Ltd, Aventis House, 50 Kings Hill Avenue, Kings Hill, West Malling, Kent, ME19 4AH, UK.
Telephone: +44 (0)1732 584000
Facsimile: +44 (0)870 5239605

Rice Steele, Eire.
Rice Steele Manufacturing Limited, Cookstown Industrial Estate, Tallaght, Dublin 24, Eire.
Telephone: +353 (0)1 451 0144/ 0108
Facsimile: +353 (0)1 452 1875

Ridgeway Biologicals, UK.
Ridgeway Biologicals, c/o Institute for animal health, Compton, Berkshire, RG20 7NN, UK.
Telephone: +44 (0)1635 579516
Facsimile: +44 (0)1635 579517

Ritter, USA.
Ritter Chemical Co, PO Box 66532, Houston, TX 77006, USA.
Telephone: +1 713 528 1818

Roche Consumer Health, UK.
Contact: Roche, UK.
Telephone: +44 (0)1707 366000
Facsimile: +44 (0)800 394353

Roche Vitamins, USA.
Roche Vitamins Inc, Roche Animal Nutrition and Health, 45 Waterview Boulevard Drive, Parsippany, NJ 07054, USA.
Telephone: +1 800 526 0189
Facsimile: +1 973 257 8416

Roche, Austral.
Roche Products Pty Ltd, Unit C2, 1-3 Rodborough Road, Frenchs Forest, NSW 2086, Australia.
Telephone: +61 (0)2 9975 8100
Facsimile: +61 (0)2 9975 5256

Roche, NZ.
Roche Products (NZ) Ltd, 8 Henderson Place, Te Papapa, Auckland, New Zealand.
Telephone: +64 (0)9 633 0741
Facsimile: +64 (0)9 633 0745

Roche, UK.
Roche Products Ltd, 40 Broadwater Road, Welwyn Garden City, Hertfordshire, AL7 3AY, UK.
Telephone: +44 (0)1707 366000
Facsimile: +44 (0)1707 338297

Rosemont, UK.
Rosemont Pharmaceuticals Ltd, Rosemont House, Yorkdale Industrial Park, Braithwaite Street, Leeds, LS11 9XE, UK.
Telephone: +44 (0)113 244 1999
Facsimile: +44 (0)113 246 0738

Royal Pigeon Racing Association
The Reddings House, Cheltenham, Gloucestershire, GL51 6RN, UK.
Telephone: +44 (0)1452 713 529
Facsimile: +44 (0)1452 857 119

RSPCA, UK.
Royal Society for Prevention of Cruelty to Animals, Head Office, Causeway, Horsham, West Sussex, RH12 1HG, UK.

Rumenco, UK.
Division of Tate & Lyle Industries Ltd, Strotten House, Derby Road, Stretton, Burton-on-Trent, Staffordshire, DE13 0DW, UK.
Telephone: +44 (0)1283 524257
Facsimile: +44 (0)1283 511013

RWR, Austral.
RWR Veterinary Products Pty Ltd, Austral.
Contact: Nature Vet, Austral.

RXV, USA.
RXV, c/o RXV Products, 6301 Deramus, Kansas City, MO 64120, USA.
Telephone: +1 816 483 9220
Facsimile: +1 816 483 9455

S & N Hlth, UK.
Smith & Nephew Healthcare Ltd, Healthcare House, Goulton Street, Hull, HU3 4DJ, UK.
Telephone: +44 (0)1482 222200
Facsimile: +44 (0)1482 222211
E-mail: advice@smith-nephew.com

Sanofi-Synthelabo, UK.
Sanofi Synthelabo, One Onslow Street, Guildford, Surrey, GU1 4YS, UK.
Telephone: +44 (0)1483 505515
Facsimile: +44 (0)1483 535432

Schering-Plough, Austral.
Schering-Plough Animal Health, 71 Epping Road, North Ryde, NSW 2113, Australia.
Telephone: +61 (0)2 9335 4000
Facsimile: +61 (0)2 9335 4085

Schering-Plough, Eire.
Schering-Plough Animal Health Ireland, Boghall Road, Bray, Co. Wicklow, Eire.
Telephone: +353 (0)1 205 0900
Facsimile: +353 (0)1 205 0924

Schering-Plough, NZ.
Schering-Plough Animal Health Ltd, 33 Whakatiki Street, Upper Hutt, New Zealand.
Telephone: +64 (0)4 528 1900
Facsimile: +64 (0)4 528 1918

Schering-Plough, UK.
Schering-Plough Animal Health, Division of Schering-Plough Ltd, Breakspear Road South, Harefield, Uxbridge, Middlesex, UB9 6LS, UK.
Telephone: +44 (0)1895 626000
Facsimile: +44 (0)1895 672429

Schering-Plough, USA.
Schering-Plough Animal Health Corporation, 1095 Morris Avenue, Union, NJ 07033, USA.
Telephone: +1 800 224 5318 or +1 800 211 3573 or +1 800 219 9286
Facsimile: +1 908 629 3316

Scottish Homing Union
231a Low Waters Road, Hamilton, Lanarkshire, ML3 7QN, UK.
Telephone: +44 (0)1698 286 983

Searle, UK.
Saerle, PO Box 53, Lane End Road, High Wycombe, Buckinghamshire, HP12 4HL, UK.
Telephone: +44 (0)1494 521124
Facsimile: +44 (0)1494 536860

Seven Seas, UK.
Seven Seas Ltd, Hedon Road, Marfleet, HU9 5NJ, UK.
Telephone: +44 (0)1482 375234
Facsimile: +44 (0)1482 374345

Shep-Fair, UK.
Shep-Fair Products, Trefecca Fawr, Trefecca, Brecon, Powys, LD3 0PW, UK.
Telephone: +44 (0)1873 890855
Facsimile: +44 (0)1873 890822

Sherley's, UK.
Sherley's Ltd, Homefield Road, Haverhill, Suffolk, CB9 8QP, UK.
Telephone: +44 (0)1440 715700
Facsimile: +44 (0)1440 713940
E-mail: sherleys@dial.pipex.com

Sinclair, UK.
Sinclair Animal and Household Care Ltd, Haycliffe Lane, Bradford, BD5 9ET, UK.
Telephone: +44 (0)1274 501001
Facsimile: +44 (0)1274 521245

SmithKline Beecham, UK.
SmithKline Beecham Pharmaceuticals, SmithKline Beecham plc, Mundells, Welwyn Garden City, Hertfordshire, AL7 1EY, UK.
Telephone: +44 (0)808 100 2228
Facsimile: +44 (0)808 100 8802
E-mail: ukpharma.customer@sb.com

Society of Greyhound Veterinarians, UK.
64 Elmroyd Avenue, Potters Bar, Hertfordshire, EN6 2EF, UK.

Sorex, UK.
Sorex Ltd, St Michael's Industrial Estate, Widnes, Cheshire, WA8 8TJ, UK.
Telephone: +44 (0)151 4207151
Facsimile: +44 (0)151 4951163
E-mail: sales@sorex.com

Sovereign, UK.
Sovereign Medical, Sovereign House, Miles Gray Road, Basildon, Essex, SS14 3FR, UK.
Telephone: +44 (0)1268 535200
Facsimile: +44 (0)1268 535299

Spencer, UK.
Brian G Spencer Ltd, 19-21 Ilkeston Road, Heanor, Derbyshire, DE75 7DT, UK.

Telephone: +44 (0)1773 533330
Facsimile: +44 (0)1773 535454

Squibb, UK.
Contact: Bristol Myers, UK.

SSAVA, Swed.
Swedish Small Animal Veterinary Association, Djurjukhuset Albano, Rinkebyvagen 23, S-18236, Sweden.
Telephone: +46 8 755 40 75

SSL International, UK.
SSL International plc, Tubiton House, Oldham, OL1 3HS, UK.
Telephone: +44 (0)161 652 2222
Facsimile: +44 (0)161 626 9090

Stafford-Miller, UK.
Stafford-Miller Ltd, Broadwater Road, Welwyn Garden City, Hertfordshire, AL7 3SP, UK.
Telephone: +44 (0)1707 331001
Facsimile: +44 (0)1707 373370

Steris, USA.
Steris Laboratories Inc, 620 N 51st Avenue, Phoenix, AZ 85043-4705, USA.
Telephone: +1 602 447 3473
Facsimile: +1 602 447 3479

Stockguard, NZ.
Stockguard Laboratories (NZ) Ltd, PO Box 10 305, Hamilton, New Zealand.
Telephone: +64 (0)7 849 6782
Facsimile: +64 (0)7 849 8783

Strakan, UK.
Strakan Ltd, Buckholm Mill, Buckholm Mill Brae, Galashiels, TD1 2HB, UK.
Telephone: +44 (0)1896 668060
Facsimile: +44 (0)1896 668 061
E-mail: medinfo@strakan.com

Stuart, UK.
Contact: Zeneca, UK.

Sungro, USA.
Sungro Chemicals Inc, 810E 18th Street, Los Angeles, CA 90021, USA.
Telephone: +1 213 747 4125
Facsimile: +1 213 747 0942

Swiss Veterinary Association
Länggasstrasse 8, CH-3001 Bern, Switzerland.
Telephone: +41 (0)31 307 35 35
Facsimile: +41 (0)31 307 35 39

Techmix, USA.
Techmix Inc, 12915 Pioneer Trail, Eden Prairie, MN 55347, USA.
Telephone: +1 612 944 7771
Facsimile: +1 612 944 7736

TechniPharm, NZ.
TechniPharm International Ltd, PO Box 959, Rotorua, New Zealand.
Telephone: +64 (0)7 349 0498
Facsimile: +64 (0)7 349 0498

Telsol, UK.
Telsol Ltd, PO Box HH7, Leeds, LS8 2YE, UK.
Telephone: +44 (0)113 2260666
Facsimile: +44 (0)113 2260999
E-mail: enquiries@telsol.co.uk

Tetra, UK.
Tetra, Division of Parke Davis & Co Ltd, Lambert Court, Chestnut Avenue, Eastleigh, Hampshire, SO53 3ZQ, UK.
Telephone: +44 (0)2380 620500
Facsimile: +44 (0)2380 629810

Thames, UK.
Contact Cortecs, UK.

Therapeutix, NZ.
Therapeutix Ltd, Ladies Mile, RD1, Queenstown, New Zealand.
Telephone: +64 (0)3 442 3143
Facsimile: +64 (0)3 442 3143

Thorne (Beehives), UK.
E H Thorne (Beehives) Ltd, Beehive Works, Wragby, Market Rasen, Lincolnshire, LN8 5LA, UK.
Telephone: +44 (0)1673 858555
Facsimile: +44 (0)1673 857004
E-mail: sales@thorne.co.uk

Thoroughbred Breeders' Association, UK.
Thoroughbred Breeders' Association, Stanstead House, The Avenue, Newmarket, Suffolk, CB8 9AA, UK.
Telephone: +44 (0)1638 661321

The Toxoplasmosis Trust, UK.
The Toxoplasmosis Trust, 61-71 Collier Street, London, N1 9BE, UK.
Telephone: +44 (0)20 7713 0599

Troy, Austral.
Troy Laboratories Pty Ltd, 98 Long Street, Smithfield, NSW 2164, Australia.
Telephone: +61 (0)2 9604 6266
Facsimile: +61 (0)2 9725 1772

TSK, UK.
TSK Animal Health Ltd, Mill Close, Patrick Brompton, Bedale, North Yorkshire, DL8 1JY, UK.
Telephone: +44 (0)1677 450585
Facsimile: +44 (0)1677 450585

Tulivin, UK.
Tulivin Laboratories Ltd, 35 Abbeydale Park, Newtownards, Co. Down, Northern Ireland, BT23 8RE, UK.
Telephone: +44 (0)28 9182 0999
Facsimile: +44 (0)28 9182 0227

UCB Pharma, UK.
UCB Pharma Ltd, 3 George Street, Watford, Hertfordshire, WD1 8UH, UK.
Telephone: +44 (0)1923 211811
Facsimile: +44 (0)1923 229002

UFAW, UK.
Universities Federation for Animal Welfare, The Old School, Brewhouse Hill, Wheathampstead, Hertfordshire, AL4 8AN, UK.
Telephone: +44 (0)1582 831818
Facsimile: +44 (0)1582 831414
E-mail: kirkwood@ufaw.org.uk

UKASTA, UK.
United Kingdom Agricultural Supply Trade Association Ltd, 4 Whitehall Court, London, SW1A 2EP, UK.
Telephone: +44 (0)20 7930 3611
Facsimile: +44 (0)20 7930 3952

Univet, Eire.
Univet Limited, Tullyvin, Cootehill, Co. Cavan, Eire.
Telephone: +353 (0)49 5553203/ 5553064
Facsimile: +353 (0)49 5553266

Valdar, USA.
Valdar LLC, 50 Clarkson Centre, Suite 400, Chesterfield, MO 63017, USA.
Telephone: +1 816 505 3277
Facsimile: +1 816 505 3627

VDS, UK.
The Veterinary Defence Society Ltd, 4 Haig Court, Park Gate Estate, Knutsford, Cheshire, WA16 8XZ, UK.
Telephone: +44 (0)1565 652737
Facsimile: +44 (0)1565 751079

Vedco, USA.
Vedco Inc, 2121 SE Bush Road, St Joseph, MO 64504, USA.
Telephone: +1 816 238 8840
Facsimile: +1 816 238 1837

Vericore AP, UK.
Vericore Aquahealth Products, Novartis Animal Health UK Ltd, New Cambridge House, Litlington, Hertfordshire, SG8 0SS, UK.
Telephone: +44 (0)1763 850 500
Facsimile: +44 (0)1763 850 600

Vericore LP, UK.
Vericore Livestock Products, Novartis Animal Health UK Ltd, New Cambridge House, Litlington, Hertfordshire, SG8 0SS, UK.
Telephone: +44 (0)1763 850 500
Facsimile: +44 (0)1763 850 600

Vericore VP, UK.
Vericore Veterinary Products, Novartis Animal Health UK Ltd, New Cambridge House, Litlington, Hertfordshire, SG8 0SS, UK.
Telephone: +44 (0)1763 850 500
Facsimile: +44 (0)1763 850 600

Vet Plus, UK.
Vet Plus Ltd, Wild Goose House, Goe Lane, Freckleton, PR4 1XH, UK.
Telephone: +44 (0)1772 631714
Facsimile: +44 (0)1772 634782

Vetafarm, Austral.
Vetafarm Pty Ltd, 3 Bye Street, Wagga Wagga, NSW 2650, Australia.
Telephone: +61 (0)2 6925 6222
Facsimile: +61 (0)2 6925 6333

Vet-A-Mix, USA.
Vet-A-Mix Division, Lloyd Inc, PO Box 130, Shenandoah, IA 51601, USA.
Telephone: +1 712 246 4000
Facsimile: +1 712 246 5245

Vetark, UK.
Vetark Products Ltd, PO Box 60, Winchester, Hampshire, SO23 7LS, UK.
Telephone: +44 (0)1962 880376
Facsimile: +44 (0)1962 881790

Vetoquinol, Austral.
Vetoquinol S.A., Austral.
Contact: Intervet, Austral.

Vetoquinol, Eire.
Vetoquinol Ireland Limited, Unit 7b, Oranmore Business Park, Co. Galway, Eire.
Telephone: +353 (0)91 792 212
Facsimile: +353 (0)91 792 214

Vétoquinol, UK.
Vétoquinol UK Ltd, Wedgwood Road, Bicester, Oxfordshire, OX6 7UL, UK.
Telephone: +44 (0)1869 241287
Facsimile: +44 (0)1869 320145
E-mail: office@vetoquinoluk.co.uk

Vetpharm, NZ.
Vetpharm (NZ) Ltd, Unit 7, 84-90 Hillside Road, Glenfield, Auckland, New Zealand.
Telephone: +64 (0)9 410 5566
Facsimile: +64 (0)9 410 6305

VetPlus, UK.
VetPlus Ltd, Wild Goose House, Goe Lane, Freckleton, Lancashire, PR4 1XH, UK.
Telephone: +44 0)1772 631714
Facsimile: +44 (0)1772 634782

Vetrepharm, Austral.
Vetrepharm (A/Asia) Pty Ltd, Level 1, Napier House, Essendon, Vic. 3040, Australia.
Telephone: +61 (0)3 9370 4974
Facsimile: +61 (0)3 9370 5290

Vetrepharm, UK.
Vetrepharm Ltd, Unit 15, Sandleheath Industrial Estate, Fordingbridge, Hampshire, SP6 1PA, UK.
Telephone: +44 (0)1425 656081
Facsimile: +44 (0)1425 655309

Vetsearch, Austral.
Vetsearch International Pty Ltd, 6 Lenton Place, North Rocks, NSW 2151, Australia.
Telephone: +61 (0)2 9683 5333
Facsimile: +61 (0)2 9683 5973

VetTek, USA.
VetTek Inc, 100 SE Magellan Drive, Blue Springs, MO 64014, USA.
Telephone: +1 816 229 9101
Facsimile: +1 816 224 3080

Vetus, USA.
Vetus Animal Health (c/o Burns Veterinary Supply), 1900 Diplomat Drive, Farmers Branch, TX 75234, USA.
Telephone: +1 972 620 9941
Facsimile: +1 972 620 1071

Virbac, Austral.
Virbac (Australia) Pty Ltd, 15 Pritchard Place, Peakhurst, NSW 2210, Australia.
Telephone: +61 (0)2 9533 2000
Facsimile: +61 (0)2 9533 1522

Virbac, Eire.
Laboratoires Virbac, B.P.27-06511 Carros Cedex, France.
Telephone: +33 (0)4 92 08 71 61
Facsimile: +33 (0)4 92 08 71 65

Virbac, NZ.
Virbac Laboratories (NZ) Ltd, 30-32 Stonedon Drive, East Tamaki, Auckland, New Zealand.
Telephone: +64 (0)9 273 3814
Facsimile: +64 (0)9 273 3815

Virbac, UK.
Virbac Ltd, Woolpit Business Park, Windmill Avenue, Woolpit, Bury St Edmunds, Suffolk, IP30 9UP, UK.
Telephone: +44 (0)1359 243243
Facsimile: +44 (0)1359 243200

Vita, UK.
Vita (Europe) Ltd, Brook House, Alencon Link, Basingstoke, Hampshire, RG21 7RD, UK.
Telephone: +44 (0)1256 473177
Facsimile: +44 (0)1256 473179

VMD, UK.
Veterinary Medicines Directorate, Woodham Lane, New Haw, Addlestone, Surrey, KT15 3LS, UK.
Telephone: +44 (0)1932 336911
Facsimile: +44 (0)1932 336618

VPIS (Leeds), UK.
VPIS (Leeds), The General Infirmary, Great George St, Leeds, LS1 3EX, UK.
Telephone: +44 (0)113 245 0530
Facsimile: +44 (0)113 244 5849

VPIS (London), UK.
Medical Toxicology Unit, Avonley Road, London, SE14 5ER, UK.
Telephone: +44 (0)20 7635 9195
Facsimile: +44 (0)20 7715 309
E-mail: vpis@gstt.sthames.nhs.uk

VPL, USA.
Veterinary Products Laboratories, 301 W Osborn Road, Phoenix, AZ

85013, USA.
Telephone: +1 888 241 9545
Facsimile: +1 800 215 5875

VRX, USA.
VRX Products, 1656 W 240th Street, Harbor City, CA 90710, USA.
Telephone: +1 310 326 2720
Facsimile: +1 310 326 8026

Wade Jones, USA.
Wade Jones Co, PO Box 309, Lowell, AR 72745, USA.
Telephone: +1 501 659 0828
Facsimile: +1 800 551 5504

Warner Lambert, UK.
Contact Parke-Davis, UK.

Wells, Austral.
W, R & D Wells Pty Ltd, 144-150 Clarendon Street, South Melbourne, Vic. 3205, Australia.
Telephone: +61 (0)3 9699 8999
Facsimile: +61 (0)3 9699 7962

Welsh Homing Union
3 Coed Cae Tir-phil, New Tredegar, Gwent, NP24 6HH, UK.
Telephone: +44 (0)1443 833 161

Wendt, USA.
Wendt Professional Laboratories Inc, 200 W Beaver Street, Belle Plaine, MN 56011, USA.
Telephone: +1 612 873 2288
Facsimile: +1 612 873 2289

Western Stock Distributors, Austral.
Western Stock Distrubutors, 17 Rheola Street, West Perth, WA 6005, Australia.
Telephone: +61 (0)8 9321 2888
Facsimile: +61 (0)8 9322 4163

Western Veterinary Supply, USA.
Western Veterinary Supply, c/o RXV Products, 6301 Deramus, Kansas City, MO 64120, USA.
Telephone: +1 816 483 9220
Facsimile: +1 816 483 9455

Whelehan, Eire.
T P Whelehan Son & Co Limited, Finglas, Dublin 11, Eire.
Telephone: +353 (0)1 834 2233
Facsimile: +353 (0)1 836 2271

Whiskas, UK.
Contact: Pedigree, UK.

Whitehall, UK.
Whitehall Laboratories Ltd, Huntercombe Lane South, Taplow, Maidenhead, Berkshire, SL6 0PJ, UK.
Telephone: +44 (0)1628 669011
Facsimile: +44 (0)1628 669846

Wildlife, USA.
Wildlife Pharmaceuticals Inc, 1512 Webster Court, Fort Collins, CO 80522, USA.
Telephone: +1 970 484 6269
Facsimile: +1 970 484 4941

WVA
World Veterinary Association, Roselunds Allé 8, DK-2720 Vanløse, Denmark.
Telephone: +45 38 71 01 56
Facsimile: +45 38 71 03 22
E-mail: wva@ddd.dk

Wyeth, UK.
Wyeth Laboratories, Huntercombe Lane South, Taplow, Maidenhead, Berkshire, SL6 0PH, UK.
Telephone: +44 (0)1628 604377
Facsimile: +44 (0)1628 666368

Yamanouchi, UK.
Yamanouchi Pharma Ltd, Yamanouchi House, Pyrford Road, West Byfleet, Surrey, KT14 6RA, UK.
Telephone: +44 (0)1932 345535
Facsimile: +44 (0)1932 353458

Young's, UK.
Young's Animal Health, Novartis Animal Health UK Ltd, New Cambridge House, Litlington, Hertfordshire, SG8 0SS, UK.
Telephone: +44 (0)1763 850 500
Facsimile: +44 (0)1763 850 600

Y-Tex, USA.
Y-Tex Corporation, 1825 Bighorn Avenue, Cody, WY 82414, USA.
Telephone: +1 307 587 5515
Facsimile: +1 307 527 6433

Zeneca, UK.
AstraZeneca, King's Court, Water Lane, Wilmslow, Cheshire, SK9 5AZ, UK.
Telephone: +44 (0)800 200123
Facsimile: +44 (0)1625 712581

Index

Drug monograph titles are listed on given on the page number in **bold** type. Proprietary names (brand names) are printed in *italic* type.

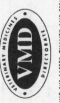

Ministry of Agriculture, Fisheries and Food
Veterinary Medicines Directorate,
FREEPOST KT4503, Woodham Lane, New Haw,
Addlestone,   Surrey KT15 3BR
Tel. No. 01932 338427   Fax : 01932 336618

Suspected Adverse Reaction Surveillance Scheme (SARSS)

Animal suspected adverse reaction report

ASSURING THE SAFETY, QUALITY AND EFFICACY OF VETERINARY MEDICINES

- This form should be completed in **BLOCK LETTERS** and sent to the **FREEPOST** address given above, whenever a suspected adverse reaction is observed in **animals** (including birds and fish) during or after the use of a veterinary medicine.

For Official Use Only

Adverse Reaction No.

SAR file

Date received

Date Ack.

All reporters MUST complete this section

Full name of product

Product number (on label)*   Batch number

This form will be copied to the Company (Marketing Authorisation holder) in order that they are aware of any reported suspected adverse reaction to their product. They may wish to contact you for further details. If you do not want the name(s) and address(es) on the form to be revealed to the Company, please tick this box ☐

Has the Company already been informed?   YES ☐   NO ☐

Your reference No. (if any)

Full name and address of person sending this form to the VMD

County:
Postcode:

Date __/__/__

Full address where reaction(s) occured

County:
Postcode:

Full name and address of veterinarian involved

County:
Postcode:

P.T.O.

MLA 252A (Rev. 1/99)

Details of animal suspected adverse reaction(s)

| | | | | Reason for using product | |

No. of animals treated on this occasion

No. of animals reacting

No. of deaths

Actual amount of product administered

Administered by (occupation)

Date of administration

Duration of treatment

Route of administration

Date of first administration

Previous use of product in this animal(s)   YES ☐ NO ☐

If YES, number of occasions products used

Date of reaction(s)	Species/Breed	Weight kg	Age	Sex (M/F)	Nature of reaction including time of onset and duration of symptoms

Full details of products given concurrently (if any)

Immediate treatment given (if any)

Vaccination history (if immunological product involved in suspected adverse reaction) product number* and batch number

Comments: If you have any comments or further information please continue on a separate sheet

Post mortem and/or laboratory tests: have any post mortems or relevant diagnostic tests been performed?   YES ☐   NO ☐

If **YES** please attach copies or forward to VMD in due course.

Extra Forms: Tick this box if extra forms are required ☐

* **The product number is preceded by PL, VM,or MA**

Receipt of this form will be acknowledged ☐

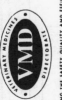

VMD
VETERINARY MEDICINES DIRECTORATE

ASSURING THE SAFETY, QUALITY AND EFFICACY OF VETERINARY MEDICINES

Ministry of Agriculture, Fisheries and Food
Veterinary Medicines Directorate,
FREEPOST KT4503, Woodham Lane, New Haw,
Addlestone,   Surrey KT15 3BR
Tel. No. 01932 338427 Fax : 01932 336618

Suspected Adverse Reaction Surveillance Scheme (SARSS)
Animal suspected adverse reaction report

- This form should be completed in **BLOCK LETTERS** and sent to the **FREEPOST**
  address given above, whenever a suspected adverse reaction is observed in **animals**
  (including birds and fish) during or after the use of a veterinary medicine.

For Official Use Only
Adverse Reaction No.

SAR file

Date received

Date Ack.

All reporters MUST complete this section

Full name of product

Product number (on label)*   Batch number

This form will be copied to the Company (Marketing
Authorisation holder) in order that they are aware of any
reported suspected adverse reaction to their product. They
may wish to contact you for further details. If you do not
want the name(s) and address(es) on the form to be revealed
to the Company, please tick this box

YES   NO

Has the Company already been informed?

Your reference No. (if any)

Full name and address of person sending this form to the VMD

County:
Postcode:

Date __/__/__

Full address where reaction(s) occured

County:
Postcode:

Full name and address of veterinarian involved

County:
Postcode:

P.T.O.

MLA 252A (Rev. 1/99)

Details of animal suspected adverse reaction(s)

No. of animals treated on this occasion [ ]
No. of animals reacting [ ]
No. of deaths [ ]

Reason for using product

Administered by (occupation) [ ]

Actual amount of product administered [ ]

Route of administration [ ]
Date of first administration [ ]
Previous use of product in this animal(s) YES [ ] NO [ ]

Duration of treatment [ ]

If YES, number of occasions products used [ ]

Date of reaction(s)	Species/Breed)	Weight kg	Age	Sex (M/F)	Nature of reaction including time of onset and duration of symptoms

Full details of products given concurrently (if any)

Immediate treatment given (if any)

Vaccination history (if immunological product involved in suspected adverse reaction) product number* and batch number

Post mortem and/or laboratory tests:
have any post mortems or relevant diagnostic tests been performed?   YES [ ]   NO [ ]
If **YES** please attach copies or forward to VMD in due course.

Comments: If you have any comments or further information please continue on a separate sheet

Extra Forms: Tick this box if extra forms are required [ ]

* **The product number is preceded by PL, VM, or MA**

Receipt of this form will be acknowledged [ ]

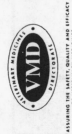

VMD
VETERINARY MEDICINES DIRECTORATE

ASSURING THE SAFETY, QUALITY AND EFFICACY OF VETERINARY MEDICINES

Ministry of Agriculture, Fisheries and Food
Veterinary Medicines Directorate,
FREEPOST KT4503, Woodham Lane, New Haw, Addlestone,
Surrey KT15 3BR
Tel. No. 01932 338427   Fax : 01932 336618

Suspected Adverse Reaction Surveillance Scheme (SARSS)
Report on suspected adverse reaction(s) in humans

- This form should be completed in **BLOCK LETTERS** and sent to the **FREEPOST** address given above, whenever a suspected adverse reaction is observed in humans during or after the use of a veterinary medicine.

All reporters MUST complete this section

Full name of product

Product number number (on label)*

Batch number

This form will be copied to the Company (Marketing Authorisation holder) in order that they are aware of any reported suspected adverse reaction to their product. They may wish to contact you for further details. If you do not want the name(s) and address(es) on the form to be revealed to the Company, please tick this box ☐

Has the Company already been informed?   YES ☐   NO ☐

*The product number is preceded by PL,VM or MA

Full name and address of person sending this form to the VMD

County:
Postcode:

Date __/__/__

Full address where reaction(s) occurred

County:

Postcode:

Your reference No. (if any)

MLA 252A (Rev. 1/99)

P.T.O.

Details of person experiencing reaction(s)

Title _____ Initials _____ Surname _____

Sex male ☐ female ☐

Age: 0-5 ☐ 6-17 ☐ 18-24 ☐ 25-44 ☐ 45-64 ☐ 65+ ☐

Occupation (e.g. farmer, vet, pet owner) _____

Details of suspected adverse reaction(s) in humans. Please use BLOCK LETTERS.

Details of exposure	Details of exposure/contact with veterinary medicine. If accidental, please give details of how accident occurred. If self injection, please give details of amount injected
	Species of animal being treated _____
	No. of animals treated _____

Date of onset of symptoms _____

Details of first symptoms

Duration of symptoms (e.g. 20 minutes 5 days, ongoing etc.)

Details of symptoms occurring afterwards

Were you suffering from any illness (e.g. flu) or taking medication prior to exposure? YES ☐ NO ☐

If **YES**, give details:

Did you seek medical advice? YES ☐ NO ☐

If **YES**, did the doctor confirm that your symptoms were associated with exposure to the veterinary medicine? YES ☐ NO ☐

Give details of any treatment received:

Receipt of this form will be acknowledged and further details may be requested

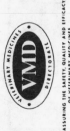

ASSURING THE SAFETY, QUALITY AND EFFICACY OF VETERINARY MEDICINES

Ministry of Agriculture, Fisheries and Food
Veterinary Medicines Directorate,
FREEPOST KT4503, Woodham Lane, New Haw, Addlestone,
Surrey KT15 3BR
Tel. No. 01932 338427   Fax : 01932 336618

Suspected Adverse Reaction Surveillance Scheme (SARSS)

Report on suspected adverse reaction(s) in humans

● This form should be completed in **BLOCK LETTERS** and sent to the **FREEPOST** address given above, whenever a suspected adverse reaction is observed in humans during or after the use of a veterinary medicine.

All reporters MUST complete this section

Full name of product

Product number number (on label)*   Batch number

This form will be copied to the Company (Marketing Authorisation holder) in order that they are aware of any reported suspected adverse reaction to their product. They may wish to contact you for further details. If you do not want the name(s) and address(es) on the form to be revealed to the Company, please tick this box

YES ☐   NO ☐

Has the Company already been informed?

*The product number is preceded by PL,VM or MA

MLA 252A (Rev. 1/99)

Full name and address of person sending this form to the VMD

County:
Postcode:

Date __ / __ / __

Full address where reaction(s) occurred

County:
Postcode:

Your reference No. (if any)

P.T.O.

Details of person experiencing reaction(s)

Title ☐ Initials ☐ Surname ☐ Sex male ☐ female ☐

Age: 0-5 ☐ 6-17 ☐ 18-24 ☐ 25-44 ☐ 45-64 ☐ 65+ ☐

Occupation (e.g. farmer, vet, pet owner) ☐

Details of suspected adverse reaction(s) in humans. Please use BLOCK LETTERS.

Date of exposure ☐

Details of exposure/contact with veterinary medicine. If accidental, please give details of how accident occurred. If self injection, please give details of amount injected ☐

Species of animal being treated ☐

No. of animals treated ☐

Date of onset of symptoms ☐

Details of first symptoms ☐

Duration of symptoms (e.g. 20 minutes 5 days, ongoing etc.) ☐

Details of symptoms occurring afterwards ☐

Were you suffering from any illness (e.g. flu) or taking medication prior to exposure? YES ☐ NO ☐
If YES, give details: ☐

Did you seek medical advice? YES ☐ NO ☐

If YES, did the doctor confirm that your symptoms were associated with exposure to the veterinary medicine? YES ☐ NO ☐
Give details of any treatment received: ☐

Receipt of this form will be acknowledged and further details may be requested